2006
Oncology Nursing Drug Handbook

2006
Oncology Nursing Drug Handbook

Gail M. Wilkes, MSN, RNC, AOCN
Oncology Nurse Practitioner and
Clinical Instructor
Boston Medical Center
Boston, Massachusetts

Margaret Barton-Burke, PhD, RN
Assistant Professor
University of Massachusetts
Amherst, Massachusetts

JONES AND BARTLETT PUBLISHERS
Sudbury, Massachusetts
BOSTON TORONTO LONDON SINGAPORE

World Headquarters
Jones and Bartlett Publishers
40 Tall Pine Drive
Sudbury, MA 01776
978-443-5000
info@jbpub.com
www.jbpub.com

Jones and Bartlett Publishers Canada
6339 Ormindale Way
Mississauga, Ontario L5V 1J2
CANADA

Jones and Bartlett Publishers International
Barb House, Barb Mews
London W6 7PA
UK

Jones and Bartlett's books and products are available through most bookstores and online booksellers. To contact Jones and Bartlett Publishers directly, call 800-832-0034, fax 978-443-8000, or visit our website at www.jbpub.com.

Substantial discounts on bulk quantities of Jones and Bartlett's publications are available to corporations, professional associations, and other qualified organizations. For details and specific discount information, contact the special sales department at Jones and Bartlett via the above contact information or send an email to specialsales@jbpub.com.

ISBN-10: 0-7637-4413-1
ISBN-13: 978-0-7637-4413-7
ISSN: 1536-0024
6048

Production Credits
Executive Publisher: Chris Davis
Associate Editor: Kathy Richardson
Production Director: Amy Rose
Production Editor: Renée Sekerak
Production Assistant: Rachel Rossi
Marketing Manager: Emily Ekle
Manufacturing and Inventory Coordinator: Amy Bacus
Composition: ATLIS Systems
Printing and Binding: Malloy, Inc.
Cover Printing: Malloy, Inc.

The drug information presented in the 2006 Oncology Nursing Drug Handbook has been derived from standard reference sources, recently published data, and respected pharmaceutical texts. The writers and publishers of this book have made every effort to ensure that the information and dosage regimens presented are accurate and in accord with current labeling at the time of publication. However, in view of the constant and rapid flow of information resulting from ongoing research and clinical experience, as well as changes in government regulations, readers are urged to check the package insert and consult with a pharmacist, if necessary, for each drug they plan to administer to be certain that changes have not been made in its indications or contraindications, or in the recommended dosage for each use. While the drugs included in this publication were chosen on the basis of frequency of use and appropriate indications, the publisher and authors do not necessarily advocate, and take no responsibility for, the use of products described herein.

Printed in the United States of America
10 09 08 07 06 10 9 8 7 6 5 4 3 2 1

Jones and Bartlett Series in Oncology

Recently Published

The Cancer Journal
Journal of the National Comprehensive Cancer Network
American Cancer Society Patient Education Guide to Oncology Drugs, Second Edition, Wilkes/Ades
American Cancer Society Consumer's Guide to Cancer Drugs, Second Edition, Wilkes/Ades/Krakoff
Biotherapy: A Comprehensive Overview, Second Edition, Reiger
Blood and Marrow Stem Cell Transplantation, Second Edition, Whedon
Cancer and HIV Clinical Nutrition Pocket Guide, Second Edition, Wilkes
Cancer Chemotherapy: A Nursing Process Approach, Third Edition, Barton-Burke/Wilkes/Ingwersen
Cancer Chemotherapy Care Plans Handbook, Third Edition, Barton-Burke/Wilkes/Ingwersen
Cancer Nursing: Principles and Practice, Sixth Edition, Yarbro/Frogge/Goodman
A Cancer Source Book for Nurses, Eighth Edition, American Cancer Society
Cancer Symptom Management, Third Edition, Yarbro/Frogge/Goodman
Cancer Symptom Management, Patient Self-Care Guides, Second Edition, Yarbro/Frogge/Goodman
Cancer Therapies, Barton-Burke/Wilkes
A Clinical Guide to Cancer Nursing, Fifth Edition, Yarbro/Frogge/Goodman
A Clinical Guide to Stem Cell and Bone Marrow Transplantation, Shapiro et al.
Clinical Handbook for Biotherapy, Rieger
Contemporary Issues in Breast Cancer: A Nursing Perspective, Second Edition, Hassey Dow
Contemporary Issues in Colorectal Cancer: A Nursing Perspective, Berg
Contemporary Contemporary Issues in Lung Cancer: A Nursing Perspective, Haas
Contemorary Issues in Lymphoma, Poniatowski et al.
Contemporary Issues in Prostate Cancer: A Nursing Perspective, Held-Warmkessel
Dx/Rx: Upper Gastrointestinal Malignancies: Cancers of the Stomach and Esophagus, Shah, Series Editor
Dx/Rx: Lung Cancer, Azzoli
Dx/Rx: Leukemia, Burke
Dx/Rx: Breast Cancer, Lake
Dx/Rx: Palliative Cancer Care, Malhotra/Moryl
Fatigue in Cancer: A Multidimensional Approach, Winningham/Barton-Burke
Glioblastoma Multiforme, Markert et al.
Handbook of Breast Cancer Risk-Assessment: Evidence-Based Guidelines for Evaluation, Prevention, Counseling, and Treatment, Vogel/Bevers
Handbook of Cancer Risk Assessment, Colditz/Stein
Handbook of Oncology Nursing, Third Edition, Johnson/Gross
Homecare Management of the Bone Marrow Transplant Patient, Third Edition, Kelley/McBride/Randolph/Leum/Lonergan
How Cancer Works, Sompayrac
Human Embryonic Stem Cells, Kiessling/Anderson

Jones and Bartlett Series in Oncology (continued)

Instruments for Clinical Health Care Research, Third Edition, Frank-Stromborg
Making the Decision: A Cancer Patient's Guide to Clinical Trials, Mulay
Malignant Liver Tumors, Second Edition, Clavien et al.
Management of Nausea and Vomiting in Cancer and Cancer Treatment, Hesketh
Memory Bank for Chemotherapy, Third Edition, Preston/Wilfinger
Molecular Oncology of Breast Cancer, Ross/Hortobagyi
Oncology Nursing in the Ambulatory Setting, Second Edition, Buchsel/Yarbro
Oncology Nursing Review, Second Edition, Yarbro/Frogge/Goodman
Outcomes in Radiation Therapy: Multidisciplinary Management, Watkins-Bruner/Moore-Higgs/Haas
Pancreatic Cancer, Von Hoff et al.
Pediatric Stem Cell Transplantation, Metha
Pocket Guide to Breast Cancer, Third Edition, Hassey Dow
Pocket Guide to Breast Cancer Drugs, Wilkes
Pocket Guide to Cancer Chemotherapy Protocols, Second Edition, Chu/DeVita
Pocket Guide to Colorectal Cancer, Berg
Pocket Guide To Colorectal Cancer Drugs and Treatment, Wilkes
Pocket Guide to Managing Cancer Fatigue, Schwartz
Pocket Guide to Prostate Cancer, Held-Warmkessel
Pocket Guide for Women and Cancer, Moore-Higgs/Almadrones/Colvin-Huff/Gossfield/Eriksson
Progress in Oncology 2004, DeVita/Hellman/Rosenberg
Quality of Life: From Nursing and Patient Perspectives, Second Edition, King/Hinds
Women and Cancer: A Gynecologic Oncology Nursing Perspective, Second Edition, Moore-Higgs/Almadrones/Colvin-Huff/Gossfield/Eriksson

Contents

Key to Abbreviations

ABV	doxorubicin (doxorubicin HCl Adriamycin) bleomycin vincristine
ac	''ante cibum;'' before meals
ADH	antidiuretic hormone
Afib	atrial fibrillation
AIDS	acquired immunodeficiency syndrome
alkphos	alkaline phosphatase
ALL	acute lymphocytic leukemia
ALT	alanine aminotransferase (formerly SGPT)
AML	acute myelocytic leukemia
ANC	absolute neutrophil count
ANLL	acute nonlymphocytic leukemia
APL	acute promyelocytic leukemia
aPTT	activated partial thromboplastin time
ARDS	adult respiratory distress syndrome
ASA	acetylsalicylic acid
AST	aspartate aminotransferase (formerly SGOT)
AUC	area under curve
bili	bilirubin
BMT	bone marrow transplant
BP	blood pressure
BRM	biologic response modifier
BTP	break through pain
BUN	blood urea nitrogen
Ca	calcium
CAPD	continuous ambulatory periotoneal dialysis
CBC	complete blood count
CFU-GEM	colony forming unit-granulocyte, erythrocyte, megakaryocyte, and macrophage
CHF	congestive heart failure
CLL	chronic lymphocytic leukemia
CPK	creatinine phosphokinase

CR	complete response, e.g., disappearance of *all* detectable tumor cells
creat	creatinine
CSF	colony-stimulating factor
CTZ	chemoreceptor trigger zone
CVA	cerebrovascular accident
CXR	chest X-ray
D5W	5% dextrose in water
DEHP	diethylhexlphthalate
DHFR	difolate reductase
DLCO	diffusion capacity of the lung for carbon monoxide, which reflects rate of gas transfer across the alveolar-capillary membrane
DMSO	dimethyl sulfoxide
DTIC	dacarbazine
DVT	deep vein thrombosis
EDTA	edetic acid, one of several salts of edetic acid used as a chelating agent
EBV	Epstein-Barr virus
EPS	extra pyramidal side-effects
FAC	fluorouracil-adriamycin-cytoxan combination chemotherapy
FSH	follicle-stimulating hormone
FUDR-MP	5-fluoro-23-deoxyuridine-53-monophosphate
FVC	forced vital capacity
GABA	gamma-aminobutyric acid
GBPS	gated blood pool scan
GFR	glomerular filtration rate
GGT (SGGT)	gamma-glutamine transferase
G6PD	glucose-6-phosphate dehydrogenase
GU	genitourinary
HACA	human anti-chimeric antibody
HAMA	human anti-murine antibody
HCl	hydrochloride
hgb	hemoglobin
5-HIAA	5-hydroxyindoleacetic acid
HIV	human immunodeficiency virus
HCT	hematocrit
hs	"hora somni;" at bedtime
HSV	herpes simplex virus
5-HT2	5-hydroxytryptamine 2
5-HT3	5-hydroxytryptamine 3
HUS	hemolytic uremic syndrome

I/O	intake/output
ICP	intracranial pressure
ICU	intensive care unit
IFN	interferon
IL	interleukin
IOP	intraocular pressure
IT	intrathecal
IVB	intravenous bolus
IVP	intravenous push; intravenous pyelogram
LAK	lymphocyte activated killer cells
LDH	lactate dehydrogenase
LFTs	liver function tests
LH	luteinizing hormone
LHRH	luteinizing hormone-releasing hormone
LVEF	left ventricular ejection fraction
lytes	electrolytes
MAC	*mycobacterium avium* complex
MAO	monoamine oxidase
MAOI	monoamine oxidase inhibitor
MCV	mean corpuscular volume
MI	myocardial infarction
MIU	milli international units
MoAbs	monoclonal antibodies
MOPP	mustard-oncovin-prednisone-procarbazine combination chemotherpy for Hodgkin's disease
MTX	methotrexate
MU	milli units
NCI	National Cancer Institute
NHL	non-Hodgkin's lymphoma
NK	natural killer cells
NK_1	Neurokinin 1 receptor for Substance P
NMDA	N-methyl-D-aspartate pain receptor
NS	normal saline
NSAIDs	nonsteroidal antiinflammatory drugs
n/v	nausea/vomiting
OTC	over-the-counter
PACs	premature atrial contractions
PBPCs	packed red blood cells for transfusion
PCA	patient controlled analgesia
PCP	pneumocystis carinii pneumonia
PFTs	pulmonary function tests
phos	phosphorus
plts	platelets

PML	polymorphonuclear leukocyte
PR	partial response, e.g., reduction in tumor mass by 50% lasting for 3 months or longer
PRN	"pro re na'ta;" as needed
PSA	prostate-specific antigen
PT	prothrombin time
PTH	parathyroid hormone
PTT	partial thromboplastin time
PVCs	premature ventricular contractions
QID	four times a day
RFTs	renal function tests
RUQ	right upper quadrant
SBP	systolic blood pressure
sed rate	sedimentation rate
SGPT	serum glutamic-pyruvic transferase
SIADH	syndrome of inappropriate antidiuretic hormone
SPF	skin protection factor
SQ	subcutaneous
SSRI	selective serotonin reuptake inhibitor
Sx	symptom
T	temperature
T4	thyroxine
TCA	tricyclic antidepressants
TFT	thyroid function tests
THC	tetrahydrocannabinol
TIL	tumor infiltrating lymphocytes
TLS	tumor lysis syndrome
TMP-SMX	trimethoprim-sulfamethoxazole
TNF	tumor necrosis factor
TTP/HUS	thrombotic thrombocytopenic purpura/hemolytic anemia syndrome
UA	urinalysis
US	ultrasound
UTI	urinary tract infection
VC	vomiting center
Vfib	ventricular fibrillation
VOD	veno-occlusive disease
VS	vital signs
VSCC	voltage-sensitive calcium channel
VZV	varicella zoster virus
WHO	World Health Organization
XRT	radiation therapy

Preface

Oncology nurses provide expert nursing care to patients with cancer and their families, as the patient moves along the disease trajectory from diagnosis to primary treatment and cure, or to remission, then relapse, and death. The nurse uses the nursing process to assess patient and family needs in the 14 high incidence problem areas identified in the Oncology Nursing Society (ONS) standards: prevention and early detection, information, coping, comfort, nutrition, protective mechanisms, mobility, elimination, sexuality, ventilation, oxygenation, complementary and alternative therapies, palliative and end-of-life care, and survivorship.

In 2003, Andrew von Eschenbach, MD, set the elimination of suffering and death due to cancer as the NCI challenge goal. He identified seven major initiatives to accomplish this goal, including developing more effective strategies for prevention and screening; early detection as well as improving our understanding of the molecular processes of carcinogenesis; and refinement of molecular targeted therapy (Miller, 2003). In this view, cancer becomes a chronic disease characterized by periods of exacerbations and remissions. As has been demonstrated in work on angiogenesis, malignant tumors must establish a blood supply when they reach a size of 1–2 mm in order to obtain oxygen and glucose, and to remove cellular waste products. Mortality is caused by metastasis in most people with cancer, and if a malignancy was confined to 1–2 mm with a combination of chemotherapy and anti-angiogenesis drug(s), then indeed, people can "live with cancer." Together, the nurse and patient, along with other members of the healthcare team, develop a plan of care. Since cancer, for many, is a chronic illness with periods of remission and relapse, nursing goals center around self-care and empowering the patient and family to live a high-quality, meaningful life outside the hospital. Nurses are involved in the pharmacologic management of disease (e.g., chemotherapy) and of symptoms that arise during the course of illness (e.g., pain, anxiety, constipation). In addition, as patients receive more aggressive treatment, nurses are deeply involved in the management of complications of disease or treatment, such as infection. As new technologies emerge, such as molecular targeted therapy, nurses need to stay abreast of newly approved agents, their mechanisms of action, and potential side effects. Finally, oncology nurses have long said that much of symptom management is in the domain of nursing practice, and they continue to advocate for effective management and symptom resolution. Knowledge of the drugs used in cancer care is critical for today's practicing nurse. In the past, pharmacists wrote drug books for nurses that did not address the application of the nursing process to potential drug toxicities. Today, as the science of cancer treatment is rapidly exploding, it is imperative to keep current with new, emerging therapies.

This book is divided into sections addressing broad areas of nursing practice. There are individual chapters within each section presenting an introductory overview. For 2006, we have also added four antineoplastic agents (clofarabine, histrelin implant, paclitaxel protein bound particles for injection, TLK 286), four antimicrobial agents (micafungin, rifaximin, gemifloxacin, tigecycline), two immunotherapy/biotherapy symptom management agents (Imiquimod 5% cream, palifermin), and eight molecularly targeted drugs (lapatanib, panitumumab, pertuzumab, sorafenib (BAY 43-9006), sunitinib malate (sutent, SU11246), temsirolimus, tipifarnib, vatalanib), and two symptom management drugs (hydromorphone extended release tablets, ziconotide intrathecal infusion). In addition, indications and additional toxicity data have been updated for individual drugs, such as bevacizumab, cetuximab, and gefitinib. Specific drugs are described in terms of their mechanism of action, metabolism, drug interactions, laboratory effects/interference, and special considerations. The most important and common drug side effects are discussed. Chapter 5, Molecularly Targeted Therapies, discusses basic cell biology, carcinogenesis, malignant flaws resulting in abnormal cell division and cell death, invasiveness, and metastases. This is intended to provide a framework for understanding the new agents that target molecular flaws. Many of these agents inhibit steps in the processes of carcinogenesis and metastases in the areas of signal transduction (growth receptor over expression, ras, tyrosine kinases), cell cycle movement (cyclin-dependent kinases, apoptosis), angiogenesis, invasion, and metastases. In addition, the processes of apoptosis and ubiquitination are further explored. Standards may change as new scientific knowledge becomes available and as dictated by governmental regulations that affect practice. This book will be updated regularly with new drugs and nursing management strategies to reflect those changes. Every effort has been made to be accurate in describing drug doses and toxicities. However, errors may occur, so the nurse is referred to original documents and manufacturer's prescribing data. Software containing indications, dosaging, adverse reactions, and toxicity for chemotherapy drugs for use with your handheld device is available.

DRUG INFORMATION sections reflect current prescribing practices in the United States, which may differ from clinical practices in Europe and the United Kingdom. (Please see disclaimer, p. iv.)

References

American Nurses' Association (2004) ANA and ONS: *Standards of Oncology Nursing Practice*. Kansas City; ANA.

Miller M (2003) 2015: A target date for eliminating suffering and death due to cancer. Available at http://cancer.gov/newscenter/benchmarks-vol3-issue2. Accessed June 10, 2004.

Contributors

Deborah Berg, BSN, RN
Genentech Oncology
North Londonderry, NH

Catherine K. Bean, BSN, RN, BA
Bone Marrow Transplant Unit
H. Lee Moffitt Center
Tampa, FL

Karen Ingwersen MS, RN
Belmont, MA

Reginald King, Pharm D
Clinical Specialist
Oncology/BMT Hahnemann
University Hospital
Philadelphia, PA

Section 1
Cancer Treatment

Chapter 1

Introduction to Chemotherapy Drugs

Chemotherapy drugs interfere with cell division, leading to cell kill, called *cytocidal effects*, or failure to replicate, called *cytostatic effects* (see Figure 1.1, Cell Cycle.) Unfortunately, drugs cannot discriminate between frequently dividing cells that are normal and those that are malignant. Consequently, normal cells as well as malignant cells are injured. Thus, anticipated acute side effects are found also in normal cell populations that divide frequently, i.e., bone marrow, gastrointestinal (GI) mucosa, gonads, and hair follicles. Since normal cells are better able to repair themselves, these side effects are usually reversible. Depending on drug properties, delayed, longer-term toxicities may occur, which may be irreversible. Properties to be aware of include route of administration, dose, excretion, and predilection for uptake by specific organ cells. Examples of toxicities are

- Lung toxicity from bleomycin, busulfan, and the nitrosureas (BCNU, CCNU)
- Cardiomyopathy from doxorubicin, daunorubicin, mitoxantrone, trastuzumab, and paclitaxel
- Renal dysfunction from cisplatin and high-dose methotrexate
- Hemorrhagic cystitis (bladder) from ifosfamide and cyclophosphamide
- Neurotoxicity from the platins, taxanes, and vinca alkaloids
- Development of second malignancies from melphalan, cyclophosphamide, and other drugs when combined with radiotherapy

Nurses play a critical role in patient education, drug administration, and minimization of toxicities. See Table 1.1 for prechemotherapy nursing assessment guidelines. Table 1.2 describes classifications of chemotherapeutic agents.

This ninth edition has been updated to include newly approved drugs as well as important investigational agents that should be approved in the near future. This section examines antineoplastic agents and classifies them by their mechanism(s) of action. As knowledge of cancer and its treatment emerges, drugs may be reclassified, such as the anthracycline antitumor antibiotics, which now appear to work by inhibiting topoisomerase II.

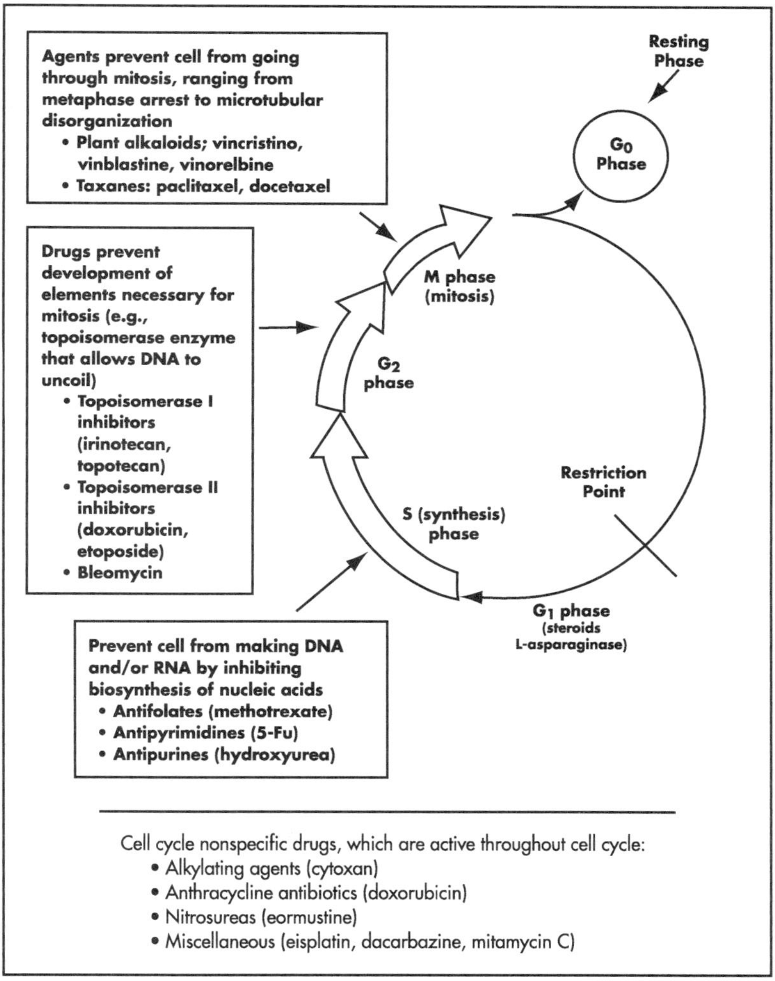

Figure 1.1 Mechanism of Action of Major Chemotherapy Drugs

As an example, the topoisomerase I inhibitors cause protein-linked DNA single-strand breaks and block DNA and RNA synthesis in dividing cells, thus preventing cells from entering mitosis. To better understand the topoisomerase inhibitors, it is important to go back to the DNA helix. The entire DNA genome consists of two strands wound into a double helix, which measures more

Table 1.1 Prechemotherapy Nursing Assessment Guidelines

Potential Problems/Nursing Diagnoses	Physical Status: Assessment Parameters/Signs and Symptoms	Drug and Dose-Limiting Factors/ Nursing Implications
Hematopoietic System		
1. Impaired tissue perfusion related to chemotherapy-induced anemia, leading to activity intolerance, changes in cardiopulmonary status due to compensatory changes	• Hgb g (norms 12–14; 14–16) • HCT% (norms 32–36; 36–40) • Vital signs (↓ BP, ↑ pulse, ↑ respiration) • Pallor (face, palms, conjunctiva) • Fatigue or weakness • Vertigo	Hgb < 8 g HCT < 20% and blood transfusions not initiated • Consider erythropoietin growth factor support when hgb < 10 g/dL (ASCO, 2002) or < 12 g/dL (Thomas, 2002) when receiving concomitant radiotherapy for cervical or head and neck cancers; also if patient is receiving anemia-causing chemotherapy, e.g. crisplatin.
2. Impaired immunocompetence and potential for infection related to chemotherapy-induced neutropenia	• WBC (norm 4500–9000/mm^3); ANC > 2000/mm^3 • Pyrexia/rigor, erythema, swelling, pain any site • Abnormal discharges, draining wounds, skin/mucous membrane lesions • Productive cough, SOB, rectal pain, urinary frequency	WBC ≤ 3,000/mm^3; ANC < 1000/mm^3 Fever > 38.3°C or 101°F • Hold all myelosuppressive agents (exceptions may include leukemia, lymphoma, and/or situations in which there is neoplastic marrow infiltration). • Consider growth factor support to prevent febrile neutropenia • Febrile neutropenia is a medical emergency

(continued)

Table 1.1 *(continued)*

Potential Problems/Nursing Diagnoses	Physical Status: Assessment Parameters/Signs and Symptoms	Drug and Dose-Limiting Factors/ Nursing Implications
		• Severe risk of infection ANC < 500 cells/ mm^3 • Protective precautions ANC < 500 cells/ mm^3
3. Potential for injury (bleeding) related to chemotherapy-induced thrombocytopenia	• Platelet count (150,000–400,000/ mm^3) • Spontaneous gingival bleeding or epistaxis • Presence of petechiae or easy bruisability • Hematuria, melena, hematemesis, hemoptysis • Hypermenorrhea • Signs and sx intracranial bleed (irritability, sensory loss, unequal pupils, headache, ataxia)	Platelet count ≤ 100,000/mm^3 • Hold all myelosuppressive agents (exceptions may include leukemia, lymphoma, and/or situations in which there is neoplastic marrow infiltration). • Platelet transfusion if bleeding • Platelet precaution: platelet count < 50,000 cells/mm^3

(continued)

Table 1.1 *(continued)*

Potential Problems/Nursing Diagnoses	Physical Status: Assessment Parameters/Signs and Symptoms	Drug and Dose-Limiting Factors/ Nursing Implications
Integumentary System		
Alteration in mucous membrane of mouth, nasopharynx, esophagus, rectum, anus, or ostomy stoma related to chemotherapy-induced tissue changes	Mucositis Scale 0 = pink, moist, intact mucosa; absence of pain or burning +1 = generalized erythema with or without pain or burning +2 = isolated small ulcerations and/or white patches +3 = confluent ulcerations with white patches on ≥ 25% mucosa +4 = hemorrhagic ulcerations	+2 mucositis • Hold antimetabolites (esp. methotrexate, 5-FU) • Hold antitumor antibiotics (esp. doxorubicin, dactinomycin) • Hold Irinotecan • In transplant settings, may require opioid analgesia, agressive antiemesis • Consider Kepivance™ before transplant chemotherapy
Gastrointestinal System		
Discomfort, nutritional deficiency, and/or fluid and electrolyte disturbances related to chemotherapy-induced:		
1. Anorexia	• Lab values: Albumin and total protein • Normal weight/present weight and % of body weight loss • Normal diet pattern/changes in diet pattern • Alterations in taste sensation • Early satiety	• Manage nutrition impact symptoms • Dietary teaching • Appetite stimulants as needed

(continued)

Table 1.1 *(continued)*

Potential Problems/Nursing Diagnoses	Physical Status: Assessment Parameters/Signs and Symptoms	Drug and Dose-Limiting Factors/ Nursing Implications
2. Nausea and vomiting	• Lab values: Electrolytes • Pattern of n/v (incidence, duration, severity) • Antiemetic plan: Drug(s), dosage(s), schedule, efficacy: Other (dietary adjustments, relaxation techniques, environmental manipulation)	Intractable n/v × 24 h if IV hydration not initiated • Consider aggressive combination antiemesis (serotonin antagonist and dexamethasone; or addition of aprepitant to serotonin-antagonist if delayed nausea and vomiting)
3. Bowel disturbances A. Diarrhea	• Normal pattern of bowel elimination • Consistency (loose, watery/bloody stools) • Frequency and duration (no./day and no. of days) • Antidiarrheal drug(s), dosage(s), efficacy	Diarrheal stools × 3/24 h above baseline • Hold antimetabolites (esp. methotrexate, 5-FU); irinotecan • Teach patient self-administration of antidiarrheal medicine • Antibiotic therapy for unresolved diarrhea per MD

(continued)

Table 1.1 *(continued)*

Potential Problems/Nursing Diagnoses	Physical Status: Assessment Parameters/Signs and Symptoms	Drug and Dose-Limiting Factors/ Nursing Implications
B. Constipation	• Normal pattern of bowel elimination • Consistency (hard, dry, small stools) • Frequency (hours or days beyond normal pattern) • Stool softener(s), laxative(s), efficacy	No BM × 48 h past normal bowel patterns • Hold vinca alkaloids (vinblastine, vincristine) • Teach patient to take stool softener with ondansetron antiemetic
4. Hepatotoxicity	• Lab values: LDH, ALT, AST, alk phos, bili • Pain/tenderness over liver, feeling of fullness • Increase in n/v or anorexia • Changes in mental status • Jaundice • High-risk factors: Hepatic metastasis Concurrent hepatotoxic drugs Viral hepatitis graft-vs.-host disease Abdominal XRT Blood transfusions	Evidence of chemical hepatitis • Hold hepatotoxic agents (esp. methotrexate, 6-MP) until differential dx established • Hold imatinib mesylate if lab thresholds exceeded • Hold oxaliplatin if venous acclusive disease suspected • Dose reduce drugs metabolized by liver if severe liver dysfunction

(continued)

Table 1.1 *(continued)*

Potential Problems/Nursing Diagnoses	Physical Status: Assessment Parameters/Signs and Symptoms	Drug and Dose-Limiting Factors/ Nursing Implications
Respiratory System		
Impaired gas exchange or ineffective breathing pattern related to chemotherapy-induced pulmonary fibrosis	• Lab values: PFTs CXR • Respirations (rate, rhythm, depth) • Chest pain • Nonproductive cough • Progressive dyspnea • Wheezing/stridor • High-risk factors: Total cumulative dose of bleomycin Age > 60 yr Preexisting lung disease Concomitant use of other pulmonary toxic drugs Prior/concomitant XRT Smoking hx	• Acute unexplained onset respiratory symptoms • Hold all antineoplastic agents until differential dx established (e.g., bleomycin, busulfan, oxaliplatin, gemcitabine) • Interstitial Lung Disease (ILD) is a class effect of EGFR antagonist (rare), eg., gefitinib, cetuximab, erlotinib. If pulmonary symptoms develop, hold drug until ILD can be ruled out.

(continued)

Table 1.1 *(continued)*

Potential Problems/Nursing Diagnoses	Physical Status: Assessment Parameters/Signs and Symptoms	Drug and Dose-Limiting Factors/ Nursing Implications
Cardiovascular System		
Decreased cardiac output related to chemotherapy-induced: 1. Cardiac arrhythmias 2. Cardiomyopathy 3. Hypertension	• Lab values: cardiac enzymes, electrolytes, ECG, ECHO, MUGA • Vital signs • Presence of arrhythmia (irregular radial/apical pulse) • Signs sx CHF (dyspnea, ankle edema, PND, decrease in LVEF, S_3 gallop, nonproductive cough, rales, cyanosis) • High-risk factors: Total cumulative dose anthracyclines Preexisting cardiac disease Prior/concurrent mediastinal XRT • Combined anthracycline, cyclophosphamide, and trastuzumab, and paclitaxel	Acute sx CHF and/or cardiac arrhythmia • Hypertension: bevacizumab • Hold all antineoplastic agents until differential dx established Total dose doxorubicin or daunorubicin > 550 mg/m^2 • Hold anthracyclines, trastuzumab, paclitaxel • Monitor baseline and serial ejection fractions (LVEF) while receiving treatment with potentially cardiotoxic drugs; evaluate any significant ↓ in LVEF. • Severe hypertension: hold bevacizumab until hypertension controlled

(continued)

Table 1.1 *(continued)*

Potential Problems/Nursing Diagnoses	Physical Status: Assessment Parameters/Signs and Symptoms	Drug and Dose-Limiting Factors/ Nursing Implications
Genitourinary System		
1. Alteration in fluid volume (excess) related to chemotherapy-induced: A. Glomerular or renal tubule damage B. Hyperuricemic nephropathy 2. Alteration in comfort related to chemotherapy-induced hemorrhagic cystitis	• Lab values: BUN, creatinine clearance, serum creatinine, uric acid, electrolytes, urinalysis, magnesium, calcium, phosphate • Color, odor, clarity of urine • 24-h fluid intake and output (estimate/actual) • Hematuria; proteinuria • Development of oliguria or anuria • High-risk factors: Preexisting renal disease Concurrent treatment with nephrotoxic drugs (esp. aminoglycoside antibiotics) • Bevacizumad: rare nephritic syndrome	• Hold cyclophosphamide, ifosfamide Serum creatinine > 2.0 and/or Creatinine clearance < 70 mL/min Hematuria • Hold cisplatin, streptozotocin Anuria × 24 h • Hold all antineoplastic agents Nephrotic syndrome (bevacizumab) • Check BUN/creatinine before treatment • 24 hour urine for protein if spilling protein • Drug dose reduction/hold if protein > 2g (e.g. Bevacizumab)

(continued)

Table 1.1 *(continued)*

Potential Problems/Nursing Diagnoses	Physical Status: Assessment Parameters/Signs and Symptoms	Drug and Dose-Limiting Factors/ Nursing Implications
Nervous System		
1. Impaired sensory/motor function related to chemotherapy-induced A. Peripheral neuropathy B. Cranial nerve neuropathy C. Acute oxliplatin neurotoxicity	• Paresthesias (numbness, tingling in feet, fingertips) • Trigeminal nerve toxicity (severe jaw pain) • Jaw or muscle spasm • Diminished or absent deep tendon reflexes (ankle and knee jerks) • Motor weakness/slapping gait/ataxia • Visual and auditory disturbances • Cold induced paresthesias and dysesthesias lasting < 14 days	Presence of any neurologic signs and symptoms or worsening: • Perform brief nursing neuro exam before each treatment focusing on symptom analysis and functional impairment; consult MD for full neuro exam if signs/symptoms or worsening of existing signs/ symptoms • Hold vinca alkaloids, cisplatin, hexamethyl melamine, oxaliplatin, procarbazine until differential dx established • Acute oxaliplation neurotoxicity: increase length of infusion time to 6 h (decreases peak serum level by 32%); teach patient to avoid cold exposure to hands/feet oral mucosa for 3–5 days after oxaliplatin drug administration.

(continued)

Table 1.1 *(continued)*

Potential Problems/Nursing Diagnoses	Physical Status: Assessment Parameters/Signs and Symptoms	Drug and Dose-Limiting Factors/ Nursing Implications
		• Assess for motor/sensory changes impact on function and ability to do ADLS prior to oxaliplatin, taxane or cisplatin administration; hold for grades 3 and 4 toxicity (see Appendix 2) • Teach avoidance of cold for 3–5 days after oxaliplatin administration
2. Impaired bowel and bladder elimination related to chemotherapy-induced autonomic nerve dysfunction	• Urinary retention • Constipation/abdominal cramping and distension • High-risk factors: Changes in diet or mobility Frequent use of opioid analgesics Obstructive disease process	Presence of any neurologic signs and symptoms • Hold vinca alkaloids until differential dx established

ALT = alanine aminotransferase; AST = aspartate aminotransferase; bili = bilirubin; BM = bowel movement; CHF = congestive heart failure; CXR = chest X-ray; dx = diagnosis; ECG = electrocardiogram; ECHO = echocardiogram; 5-FU = 5-fluorouracil; hx = history; LDH = lactate dehydrogenase; LVEF = left ventricular ejection fraction; MUGA = multigated acquisition (MUGA heart scan); n/v = nausea and vomiting; PFT = pulmonary function test; 6-MP = 6-mercaptopurine; SOB = shortness of breath; sx = symptoms; XRT = radiation therapy *Modified from:* Engleking C 1988 Prechemotherapy Nursing Assessment in Outpatient Settings. *Outpatient Chemotherapy* 3(1):10–11.

Table 1.2 Classifications of Antineoplastic Drugs

Classification	Mechanism of Action	Examples
	Cell Cycle Specific Agents	
Antimetabolites	Interfere with DNA and RNA synthesis by acting as false metabolites, which are incorporated into the DNA strand, or block essential enzymes, so that DNA synthesis is prevented.	Pemetraxate (slinta) Cytosine arabinoside (ara-C, Cytosar-U) Eniluracil 5-Fluorouracil (5-FU) Floxuridine (FUDR, 5-FUDR) Hydroxyurea (Hydrea) 6-Mercaptopurine (6-MP, Purinethol) Methotrexate (Amethopterin, Mexate, Folex) 6-Thioguanine (6-TG) Gemcitabine (Gemzar®) Fludarabine (Fludara®) Capecitabine (Xeloda®) Deoxycoformycin (Pentostatin)
Vinca Alkaloids	Crystallize microtubules of mitotic spindle causing metaphase arrest (vincristine, vinblastine, vindesine), role in blocking DNA and preventing cell division in M phase (vinorelbine).	Vincristine (VCR, Oncovin) Vinblastine (VLB, Velban) Vinorelbine (Navelbine®)
Epipodophyllotoxins	Damage the cell prior to mitosis, late S and G_2 phase; inhibit topoisomerase II.	Etoposide (VP-16, Vepesid) Teniposide (VM-26, Vumon)

(continued)

Table 1.2 *(continued)*

Classification	Mechanism of Action	Examples
	Cell Cycle Specific Agents	
Taxanes	Promotes early microtubule assembly. Prevents depolymerization, causing cell death (paclitaxel); enhances microtubule assembly and inhibits tubulin depolymerization, thus arresting cell division in metaphase (docetaxel).	Paclitaxel (Taxol®) Docetaxel (Taxotere®) Paclitaxe) protein bound
Camptothecins	Act in S phase to inhibit topoisomerase I and cause cell death.	Topotecan (Hycamtin®) Irinotecan (CPT-11, Camptosar®)
Miscellaneous		G_1 phase: L-asparaginase (ELSPAR), Prednisone G_2 phase: Bleomycin (Bleo, Blenoxane)
	Cell Cycle Non-Specific Agents	
Alkylating Agents	Substitute alkyl group for H+ ion causing single- and double-strand breaks in DNA, as well as cross-linkages; thus DNA strands are unable to separate during DNA replication.	Busulfan (Myleran®, oral; Busulfex®, IV) Carboplatin (Paraplatin) *Carmustine (BiCNU, BCNU) Chlorambucil (Leukeran) Cisplatin (*Cis*-Platinum, CDDP, Platinol) Cyclophosphamide (Cytoxan, CTX, Neosar) Dacarbazine (DTIC-Dome, Imidazole) Estramustine phosphate (Estracyte, Emcyt) Oxaliplatin (Eloxatin®)

(continued)

Table 1.2 *(continued)*

Classification	Mechanism of Action	Examples
	Cell Cycle Non-Specific Agents	
		Ifosfamide (IFEX) *Lomustine (CCNU) Mechlorethamine hydrochloride (nitrogen mustard, mustargen, HN_2) Melphalan (Alkeran, 1-PAM, Phenylalanine Mustard) Oxaliplatin (Eloxatin) *Streptozocin (Streptozotocin, Zanosar) Thiotepa (Triethylene Thiophosphoramide, TSPA)
Antibiotics	Use a variety of mechanisms to prevent cell division and death (DNA strand breakage, intercalation of base pairs, inhibition of RNA and DNA synthesis).	Dactinomycin (Actinomycin D, Cosmegan) Daunorubicin hydrochloride (Daunomycin, Cerubidine) Doxorubicin hydrochloride (Adria, Adriamycin) Epirubicin HCl (Ellenee) Indarubicin (Idamycin) Mithramycin (Mithramycin, Plicamycin) Mitomycin C (Mito, Mutamycin) Mitoxantrone (Novantrone)

*Nitrosoureas (cross blood-brain barrier)

Table 1.3 Common Agents Used in Dose-Intensive/High-Dose Chemotherapy and Associated Toxicities

Drug	Toxicity
Doxorubicin	1. Cardiotoxicity leading to degenerative cardiomyopathy over time Standard dose: 60–75 mg/m^2 Current lifetime dose: 450–550 mg/m^2 Current protocol dose ranges: 430–650 mg/m^2 (lifetime) When given over 96 hours in a dilute solution or at low weekly doses, cardiotoxicity appears to decrease. Prior radiation therapy to the chest or prior anthracycline therapy may predispose patient to or enhance cardiotoxicity. 2. Severe mucositis 3. Acute myelosuppression; late onset in children, even at low cumulative doses
Cyclophosphamide	1. Standard dose: 400–1600 mg/m^2 IV; high dose: up to 200 mg/kg 2. High dose: Cardiotoxicity, acute cardiomyopathy Diminished QRS complex on ECG Pulmonary congestion and pleural effusions Cardiomegaly Prior radiation therapy to the chest or prior anthracycline therapy may predispose patient to or enhance cardiotoxicity. Ejection fraction of > 50% not predictive of reduced risk for cardiotoxicity. 3. Hemorrhagic cystitis (occasionally chronic, severe) 5. Acral erythema and sloughing of skin on palms of hands and soles of feet 6. Diffuse hyperpigmentation 7. Gonadal dysfunction Delayed pubertal development Diminished testicular volume in adult males
Cisplatin	1. Standard dose: 15–120 mg/m^2; high dose: 160–200 mg/m^2 2. Renal and hepatic toxicity 3. Eighth cranial nerve damage and ototoxicity 4. Myelosuppression 5. Peripheral neuropathy 6. Intense nausea and vomiting

(continued)

Table 1.3 *(continued)*

Drug	Toxicity
Carboplatin	1. Standard dose: 400–500 mg/m^2; high dose: 800–1600 mg/m^2 2. Myelosuppression (dose-limiting); pronounced thrombocytopenia 3. Severe nausea and vomiting 4. Hepatotoxicity 5. Auditory toxicity 6. Mild renal toxicity
Cytosine arabinoside	1. Standard dose: 100–200 mg/m^2; high dose: 2–3 g/m^2 2. Acute neurotoxicity: cerebellar toxicity Those over 50 at highest risk for minimal recovery from symptoms. Assess prior to each dose for ataxia, nystagmus, and slurred speech; hold dose if any indication of symptomatology (over baseline assessment). 3. Acral erythema and possible sloughing of skin on palms of hands and soles of feet 4. Conjunctivitis, Steroid eye drops may prevent or alleviate 5. Intense diarrhea, up to 2–3 liters/24 hours
Busulfan	1. Standard dose: 1–4 mg/m^2; high dose: 16 mg/kg 2. Myelosuppression 3. Severe nausea and vomiting 4. Severe mucositis 5. Pneumonitis, pulmonary fibrosis; "busulfan lung" 6. Hepatic dysfunction leading to veno-occlusive disease 7. Diffuse hyperpigmentation; rare: development of bullae 8. Chronic alopecia
Etoposide	1. Standard dose: 60 mg/m^2; high dose: 60 mg/kg or 80–250 mg/m^2 2. Severe mucositis 3. Acral erythema and sloughing of skin or palms of hands and soles of feet 4. Myelosuppression 5. Severe blood pressure fluctuations 6. Fever and chills during infusion
Methotrexate	1. Standard dose: 10–500 mg/m^2; high dose: 500 mg/m^2 and greater 2. Photosensitivity 3. Diffuse hyperpigmentation

(continued)

Table 1.3 *(continued)*

Drug	Toxicity
	4. Neurotoxicity: seizures, aphasia, cerebellar toxicity (rare; see cytosine arabinoside) 5. Severe diarrhea 6. Renal toxicity 7. Hepatotoxicity and coagulopathies 8. Thrombocytopenia 9. Pulmonary toxicities
Melphalan	1. Standard dose: 6–8 mg/m^2; high dose: 80–140 mg/m^2 2. Severe mucositis 3. Diarrhea 4. Severe nausea, especially in combination with another emetogenic drug 5. Renal toxicity 6. Profound myelosuppression 7. Severe liver toxicity
Carmustine	1. Standard dose: 200–240 mg/m^2; high dose: 600–1200 mg/m^2 2. Hepatic dysfunction leading to veno-occlusive disease 3. Central nervous system changes, including diffuse encephalopathy 4. Mild alopecia
5-Fluorouracil	1. Standard dose: 7–15 mg/kg for five days; high dose: 255–300 mg/m^2 continuous infusion weekly 2. Cardiotoxicity mimicking acute myocardial infarction, angina, cardiogenic shock 3. Photosensitivity and hyperpigmentation 4. Severe diarrhea 5. Cerebellar toxicity

Source: Brown KA, Esper P, Kelleher LO, et al (2001) *Chemotherapy and Biotherapy Guidelines and Recommendations for Practice*. Pittsburgh, Oncology Nursing Soc, pp 60–63. Reproduced with permission from Oncology Nursing Society Publishing.

than 3 feet and is condensed into chromosomes by torsion of the helix. During cell replication, the DNA strands that are coiled in the double helix need to unwind so that they can separate and be copied. This is made possible by the topoisomerase I and II enzymes (Chen and Liu, 1994).

Topoisomerase I relaxes tension in the DNA helix torsion by causing a transient single-strand break or nick in the DNA when it covalently bonds to the end of one of the DNA strands. The other, intact strand then passes through the break, and relaxation of the DNA helix occurs as the strands swivel at the strand break. The topoisomerase I enzyme then reseals the cleaved strand (religation step), and the enzyme is released from the DNA strand. Transcription (copying of the strands) is then initiated. Interestingly, topoisomerase I is found in greater concentrations in patients with cancers of the colon, non-Hodgkin's lymphoma, and some leukemias (Husain et al, 1994). Drugs developed within this decade, such as topotecan and irinotecan, work by inhibiting the religation or repair of the single-strand break by binding to topoisomerase I, and cells are arrested in G_2 phase.

Topoisomerase II is also involved in the relaxation of the helix torsion, but it causes a double-strand break to allow crossing of two double-stranded DNA segments. It then causes the closing of the two DNA strand breaks. This permits assembly of chromatin, as well as condensation and decondensation of the chromosomes, and separation of the DNA in the daughter cells during mitosis (Lui et al, 1980). Drugs that are well known to interfere with topoisomerase II are etoposide (nonintercalator, and cell cycle specific for M phase) and doxorubicin (intercalator of base pairs and cell cycle nonspecific) (Eber, 1996).

Descriptions of the drugs in the chapter have been updated to reflect new indications. Agents that have now been approved by the Food and Drug Administration (FDA) for use in cancer treatment have been updated, and investigational agents that are nearing FDA application or appear very promising, are included.

With the promise of increased survival in patients with solid tumors, standard chemotherapy agents are being combined at higher doses for marrow ablation, with subsequent stem cell rescue. However, more severe toxicity is seen (see Table 1.3). In addition, there have been advances in the approval of agents that provide organ protection from drug toxicity (cytoprotectants) which is discussed in Chapter 4.

New technology has permitted a reduction in toxicity from a number of drugs. For instance, the use of nanotechnology to manufacture liposomal delivery vehicles for doxorubicin, daunorubicin, cytarabine, amphotericin, paclitaxel and camptothecins are currently available or being studied. The liposomal "wrapping" of water-soluble or insoluble drugs permits the drug to be preferentially delivered to sites of infection, inflammation, or tumor. Liposomes may pass through gaps in the endothelial lining of blood capillaries within the tumor, where the drug may be unpackaged and released within the tumor. Healthy tissues, on the other hand, have capillary walls that prevent the leakage of liposomes into the tissues, so that toxicity is reduced. The targeting of liposomes for specific tissues or disease sites is accomplished by variation in the number of lipid layers, and the size, charge, and permeability of the layers (Bangham, 1992). In addition, oral formulations of intravenous drugs are being studied, such as topotecan, and the investigational camptothecins rubitecan and liposomal karenitecin. Efforts are being made to try to find agents offering equal efficacy but that can improve quality of life, such as new oral antineoplastic agents, by minimizing trips to the hospital or intrusive administration techniques.

Within the last few years, interest and clinical testing of new approaches to old drugs has occurred. 5-fluorouracil (5-FU) is an old drug that has good efficacy in colorectal cancer and other gastrointestinal cancers. However, it is limited, and increased doses are not necessarily more effective. Also, given by continuous infusion, 5-FU is often more effective because, being cell cycle specific for the S phase, more malignant cells are likely to be exposed to continuous infusion of chemotherapy than if the drug is given by bolus injection.

In an effort to improve the efficacy, new oral fluoropyrimidines have been developed, along with other agents that decrease the breakdown of 5-FU, so that serum drug levels are higher and more sustained, mimicking a continuous infusion. An example of a prodrug is tegafur, and an inhibitor of DPD is uracil, and also eniluracil. In an effort to reduce the toxicity of bolus 5FU/LV deGramont et al (1997) showed that infusional 5FU/LV was equivalent in efficacy but significantly less toxic. This has become the standard way to administer 5FU/LV in the United States at this time.

Capecitabine (Xeloda), a 5-FU prodrug that is preferentially taken up by tumor cells. The drug has been approved for both the adjuvant treatment of patients with colon cancer as well as patients with advanced metastatic breast and colon cancers. Capecitabine has been shown to be equivalent to 5FU/LV and is being studied as a replacement in combination with oxaliplatin, irinotecan, or alone during radiotherapy. It simulates a continuous infusion of 5-FU, and has been shown equivalent to 5FU/LV in both adjuvant and metastatic settings (Cassidy et al, 2004). Ideally, these oral agents could be used to provide radiosensitization for patients with gastrointestinal tumors undergoing external beam radiotherapy.

Antineoplastic agents are classified by mechanism of action (see Table 1.2). Cell cycle specific agents are most active during specific phases of the cell cycle and include antimetabolites (synthesis phase), vinca alkaloids (mitotic phase), and miscellaneous drugs. Examples of these include L-asparaginase and prednisone (G_1 phase) and bleomycin and etoposide (G_2 phase). In addition, effective drugs such as the taxanes, that have a clear mechanism of action at therapeutic doses, may in fact, have an antiangiogenic effect at lower, more frequent dosing. Endothelial cells appear to be very sensitive to the taxanes. Seidman et al (2004) demonstrated that paclitaxel given weekly at a lower dose (dose density) was superior to an increased dose given every 3 weeks.

Cell cycle nonspecific agents can damage cells in all phases of the cell cycle and include alkylating agents (cyclophosphamide, cisplatin), antitumor/antibiotics (doxorubicin, mitomycin-C), the nitrosureas (carmustine, lomustine), and others (dacarbazine, procarbazine) (see Table 1.2).

Antineoplastic agents are effective because they interfere with cellular metabolism and replication, resulting in cell death. When malignant cells evade programmed cell death, the tumor cells no longer are controlled by apoptosis, and resistance emerges. However, it is critical that nurses protect themselves when handling these drugs so that they are not exposed to the potential drug hazards. These drugs can be:

- *Mutagenic*: capable of causing a change in the genetic material within a cell that can be passed on to future cell generations;
- *Teratogenic*: capable of causing damage to a developing fetus exposed to the drug; the greatest risk is during the first trimester of pregnancy when the fetal organ systems are developing;
- *Carcinogenic*: capable of causing malignant change in a cell.

In 1985, the Occupational Safety and Health Administration (OSHA) developed guidelines for the safe handling of antineoplastic agents. These guidelines were revised in 1995 and then in 2004 to include all hazardous drugs (see Appendix I). NIOSH has updated recommendations as of March 2004.

Hormones are used in the management of hormonally sensitive cancers, such as breast and prostate cancers. The hormone changes the hormonal environment, probably affecting growth factors, so that the stimulus for tumor growth is suppressed or removed (see Table 1.4). New SERMs and aromatase inhibitors are being developed to improve on the demonstrated success of tamoxifen.

COMPLICATIONS OF DRUG ADMINISTRATION

All drugs can cause hypersensitivity reactions including anaphylaxis, but only a few drugs cause severe problems. These include:

- L-asparaginase
- Paclitaxel (related to carrier vehicle solution CR cremefor)
- Docetaxel (related to delivery vehicle solution Tween)
- Cisplatin
- Teniposide (Vumon, VM-26)
- Bleomycin (less common; 2% incidence in lymphoma patients)
- Cetuximab (Erbitux, discussed in Chapter 5), rare but may be fatal.
- Rituximab (Rituxan, discussed in Chapter 5)

In addition, certain drugs can cause delayed hypersensitivity, such as carboplatin and oxaliplatin, where the patient develops a range of signs and symptoms of hypersensitivity after receiving a number of cycles of the drug, such as 7 cycles of carboplatin (Markman et al. 2003). For nursing management of patients

Table 1.4 Common Hormonal Agents

Classification	Examples
Adrenocorticoids	cortisone hydrocortisone dexamethasone methylprednisone methylprednisolone prednisone prednisolone
Androgens	testosterone propionate (Neo-hombreol, Oreton) fluoxymesterone (Halotestin, Ora-Testryl) testolactone
Estrogens	chlorotrianisene (TACE) diethylstilbestrol (DES) diethylstilbestrol diphosphate (Stilphostrol) ethinyl estradiol (Estinyl) conjugated estrogen (Premarin) Stradiol
Selective Estrogen Receptor	tamoxifen citrate (Nolvadex)
Modulators (SERM)	toremifene citrate (Fareston) raloxifene (Evista)
Selective aromatase inhibitors	
• Reversible	Anastrozole (Arimidex) Letrozole (Femara)
• Irreversible	Exemestane (Aromasin)
Progesterones	medroxyprogesterone acetate (Provera, Depo-Provera) megestrol acetate (Megace, Pallace)
Antitestosterone	leuprolide acetate (Lupron) bicalutamide (Casodex) flutamide (Eulexin) nilutamide (Nilandron)

experiencing hypersensitivity or anaphylaxis, as recommended by the Oncology Nursing Society Practice Committee, see Table 1.5.

Table 1.5 Management of Hypersensitivity and Anaphylactic Reactions

1. Review the patient's allergy history.
2. Consider prophylactic medications with hydrocortisone or an antihistamine in atopic/allergic individuals. (This requires a physician's order.)
3. *Patient and family education:* Assess the patient's readiness to learn. Inform patient of the potential for an allergic reaction and instruct to report any unusual symptoms such as:
   A. Uneasiness or agitation
   B. Abdominal cramping
   C. Itching
   D. Chest tightness
   E. Light-headedness or dizziness
   F. Chills
4. Ensure that emergency equipment and medications are readily available.
5. Obtain baseline vital signs and note patient's mental status.
6. As appropriate, perform a scratch test, intradermal skin test, or test dose before administering the full dosage (this requires a physician's order). If there is no reaction, the remaining dose can be administered. If an allergic response is suspected, discontinue the test dose (unless it has been completed), maintain the intravenous line, and notify the physician.
7. For a *localized allergic response:*
   A. Evaluate symptoms; observe for urticaria, wheals, localized erythema.
   B. Administer diphenhydramine or hydrocortisone as per physician's order.
   C. Monitor vital signs every 15 minutes for 1 hour.
   D. Continue subsequent dosing or desensitization program according to a physician's order.
   E. If a "flare" reaction appears along the vein with doxorubicin (Adriamycin) or daunorubicin, flush the line with saline.
      a. Insure that extravasation has not occurred.
      b. Administer hydrocortisone 25–50 mg intravenously with a physician's order, followed by a 0.9% NS flush. This may be adequate to resolve the "flare" reaction.
      c. Once the "flare" reaction has resolved, continue slow infusion of the drug.
      d. Monitor for repeated "flare" episodes. It is preferable to change the intravenous site if possible.
8. For a generalized allergic response, *anaphylaxis* may be suspected if the following signs or symptoms occur (usually within the first 15 minutes of the start of the infusion or injection):
   A. Subjective signs and symptoms
      a. Generalized itching
      b. Chest tightness
      c. Agitation
      d. Uneasiness
      e. Dizziness
      f. Nausea
      g. Crampy abdominal pain
      h. Anxiety

Table 1.5 *(continued)*

i. Sense of impending doom
j. Desire to urinate or defecate
k. Chills

B. Objective signs
a. Flushed appearance (edema of face, hands, or feet)
b. Localized or generalized urticaria
c. Respiratory distress with or without wheezing
d. Hypotension
e. Cyanosis
f. Difficulty speaking

9. For a *generalized allergic response:*
A. Stop the infusion immediately and notify the physician.
B. Maintain the intravenous line with appropriate solution to expand the vascular space, e.g., NS.
C. If not contraindicated, ensure maximum rate of infusion if the patient is hypotensive.
D. Position the patient to promote perfusion of the vital organs; the supine position is preferred.
E. Monitor vital signs every 2 minutes until stable, then every 5 minutes for 30 minutes, then every 15 minutes as ordered.
F. Reassure the patient and the family.
G. Maintain the airway and anticipate the need for cardiopulmonary resuscitation.
H. All medications must be administered with a physician's order.
I. Anticipate administering the following medications for the following effects:
a) Vasoconstriction to increase cardiac output and blood pressure:
1) epinephrine (1:1000, 0.3–0.5 mL or 0.3–0.5 mg IM or SQ q 10–15 min; or if hypotensive, 1:10,000 concentration giving 0.5–1.0 mL (0.1 mg) IVP in Adults; in pediatrics, 1:1000 IM 0.01 mL/kg (up to 0.3 mL)
2) dopamine 2–20 micrograms/kg/min (adults)
b) Antihistamines to stop allergic release of histamines:
1) H1: diphenhydramine: 25–50 mg IVP (adults), 1 mg/kg (max 50 mg, pediatrics)
2) H2: ranitidine 50 mg IV or famotidine 20 mg IV (adults)
c) Bronchodilation: aminophylline 5 mg/kg IV over 30 min (adults)
d) Anti-inflammation/Bronchodilation: steroids. Methylprednisolone 30–50 mg IV (peds 0.3–0.5 mg/kg); or dexamethasone 10–20 mg IVP (peds 1–2 mg/kg); or hydrocortisone 100–500 mg IV (peds 1–2 mg/kg)

10. Document the incident in the medical record according to institution policy and procedures.
11. Physician-guided desensitization may be necessary for subsequent dosing.

References: Polovich M, White JM, Kelleher LC, (eds), *Chemotherapy and Biotherapy Guidelines and Recommendations for Practice.* 2nd ed. Pittsburgh, PA: ONS; 2005;86. Barton-Burke, M, Wilkes GM, Ingwersen K. *Cancer Chemotherapy: A Nursing process Approach,* 3rd ed. Sudbury, MA: Jones and Bartlett Publishers Inc.; 2001. Ellis AK and Day JH. Diagnosis and Management of Anaphylaxis. *Canadian Medical Association Journal* 2003;169(4): 307—312. Sheperd GM. Hypersensitivity Reactions to Chemotherapeutic Drugs. *Allergy and Immunology* 2003;24:253–262.

Table 1.6 Vesicants and Irritants

Vesicants				
Chemotherapeutic Agents	**Antidote**	**Antidote Preparation**	**Local Care**	**Comments**
Alkylating agents				
Mechlorethamine (nitrogen mustard)	Isotonic sodium (NA) thiosulfate	Prepare 1/6 molar solution: 1. If 10% Na thiosulfate solution, mix 4 mL with 6 ml sterile water for injection. 2. If 25% Na thiosufate solution, mix 1.6 mL with 8.4 ml sterile water.	1. Immediately inject Na thiosulfate through IV cannula, 2 mL for every mg extravasated. 2. Remove needle. 3. Inject antidote into subcutaneous (SC) tissue.	1. Na thiosulfate neutralizes nitrogen mustard, which then is excreted via the kidneys. 2. Time is essential in treating extravasation. 3. Heat and cold not proven effective. 4. Although clinically accepted, reports of the benefits are scant.
Cisplatin (Platinol®[a])	Same as above	Same as above	1. Use 2 ml of the 10% Na thiosulfate for each 100 mg of cisplatin. 2. Remove needle. 3. Inject SC.	1. Vesicant potential seen with a concentration of more than 20 cc of 0.5 mg/ml extravasates. If less than this, drug is an irritant; no treatment recommended.

(continued)

Table 1.6 *(continued)*

Vesicants				
Chemotherapeutic Agents	**Antidote**	**Antidote Preparation**	**Local Care**	**Comments**
Antitumor antibiotics				
Doxorubicin (Adriamycin®[b])	None		1. Apply cold pad with circulating ice water, ice pack, or cryogel pack for 15–20 minutes at least four times per day for the first 24–48 hours. Elevate site for 48 hrs, then resume normal activity	1. Extravasations of less than 1–2 cc often will heal spontaneously. If greater than 3 cc, ulceration often results. 2. Protect area from sunlight and heat. 3. Studies suggest benefit of 99% dimethyl sulfoxide (DMSO) 1–2 mL applied to site every 6 hours. Other studies show delayed healing with DMSO.
Daunorubicin (Cerubidine®[c])	None			1. Little information known. 2. In mouse experiments, some benefit from topical DMSO.
Mitomycin-C (mitamycin)	None			1. Protect from sunlight. 2. Delayed skin reactions have occurred in areas far from original IV site.

(continued)

Table 1.6 *(continued)*

Vesicants				
Chemotherapeutic Agents	**Antidote**	**Antidote Preparation**	**Local Care**	**Comments**
				3. Some research studies show benefit with use of 99% DMSO 1–2 mL applied to site every 6 hours for 14 days. More studies needed.
Dactinomycin (actinomycin-D)	None		1. Apply ice to increase comfort at the site. 2. Elevate for 48 hours then resume normal activity.	1. Heat may enhance tissue damage.
Mitoxantrone (concentrated dose)	Unknown			1. Antidote and local care measures unknown. 2. Ulceration rare unless concentrated dose infiltrates.
Epirubicin (Ellence®[d])	None			1. Antidote and local care measures unknown. 2. Cold, DMSO, and corticosteriods ineffective in experiments with mice.

(continued)

Table 1.6 *(continued)*

Vesicants				
Chemotherapeutic Agents	**Antidote**	**Antidote Preparation**	**Local Care**	**Comments**
Vinca alkaloids/microtubular inhibiting agents				
Vincristine (Oncovin®[e])			1. Apply warm pack for 15–20 minutes at least four times per day for the first 24–48 hours and elevate.	Apply heat for 15–20 minutes at least four times per day for the first 24–48 hours. 1. These two methods of treatment are very effective for rapid absorption of drug.
Vinblastine (Velban®[e])			Same as above.	Same as above.
Vindesine (Eblisine®)				Same as above.
Vinorebine (Navelbine®[f])			Same as above.	1. Same treatment as vincristine/vinblastine. 2. Moderate vesicant. 3. Manufacturer recommends administering drug over 6–10 minutes into side port of free-flowing IV closest to the IV bag, followed by flush of 75–125 mL of IV solution to reduce incidence of phlebitis and severe back pain.

(continued)

Table 1.6 *(continued)*

Chemotherapeutic Agents	Antidote	Antidote Preparation	Local Care	Comments
Vesicants				
Taxanes				
Paclitaxel (Taxol®[a]) (concentrated solution)	Ice		Apply ice pack for 15–20 minutes at least four times per day for the first 24 hours.	1. Paclitaxel may have rare vesicant potential (probably due to dilution in 500 cc diluent. 2. Ice and hyaluronidase have been effective in decreasing local tissue damage in a mouse model.
Irritants				
Alkylating agents				
Dacarbazine (DTIC)				1. May cause phlebitis. 2. Protect drug from sunlight.
Ifosfamide Carboplatin				1. May cause phlebitis. 2. Antidote or local care measures unknown.

(continued)

Table 1.6 *(continued)*

Chemotherapeutic Agents	Antidote	Antidote Preparation	Local Care	Comments
Irritants *(continued)*				
Oxaliplatin (however, has vesicant potential)				1. Oxaliplatin has vesicant potential so is best given via CL. If oxaliplatin given via peripheral line, drug can be diluted in 500 mL D5W (Sanofi Synthelabo, 2004) and infused over 6 hours to decrease discomfort. 2. High dose dexamethasone should be considered as a therapeutic intervention (Kretzschman et al., 2003)
Antitumor Antibiotics Daunorubicin citrace (DaunoXone®				
Nitrosoureas				
Carmustine (BCNU)				1. May cause phlebitis Local care measures are unknown. 2. Antidote or local care measures unknown.
Antitumor antibiotics				
Doxorubicin liposome (Doxil)®)				1. May produce redness and tissue edema. 2. Low ulceration potential. 3. If ulceration begins or pain, redness, or swelling persist, treat like doxorubicin.
Bleomycin (Blenoxan®)				1. May cause irritation to tissue. 2. Little information known.

(continued)

Table 1.6 *(continued)*

Irritants *(continued)*				
Chemotherapeutic Agents	**Antidote**	**Antidote Preparation**	**Local Care**	**Comments**
Epipodophyl-lotoxin				
Etoposide (VP-16)			1. Apply warm pack.	1. Treatment necessary only if large amount of a concentrated solution extravasates. In this case, treat like vincristine or vinblastine. 2. May cause phlebitis, urticaria, and redness.
Teniposide (VM-26)				Same as above.

[a]*Bristol-Myers-Squibb Oncology, Princeton, NJ;*
[b]*Pharmacia & Upjohn Co, Kalamazoo, MI;*
[c]*Chiron Therapeutics, Emeryville, CA;*
[d]*Andria Laboratories, Dublin, OH;*
[e]*Eli Lilly and Co., Indianapolis, IN;*
[f]*Glaxo Wellcome Oncology/HIV, Research Triangle Park, NC*

Note: Based on information from Bertelli, G., Gozzo, A., Forno, G.B., Vidili, M.G., Silvestro, S., Venturini, M., DelMastro, L., Garrone, O., Rosso, R., and Dini, D., 1995. Topical Dimethylsulfoxide for the Prevention of Soft Tissue Injury after Extravasation of Vesicant Cytotoxic Drugs: A Prospective Clinical Study. *Journal of Clinical Oncology,* 13(11):2851–2855; Lebredo, L., Barrie, R., and Woltering, E.A., 1992. DMSO Protection Against Adriamycin-induced Tissue Necrosis. *Journal of Surgery Research,* 53(1):62–65; Rospond, E.M., and Engel, L.M., 1993. Dimethyl Sulfoxide for Treating Anthracycline Extravesation. *Clinical Pharmatherapeutics* 12(8):560–561. *Source:* Brown KA, Esper P, Kellher LO, et al (2001) *Cancer Chemotherapy Guidelines and Recommendations for Practice,* pp 46–47. Reproduced with permission from Oncology Nursing Society Publishing.

Modified from Polovich M, White Jim, Kellner LO (Eds) (2005) *Chemotherapy and Biotherapy Guidelines and Recommendations for Practice*, 2nd Ed, pp. 79-81. Reproduced with permission from Oncology Nursing Society.

Table 1.7 Standardized Nursing Care Plan for Management of the Patient Experiencing Extravasation (Based on Oncology Nursing Press Cancer Chemotherapy Guidelines)

Nursing Diagnosis	Defining Characteristics	Expected Outcomes	Nursing Interventions
I. Potential alteration in skin integrity related to extravasation.	I. Vesicant drugs may cause erythema, burning, tissue necrosis, tissue sloughing.	I. Extravasation, if it occurs, is detected early with early intervention.	I. Careful technique is used during venipuncture. A. Select venipuncture site away from underlying tendons and blood vessels. B. Secure IV so that catheter/needle site is visible at all times. C. Administer vesicant through freely flowing IV, constantly monitoring IV site and patient response. Nurse should be thoroughly familiar with institutional policy and procedure for administration of a vesicant agent. D. If vesicant drug is administered as a continuous infusion, drug must be given through a patent central line and monitored closely.
II. Potential pain at site of extravasation.	II. Vesicant drugs include: A. Commercial agents 1. dactinomycin 2. daunorubicin 3. doxorubicin 4. mitomycin C	II. Skin and underlying tissue damage is minimized.	II. If extravasation is suspected: A. Stop drug administration. B. Aspirate any residual drug and blood from IV tubing, IV catheter/needle IV site if possible.

(continued)

Table 1.7 *(continued)*

Nursing Diagnosis	Defining Characteristics	Expected Outcomes	Nursing Interventions
	5. estramustine 6. mechlorethamine 7. vinblastine 8. vincristine 9. vinorelbine 10. idarubicin 11. vindesine 12. epirubicin 13. esorubicin 14. cisplatin (concentrated) 15. mitoxantrone 16. paclitaxel (concentrated) 17. fluorouracil (concentrated) B. Investigational agents 1. amsacrine 2. maytansine 3. bisantrene 4. pyrazofurin 5. adozelesin 6. anti-B4-blocked ricin		C. Instill antidote, if one exists, through needle if able to remove remaining drug in previous step. If standing orders are not available, notify MD and obtain order. D. Remove needle. E. Inject antidote into area of apparent infiltration, if antidote is recommended, using 25-gauge needle into subcutaneous tissue. F. Apply topical cream if recommended. G. Cover lightly with occlusive sterile dressing. H. Apply warm or cold applications as prescribed. I. Elevate arm. J. Assess site regularly for pain, progression of erythema, induration, and for evidence of necrosis: 1. If outpatient, arrange to assess site or teach patient to and to notify provider if condition worsens. Arrange next visit for assessment of site depending on drug, amount infiltrated, extent of potential injury, and patient variables.

(continued)

Table 1.7 *(continued)*

Nursing Diagnosis	Defining Characteristics	Expected Outcomes	Nursing Interventions
			2. Discuss with MD the need for plastic-surgical consult if erythema, induration, pain, tissue breakdown occurs. K. When in doubt about whether drug is infiltrating, treat as an infiltration. L. Document precise, concise information in patient's medical record: 1. Date, time 2. Insertion site, needle size and type 3. Drug administration technique, drug sequence, and approximate amount of drug extravasated 4. Appearance of site, patient's subjective response 5. Nursing interventions performed to manage extravasation, and notification of MD 6. Photo documentation if possible 7. Follow-up plan 8. Nurse's signature 9. Institutional policy and procedure for documentation should be adhered to
III. Potential loss of function of extremity related to extravasation			
IV. Potential infection related to skin breakdown			

Source: Barton-Burke M et al (2001) *Cancer Chemotherapy: A Nursing Process Approach,* pp 628–629. Reprinted with permission from Jones and Bartlett Publishers, Inc.

EXTRAVASATION

Specific chemotherapeutic drugs called *vesicants* may cause severe tissue necrosis if extravasated. Some of these drugs have antidotes that will minimize or prevent local tissue damage. These are shown in Table 1.6. For a Standardized Nursing Care Plan for management of patients experiencing extravasation, see Table 1.7.

When vesicants are administered as a continuous infusion, a central line is required. In addition, it is imperative that the IV insertion site be checked for signs/symptoms of extravasation at least hourly, and that the patient be instructed to tell the nurse immediately if stinging or burning is felt. As many continuous infusions of vesicant chemotherapy occur when the patient is at home, it is again imperative to instruct the patient to pay attention to any changes in sensation at the site, and to call the nurse if any discomfort, stinging, or burning is felt. A number of patients have had extravasation of drug from a needle dislodged from an implanted port onto the surrounding skin, which then caused a necrotic ulcer and necessitated explantation of the subcutaneous port.

Within the last decade, oncology nurses have been humbled by the reports of significant and lethal errors that have occurred during the chemotherapy prescription, admixing, and administration processes. It is clear that institutional and physician office practices must have systematic review of the entire linked process and steps taken to prevent the occurrence of these errors and tragic consequences through competent checks and balances (Fisher et al, 1996). Fortunately, the series of well-publicized errors have been a "wake-up" call, and oncology nurses, pharmacists, and physicians have worked together to develop safe environments for clinical practice. The Oncology Nursing Society position paper, "Regarding the Preparation of the Professional Registered Nurse Who Administers and Cares for the Individual Receiving Chemotherapy", states that the nurse administering chemotherapy and caring for patients receiving chemotherapy should complete a chemotherapy course and clinical practicum to safely and competently deliver chemotherapy. The course topics should include history of cancer chemotherapy; drug development; principles of cancer chemotherapy; chemotherapy preparation, storage, and transport; nursing assessment; chemotherapy administration; safety precautions during chemotherapy administration; disposal/accidental exposure and spills; and, finally, institutional considerations (ONS Position Paper, revised 6/99: ONS Safe Handeling of Hazardous Drugs, 2003; NISOH Safe Handeling of Hazardous Drugs, June 2004).

References

Ajani JA, Dodd LS, Daughtery K, et al. Taxol-Induced Soft-Tissue Injury Secondary to Extravasation: Characterization by Histo-Pathology and Clinical Course. *JNCI* 1994;86:51–53

Alberts DS, Dorr RT. Case Report: Topical DMSO for Mitomycin-C-Induced Skin Ulceration. *Oncol Nurs Forum* 1991;18:693–695

Andre T, Boni C, Mounedji-Boudiaf L, et al. Oxaliplatin, fluorouracil and leucovorin as adjuvant treatment for colon cancer. *N Engl J Med* 2004;350(23):2342–2351

Anttila M, Laakso S, Nylanden P, Sotaniemi EA. Pharmacokinetics of the Novel Antiestrogenic Agent Toremifene in Subjects with Altered Liver and Kidney Function. *Clin Pharmacol Ther* 1995;57(6):628–635

AstraZeneca Pharmaceuticals LP. Prescribing Package Insert: Faslodex. Wilmington, DE:, AstraZeneca Pharmaceuticals LP; 2002

Aventis. Nilandron (Nilutamide) Product Information Center for Prostate Cancer. 2001; available at http://www.aventis-us.com/pls/nilandron_TXT.html. Accessed June 2004

Ayash LJ, Hunt M, Antman K. Hepatic Occlusive Disease in Autologous Bone Marrow Transplantition of Solid Tumor and Lymphomas. *J Clin Oncol* 1990;8:1699–1706

Bangham AC. Liposomes: Realizing Their Promise. *Hosp Pract* 1992;27(12):51–62

Barton-Burke M, Wilkes G, Berg D, et al. *Cancer Chemotherapy: A Nursing Process Approach,* 3rd ed Sudbury, MA: Jones and Bartlett; 2001

Baylin SB, Herman JG, Graff JR, et al. Alterations in DNA Methylation—A Fundamental Aspect of Neoplasia. *Adv Cancer Res* 1998;72:141–196

Berenson JR, et al. Efficacy of Pamidronate in Reducing Skeletal Events in Patients with Advanced Multiple Myeloma. *N Engl J Med* 1996;334:488–493

Bower M, Newlands ES, Bleehan NM, et al. Multicenter CRC Phase II Trial of Temozolomide in Recurrent or Progressive High Grade Glioma. *Cancer Chemother Pharmacol* 1997;40:484–488

Bristol-Myers Squibb Pharmaceutical Research Institute. Investigator Brochure for UFT (Uracil:Ftorafur in a molar ratio of 4:1); 1996

Brogden JM, Nevidjon B. Vinorelbine Tartare (Navelbine®): Drug Profile and Nursing Implications of a New Vinca Alkaloid. *Oncol Nurs Forum* 1995;22(4):635–646

Burris HA, Edelman MJ, Stewart F, et al. Phase II dose-ranging study of TLK286 (Telcyta), a novel glutathione analog prodrug, in combination with cisplatin as first-line treatment in locally advanced or metastatic non-small cell lung cancer (NSCLC). *Proc Am Soc Clin Oncol* 2005; abstract 7126, 41st Am Soc Clin Oncol Meeting, Orlando, FL

Camp-Sorrell D. Chemotherapy-Toxicity Management. Groenwald SL, Frogge MH, Goodman M, Yarbro CH, (eds), *Cancer Nursing: Principles and Practice.* Sudbury, MA: Jones and Bartlett; 1993

Cassidy J, Scheithauer W, McKendrick J, et al. *Capecitabine (X) vs bolus 5-FU/leucovorin (LV) as adjuvant therapy for colon cancer (the X-ACT study): efficacy results of a phase III trial J Clin Oncol 2004 ASCO Meeting Proceedings,* (Post-Meeting edition) 2004;22(14S):3509

Chabner BA, Longo DL. *Cancer Chemotherapy and Biotherapy: Principles and Practice,* 3rd ed. Philadelphia, Lippincott-Raven; 2001

Chang AY, Kuebler JP, Pandya KJ, et al. Pulmonary Toxicity Induced by Mitomycin C Is Highly Responsive to Glucocorticoids. *Cancer* 1986;57:2285–2290

Chen AY, Liu LF. Topoisomerases: Essential Enzymes and Lethal Targets. *Annu Rev Pharmacol Toxicol* 1994;34:191–218

Cheson BD, Vena DA, Foss FM, Sorenson JM. Neurotoxicity of Purine Analogs: A Review. *J Clin Oncol* 1994;12(10):2216–2228

Chew T, Jacobs M. Pharmacology of Liposomal Daunorubicin and Its Use in Kaposi's Sarcoma. *Oncology* 1996;10(6):28–34

Chiron Therapeutics. Depocyt Package Insert. *Emeryville, CA, Chiron Therapeutics* 1999

Clinical Trials. *Colorectal Cancer Trials involving Irinotecan and the Saltz Regimen are Temporarily Suspended.* 2001; http://www.cancer.gov/clinicaltrials

Coombes RC, Haynes BP, Dowsett M, et al. Idoxifene: Report of a Phase I Study in Patients with Metastatic Breast Cancer. *Cancer Res* 1995;55:1070–1074

de Gramont A, Bossett JF, Milan C, et al. Randomized trial comparing monthly low-dose leucovorin and fluorouracil bolus with bimonthly high-dose leucovorin and fluorouracil bolus plus continuous infusion for advanced colorectal cancer: A French Intergroup study. *J Clin Oncol* 1997;15:808–815

de Gramont A, Banzi M, Navarro M, et al. Oxaliplatin/5-FU/LV in Adjuvant Colon Cancer: Results of the International Randomized Mosaic Trial. *Proc Am Society Clin Oncol* 2003; abstract 101,522:253

de Gramont A, Boni C, Navarro M, et al. Oxaliplatin/5FU/LV in the adjuvant treatment of stage II and stage III colon cancer: Efficacy results with a median follow-up of 4 years. Oral abstract presented at: ASCO 2005 Gastrointestinal Cancers Symposium; January 27–29, 2005; Hollywood, FL

Dorr R. Personal Communication, 8/22/95. 1995

Dorr RT. Antidotes to Vesicant Chemotherapy. *Blood Reviews* 1990;4(1):41–60

Dorr RT, Von Hoff DD. *Cancer Chemotherapy Handbook,* 2nd ed. Norwalk, CT: Appleton & Lange; 1994

Dowlati, et al. Phase 1 Clinical and Pharmacokinetic Study of Rebeccamycin Analog NSC 655649 Given Daily for Five Consecutive Days. *J Clin Oncol* 2001;19(8): 2309–2318

Eber JP. Camptothecins: New Traditionalists. *Adv Oncol* 1996;12(2):11–16

Ellis AK, Day JH. Diagnosis and Management of Anaphylaxis. *Canadian Medical Association Journal* 2003169(4):307–312

Fabian CJ, Molina R, Slavik M, et al. Pyridoxine Therapy for Palmar-Plantar Erythrodysesthesia Associated with Continuous 5-Fluorouracil Infusion. *Invest New Drugs* 1990;8(1):57–63

Fischer DS, Alfano S, Knof MT, et al. Improving the Cancer Chemotherapy Use Process. *J Clin Oncol* 1996;14(12):3148–3155

Fischer DS, Knobf MT, Durivage HJ, Beaulieu NJ. *The Cancer Chemotherapy Handbook,* 6th ed. St. Louis: Mosby Year-Book; 2003

Fishman M, Mrozek-Orlowski M. *Cancer Chemotherapy Guidelines and Recommendations for Practice,* 2nd ed. Pittsburgh, PA: Oncology Nursing Press; 1999

Franks AL, Steinberg KK. Encouraging News from the SERM Frontier: Selective Estrogen Receptor Modulators. *JAMA* 1999;281(23):2243–2244

Gianni L, Dombernowsky P, Sledge G, et al. Cardiac Function Following Combination Therapy with Taxol (T) and Doxorubicin (D) for Advanced Breast Cancer (ABC). *Proc Am SocClin Oncol* 1998;17:115a

Goodman M, Ladd LA, Pune S. Integumentary and Mucous Membrane Alterations. In Groenwald SL, Frogge M, Goodman M, Yarbro CH, (eds), *Cancer Nursing: Principles and Practice,* 3rd ed. Sudbury, MA: Jones and Bartlett; 1993;734–800

Harwood KV, Govin K. Short-Term vs Long-Term Local Cooling after Doxorubicin Extravasations: An Eastern Cooperative Oncology Group (ECOG) Study [abstract]. *Proceedings of the American Society of Clinical Oncology* 1994;13:447

Hortobagyi GM, et al. New Cytotoxic Agents for the Treatment of Breast Cancer. *Oncology* 1996;10(Suppl):21–29

Hortobagyi GM, et al. Reduction of Skeletal Related Complications in Breast Cancer Patients with Osteolytic Bone Metastases Receiving Chemotherapy by Monthly Pamidronate Sodium Infusion. Proceedings of 32nd Annual ASCO Meeting, Philadelphia, ASCO 1996; abstract 99

Hossan E, Logothetis CJ. The Medical Managment of Progressive Prostate Cancer. *Oncology Special Edition* 1999;2:13–16

Husain I, Mohler JL, Seigler HF, et al. Elevation of Topoisomerase I Messenger RNA, Protein, and Catalytic Activity in Human Tumors: Demonstration of Tumor-Type Specificity and Implications for Cancer Chemotherapy. *Cancer Res* 1994;54: 539–546

Ibrahim NK, Desai N, Legha S, et al. Phase I and pharmacokinetic study of ABI-007, a cremaphor-free protein-stabilized, nanoparticle formulation of paclitaxel. *Clin Cancer Res* 2002;8:1038–1044

Kaisery AV. Current Clinical Studies with a New Nonsteroidal Antiandrogen, CasodeX. *Prostate Suppl* 1994;5:27–33

Kaufmann M, Bajetta E, Dirix LY, et al. Exemestane Is Superior to Megestrol Acetate after Tamoxifen Failure in Postmenopausal Women with Advanced Breast Cancer: Results of a Phase III Randomized Double-blind Trial. The Exemestance Study Group. *J Clin Oncol* 2000;18(7):1399–1411

Kelland LR, Jarman M. Idoxifene. *Drugs of the Future* 1995;20(7):666–669

Larson DK. What Is the Appropriate Treatment for Tissue Extravasation by Antitumor Agents?. *Plastic and Reconstructive Surgery* 1985;75:397–405

Lathia C, Fleming G, Meyer M, Whitfield L. Pentostatin Pharmacokinetics and Dosing Guidelines in Patients with Renal Impairment. *PharmSci* 1998;1(1):Abstract 3360 American Association of Pharmaceutical Scientists Supplement, 1998 AAPS Annual Meeting, San Francisco, CA, November 1998

Laurie SW, Wilson KL, Keinahan DA, et al. Intravenous Extravasation Injuries: The Effectiveness of Hyaluronidase in Their Treatment. *Annals of Plastic Surgery* 1984; 13(3):191–194

Ligand Pharmaceuticals. Panretin Package Insert. San Diego, Ligand Pharmaceuticals 1999

Loprinzi CL, Pisansky TM, Fonseca R, et al. Pilot Evaluation of Venlafaxine Hydrochloride for the Therapy of Hot Flashes in Cancer Survivors. *J Clin Oncol* 1998;16: 2377–2381

Loprinzi CL, Sloane JA, Perez EA, et al. Phase III Evaluation of Fluoxetine for Treatment of Hot Flashes. *J Clin Oncol* 2002;20(6):1578–1583

Lui LF, Lui CC, Alberts BM. Type 2 DNA Topoisomerases: Enzymes That Can Unknot a Topologically Knotted DNA Molecule via a Reversible Double-Strand Break. *Cell* 1980;19:697–707

Mandelli F. Introduction to the Workshop on DNA Methyltransferase Inhibitors. *Leukemia* 1993;7(Suppl 1):1–2

Markman M. Prevention of paclitaxel-associated arthralgias and myalgias. *J Support Oncol* 2003;1:233–234

Markman M, Zanotti L, Peterson G, et al. Expanded experience with an intradermal skin test to predict for the presence or absence of carboplatin sensitivity. *J Clin Oncol* 2003;21:4611–4614

Matsuura T, Fukuda Y, Fujitaka T, et al. Preoperative Treatment with Tegafur Suppositories Enhances Apoptosis and Reduces the Intratumoral Microvessel Density of Human Colorectal Carcinoma. *Cancer* 2000;88(5):1007–1015

McEvoy GK, (ed). *AHFS 96 Drug Information.* Bethesda, MD: American Society of Health-System Pharmacists, Inc.; 1996

McFarland HM. Guide for the Administration and Use of Cancer Chemotherapeutic Agents. *Oncology Special Edition* 1999;2:82–87

Mouridsen H, Gershanovich M, Sun Y, et al. Superior Efficacy of Letrozole Versus Tamoxifen as First-line Therapy for Postmenopausal Women with Advanced Breast Cancer: Results of a Phase III Study of the International Letrozole Breast Cancer Group. *J Clin Oncol* 2001;19(10):2596–2606

Natelson EA, Giovanella BC, Verschraegen CF, et al. Phase I Clinical and Pharmacological Studies of 20-(S)-Camptothecin and 20-(S)-9-Nitrocamptothecin as Anticancer Agents. *Ann New York Acad Sci* 1996;803:224–230

Newlands ES, Stevens MFG, Wedge SR, et al. Temozolomide: A Review of Its Discovery, Chemical Properties, Pre-clinical Development and Clinical Trials. *Cancer Treat Rev* 1997;23:35–61

Niitsu N, Yamaguchi Y, Umeda M, Honma Y. Human Monocytoid Leukemia Cells Are Highly Sensitive to Apoptosis Induced by 2′-Deoxycoformycin and 2′-Deoxyadenosine: Association with dATP-dependent Activation of Caspase-3. *Blood* 1998;92(9): 3368–3375

Ninomoto J. Personal communication re rubitecan, decitabine, and pentostatin. San Ramon, CA: SuperGen; 2000

Novartis Pharmaceuticals. Aredia Package Insert. East Hanover, NJ: Novartis; 1998

Novotny WF, Holmgren E, Nelson B, et al. Bevacizumab (a monocolonal antibody to vascular endothelial growth factor) does not increase the incidence of venous thromboembolism when added to first-line chemotherapy to treat metastatic colorectal cancer. *Proc Am Soc Clin Oncol* 2004;23:252, abstract 3529

Occupational Safety and Health Administration. *Controlling Occupational Exposure to Hazardous Drugs.* 1995; Washington (OSHA Instruction CPL 2-2.20B)

Oktay, et al. JCO 2005

Oncology Nursing Society Board of Directors. *ONS Position Paper: Regarding the Preparation of the Professional Registered Nurse who Administers and Cares for the Individual Receiving Chemotherapy.* Pittsburgh, PA: Oncology Nursing Society; 1999

Orphan Medical. Busulfex (Busulfan) for Injection: Prescribing Information, 1999; available at http://www.orphan.com. Accessed June 2004

Perry MC, (ed). *The Chemotherapy Source Book,* 2nd ed. Baltimore: Williams & Wilkins; 1997

Pharmacia and Upjohn Company. *Patient Instructions for Management of Diarrhea Resulting from Camptosar®.* Kalamazoo, MI, Pharmacia and Upjohn Company 1996

Praecis Pharmaceuticals Incorporated. Plenaxis Package Insert. Waltham, MA: Praecis Pharmaceuticals Inc.; 2001

Polovich M, White JM, Kelleher LO, (eds), *Chemotherapy and Biotherapy Guidelines and Recommendations for Practice* 2nd ed. Pittsburgh, PA: Oncology Nursing Society; 2005

Rhone-Poulenc Rorer Pharmaceutical. Gliadel Package Insert. Collegeville, PA: Rhone-Poulenc Rorer 1997

Rittenberg CN, Gralla RJ, Rehmeyer TA. Assessing and Managing Venous Irritation Associated with Vinorelbine Tartare (Navelbine®). *Oncol Nurs Forum* 1995;22(4): 707–710

Sacchi S, Kantarjian HM, O'Brien S, et al. Chronic Myelogenous Leukemia in Nonlymphoid Blastic Phase: Analysis of the Results of First Salvage Therapy with Three Different Treatment Approaches for 162 Patients. *Cancer* 1999;86(12):2632–2641

Sanofi Synthelabo. Eloxatin Package Insert. New York: Sanofi Synthelabo, Inc.; 2004

Seidman AD, Berry D, Cirrincione L, et al. CALGB 9840: Phase III study of weekly (W) paclitaxel (P) via 1-hour (h) infusion versus standard (S) 3 h infusion every third week in the treatment of metastatic breast cancer (MBC), with trastuzumab (T) for HER2 positive MBC and randomized for T in HER2 normal MBC. *Proc Am Soc Clin Oncol* 2004;23:6, abstract 512

Sheperd GM. Hypersensitivity Reactions to Chemotherapeutic Drugs. *Allergy and Immunology* 2003;24:253–262

Shifflett SL, Harvey RD, Pfeiffer D, et al. Cancer Chemotherapeutic Regimens. *Oncology Special Edition* 1999;2:59–66

Slichenmyer WJ, Rowinsky EK, Donehower RC, Kaufmann SH. The Current Status of Camptothecin Analogues as Antitumor Agents. *J Natl Cancer Instit* 1993;85(4): 271–291

Smith IE, Johnston SRD, O'Brien MER, et al. Low-Dose Oral Fluorouracil with Eniluracil as First-Line Chemotherapy Against Advanced Breast Cancer: A Phase I Study. *J Clin Oncol* 2000;18(12):2378–2384

Solimando DA, Bressler L, Kintzel PE, Geraci MC. *Drug Information Handbook for Oncology,* 2nd ed. Cleveland, Ohio: Lexi-Comp, Inc.; 2000

Suwanawiboon B, Sumida KN. 5-azacitidine: An alternative treatment of myeloplastic syndromes in patient with refractory response to hematopoietic growth factor, a case report and review of the literature. *Hawaii Med J* 2004;63(1):14–16, 25

Taylor SCM. Raltitrexed for Advanced Colorectal Cancer: The Story So Far. *Cancer Practice* 2000;8(1):51–54

Thomas GM. Raising Hemoglobin: An Opportunity for Increasing Survival. *Oncology* 2002;63 Suppl 2:19–28

Trissel LA, Saenz CA, Ingram DS, Ogundele AB. Compatibility Screening of Oxaliplatin during Simulated Y-site Administration with Other Drugs. *J Oncol Pharm Practice* 2002;8(1):33–37

Venook AP, Egorin MJ, Rosner GL, et al. Phase I and Pharmacokinetic Trial of Paclitaxel in Patients with Hepatic Dysfunction: Cancer and Leukemia Group B 9264. *J Clin Oncol* 1998;16:1811–1819

Verschraegen CF, Hupta E, Loyer E, et al. A Phase II Clinical and Pharmacological Study of Oral 9-Nitrocamptothecin in Patients with Refractory Epithelial Ovarian, Tubal or Peritoneal Cancer. *Anti-Cancer Drugs* 1999;10:373–383

Verschraegen CF, Nateson E, Giovanella BC, et al. A Phase I Clinical and Pharmacological Study of Oral 9-Nitrocamptothecin, a Novel Water-Insoluble Topoisomerase I Inhibitor. *Anti Cancer Drugs* 1998;9:36–44

Vukelja SJ, Lombardo FA, James WD, Weiss RB. Pyridoxine for the Palmar-Plantar Erythrodysesthesia Syndrome [letter]. *Ann Intern Med* 1989;111:688–689

Wijermans P, Lubbert M, Verhoef G, et al. Low Dose 5-aza-2′-Deoxycytidine, a DNA Hypomethylating Agent, for the Treatment of High-Risk Myelodysplastic Syndrome: A Multicenter Phase II Study in Elderly Patients. *J Clin Oncol* 2000;18(5): 956–967

Wilkes GM. New Therapeutic Options in Colon Cancer: Focus on Oxaliplatin. *Clinical Journal of Oncology Nursing* 2002;3:131–137

Wilkes GM. Therapeutic Options in the Management of Colon Cancer: 2005 Update. *Clinical Journal of Oncology Nursing* 2005;9(1):31–44

Drug: abarelix for injectable suspension (Plenaxis)

Class: Gonadotropin releasing-hormone (GnRH) antagonist.

Mechanism of Action: Directly and competitively blocks GnRH receptors in the pituitary: suppresses luteinizing hormone (LH) and follicle stimulating hormone (FSH) secretion, and thereby reduces the secretion of testosterone by the testes. There is no initial increase in serum testosterone concentrations.

Metabolism: Following IM administration, drug is slowly absorbed with a mean peak concentration 3 days after injection, and distributes extensively within the body. Drug is highly protein bound (96–99%), and is excreted in the urine, with 13% of drug unchanged.

Dosage/Range:

- 100 mg IM in the buttock days 1, 15, 29 (week 4), and every 4 weeks thereafter
- Assess efficacy by monitoring serum testosterone levels baseline, day 29, and then every 8 weeks thereafter

Drug Preparation/Administration:

- Reconstitute drug following manufacturer's recommendations to yield 50 mg/mL
- Administer in the buttock, and rotate sites

Drug Interactions:

Lab Effects/Interference:

- LFTs: transaminases may become elevated
- Serum testosterone levels should decrease to < 50 ng/dL. Slight decrease in hemoglobin
- Increase in serum triglycerides by 10%

Special Considerations:

- Drug is indicated for the palliative treatment of men with advanced symptomatic prostate cancer, in whom LHRH agonist therapy is not appropriate and who refuse surgical castration, and have one or more of the following:
  1) risk of neurological compromise due to metastases,
  2) ureteral or bladder outlet obstruction due to local encroachment of metastatic disease, or
  3) severe bone pain from skeletal metastases persisting on opioid analgesia
- Drug achieves castration levels of testosterone 24 hours after IM injection
- The effectiveness of abarelix in suppressing serum testosterone to castration levels decreases with continued dosing in patients weighing > 225 lbs, and effectiveness beyond 12 months has not been established. Assess total serum testosterone levels just prior to drug administration on day 29, and every 8 weeks thereafter to assure continued response in all patients. Periodic measurement of serum PSA will assist in assessing response.
- Immediate-onset systemic allergic reactions, with hypotension and syncope, may occur; risk increases with increased cumulative dose so patients should be observed for at least 30 minutes following the injection.
- Drug may cause QT interval prolongation in 20% of patients (changes from baseline of > 30 msec, or end-of-treatment QTc values > 450 msec; use cautiously if at all in patients taking class IA (quinidine, procainamide) or class III (amiodarone, sotalol) antiarrhythmic medications.
- Drug is not indicated for women or children; drug may cause fetal harm if administered to a pregnant woman.
- Transaminase levels became clinically significantly elevated in some patients, so levels should be assessed baseline, and periodically during treatment.
- Bone mineral density may decrease with extended treatment with GnRH antagonists and LHRH agonists.

Potential Toxicities/Side Effects and the Nursing Process

I. POTENTIAL FOR INJURY related to HYPERSENSITIVITY REACTION

Defining Characteristics: Allergic reactions can occur immediately after injection, and may result in hypotension and syncope, starting with the initial dose, or occurring later in the course of treatment. Risk increases with the duration of treatment.

Nursing Implications: Assess baseline VS and mental status prior to drug administration, and observe patient for 30 minutes following injection. Recall signs/symptoms of anaphylaxis, and if these occur, notify physician, and assess patient's vital signs. Subjective symptoms are generalized itching, nausea, chest tightness, crampy abdominal pain, difficulty speaking, anxiety, agitation, sense of impending doom, uneasiness, desire to urinate/defecate, dizziness, and chills. Objective signs are flushed appearance; angioedema of face, neck, eyelids, hands, and feet; localized or generalized urticaria; respiratory distress with or without wheezing; hypotension; and cyanosis. Review standing orders or nursing procedures for patient management of anaphylaxis, and be prepared to administer ordered medications, which may include epinephrine 1:1000, hydrocortisone sodium succinate, and diphenhydramine. Teach patient to report any unusual symptoms.

II. ALTERATION IN COMFORT related to HOT FLUSHES, SLEEP DISTURBANCES, PAIN, BREAST ENLARGEMENT/TENDERNESS, HEADACHE, EDEMA, AND DIZZINESS

Defining Characteristics: Signs and symptoms of androgen deprivation are: Hot flushes (79%), sleep deprivation (44%), breast enlargement (30%), breast pain/nipple tenderness (20%). Pain in general occurs in about 31% of patients, as well as back pain (17%).

Nursing Implications: Teach patient that symptoms may occur. Encourage patient to report symptoms early. Develop symptom management plan with patient and physician.

III. ALTERATION IN BOWEL AND BLADDER ELIMINATION related to HORMONAL CHANGES

Defining Characteristics: Diarrhea occurs in about 11% of patients, while constipation occurs in 15%. 10% of patients develop dysuria, micturition frequency, urinary retention, or urinary tract infection.

Nursing Implications: Assess baseline bowel and bladder elimination pattern, and teach patient to report any changes. Teach patient to modify diet to minimize either diarrhea or constipation. Discuss need for referral to urologist if dysuria, urinary retention, or urinary tract infections persist.

Drug: adrenocorticoids (Cortisone, Dexamethasone, Hydrocortisone, Methylprednisolone, Prednisolone, Prednisone)

Class: Hormones.

Mechanism of Action: Cause lysis of lymphoid cells, which leads to their use against lymphatic leukemia, myeloma, malignant lymphoma. May also recruit malignant cells out of G_0 phase, making them vulnerable to damage caused by cell-cycle-phase-specific agents.

Metabolism: Metabolized by the liver, excreted in urine. Prednisone is activated by the liver in its active form, prednisolone.

Dosage/Range:
- Varies according to which preparation is used. Dexamethasone is 25 times the potency of hydrocortisone.
- Cortisone 25 mg.
- Dexamethasone 0.75 mg.
- Hydrocortisone 20 mg.
- Methylprednisolone 4 mg.
- Prednisone, Prednisolone 5 mg.

Drug Preparation:
- None.

Drug Administration:
- Oral.

Drug Interactions:
- May increase K+ loss and hypokalemia when combined with amphotericin B or potassium-depleting diuretics.
- Warfarin (Coumadin) dose may need to be increased.
- Insulin or oral hypoglycemia dose may need to be increased.
- Oral contraceptives may inhibit steroid metabolism.

Lab Effects/Interference:
- Increased Na, decreased K with hypokalemic alkalosis.
- Decreased I^{131} uptake and protein-bound iodine concentration. May cause difficulty monitoring therapeutic response of patients treated for thyroid conditions.
- False-negative results in nitroblue tetrazolium test for systemic bacterial infections.
- May suppress reactions to skin tests.

Special Considerations:
- Chronic steroid use is associated with numerous side effects. Intermittent therapy is safer and in some conditions just as effective as daily therapy.

Potential Toxicities/Side Effects and the Nursing Process

I. ALTERATION IN NUTRITION, LESS THAN BODY REQUIREMENTS, related to GASTRIC IRRITATION, DECREASED CARBOHYDRATE METABOLISM, AND HYPERGLYCEMIA

Defining Characteristics: Steroids can cause increased secretion of hydrochloric acid and decreased secretion of protective gastric mucus, which can exacerbate an existing gastric ulcer. They are insulin antagonists and may cause gluconeogenesis. In addition, steroids may increase appetite and cause weight gain.

Nursing Implications: Administer drugs with meals or an antacid. Instruct patient to report evidence of gastric distress immediately; teach patient to take steroids prior to a meal or with milk or food. Obtain baseline glucose levels and monitor periodic blood sugars throughout therapy. Teach patient to recognize signs/symptoms of hyperglycemia (polyuria, polydipsia, polyphagia), and to report these to the doctor or nurse.

II. POTENTIAL FOR INJURY related to SODIUM AND WATER RETENTION, ALTERATIONS IN FLUID AND ELECTROLYTE BALANCE, AND STEROIDINDUCED IMMUNOSUPPRESSION

Defining Characteristics: Sodium and water retention may occur and lead to CHF, hypertension, and edema in susceptible individuals; hypokalemia and hypocalcemia may occur due to increased excretion of potassium and calcium. Osteoporosis may occur with long-term therapy. Steroids increase susceptibility to infections and tuberculosis, may mask or aggravate infection, and may prolong or delay healing of injuries.

Nursing Implications: Identify patients at risk for complications associated with fluid/sodium retention (i.e., patients with preexisting cardiac, renal, hepatic dysfunction); monitor fluid and electrolyte balance and assess for imbalance. Document baseline cardiac status and monitor through therapy. Instruct patient to report signs/symptoms of hypokalemia (anorexia, muscle twitching, tetany, polyuria, polydipsia) and of hypocalcemia (leg cramps, tingling in fingertips, muscle twitching); monitor electrolytes regularly and discuss abnormal values with physician. Encourage high-potassium, high-calcium diet, and instruct patient in safety measures as needed. Teach patient to report slow healing of wounds, signs/symptoms of infection (erythema, warmth, purulence) of skin areas, as well as sore throat and burning on urination. Reinforce/teach patient hygiene measures for mouth, perineum, and skin.

III. POTENTIAL FOR INJURY related to RAPID WITHDRAWAL OF THERAPY

Defining Characteristics: Long-term therapy leads to suppression of normal adrenal function. Rapid cessation of therapy will lead to adrenal insufficiency, characterized by anorexia, nausea, orthostatic hypotension, dizziness, depression, dyspnea, hypoglycemia, and rebound inflammation (fever, myalgias, arthralgia, malaise). It can be fatal.

Nursing Implications: Discuss with physician the taper of steroids and instruct patient/family carefully. Teach patient to report symptoms of rapid withdrawal to nurse or physician.

IV. POTENTIAL FOR BODY IMAGE DISTURBANCE related to CUSHINGOID CHANGES

Defining Characteristics: Cushingoid state may occur with prolonged use and may be diminished by every-other-day dosing. Changes include moonface, striae, purpura, acne, hirsutism. In addition, increased appetite from steroids may lead to weight gain.

Nursing Implications: Teach patient about potential changes and provide reassurance that they will resolve once therapy ceases; encourage patient to verbalize feelings and provide emotional support.

V. POTENTIAL FOR SENSORY/PERCEPTUAL ALTERATIONS related to CATARACTS OR GLAUCOMA, AND OCULAR INFECTIONS (increased risk)

Defining Characteristics: Cataracts or glaucoma may develop with prolonged steroid use; risk of ocular infections from virus or fungi is increased.

Nursing Implications: Teach patient to report signs/symptoms of eye infection, such as discharge, erythema, or visual changes; ophthalmologic exams are recommended every two to three months.

VI. INEFFECTIVE COPING related to AFFECTIVE/BEHAVIORAL CHANGES

Defining Characteristics: Emotional lability, insomnia, mood swings, euphoria, and psychosis may occur, causing ineffective coping and role-relationship problems if unprepared.

Nursing Implications: Teach patient and family that affective/behavioral changes may occur and that they will resolve once therapy is discontinued. Encourage patient and family to report these changes, especially if troublesome.

VII. IMPAIRED PHYSICAL MOBILITY related to MUSCULOSKELETAL CHANGES

Defining Characteristics: With chronic, high-dose usage, loss of muscle mass, muscle weakness (steroid myopathy), tendon rupture, osteoporosis, pathologic fractures, and aseptic necrosis of the heads of the humerus and femur can occur.

Nursing Implications: Teach patient that muscle weakness and other effects can occur with therapy and that muscle cramping may occur with discontinuation of therapy. Teach patient to report weakness, cramping, and any musculoskeletal changes. If weakness occurs, therapy may be discontinued.

Drug: altretamine (Hexalen, Hexamethylmelamine)

Class: Alkylating agent.

Mechanism of Action: The exact mechanism of action is unknown. May inhibit incorporation of thymidine and uridine into DNA and RNA, respectively. Altretamine is believed not to act as an alkylating agent in vitro, but it may be activated to an alkylating agent in vivo. Also may act as an antimetabolite with activity in S phase.

Metabolism: Well absorbed orally although bioavailability is variable. Peak plasma concentration in 1 hour. Metabolized extensively in the liver, with majority excreted in the urine. Some of the drug is excreted as respiratory CO_2. Half-life of the parent compound is 4.7–10.2 hours.

Dosage/Range:
- 4–12 mg/kg/day (divided in 3 or 4 doses) × 21–90 days, or
- 240 mg/m^2 (6 mg/kg)–320 mg/m^2 (8 mg/kg) daily × 21 days, repeated every 6 weeks.

Drug Preparation:
- Available in 50-mg and 100-mg capsules.

Drug Administration:
- Oral.

Drug Interactions:
- Concurrent administration of drug with monoamine oxidase inhibitor (MAO) antidepressants may cause severe orthostatic hypotension.

Lab Effects/Interference:
- Decreased CBC.
- Increased BUN, creatinine.

Special Considerations:

- Nausea and vomiting can be minimized if patient takes dose two hours after meals and at bedtime.
- Nadir three to four weeks after treatment.

Potential Toxicities/Side Effects and the Nursing Process

I. INFECTION AND BLEEDING related to BONE MARROW DEPRESSION

Defining Characteristics: Causes mild to moderate bone marrow suppression, with nadir occurring 21–28 days after beginning treatment, and rapid recovery within one week of cessation of drug. Anemia occurs in 33% of patients and is moderate to severe in 9% of patients.

Nursing Implications: Assess CBC, WBC, differential, and platelet count prior to drug administration, as well as for signs/symptoms of infection or bleeding. Teach patient signs/symptoms of infection and bleeding, and instruct to report them immediately. Teach self-care measures to minimize risk of infection and bleeding, including avoidance of OTC aspirin-containing medications. Assess energy and activity tolerance; discuss blood transfusion with physician as appropriate. Discuss with physician dose interruption and reduction if WBC $< 2000/mm^3$, ANC $< 1000/mm^3$, or platelet count $< 75,000/mm^3$.

II. SENSORY/PERCEPTUAL ALTERATIONS related to PERIPHERAL NEUROPATHY AND CNS EFFECTS

Defining Characteristics: Peripheral sensory neuropathy occurs in 31% of patients and is moderate to severe in 9% of patients. Paresthesia, hyperesthesia, hyperreflexia, and numbness may occur and are reversible. CNS effects of agitation, confusion, hallucinations, depression, mood disorders, and Parkinson-like symptoms may occur, and usually are reversible. Neurologic effects are more common with continuous dosing > 3 months, rather than pulse dosing.

Nursing Implications: Assess baseline neurologic status. Teach patient that possible side effects may occur, and instruct to report them. If neurologic toxicity is severe, drug should be dose reduced, then discontinued if symptoms do not improve.

III. ALTERATION IN NUTRITION, LESS THAN BODY REQUIREMENTS, related to NAUSEA AND VOMITING, DIARRHEA, ABDOMINAL CRAMPS, ANOREXIA

Defining Characteristics: Nausea occurs in 33% of patients and is dose related. Tolerance may develop after three weeks of drug administration. Diarrhea and cramps may be dose-limiting. Anorexia may occur.

Nursing Implications: Premedicate with antiemetics (phenothiazines are usually effective) at least initially, then as needed. Divide dose into four doses, and give 1–2 hours after meals and at bedtime. Instruct patient to report nausea/vomiting, diarrhea, abdominal cramping. Teach self-administration of prescribed antidiarrheals and self-care techniques to manage cramps, e.g., heat pads or position change. If GI side effects are refractory to symptom management, discuss interrupting dose and then dose reduction with physician.

IV. ALTERATION IN SKIN INTEGRITY related to SKIN RASHES

Defining Characteristics: Skin rashes, pruritus, eczematous skin lesions may occur but are rare.

Nursing Implications: Assess for changes in skin color, texture, and integrity. Teach patient to report any changes in skin, and discuss measures to minimize discomfort.

V. ALTERATION IN ELIMINATION related to RENAL DYSFUNCTION

Defining Characteristics: Elevations in BUN (9% of patients) or creatinine (7%) can occur.

Nursing Implications: Assess baseline renal status and monitor renal function studies throughout treatment.

VI. POTENTIAL SEXUAL DYSFUNCTION related to DRUG EFFECTS

Defining Characteristics: Drug is mutagenic, carcinogenic, and teratogenic. Drug causes testicular atrophy and decreased spermatogenesis. It is unknown whether drug is excreted in human milk.

Nursing Implications: Discuss with patient and partner normal sexual patterns and anticipated dysfunction resulting from drug or disease. Provide information, emotional support, and referral for counseling as appropriate.

Drug: 9-aminocamptothecin (9-AC) (investigational)

Class: Topoisomerase inhibitor.

Mechanism of Action: Induces protein-linked DNA single-strand breaks and blocks DNA and RNA synthesis in dividing cells, preventing cells from entering mitosis. Cell cycle specific.

Metabolism: 32% of the drug is excreted in the urine as unchanged drug at 96 hours.

Dosage/Range:
- 35 μg/m²/h every 2 weeks or 45 μg/m²/h every 3 weeks (Phase II trials) as 72-hour infusion.
- Prolonged infusion studies under way.

Drug Preparation:
- Per protocol.

Drug Administration:
- IV infusion over 72 hours.

Drug Interactions:
- Unknown.

Lab Effects/Interference:
- Decreased CBC.

Special Considerations:
- Neutropenia is dose-limiting toxicity.

Potential Toxicities/Side Effects and the Nursing Process

I. INFECTION AND BLEEDING related to BONE MARROW DEPRESSION

Defining Characteristics: Causes neutropenia (dose-limiting), thrombocytopenia, and anemia.

Nursing Implications: Assess CBC, WBC, differential, and platelet count prior to drug administration, as well as signs/symptoms of infection or bleeding. Teach patient signs/symptoms of infection and bleeding, and instruct to report them immediately. Teach self-care measures to minimize risk of infection and bleeding, including avoidance of OTC aspirin-containing medications. Assess energy and activity tolerance; discuss blood transfusion with physician as appropriate. Discuss with physician dose interruption and reduction if WBC $< 2000/mm^3$ or absolute neutrophil count $< 1000/mm^3$, platelet count $< 75,000/mm^3$.

II. ALTERATION IN NUTRITION, LESS THAN BODY REQUIREMENTS, related to NAUSEA AND VOMITING, DIARRHEA

Defining Characteristics: Nausea, vomiting, diarrhea, mucositis may occur.

Nursing Implications: Premedicate with antiemetics. Teach patient to report nausea/vomiting, diarrhea, and changes in oral mucosa. Teach self-administration of prescribed antidiarrheals, and self-care techniques for discomfort and mucosal integrity. Teach oral hygiene self-care measures, including self-assessment, and systematic oral cleansing. Refer to clinical protocol.

III. ALTERATION IN SKIN INTEGRITY related to ALOPECIA

Defining Characteristics: Alopecia may occur.

Nursing Implications: Teach patient about possible side effects and self-care measures, including obtaining a wig or cap as appropriate prior to hair loss. Encourage patient to verbalize feelings and provide patient emotional support.

IV. POTENTIAL FOR ACTIVITY INTOLERANCE related to FATIGUE

Defining Characteristics: Fatigue and anemia are common.

Nursing Implications: Teach patient to report increasing fatigue, signs of severe anemia (shortness of breath, chest pain/angina, headaches). Monitor hemoglobin/hematocrit; discuss transfusion with physician if signs/symptoms develop or hematocrit falls (refer to protocol).

Drug: aminoglutethimide (Cytadren, Elipten)

Class: Adrenal steroid inhibitor.

Mechanism of Action: Causes "chemical adrenalectomy." Blocks adrenal production of steroids, reducing levels of glucocorticoids, mineralocorticoids, and estrogens. Also inhibits peripheral aromatization of androgens to estrogens.

Metabolism: Well-absorbed orally. Hydroxylated in liver; undergoes enterohepatic circulation. Most of drug is excreted in urine.

Dosage/Range:
- 750–2000 mg PO daily in divided doses.
- 40 mg hydrocortisone daily given to replace glucocorticoid deficiencies.

Drug Preparation:
- None.

Drug Administration:
- Oral.

Drug Interactions:
- Drug enhances dexamethasone metabolism, so hydrocortisone should be used for glucocorticoid replacement.
- Warfarin (Coumadin) dose may need to be increased.
- Alcohol potentiates drug side effects.
- May need to increase doses of theophylline, digitoxin, or medroxyprogesterone.

Lab Effects/Interference:
- Hypothyroidism: monitor TFT.
- Elevated LFTs, especially SGOT, alk phos, bili.

Special Considerations:

- Skin rash may develop within 5–7 days, lasting 8 days, often with malaise and fever (37.7–39°C [100–102°F]). If not resolved in 7–14 days, drug should be discontinued.
- Adjuvant corticosteroids need to be administered.

Potential Toxicities/Side Effects and the Nursing Process

I. ALTERATION IN ENDOCRINE FUNCTION related to ADRENAL INSUFFICIENCY

Defining Characteristics: Drug causes reversible chemical adrenalectomy by blockade of steroid hormone production. Patient will experience signs/symptoms of adrenal insufficiency if enough replacement glucocorticoid steroids are not received. Signs/symptoms of adrenal insufficiency include hyponatremia, hypoglycemia, dizziness, and postural hypotension. In addition, possible ovarian blockade may result in virilization.

Nursing Implications: Teach patient about self-administration of hydrocortisone replacement therapy (i.e., administer in A.M. with breakfast), potential side effects, and tapering schedule; refer to section on adrenocorticoids. Teach patient side effects of hormone replacement and self-assessment techniques, including weekly weights and signs/symptoms of infection. Monitor electrolytes, especially Na+, K+, and Ca++. Assess for signs/symptoms of adrenal insufficiency (fatigue, anorexia, nausea, vomiting, diarrhea, weight loss, weakness, dizziness, and low blood sugar). As appropriate, explore with patient/significant other reproductive and sexuality patterns and impact chemotherapy may have. Recognize that patient may need increased hydrocortisone and mineralocorticoid support if surgery is needed (increased stress requirement).

II. IMPAIRED SKIN INTEGRITY related to DRUG RASH

Defining Characteristics: Area of erythema, pruritus, and unexplained dermatitis may appear within one week of treatment and disappear in 5–8 days. May be accompanied by malaise and low-grade fever.

Nursing Implications: Teach patient to report symptoms and to avoid scratching involved areas if rash develops. Assess skin for any changes and rash development. Consider use of Sarna cream, and use of OTC diphenhydramine.

III. SENSORY/PERCEPTUAL ALTERATIONS related to TRANSIENT SYMPTOMS

Defining Characteristics: Transient symptoms such as drowsiness, lethargy, somnolence, visual blurring, vertigo, and ataxia may occur, as may nystagmus. Lethargy may be severe in elderly patients.

Nursing Implications: Document baseline neurological function and general health assessment. Teach patient possible side effects, self-assessment, and to report symptoms. Discuss with physician possible dose reduction for significant symptoms.

IV. ALTERATION IN NUTRITION related to NAUSEA/VOMITING AND ANOREXIA

Defining Characteristics: Nausea/vomiting and anorexia occur in approximately 10–13% of patients and are mild.

Nursing Implications: Initially, premedicate (and teach patient to) with antiemetics prior to drug administration. Usually symptoms subside within two weeks. Encourage small, frequent feedings.

V. ALTERATION IN OXYGENATION/PERFUSION related to HYPOTENSION

Defining Characteristics: Drug may block aldosterone production leading to orthostatic or persistent hypotension. This is not usually a problem when hydrocortisone replacement is given.

Nursing Implications: Monitor BP regularly. Instruct patient to change position slowly and to report dizziness.

Drug: anastrozole (Arimidex)

Class: Nonsteroidal aromatase inhibitor.

Mechanism of Action: Inhibits the enzyme aromatase. Aromatase is one of the P-450 enzymes and is involved in estrogen biosynthesis. Circulating estrogen in postmenopausal women (mainly estradiol) arises from the aromatase-mediated conversion of androstenedione (made by the adrenals) to estrone, then estrone to estradiol, in the peripheral tissues, such as adipose tissue. Anastrozole is highly selective for this enzyme and does not affect steroid synthesis, so that estradiol synthesis is potently suppressed (to undetectable levels) while cortisol and aldosterone levels are unchanged.

Metabolism: Extensively metabolized, with 85% of the drug metabolized by the liver. About 10% of the unchanged drug and 60% of the drug as metabolites are excreted in the urine within 72 hours of drug administration.

Dosage/Range:

- 1 mg PO qd. No dosage adjustment required for mild to moderate hepatic impairment.

Drug Preparation:
- None. Available as 1-mg tablet.

Drug Administration:
- Take orally with or without food, at approximately the same time daily.

Lab Effects/Interference:
- Elevated GGT, especially in patients with liver metastases.

Special Considerations:
- Indicated for the adjuvant treatment of postmenopausal women with hormone receptor positive early breast cancer; as first-line therapy for postmenopausal women with hormone receptor-positive or hormone receptor-unknown locally advanced or metastatic breast cancer; and for treatment of advanced breast cancer in postmenopausal women with disease progression following tamoxifen therapy.
- In the large Arimidex Tamoxifen Alone or in Combination (ATAC) clinical trial, anastrozole was shown to reduce the relative risk of breast cancer recurrence by 17% over tamoxifen in hormone receptor-positive patients in the adjuvant setting.
- Well-tolerated with low toxicity profile.
- Coadministration of corticosteroids is not necessary.
- Absolutely contraindicated during pregnancy.

Potential Toxicities/Side Effects and the Nursing Process

I. SEXUAL DYSFUNCTION related to DECREASED ESTROGEN LEVELS

Defining Characteristics: Hot flashes (12%), asthenia or loss of energy (16%), and vaginal dryness may occur.

Nursing Implications: As appropriate, explore with patient and partner patterns of sexuality and impact therapy may have. Discuss strategies to preserve sexual health. Teach patient that the vaginal dryness may be from menopause, not the drug, and that the patient SHOULD NOT use estrogen creams. Teach patient to use lubricants.

II. POTENTIAL ALTERATION IN CARDIAC OUTPUT related to THROMBOPHLEBITIS

Defining Characteristics: Thrombophlebitis may occur, but is uncommon.

Nursing Implications: Identify patients at risk. Teach patients to report/come to emergency room for pain, redness, or marked swelling in arms or legs, or if shortness of breath or dizziness occur.

III. ALTERATION IN COMFORT related to HEADACHES, WEAKNESS

Defining Characteristics: Headaches are mild and occur in about 13% of patients. Decreased energy and weakness is common. Mild swelling of arms/legs may occur and is mild.

Nursing Implications: Teach patient that headache is usually relieved by nonprescription analgesics, and to report headaches that are unrelieved. Teach patient to elevate extremities when at rest, as needed.

IV. POTENTIAL ALTERATION IN NUTRITION, LESS THAN BODY REQUIREMENTS, related to NAUSEA

Defining Characteristics: Nausea is mild, with a 15% incidence.

Nursing Implications: Determine baseline weight, and monitor at each visit. Teach patient that nausea may occur, and to report this. Discuss strategies to minimize nausea, including diet and dosing time.

V. POTENTIAL ALTERATION IN BOWEL ELIMINATION related to DIARRHEA

Defining Characteristics: Diarrhea is uncommon (9% incidence) and mild.

Nursing Implications: Assess for change in bowel patterns and teach patient to report diarrhea. If diarrhea occurs, teach patient that diarrhea is usually relieved by nonprescription medications, such as loperamide HCl and kaopectate, and to report unrelieved diarrhea.

Drug: androgens: testosterone propionate (Testex), obfluoxymesterone (Halotestin), obtestolactone (Teslac)

Class: Hormones.

Mechanism of Action: Has stimulatory effect on red blood cells that results in an increased HCT. Other mechanism of action unknown.

Metabolism: Metabolized by the liver; excreted in the urine and feces.

Dosage/Range:
- Fluoxymesterone: 10–30 mg PO daily (3–4 divided doses).
- Testolactone: 100 mg IM 3 × weekly or 250 mg PO 4 × daily.
- Testosterone Propionate: 50–100 mg IM 3 × weekly.

Drug Preparation:
- Drug comes in ready-to-use vials or tablets.

Drug Administration:
- Before IM administration, shake vial vigorously and give injection immediately to avoid solution settling.

Drug Interactions:
- Pharmacological effects of oral anticoagulants may be enhanced; monitor patient and adjust dose.

Lab Effects/Interference:
- LFTs: possible hepatic dysfunction with long-term use.
- Increased serum Ca.
- May cause decreased total serum thyroxine (T_4) concentrations and increased T_3 and T_4.

Special Considerations:
- Fluoxymesterone may increase sensitivity to oral anticoagulants. Should be administered in divided doses because of its short action.

Potential Toxicities/Side Effects and the Nursing Process

I. POTENTIAL FOR INJURY related to SODIUM AND WATER RETENTION, HYPERCALCEMIA, AND OBSTRUCTIVE JAUNDICE

Defining Characteristics: Sodium and water retention may occur, necessitating dose reduction or diuretic use; hypercalcemia may occur initially in patients with bony metastases and needs to be distinguished from disease progression. Obstructive jaundice has occurred with methyltesterone, fluoxymesterone, and oxymethalone.

Nursing Implications: Identify patients most at risk for injury related to sodium and water retention: patients with cardiac, renal, or hepatic dysfunction, as well as patients with low serum albumin. Teach patient about potential side effects and instruct to report any changes to physician or nurse; assess patient at each visit for signs/symptoms of fluid and electrolyte imbalance. Identify patients at risk for hypercalcemia (those with bony metastases) and monitor serum calcium during first few weeks of therapy; hypercalcemia is an indication to discontinue therapy. Teach patient/family signs/symptoms of hypercalcemia (drowsiness, increased thirst, constipation, polyuria) and to notify physician. Monitor LFTs and instruct patient/family to report signs/symptoms of GI distress, diarrhea, jaundice.

II. POTENTIAL FOR SEXUAL DYSFUNCTION related to MASCULINIZATION

Defining Characteristics: Commonly occurs in women receiving drug for > 3 months; with prolonged use masculinization may be irreversible. Symptoms include increased libido, deepening of voice, excessive growth of body (face) hair, acne, and clitoral hypertrophy. In men, priapism (sustained and often painful erections) and reduced ejaculatory volume may occur.

Nursing Implications: Instruct patient to report symptoms of changes in sexual health. Discuss strategies to preserve sexual health; if unacceptable, discuss alternative medications with physician.

III. ALTERATION IN NUTRITION, LESS THAN BODY REQUIREMENTS, related to NAUSEA AND VOMITING

Defining Characteristics: Nausea may occur.

Nursing Implications: Teach patient about possible side effects and administer antiemetics as ordered. Encourage small, frequent feedings and dietary modifications as appropriate.

Drug: arsenic trioxide (Trisenox)

Class: Miscellaneous antineoplastic agent.

Mechanism of Action: Not completely understood, but drug appears to cause changes in DNA with fragmentation typical of apoptosis or programmed cell death. Drug also damages and causes degradation of the fusion protein PMLRAR alpha characteristic of acute promyelocytic leukemia. The gene responsible for the fusion protein is corrected in many cases (cytogenetic complete response), so that immature malignant myelocytic cells mature into normal white blood cells.

Metabolism: Pharmacokinetics continue to be characterized. Drug is metabolized by methylation, primarily in the liver. Arsenic is stored primarily in the liver, kidney, heart, lung, hair, and nails. Drug appears to be excreted in the urine.

Dosage/Range:

Adult:

- Induction dose of 0.15 mg/kg/d IV until bone marrow remission, not to exceed 60 doses.
- Consolidation begins 3–6 weeks after induction therapy is completed, at a dose of 0.15 mg/kg/d IV for 25 doses over a period of up to 5 weeks.

Drug Preparation/Administration:

- Drug is available in 10 mL, single-use ampules containing 10 mg of arsenic trioxide, with a concentration of 1 mg/mL.
- Further dilute prescribed dose immediately in 100–250 ml 5% dextrose injection, USP or 0.9% Sodium Chloride Injection, USP.

- Administer IV over 1–2 hours, or up to 4 hours if acute vasomotor reactions occur (does not require a central line).
- Drug is chemically and physically stable for 24 hours at room temperature and 48 hours when refrigerated.
- Drug does not contain any preservatives, so unused portions should be discarded.
- Overdosage: If symptoms of serious acute arsenic toxicity appear (seizures, muscle weakness, confusion), discontinue drug immediately and chelation therapy should be considered: dimercaprol 3 mg/kg IMq 4 hours until immediate life-threatening toxicity has subsided, then give penicillamine 250 mg PO up to qid (1 Gm per day).

Drug Interactions:

- Unknown; do not mix with any other medications.
- Drugs that can prolong the QT interval (e.g., certain antiarrhythmics or thioridazine) or lead to electrolyte abnormalities (e.g., diuretics or amphotericin B) should be avoided if possible; otherwise, scrupulous monitoring and correction of abnormalities is critical.

Lab Effects/Interference:

- Hyperkalemia or hypokalemia.
- Hypomagnesemia.
- Hyperglycemia or hypoglycemia.
- Hypocalcemia.
- Increased hepatic transaminases ALT and AST.
- Leukocytosis (50% of patients).
- Anemia (14% of patients).
- Thrombocytopenia (19% of patients).
- Neutropenia (10% of patients).
- Disseminated intravascular coagulation (DIC) (8% of patients).

Special Considerations:

- Drug is indicated for induction of remission and consolidation in paients with acute promyelocytic leukemia (APL) who are refractory to, or have relapsed from, retinoid and anthracycline chemotherapy, and whose APL is characterized by the presence of the t(15;17) translocation or PML/RAR-alpha gene expression.
- Arsenic has been used in medical care for the last 2000 years, and 100 years ago it was used to treat leukemia and infections. However, it was replaced with current chemotherapy and antibiotics. Certain traditional Chinese medicines were found to be anti-leukemic, and the active ingredient was shown to be arsenic trioxide.
- Preliminary studies showed high hematologic complete response rate (55–82%) and cytogenetic conversion to no detection of APL chromosome

rearrangement (29–100%) depending on response criteria. This led to a fast track status and early FDA approval. Additional post-approval toxicity reports will help clarify full toxicity profile of this drug.

- Drug may cause APL Differentiation Syndrome similar to the retinoicacidacute Promyelocytic Leukemia (RA-APL), which is characterized by fever, dyspnea, weight gain, pulmonary infiltrates, and pleural or pericardial effusions, with or without leukocytosis. This syndrome can be fatal, and, at the first suggestion, high-dose steroids should be instituted (dexamethasone 10 mg IV bid) for at least 3 days or longer until signs and symptoms abate. The drug manufacturer states that the majority of patients do not require termination of arsenic trioxide therapy during treatment of the syndrome (Cell Therapeutics, Inc., Trisenox package insert, 9/2000).
- Drug can cause QT interval prolongation and complete atrioventricular block. Prolonged QT interval can progress to a torsade de pointes-type fatal ventricular arrythmia. Risk factors for development of torsade de pointes are: significant QT prolongation; concomitant administraton of drugs that prolong the QT interval; history of torsades de pointes; preexisting QT prolongation; CHF; administration of potassium-wasting diuretics; conditions resulting in hypokalemia or hypomagnesemia, such as concurrent administration of amphotericin B.
- The manufacturer recommends the following: Prior to treatment with arsenic trioxide, the patient should have a baseline 12-lead EKG as well as serum electrolytes and renal function tests. Electrolyte abnormalities should be corrected. Any drugs that prolong the QT interval should be discontinued. If the QT interval prolongation is > 500 msec, this should be corrected prior to drug administration. During arsenic trioxide therapy, serum potassium should be kept > 4.0 mEq/dL and serum magnesium > 1.8 mg/dL. If the QT interval exceeds 500 msec, reassessment and correction of risk factors should occur. The patient should be hospitalized for monitoring if syncope, or rapid or irregular heart rate occurs, and serum electrolytes assessed and any abnormalities corrected. Drug should be stopped until QT interval falls below 460 msec, electrolyte abnormalities corrected, and symptoms resolve.
- Drug is a human carcinogen. Drug should not be used by pregnant or breast-feeding women.
- Standard monitoring: At least 2 times a week, the patient should have electrolyte, hematologic, and coagulation assessed; more frequently if abnormal during the induction phase, and at least weekly during the consolidation phase. EKGs should be done weekly; more frequently if abnormal.
- Most common side effects are manageable, are reversible, and include: leukocytosis, nausea, vomiting, diarrhea, abdominal pain, fatigue, edema, hyperglycemia, dyspnea, cough, rash, itching, headaches, and dizziness.

Potential Toxicities/Side Effects and the Nursing Process

I. ALTERATION IN OXYGENATION, POTENTIAL, related to APL DIFFERENTIATION SYNDROME

Defining Characteristics: Drug may cause APL Differentiation Syndrome similar to the retinoic-acid-acute Promyelocytic Leukemia (RA-APL), which is characterized by fever, dyspnea, weight gain, pulmonary infiltrates, and pleural or pericardial effusions, with or without leukocytosis. This syndrome develops in response to the differentiation of immature malignant cells into mature normal white blood cells and the increased white blood cell count. The body's response is an inflammatory reaction with fluid retention in the lining of the lungs and heart.) This syndrome can be fatal, and at the first suggestion, high-dose steroids should be instituted (dexamethasone 10 mg IV bid) for at least 3 days or longer until signs and symptoms abate. The drug manufacturer states that the majority of patients do not require termination of arsenic trioxide therapy during treatment of the syndrome. The reported incidence is 20%. Leucocytosis, if it occurs, at levels $> 10 \times 10^3/\mu L$ is unrelated to baseline or peak white blood cell counts. Leukocytosis was not treated with chemotherapy, and levels were lower during consolidation than during induction.

Nursing Implications: Assess temperature and VS, oxygen saturation, cardiopulmonary status baseline and at each visit. Assess weight daily, and teach patient to report any SOB, fever, or weight gain immediately. If signs or symptoms develop, notify physician immediately and discuss obtaining CXR, cardiac echo, and focused exam. Discuss CXR, ECHO, and laboratory findings with physician. Be prepared to administer high-dose steroids (e.g., dexamethasone 10 mg IV bid × 3 days or longer depending on symptom resolution). Provide pulmonary and hemodynamic support as necessary. Assess CBC, with focus on white blood cell count and presence of leukocytosis.

II. POTENTIAL ALTERATION IN CARDIAC FUNCTION related to QT PROLONGATION AND ARRYTHMIA

Defining Characteristics: Drug can cause QT interval prolongation and complete atrioventricular block. Prolonged QT interval can progress to a torsade de pointes-type fatal ventricular arrythmia. Risk factors for development of torsade de pointes are significant QT prolongation, concomitant administraton of drugs that prolong the QT interval, history of torsades de pointes, preexisting QT prolongation, CHF, administration of potassium-wasting diuretics, and conditions resulting in hypokalemia or hypomagnesemia such as concurrent administration of amphotericin B.

Nursing Implications: Assess baseline risk, cardiovascular status, EKG determined QT interval, electrolyte and renal blood studies, and medications the patient is taking that may prolong QT interval, such as serotonin antagonist antiemetics. At least 2 times a week, the patient should have electrolyte, hematologic and coagulation assessed; more frequently if abnormal during the induction phase, and at least weekly during the consolidation phase. EKGs should be done weekly, and more frequently if abnormal. Discuss correction of any electrolyte abnormalities, as well as other risk factors, with physician. Any drugs that prolong the QT interval should be discontinued. If the QT interval prolongation is > 500 msec, this should be corrected prior to drug administration. During arsenic trioxide therapy, serum potassium should be kept > 4.0 mEq/dL and serum magnesium > 1.8 mg/dL. If the QT interval exceeds 500 msec, reassessment and correction of risk factors should occur. The patient should be hospitalized for monitoring if syncope or rapid or irregular heart rate occurs, and serum electrolytes assessed and any abnormalities corrected. Drug should be stopped until QT interval falls below 460 msec, electrolyte abnormalities corrected, and symptoms resolve.

III. ALTERATION IN NUTRITION, LESS THAN BODY REQUIREMENTS related to GI DYSFUNCTION

Defining Characteristics: Nausea is most common (incidence 75%), followed by vomiting (58%), abdominal pain (58%), diarrhea (53%), constipation (28%), anorexia (23%), dyspepsia (10%), abdominal tenderness or distention (8%), and dry mouth (8%).

Nursing Implications: Assess GI and nutrition status and presence of GI dysfunction baseline, and with each visit. Administer antiemetics, and teach patient self-administration. Discuss risk of serotonin antagonists to prolong QT interval, and contraindication with physician. Teach patient to report signs and symptoms, and evaluate symptom management plan based on effectiveness of symptom control. Assess presence of pain, and discuss pharmacologic and nonpharmacologic analgesic plan with physician.

IV. ALTERATION IN PROTECTIVE MECHANISMS, related to FEVER, ANEMIA, DIC, BLEEDING

Defining Characteristics: Fever affects 63% of patients (13% febrile neutropenia), with 38% of patients having rigors. In clinical studies, 8% of patients had hemorrhage, 14% anemia, 19% thrombocytopenia, 10% neutropenia, and 8% DIC. Patients may develop infections, and in clinical studies, most commonly these were: sinusitis 20%, herpes simplex 13%, upper respiratory tract infection 13%, nonspecific bacterial 8%, herpes zoster 8%, oral candidiasis 5%, and (rarely) sepsis 5%.

Nursing Implications: At least 2 times a week, the patient should have electrolyte, hematologic and coagulation assessed; more frequently if abnormal during the induction phase, and at least weekly during the consolidation phase.

Monitor laboratory results, and discuss abnormalities with physician. Assess patient for fever, signs and symptoms of infection, rigors, and bleeding, and implement management plan to assure patient safety. Transfuse patient as ordered, and monitor closely.

V. ALTERATION IN COMFORT related to HEADACHE, CHEST PAIN, AND INJECTION SITE CHANGES

Defining Characteristics: Headache occurred in approximately 60% of patients while chest pain occurred in 25%. Injection site reactions of pain, erythema, and edema occurred in 20%, 13%, and 10% of patients, respectively.

Nursing Implications: Assess level of comfort, and develop plan for comfort, including pharmacologic, and non-pharmacologic measures. Assess effectiveness, and revise plan as needed. Assess patency of IV site and need for IV catheter change. Assess need for central line. Although not necessary for drug delivery, if patient venous access is limited this may provide enhanced patient comfort.

VI. ALTERATION IN ACTIVITY TOLERANCE related to FATIGUE, MUSCULOSKELETAL PROBLEMS

Defining Characteristics: 63% of patients reported fatigue. In clinical studies, musculoskeletal events were: arthralgias (33%), myalgias (25%), bone pain (23%), back pain (18%), neck pain, and pain in limbs (13%).

Nursing Implications: Assess baseline energy and activity level, and level of comfort. Assess need for assistance with ADLs and home assistance. Assess need for analgesics or local measures to relieve pain and discomfort. Teach patient self-care strategies to minimize exertion and maximize activity, such as clustering activity during shopping, alternating rest and activity periods, diet, gentle exercise. Evaluate success of plan and need for revisions.

VII. ALTERATION IN FLUID AND ELECTROLYTE BALANCE related to HYPOKALEMIA, HYPOMAGNESEMIA, HYPERGLYCEMIA, EDEMA

Defining Characteristics: Hypokalemia occurs in about 50% of patients, hypomagnesemia (45%), hyperglycemia (45%), and edema (40%). Other electrolyte abnormalities are hyperkalemia (18%), hypocalcemia (10%), hypoglycemia (8%), acidosis (5%), and increased transaminases (13–20%).

Nursing Implications: At least 2 times a week, the patient should have electrolyte, hematologic and coagulation assessed; more frequently if abnormal during the induction phase, and at least weekly during the consolidation phase. EKGs should be done weekly, and more frequently if abnormal. Teach patient that edema may occur, and to report it. Assess patient baseline and before each treatment for weight and presence of edema. Discuss abnormalities with physician, correct as ordered, and monitor closely for signs and symptoms of imbalance.

VIII. SENSORY/PERCEPTUAL ALTERATIONS, POTENTIAL related to PARESTHESIA, DIZZINESS, TREMOR, INSOMNIA

Defining Characteristics: Insomnia occurs in 43% of patients, paresthesia (33%), dizziness (23%), tremor (13%), seizures (8%), somnolence (8%), and (rarely) coma (5%).

Nursing Implications: Assess baseline mental and neurological status, and monitor frequently during therapy. Assess sensory function, and teach patient to report numbness, tingling, dizziness, tremor, seizure, decrease in alertness, and changes in sleep. Assess presence of paresthesias, and motor and sensory function prior to each treatment; discuss presence or worsening with physician. Teach patient self-care strategies, including maintaining safety when walking, getting up, taking a bath, or washing dishes if unable to feel temperature changes. Teach self-care measures to manage sleep problems, and discuss possible need for sleeping medication.

IX. ALTERATION IN GAS EXCHANGE, POTENTIAL, related to COUGH, DYSPNEA, HYPOXIA, PLEURAL EFFUSION

Defining Characteristics: Cough is common, affecting 65% of patients, followed by dyspnea (53%), epistaxis (25%), hypoxia (23%), pleural effusion (20%), postnasal drip (13%), wheezing (13%), decreased breath sounds (10%), crepitations (10%), rales (crackles) (10%), hemoptysis (8%), tachypnea (8%), and rhonchi (8%).

Nursing Implications: Assess baseline pulmonary status, including breath sounds and oxygen saturation, and monitor at least daily during treatment. Teach patient that symptoms may occur and to report them. Discuss management of patients experiencing cough, dyspnea, and other symptoms with physician, and develop individualized management plan.

X. ALTERATION IN SKIN INTEGRITY, POTENTIAL, related to SKIN IRRITATION

Defining Characteristics: Dermatitis affects about 43% of patients, pruritis (33%), ecchymosis (20%), dry skin (13%), erythema (10%), hyperpigmentation (8%), and urticaria (8%).

Nursing Implications: Assess baseline skin integrity and monitor at each visit. Teach patient to report any skin changes or itching. Teach patient symptomatic local measures to manage dermatitis, itch, or other changes. If plan ineffective, discuss other measures with physician.

Drug: asparaginase (Elspar)

Class: Miscellaneous agents (enzyme).

Mechanism of Action: Hydrolyzes serum asparagine, which deprives leukemia cells of the required amino acid. Normal cells are spared because they generally have the ability to synthesize their own asparagine. Cell cycle specific for G1 postmitotic phase. Some leukemic cells are unable to synthesize asparagine. These cells must obtain asparagine from an exogenous source, the patient's serum. Administration of the enzyme L-asparaginase causes hydrolysis of asparagine to aspartate, resulting in rapid depletion of the asparagine concentration in the patient's serum.

Metabolism: Metabolism of L-asparaginase is independent of renal and hepatic function. The drug is not recovered in the urine and does not appear to cross the blood-brain barrier.

Dosage/Range:

- IM or IV varies with protocol. Typical dosing is 200 IU/kg IV qd × 28 days (ALL).

Drug Preparation:

- IV injection: reconstitute with sterile water for injection or 0.9% Sodium Chloride injection (without preservative) and use within 8 hours of restoration.
- IV infusion: dilute with 0.9% Sodium Chloride injection or 5% Dextrose injection and use within 8 hours, only if clear; if gelatinous particles develop, filter through a 5.0-μm filter.
- The lyophilized powder must be stored under refrigeration. The reconstituted solution must also be stored under refrigeration if it is not used immediately. The solution must be discarded 8 hours after preparation.

Drug Administration:

- Use in a hospital setting. Make preparations to treat anaphylaxis at each administration of the drug.

Drug Interactions:

- Prednisone: potential additive hyperglycemic effect; monitor blood glucose levels.
- Cyclophosphamide, vincristine, 6-mercaptopurine: may increase or decrease drug's effect (CTX, VCR, 6-MP).
- 6-mercaptopurine: Enhanced hepatotoxicity; monitor LFTs closely.

- Methotrexate: Antagonism if administered immediately prior to methotrexate; when administered some time after methotrexate, may enhance methotrexate activity.
- Synergy with cytosine arabinoside.
- Increased hyperglycemia when given together with prednisone.
- Reduced hypersensitivity when given with 6-mercaptopurine or prednisone.
- Additive neurotoxicity when given with vincristine.

Lab Effects/Interference:
- Increased LFTs.
- Decreased hepatically derived clotting factors.
- Interferes with thyroid function tests after first two days of therapy: effect lasts four weeks.

Special Considerations:
- Potential reduction in antineoplastic effect of methotrexate when given in combination.
- Anaphylaxis is associated with the administration of this drug.
- Intravenous administration of L-asparaginase concurrently with or immediately before prednisone and vincristine administration may be associated with increased toxicity.

Potential Toxicities/Side Effects and the Nursing Process

I. POTENTIAL FOR INJURY related to HYPERSENSITIVITY OR ANAPHYLACTIC REACTIONS

Defining Characteristics: Occurs in 20–30% of patients. Increased incidence after several doses administered, but may occur with first dose. Occurs less often with IM route of administration. May be life-threatening reaction, but is usually mild.

Nursing Implications: Discuss with physician use of test dose prior to drug administration. Assess baseline vital signs and mental status prior to drug administration. Review standing orders or nursing procedure for management of anaphylaxis and be prepared to stop drug immediately if signs/symptoms occur; keep IV line open with 0.9% Sodium Chloride, notify physician, monitor vital signs, and administer ordered medications, which may include epinephrine 1:1000, hydrocortisone sodium succinate, and diphenhydramine. Teach patient the potential of a hypersensitivity or anaphylactic reaction and to immediately report any unusual symptoms. *Escherichia coli* preparation of L-asparaginase and *Erwinia carotovora* preparation are non-cross-resistant, so if an anaphylactic reaction occurs with one, the other preparation may be used.

II. POTENTIAL FOR INJURY related to HEPATIC DYSFUNCTION OR THROMBOEMBOLISM

Defining Characteristics: Two-thirds of patients have elevated LFTs starting within the first two weeks of treatment: e.g., SGOT, bili, and alk phos. Hepatically derived clotting factors may be depressed, resulting in excessive bleeding or blood clotting. Relatively uncommon.

Nursing Implications: Monitor SGOT, bili, alk phos, albumin, and clotting factors CPT, PTT, fibrinogen. Teach patient of the potential of excessive bleeding or blood clotting, and instruct to report any unusual symptoms. Assess patient for signs/symptoms of bleeding.

III. ALTERED NUTRITION, LESS THAN BODY REQUIREMENTS related to NAUSEA/VOMITING, ANOREXIA, HYPERGLYCEMIA

Defining Characteristics: 50–60% of patients experience mild to severe nausea and vomiting starting within 4–6 hours after treatment. Anorexia commonly occurs. Hyperglycemia is a transient reaction caused by effects on the pancreas with decreased insulin synthesis. Pancreatitis occurs in 5% of patients.

Nursing Implications: Premedicate with antiemetics and continue prophylactically for 24 hours to prevent nausea and vomiting. Encourage small, frequent meals of cool, bland foods and liquids, as well as favorite foods, especially high-calorie, high-protein foods. Encourage use of spices and do weekly weights. Teach patient about the potential of hyperglycemia and pancreatitis, and instruct to report any unusual symptoms, e.g., increased thirst, urination, and appetite. Monitor serum glucose, amylase, and lipase levels periodically during treatment. Report any laboratory elevations to physician. Treat hyperglycemia issues with diet or insulin as ordered by physician. Treat pancreatitis per physician orders.

IV. SENSORY/PERCEPTUAL ALTERATIONS related to CHANGES IN MENTAL STATUS

Defining Characteristics: 25% of patients experience some changes in mental status—commonly, lethargy, drowsiness, and somnolence; rarely coma. Predominantly seen in adults. Malaise (feeling "blah") occurs in most patients, and generally gets worse with subsequent doses. Drug does not cross BBB.

Nursing Implications: Teach patient about the potential of CNS toxicity, and instruct to report any unusual symptoms. Obtain baseline neurologic and mental function. Assess patient for any neurologic abnormalities and report changes to physician. Discuss with patient the impact of malaise on his/her general sense of well-being and strategies to minimize the distress.

V. POTENTIAL FOR SEXUAL DYSFUNCTION related to REPRODUCTION HAZARD

Defining Characteristics: Drug is teratogenic.

Nursing Implications: As appropriate, explore with patient and partner issues of reproductive and sexual patterns and impact chemotherapy will have. Discuss strategies to preserve sexuality and reproductive health (e.g., sperm banking, contraception).

VI. INFECTION, BLEEDING, AND FATIGUE related to BONE MARROW DEPRESSION

Defining Characteristics: Bone marrow depression is not common. Mild anemia may occur. Serious leukopenia and thrombocytopenia are rare.

Nursing Implications: Monitor CBC, platelet count prior to drug administration, as well as signs/symptoms of infection, bleeding, or anemia. Instruct patient in self-assessment of signs/symptoms of infection, bleeding, or anemia and to report immediately.

Drug: 5-azacytidine (Vidaza)

Class: Antimetabolite.

Mechanism of Action: Azacytidine causes hypomethylation of DNA, which may restore normal gene function to genes responsible for cell division and differentiation of the bone marrow. At higher doses, it also interferes with nucleic acid metabolism by acting as a false metabolite when incorporated into DNA and RNA; cell cycle phase specific for S phase.

Metabolism: Rapidly absorbed following subcutaneous administration, with peak plasma level in 30 minutes. Bioavailability of subcutaneously administered drug is 89% of IV dose. 85% of the total administered dose is excreted in the urine, and $< 1\%$ in feces. Mean elimination half-life is about 4 hours in both subcutaneous and IV administered drug.

Dosage/Range:

- 75 mg/m^2 Subcutaneous injection qd × 7 days, repeated q 4 weeks for at least 4 cycles
- Dose may be increased to 100 mg/m^2 after 2 cycles if initial dose ineffective and toxicity manageable (no toxicity except nausea and vomiting)
- Decrease or hold dose if significant bone marrow depression
- If baseline WBC $> 3000/mm^3$, ANC $> 1500/mm^3$, and platelets $> 75{,}000/mm^3$, modify dose based on nadir counts:
- ANC $< 500/mm^3$, platelets $< 25{,}000/mm^3$ = 50% dose next course

- ANC 500–1500/mm^3, platelets 25,000–50,000/mm^3 = 67% of dose next course
- ANC > 1500/mm^3, platelets > 50,000/mm^3 = 100% dose
- If baseline WBC < 3000/mm^3, ANC < 1500/mm^3, or platelets < 75,000/mm^3, dose modifications and bone marrow biopsy cellularity at time of nadir used, unless there is clear improvement in differentiation (% mature granulocytes is higher with ANC higher than at onset of treatment)- see package insert.
- Dose modification based on renal function and serum electrolytes
- If unexplained decreases in serum bicarbonate < 20 mEq/L, dose reduce 50% in next cycle
- If elevations of BUN or serum creatinine occur, delay next dose until values return to normal or baseline, and reduce dose by 50% in next cycle.

Drug Preparation:
- Drug is a lyophilized powder in 100 mg single-use vials
- Reconstitute asceptically with 4 mL sterile water for injection, adding diluent slowly into the vial
- Invert vial 2–3 times and gently rotate, yielding a cloudy suspension containing 25 mg/mL
- Divide doses greater than 4 mL into 2 syringes and administer within 1 hour of reconstitution at room temperature
- Reconstituted solution may be kept in the vial or drawn in a syringe(s) and refrigerated immediately for later use for up to 8 hours. After removal from the refrigerator, the suspension may be allowed to equilibrate to room temperature for up to 30 minutes prior to administration

Drug Administration:
- Invert syringe(s) 2–3 times and gently roll syringe(s) between palms for 30 seconds immediately prior to administration to provide a homogenous suspension.
- Rotate sites for each subcutaneous injection (thigh, abdomen, or upper arm), and give new injection at least 1 inch from old site, and never into areas where site is tender, bruised, red or hard.

Drug Interactions:
- None significant.

Lab Effects/Interference:
- Decreased ANC, platelets, red blood cell counts.
- Renal tubular acidosis
- Increased BUN and creatinine
- Hypokalemia

Special Considerations:

- Azacytidine is indicated for treatment of patients with all five Myelodysplastic subtypes: refractory anemia (RA) or refractory anemia with ringed sideroblasts (RARS) (if accompanied by neutropenia or thrombocytopenia or requiring transfusions), refractory anemia with excess blasts (RAEB), refractory anemia with excess blasts in transformation (RAEB-T), and chronic myelomonocytic leukemia (CMMoL).
- Overall response rate of patients with all patients except those with AML was 15.7% (Complete and partial responders).
- Drug is contraindicated in patients with hypersensitivity to mannitol, and in patients with advanced malignant hepatic tumors.
- Drug is fetotoxic and embryotoxic. Women of child-bearing age must use effective contraception methods; men should be advised not to father a child while receiving treatment with azacitidine. Women who are receiving azacitidine should not breast feed their infant as drug causes tumors in animals, and has the potential for severe toxicity.
- Monitor renal function closely in elderly patients.
- Use cautiously in patients with pre-existing hepatic disease as patients with extensive liver metastases have rarely been reported to develop coma and death.

Potential Toxicities/Side Effects and the Nursing Process

I. INFECTION AND BLEEDING related to BONE MARROW DEPRESSION

Defining Characteristics: Leukopenia is dose-limiting, with nadir occurring from days 14–17; lasts two weeks, with recovery in 14 days. Thrombocytopenia and anemia also occur. Bone marrow depression lessens once patient has a response to therapy.

Nursing Implications: Monitor CBC, neutrophil, and platelet count prior to drug administration and postchemotherapy; assess for signs/symptoms of infection, bleeding, and anemia. Teach patient/family signs/symptoms of infection, bleeding, and anemia, and instruct to report them to nurse or physician immediately. Teach patient to avoid aspirin-containing OTC medications.

II. ALTERATION IN NUTRITION, LESS THAN BODY REQUIREMENTS, related to NAUSEA AND VOMITING, ANOREXIA, STOMATITIS, CONSTIPATION and DIARRHEA

Defining Characteristics: Nausea/vomiting is dose-related, and occurs in about 70.5%/54.1% of patients, respectively, beginning 1–3 hours postchemotherapy. This tends to be worse in the first 1–2 cycles, and increases in incidence with increasing doses. Diarrhea develops in 36.4% of patients, with incidence increasing as dose increases. Constipation occurs in about 33% of patients and is worse during the first 2 cycles of therapy. Anorexia affects 20% of patients, and stomatitis occurs in 7% of patients.

Nursing Implications: Assess baseline nutritional status, and periodically at visits. Premedicate with antiemetics before injection, and teach patient self-administration of antiemetics at home; encourage small, frequent feedings as tolerated; if severe vomiting occurs, treat with alternative antiemetics and assess for signs/symptoms of fluid and electrolyte imbalance. Monitor serum potassium, as hypokalemia may be a side effect of treatment. Assess baseline bowel elimination stastus. Instruct patient to report onset of diarrhea and administer antidiarrheals as ordered. If diarrhea is protracted, ensure adequate hydration, monitor total body fluid balance, and teach/reinforce perineal hygiene. Instruct patient to monitor for constipation, and to use measures to prevent constipation if that is a problem. If patient has anorexia, teach patient to identify nutrient-dense foods and to eat small frequent meals, including a bedtime snack. Teach patient strategies to increase appetite, depending upon an individualized assessment. Teach patient to self-assess oral mucosa, and to use a systematic cleansing of teeth/mouth after meals and at bedtime. Monitor LFTs periodically during therapy and discuss abnormalities with physician.

III. ALTERATION IN COMFORT related to FEVER, FATIGUE, ARTHRALGIAS, and INJECTION SITE IRRITATION

Defining Characteristics: Fever occurs in 54% of patients, with rigors affecting about 25%; fatigue in 36% of patients; arthralgias in 22%; and injection site erythema (35%), injection site pain (23%), injection site bruising (14%), injection site reaction (14%). Injection site discomfort was more pronounced during the 1st and 2nd cycles of therapy.

Nursing Implications: Monitor temperature and teach patient to self-assess temperature. Teach patient that pyrexia may occur, and how to self-administer antipyretics. Teach patient to notify nurse/MD if rigors occur and are severe. Teach measures to reduce discomfort related to myalgias if they occur, such as application of heat and NSAIDs. Teach patient strategies to conserve energy, such as alternating activity with reset. Teach patient to rotate sites used for injection, and local measures to increase comfort.

Drug: bicalutamide (Casodex)

Class: Nonsteroidal antiandrogen.

Mechanism of Action: Binds to androgen receptors in the prostate; affinity is four times greater than that of flutamide.

Metabolism: Extensively metabolized in the liver. Decreased drug excretion in patients with moderate to severe hepatic dysfunction.

Dosage/Range:

- 50 mg PO qd.

Drug Preparation:

- None.

Drug Administration:

- Orally.

Drug Interactions:

- None known.

Lab Effects/Interference:

- Increased LFTs.

Special Considerations:

- Use cautiously in patients with moderate to severe hepatic dysfunction. Observe closely for toxicity, as dosage adjustment may be required.
- No dose modification needed for renal dysfunction.

Potential Toxicities/Side Effects and the Nursing Process

I. ALTERATION IN COMFORT, POTENTIAL related to GYNECOMASTIA AND HOT FLASHES

Defining Characteristics: Gynecomastia occurs in 23% of patients, breast tenderness in 26%, and hot flashes in 9.3%.

Nursing Implications: Teach patient that these side effects may occur, and discuss measures that may offer symptomatic relief.

II. ALTERATION IN NUTRITION, LESS THAN BODY REQUIREMENTS, related to NAUSEA, POTENTIAL

Defining Characteristics: Nausea may occur in 6% of patients.

Nursing Implications: Teach patient that nausea may occur, and instruct to report nausea. Determine baseline weight, and monitor at each visit. Discuss strategies to minimize nausea, including diet modification and time of dosing.

III. ALTERATION IN ELIMINATION, POTENTIAL, related to CONSTIPATION OR DIARRHEA

Defining Characteristics: Incidence of constipation is 6%, while that of diarrhea is 2.5%.

Nursing Implications: Assess baseline elimination pattern. Teach patient that alterations may occur, and instruct to report them if changes do not respond to usual nonprescription management strategies (OTC medications, dietary modifications).

Drug: bleomycin sulfate (Blenoxane)

Class: Antitumor action of bleomycin; isolated from fungus *Streptomyces verticullus*. Possesses both antitumor and antimicrobial actions.

Mechanism of Action: Induces single-strand and double-strand breaks in DNA. DNA synthesis is inhibited.

Metabolism: Excreted via the renal system. About 70% is excreted unchanged in urine; 30–60 minutes after IV infusion, urine levels are 10 times the serum level.

Dosage/Range:
- 5–20 U/m^2 once a week.
- 10–20 U/m^2 twice a week.
- Frequency and schedule may vary according to protocol and age.

Drug Preparation:
- Dilute powder in 0.9% Sodium Chloride or sterile water.

Drug Administration:
- IV, IM, or SQ doses may be administered. Some clinical trial protocols may use 24-hour infusions. There is a risk for anaphylaxis in lymphoma patients and hypotension with higher doses of drug. It may be recommended that a test dose be given before the first dose to detect hypersensitivity.

Drug Interactions:
- Digoxin dose may need to be increased.
- Phenytoin dose may need to be increased.

Lab Effects/Interference:
- None.

Special Considerations:
- Because of pulmonary toxicities with increasing dose, pulmonary function tests (PFTs) and CXR should be obtained before each course or as outlined by protocol.
- Maximum cumulative lifetime dose: 400 U.
- Oxygen (FIO2) increases risk of pulmonary toxicity.
- Reduce dose for impaired renal function (urinary creatinine clearance $<$40–60 mL/min).
- Risk of pulmonary toxicity increased in elderly ($>$70 years old); renal impairment; pulmonary disease or prior chest XRT; exposure to high oxygen concentration (i.e., surgery); cumulative doses $>$400 U lifetime.

- May cause chemical fevers up to 39.4–40.5°C (103–105°F) in up to 60% of patients. May need to administer premedications such as acetaminophen, antihistamines, or in some cases steroids.
- Watch for signs/symptoms of hypotension and anaphylaxis with high drug doses; physician may order test dose in patients with lymphoma.
- May cause irritation at site of injection (is considered an irritant, not a vesicant).
- Decreases the oral bioavailability of digoxin when given together.
- Decreases the pharmacologic effects of phenytoin when given in combination.

Potential Toxicities/Side Effects and the Nursing Process

I. POTENTIAL FOR IMPAIRED GAS EXCHANGE related to PULMONARY TOXICITY

Defining Characteristics: Pneumonitis occurs in 10% of patients and is characterized by rales, dyspnea, infiltrate on CXR; in 1% may progress to irreversible pulmonary fibrosis. Risk factors include age > 70, dose > 400 U (but may occur at much lower doses), and concurrent or prior radiotherapy to the chest. Slower, continuous infusion may lower the risk.

Nursing Implications: Discuss with physician the need for PFTs and CXR prior to initiating therapy and monthly during therapy. Assess pulmonary status prior to each treatment (early symptom is dyspnea, and earliest sign is fine crackles). Instruct patient to report cough, dyspnea, shortness of breath. If patient needs surgery, discuss with physician the need to use low FIO2 during surgery since the lung tissue has been sensitized to bleomycin, and high concentrations of oxygen will cause further lung damage.

II. POTENTIAL FOR INJURY related to ANAPHYLAXIS

Defining Characteristics: Anaphylactoid reaction may occur in 1% of lymphoma patients, characterized by hypotension, confusion, tachycardia, wheezing, and facial edema. Reaction may be immediate or delayed for several hours and may occur after the first or second drug administration.

Nursing Implications: Discuss with physician the use of test dose prior to drug administration in lymphoma patients. Assess baseline vital signs (VS) and mental status prior to drug administration. Review standing orders or nursing procedure for patient management of anaphylaxis, and be prepared to stop drug immediately if signs/symptoms occur. Keep IV line open with 0.9% Sodium Chloride; notify physician, monitor VS, and administer ordered medications, which may include epinephrine 1:1000, hydrocortisone sodium succinate, and diphenhydramine.

III. POTENTIAL ALTERATION IN COMFORT related to FEVER AND CHILLS AND PAIN AT TUMOR SITE

Defining Characteristics: Fever (up to 39.4°–40.5°C [103°–105°F]) and chills, occurring in up to 60% of patients, begin 4–10 hours after drug administration and may last 24 hours. There appears to be tolerance with successive doses of bleomycin. Pain may occur at tumor site due to chemotherapy-induced cellular damage.

Nursing Implications: Teach patient that these side effects may occur, and assess patient during and postadministration. If fever occurs, notify physician and administer ordered acetaminophen, antihistamine, or steroid. If tumor pain occurs, reassure patient and discuss with physician the use of acetaminophen as analgesic.

IV. POTENTIAL FOR IMPAIRED SKIN INTEGRITY related to ALOPECIA, SKIN CHANGES, AND NAIL CHANGES

Defining Characteristics: Dose-related alopecia begins 3–4 weeks after first dose and is reversible. Skin changes occur in 50% of patients and include erythema, rash, striae, hyperpigmentation, skin peeling of fingertips, and hyperkeratosis; these are dose-related and begin after 150–200 U have been administered. Skin eruptions include a macular rash over hands and elbows, urticaria, and vesiculations. Pruritus may occur. Nail changes and possible nail loss may occur. Phlebitis at the IV site may occur.

Nursing Implications: Teach patient about possible side effects and self-care measures, including obtaining a wig or cap as appropriate prior to hair loss. Encourage patient to verbalize feelings and provide patient emotional support. Discuss with physician symptomatic treatment of skin changes. Assess IV site for phlebitis and restart IV at alternate site if phlebitis develops.

V. POTENTIAL ALTERATION IN NUTRITION, LESS THAN BODY REQUIREMENTS, related to NAUSEA AND VOMITING, ANOREXIA AND WEIGHT LOSS, AND STOMATITIS

Defining Characteristics: Nausea with or without vomiting may occur; anorexia and weight loss may occur and may continue after treatment is completed; stomatitis may occur and decrease ability and desire to eat.

Nursing Implications: Administer antiemetic prior to initial treatment and revise plan for successive treatments if no nausea/vomiting. Teach patient about possible anorexia and encourage patient to eat high-calorie, high-protein foods. Assess oral mucosa prior to drug administration; teach patient self-assessment and instruct to notify nurse or physician if stomatitis develops. Teach patient oral care prior to drug administration.

VI. POTENTIAL FOR SEXUAL DYSFUNCTION related to REPRODUCTIVE HAZARDS

Defining Characteristics: Drug is mutagenic and probably teratogenic.

Nursing Implications: Discuss with patient and partner both sexuality and reproductive goals, as well as possible impact of chemotherapy. Discuss contraception and sperm banking if appropriate.

Drug: busulfan (Myleran)

Class: Alkylating agent.

Mechanism of Action: Forms carbonium ions through the release of a methane sulfonate group, resulting in the alkylation of DNA. Acts primarily on granulocyte precursors in the bone marrow and is cell cycle phase nonspecific.

Metabolism: Well absorbed orally; almost all metabolites are excreted in the urine. Has a very short half-life.

Dosage/Range:

Chronic myelogenous leukemia:

- 4–8 mg/day PO for 2–3 weeks initially, then maintenance dose of 1–3 mg/m^2 PO qd or 0.05 mg/kg orally qd. Dose titrated based on leukocyte counts. Drug witheld when leukocyte count reaches 15,000/μL; resume when total leukocyte count is 50,000/μL; maintenance dose of 1–3 mg qd used if remission lasts < 3 months.

High doses with bone marrow transplantation:

- See Busulfan for Injection.

Drug Preparation:

- None.

Drug Administration:

- Available in 2-mg scored tablets given orally.

Drug Interactions:

- Combination treatment with thioguanine may cause hepatic dysfunction and the development of esophageal varices in a small number of patients.

Lab Effects/Interference:

- Decreased CBC.
- Increased LFTs.

Special Considerations:

Regular dose:

- If WBC is high, patient is at risk for hyperuricemia. Allopurinol and hydration may be indicated.

- Follow weekly CBC and platelet count initially, then monthly. Dose is decreased to maintenance level when leukocyte count falls below 50,000 mm^3.
- Hyperpigmentation of skin creases may occur due to increased melanin production.
- If given according to accepted guidelines, patients should have minimal side effects.

High dose:

- See Busulfan for Injection.

Potential Toxicities/Side Effects and the Nursing Process

I. POTENTIAL FOR INFECTION, BLEEDING, AND FATIGUE related to BONE MARROW DEPRESSION

Defining Characteristics: The nadir is at 11–30 days following initial drug administration, with recovery in 24–54 days; however, delayed, refractory pancytopenia has occurred.

Nursing Implications: Monitor CBC, WBC differential, and platelets, initially weekly, then at least monthly. Expect drug will be interrupted if counts fall rapidly or steeply. Teach patient to self-assess for signs/symptoms of infection, bleeding, or severe fatigue, and to notify nurse or physician immediately. Teach patient to avoid aspirin-containing OTC medications.

II. POTENTIAL FOR IMPAIRED GAS EXCHANGE related to INTERSTITIAL PULMONARY FIBROSIS

Defining Characteristics: Rarely, bronchopulmonary dysplasia progressing to pulmonary fibrosis can occur, beginning one to many years posttherapy. Symptoms are usually delayed (occurring after four years) and include anorexia, cough, dyspnea, and fever. High-dose corticosteroids may be helpful, but condition may be fatal due to rapid, diffuse fibrosis.

Nursing Implications: Assess pulmonary status routinely in all patients receiving long-term therapy. Discuss plan for regular pulmonary function studies with physician.

III. POTENTIAL FOR SEXUAL AND REPRODUCTIVE DYSFUNCTION related to REPRODUCTIVE HAZARDS

Defining Characteristics: Premenopausal female patients commonly experience ovarian suppression and amenorrhea with menopausal symptoms; men experience sterility, azoospermia, and testicular atrophy. Although successful pregnancies have occurred following busulfan therapy, the drug is potentially teratogenic.

Nursing Implications: Assess patient's/partner's sexual patterns and reproductive goals. Provide information, supportive counseling, and referral as needed. Teach importance of birth control measures as appropriate.

Drug: busulfan for injection (Busulfex)

Class: Alkylating agent.

Mechanism of Action: Forms carbonium ions through the release of a methane sulfonate group, resulting in the alkylation of DNA. Acts primarily on granulocyte precursors in the bone marrow, and is cell cycle, phase nonspecific.

Metabolism: After IV administration, drug achieves equal concentrations in the plasma and CSF. Drug is 32% protein-bound. Metabolized in the liver, and excreted in the urine (30%). Appears metabolites may be long-lived.

Dosage/Range:
Conditioning regimen:
- Indicated in combination with cyclophosphamide prior to allogeneic hematopoietic progenitor cell transplantation for chronic myelogenous leukemia.
- 0.8 mg/kg (IBW or actual weight, whichever is lower, or adjusted IBW) IV q6h × 4 days (total of 16 doses).
- Cyclophosphamide dose is given on each of 2 days as a 1-hour infusion at a dose of 60 mg/kg beginning on BMT day −3, 6 hours following the 16th dose of IV busulfan.

Drug Preparation:
- Asceptically open ampule, and using the 25-mm, 5-micron nylon membrane syringe filter provided, remove the ordered, calculated drug dose.
- Remove the syringe/filter, replace with a new needle, and dispense the syringe contents into a bag or syringe containing 10 times the volume of the drug, either 0.9% NS Injection or 5% Dextrose Injection. The final concentration of drug should be ≥ 0.5 mg/mL. For example, a 70-kg patient at a dose of 0.8 mg/kg given a concentration of 6 mg/mL would require 9.3 mL (56 mg) busulfan total dose. 9.3 mL of drug × 10 = 93 mL. As the further diluent needed is 0.9% NS Inj or D%W Inj, the total volume is 9.3 mL + 93 mL = 102.3 mL.
- Mix contents thoroughly.
- Ensure that this meets the recommended drug concentration, e.g., (9.3 mL × 6 mg/mL)/102.3 mL = 0.54 mg/mL.
- Unopened ampules must be refrigerated at 2–8°C (36–46°F).
- Diluted drug is stable at room temperature (25°C) for up to 8 hours, but infusion must be completed within this time. Drug diluted in 0.9% NS Inj,

USP, is stable refrigerated (2–8°C) for up to 12 hours, but the infusion must be completed within that time.

Drug Administration:

- Available in a 10-mL, single-use ampule containing 60 mg (6 mg/mL).
- Dilute in 0.9% NS Injection or 5% Dextrose Injection to 10 times volume of drug (see example in Preparation) prior to IV infusion.
- Infuse dose over 2 hours via infusion pump.
- Drug should be administered through a central line.
- All patients should be premedicated with phenytoin, as drug crosses BBB and causes seizures (see Drug Interactions).

Drug Interactions:

- Phenytoin decreases busulfan AUC by 15%, resulting in the target dose. If phenytoin is not used concomitantly, AUC and drug exposure may be greater.
- Other anticonvulsants may increase busulfan AUC, increasing the risk of veno-occlusive disease or seizures. Monitor busulfan exposure and toxicity closely.
- Itraconazole decreases busulfan clearance by up to 25% with potential significant increases in serum busulfan levels.
- Acetaminophen prior to (< 72 hours) or concurrent with busulfan may result in decreased drug clearance and increased serum busulfan levels.

Lab Effects/Interference:

- Profound myelosuppression/aplasia with decreased WBC, neutrophils, Hgb/HCT, and platelet counts.
- If liver veno-occlusive disease develops, increased serum transaminases, alk phos, and bili.
- Creatinine is elevated in 21% of patients.

Special Considerations:

- Drug clearance is best predicted when the busulfan dose is based on adjusted ideal body weight (AIBW).
- Ideal body weight (IBW in kg): men = 50 + 0.91 × (height in cm − 152); Women = 45 + 0.91 × (height in cm − 152).
- AIBW = IBW + 0.25 × (actual weight − IBW).
- No known antidote if overdose occurs; one report says that drug is dialyzable.

Drug is metabolized by conjugation with glutathione, so consider administration of same. Drug should only be given in combination with hematopoietic progenitor cell transplantation, as expected toxicity is profound myelosuppression.

CNS effects including seizures, hepatic veno-occlusive disease (VOD), cardiac tamponade, bronchopulmonary dysplasia with pulmonary fibrosis four months to ten years after therapy.

- Contraindicated in patients with a history of hypersensitivity to drug or its components.
- Women of childbearing age should use effective birth control measures; nursing mothers should interrupt breast-feeding during therapy.
- Drug is for adult use, and has not been studied in patients with hepatic insufficiency.
- Drug may cause cellular dysplasia in many organs (characterized by giant, hyperchromatic nuclei in lymph nodes, pancreas, thyroid, adrenal glands, liver, lungs, and bone marrow), which may cause difficult interpretation of subsequent cytologic examinations in lungs, bladder, and uterine cervix.
- Factors that may increase risk of veno-occlusive disease are history of XRT, more than three cycles of chemotherapy, prior progenitor cell transplantation, or busulfex dose AUC concentrations of > 1500 μm/min.

Potential Toxicities/Side Effects and the Nursing Process

I. POTENTIAL FOR INFECTION, BLEEDING, AND ANEMIA related to BONE MARROW DEPRESSION

Defining Characteristics: Myelosuppression is profound in 100% of patients. ANC < 500/mm^3 occurred a median of four days posttransplant in 100% of patients. Following progenitor cell infusion, the median recovery of neutrophil count to ≥ 500 cells/mm^3 was day 13 when prophylactic G-CSF was given. 51% of patients experienced 1+ episodes of infection; fever occurred in 80% of patients, with chills in 33%. Thrombocytopenia (< 25,000/mm^3 or requiring platelet transfusion) occurred in 5–6 days in 98% of patients. There was a median of six platelet transfusions per patient in clinical trials. Anemia affected 50% of patients, and the median number of red blood cell transfusions on clinical trials was 4 per patient.

Nursing Implications: Assess WBC, with differential, Hgb/HCT, and platelet count prior to drug administration, and at least daily during treatment. Discuss any abnormalities with physician. Monitor continuously for signs/symptoms of infection or bleeding. Teach patient signs/symptoms of infection and bleeding, self-assessment, and to report signs/symptoms immediately. Teach self-care measures to minimize infection and bleeding, including avoidance of OTC aspirin-containing medications. Discuss with physician use of granulocyte-colony stimulating factor (G-CSF) to prevent febrile neutropenia. Transfuse platelets and red blood cells per physician order.

II. ALTERATION IN CARDIAC OUTPUT, POTENTIAL related to TACHYCARDIA, THROMBOSIS, HYPERTENSION, VASODILATION

Defining Characteristics: Mild-to-moderate tachycardia has been noted in 44% of patients (11% during drug infusion), and, less commonly, other rhythm disturbances such as arrhythmia (5%), atrial fibrillation (2%), ventricular extrasystoles (2%), and third-degree heart block (2%). Mild-to-moderate thrombosis may occur in 33% of patients, usually associated with a central venous catheter. Hypertension has been seen in 36% of patients and grade ¾ in 3%. Mild vasodilation (flushing and hot flashes) occurs in 25% of patients. In clinical trials, most commonly in the postcyclophosphamide phase, other less common events were cardiomegaly (5%), mild EKG changes (2%), grades 3 and 4 CHF (2%), and moderate pericardial effusion (2%).

Nursing Implications: Assess baseline cardiac status and frequently during shift/care depending upon patient condition, including HR, BP, EKG, and total body fluid balance. Monitor patient for changes in cardiac function throughout treatment course, and report changes immediately. Monitor central venous lines for patency, and use scrupulous care in maintaining catheters; assess for signs/symptoms of venous thrombosis, and discuss management with physician as soon as it is discovered.

III. ALTERATION IN FLUID AND ELECTROLYTE BALANCE, POTENTIAL related to TREATMENT, CARDIAC RESPONSE

Defining Characteristics: 79% of patients develop edema, hypervolemia, or weight increase, mild or moderate.

Nursing Implications: Assess baseline fluid volume status, weight, orthostatic vital signs, and presence/absence of edema, and assess at least daily, especially after fluid or blood product infusion. Closely monitor I/O and daily total body balance, and discuss abnormalities with physician. Assess renal status, as BUN and creatinine can become elevated in 21% of patients. Assess patient for signs/symptoms of dysuria, oliguria, and hematuria, as hemorrhagic cystis may occur with cyclophosphamide.

IV. POTENTIAL FOR IMPAIRED GAS EXCHANGE related to DYSPNEA AND INTERSTITIAL PULMONARY FIBROSIS

Defining Characteristics: Mild or moderate dyspnea was seen in 25% of study patients, and was severe in 2% (severe hyperventilation). 5% of patients in the study developed alveolar hemorrhage and died. One patient developed nonspecific interstitial fibrosis and died from respiratory failure on BMT day +98. Other reported pulmonary events were mild or moderate, including pharyngitis (18%), hiccup (18%), asthma (8%), atelectasis (2%), pleural effusion

(3%), hypoxia (2%), hemoptysis (3%), and sinusitis (3%). As with oral busulfan, pulmonary fibrosis can occur one to many years post-therapy, with the average onset of symptoms four years after therapy (range 4 months to 10 years).

Nursing Implications: Assess pulmonary status, including breath sounds, rate, oxygen saturation, at baseline, and regularly during care. Assess for any underlying problems, such as infection, effusions, and leukemic infiltrates. Teach patient to report any dyspnea, SOB, or other change, and monitor closely. Provide oxygen and support and discuss management plan with physician and implement promptly. After therapy is completed, remind patient that pulmonary fibrosis may develop as a late effect. The patient should have long-term follow-up, and report any dyspnea or SOB, especially in the cold.

V. POTENTIAL FOR ALTERATION IN NUTRITION, LESS THAN BODY REQUIREMENTS, related to NAUSEA/VOMITING, ANOREXIA, STOMATITIS, DIARRHEA, AND ELECTROLYTE ABNORMALITIES

Defining Characteristics: The incidence of GI toxicities is high, but manageable: nausea 98%, vomiting 95%, stomatitis 97%, diarrhea 84%, anorexia 85%, dyspepsia 44%, and mild-to-moderate constipation 38%. Grade ¾ stomatitis occurred in 26% of patients, severe anorexia in 21%, and grade ¾ diarrhea in 5%. Additionally, hyperglycemia was seen in 67% of patients, with grade 3/4 in 15%. Hypomagnesemia was mild/moderate in 62%, and severe in 2%; hypokalemia was mild/moderate in 62% and severe in 2%; hypocalcemia was mild/moderate in 46%, and severe in 3%; hypophosphatemia was mild/moderate in 17%, and hyponatremia occurred in 2%.

Nursing Implications: Assess baseline weight, usual weight, and any changes. Assess appetite, and favorite foods. Assess baseline glucose, electrolytes, and minerals, and monitor throughout therapy. Premedicate with aggressive antiemetics (serotonin antagonist) and continue protection throughout treatment. Assess efficacy and modify regimen as needed. Assess oral mucosa and teach patient self-care strategies, including assessment, what to report, oral hygiene regimen. Encourage dietary modifications as needed. Assess bowel elimination pattern baseline and daily during therapy. Teach patient to report diarrhea, and discuss management with physician. Provide comfort measures, and teach patient scrupulous hygiene to prevent infection. Discuss abnormal lab values with physician, correct hyperglycemia, and replete magnesium, potassium, phosphate, calcium, and sodium as ordered.

VI. POTENTIAL FOR SENSORY/PERCEPTUAL ALTERATIONS related to NEUROLOGICAL TOXICITY

Defining Characteristics: Drug crosses BBB, achieving levels equivalent to plasma concentration. Neurologic changes observed in clinical testing were insomnia (84%), anxiety (75%), headaches (65%), dizziness (30%), depression (23%), confusion (11%), lethargy (7%), and hallucinations (5%). Less commonly, delirium occurred in 2%, agitation in 2%, encephalopathy in 2%, and somnolence in 2%. Despite prophylaxis with phenytoin, one patient developed seizures while receiving cyclophosphamide. Especial caution should be used when patients with a history of seizure disorder or head trauma receive the drug.

Nursing Implications: Assess baseline neurologic status and continue to monitor status throughout. Closely monitor patients who have a history of seizure disorder, or head trauma for the development of seizures (seizure precautions). Teach patient to report any changes in usual patterns. Discuss any abnormalities with physician, and develop collaborative symptom-management strategies, including medications. Assess patient interest in relaxation exercises or imagery, or other techniques, and teach self-care strategies. Be prepared to manage seizures as needed.

VII. ALTERATION IN HEPATIC FUNCTION, POTENTIAL related to VENOOCCLUSIVE DISEASE (VOD) AND GRAFT-VERSUS-HOST DISEASE (GVHD)

Defining Characteristics: Increased bilirubin occurred in 49% of patients, and grade ¾ hyperbilirubinemia occurred in 30% within 28 days of transplantation. This was associated with graft-versus-host disease in 6 patients in clinical studies, and with VOD in 8% of patients (5). Severe increases in SGPT occurred in 7%, while mild increases in alkaline phosphatase occurred in 15% of patients. Jaundice occurred in 12%, while hepatomegaly developed in 6%. VOD is a complication of conditioning therapy prior to transplant and occurred in 8% of patients (fatal in 2 of the 5 patients). Factors that may increase risk of venoocclusive disease are history of XRT, more than three cycles of chemotherapy, prior progenitor cell transplantation, or busulfex dose AUC concentrations of > 1500 μm/min. Use Jones' criteria to diagnose VOD hyperbilirubinemia, and two of the following: painful hepatomegaly, weight gain > 5%, or ascites. GVHD developed in 18% of patients (severe 3%, mild/moderate 15%, fatal in 3 patients).

Nursing Implications: Assess hepatic function baseline and daily during treatment. Discuss any abnormalities with physician. Teach the patient to report RUQ pain, weight gain, increasing girth, or yellowing of eyes or skin.

VIII. ALTERATION INCOMFORT, POTENTIAL, related to ASTHENIA, PAIN, INJECTION SITE INFLAMMATION, ARTHRALGIAS

Defining Characteristics: Symptoms leading to discomfort include: abdominal pain (mild/moderate 69%, severe 3%), asthenia (mild/moderate 49%, severe 2%), general pain (45%), injection site inflammation or pain (25%), chest or back pain (23–26%), and arthralgia (13%).

Nursing Implications: Assess baseline comfort, and usual strategies to promote comfort. Teach patient to report any pain, weakness, listlessness, injection site discomfort, or any other changes. Discuss strategies to promote comfort, such as use of heat or cold. If discomfort persists, discuss pharmacologic management to reduce symptom distress.

IX. POTENTIAL SEXUAL DYSFUNCTION related to DRUG EFFECTS

Defining Characteristics: Similar to oral busulfan: premenopausal female patients commonly experience ovarian suppression and amenorrhea with menopausal symptoms; men experience sterility, azoospermia, and testicular atrophy. The drug is potentially teratogenic.

Nursing Implications: Assess patient's signs/symptoms and partner's patterns of sexuality and reproductive goals. Teach patient/partner about need for effective contraception and provide other information as appropriate. Provide emotional support, supportive counseling, and referral as needed.

X. ALTERATION IN SKIN INTEGRITY, POTENTIAL related to SKIN RASH, ALOPECIA

Defining Characteristics: Rash is common (57%) and pruritus less so (28%). Alopecia occurred in 15% of patients. Character of rash ranged from mild vesicular rash (10%), mild/moderate maculopapular rash (8%), vesiculo-bullous rash (10%), and exfoliative dermatitis (5%). Other skin abnormalities described were erythema nodosum (2%).

Nursing Implications: Assess baseline skin integrity, presence of rashes, itching, and repeat qd. Teach patient skin changes may occur, and to report them. Discuss use of topical agents and antipruritic medications with physician.

Drug: capecitabine (Xeloda, N4-Pentoxycarbonyl-5-deoxy-5-fluorocytidine)

Class: Fluoropyrimidine carbamate.

Mechanism of Action: Metabolites bind to thymidylate synthetase, inhibiting the formation of uracil from thymidylate, and reducing the cell's ability to produce DNA. It also prevents cell division by hindering the formation of RNA, by causing nuclear transcription enzymes to mistakenly incorporate its metabolites in the process of RNA transcription.

Metabolism: Absorbed from the intestinal mucosa as an intact molecule, metabolized in the liver to intermediary metabolite, and then in the liver and tumor tissue to 5-FU precursor. It is then converted through catalytic activation to 5-FU at the tumor site. Metabolites are cleared in the urine.

Dosage/Range:
- 2500 mg/m^2/d PO in two divided doses with food for two weeks, although some patients require starting at 75% of the recommended dose.
- Two-week treatment followed by a one-week rest period and repeated every three weeks.
- Interrupt for grade 2 nausea, vomiting, diarrhea, stomatitis, or hand-foot syndrome.
- Dose reduce for renal dysfunction.
- Adjuvant colon regimen: 1250 mg/m2 po bid d1-14 repeated q 21 days × 8 cycles (24 weeks).
- In combination with docetaxel: 1250 mg/m^2 po bid × 14 days, followed by a 7 day rest period, repeated q 3 weeks, with docetaxel 75 mg/m^2 IV over 1 hr day 1, repeated q 3 weeks.

Drug Preparation/Administration:
- Oral.
- Administer within 30 min of a meal with plenty of water.
- Divide daily dose in half; take 12 hours apart.

Drug Interactions:
- Warfarin: ↑ INR, monitor closely and adjust warfarin dose as needed.
- Phenytoin: monitor phenytoin serum level closely and adjust dose as needed.
- Docetaxel: synergy due to up regulation of 5-FU enzyme.
- Leucovorin: synergy and ↑ toxicity; monitor closely.

Lab Effects/Interference:
- Increased bili, alk phos.

Special Considerations:
- Indications:

Adjuvant Colon Cancer: In patients who have undergone complete resection of the primary tumor when fluoropyrimidine therapy alone is preferred.
Metastatic Colorectal Cancer: First line treatment when treatment with fluropyrimidine therapy alone preferred.
Breast Cancer (metastatic): In patients who are resistant to both paclitaxel and an anthracycline-containing regimen, or resistant to paclitaxel in women who cannot receive anthracycline therapy.
Breast Cancer (metastatic): In combination with docetaxel, capecitabine is indicated for the treatment of patients after failure of prior anthracycline-containing chemotherapy.

- Many oncologists begin dosing at 1500 mg/m^2–1875 $mg/m^2/d \times 14$ days.
- Monitor bili baseline and before each cycle, as dose modifications are necessary with hyperbilirubinemia.
- Folic acid should be avoided while taking drug.
- Contraindicated in patients hypersensitive to 5-fluorouracil or patients with creatinine clearance < 30 mL/mm.

Potential Toxicities/Side Effects and the Nursing Process

I. POTENTIAL FOR INFECTION AND BLEEDING related to BONE MARROW DEPRESSION

Defining Characteristics: Commonly causes anemia, neutropenia, and thrombocytopenia.

Nursing Implications: Assess baseline CBC, WBC with differential, and platelet count prior to chemotherapy, as well as for signs/symptoms of infection or bleeding. Teach patient signs/symptoms of infection and bleeding and instruct to report these immediately; teach patient self-care measures to minimize risk of infection and bleeding. This includes avoidance of crowds, proximity to people with infections, and avoidance of OTC aspirin-containing medications.

II. ALTERED NUTRITION, LESS THAN BODY REQUIREMENTS, related to NAUSEA AND VOMITING, STOMATITIS, AND DIARRHEA

Defining Characteristics: Nausea and vomiting occur in 30–50% of patients. Stomatitis and diarrhea also occur in about 50% of patients. Less common with reduced doses. Abdominal pain (35%), constipation (14%), anorexia (26%), dehydration (7%) also occur. Side effects are increased in the old elderly (≥ 80 yrs old).

Nursing Implications: Premedicate patient with antiemetics (phenothiazines usually effective), and continue for 24 hours, at least for first cycle. Encourage small, frequent meals of cool, bland foods. Assess oral mucosa prior to drug administration and teach patient to report changes. Teach patient oral hygiene measures and self-assessment. Instruct patient to report diarrhea, to self-administer prescribed antidiarrheal medications, and to drink adequate fluids. Moderate to severe stomatitis, diarrhea, or nausea and vomiting is an indication to interrupt therapy.

III. ALTERATION IN SKIN INTEGRITY/COMFORT related to HAND/FOOT SYNDROME

Defining Characteristics: Hand and foot syndrome occurs in more than half of patients and is characterized by tingling, numbness, pain, erythema, dryness, rash, swelling, and/or pruritus of hands and feet. Less common with reduced doses.

Nursing Implications: Teach patient about the possibility of this side effect and instruct to inform physician immediately should it occur. If patient has pain, expect dose interruption, with dose reduction if this is 2nd or subsequent episode at current dose. Teach patient self-assessment of soles of feet and palms of hands daily for erythema, pain, dry desquamation, and to report pain right away. Teach patients to avoid hot showers, whirlpools, paraffin treatments of nails, vigorous repetitive movements of hands, feet, as well as other body areas; avoid tight fitting shoes and clothes. Teach patients to take cool showers, keep skin surfaces intact and soft with skin emollients. Studies ongoing establishing evidence base for prophylaxis or treatment: vitamin B_6, urea moisturizers, nicotine patch.

IV. ALTERATION IN COMFORT related to FATIGUE, WEAKNESS, DIZZINESS, HEADACHE, FEVER, MYALGIAS, INSOMNIA, AND TASTE PROBLEMS

Defining Characteristics: Fatigue affects approximately 43% of patients, while 42% of patients complained of weakness. Fever was reported in 18% of patients, headache 10%, dizziness 8%, insomnia 7%, and taste problems 6%. Eye irritation was reported by 13% of patients and is related to the drug's excretion via tears.

Nursing Implications: Assess baseline comfort, and teach patient that these symptoms may occur. Teach patient strategies to manage fatigue, such as alternating rest and activity periods, and consolidating tasks. Teach patient to report fever, headache, and eye irritation, and discuss management plan with physician.

Drug: carboplatin (Paraplatin)

Class: Alkylating agent (heavy metal complex).

Mechanism of Action: A second-generation platinum analog. The cytotoxicity is identical to that of the parent, cisplatin, and it is cell cycle phase nonspecific. It reacts with nucleophilic sites on DNA, causing predominantly intrastrand and interstrand crosslinks rather than DNA-protein crosslinks. These crosslinks are similar to those formed with cisplatin but are formed later.

Metabolism: At 24 hours postadministration, approximately 70% of carboplatin is excreted in the urine. The mean half-life is roughly 100 minutes.

Dosage/Range:
- Dose usually given as a function of Area Under the Curve (AUC). Since carboplatin has predictable pharmokinetics based on the drug's excretion by the kidneys, area under the curve (AUC) dosing is recommended for this drug. This allows tailoring the drug dose precisely to the individual patient's excretion of the drug (renal function). The Calvert formula is used where the total dose (mg) = target AUC × GFR or glomerular filtration rate + 25. The GFR is approximated by the urine creatinine clearance, either estimated or actual, and can be calculated by hand. The target AUC is determined by the treatment plan depending upon the type of malignancy, such as an AUC of 6 for cancer of unknown primary. Then the dose calculation can be done by hand. Additionally, the manufacturer (Bristol-Myers-Squibb Oncology) distributes a calculator to determine dose.
- As a single agent, 360 mg/m^2 every 4 weeks, or 300 mg/m^2 when combined with cyclophosphamide for advanced ovarian cancer. Delay drug for neutrophil count $< 2000/mm^2$ or platelets $< 100{,}000/mm^2$.
- Drug dose reduction for urine creatinine clearance < 60 mL/minute.

Drug Preparation:
- Available as a white powder in amber vial.
- Reconstitute with sterile water for injection, 5% Dextrose, or 0.9% Sodium Chloride solution.
- Dilute further in 5% Dextrose or 0.9% Sodium Chloride.
- The solution is chemically stable for 24 hours; discard solution after 8 hours because of the lack of bacteriostatic preservative.

Drug Administration:
- Administered by IV bolus over 15 minutes to 1 hour.
- May also be given as a continuous infusion over 24 hours.
- May be administered intraperitoneally in patients with advanced ovarian cancer.

Drug Interactions:
- Increases in renal toxicity when combined with cisplatin.
- Increases in bone marrow depression when combined with myelosuppressive drugs.
- Avoid aluminum needles in drug handling.
- Taxol: administer following taxol to maximize cell kill.

Lab Effects/Interference:
- Increased LFTs, RFTs.

Special Considerations:

- Does not have the renal toxicity seen with cisplatin.
- Thrombocytopenia is dose-limiting toxicity, and correlates with GFR.
- Monitor urine creatinine clearance.
- Calculators that facilitate AUC dosing are available from Bristol-Myers-Squibb (Princeton, NJ) along with a helpful booklet entitled, *Individualized Dosing of Paraplatin Using Area Under the Curve (AUC).*

Potential Toxicities/Side Effects and the Nursing Process

I. POTENTIAL FOR INFECTION AND BLEEDING related to BONE MARROW DEPRESSION

Defining Characteristics: Myelosuppression is dose-limiting toxicity; platelet nadir is 14–21 days, with usual recovery by day 28; WBC nadir follows 1 week later, but recovery may take 5–6 weeks. The risk of thrombocytopenia is severe, especially when the drug is combined with other myelosuppressive drugs, or if the patient has renal compromise. Anemia may occur with prolonged treatment.

Nursing Implications: Assess CBC, WBC, with differential, and platelet count prior to drug administration. Monitor for signs/symptoms of infection or bleeding. Drug dosage should be reduced if urine creatinine clearance is < 60 mL/min. Drug should be held or dose reduced if absolute neutrophil count (ANC) and/or platelet count is low. Teach the patient signs/symptoms of infection and bleeding, and instruct to report them immediately if they occur. Teach self-care measures to minimize infection and bleeding. Discuss with physician use of granulocyte-colony stimulating factor (G-CSF) to prevent neutropenia in heavily pretreated patients.

II. POTENTIAL FOR ALTERED URINARY ELIMINATION related to NEPHROTOXICITY

Defining Characteristics: The drug does not have the renal toxicity seen with cisplatin (Platinol), so that only minimal hydration is needed. However, the drug is excreted by the kidneys, and concomitant treatment with drugs causing nephrotoxicity (i.e., aminoglycoside antibiotics) can alter renal function studies. Nephrotoxicity does occur at high doses, and patients with renal dysfunction are at risk. In addition, serum electrolyte loss can occur (K^+, Mg^{++}, rarely Ca^{++}). Monitor serum electrolytes prior to treatment and periodically after treatment. Replete electrolytes as ordered.

Nursing Implications: Assess renal function studies, (i.e., urine creatinine clearance, serum blood urea nitrogen [BUN], and creatinine) prior to drug administration. Discuss drug dose modification if creatinine clearance < 60 cc/min, or if other values are abnormal.

III. POTENTIAL FOR ALTERATION IN NUTRITION, LESS THAN BODY REQUIREMENTS, related to NAUSEA/VOMITING, ANOREXIA, STOMATITIS, DIARRHEA, AND HEPATIC DYSFUNCTION

Defining Characteristics: Nausea and vomiting begin 6+ hours after administration and last for <24 hours, but may be easily prevented by available antiemetics. Anorexia occurs in 10% of patients but is usually mild, lasting 1–2 days. Diarrhea occurs in 10% of patients and is mild. Reversible hepatic dysfunction is mild to moderate, as evidenced by changes in alk phos and SGOT and, rarely, serum glutamic pyruvic transaminase (SGPT) and bili.

Nursing Implications: Premedicate with antiemetics and continue protection for 24 hours, at least for the first cycle. Encourage dietary modifications as needed. Monitor LFTs prior to and periodically during treatment.

IV. POTENTIAL FOR SENSORY/PERCEPTUAL ALTERATIONS related to NEUROLOGICAL CHANGES

Defining Characteristics: Neurologic dysfunction is infrequent, but there is increased risk in patients >65 years old, or if previously treated with cisplatin and receiving prolonged carboplatin treatment.

Nursing Implications: Assess baseline neurologic status and continue to monitor status throughout treatment, looking for dizziness, confusion, peripheral neuropathy, ototoxicity, visual changes, and changes in taste. Teach patient the potential for side effects, and to report any changes.

V. POTENTIAL SEXUAL DYSFUNCTION related to DRUG EFFECTS

Defining Characteristics: Drug is mutagenic and probably teratogenic. It is unknown whether drug is excreted in breast milk.

Nursing Implications: Assess patient's signs/symptoms and partner's patterns of sexuality and reproductive goals. Teach patient/partner about need for contraception and provide other information as appropriate. Provide emotional support.

VI. POTENTIAL FOR INJURY related to HYPERSENSITIVITY REACTIONS

Defining Characteristics: Drug may cause allergic reactions, ranging from rash, urticaria, erythema, and pruritus to anaphylaxis; they can occur within minutes of drug administration.

Nursing Implications: Assess baseline VS. During drug administration, observe for signs/symptoms of hypersensitivity reaction. If signs/symptoms of anaphylaxis (tachycardia, wheezing, hypotension, facial edema) occur, stop drug immediately. Keep IV patent with 0.9% Sodium Chloride, notify physician, monitor VS, and be prepared to administer ordered drugs (i.e., steroid, epinephrine, or antihistamines).

Drug: carmustine (BCNU, BiCNU)

Class: Nitrosourea.

Mechanism of Action: Alkylates DNA by causing crosslinks and strand breaks in the same manner as classic mustard agents; it also carbamoylates cellular proteins, thus inhibiting DNA repair. Cell cycle phase nonspecific.

Metabolism: Rapidly distributed and metabolized with a plasma half-life of 1 hour; 70% of IV dose is excreted in urine within 96 hours. Significant concentrations of drug remain in cerebrospinal fluid for 9 hours due to lipid solubility of drug.

Dosage/Range:

Usual:

- 75–100 mg/m^2 IV/day × 2 days, OR
- 200–225 mg/m^2 every 6 weeks, OR
- 40 mg/m^2/day on 5 successive days, repeating cycle every 6–8 weeks.

High dose with autologous BMT (*investigational*):

- 450–600 mg/m^2 IV; however, doses of 900 mg/m^2 (in combination with cyclophosphamide) or 1200 mg/m^2 as single agent have been reported.
- These doses are fatal and require AUTOLOGOUS BMT after drug administration.
- Refer to protocol for exact dosages.

Drug Preparation/Administration:

- Add sterile alcohol (provided with drug) to vial, then add sterile water for injection.
- May be further diluted with 100–250 mL 5% Dextrose or 0.9% Sodium Chloride.

High dose (*investigational*):

- IV bolus in at least 500 mL of 5% Dextrose over 2 hours; can also divide dose into two equal fractions administered 12 hours apart. Refer to protocol for exact information.
- When given for gliomas as a single agent, administer with dexamethasone or mannitol infusion to reduce cerebral edema.
- Usually given in combination with other cytotoxic agents in BMT protocols.

Mycosis fungoides:

- Carmustine topical solution 0.5–3.0 mg/mL may be painted on body after showering, qd × 14 days (investigational).

Drug Interactions:
- Cimetidine may increase myelosuppression when given concurrently. AVOID IF POSSIBLE.
- Possible increased cellular uptake of drug when administered in combination with amphotericin B.
- Carmustine may decrease the pharmacologic effects of phenytoin.

Lab Effects/Interference:
- Pulmonary, hepatic, and renal function tests.

Special Considerations:
- Drug is an irritant; avoid extravasation.
- Pain at the injection site or along the vein is common. Treat by applying ice pack above the injection site and decreasing the infusion flow rate.
- Patient may act inebriated related to the alcohol diluent and may experience flushing.

High dose:
- Pulmonary toxicity related to higher systemic levels (higher AUC).

Potential Toxicities/Side Effects and the Nursing Process

I. POTENTIAL FOR INFECTION AND BLEEDING related to BONE MARROW DEPRESSION

Defining Characteristics: Delayed myelosuppression is dose-limiting toxicity and is cumulative. WBC nadir 3–5 weeks after dose and persists 1–2 weeks; platelet nadir at 4 weeks, persisting 1–2 weeks. Drug should not be dosed more frequently than once every 6 weeks.

Nursing Implications: Assess baseline CBC, WBC with differential, and platelet count prior to chemotherapy and at least weekly postchemotherapy for the first cycle. Discuss dose reductions with physician for subsequent cycles if counts are lower than normal since bone marrow depression is cumulative. Teach patient and family self-assessment for signs/symptoms of infection and bleeding, and instruct to report them immediately. Teach self-care measures to minimize risk of infection and bleeding, including avoidance of aspirin-containing medicines.

II. POTENTIAL FOR IMPAIRED GAS EXCHANGE related to PULMONARY FIBROSIS

Defining Characteristics: Pulmonary toxicity appears to be dose-related, with risk greatest in patients receiving total doses > 1400 mg (although it can occur at lower doses). Other risk factors include patients with abnormal PFTs prior to drug administration; i.e., baseline forced vital capacity (FVC) < 70% of predicted; carbon monoxide diffusion capacity (DLCO) < 70% of predicted; or if patient is receiving concurrent cyclophosphamide or thoracic radiation. Presents as insidious cough and dyspnea, or may be the sudden onset of respiratory failure. CXR shows interstitial infiltrates. Incidence is 20–30% of patients, with a mortality of 24–80%.

Nursing Implications: Assess patient's risk and baseline pulmonary function prior to chemotherapy, as well as the results of pulmonary function testing periodically during treatment, for evidence of pulmonary dysfunction. Teach patient to report any changes in respiratory pattern.

III. ALTERATION IN NUTRITION, LESS THAN BODY REQUIREMENTS, related to NAUSEA/VOMITING AND LIVER DYSFUNCTION

Defining Characteristics: Severe nausea and vomiting may occur 2 hours after administration and last 4–6 hours. Reversible liver dysfunction, although rare, is related to subacute hepatitis and is characterized by abnormal LFTs, painless jaundice, and (rarely) coma.

Nursing Implications: Premedicate with antiemetics and continue antiemetic protection for 24 hours, at least for the first treatment. Encourage small, frequent feedings of cool, bland foods, and liquids. Infuse drug over 60–120 minutes. Monitor LFTs (SGOT, SGPT, lactic dehydrogenase [LDH], alk phos, bili) during treatment and discuss any abnormalities with physician.

IV. ALTERATION IN COMFORT related to DRUG ADMINISTRATION

Defining Characteristics: Drug diluent is absolute alcohol, so irritation may result in pain along the vein path. Thrombosis is rare, but venospasms and flushing of skin or burning of the eyes can occur with rapid drug infusion.

Nursing Implications: Administer drug only through patent IV and dilute drug in 250 mL of 5% Dextrose or 0.9% Sodium Chloride and infuse over 1–2 hours. If pain along vein occurs, use ice packs above injection site, decrease infusion rate, or further dilute drug. If patient will receive ongoing therapy, consider venous access device.

V. ALTERED URINARY ELIMINATION related to NEPHROTOXICITY

Defining Characteristics: Increase in BUN occurs in 10% of patients and is usually reversible. However, decreased kidney size, progressive azotemia, and renal failure have occurred in patients receiving large cumulative doses over long periods.

Nursing Implications: Assess baseline renal function and monitor BUN and creatinine prior to each successive cycle. Since drug is excreted by the kidneys, drug dosage should be reduced if renal dysfunction exists. If abnormalities occur and persist, discuss discontinuing drug with physician.

VI. POTENTIAL SEXUAL DYSFUNCTION related to DRUG EFFECTS

Defining Characteristics: Drug is mutagenic and teratogenic.

Nursing Implications: Assess patient's and partner's pattern of sexuality and reproductive goals. Teach patient and partner the need for contraception as appropriate. Provide emotional support and counseling, or referral as appropriate.

VII. SENSORY/PERCEPTUAL ALTERATIONS related to OCULAR TOXICITY

Defining Characteristics: Infarcts of optic nerve fiber, retinal hemorrhage, and neuroretinitis have been associated with high-dose therapy.

Nursing Implications: Assess baseline vision and appearance of eyes. Instruct patient to report any visual changes to physician or nurse.

Drug: chlorambucil (Leukeran)

Class: Alkylating agent.

Mechanism of Action: Alkylates DNA by causing strand breaks and cross-links in the DNA. The drug is a derivative of a nitrogen mustard.

Metabolism: Pharmacokinetics are poorly understood. It is well absorbed orally, with a plasma half-life of 1.5 hours. Degradation is slow; it appears to be eliminated by metabolic transformation, with 60% excreted in urine in 24 hours.

Dosage/Range:
- 0.1–0.2 mg/kg/day (equals 4–8 mg/m^2/day) to initiate treatment, OR
- 14 mg/m^2/day × 5 days with a repeat every 21–28 days, depending on platelet count and WBC.

Drug Preparation:
- 2-mg tablets.

Drug Administration:
- Oral.

Drug Interactions:
- None significant.
- Simultaneous administration of barbiturates may increase toxicity of chlorambucil due to hepatic drug activation.

Lab Effects/Interference:
- BUN, uric acid.
- LFTs, especially alk phos and AST (SGOT).
- CBC, especially WBC with differential.

Special Considerations:
- None.

Potential Toxicities/Side Effects and the Nursing Process

I. POTENTIAL FOR INFECTION related to BONE MARROW DEPRESSION

Defining Characteristics: Neutropenia after third week of treatment lasting for 10 days after the last dose. Neutropenia and thrombocytopenia occur with prolonged use and may be irreversible occasionally (especially if high total doses are given; i.e., > 6.5 mg/kg). Increased toxicity may occur with prior barbiturate use.

Nursing Implications: Assess baseline CBC, including WBC with differential, and platelet count prior to dosing, as well as weekly for the first cycle of therapy. Discuss dose reduction with physician if blood values are abnormal. Teach patient self-assessment of signs/symptoms of infection and bleeding and instruct to report them immediately. Teach self-care measures to minimize risk of infection and bleeding, including avoidance of OTC aspirin-containing medications.

II. POTENTIAL FOR SEXUAL DYSFUNCTION related to REPRODUCTIVE HAZARD

Defining Characteristics: Drug is mutagenic, teratogenic, and suppresses gonadal function with consequent temporary or permanent sterility. Amenorrhea occurs in females, and oligospermia/azoospermia occur in males.

Nursing Implications: Assess patient's and partner's sexual patterns and reproductive goals. Provide teaching and emotional support; encourage birth control measures as appropriate.

III. POTENTIAL FOR ALTERATION IN NUTRITION, LESS THAN BODY REQUIREMENTS, related to NAUSEA/VOMITING, ANOREXIA/WEIGHT LOSS, AND HEPATIC DYSFUNCTION

Defining Characteristics: Nausea and vomiting are rare. Anorexia and weight loss may occur and be prolonged. Hepatotoxicity with jaundice is rare, but abnormal LFTs may occur.

Nursing Implications: Administer antiemetics as needed and instruct patient in self-administration. Suggest weekly weights and dietary instruction if patient develops anorexia and weight loss. Monitor LFTs baseline and periodically during treatment. Discuss any abnormalities with physician and consider dose modification.

IV. POTENTIAL FOR IMPAIRED GAS EXCHANGE related to PULMONARY FIBROSIS

Defining Characteristics: Bronchopulmonary dysplasia and pulmonary fibrosis may occur rarely with long-term use.

Nursing Implications: Assess patients at risk: increased risk with cumulative dose > 1 g/m^2, preexisting lung disease, concurrent treatment with cyclophosphamide or thoracic radiation. Assess pulmonary status prior to chemotherapy and at each visit, notifying physician of dyspnea. Monitor PFTs periodically for evidence of pulmonary dysfunction. Teach patient to report any changes in pulmonary pattern, such as dyspnea.

V. POTENTIAL FOR SENSORY/PERCEPTUAL ALTERATIONS related to OCULAR DISTURBANCES, CNS ABNORMALITIES

Defining Characteristics: Ocular disturbances may occur, e.g., diplopia, papilledema, retinal hemorrhage. Tremors, muscular twitching, confusion, agitation, ataxia, flaccid paresis, and hallucinations have been described. Seizures, although uncommon, have occurred in adults and children during normal dosing, as well as with overdosing.

Nursing Implications: Assess baseline neurologic status prior to treatment and at each visit. Instruct patient to report any abnormalities.

Drug: cisplatin (Platinol)

Class: Heavy metal that acts like alkylating agent.

Mechanism of Action: Inhibits DNA synthesis by forming inter- and intrastrand crosslinks and by denaturing the double helix, preventing cell replication. Cell cycle phase nonspecific; the chemical properties are similar to those of bifunctional alkylating agents.

Metabolism: Rapidly distributed to tissues (predominately the liver and kidneys) with less than 10% in the plasma 1 hour after infusion. Clearance from plasma proceeds slowly after the first 2 hours due to platinum's covalent bonding with serum proteins; 20–74% of administered drug is excreted in the urine within 24 hours.

Dosage/Range:
- 50–120 mg/m^2 every 3–4 weeks, OR

- 15–20 mg/m^2 × 5 repeated every 3–4 weeks.
- Radiosensitizing effect: Administer 1–3 times per week at doses of 15–50 mg/m^2 (total weekly dose 50 mg/m^2) with concomitant radiotherapy.

High dose (investigational):
- 200 mg/m^2 given in 250 mL of 3% Sodium Chloride (hypertonic).

Drug Preparation:
- 10-mg and 50-mg vials. Add sterile water to develop a concentration of 1 mg/mL.
- Further dilute solution with 250 mL or more of 0.9% Sodium Chloride (recommended) or 5% Dextrose (D_5 ½ NS) Sodium Chloride.
- Never mix with 5% Dextrose, as a precipitate will form. Drug stability increased in 0.9% Sodium Chloride.
- Available as an aqueous solution.
- Do not refrigerate.

Drug Administration:
- Avoid aluminum needles when administering, as precipitate will form.

Drug Interactions:
- Decreases pharmacologic effect of phenytoin, so dose may need to be increased.
- Possible increase in ototoxicity when combined with loop diuretics.
- Increased renal toxicity with concurrent use of aminoglycosides, amphotericin B.
- Cisplatin reduces drug clearance of high-dose methotrexate (MTX) and standard-dose bleomycin by increasing the drugs' half-life; enhances toxicity of ifosfamide (myelosuppression) and etoposide.
- Synergy when cisplatin is combined with etoposide.
- Radiosensitizing effect.
- Sodium thiosulfate and mesna: Each directly inactivates cisplatin.
- Taxol: Administer cisplatin *after* taxol to prevent delayed taxol excretion with subsequent increased bone marrow depression.

Lab Effects/Interference:
- Decreased Mg, K, Ca, Na, phos.
- Increased creatinine, uric acid.

Special Considerations:
- Administer cautiously, if at all, to patients with renal dysfunction, hearing impairment, peripheral neuropathy, or prior allergic reaction to cisplatin.
- Hydrate vigorously before and after administering drug. Urine output should be at least 100–150 mL/hour. Mannitol or furosemide diuresis may be needed to ensure this output.

- Hypersensitivity reactions have occurred, manifested by wheezing, flushing, hypotension, tachycardia. Usually occurs within minutes of starting infusion. Treat with epinephrine, corticosteroids, antihistamines.
- Drug causes potassium and magnesium wasting. Some ideas to help increase magnesium follow.
- To help increase absorption, it is recommended that excessive milk, cheese, or other high-calcium products be limited when eating foods high in magnesium.

Calcium and magnesium compete to gain entrance to the body in the intestines, so a high-calcium diet increases requirements for dietary magnesium. Foods high in magnesium are those with 100 mg or greater per 100 grams, including

Nuts:
Almonds
Brazil nuts
Cashews
Peanut butter
Peanuts
Pecans
Walnuts

Peas and beans:
Red beans
Split peas
White beans

Other good sources:
Blackstrap molasses
Brewer's yeast
Chocolate (bitter)
Cocoa (dry breakfast)
Cornmeal
Instant coffee and tea
Oatmeal
Shredded wheat
Wheat germ
Whole wheat breads and cereals

- Phase I studies are ongoing, evaluating an oral platinum (JM-216) agent in small-cell lung cancer.
- Amifostine has been shown to be renally protective in patients at risk for renal toxicity from cisplatin; in addition, drug offers protection from neurotoxicity. Other agents being studied, e.g., BNP7787.

Potential Toxicities/Side Effects and the Nursing Process

I. POTENTIAL ALTERATION IN URINARY ELIMINATION related to DRUG-INDUCED RENAL DAMAGE

Defining Characteristics: Dose-limiting toxicity, which may be cumulative. The drug accumulates in the kidneys, causing necrosis of proximal and distal renal tubules. Damage to renal tubules prevents reabsorption of Mg++, Ca++, and K+, with resultant decreased serum levels. Renal damage becomes most obvious 10–20 days after treatment, is reversible, and can be prevented by adequate hydration and diuresis, as well as slower infusion time. Hyperuricemia may occur due to impaired tubular transport of uric acid, but it is responsive to allopurinol. Concurrent administration of nephrotoxic agents is not recommended.

Nursing Implications: Assess renal function studies prior to administration (BUN, creatinine, 24-hour creatinine clearance) and discuss any abnormalities with physician. Assess cardiac and pulmonary status in terms of tolerance of aggressive hydration. Anticipate vigorous hydration regimen with or without forced diuresis (i.e., mannitol, lasix). The typical hydration schedule is 0.9% Sodium Chloride or D_5 ½ NS at 250 mL/hr × 3–5 hours prechemotherapy and 3–5 hours postchemotherapy (total hydration 3 L). Outpatient hydration of 1–2 L over 1–2 hours prechemotherapy and 1 L postchemotherapy, is typical. Strictly monitor I/O and total body fluid balance. Assess for signs/symptoms of fluid overload and notify physician for supplemental furosemide or other diuretic as needed. Monitor serum electrolytes (Na+, K+, Mg++, Ca++, PO_4) and replete as ordered by physician. Teach patient and family the need for increased oral fluids on discharge—up to 3 L or more for 5 days posttherapy.

II. ALTERATION IN NUTRITION, LESS THAN BODY REQUIREMENTS, related to SEVERE NAUSEA AND VOMITING, TASTE ALTERATIONS

Defining Characteristics: Nausea and vomiting may be severe and will occur in 100% of patients if antiemetics are not given. They begin 1 or more hours postchemotherapy and last 8–24 hours. Since the drug is slowly excreted over five days, delayed nausea and vomiting may occur 24–72 hours after dose. Taste alterations and anorexia occur with long-term use.

Nursing Implications: Premedicate with combination antiemetics (i.e., serotonin antagonist plus dexamethasone), especially for high-dose cisplatin, and continue antiemetics for up to five days with dopamine antagonist. Encourage small, frequent intake of cool, bland foods as tolerated. Infuse cisplatin over at least 1 hour to minimize emesis, since slower infusion rates decrease emesis. Taste alterations may be improved with the use of spices and zinc dietary supplementation. Refer the patient for dietary consultation as needed.

III. POTENTIAL FOR INJURY related to ANAPHYLAXIS

Defining Characteristics: Anaphylaxis has occurred, characterized by wheezing, bronchoconstriction, tachycardia, hypotension, and facial edema, in patients who have previously received the drug.

Nursing Implications: Assess baseline VS and continue to assess patient during infusion. Prior to drug administration, review standing orders or protocols for nursing management of anaphylaxis: stop infusion; keep line open with 0.9% Sodium Chloride; notify physician; monitor VS; be prepared to administer epinephrine, antihistamines, corticosteroids.

IV. POTENTIAL FOR SENSORY/PERCEPTUAL ALTERATIONS related to NEUROLOGIC TOXICITY

Defining Characteristics: Severe neuropathy may occur in patients receiving high doses or prolonged treatment and may be irreversible and is seen in stocking-and-glove distribution, with numbness, tingling, and sensory loss in arms and legs. Areflexia, loss of proprioception and vibratory sense, and loss of motor function can occur. Ototoxicity, beginning with loss of high-frequency hearing, affects > 30% of patients. It may be preceded by tinnitus, is doserelated, and can be unilateral or bilateral. The damage results from destruction of hair cells lining the organ of Corti and is cumulative and may be permanent. Rarely, ocular toxicity has occurred, but it is reversible (optic neuritis, papilledema, cerebral blindness).

Nursing Implications: Assess baseline neurologic, motor, and sensory functions prior to drug administration. Discuss use of neuroprotector in high-risk patients. Discuss baseline audiogram with physician as appropriate. Instruct patient to report changes in function or sensation, as well as diminished hearing. Discuss with physician risks vs benefits of continuing therapy if/when symptoms develop. If severe neuropathies develop, provide teaching related to activity, emotional support, and referral to physical/occupational therapy as appropriate. Discuss use of neuroprotector in high-risk patients.

V. POTENTIAL FOR ACTIVITY INTOLERANCE related to ANEMIA

Defining Characteristics: Drug may interfere with renal erythropoietin production, resulting in late development of anemia.

Nursing Implications: Teach patient to report increasing fatigue, signs of severe anemia (shortness of breath, chest pain/angina, headaches). Monitor hemoglobin/hematocrit; discuss transfusion with physician if signs/symptoms develop or hematocrit falls < 25 mg/dL. Teach patient about diet high in iron. Exogenous erythropoietin (epoetin alpha) may be helpful.

VI. INFECTION AND BLEEDING related to BONE MARROW DEPRESSION

Defining Characteristics: Bone marrow depression is mild with low to moderate doses, but may be significant when high doses are used, or when drug is given in combination with radiation as a radiation-sensitizer. Nadir is in 2–3 weeks, with recovery in 4–5 weeks.

Nursing Implications: Assess CBC, WBC, differential, and platelet count, as well as any signs/symptoms of infection or bleeding, prior to drug administration. Teach patient to self-assess for signs/symptoms of infection and bleeding. Teach self-care measures to minimize infection and bleeding, including avoidance of aspirin-containing medications.

VII. POTENTIAL SEXUAL DYSFUNCTION related to DRUG EFFECTS

Defining Characteristics: Drug is mutagenic and probably teratogenic.

Nursing Implications: Assess patient's and partner's sexual patterns and reproductive goals. Provide emotional support and discuss strategies to preserve sexual and reproductive health (i.e., contraception and sperm banking).

VIII. POTENTIAL FOR ALTERATIONS IN CARDIOVASCULAR FUNCTION related to CISPLATIN-CONTAINING COMBINATION CHEMOTHERAPY

Defining Characteristics: Angina, myocardial infarction, cerebrovascular accident, thrombotic microangiopathy, cerebral arteritis, and Raynaud's phenomenon have occurred, although they are uncommon. Combination drugs include bleomycin, vinblastine, vincristine, and etoposide.

Nursing Implications: Assess cardiopulmonary status, especially if patient has preexisting cardiac disease, both prior to and throughout treatment.

Drug: cladribine (Leustatin, 2-CdA)

Class: Antimetabolite.

Mechanism of Action: Selectively damages normal and malignant lymphocytes and monocytes that have large amounts of deoxycytidine kinase but small amounts of deoxynucleotidase. The drug, a chlorinated purine nucleoside, enters passively through the cell membrane, is phosphorylated into the active metabolite 2-CdATP, and accumulates in the cell. 2-CdATP interferes with DNA synthesis and prevents repair of DNA strand breaks in both actively dividing and normal cells. The process may also involve programmed cell death (apoptosis).

Metabolism: Drug is 20% protein-bound and is cleared from the plasma within 1–3 days after cessation of treatment.

Dosage/Range:

- 0.09 mg/kg/day IV as a continuous infusion for 7 days for one course of therapy of hairy-cell leukemia.

Drug Preparation:

- Available in 10 mg/10 mL preservative-free, single-use vials (1 mg/mL), which must be further diluted in 0.9% Sodium Chloride injection. Diluted drug stable at room temperature for at least 24 hours in normal light. Once prepared, the solution may be refrigerated up to 8 hours prior to use.
- Single daily dose: add calculated drug dose to 500 mL of 0.9% Sodium Chloride injection, and administer over 24 hours; repeat daily for a total of 7 days.
- 7-day continuous infusion by ambulatory infusion pump: add calculated drug dose for 7 days to infusion reservoir using a sterile 0.22-μm hydrophilic syringe filter. Then add, again using 0.22-μm filter, sufficient sterile bacteriostatic 0.9% Sodium Chloride injection containing 0.9% benzyl alcohol to produce 100 mL in the infusion reservoir.
- Do not use 5% Dextrose, as it accelerates degradation of drug.

Drug Administration:

- Dilute in minimum of 100 mL.
- Administer as continuous infusion over 24 hours for 7 days.

Drug Interactions:

- None known.

Lab Effects/Interference:

- Decreased CBC, platelets.
- Increased LFTs, RFTs.

Special Considerations:

- Indicated for the treatment of active hairy-cell leukemia.
- Unstable in 5% Dextrose; should not be used as diluent or infusion fluid.
- Store unopened vials in refrigerator and protect from light.
- Drug may precipitate when exposed to low temperatures. Allow solution to warm to room temperature and shake vigorously. DO NOT HEAT OR MICROWAVE.
- Drug is structurally similar to pentostatin and fludarabine.
- Contraindicated in patients who are hypersensitive to the drug.
- Administer with caution in patients with renal or hepatic insufficiency.
- Embryotoxic; women of childbearing age should use contraception.

Potential Toxicities/Side Effects and the Nursing Process

I. INFECTION AND BLEEDING related to BONE MARROW DEPRESSION

Defining Characteristics: Neutropenia occurs in 70% of patients with nadir 1–2 weeks after infusion, recovery by weeks 4–5. Incidence of infection 28%, with 40% caused by bacterial infection of lungs and venous access sites. Prolonged hypocellularity of bone marrow occurs in 34% of patients, and may last for at least four months. Infections most common in patients with pancytopenia and lymphopenia due to hairy-cell leukemia. Lymphopenia is common with decreased CD4 (helper T cells) and CD8 (suppressor T cells), with recovery by weeks 26–34. Common infectious agents are viral (20%) and fungal (20%). Thrombocytopenia occurs commonly, along with purpura (10%), petechiae (8%), and epistaxis (5%). Platelet recovery occurs by day 12, but 14% of patients require platelet support.

Nursing Implications: Monitor CBC, platelet count prior to therapy, and periodically posttherapy at expected time of nadir. Monitor for, and teach patient self-assessment of signs/symptoms of infection, bleeding. Instruct patient to call physician or nurse or go to emergency room if temperature (T) is greater than 101°F (38.3°C) or bleeding. Transfuse platelets per physician order.

II. ALTERATION IN COMFORT related to FEVER, HEADACHES

Defining Characteristics: Fever (> 100°F [37.5°C]) occurs in 66% of patients during the month following treatment due either to infection (47%) or the release of endogenous pyrogen from lysed lymphocytes. Other symptoms include chills (9%), diaphoresis (9%), malaise (7%), dizziness (9%), insomnia (7%), myalgia (7%), arthralgias (5%). Headaches occur in 22% of patients.

Nursing Implications: Assess patient for fever, chills, diaphoresis during visits; assess signs/symptoms of infection. Teach patient self-assessment, how to report this, and measures to reduce fever. Anticipate laboratory and X-ray tests to rule out infection and perform according to physician order.

III. POTENTIAL IMPAIRMENT OF SKIN INTEGRITY related to RASH

Defining Characteristics: Rash occurs in 27–50% of patients. Other symptoms include pruritus (6%), erythema (6%), injection site reactions (erythema, swelling, pain, phlebitis).

Nursing Implications: Assess skin for any cutaneous changes, such as rash or changes at injection site, and any associated symptoms such as pruritus; discuss with physician. Instruct patient in self-care measures, including avoiding abrasive skin products and clothing; avoiding tight-fitting clothing; use of skin emolients appropriate to specific skin alteration; measures to avoid scratching involved areas. Consider venous access device if skin is at risk for reaction.

IV. FATIGUE related to ANEMIA

Defining Characteristics: Fatigue occurs in 45% of patients. Red cell recovery is by week 8, but 40% of patients require red cell transfusion.

Nursing Implications: Monitor Hgb and HCT and transfuse per physician order. Administer erythropoietin per physician order and teach patient selfadministration. Teach patient about diet and instruct to alternate rest and activity; stress reduction/relaxation techniques may improve energy level.

V. ALTERATION IN ELIMINATION related to DIARRHEA, CONSTIPATION

Defining Characteristics: Diarrhea occurs in 10% of patients while constipation occurs in 9%. Abdominal pain affects 6% of patients.

Nursing Implications: Encourage patient to report onset of change in bowel habits (diarrhea or constipation) and assess factors contributing to changes. Administer or teach patient self-administration of antidiarrheal medication or cathartic as ordered. Teach patient diet modification regarding foods that minimize diarrhea or constipation.

VI. POTENTIAL FOR IMPAIRED GAS EXCHANGE related to COUGH

Defining Characteristics: Cough affects 10%, while abnormal breath sounds occur in 11% and shortness of breath in 7%.

Nursing Implications: Assess baseline pulmonary status, including breath sounds, presence of cough, shortness of breath. Instruct patient to report symptoms of cough, shortness of breath, other abnormalities.

VII. ALTERATION IN NUTRITION, LESS THAN BODY REQUIREMENTS, related to NAUSEA, VOMITING

Defining Characteristics: Nausea is mild and occurs in 28% of patients, while vomiting may occur in 13%. If antiemetics are required, nausea/vomiting is easily controlled by phenothiazines. Renal and hepatic function studies are rarely affected.

Nursing Implications: Premedicate with antiemetics. If nausea and/or vomiting occur, teach patient to self-administer antiemetics per physician order. Encourage small, frequent feedings of cool, bland foods and liquids. Teach patient to record diet history for 2–3 days and weekly weights. If patient has decreased appetite, assess food preferences (encourage or discourage) and suggest use of spices.

VIII. POTENTIAL ALTERATION IN CARDIAC OUTPUT related to TACHYCARDIA

Defining Characteristics: Occurs rarely, with edema and tachycardia each affecting 6% of patients.

Nursing Implications: Assess baseline cardiac status, including apical heart rate, presence of peripheral edema. Instruct patient to report rapid heartbeat or swelling of ankles.

Drug: clofarabine

Class: Purine nucleoside anti-metabolite.

Mechanism of Action: Drug inhibits DNA and DNA repair, causing cell death of both cycling and quiescent cancer cells. In addition, it breaks down the mitochondrial membranes, releasing cytochrome C and apoptosis-inducing factor, leading to programmed cell death.

Metabolism: Drug is 47% protein bound (mostly to albumin), with a terminal half-life of 5.2 hours. 49–60% of the dose is excreted unchanged in the urine. Other non-renal excretion is unknown.

Dosage/Range:
52 mg/m2 IV over 2 hr qd × 5, to be repeated after recovery of all baseline organ function, about q 2–6 weeks. IV hydration should be continued during the 5 days of treatment.

Drug Preparation: Drug is supplied as a 20 mg in 20 mL vial. Withdraw drug using a sterile 0.2 μm syringe filter and then further diluted with 5% dextrose injection USP or 0.9% sodium chloride injection USP prior to IV infusion. This admixture may be stored at room temperature but must be used within 24 hr of preparation.

Drug Administration: Administer IV over 2 hours; if hyperuricemia (tumor lysis syndrome), patient should receive allopurinol, and may need urine alkalinization and aggressive hydration as well.

Drug Interactions: Concurrent administration with other renally cleared drugs may alter drug levels so should be avoided during the 5 days of treatment; avoid other hepatotoxic drugs, as well as those affecting blood pressure or cardiac function if possible during drug administration.

Lab Effects/Interference: Severe bone marrow depression with decreased white blood cells, neutrophils, red blood cells and platelets. Drug may cause tumor lysis syndrome with increased levels of potassium, phosphate, uric acid, creatinine, and changes in other electrolyte values. Renal and hepatic function studies should be monitored during the 5 days of drug treatment.

Special Considerations:

- Drug is indicated for the treatment of pediatric patients aged 1–21 years old with relapsed or refractory acute lymphoblastic leukemia after at least 2 prior regimens.
- Treatment results in the rapid lysis of peripheral leukemia cells.
- Drug is fetotoxic so all patients should be taught to use effective contraceptive measures to prevent pregnancy; female patients shold be taught not to breast feed during treatment.
- Drug may cause dehydration, hypotension, capillary leak syndrome.

Potential Toxicities/Side Effects and the Nursing Process

I. INFECTION AND BLEEDING related to BONE MARROW DEPRESSION

Defining Characteristics: Bone marrow depression is dose limiting. Febrile neutropenia occurs in 57% of patients. Pyrexia affects 41% of patients, while 38% experience rigors. Infections include bacteremia, cellulites, herpes simplex, oral candidiasis, pneumonia, sepsis, and staphylococcal infections.

Nursing Implications: Assess WBC, neutrophil, and platelet count, and discuss any abnormalities with physician prior to drug administration; assess for signs/symptoms of skin infections (all mucosal surfaces, body orifices) and bleeding; instruct patient in signs/symptoms of infection and bleeding, as well as to report them or come to emergency room. Teach patient self-care measures to minimize risk of infection and bleeding, including avoidance of OTC aspirin-containing medications. Assess patient's Hgb/HCT and signs/symptoms of fatigue; teach patient self-assessment and to alternate rest and activity as needed.

II. ALTERED NUTRITION, LESS THAN BODY REQUIREMENTS, related to NAUSEA AND VOMITING, ANOREXIA, DIARRHEA, and HEPATOTOXICITY

Defining Characteristics: Nausea and vomiting occur in 75% and 83% of patients respectively. Can be successfully prevented with combination antiemetics. Anorexia occurs in about 1/3 of patients. Diarrhea is frequent, affecting about 50% of patients. Constipation affects 21% of patients. Hepatotoxicity and jaundice occur in 15% of patients.

Nursing Implications: Premedicate with antiemetics depending on dose, using aggressive, combination antiemetics, and continue throughout chemotherapy. If patient develops nausea/vomiting, assess fluid and electrolyte balance and the need for replacements. Assess oral mucosa prior to chemotherapy and teach patient oral hygiene regimen and self-assessment; encourage patient to report diarrhea, discuss use of antidiarrheals with physician, and teach self-care PRN. Since patients become neutropenic, all mucosal surfaces need to be assessed for infection, and patients must be taught scrupulous perineal hygiene. Monitor LFTs prior to, during, and posttherapy.

III. IMPAIRED SKIN/MUCOSAL INTEGRITY related to RASH, ANAL INFLAMMATION/ULCERATION, ALOPECIA

Defining Characteristics: Maculopapular rash, with or without fever, myalgia, bone pain, occasional chest pain, conjunctivitis, and malaise (cytarabine syndrome) may occur. Syndrome is not common, but occurs 6–12 hours after drug administration; corticosteroids have been helpful in treating/preventing syndrome. Mucosal inflammation and ulceration of anus/rectum may occur, especially in patients with prior hemorrhoids or history of abscesses. Alopecia occurs less frequently.

Nursing Implications: Assess baseline skin and mucous membranes prior to chemotherapy and identify patients at risk for problems. Consider including corticosteroid in antiemetic regimen, especially for high-dose therapy, and discuss with physician prophylactic use of dexamethasone eye drops to prevent conjunctivitis. Teach patient scrupulous perineal hygiene, instruct to report any rectal discomfort, and assess rectal mucosa daily with high-dose therapy. Discuss with patient potential coping strategies if alopecia occurs (i.e., wig, scarves).

IV. ALTERATION IN COMFORT, POTENTIAL, related to EDEMA, FATIGUE, LETHARGY, PAIN

Defining Characteristics: In clinical studies, the frequency of occurrence of these symptoms was: edema 20%, fatigue 36%, injection site pain 14%, pain 19%, arthralgia 11%, back pain 13%, myalgia 14%, pain in limb 29%, dermatitis 41%, erythema 18%, pruritis 47%, palmar plantar erythrodyesthesia syndrome (PPE) 13%, and flushing 18%.

Nursing Implications: Teach patient that these symptoms may occur and to report them. Teach patient self-care measures to reduce discomfort, such as application of heat or cold for pain, arthralgias and myalgias. Teach patient to report redness and pain on palms of hands or soles of feet as this may be PPE, and would require close monitoring and follow-up to prevent moist desquamation. Instruct patient to report any symptoms that do not resolve or improve with self-care measures.

Drug: cyclophosphamide (Cytoxan)

Class: Alkylating agent.

Mechanism of Action: Causes crosslinkage in DNA strands, thus preventing DNA synthesis and cell division. Cell cycle phase nonspecific.

Metabolism: Inactive until converted by microsomes in liver and serum enzymes (phosphamidases). Both cyclophosphamide and its metabolites are excreted by the kidneys. Plasma half-life: 6–12 hours, with 25% of drug excreted after 8 hours. Prolonged plasma half-life in patients with renal failure results in increased myelosuppression.

Dosage/Range:
- 400 mg/m^2 IV × 5 days.
- 100 mg/m^2 PO × 14 days.
- 500–1500 mg/m^2 IV q3–4 weeks.

High dose with BMT (*investigational*):
- 1.8–7 gm/m^2 in combination with other cytotoxic agents.

Drug Preparation:
- Dilute vials with sterile water. Shake well. Allow solution to clear if lyophilized preparation is not used. Do not use solution unless crystals are fully dissolved. Available in 25- and 50-mg tablets.

Drug Administration:
- Oral use: Administer in morning or early afternoon to allow adequate excretion time. Should be taken with meals.
- IV use: For doses > 500 mg, pre- and posthydration to total 500–3000 mL is needed to ensure adequate urine output and to avoid hemorrhagic cystitis. Administer drug over at least 20 minutes for doses > 500 mg.
- Mesna given with high-dose cyclophosphamide to prevent hemorrhagic cystitis.
- Solution is stable for 24 hours at room temperature, 6 days if refrigerated.
- Rapid infusion may result in dizziness, nasal stuffiness, rhinorrhea, sinus congestion during or soon after infusion.

Drug Interactions:
- Increases chloramphenicol half-life.
- Increases duration of leukopenia when given in combination with thiazide diuretics.
- Increases effect of anticoagulant drugs.

- Decreases digoxin level, so dose may need to be increased.
- Potentiation of doxorubicin-induced cardiomyopathy.
- Increased succinylcholine action with prolonged neuromuscular blockage.
- Increased drug action of barbiturates; induction of hepatic microsomes.

Lab Effects/Interference:

- Increased K, uric acid secondary to tumor lysis.
- Monitor electrolytes for symptoms of SIADH.
- Decreased CBC, platelets.

Special Considerations:

- Metabolic and leukopenic toxicity is increased by simultaneous administration of barbiturates, corticosteroids, phenytoin, and sulfonamides.
- Activity and toxicity of both cyclophosphamide and the specific drug may be altered by allopurinol, chloroquine, phenothiazides, potassium iodide, chloramphenicol, imipramine, vitamin A, warfarin, succinylcholine, digoxin, thiazide diuretics.
- Test urine for occult blood.
- High-dose cyclophosphamide therapy may require catheterization and constant bladder irrigation. Mesna should be given, either as a continuous infusion or in bolus doses, around drug administration. Consult protocol. See Chapter 4.

Potential Toxicities/Side Effects and the Nursing Process

I. INFECTION AND BLEEDING related to BONE MARROW DEPRESSION

Defining Characteristics: Leukopenia nadir occurs days 7–14, with recovery in 1–2 weeks; thrombocytopenia is less frequent and anemia is mild. Drug is a potent immunosuppressant.

Nursing Implications: Assess CBC, WBC with differential, platelet count, and signs/symptoms of infection and bleeding prior to treatment. Teach patient signs/symptoms of infection and instruct to report them if they occur. Teach patient self-care measures to minimize infection and bleeding. Increased risk of bone marrow depression in patients with prior radiation or chemotherapy.

II. ALTERED URINARY ELIMINATION related to HEMORRHAGIC CYSTITIS

Defining Characteristics: Metabolites of drug, if allowed to accumulate in the bladder, irritate bladder wall capillaries, causing hemorrhagic cystitis. This occurs in 7–40% of patients, is evidenced by microscopic or gross hematuria, is common with high doses, and is preventable. Long-term drug exposure may lead to bladder fibrosis.

Nursing Implications: Monitor BUN and creatinine prior to drug dose and as drug is excreted by the kidneys. Assess for signs/symptoms of hematuria, urinary frequency, or dysuria; instruct patient to report these if they occur. Instruct patient to take in at least 3 L of fluid per day and to empty bladder every 2–3 hours, as well as at bedtime. If patient is receiving a high dose, ensure vigorous hydration prior to drug administration. Bladder irrigation per protocol. Instruct patient to take oral cyclophosphamide early in the day to prevent drug accumulation in bladder during the night.

III. ALTERATION IN NUTRITION, LESS THAN BODY REQUIREMENTS, related to NAUSEA AND VOMITING, ANOREXIA, STOMATITIS, DIARRHEA, AND HEPATOTOXICITY

Defining Characteristics: Nausea and vomiting are dose-related and begin 2–4 hours after dose, peak in 12 hours, and may last 24 hours. Anorexia is common; stomatitis, if it occurs, is mild; and diarrhea is mild and infrequent. Hepatotoxicity is rare.

Nursing Implications: Premedicate with antiemetics prior to drug administration and continue prophylactically for 24 hours, at least for the first cycle. Encourage small feedings of bland foods and liquids. Encourage favorite foods and consult dietitian regarding anorexia if needed. Assess oral mucosa prior to drug administration; teach patient self-assessment techniques and oral care. Monitor LFTs before, during, and after therapy.

IV. ALTERED BODY IMAGE related to ALOPECIA, CHANGES IN NAILS AND SKIN

Defining Characteristics: Alopecia occurs in 30–50% of patients, especially with IV dosing, but some degree of hair loss occurs in all patients. Hair loss begins after 3+ weeks; hair may grow back while on therapy, but will grow back after therapy is discontinued (may be softer in texture). Hyperpigmentation of nails and skin, as well as transverse ridging of nails (banding), may occur.

Nursing Implications: Teach patient about potential hair loss and other changes. Discuss impact of hair loss on patient and strategies to minimize it (i.e., wig, scarf, cap) prior to drug administration. Assess ongoing coping during treatment. If nail changes are distressing, discuss the use of nail polish or other measures.

V. POTENTIAL SEXUAL DYSFUNCTION related to DRUG EFFECTS

Defining Characteristics: Drug is mutagenic and teratogenic. Amenorrhea often occurs in females, and testicular atrophy, possibly with reversible oligospermia/azoospermia, occurs in males. Drug is excreted in breast milk.

Nursing Implications: Assess patient's/partner's sexual patterns and reproductive goals. Discuss strategies to preserve sexual and reproductive health, including contraception and sperm banking, as appropriate. Mothers receiving cyclophosphamide should not breast-feed.

VI. POTENTIAL FOR INJURY related to ACUTE WATER INTOXICATION (SIADH) AND SECOND MALIGNANCY

Defining Characteristics: SIADH may occur with high-dose administration (> 50 mg/kg). Prolonged therapy may cause bladder cancer and acute leukemia.

Nursing Implications: Assess patients receiving high-dose cyclophosphamide: monitor serum Na+, osmolality, and urine osmolality and electrolytes; strictly monitor I/O, total body fluid balance, and daily weight. Screen patients who are receiving prolonged cyclophosphamide therapy for secondary malignancies.

VII. ALTERATION IN CARDIAC OUTPUT related to HIGH-DOSE CYCLOPHOSPHAMIDE

Defining Characteristics: Cardiomyopathy may occur with high doses as well as hemorrhagic cardiac necrosis, transmural hemorrhage, and coronary artery vasculitis at doses of 120–240 mg/kg. The mechanism is endothelial injury with subsequent hemorrhagic necrosis. The incidence is 22%, with 11% mortality, which may be decreased by dividing the dose into two split daily infusions. The risk at standard doses is increased by coadministration of doxorubicin (Adriamycin).

Nursing Implications: Assess cardiac status, especially if patient is receiving a high dose. Discuss baseline cardiac function test (GBPS) and assess for signs/symptoms of cardiomyopathy as treatment continues. Instruct patient to report dyspnea, shortness of breath, or other changes.

VIII. POTENTIAL FOR IMPAIRED GAS EXCHANGE related to PULMONARY TOXICITY

Defining Characteristics: Rare, but may occur with prolonged, high-dose therapy or continuous, low-dose therapy. Onset is insidious and appears as interstitial pneumonitis, which may progress to fibrosis. May respond to steroids.

Nursing Implications: Assess patients receiving high-dose or continuous low-dose cyclophosphamide for signs/symptoms of pulmonary dysfunction. Discuss pulmonary function studies with physician. Assess lung sounds prior to drug administration and periodically during treatment. Teach patient to report dyspnea, cough, or any abnormalities.

Drug: cytarabine, cytosine arabinoside (Ara-C, Cytosar-U)

Class: Antimetabolite.

Mechanism of Action: Incorporated into DNA, slowing its synthesis and causing defects in the linkages to new DNA fragments. Also, cells exposed to cytarabine in the S phase reinitiate DNA synthesis when the drug, a pyrimidine analogue, is removed, resulting in erroneous duplication of the early portions of the DNA strands. Most effective when cells are undergoing rapid DNA synthesis.

Metabolism: Inactivated by liver enzymes in biphasic manner: half-lives 10–15 minutes and 2–3 hours. Crosses the BBB with cerebrospinal fluid concentration of 50% that of plasma; 70% of dose excreted in urine as Ara-U; 4–10% excreted 12–24 hours after administration.

Dosage/Range:
- Varies depending on disease.
- Leukemia: 100 mg/m^2/day IV continuous infusion × 5–10 days; 100 mg/m^2 q12h × 1–3 weeks IV or SQ.
- Head and neck: 1 mg/kg q12h × 5–7 days IV or SQ.
- High dose: 2–3 g/m^2 IV q12h × 4–12 doses to treat refractory acute leukemia.
- Differentiation: 10 mg/m^2 SQ q12h × 15–21 days.
- Intrathecal: 20–30 mg/m^2.

Drug Preparation:
- 100-mg vials: add water with benzyl alcohol then dilute with 0.9% Sodium Chloride or 5% Dextrose.
- 500-mg vials: add water with benzyl alcohol then dilute with 0.9% Sodium Chloride or 5% Dextrose.
- For intrathecal use and high dose: use preservative-free diluent.
- Reconstituted drug is stable 48 hours at room temperature and 7 days refrigerated.

Drug Administration:
- Doses of 100–200 mg can be given SQ.
- Doses less than 1 g: Administer via pump over 10–20 minutes.
- Doses over 1 g: Administer over 2 hours.

Drug Interactions:
- May be a decreased bioavailability of digoxin when given in combination.

Lab Effects/Interference:
- Decreased CBC.
- Increased LFTs, RFTs.
- Increased uric acid due to tumor lysis.

Special Considerations:

- Thrombophlebitis, pain at the injection site, should be treated with warm compresses.
- Dizziness has occurred with too rapid IV infusions.
- Use with caution if hepatic dysfunction exists.
- Drug is excreted in tears requiring protection of eye conjunctiva with high-dose therapy.

Potential Toxicities/Side Effects and the Nursing Process

I. INFECTION AND BLEEDING related to BONE MARROW DEPRESSION

Defining Characteristics: Bone marrow depression is related to dose and duration of therapy. WBC depression is biphasic. After a 5-day continuous infusion at doses of 50–600 mg/m^2, WBC begins to fall within 24 hours, reaching nadir in 7–9 days, briefly rises around day 12, and begins to fall again, reaching nadir at days 15–24, with recovery within 10 days. Platelet drop begins day 5, reaching nadir at days 12–15, with recovery within 10 days. Anemia is seen frequently, with megaloblastic changes common in the bone marrow. Potent but transient suppression of primary and secondary antibody responses occur.

Nursing Implications: Assess WBC, neutrophil, and platelet count, and discuss any abnormalities with physician prior to drug administration; assess for signs/symptoms of skin infections (all mucosal surfaces, body orifices) and bleeding; instruct patient in signs/symptoms of infection and bleeding, as well as to report them or come to emergency room. Teach patient self-care measures to minimize risk of infection and bleeding, including avoidance of OTC aspirin-containing medications. Assess patient's Hgb/HCT and signs/symptoms of fatigue; teach patient self-assessment and to alternate rest and activity as needed.

II. ALTERED NUTRITION, LESS THAN BODY REQUIREMENTS, related to NAUSEA AND VOMITING, ANOREXIA, STOMATITIS, DIARRHEA, HEPATOTOXICITY

Defining Characteristics: Nausea and vomiting occurs in 50% of patients, is dose related, and lasts for several hours. Can be successfully prevented with combination antiemetics. Anorexia commonly occurs. Stomatitis occurs 7–10 days after therapy is initiated, occurs in 15% of patients, and is dose related. May be preceded by angular stomatitis (reddened area at juncture of lips). Diarrhea is infrequent and mild. Hepatotoxicity is usually mild and reversible, but drug should be used cautiously in patients with impaired hepatic function.

Nursing Implications: Premedicate with antiemetics depending on dose, using aggressive, combination antiemetics for high-dose therapy, and continue throughout chemotherapy. If patient develops nausea/vomiting, assess fluid and electrolyte balance and the need for replacements. Assess oral mucosa prior to chemotherapy and teach patient oral hygiene regimen and self-assessment; encourage patient to report diarrhea, discuss use of antidiarrheals with physician, and teach self-care PRN. Since patients become neutropenic, all mucosal surfaces need to be assessed for infection, and patients must be taught scrupulous perineal hygiene. Monitor LFTs prior to, during, and posttherapy.

III. IMPAIRED SKIN/MUCOSAL INTEGRITY related to RASH, ANAL INFLAMMATION/ULCERATION, ALOPECIA

Defining Characteristics: Maculopapular rash, with or without fever, myalgia, bone pain, occasional chest pain, conjunctivitis, and malaise (cytarabine syndrome) may occur. Syndrome is not common, but occurs 6–12 hours after drug administration; corticosteroids have been helpful in treating/preventing syndrome. Mucosal inflammation and ulceration of anus/rectum may occur, especially in patients with prior hemorrhoids or history of abscesses. Alopecia occurs less frequently.

Nursing Implications: Assess baseline skin and mucous membranes prior to chemotherapy and identify patients at risk for problems. Consider including corticosteroid in antiemetic regimen, especially for high-dose therapy, and discuss with physician prophylactic use of dexamethasone eye drops to prevent conjunctivitis. Teach patient scrupulous perineal hygiene, instruct to report any rectal discomfort, and assess rectal mucosa daily with high-dose therapy. Discuss with patient potential coping strategies if alopecia occurs (i.e., wig, scarves).

IV. POTENTIAL FOR INJURY related to NEUROTOXICITY

Defining Characteristics: Neurotoxicity can occur at high doses. If cerebellar toxicity (characterized by nystagmus, dysarthria, ataxia, slurred speech, and/or disdiadochokinesia or inability to make fine, coordinated movements) develops, it is an indication to terminate therapy. Onset usually 6–8 days after first dose, lasts 3–7 days. Lethargy and somnolence have resulted from rapid infusion of the drug. Incidence of CNS toxicity is 10% and may be related to total cumulative drug dose, impaired renal function, and/or age > 50 years old. Ocular toxicity may occur, characterized by injection of conjunctive, corneal opacities, decreased visual acuity. This may be a result of inhibition of DNA synthesis of corneal epithelium. Conjunctivitis occurs due to excretion of drug in lacrimal tearing and can be prevented by corticosteroid eye drops. Other visual symptoms that may occur are increased lacrimation, blurred vision, photophobia, eye pain.

Nursing Implications: Assess baseline neurologic status and cerebellar function (coordinated movements such as handwriting and gait) prior to and during therapy. Teach patient to self-assess and report changes in coordination, control of eye movement, handwriting. Monitor patient for somnolence and lethargy during infusion, and infuse drug according to established guidelines. With high-dose therapy, discuss with physician use of prophylactic corticosteroid eye drops. Assess and teach patient self-assessment of eyes and instruct to report increased lacrimation, blurred vision, photophobia, eye pain.

V. POTENTIAL FOR INJURY related to TUMOR LYSIS SYNDROME (TLS)

Defining Characteristics: May develop with initial therapy if patient has a large tumor burden; results from rapid lysis of tumor cells. This usually begins 1–5 days after initiation of therapy and causes elevations in serum uric acid, potassium, phosphorus, BUN, creatinine.

Nursing Implications: If this is induction therapy for a patient with acute leukemia or high tumor burden, expect medical orders to include IV hydration at 150 mL/hour with or without alkalinization, oral allopurinol, strict monitoring of I/O, daily weight, and total body fluid balance determination. Monitor baseline and daily BUN, creatinine, K+, phosphorus, uric acid, and calcium. Monitor for renal, cardiac, neuromuscular signs/symptoms of TLS.

VI. POTENTIAL SEXUAL DYSFUNCTION related to DRUG EFFECTS

Defining Characteristics: Drug is mutagenic and probably teratogenic. Although normal babies have been delivered by mothers receiving drug in first trimester, other babies have had congenital defects. It is unknown whether the drug is excreted in breast milk.

Nursing Implications: Discuss with patient and partner sexuality and reproductive goals and possible impact of chemotherapy. Discuss contraception and sperm banking if appropriate. Discourage breast-feeding if the mother is receiving chemotherapy.

Drug: cytarabine, liposome injection (DepoCyt)

Class: Antimetabolite.

Mechanism of Action: Drug is converted to the metabolite ara-CTP intracellularly. Ara-CTP is thought to inhibit DNA polymerase, thereby affecting DNA synthesis. Incorporation into DNA and RNA may also contribute to cytarabine cellular toxicity.

Metabolism: With systemically administered cytarabine, the drug is metabolized to an inactive compound, ara-U, and is then renally excreted. In the CSF, however, conversion to the ara-U is negligible, because CNS tissue and CSF lack the enzyme necessary for the conversion to occur. Liposomal formulation gives sustained effect over 2 weeks.

Dosage/Range:

Indicated for the intrathecal treatment of lymphomatous meningitis only. To be given as follows:

- Induction therapy: DepoCyt, 50 mg, administered intrathecally (intraventricular or lumbar puncture) every 14 days for 2 doses (weeks 1 and 3).
- Consolidation therapy: DepoCyt, 50 mg, administered intrathecally (intraventricular or lumbar puncture) every 14 days for 3 doses (weeks 5, 7, and 9) followed by 1 additional dose at week 13.
- Maintenance therapy: DepoCyt, 50 mg, administered intrathecally (intraventricular or lumbar puncture) every 28 days for 4 doses (weeks 17, 21, 25, and 29).
- If drug-related neurotoxicty develops, the dose should be reduced to 25 mg. If toxicity persists, treatment with DepoCyt should be terminated.

Drug Preparation/Administration:

- Drug is supplied in single-use vials and comes as a white to off-white suspension in 5 mL of fluid.
- Drug is to be withdrawn immediately before use and should not be used later than 4 hours from the time of withdrawal from vial.
- DepoCyt should be administered directly into the CSF over 1–5 minutes. Patients should lie flat for 1 hour after administration.
- Patients should be started on dexamethasone 4 mg bid either PO or IV for 5 days beginning on the day of DepoCyt injection.

Drug Interactions:

- No formal drug interaction studies of DepoCyt and other drugs have been done.
- Expect increased neurotoxicity if drug is administered at same time as other intrathecal, cytotoxic agents.

Lab Effects/Interference:

- DepoCyt particles are similar in size and appearance to white blood cells, so care must be taken when interpreting CSF samples.

Special Considerations:

- Do not use inline filters with DepoCyt; administer directly into CSF.
- Must be administered with concurrent dexamethasone as described above.
- FDA indication based on controlled clinical trial showing superior CR rate (41%) compared to standard intrathecal cytarabine.

Potential Toxicities/Side Effects and the Nursing Process

I. ALTERATION IN NUTRITION, LESS THAN BODY REQUIREMENTS, related to NAUSEA AND VOMITING

Defining Characteristics: Nausea, vomiting, and headache are common, and are physical manifestations of chemical arachnoiditis.

Nursing Implications: Administer dexamethasone throughout treatment course as described above. Observe patient for at least 1 hour after administration for toxicity. Administer antiemetics as ordered. Encourage small, frequent feedings of cool, bland foods. Instruct patient to report nausea and vomiting and to self-administer antiemetics as ordered.

II. ALTERATION IN COMFORT related to HEADACHE, NECK AND/OR BACK PAIN, FEVER, NAUSEA, AND VOMITING

Defining Characteristics: Some degree of chemical arachnoiditis is expected in about one-third of patients: incidence approaches 100% of patients when dexamethasone is NOT given with DepoCyt. Causes headache, neck pain, and/or rigidity, back pain, fever, nausea, and vomiting, which are reversible.

Nursing Implications: Instruct patient in dexamethasone self-administration and to report to physician if oral doses are not tolerated. Patients should lie flat for one hour after lumbar puncture and should be observed for immediate toxic reactions. Administer medications to treat pain.

Drug: dacarbazine (DTIC-Dome, Dimethyl-triazeno-imidazolecarboximide)

Class: Alkylating agent.

Mechanism of Action: Appears to methylate nucleic acids (particularly DNA) causing crosslinkage and breaks in DNA strands, which inhibits RNA and DNA synthesis. Also interacts with sulfhydral groups in proteins. Generally, cell cycle phase nonspecific.

Metabolism: Thought to be activated by liver microsomes. Excreted renally, with a plasma half-life of 0.65 hour, and terminal half-life of 5 hours.

Dosage/Range:
- 375 mg/m^2 every 3–4 weeks, OR
- 150–250 mg/m^2/day × 5 days, repeat every 3–4 weeks, OR
- 800–900 mg/m^2 as a single dose every 3–4 weeks.

High dose (investigational):
- 350 mg/m^2–2.5 g/m^2 IV as 24-hour infusion with hemibody radiotherapy.

Drug Preparation:
- Add sterile water or 0.9% Sodium Chloride to vial.

Drug Administration:
- Administer via pump over 20 minutes or give via IV push over 2–3 minutes.
- Stable for 8 hours at room temperature, for 72 hours if refrigerated. Store lyophilized drug in refrigerator and protect from light. Drug decomposition is denoted by a change in color from yellow to pink.

Drug Interactions:
- Increased drug metabolism with concurrent administration of dilantin, phenobarbital; potential increased toxicity with (Imuran) and 6-MP.

Lab Effects/Interference:
- Decreased CBC.
- Increased LFTs.

Special Considerations:
- Irritant—avoid extravasation.
- Pain may occur above site: Usually unrelieved by slowing IV, but may be relieved by applying ice to painful area. May cause venospasm; slow rate if this occurs.
- Anaphylaxis has occurred with infusion of dacarbazine.

Potential Toxicities/Side Effects and the Nursing Process

I. INFECTION AND BLEEDING related to BONE MARROW DEPRESSION

Defining Characteristics: Nadir occurs days 14–28 following drug administration; anemia may occur with long-term treatment.

Nursing Implications: Evaluate WBC, neutrophil, and platelet count and discuss any abnormalities with physician prior to drug administration; assess for signs/symptoms of infection or bleeding; instruct patient in identifying signs/symptoms of infection and bleeding, and to report them. Teach patient selfcare measures to minimize risk of infection and bleeding, including avoidance of OTC aspirin-containing medications. Assess patient's Hgb/HCT and signs/symptoms of fatigue; teach patient self-assessment and instruct to alternate rest and activity as needed.

II. ALTERATION IN NUTRITION, LESS THAN BODY REQUIREMENTS, related to NAUSEA AND VOMITING, DIARRHEA, ANOREXIA, HEPATOTOXICITY

Defining Characteristics: Nausea/vomiting occurs in 90% of patients and is moderate to severe, beginning 1–3 hours after dose. Nausea and vomiting decrease with each consecutive day the drug is given. Preventable by aggressive combination antiemetics. Diarrhea is uncommon. Anorexia is common, occurring in 90% of patients; drug may also cause a metallic taste. Hepatotoxicity is rare, but hepatic venoocclusive disease has been described (hepatic vein thrombosis and hepatocellular necrosis).

Nursing Implications: Premedicate with combination antiemetics and continue protection during infusions. Administer drug over at least one hour. Use relaxation exercises, imagery, or other techniques; teach patient exercises prior to drug treatment. Teach patient to report diarrhea and administer antidiarrheal medication as ordered, or teach patient self-administration as appropriate. Encourage small, frequent feedings of favorite foods; teach patient/caregiver to make foods ahead of time so patient will have them ready for snacks when hungry; encourage use of spices if food tastes bland; encourage patient to weigh self weekly. Monitor LFTs and discuss abnormalities with physician.

III. ALTERATION IN COMFORT related to FLULIKE SYNDROME, PAIN AT INJECTION SITE

Defining Characteristics: Flulike syndrome may occur, characterized by malaise, headache, myalgia, hypotension; may occur up to 7 days after first dose, lasting 7–21 days, and may recur with subsequent doses of drug. Drug is an irritant and may cause phlebitis of vein.

Nursing Implications: Teach patient flulike symptoms may occur; suggest symptom management using acetaminophen as needed; encourage fluid intake of > 3 L/day and rest, as determined by healthcare team. Assess patient vein selection prior to drug administration and suggest venous access device early on if patient is to receive ongoing treatment with dacarbazine (DTIC). Administer drug in 100–250-mL IV fluid and infuse slowly over 1 hour. Consider premedications when drug is given peripherally and discuss with physician: hydrocortisone IVP (DTIC forms precipitate with hydrocortisone sodium succinate [Solucortef] but not with hydrocortisone), lidocaine 1–2% IVP, or heparin IVP to minimize vein trauma prior to DTIC infusion. Apply heat or ice above injection site to reduce venous burning.

IV. IMPAIRED SKIN INTEGRITY related to ALOPECIA, FACIAL FLUSHING, ERYTHEMA, URTICARIA

Defining Characteristics: Alopecia occurs in 90% of patients. Facial flushing occurs rarely and is self-limiting; erythema and urticaria may occur around injection site. High dose-related photosensitization may occur, with resulting severe reaction to sunlight, e.g., burning, pain.

Nursing Implications: Teach patient about expected hair loss; encourage patient to verbalize feelings regarding anticipated/actual hair loss and discuss strategies to minimize impact of alopecia. Encourage female patients to obtain wig prior to hair loss; ask male patients to identify how they will manage hair loss. Provide emotional support. In cold climates, encourage patient to wear cap at night to prevent loss of body heat. Teach patient receiving high-dose therapy to cover body, head, and hands when exposed to sunlight, or to avoid direct sunlight. Patient should also use sunblock.

V. POTENTIAL FOR SENSORY/PERCEPTUAL ALTERATIONS related to FACIAL PARESTHESIA, PHOTOSENSITIVITY

Defining Characteristics: Photosensitivity may occur in bright sunlight or ultraviolet light. Facial paresthesias may occur.

Nursing Implications: Instruct patient to report facial paresthesias and in self-care measures if sensory changes occur: wear sunglasses in strong sunlight; wear sunscreens when out in the sun; as well as protective clothing, including a hat, avoid UV or strong sunlight exposure if possible.

VI. POTENTIAL SEXUAL DYSFUNCTION related to DRUG EFFECTS

Defining Characteristics: Drug is teratogenic. It is unknown whether drug is excreted in breast milk. Drug is probably carcinogenic.

Nursing Implications: Assess patient's and partner's patterns of sexuality and reproductive goals. Teach need for contraception and provide information and referral as appropriate. Encourage verbalization of feelings and provide emotional support. Discourage breast-feeding if patient is a lactating mother.

Drug: dactinomycin (Actinomycin D, Cosmegen)

Class: Antitumor antibiotic isolated from *Streptomyces* fungus.

Mechanism of Action: Binds to guanine portion of DNA and blocks the ability of DNA to act as a template for both DNA and RNA. At lower drug doses, the predominant action inhibits RNA, whereas at higher doses both RNA and DNA are inhibited. Cell cycle specific for G1 and S phases.

Metabolism: Most of drug is excreted unchanged in bile and urine. There is a rapid clearance of drug from plasma (approximately 36 hours). Dose reduction in the presence of liver or renal failure may be needed.

Dosage/Range:
- 10–15 μg/kg/day × 5 days q3–4 weeks.
- 15–30 μg/kg/week, 400–600 μg/m^2 day for 5 days IV.
- Frequency and schedule may vary according to protocol and age.

Drug Preparation:

- Add sterile water for a concentration of 500 μg/mL. Use preservative-free water, as precipitate may develop otherwise.

Drug Administration:

- IV: Drug is a vesicant and should be given through a running IV to avoid extravasation, which can lead to ulceration, pain, and necrosis. Be sure to check the nursing policy and procedure for administration of vesicants.

Drug Interactions:

- None significant.

Lab Effects/Interference:

- Decreased CBC.
- Increased LFTs.
- Decreased calcium.

Special Considerations:

- Drug is a vesicant. Give through a running IV to avoid extravasation, which may develop into ulceration, necrosis, and pain.
- Nausea and vomiting are moderate to severe. Usually occurs 2–5 hours after administration; may persist up to 24 hours.
- Potent myelosuppressive agent: Severity of nadir is dose-limiting toxicity.
- GI toxicity: Mucositis, diarrhea, and abdominal pain.
- Skin changes: Radiation recall phenomenon. Skin discoloration along vein used for injection.
- Alopecia.
- Malaise, fatigue, mental depression.
- Contraindicated in patients with chickenpox or herpes zoster, as life-threatening systemic disease may develop.

Potential Toxicities/Side Effects and the Nursing Process

I. POTENTIAL FOR INFECTION AND BLEEDING related to BONE MARROW DEPRESSION

Defining Characteristics: Myelosuppression often dose-limiting toxicity. Onset of decreasing WBC and platelets in 7–10 days, with nadir 14–21 days after dose and recovery in 21–28 days. Delayed anemia.

Nursing Implications: Assess CBC, WBC, differential, and platelet count prior to drug administration, as well as for signs/symptoms of infection and bleeding, and discuss any abnormalities with physician prior to drug administration. Instruct patient in signs/symptoms of infection and bleeding and instruct to report this; teach patient self-care measures to minimize risk of infection and bleeding, including avoidance of OTC aspirin-containing medications. Assess patient's Hgb/HCT and signs/symptoms of fatigue; teach patient self-assessment and instruct to alternate rest and activity as needed.

II. ALTERATION IN NUTRITION, LESS THAN BODY REQUIREMENTS, related to NAUSEA/VOMITING, DIARRHEA, ANOREXIA

Defining Characteristics: Nausea/vomiting may be severe and begins 2–5 hours after dose, lasting 24 hours. Diarrhea with/without cramps occurs in 30% of patients. Anorexia occurs frequently.

Nursing Implications: Use combination antiemetics to prevent nausea and vomiting. Nausea/vomiting may be prevented by aggressive, combination antiemetics, such as serotonin antagonist plus dexamethasone. Encourage small, frequent feedings of bland foods. Encourage patient to eat favorite foods and use seasonings on foods if anorexia persists; refer to dietitian as needed.

III. ALTERATION IN MUCOUS MEMBRANES related to STOMATITIS, ESOPHAGITIS, AND PROCTITIS

Defining Characteristics: Irritation and ulceration may occur along the entire GI mucosa.

Nursing Implications: Assess baseline oral mucosa and presence of irritation along GI tract. Instruct patient in self-assessment and teach patient to report irritation; instruct regarding oral hygiene regimen.

IV. POTENTIAL IMPAIRED SKIN INTEGRITY related to RADIATION RECALL, RASH, ALOPECIA, AND DRUG EXTRAVASATION

Defining Characteristics: Recalls damage to skin from previous radiation, resulting in erythema or increased pigmentation at the radiation site. Acnelike rash and alopecia can occur in 47% of patients. Drug is a potent vesicant.

Nursing Implications: Conduct baseline skin, hair assessment. Discuss with patient impact of potential changes on body image, as well as possible coping/adaptive strategies (e.g., obtain wig prior to hair loss). When administering the drug, ensure use of a patent vein to avoid extravasation; consider the use of venous access device early. Be familiar with institution's policy and procedure for administration of a vesicant and management of extravasation.

V. ALTERATION IN COMFORT related to FLULIKE SYMPTOMS

Defining Characteristics: Flulike symptoms can occur, including symptoms of malaise, myalgia, fever, depression.

Nursing Implications: Inform patient this may occur. Assess for occurrence during and after treatment. Discuss with physician symptomatic management.

VI. POTENTIAL FOR ALTERATION IN METABOLISM related to HEPATOTOXICITY AND RENAL TOXICITY

Defining Characteristics: Hepatotoxicity is related to drug metabolism in liver; renal toxicity is related to drug excretion by kidneys.

Nursing Implications: Monitor LFTs, BUN, and creatinine. Discuss abnormalities with physician, as drug doses may need to be reduced.

VII. POTENTIAL FOR SEXUAL DYSFUNCTION

Defining Characteristics: Drug is carcinogenic, mutagenic, and teratogenic. It is unknown if drug is excreted in breast milk.

Nursing Implications: Assess patient's/partner's sexual patterns and reproductive goals. Provide information, supportive counseling, and referral as needed. Teach importance of birth control measures as appropriate. Discourage breast-feeding if patient is a lactating mother.

Drug: daunorubicin citrate liposome injection (DaunoXome)

Class: Anthracycline antibiotic that is isolated from streptomycin products, in particular the rhodomycin products, and encapsulated in a liposome.

Mechanism of Action: No clearly defined mechanism. Intercalates DNA, therefore blocking DNA, RNA, and protein synthesis. Binds to DNA and inhibits DNA replication and DNA-dependent RNA synthesis. Drug is encapsulated within liposomes (lipid vesicles) and is preferentially delivered to solid tumor sites. The liposomal encapsulated drug is protected from chemical and enzymatic degradation, protein binding, and uptake by normal tissues while circulating in the blood. The exact mechanism for selective targeting of tumor sites is unknown but is believed to be related to increased permeability of the tumor neovasculature. Once delivered to the tumor, the drug is slowly released and exerts its antineoplastic action.

Metabolism: Cleared from the plasma at 17 mL/min with a small steady-state volume of distribution. As compared to standard IV daunorubicin, the liposomal encapsulated daunorubicin has higher daunorubicin exposure (plasma area under the curve, ARC). The elimination half-life (4.4 hours) is shorter than standard daunorubicin.

Dosage/Range:

- 40 mg/m^2/day IV bolus over 60 minutes every 2 weeks.

Drug Preparation:

- Drug is available as 50 mg of daunorubicin base in a total volume of 25 mL (2 mg/mL).

- Visually inspect for particulate matter and discoloration (drug appears as a translucent dispersion of liposomes that scatters light, but should not be opaque or have precipitate or foreign matter present).
- Withdraw the calculated volume of drug and add to an equal volume of 5% Dextrose to deliver a 1:1, or 1 mg/mL solution.
- Administer immediately, or may be stored in the refrigerator at 2–8°C (36–46°F) for 6 hours.
- Use ONLY 5% Dextrose, NOT 0.9% Sodium Chloride or any other solution.
- Drug contains no preservatives.
- Unopened drug vials should be stored in the refrigerator at 2–8°C (36–46°F), but should not be frozen. Protect from light.

Drug Administration:
- IV bolus over 60 minutes, repeated every 2 weeks.
- Do not use an inline filter.
- Drug is an irritant, not a vesicant.
- Dose should be reduced in patients with renal or hepatic dysfunction.
- Hold dose if absolute granulocyte count is < 750 cells/mm^3.

Drug Interactions:
- Unknown at this time, so do not mix with any other drugs.

Lab Effects/Interference:
- Increased LFTs, RFTs (especially if elevated prior to administration).
- Increased uric acid secondary to tumor lysis.

Special Considerations:
- Drug is embryotoxic, so female patients should use contraceptive measures as appropriate.
- Back pain, flushing, and chest tightness may occur during the first 5 minutes of drug administration and resolve with cessation of the infusion. Most patients do not experience recurrence when the infusion is restarted at a slower rate.
- Drug indicated in the treatment of Kaposi's sarcoma. Activity reported to be equivalent to treatment with ABV (doxorubicin, vincristine, bleomycin) but with less alopecia, cardiotoxicity, and neurotoxicity.

Potential Toxicities/Side Effects and the Nursing Process

I. POTENTIAL FOR INFECTION AND BLEEDING related to BONE MARROW DEPRESSION

Defining Characteristics: Myelosuppression can be severe and affects the granulocytes primarily. Incidence of neutropenia of 36% is similar to that of patients receiving ABV (doxorubicin, vincristine, bleomycin), which is 35%.

Neutropenia with < 500 cells/mm^3 occurs in 15% of patients (vs 5% in patients receiving ABV). Fever incidence is 47%. Concurrent antiretroviral and antiviral agents received for HIV infection may enhance this. Patients are immunocompromised; therefore, monitoring for opportunistic infection is essential. Platelets and RBCs are less affected.

Nursing Implications: Monitor CBC, WBC, differential, and platelet count prior to drug administration, and discuss any abnormalities with physician. Drug should not be given if ANC is < 750 cells/mm^3. Assess for signs/symptoms of infection or bleeding, and instruct patient in self-assessment and to report signs/symptoms immediately. Teach patient self-care measures to minimize risk of infection and bleeding, including avoidance of OTC aspirin-containing medications. Drug dosage must be reduced if patient has hepatic dysfunction: 75% of drug dose if serum bili 1.2–3.0 mg/dL, 50% reduction if bili is > 3.0 mg/dL. Drug dosage must be reduced if patient has renal impairment: creatinine > 3 mg/dL, give 50% of normal dose.

II. ALTERATION IN COMFORT related to TRIAD OF BACK PAIN, FLUSHING, CHEST TIGHTNESS

Defining Characteristics: This occurs in 13.8% of patients and is mild to moderate. The syndrome resolves with cessation of the infusion, and does not usually recur when the infusion is resumed at a slower infusion rate.

Nursing Implications: Infuse drug at prescribed rate over 60 minutes. Assess for, and teach patient to report, back pain, flushing, and chest tightness. Stop infusion if this occurs, and once symptoms subside, resume infusion at a slower rate.

III. POTENTIAL FOR ALTERATION IN SKIN INTEGRITY related to ALOPECIA, CHANGES IN SKIN

Defining Characteristics: Mild alopecia occurs in 6% of patients and moderate alopecia in 2% of patients, as compared to 36% of patients receiving ABV chemotherapy. The drug is considered an irritant, NOT a vesicant. Folliculitis, seborrhea, and dry skin occur in < 5% of patients.

Nursing Implications: Teach patient that hair loss is unlikely, and to report this or any skin changes.

IV. POTENTIAL FOR ALTERATION IN NUTRITION, LESS THAN BODY REQUIREMENTS, related to NAUSEA AND VOMITING, ANOREXIA, DIARRHEA

Defining Characteristics: Mild nausea occurs in 35% of patients, moderate nausea in 16% of patients, and severe nausea in 3% of patients. Vomiting is less common, with 10% experiencing mild, 10% experiencing moderate, and 3% experiencing severe vomiting. Anorexia may occur (21%) or increased appetite may occur in < 5% of patients. Diarrhea may occur in 38% of patients. Other GI problems, occurring < 5% of the time, are dysphagia, gastritis, hemorrhoids, hepatomegaly, dry mouth, and tooth caries.

Nursing Implications: Premedicate with antiemetics. Encourage small, frequent feedings of bland foods. If patient has anorexia, teach patient or caregiver to make foods ahead of time, use spices, and encourage weekly weights. Instruct patient to report diarrhea, and to use self-management strategies (medications as ordered, diet modification). Instruct patient to report other GI problems.

V. POTENTIAL FOR ALTERATION IN CARDIAC OUTPUT related to CARDIAC CHANGES

Defining Characteristics: Daunorubicin may cause cardiotoxicity and CHF, but studies with liposomal daunorubicin show rare clinical cardiotoxicity at cumulative doses > 600 mg/m^2. However, especially in patients with preexisting cardiac disease or prior anthracycline treatment, assessment of cardiac function (history and physical) should be performed prior to each dose. In addition, testing of cardiac ejection fraction and echocardiogram should be performed at cumulative doses of 320 mg/m^2, 480 mg/m^2, and every 160 mg/m^2 thereafter.

Nursing Implications: Assess cardiac status prior to chemotherapy administration: signs/symptoms of CHF, quality/regularity and rate of heartbeat, results of prior tests of left ventricular ejection fraction (LVEF) or echocardiogram, if performed. Instruct patient to report dyspnea, palpitations, swelling in extremities. Maintain accurate records of total dose, and expect GBPS to be repeated periodically during treatment and the drug to be discontinued if there is a significant drop in heart function.

VI. POTENTIAL FOR ACTIVITY INTOLERANCE related to FATIGUE

Defining Characteristics: Fatigue occurs in 49% of patients.

Nursing Implications: Assess baseline activity level. Instruct patient to report fatigue and activity intolerance. Teach self-management strategies, including alternating rest and activity periods, and stress reduction.

Drug: daunorubicin hydrochloride (Cerubidine, Daunomycin HCl, Rubidomycin)

Class: Anthracycline antibiotic isolated from streptomycin products, in particular the rhodomycin products.

Mechanism of Action: No clearly defined mechanism. Intercalates DNA, therefore blocking DNA, RNA, and protein synthesis. Binds to DNA and inhibits DNA replication and DNA-dependent RNA synthesis.

Metabolism: Site of significant metabolism is in the liver. Doses need to be modified in presence of abnormal liver function. Excreted in urine and bile.

Dosage/Range:

- 30–60 mg/m^2/day IV for 3 consecutive days.

Drug Preparation:

- Add sterile water to produce liquid. Drug will form a precipitate when mixed with heparin and is incompatible with dexamethasone.

Drug Administration:

- IV: This drug is a potent vesicant. Give through a running IV to avoid extravasation, which can lead to ulceration, pain, and necrosis. Check individual hospital policy and procedure on administration of a vesicant.

Drug Interactions:

- Incompatible with heparin (forms a precipitate).

Lab Effects/Interference:

- Increased bili, AST, alk phos.
- Increased uric acid secondary to tumor lysis.

Special Considerations:

- Drug is a potent vesicant. Give through running IV to avoid/minimize effects of extravasation.
- Moderate to severe nausea and vomiting occur in 50% of patients within first 24 hours.
- Causes discoloration of urine (pink to red for up to 48 hours after administration).
- Potent myelosuppressive agent. Nadir occurs within 10–14 days.
- Alopecia.
- Cardiac toxicity: Dose limit at 550 mg/m^2. Patients may exhibit irreversible CHF. Acute toxicity may be seen within hours after administration. This is unrelated to cumulative dose and may manifest symptoms of pump or conduction dysfunction. Rarely, transient EKG abnormalities, CHF; pericardial effusion (whole syndrome referred to as myocarditis-pericarditis syndrome) may occur, which may lead to death.
- Dose reduction necessary in patients with impaired liver function.

- Available in liposomal encapsulated vehicle (Daunoxome) that has less myelosuppression and cardiotoxicity. Drug is currently approved for therapy of Kaposi's sarcoma.

Potential Toxicities/Side Effects and the Nursing Process

I. POTENTIAL FOR INFECTION AND BLEEDING related to BONE MARROW DEPRESSION

Defining Characteristics: WBC and platelet counts begin to decrease in 7 days, with nadir 10–14 days after drug dose; recovery in 21–28 days. Dose reduction indicated with renal or hepatic dysfunction as drug is excreted by these routes.

Nursing Implications: Evaluate WBC, neutrophil, and platelet count and discuss any abnormalities with physician prior to drug administration; assess for signs/symptoms of infection and bleeding; instruct patient in signs/symptoms of infection and bleeding and to report these immediately. Teach patient self-care measures to minimize risk of infection and bleeding, including avoidance of OTC aspirin-containing medications.

II. POTENTIAL FOR ALTERATION IN CARDIAC OUTPUT related to ACUTE AND CHRONIC CARDIAC CHANGES

Defining Characteristics: Acute effects (i.e., EKG changes, atrial arrhythmias) occur in 6–30% of patients 1–3 days after dose and are not life-threatening. Chronic myofibril damage resulting in irreversible cardiomyopathy is life-threatening and dose-related. Cumulative dose should not exceed 550 mg/m^2 or 450 mg/m^2 if patient is receiving/has received radiation to chest or with concurrent administration of cyclophosphamide or other cardiotoxic agent. CHF may develop 1–16 months after therapy ceases if cumulative dose is exceeded.

Nursing Implications: Assess baseline cardiac status, quality and regularity of heartbeat, and baseline EKG. Patient should have baseline GBPS or other measure of left ventricular ejection fraction at baseline, and periodically during treatment. If there is a significant drop in ejection fraction, then drug should be stopped. Maintain accurate documentation of doses administered so that cumulative dose is known. Instruct patient to report dyspnea, shortness of breath, edema, orthopnea.

III. ALTERATION IN NUTRITION, LESS THAN BODY REQUIREMENTS, related to NAUSEA AND VOMITING, STOMATITIS

Defining Characteristics: Mild nausea and vomiting on the day of therapy occur in 50% of patients and can be prevented with antiemetics. Stomatitis is infrequent but may occur 3–7 days after dose.

Nursing Implications: Premedicate with antiemetics, and continue for 24 hours for protection. Assess oral mucosa prior to chemotherapy, teach patient oral hygiene regimen and self-assessment; encourage patient to report burning or oral irritation. Assess pain in mouth, and administer analgesics as needed and ordered.

IV. POTENTIAL FOR IMPAIRED SKIN INTEGRITY related to ALOPECIA, HYPERPIGMENTATION OF FINGERNAILS AND TOENAILS, RADIATION RECALL, AND DRUG EXTRAVASATION

Defining Characteristics: Reversible total alopecia occurs 3–4 weeks after treatment begins; nail beds become hyperpigmented. Drug is a potent vesicant and will result in severe soft tissue damage if extravasated. Damage to skin from prior irradiation may be reactivated (radiation recall). Rash may occur, as may onycholysis (nail loosening from nail bed).

Nursing Implications: Teach patient that alopecia will occur and discuss impact hair loss will have on body image. Discuss coping strategies, including obtaining wig or cap prior to hair loss. Encourage patient to verbalize feelings and provide patient with emotional support. Drug dose may be decreased with prior irradiation; assess for skin changes from radiation recall. Hyperpigmentation of nail beds may cause body image problem; discuss with patient and identify measures to minimize distress. Ensure that drug is administered only through a patent IV and that nurse is familiar with institution's policy for vesicant administration and management of extravasation. Manufacturer recommends aspiration of any remaining drug from IV tubing, discontinuing IV, and applying ice. Assess need for venous access device early.

V. POTENTIAL SEXUAL DYSFUNCTION related to DRUG EFFECTS

Defining Characteristics: Drug is mutagenic and teratogenic. Drug may cause testicular atrophy and azoospermia. It is unknown whether drug is excreted in breast milk.

Nursing Implications: Assess patient's and partner's sexual patterns and reproductive goals. Provide information, supportive counseling, and referral as needed. Male patients may wish to try sperm banking. Teach importance of birth control measures as appropriate. Women receiving the drug should not breast-feed.

VI. POTENTIAL FOR ALTERATION IN COMFORT related to ABDOMINAL PAIN, FEVER, CHILLS

Defining Characteristics: Abdominal pain may occur but is uncommon. Fever and chills, with or without rash, occur rarely.

Nursing Implications: Assess patient for occurrence and provide symptomatic management.

Drug: decitabine (5-Aza-2-deoxycytidine) (investigational)

Class: Antimetabolite, molecular/genetic modulator.

Mechanism of Action: Drug is a pyrimidine analogue, and prevents DNA synthesis in the S phase, leading to cell death. In addition, and more important, drug inhibits methyltransferase, an enzyme necessary for the expression of cellular genes. The cells in tumors that have progressed or that are resistant to therapy, characteristically have DNA *hyper*methylation. Decitabine "traps" DNA methyltranferase, thus greatly reducing its activity, which results in the synthesis of DNA that is *hypo*methylated. DNA hypomethylation results in activating genes that have been silent, causing the cell to differentiate, and then to die (cell death through disorganized gene expression or extinction of clones of cells that were terminally differentiated). Research has shown that the drug modulates Tumor Suppressor Genes (TSG), the expression of tumor antigens, other genes, and overall cell differentiation. (Mandelli, 1993; Wijermans et al, 2000; Ninomoto, 2000; Baylin et al, 1998).

Metabolism: Unknown.

Dosage/Range:
- Per protocol.
- Myelodysplastic syndrome: 15 mg/m^2 IV q4h q8h × 3 days (total dose 45 mg/m^2/d), repeated q6 weeks.
- Chronic myelogenous leukemia: 25–50 mg/m^2 IV over 6 h q12h × 5 days (reduce dose 25–50% to permit drug delivery q4–5 weeks).

Drug Preparation:
- Per protocol.

Drug Administration:
- Intravenously, per protocol.

Drug Interactions:
- Appears to be synergistic with biological agents such as interferons and reinoids (retinoic acid).
- Synergistic cytotoxic effects when given together with each of the following: cisplatin, 4-hydroperoxycyclophosphamide, 3-deazauridine, cyclopentenyl cytosine, cytosine arabinoside, topotecan, and thymidine.

Lab Effects/Interference:
- Unknown.

Special Considerations:
- Contraindicated in patients with a history of hypersensitivity reactions to the drug or any of its components.
- Current clinical trials (phase): Myelodysplastic syndrome (II), CML (II), relapse postautoBMT (I/II), alloBMT for acute myelogenous leukemia and CML (I/II), metastatic breast cancer (II), lung cancer (I), stage III/IV melanoma (I), advanced solid malignancies (I).

Potential Toxicities/Side Effects and the Nursing Process

I. POTENTIAL FOR INFECTION AND BLEEDING related to BONE MARROW DEPRESSION

Defining Characteristics: Dose-limiting factor is bone marrow suppression. In one study of patients with CML blast crisis, the incidence of neutropenia was 85% with most patients experiencing fever. Nadir is delayed, occurring on day 21, with recovery on day 35. Thrombocytopenia occurs, with nadir platelet count on day 15, and recovery by day 21.

Nursing Implications: Assess baseline CBC and differential, and platelet count prior to chemotherapy, as well as for signs/symptoms of infection or bleeding. Teach patient signs/symptoms of infection or bleeding, to report these immediately, and to come to the emergency room or clinic if febrile, and teach patient self-care measures to minimize risk of infection and bleeding. This includes avoidance of crowds and proximity to people with infections, and avoidance of OTC aspirin-containing medications.

II. ALTERED NUTRITION, LESS THAN BODY REQUIREMENTS, RELATED TO NAUSEA AND VOMITING, STOMATITIS

Defining Characteristics: Nausea and vomiting occur commonly, are mild to moderate, and preventable by antiemetic medicines.

Nursing Implications: Premedicate patient with antiemetic. If patient develops nausea and/or vomiting, encourage small, frequent intake of cool, bland foods. Instruct patient to report nausea, and teach self-administration of antiemetic medications. If nausea/vomiting occur and are severe, assess for signs/

symptoms of fluid/electrolyte imbalance. Teach patient to self-administer anti-diarrheal medications if needed. Assess baseline oral mucous membranes. Teach patient oral assessment, hygiene measures, and to report any alterations.

Drug: docetaxel (Taxotere)

Class: Taxoid, mitotic spindle poison.

Mechanism of Action: Enhances microtubule assembly and inhibits disassembly. Disrupts microtubule network that is essential for mitotic and interphase cellular function. Stabilization of microtubules inhibits mitosis.

Metabolism: Drug is extensively protein-bound (94–97%). Triphasic elimination. Metabolism involves P-450 3A (CYP3A4) isoenzyme system (in vitro testing). Fecal elimination is main route, accounting for excretion of 75% of the drug and its metabolites within seven days; 80% of the fecal excretion occurs during the first 48 hours. Mild to moderate liver impairment (SGOT and/or SGPT > 1.5 times normal and alk phos > 2.5 times normal) results in decreased clearance of drug by an average of 27%, resulting in a 38% increase in systemic exposure (AUC).

Dosage/Range:

- Adjuvant breast cancer: docetaxel 75 mg/m^2 IV 1-hour after doxorubicin 50 mg/m^2 IVP and cyclophamide 500 mg/m^2 IV q3 weeks × 6 courses, with G-CSF support PRN.
- Breast cancer: 60–100 mg/m^2 IV as a 1-hour infusion every 3 weeks.
- Non-small-cell lung cancer: 1) 75 mg/m^2 as a 1-hour infusion as a single agent, 2) 75 mg/m^2 as a 1-hour infusion, followed by cisplatin over 30–60 minutes every 3 weeks.
- Prostate cancer: docetaxel 75 mg/m^2 day 1 repeated q 21 days, in combination with prednisone 5 mg PO bid continuously, to be repeated for 10 cycles.
- Dose reductions for nadir ANC < 500 cells/mm^3 for > 1 week, or severe and cumulative cutaneous reactions, or moderate neurosensory signs and/or symptoms, should have a dose reduction when symptoms resolve (see package insert).
- Premedication regimen with corticosteroids: e.g., dexamethasone 8 mg bid × 3 days, starting 1 day prior to docetaxel to reduce the incidence and severity of fluid retention and hypersensitivity reactions. For patients with prostate cancer receiving prednisone, the doses of oral dexamethasone are: 8 mg at 12 hours, 3 hours, and 1 hour prior to docetaxel dose.

Drug Preparation: (requires 2 dilutions prior to administration):

- Vials available as 80-mg and 20-mg concentrate as single-dose blister packs with diluent. Do not reuse single-dose vials. Drug contains polysorbate 80.
- Unopened vials require protection from bright light. May be stored at room temperature or in refrigerator (36–77°F). Allow to stand at room temperature for at least 5 minutes prior to reconstitution.
- Reconstitute 20-mg and 80-mg vials with the entire contents of accompanying diluent vial (13% Ethanol in water for injection). Reconstituted vials contain 10 mg/mL docetaxel (initial diluted solution).
- Gently invert repeatedly, but do not shake the initial diluted solution for approximately 45 seconds.
- Reconstituted vials (10 mg/mL initial diluted solution) are stable for 8 hours at either room temperature or under refrigeration.
- Use only glass or polypropylene or polyolefin plastic (bag) IV containers.
- Withdraw ordered dose, and further dilute in 250 mL volume of 5% Dextrose or 0.9% Sodium Chloride to a final concentration of 0.3–0.74 mg/mL. Thoroughly mix by manual rotation.
- Inspect for any particulate matter or discoloration, and if found, discard.
- Use infusion solution immediately or within 4 hrs.

Drug Administration:

- Assess patient's ANC and liver function studies, and if abnormal, discuss with physician. See Special Considerations.
- Use only glass or polypropylene bottles, or polypropylene or polyolefin plastic bags for drug infusion, and administer infusion ONLY through polyethylenelined administration sets.
- Patient should receive corticosteroid premedication (e.g., dexamethasone 8 mg bid) for 3 days beginning 1 day before drug administration to reduce the incidence and severity of fluid retention and hypersensitivity reactions.
- Infuse drug over 1 hour.

Drug Interactions:

- Radiosensitizing effect.
- Theoretically, CYP3A4 inhibitors, such as ketoconazole, erythromycin, troleandomycin, cyclosporine, terfenadine, and nifedipine, can inhibit docetaxel metabolism and result in elevated serum levels of docetaxel; use together with caution or not at all.
- Theoretically, CYP3A4 inducers, such as anticonvulsants and St. John's Wort, may increase metabolism, and decrease serum levels of docetaxel.
- Capecitabine.

Lab Effects/Interference:

- Decreased CBC.

Special Considerations:

- Indicated for the treatment of (1) adjuvant treatment of operable node-positive breast cancer; (2) locally advanced or metastatic breast cancer after failure of prior chemotherapy; (3) as a single agent in locally advanced or metastatic non-small-cell lung cancer (NSCLC) after failure of prior platinum-based chemotherapy; (4) in combination with cisplatin, in patients with unresectable locally advanced or metastatic NSCLC who have not received prior chemotherapy; and (5) in combination with prednisone for the treatment of androgen-independent (hormone-refractory) metastatic prostate.
- Contraindicated in patients with history of severe hypersensitivity reactions to docetaxel or to other drugs formulated with polysorbate 80; drug should not be used in patients with neutrophil counts of < 1500 cells/mm^3. Drug should not be used in pregnant or breast-feeding women; women of child-bearing age should use effective birth control measures.
- Docetaxel generally should not be administered to patients with bilirubin $>$ upper limit of normal (ULN) or to patients with SGOT and/or SGPT $> 1.5 \times$ ULN concomitant with alkaline phosphatase $> 2.5 \times$ ULN. Patients treated with elevated bilirubin or abnormal transaminases plus alkaline phosphatase have an increased risk of grade 4 neutropenia, febrile neutropenia, severe stomatitis, infections, severe thrombocytopenia, severe skin toxicity, and toxic death. Serum bilirubin, SGOT or SGPT, and alkaline phosphatase should be obtained and reviewed by the treating physician before each cycle of docetaxel treatment.
- Dose modifications during treatment: (1) Patients with breast cancer dosed initially at 100 mg/m^2 who experience either febrile neutropenia, ANC < 500/mm^3 for > 1 week, or severe or cumulative cutaneous reactions, or other grade ¾ non-hematologic toxicity, should have dose reduced to 75 mg/m^2. If reactions continue at the reduced dose, further reduce to 55 mg/m^2 or discontinue drug. Patients dosed initially at 60 mg/m^2 who do not experience febrile neutropenia, ANC < 500/mm^3 for > 1 week, nadir platelets $< 25{,}000$ cells/mm^3, or severe cutaneous reactions, or severe peripheral neuropathy during drug therapy may tolerate higher drug doses and may be dose-escalated. Patients who develop $\geq$ grade 3 peripheral neuropathy should have drug discontinued. (2) Patients with NSCLC dosed initially at 75 mg/m^2 who experience febrile neutropenia, ANC < 500 mg/m^2 for > 1 week, nadir platelets $< 25{,}000$ cells/mm^3, or severe or cumulative cutaneous reactions, or other nonhematologic toxicity grades 3 or 4 should have treatment withheld until toxicity resolves and then have dose reduced to 55 mg/m^2; patients who developμgrade 3 peripheral neuropathy should discontinue docetaxel chemotherapy. (3) Patients with Prostate cancer who experience febrile neutropenia, ANC < 500/mm^3 for > 1 week, or severe or

cumulative cutaneous reactions, or moderate neuro-sensory signs and/or symptoms during docetaxel therapy should have dose reduced from 75mg/m^2 to 60 mg/m^2. If the same symptoms arise at the reduced dosage, the drug should be discontinued.

- Patients should receive dexamethasone premedication (such as 8 mg bid × 3 days starting 1 day prior to taxotere).
- Administration of docetaxel in Europe is not subject to United States Federal Drug Administration recommendations—non-PVC containers and tubing are not required.
- Incomplete cross-resistance between paclitaxel and docetaxel in many tumor types.
- Studies are ongoing to determine the effectiveness of docetaxel 25–40 mg/m^2 weekly in breast cancer, lung cancer, prostate cancer, and other cancers as drug given in this "dose-dense" fashion may act as an antiangiogenesis agent, and may provide less opportunity for malignant cells to develop resistant clones. Weekly dose schedules being studied include 3 weeks of treatment followed by 1 week of rest every 4 weeks, and 6 weekly treatments followed by 2 weeks off every 8 weeks. Docetaxel is administered as a 15–30-minute infusion. Hematologic side effects are uncommon with these schedules. Nonhematologic side effects of weekly therapy include asthenia, fluid retention, nail changes, and tearing. Corticosteroid premedication is often dexamethasone 4 or 8 mg PO q12h × 3 doses beginning the day before treatment.

Potential Toxicities/Side Effects and the Nursing Process

I. POTENTIAL FOR INJURY related to HYPERSENSITIVITY OR ANAPHYLAXIS REACTIONS

Defining Characteristics: Severe hypersensitivity reactions characterized by hypotension, dyspnea and/or bronchospasm, or generalized rash/erythema occurred in 2.2% (2/92) patients who received 3-day dexamethasone premedication. If patient experiences a severe hypersensitivity reaction, patient should not be rechallenged with docetaxel (e.g., patients with bronchospasm, angioedema, systolic BP < 80 mmHg, generalized urticaria). Minor allergic reactions are characterized by flushing, chest tightness, or low back pain.

Nursing Implications: Ensure that patient has taken premedication (e.g., dexamethasone 8 mg bid starting 1 day prior to chemotherapy). Assess baseline VS and mental status prior to drug administration, especially first and second doses of the drug. Monitor VS every 15 minutes, and remain with patient during first 15 minutes of drug infusion, as most reactions occur during the first 10 minutes. Stop drug if cardiac arrhythmia (irregular apical pulse) or hypo- or hypertension occur and discuss continuance of infusion with physician. Recall signs/symptoms of anaphylaxis, and if these occur, stop drug immediately and notify physician. Subjective symptoms are generalized itching, nausea, chest tightness, crampy abdominal pain, difficulty speaking, anxiety, agitation, sense of impending doom, uneasiness, desire to urinate/defecate, dizziness, chills. Objective signs are flushed appearance; angioedema of face, neck, eyelids, hands, feet; localized or generalized urticaria; respiratory distress with or without wheezing, hypotension, cyanosis. Review standing orders or nursing procedure for patient management of anaphylaxis, and be prepared to stop drug immediately if signs/symptoms occur, keep IV line open with 0.9% Sodium Chloride, notify physician, monitor VS, and administer ordered medications, which may include epinephrine 1:1000, hydrocortisone sodium succinate, and diphenhydramine. Teach patient the potential of a hypersensitivity or anaphylactic reaction and to immediately report any unusual symptoms. Depending upon severity of reaction, when planning subsequent treatment discuss with physician administration of antihistamine prior to docetaxel and also gradual increase in infusion rate, e.g., starting at 8-hour rate × 5 minutes, then increasing to 4-hour rate × 5 minutes, then 2-hour rate × 5 minutes, and finally 1-hour infusion rate.

II. POTENTIAL FOR INFECTION AND BLEEDING related to BONE MARROW DEPRESSION

Defining Characteristics: Neutropenia may be severe, is dose-related, is the dose-limiting toxicity, and is noncumulative. Nadir is day 7, with recovery by day 15. Incidence of grade 4 neutropenia (ANC < 500 mm^3) in 2045 patients (any tumor type) with normal hepatic function was 75% at a dose of 100 mg/m^2. Incidence of febrile neutropenia requiring IV antibiotics and/or hospitalization in these patients was 11% and the incidence of septic deaths was 1.6%. Severe thrombocytopenia was less common (8%). However, fatal GI bleeding has been reported in patients with severe hepatic impairment who received docetaxel.

Nursing Implications: Assess LFTs, as dose generally should not be given if SGOT, SGPT, alk phos, or bili suggest moderate to severe hepatic dysfunction (see Special Considerations section). Assess baseline CBC and differential to ensure that ANC is $> 1500/mm^3$, and platelet count is $> 100{,}000/mm^3$ prior to chemotherapy, as well as for signs/symptoms of infection or bleeding. Teach patient signs/symptoms of infection or bleeding and to report these immediately, and teach patient self-care measures to minimize risk of infection and bleeding. This includes avoidance of crowds and proximity to people with infections, and avoidance of OTC aspirin-containing medications. Teach patient self-administration of G-CSF as ordered to prevent severe neutropenia, and EPO as ordered to prevent severe anemia/transfusion requirements. Instruct patient to alternate rest and activity periods, and to report increased fatigue, shortness of breath, or chest pain that might herald severe anemia.

III. POTENTIAL ALTERATION IN ACTIVITY TOLERANCE related to ASTHENIA, FATIGUE

Defining Characteristics: Fatigue, weakness, and malaise may last from a few days to several weeks, but is rarely severe enough to be dose-limiting. Incidence of asthenia (all grades) is 50–66%. Incidence of anemia is 90%, with grades of 3 and 4 occurring in 8% at doses of 100 mg/m^2 and in 9% at doses of 75 mg/m^2.

Nursing Implications: Assess Hgb/HCT prior to each treatment and at nadir counts. Assess patient activity tolerance and ability to do ADLs. Teach patient self-care strategies to minimize exertion, and maximize activity, such as clustering activity during shopping, alternating rest and activity periods, diet, gentle exercise. Teach self-administration of EPO, if ordered, to prevent severe anemia/transfusion requirements. Instruct patient to alternate rest and activity periods, and to report increased fatigue, shortness of breath, or chest pain that might herald severe anemia.

IV. POTENTIAL ALTERATION IN FLUID BALANCE related to FLUID RETENTION

Defining Characteristics: Fluid retention is a cumulative toxicity that may occur in docetaxel treated patients. Peripheral edema usually begins in the lower extremities and may become generalized with weight gain (2kg avg). Fluid retention is not associated with cardiac, renal, or hepatic impairment and may be minimized by use of dexamethasone 8 mg bid for 3 days beginning the day prior to therapy. Severe fluid retention may occur in up to 6.5% of patients despite premedication, and is characterized by generalized edema, poorly tolerated peripheral edema, pleural effusion requiring drainage, dyspnea at rest, cardiac tamponade, or abdominal distention (due to ascites). Fluid retention usually resolves completely within 16 weeks of last docetaxel dose (range, 0–42+ weeks).

Nursing Implications: Ensure that patient takes corticosteroids as ordered to minimize risk of developing fluid retention. Assess baseline weight and skin turgor, especially in the extremities. Assess respiratory status, including breath sounds. Instruct patient to report any alterations in breathing patterns, swelling in the extremities, and weight gain. If patient has preexisting effusion, monitor effusion closely during treatment. If fluid retention occurs, instruct patient to elevate extremities while at rest. Teach patient not to use added salt when eating or cooking. Discuss with physician use of diuretics for new-onset edema, progression of edema, and weight gain, e.g., > 2 lb.

V. POTENTIAL IMPAIRMENT OF SKIN INTEGRITY related to RASH, ALOPECIA, NAIL CHANGES

Defining Characteristics: Maculopapular, violaceous/erythematous, and pruritic rash may occur, usually on the feet and/or hands, but may also occur on arms, face, or thorax. These localized eruptions usually occur within one week of last docetaxel treatment, and are reversible and usually resolve prior to next treatment. Overall, about 50% of patients experience skin problems. Palmar-plantar erythrodysesthia (hand-foot syndrome) may occur but can be minimized by adherence to three-day corticosteroid premedication. Drug extravasation may cause skin discoloration, but no necrosis. Most patients on every-3-week schedules experience alopecia (75% at dose of 100 mg/m^2 and 56% at dose of 75%). Changes in nails may occur in 11–40% of patients, and be severe in 1–2% of patients (hypo- or hyperpigmentation, onycholysis [loss of nail]).

Nursing Implications: Assess skin for any cutaneous changes, such as rash, and any associated symptoms, such as pruritus, and discuss management with physician. If patient develops severe or cumulative skin toxicity, docetaxel dose should be reduced (see Special Considerations). Instruct patient in self-care measures such as avoidance of abrasive skin products and clothing, avoidance of tight-fitting clothes, use of skin emollients appropriate for skin problem, and measures to prevent itching. Discuss potential impact of hair loss prior to drug administration, coping strategies, and plan to minimize body image distortion (e.g., wig, scarf, cap). Assess patient for signs/symptoms of hair loss. Assess patient's response and use of coping strategies; help patient to build on effective strategies. Teach patient self-care measures to preserve hair, such as washing hair with warm water, use of a gentle shampoo and conditioner, use of a softbristle brush, cutting hair short to reduce pressure on hair shaft, and use of a satin pillowcase to minimize friction on hair shaft. Teach patient to wear a wide-brimmed hat and sunglasses when outside, and to use sunscreen (at least SPF 15) on scalp when outdoors without a hat. Assess nails baseline, and teach patient to report changes. Teach patient to keep nails clean and trimmed, not to wear nail polish or imitation nails, and to wear protective gloves when doing house cleaning, and gardening. Teach patient to use a nail hardener if nails appear soft, and to use Lotrimin cream if ordered.

VI. SENSORY/PERCEPTUAL ALTERATIONS related to SENSORY NEUROPATHY

Defining Characteristics: Grade 1–4 Peripheral neuropathy may affect up to 49% of patients (severe 5.5%). Sensory alterations are paresthesias in a glove and stocking distribution, and numbness. There may be loss of sensation symmetrically, of vibration, and of proprioception. Risk is increased in patients receiving both docetaxel and cisplatin, or in patients with prior neuropathy from diabetes mellitus or alcohol. Extremity weakness or transient myalgia may also occur. Patients described spontaneous reversal of symptoms in a median of 9 weeks from onset (range 0–106).

Nursing Implications: Assess baseline neurologic status. Instruct patient to report signs/symptoms of pins and needle sensation, numbness, pain, increased discomfort with certain sensations, especially in the extremities, or motor weakness. Identify patients at risk: prior cisplatin, or having preexisting neuropathies (ethanol- and diabetes mellitus-related). Assess sensory and motor function prior to each treatment, and if abnormality found, assess impact on patient function, safety, independence, and quality of life. Test patient's ability to button a shirt, or pick up a dime from a flat surface. If severely impacting safety or quality of life, discuss with patient and physician drug discontinuance or use of cytoprotective agent. Teach self-care strategies, including maintaining safety when walking, getting up, taking bath, or washing dishes and unable to sense temperature, and the need to keep extremities warm in cold weather. Docetaxel should be discontinued if patient develops grades 3 or 4 peripheral neuropathy (see NCI Common Toxicity Criteria, Appendix II). Grade 3 motor = objective weakness, interfering with ADLs; grade 3 sensory = sensory loss or paresthesia interfering with ADLs; grade 4 motor = paralysis; grade 4 sensory = permanent sensory loss that interferes with function.

VII. ALTERED NUTRITION, LESS THAN BODY REQUIREMENTS, related to NAUSEA AND VOMITING, DIARRHEA, STOMATITIS

Defining Characteristics: Nausea and vomiting may occur, but are mild and preventable with antiemetics. Diarrhea occurs and is mild; incidence of any grade of nausea is 33–42%, vomiting 22%, and diarrhea 22–42%. Incidence of stomatitis is 26–51% (severe 5.5%). Only 1.1% of breast cancer patients who received three-day corticosteroid treatment developed severe mucositis.

Nursing Implications: Premedicate patient with antiemetic. If patient develops nausea and/or vomiting, encourage small, frequent intake of cool, bland foods. Instruct patient to report nausea, and teach self-administration of antiemetic medications. If nausea/vomiting occur and are severe, assess for signs/symptoms of fluid/electrolyte imbalance. Encourage patient to report onset of diarrhea. Teach patient to self-administer antidiarrheal medications if needed. Assess baseline oral mucous membranes. Ensure that patient takes three-day corticosteroid regimen. Teach patient oral assessment, hygiene measures, and to report any alterations.

VIII. ALTERATION IN VISION, POTENTIAL, related to HYPERLACRIMATION

Defining Characteristics: Epiphora or hyperlacrimation occurs as a result of lacrimal duct stenosis. There is inflammation of the conjunctiva and ductal epithelium, which occurs chronically, especially with weekly docetaxel therapy. This appears related to cumulative dose, usually about 300 mg/m^2 and resolves after treatment is stopped. Stenosis of tear ducts is reversible.

Nursing Implications: Assess baseline vision and function of tear ducts. Teach patient that this may occur, and to report it. If this occurs, teach patient to use "Artificial Tears" frequently throughout day, or saline eyewash. Discuss with physician use of prophylactic steroid ophthalmic solution, such as prednisolone acetate 2 gtt bid × 3 days, beginning the day before docetaxel treatment, if patient does not have a history of herpetic eye infection. If the patient is on weekly therapy, discuss with physician treatment break × 2 weeks for symptoms to resolve, and resumption of therapy on a three-week-on, one-week-off schedule.

Drug: doxorubicin hydrochloride (Adriamycin)

Class: Anthracycline antibiotic isolated from streptomycin products, in particular from the rhodomycin products.

Mechanism of Action: Topoisomerase-inhibitor; antitumor antibiotic binds directly to DNA base pairs (intercalates) and inhibits DNA and DNA-dependent RNA synthesis, as well as protein synthesis. Cell cycle specific for S phase.

Metabolism: Excretion of drug predominates in the liver; renal clearance is minor. Alteration in liver function requires modification of doses, whereas with renal failure there is no need to alter doses. Drug is excreted through urine and may discolor urine from 1–48 hours after administration.

Dosage/Range:

- 30–75 mg/m^2 every 3–4 weeks.
- 20–45 mg/m^2/IV for 3 consecutive days.
- For bladder instillation: 3–60 mg/m^2.
- For interperitoneal instillation: 40 mg in 2 L dialysate (no heparin).
- Continuous infusion: Varies with individual protocol.

Drug Preparation:

- Drug will form a precipitate if mixed with heparin or 5-FU. Dilute with 0.9% Sodium Chloride (preservative-free) to produce 2-mg/mL concentration.

Drug Administration:

- This drug is a potent vesicant. Give through a running IV to avoid extravasation, which may lead to ulceration, pain, and necrosis. Be sure to check nursing procedure for administration of a vesicant.

Drug Interactions:

- When given with barbituates there is increased plasma clearance of doxorubicin.
- When given with cyclophosphamide there is risk of hemorrhage and cardiotoxicity.
- When given with mitomycin there is increased risk of cardiotoxicity.
- There is decreased oral bioavailability (decreased serum levels) of digoxin when given together.
- When given with mercaptopurine there is increased risk of hepatotoxicity.
- Incompatible with heparin, forming a precipitate.

Lab Effects/Interference:

- Decreased CBC.
- Increased LFTs.
- Increased uric acid secondary to tumor lysis.

Special Considerations:

- Drug is a potent vesicant. Give through running IV to avoid extravasation and tissue necrosis.
- Give through central line if drug is to be given by continuous infusion.
- Nausea and vomiting are dose-related. Occur in 50% of patients and begin 1–3 hours after administration.
- Causes discoloration of urine (from pink to red for up to 48 hours).
- Skin changes: May cause radiation recall phenomenon—recalls reaction in previously irradiated tissue.
- Potent myelosuppressive agent causes GI toxicities: mucositis, esophagitis, and diarrhea.
- Cardiac toxicity: Dose limit at 550 mg/m^2. Patients may exhibit irreversible CHF. Acute toxicity may be seen within hours after administration. This is unrelated to cumulative dose and may manifest symptoms of pump or conduction dysfunction. Rarely, transient EKG abnormalities, CHF, pericardial effusion (whole syndrome referred to as *myocarditis-pericarditis syndrome*) may occur, which may lead to death of patient.
- Vein discoloration.
- Increased pigmentation in black patients.
- Drug dosage reductions necessary for hepatic dysfunction: 50% dose given for serum bili 1.2–2.9 mg/dL, 25% dose given for serum bili 3 mg/dL.
- Prior chest radiation therapy (XRT): reduce total lifetime dose to 300–350 mg/m^2.

- Concomitant cyclophosphamide administration: may limit to 450 mg/m^2.
- Obesity: use ideal body weight table found in nutrition books to calculate dose.
- Dexrazoxane available for patients at risk for cardiotoxicity but for whom doxorubicin continues to be effective. See Chapter 4.

Potential Toxicities/Side Effects and the Nursing Process

I. POTENTIAL FOR INFECTION AND BLEEDING related to BONE MARROW DEPRESSION

Defining Characteristics: WBC and platelet nadir 10–14 days after drug dose, with recovery from days 15–21. Myelosuppression may be severe but is less severe with weekly dosing.

Nursing Implications: Monitor CBC, WBC, differential, and platelet count prior to drug administration; discuss any abnormalities with physician. Assess for signs/symptoms of infection or bleeding; instruct patient in self-assessment and to report signs/symptoms immediately. Teach patient self-care measures to minimize risk of infection and bleeding, including avoidance of OTC aspirin-containing medications. Drug dosage must be reduced if patient has hepatic dysfunction: 50% reduction of drug dose if bili is 1.2–3.0 mg/dL; 75% reduction if bili is > 3.0 mg/dL.

II. POTENTIAL FOR ALTERATION IN CARDIAC OUTPUT related to ACUTE AND CHRONIC CARDIAC CHANGES

Defining Characteristics: Acutely, pericarditis-myocarditis syndrome may occur during infusion or immediately after (non–life-threatening EKG changes of flat T waves, ST segment, PVCs). With high cumulative doses > 550 mg/m^2 (450 mg/m^2 if concurrent treatment with cardiotoxic drugs or radiation to the chest), cardiomyopathy may occur. Risk is decreased if drug given as continuous infusion.

Nursing Implications: Assess cardiac status prior to chemotherapy administration: signs/symptoms of CHF, quality/regularity and rate of heartbeat, results of prior GBPS or other test of LVEF. Instruct patient to report dyspnea, palpitations, swelling in extremities. Maintain accurate records of total dose; expect GBPS to be repeated periodically during treatment and the drug to be discontinued if there is a significant drop in heart function.

III. POTENTIAL FOR ALTERATION IN NUTRITION, LESS THAN BODY REQUIREMENTS, related to NAUSEA AND VOMITING, ANOREXIA, STOMATITIS

Defining Characteristics: Nausea/vomiting occurs in 50% of patients, is moderate to severe, and is preventable with combination antiemetics. Onset 1–3 hours after drug dose and lasts 24 hours. Anorexia occurs frequently, and stomatitis occurs in 10% of patients.

Nursing Implications: Premedicate with combination antiemetics and continue protection for 24 hours. If patient has a central line, slower infusion of drug over 1 hour decreases nausea/vomiting. Encourage small, frequent feedings of bland foods. Anorexia occurs frequently: teach patient or caregiver to make foods ahead of time and use spices; encourage taking weekly weight. Stomatitis occurs in 10% of patients, and esophagitis may occur in patients who have received prior radiation to the chest. Perform oral assessment prior to drug administration and during posttreatment visits. Teach patient oral hygiene and self-assessment techniques.

IV. POTENTIAL ALTERATION IN SKIN INTEGRITY related to ALOPECIA, RADIATION RECALL, NAIL AND SKIN CHANGES, AND DRUG EXTRAVASATION

Defining Characteristics: Complete alopecia occurs with doses > 50 mg/m^2, occurring after therapy begins. Regrowth usually begins a few months after drug is stopped. Hyperpigmentation of nail beds and dermal creases of hands is greatest in dark-skinned individuals. Skin damage from prior radiation may be reactivated. Adriamycin "flare" may occur during peripheral drug administration, often with urticaria and pruritus, and is due to local allergic reaction. Drug is a potent vesicant and causes SEVERE tissue destruction if drug extravasates.

Nursing Implications: Discuss with patient hair loss, anticipated impact, and strategies to decrease distress, e.g., obtaining wig prior to hair loss. Assess body disturbance from hyperpigmentation and discuss strategies to minimize this, e.g., nail polish for dark nail beds. Drug must be administered via patent IV. If flare occurs, this must be distinguished from extravasation, where there is leakage of drug into the perivascular tissue. Stop or slow drug injection and flush with plain IV solution. Wait to see whether reaction will resolve. If confirmed flare, consider diphenhydramine 25 mg IVP to resolve pruritus and/or urticaria, and then resume administration of drug slowly into freely flowing IV. Assess need for venous access device early. If drug administered as a continuous infusion, IT MUST BE GIVEN VIA A CENTRAL LINE.

V. POTENTIAL SEXUAL DYSFUNCTION related to DRUG EFFECT

Defining Characteristics: Drug is teratogenic, mutagenic, and carcinogenic.

Nursing Implications: Assess patient's/partner's sexual patterns and reproductive goals. Provide information, supportive counseling, and referral as needed. Teach importance of birth control measures as appropriate. Male patients may wish to use a sperm bank prior to therapy.

Drug: doxorubicin hydrochloride liposome injection (Doxil)

Class: Anthracycline antibiotic isolated from streptomycin products.

Mechanism of Action: Topoisomerase-inhibitor; antitumor antibiotic binds directly to DNA base pairs (intercalates) and inhibits DNA and DNA-dependent RNA synthesis, as well as protein synthesis. Cytotoxic in all phases of cell cycle but maximally in S phase. Cell cycle nonspecific. Drug is encapsulated in STEALTH liposomes, which have surface-bound methoxypolyethylene glycol to protect the liposome from detection by blood phagocytes, and thus prolong circulation time. It is believed that the liposomal-encapsulated drug is able to penetrate the tumor through abnormal capillaries (tumor neovasculature) and then, once inside the tumor, accumulates and the drug is released.

Metabolism: Slower clearance from the body than doxorubicin (0.041 L/h/m^2 vs 24–35 L/h/m^2) with resulting larger AUC than a similar dose of doxorubicin. Half-life is approximately 55 hours. Has preferential uptake in Kaposi's sarcoma tumors.

Dosage/Range:
- Treatment of metastic carcinoma of the ovary refractory to both paclitaxel and platinum-based chemotherapy: 50 mg/m^2 every 4 weeks × at least 4 cycles (in clinical trials, median time to response was 4 months).
- AIDS/Kaposi's sarcoma: 20 mg/m^2 IV over 30 minutes once every 3 weeks.
- Dose-reduce for palmar-plantar erythrodysesthesia, hematologic toxicity, or stomatitis.

Drug Preparation:
- Drug is available as 20-mg doxorubicin HCl in a 2-mg/mL concentration.
- Inspect drug for any particulate matter or discoloration; drug is translucent, with red liposomal dispersion.
- Further dilute drug (dose up to 90 mg) in 250 mL 5% Dextrose USP ONLY; use 500 mL 5% Dextrose USP for doses > 90 mg.
- Administer at once or store diluted drug for 24 hours refrigerated at 2–8°C (36–46°F).

Drug Administration:
- Ovarian cancer: Administer IV at an initial rate of 1 mg/min to minimize risk of infusion reaction; if no reaction, increase rate to complete administration over 1 hour.
- AIDS/Kaposi's sarcoma: Administer IV over 30 minutes through patent IV.
- Dose-reduce for hepatic dysfunction: 50% dose reduction for bilirubin 1.2–3.0 mg/dL; 75% dose reduction if bilirubin > 3.0 mg/dL.
- Do not use inline filter.
- Monitor for infusion reactions if drug is infused too rapidly.
- DO NOT ADMINISTER IM OR SQ.

Drug Interactions:
- Doxorubicin may potentiate the toxicity of (1) cyclophosphamide-induced hemorrhagic cystitis; (2) hepatotoxicity of 6-mercaptopurine; (3) radiation toxicity to heart, mucous membranes, skin, liver.

Lab Effects/Interference:
- Decreased CBC.

Special Considerations:
- Drug is an irritant, not a vesicant.
- Acute, infusion-associated reactions may occur (7% incidence) during drug infusion, characterized by flushing, shortness of breath, facial swelling, headache, chills, back pain, chest or throat tightness, and/or hypotension. Infusion should be stopped. If symptoms are minor, infusion may be resumed at a slower rate, but discontinue if symptoms resume.
- Assessment for cardiac toxicity similar to that for doxorubicin should be done since limited information is available as to cardiotoxicity of liposomal doxorubicin at high cumulative doses.
- Drug dosage reductions.
- FDA-approved at this time for treatment of progressive AIDS-related Kaposi's sarcoma after treatment with combination chemotherapy or in patients unable to tolerate combination chemotherapy, and FDA indicated for the treatment of refractory ovarian cancer.
- Drug has been used for the treatment of breast cancer.

Potential Toxicities/Side Effects and the Nursing Process

I. POTENTIAL FOR INFECTION AND BLEEDING related to BONE MARROW DEPRESSION

Defining Characteristics: Dose-limiting toxicity in the treatment of HIV-infected patients, possibly due to HIV disease and/or concomitant medications. Leukopenia occurs in 91% of patients, with anemia and thrombocytopenia (< 150,000/mm^3) less common (55% and 60%, respectively). Neutropenia (< 2000/mm^3) occurred in 85% and ANC (< 500/mm^3) occurred in 13% of patients. In ovarian cancer patients, incidence of neutropenia (<2000cells/mm^3) was 51%, but ANC <500 cells/mm^3 was only 8.3%. Thrombocytopenia ($<150{,}000/mm^3$) occurred in 24%, while severe ($<25{,}000/mm^3$) occurred in 1.1% of patients with ovarian cancer.

Nursing Implications: Monitor CBC, WBC, differential, and platelet count prior to drug administration, and discuss any abnormalities with physician. Assess for signs/symptoms of infection or bleeding, and instruct patient in self-assessment and to report signs/symptoms immediately. Teach patient self-care measures to minimize risk of infection and bleeding, including avoidance of OTC aspirin-containing medications. See drug dosage reductions in Special Considerations section.

II. POTENTIAL FOR ALTERATION IN CARDIAC OUTPUT related to ACUTE AND CHRONIC CARDIAC CHANGES

Defining Characteristics: Experience and data is limited in the cardiotoxicity of liposomal doxorubicin at high cumulative doses. Therefore, the manufacturer recommends the adoption of cardiotoxicity warnings made for doxorubicin HCl. With high cumulative doses >550 mg/m^2 (400 mg/m^2 if concurrent treatment with cardiotoxic drugs such as cyclophosphamide, or radiation to the chest), cardiomyopathy may occur. In clinical trials, the incidence of "possibly or probably related" cardiac-related adverse events, including cardiomyopathy, arrhythmia, heart failure, pericardial effusion, and tachycardia, was 1–5% in patients with AIDS/Kaposi's sarcoma and $<1\%$ in ovarian cancer patients.

Nursing Implications: Assess patient risk (history of prior anthracycline chemotherapy, history of cardiovascular disease). Assess cardiac status prior to chemotherapy administration: signs/symptoms of CHF, quality/regularity and rate of heart beat, results of prior GBPS or other test of LVEF. Instruct patient to report dyspnea, palpitations, swelling in extremities. Maintain accurate records of total dose. Expect GBPS to be repeated periodically during treatment and the drug to be discontinued if there is a significant drop in heart function.

III. POTENTIAL FOR INJURY related to ALLERGIC INFUSION REACTION TO LIPOSOMAL COMPONENT(S)

Defining Characteristics: During the initial infusion, patients may experience an acute reaction characterized by flushing, shortness of breath, facial swelling, headache, chills, back pain, chest or throat tightness, and/or hypotension. Incidence is 5–6%. Reactions generally resolve after the immediate termination of the infusion in several hours to a day, or in some patients, after slowing of the infusion rate. Of those patients who experienced reactions, many were able to tolerate subsequent treatment without problem; however, some patients terminated therapy with liposomal doxorubicin because of the reaction.

Nursing Implications: Assess baseline comfort, vital signs, general condition. Infuse liposomal doxorubicin at 1 mg/min to minimize risk of acute reaction. Teach patient to report signs/symptoms of reaction immediately during infusion, and assess patient frequently during initial infusion. If signs/symptoms occur, stop infusion immediately. Discuss with the physician, but anticipate that if signs/symptoms are mild, infusion will resume at slower rate, and if signs/symptoms are severe, patient may not receive additional liposomal doxorubicin.

IV. POTENTIAL ALTERATIONS IN COMFORT AND ACTIVITY related to PALMAR-PLANTAR ERYTHRODYSESTHESIA (HAND-FOOT SYNDROME)

Defining Characteristics: Incidence is approximately 3.4% in patients receiving a dose of 20 mg/m^2 and 37% in patients with ovarian cancer (16% grades 3 and 4). Toxicity becomes dose-limiting in clinical studies at doses of 60 mg/m^2, or when treatment is administered more frequently than every three weeks. signs/symptoms are swelling, pain, erythema, possibly progressing to desquamation of the skin on hands and feet, and usually occur after six weeks of treatment. Reaction is generally mild, not requiring treatment delays. However, in some patients, reaction can be severe and debilitating, necessitating discontinuance of treatment.

Nursing Implications: Assess baseline skin of patients' hands and feet, and in women with ovarian cancer, skin under areas of pressure, such as under the breasts of women with large breasts or skin folds, before each treatment. Teach patient to report signs/symptoms of reaction (e.g., tingling or burning, redness, flaking of skin in areas of pressure such as soles of feet, under breasts in large-breasted women, small blisters, or small sores on the palms of hands or soles of feet). If signs/symptoms occur, discuss treatment, treatment delays, or discontinuance. Do not use hydrocortisone cream as this will cause greater desquamation of skin.

V. POTENTIAL FOR ALTERATION IN NUTRITION, LESS THAN BODY REQUIREMENTS, related to NAUSEA AND VOMITING, STOMATITIS, DIARRHEA, ANOREXIA

Defining Characteristics: Nausea and/or vomiting occur in 17% and 8% of patients, respectively, are mild to moderate, and are preventable with antiemetics. Stomatitis occurs in 7% of patients. Incidence of diarrhea is 8%. Anorexia may affect 1–5% of patients.

Nursing Implications: Premedicate with antiemetic (dopamine antagonist or serotonin antagonist). Encourage small, frequent feeding of bland foods. Stomatitis occurs in 7% of patients. Perform oral assessment prior to drug administration, and during posttreatment visits. Dose reductions or delay necessary for grades 2–4 stomatitis. Teach patient oral hygiene, and self-assessment techniques. Instruct patient to report diarrhea, and teach self-management strategies for diarrhea.

VI. POTENTIAL FOR ALTERATION IN SKIN INTEGRITY related to ALOPECIA, RASH, PRURITUS, AND RADIATION RECALL

Defining Characteristics: Incidence of alopecia significantly less with liposomal delivery of doxorubicin, and is about 9% in AIDS/Kaposi's sarcoma patients and 15% in women with ovarian cancer. Skin damage from prior radiation may be reactivated. Rash and itching occur in 1–5% of the patients. Rarely, significant skin reactions may occur, such as exfoliative dermatitis. Drug is an irritant, but extravasation should be avoided.

Nursing Implications: Discuss with patient low incidence of hair loss, and to report hair thinning if it occurs. At that time, discuss impact and strategies to decrease distress. Instruct patient to report skin rash or itching, and discuss significance and management with physician. Teach patient to assess for skin changes in prior radiated sites, including mucous membranes, and to report this immediately. Assess and develop management strategies depending on site and extent. Use caution to avoid drug extravasation; if infiltration occurs, stop infusion, apply ice for 30 minutes, and restart a new IV elsewhere.

VII. POTENTIAL ALTERATION IN NUTRITION related to NAUSEA AND/OR VOMITING, STOMATITIS

Defining Characteristics: Nausea occurs in 37% (severe, grade ¾ in 8%) of ovarian cancer patients and 17% of AIDS/Kaposi's sarcoma patients. Vomiting occurs in 22% of ovarian cancer patients and 7.8% of patients with AIDS/Kaposi's sarcoma. Stomatitis occurs in 37% of women with ovarian cancer and is severe in 7.7%; overall incidence in AIDS/Kaposi's sarcoma patients is 6.8%.

Nursing Implications: Assess baseline nutritional status. Teach patient that these side effects may occur and teach self-care measures, including self-assessment, oral hygiene regimen, and to report occurrence of symptoms. Administer antiemetic prior to chemotherapy, especially in ovarian cancer patients, and assess efficacy after treatment. Revise antiemetic regimen as needed to provide complete protection from nausea and/or vomiting. Assess oral mucosa prior to each treatment. If stomatitis develops, dose reduction be considered.

VIII. POTENTIAL SEXUAL DYSFUNCTION related to DRUG EFFECTS

Defining Characteristics: Drug is embryotoxic. Doxorubicin has been shown to be carcinogenic and mutagenic.

Nursing Implications: Assess patient's/partner's sexual pattern and reproductive goals. Provide information, supportive counseling, and referral as needed. Teach importance of birth control measures for female patients of childbearing age. Mothers who are nursing should discontinue nursing during treatment.

IX. ACTIVITY INTOLERANCE related to ASTHENIA AND FATIGUE

Defining Characteristics: Anemia is the most common hematologic event, affecting 52.6% of women with ovarian cancer, but only 25% experienced severe anemia (Hgb < 8 gm/dL). Incidence for patients with AIDS/Kaposi's syndrome overall is 55%, with 4% experiencing severe anemia. Asthenia is more common in women with ovarian cancer, affecting 33%, while patients with AIDS/Kaposi's syndrome had an incidence of 9.9%.

Nursing Implications: Assess activity tolerance, and HCT/Hgb baseline, and prior to each treatment. Teach patients to report any changes in energy and activity level. Teach patients self-care strategies to maximize energy use and conservation. Evaluate efficacy of strategies at each visit, and if ineffective, assist patient to problem solve other alternative solutions, such as friends, volunteers, to help with activities such as shopping, food preparation.

Drug: eniluracil (776C85) (investigational)

Class: Dihydropyrimidine dehydrogenase inhibitor. When used with 5-fluorouracil (5-FU), together they become dihydropyrimidine dehydrogenase inhibitory fluoropyrimidines.

Mechanism of Action: Dihydropyrimidine dehydrogenase (DPD) is the ratelimiting enzyme in the degradation of 5-FU. By inhibiting DPD, eniluracil permits higher and longer sustained serum levels of 5-FU. In early studies, a single dose of eniluracil increased plasma half-life of oral 5-FU 6 times, and produced 100% bioavailability (Smith et al, 2000).

Metabolism: Unclear.

Dosage/Range:
- Per protocol.
- Advanced breast cancer: 10 mg/m^2 bid qd × 28 days, with oral 5-FU 1.0 mg/m^2 bid qd × 28 days, then rest × 7 days, cycle repeated q35 days.
- Dose reduce for hematologic or gastrointestinal toxicity.

Drug Preparation:
- None, oral, available as 2.5-mg and 10-mg tablets.

Drug Administration:

- Take with large amount of water (e.g., 180 mL) at least 1 hour before or after eating.

Drug Interactions:

- Significantly increases 5-FU serum level and half-life, mimicking continuous 5-FU infusions.

Lab Effects/Interference:

- Unknown.

Special Considerations:

- Eniluracil dose is in 10:1 ratio with 5-FU.
- In study of patients with advanced breast cancer, using oral 5-FU concurrently with eniluracil, incidence of grade 1 hand-foot syndrome was 15% and neuropathy 9%, grade 1 only.
- Concurrent oral eniluracil and oral 5-FU well tolerated with low toxicity profile.

Potential Toxicities/Side Effects and the Nursing Process (when used together with oral 5-FU in study on advanced breast cancer)

I. POTENTIAL FOR INFECTION AND BLEEDING related to BONE MARROW DEPRESSION

Defining Characteristics: Neutropenia and thrombocytopenia are dose-related and occur rarely. In the advanced breast cancer trial of oral eniluracil and 5-FU, 30% of patients had granulocytopenia (6% grade 3, 1 patient had neutropenic sepsis), and 42% had thrombocytopenia (3% grade 3). 36% of patients had anemia. Toxicity is enhanced when combined with leucovorin calcium.

Nursing Implications: Assess baseline CBC, WBC, differential, and platelet count prior to chemotherapy, as well as for signs/symptoms of infection or bleeding. Teach patient signs/symptoms of infection or bleeding, and instruct to report these immediately. Teach patient self-care measures to minimize risk of infection and bleeding, including avoidance of crowds, proximity to people with infections, and OTC aspirin-containing medications.

II. ACTIVITY INTOLERANCE, POTENTIAL, related to ASTHENIA, FATIGUE, MALAISE

Defining Characteristics: Malaise and fatigue were reported in 45% of patients, grades 1–2. Anemia occurred in 36% of patients, all grades 1–2.

Nursing Implications: Assess baseline activity level, tolerance, and self-care ability. Teach patients that these side effects are common, but manageable. Assess need for home care assistance and arrange if possible. If not, and needed, involve social worker to assist in coordinating care. Teach patient to alternate rest and activity periods, and strategies to conserve energy.

III. ALTERED NUTRITION, LESS THAN BODY REQUIREMENTS, related to NAUSEA AND VOMITING, STOMATITIS, AND DIARRHEA

Defining Characteristics: Nausea occurred in 27% and vomiting in 12% of patients but was mild. Mucositis was uncommon, affecting 6% of patients, all grades 1–2. Diarrhea can be severe, and in prolonged courses is the dose-limiting toxicity.

Nursing Implications: Premedicate patient with antiemetics (phenothiazines are usually effective), and continue for 24 hours, at least for the first cycle. Encourage small, frequent meals of cool, bland foods. Assess oral mucosa prior to drug administration and instruct patient to report changes. Teach patient oral hygiene measures and self-assessment. Instruct patient to report diarrhea, to self-administer prescribed antidiarrheal medications, and to drink adequate fluids.

Drug: epirubicin HCl (Ellence, Farmorubicin(e), Farmorubicina, Pharmorubicin)

Class: Anthracycline antitumor antibiotic analogue.

Mechanism of Action: Drug complexes with DNA by intercalation of planar rings between DNA base pairs; this inhibits nucleic acid (DNA and RNA) and protein synthesis. This also causes cleavage of DNA by topoisomerase II, causing cell death. Drug also prevents enzymatic separation of DNA, interfering with replication and transcription. Drug also causes the production of cytotoxic free radicals.

Metabolism: Following IV administration, drug rapidly disperses into body tissues and into red blood cells; drug is 77% bound to plasma proteins. Drug is rapidly and extensively metabolized in the liver, excreted primarily through the bilary system, and to a lesser extent in the urine. Drug clearance is reduced in elderly women (35% lower in women aged ≥ 70 years old). Drug clearance is reduced 30% in mild hepatic dysfunction, and 50% in moderate hepatic dysfunction. Drug clearance is reduced (50%) in patients with severe renal impairment (serum creatinine ≥ 5 mg/dL). Dose reductions should be made for patients with hepatic dysfunction and patients with severe renal dysfunction.

Dosage/Range:
FDA indication:

Starting dose as part of adjuvant therapy in patients with axillary node positive breast cancer: 100 mg/m² to 120 mg/m² IV every 3–4 weeks.

- Drug dose may be given in one day, or divided equally and given on day 1 and day 8.
- Other dosing schedules that have been studied: 60–90 mg/m² IV as a single dose q3weeks (dose divided over 2–3 days; 45 mg/m² IV qd × 3 repeated q3weeks; 20 mg IV qweek; intravesicular dose of 50 mg weekly as a 0.1% solution × 8 weeks, with dose reduction for chemical cystitis.

Dose modifications:

- Bone marrow dysfunction: Consider dose of 75–90 mg/m² if patient heavily pretreated (e.g., with existing BMD or bone marrow infiltration by tumor).
- Hepatic dysfunction: Bilirubin 1.2–3 mg/dL or AST 2–4 × Upper Limit of Normal (ULN) = 50% of recommended starting dose; bilirubin > 3 mg/dL or AST > 4 × ULN = 25% of recommended starting dose.
- Renal dysfunction: Consider lower doses if serum creatinine > 5 mg/dL.
- Dosage adjustment after first treatment cycle: Platelet count < 50,000/mm³, ANC < 250/mm³, neutropenic fever, or grades ¾ nonhematologic toxicity: day 1 dose should be 75% of prior day 1 dose. Delay day 1 chemo until platelet count ≥ 100,000/mm³, ANC ≥ 1500/mm³, and nonhematologic toxicities have recovered to ≤ grade 1. If patient is receiving dose divided into day 1 and 8, day 8 dose should be 75% of day 1 dose if platelet counts are 75,000/mm³–100,000/mm³ and ANC is 1000–1499/mm³. If day 8 platelet counts are < 75,000/mm³, ANC < 1000, or grade ¾ nonhematologic toxicity has occurred, omit the day 8 dose.
- Patients receiving dose of 120 mg/m² regimen should also receive prophylactic antibiotic therapy with trimethoprim-sulfamethoxazole or a fluoroquinolone.

Drug Preparation:

- Drug is provided as a preservative-free, ready-to-use solution (50-mg/25-mL and 200-mg/100-mL single-use vials).
- Use within 24 hours of penetration of rubber stopper; discard any unused drug.
- Store unopened vials in refrigerator between 36–46°F (2–8°C).

Drug Administration:

- Drug is a vesicant, so vesicant precautions should be used (check nursing procedure for administration of a vesicant).
- Administer via slow IVP into the tubing of a freely flowing IV infusion of 0.9% NS or 5% Glucose solution over 3–5 minutes, checking blood return every few ml of drug.

Drug Interactions:

- Cytotoxic drugs: Additive toxicity (hematologic and gastrointestinal).

- Cardioactive drugs (e.g., calcium channel blockers): May increase risk of congestive heart failure; use together cautiously, and monitor cardiac function closely during treatment.
- Radiation therapy: Tissue sensitization to cytotoxic effects of radiation therapy; when drug is given after prior radiation therapy, a radiation recall inflammatory reaction may occur at site of prior radiation.
- Cimetidine: Increases drug AUC by 50%, DO NOT use together. Hold cimetidine during treatment with epirubicin.
- Other drugs extensively metabolized by the liver: Changes in hepatic function caused by concomitant therapies may affect clearance of epirubicin; use together with caution, if at all, and monitor for hematologic and gastrointestinal toxicity closely during treatment.

Lab Effects/Interference:
- Decreased white blood and neutrophil cell counts, platelet counts.

Special Considerations:
- Drug is a vesicant, and severe local tissue necrosis will occur if drug infiltrates; avoid IV sites over joints, into small veins, or in veins on arms that have compromised venous or lymphatic drainage.
- Drug should never be given intramuscularly.
- Myocardial toxicity (e.g., CHF) may occur during therapy or months to years after cessation of therapy, and risk increases according to dose. Cumulative doses >900 mg/m^2 should generally not be exceeded. Risk increases with prior anthracycline or anthracenedione therapy, past or concurrent radiation therapy to mediastinal/pericardial area, active or history of cardiovascular disease, or concomitant use of other cardiotoxic drugs.
- Rarely, secondary cancers (e.g., acute myelogenous leukemia) have been reported, and risk is increased when given in combination with other cytotoxic drugs or when doses of anthracycline chemotherapy have been escalated. The estimated risk is 0.2% at three years, and 0.8% at five years.
- Myelosuppression is the dose-limiting toxicity, and severe myelosuppression may occur.
- Doses must be reduced in patients with hepatic dysfunction.
- Drug is mutagenic, carcinogenic, and genotoxic. Men and women of childbearing age should use effective birth control measures.
- Nursing mothers should not breast-feed during chemotherapy treatment.
- Teach patients that urine will be pink-red for the first 1–2 days following drug administration.

Potential Toxicities/Side Effects and the Nursing Process

I. POTENTIAL FOR INFECTION, BLEEDING, FATIGUE related to BONE MARROW DEPRESSION

Defining Characteristics: WBC and platelet nadir 10–14 days after drug dose, with recovery by day 21. Leukopenia and neutropenia may be severe, especially when given with other myelosuppressive chemotherapy. Thrombocytopenia may be severe, and anemia may occur.

Nursing Implications: Monitor CBC, WBC, differential, and platelet count prior to drug administration; discuss any abnormalities with physician. Assess for signs/symptoms of infection or bleeding; instruct patient in self-assessment and to report signs/symptoms immediately. Teach patient self-care measures to minimize risk of infection and bleeding, including avoidance of company of people with colds and OTC aspirin-containing medications. Dose reduction necessary in patients with hepatic dysfunction, as decreased metabolism of drug results in increased serum levels of drug and hematologic toxicity. Patients receiving 120 mg/m^2 dose should also receive prophylactic antibiotic therapy with trimethoprim-sulfamethoxazole or a fluoroquinolone antibiotic.

II. POTENTIAL FOR ALTERATION IN CARDIAC OUTPUT related to ACUTE AND CHRONIC CARDIAC CHANGES

Defining Characteristics: Cardiotoxicity is dose-related, cumulative, and may occur during or months to years after cessation of therapy. The estimated probability of developing clinically evident CHF is 0.9% at a cumulative dose of 500 mg/m^2, 1.6% at 700 mg/m^2, and 3.3% at a cumulative dose of 900 mg/m^2. The risk of CHF increases rapidly with cumulative doses in excess of 900 mg/m^2. Risk of developing cardiotoxicity is increased by history of cardiovascular disease, prior anthracycline or anthrocenedione therapy, prior or concomitant radiation therapy to mediastinum and/or pericardial area, and concomitant use of other cardiotoxic drugs. Cardiotoxicity may be acute (early) or delayed (late). signs/symptoms of early toxicity are not usually of clinical significance, do not predict late cardiotoxicity, and usually do not require change in epirubicin therapy. These include: sinus tachycardia and EKG abnormalities (nonspecific ST–T wave changes, and, rarely, PVCs, VT, bradycardia, atrioventricular and bundle branch block). Delayed cardiotoxocity is related to cardiomyopathy, characterized by decreased left ventricular ejection fraction (LVEF) and classic signs/symptoms of CHF (tachycardia, dyspnea, pulmonary edema, dependent edema, hepatomegaly, ascites, pleural effusion, gallop rhythm). If late cardiotoxicity occurs, it is in the late stages of treatment or within months following treatment, and is cumulative dose-related.

Nursing Implications: Assess cardiac status prior to chemotherapy administration: risk factors and signs/symptoms of CHF, quality/regularity and rate of heartbeat, results of baseline and periodic prior gated blood pool scan (GBPS), multigated radionuclide angiography (MUGA), echocardiogram (ECHO), or other test of LVEF. Instruct patient to report dyspnea, palpitations, and swelling in extremities. Maintain accurate records of total dose; expect GBPS or measure of LVEF to be repeated periodically during treatment and the drug to be discontinued if there is a significant drop in heart function as evidenced by LVEF falling below normal range.

III. POTENTIAL FOR ALTERATION IN NUTRITION, LESS THAN BODY REQUIREMENTS, related to NAUSEA AND VOMITING, DIARRHEA, STOMATITIS

Defining Characteristics: Nausea/vomiting occurs in > 90% of patients, can moderate to severe especially when drug is given together with other emetogenic chemotherapy, and is preventable with combination antiemetics. Onset 1–3 hours after drug dose and lasts 24 hours. Mucositis may occur; stomatitis is most common. Esophagitis is less common but may occur, especially if patient has had prior radiotherapy to the chest. Drug dose must be reduced in patients with hepatic dysfunction; otherwise, increased gastrointestinal toxicity will occur.

Nursing Implications: Assess baseline LFTs, and discuss with physician dose reduction if abnormal. Premedicate with combination antiemetics and continue protection for 24 hours. If patient has a central line, slower infusion of drug over 1 hour decreases nausea/vomiting. Encourage small, frequent feedings of bland foods. Perform oral assessment prior to drug administration and during posttreatment visits. Teach patient oral hygiene and self-assessment techniques. Teach patient to report pain, burning sensation, erythema, erosions, ulcerations, bleeding, or oral infections.

IV. POTENTIAL ALTERATION IN SKIN INTEGRITY related to ALOPECIA, RADIATION RECALL, FACIAL FLUSHING, FLARE REACTION, NAIL/SKIN/ORAL MUCOUS MEMBRANE HYPERPIGMENTATION, AND DRUG EXTRAVASATION

Defining Characteristics: Alopecia is universal, but is reversible, with hair regrowth in two to three months following cessation of therapy. Skin damage and inflammation from prior radiation may be reactivated when drug is given. Drug may cause "flare" reaction or streaking along vein during peripheral drug administration, often with facial flushing, and may be related to excessively rapid drug administration. If it occurs, slow drug administration time, flush line with plain IV solution, and slowly complete therapy. This must be distinguished from extravasation, where there is leakage of drug into the perivascular tissue. Skin and nail hyperpigmentation may occur.

Nursing Implications: Discuss with patient hair loss, anticipated impact, and strategies to decrease distress, e.g., obtaining wig prior to hair loss. Assess body disturbance from hyperpigmentation and discuss strategies to minimize this, e.g., nail polish for dark nail beds. Drug must be administered via patent IV. Local phlebitis or thrombophlebitis may follow a flare reaction, so assess vein path closely, and teach patient to report any pain, erythema, or swelling following drug administration. Drug is a potent vesicant and causes SEVERE tissue destruction if drug extravasates. Teach patient to report any stinging or burning during drug administration, and stop administration if there is any question at all. Assess need for venous access device early.

V. POTENTIAL FOR SEXUAL DYSFUNCTION related to REPRODUCTIVE HAZARD

Defining Characteristics: Drug is genotoxic, mutagenic, and carcinogenic. In laboratory animals receiving very high doses of the drug, testicular atrophy occurred. Drug may cause irreversible amenorrhea in premenopausal women (premature menopause).

Nursing Implications: Assess patient's/partner's sexual patterns and reproductive goals. Provide information, supportive counseling, and referral as needed. Teach importance of birth control measures as appropriate. Male patients may wish to use a sperm bank, and women may wish to investigate cryopreservation of oocytes prior to therapy.

Drug: estramustine (Estracyte, Emcyt)

Class: Alkylating agent.

Mechanism of Action: Acts as a weak alkylator at usual therapeutic concentrations. A chemical combination of mechlorethamine and estradiol phosphate, estramustine is believed to selectively enter cells with estrogen receptors, where the drug acts as an alkylating agent due to bischlorethyl side-chain and liberated estrogens. Believed to have antimicrotubule activity. Cell cycle nonspecific.

Metabolism: Well-absorbed orally, metabolized in liver, partly excreted in urine. Induces a marked decline in serum calcium and phosphate levels.

Dosage/Range:
- 600 mg/m^2 (15 mg/kg) orally daily in three divided doses (range, 10–16 mg/kg/day in most studies with evaluation after 30–90 days).
- IV: Available for investigational use; 150 mg IV initially, then may increase to 300 mg/day per protocol.

Drug Preparation:
- Available in 140-mg capsules.
- Store in refrigerator (2–8°C [36–46°F]); may be stored at room temperature for 24–48 hours.
- IV: Dissolve in at least 10 mL sterile water.

Drug Administration:
- Oral with water, at least 1 hour before or 2 hours after meals.
- IV (investigational): Slow IVP via IV containing 5% Dextrose.

Drug Interactions:
- Drug/food: milk, milk products, and Ca++ rich foods may decrease drug absorption.
- Synergy with vinblastine.

Lab Effects/Interference:
- Changes in Ca.
- Increased LFTs, RFTs.
- May affect certain endocrine and LFTs because it contains estrogen.

Special Considerations:
- Avoid taking drug with milk, milk products, and calcium-rich foods (i.e., antacids), as this will delay or impair drug absorption.
- Contraindicated or to be used with great caution in patients who are children or who have thrombophlebitis or thromboembolic disorders, peptic ulcers, severe hepatic dysfunction, cardiac disease, hypertension, or diabetes.
- IV preparation is a vesicant; avoid extravasation.
- Transient perineal itching and pain after IV administration.

Potential Toxicities/Side Effects and the Nursing Process

I. POTENTIAL ALTERATION IN TISSUE PERFUSION related to THROMBOPHLEBITIS, THROMBOSIS

Defining Characteristics: Increased risk of clot formation, with risk for development of thrombophlebitis, pulmonary emboli, myocardial infarction, and cerebrovascular accident.

Nursing Implications: Assess patient risk; drug is contraindicated in patients with thrombophlebitis or thromboembolic disorders, unless caused by the malignancy. Should be used cautiously in these patients, and in those patients with coronary artery disease. Drug may worsen CHF. Assess baseline cardiac and peripheral vascular status, including signs/symptoms of CHF. Monitor blood pressure and glucose tolerance during therapy. Instruct patient to report immediately any signs/symptoms, e.g., dyspnea, edema, pain, and erythema in legs.

II. BODY IMAGE DISTURBANCE related to GYNECOMASTIA

Defining Characteristics: Mild to moderate breast enlargement may occur, with nipple tenderness initially.

Nursing Implications: Teach patient about potential side effects; discuss potential impact on body image and comfort. Encourage patient to verbalize feelings; provide information and emotional support.

III. POTENTIAL ALTERATION IN COMFORT related to PERINEAL SYMPTOMS, HEADACHE, RASH, URTICARIA, TRANSIENT PARESTHESIAS (IV)

Defining Characteristics: Perineal itching and pain, as well as transient paresthesias of the mouth, may occur after IV administration (investigational). Other symptoms that may accompany oral dosing are rash, pruritus, dry skin, peeling skin of fingertips, thinning hair, night sweats, lethargy, pain in eyes, and breast tenderness.

Nursing Implications: Assess patient for occurrence of symptoms and discuss measures for symptomatic relief.

IV. POTENTIAL FOR ALTERATION IN NUTRITION, LESS THAN BODY REQUIREMENTS, related to NAUSEA AND VOMITING, DIARRHEA, HEPATIC DYSFUNCTION

Defining Characteristics: Nausea and vomiting occur at higher dosing; tolerance may develop, but dose may need to be reduced. Nausea and vomiting may be delayed but become intractable and necessitate discontinuance of the drug. Diarrhea occurs occasionally. Mild elevations in liver function tests may occur (LDH, SGOT, bili) with or without jaundice, but are usually self-limiting. Abnormal Ca++ and P levels may occur.

Nursing Implications: Assess baseline nutritional fluid and electrolyte status. Premedicate with antiemetics prior to drug administration and continue through treatment. Assess baseline LFTs and Ca++ and P levels; monitor during therapy and discuss any abnormalities with physician. Monitor daily or weekly weights.

Drug: estrogens: diethylstilbestrol (DES), ethinyl estradiol (Estinyl), conjugated estrogen (Premarin), chlorotrianisene (Tace)

Class: Hormones.

Mechanism of Action: Unknown; estrogens change the hormonal milieu of the body.

Metabolism: Metabolized mainly in the liver. Undergoes enterohepatic recirculation. DES is metabolized more slowly than natural estrogens.

Dosage/Range:
- DES: Prostate cancer: 1–3 mg PO daily; breast cancer: 5 mg PO tid.
- Diethylstilbestrol diphosphate: Prostate cancer: 50–200 mg PO tid, 0.5–1.0 g IV daily × 5 days, then 250–1000 mg each week.
- Chlorotrianisene: 1–10 mg PO tid.
- Ethinyl estradiol: 0.5–1.0 mg PO tid.

Drug Preparation:
- None.

Drug Administration:
- Oral.

Drug Interactions:
- None significant.

Lab Effects/Interference:
- Increased Ca.
- Increased T_4 levels.
- Increased clotting factors.
- Decreased serum folate.

Special Considerations:
- Long-term dosage of DES in men has been associated with cardiovascular deaths. Maximum dose should be 1 mg tid for prostate cancer.
- Can cause inaccurate laboratory results (liver, adrenal, thyroid).
- Causes rapid rise in serum calcium in patients with bony metastases; watch for symptoms of hypercalcemia.

Potential Toxicities/Side Effects and the Nursing Process

I. POTENTIAL FOR INJURY related to THROMBOEMBOLIC COMPLICATIONS, HYPERCALCEMIA, SODIUM AND WATER RETENTION, AND CARDIOTOXICITY

Defining Characteristics: Thromboembolic complications are infrequent but serious, and increased risk occurs with long-term use and higher doses. Hypercalcemia occurs in 5–10% of women with breast cancer metastatic to bone, appears in first two weeks of therapy, and is aggravated by preexisting renal disease. There is an increased risk of cardiovascular-related deaths, especially in men on high-dose estrogens for prostate cancer. Drug should be used cautiously, if at all, in patients with underlying cardiac, renal, or hepatic disease.

Nursing Implications: Assess risk (preexisting cardiac, hepatic, and renal disease), baseline cardiac, and vascular status; discuss abnormalities with physician. Monitor status during therapy. Teach patient to report signs/symptoms of edema, dyspnea, localized swelling, pain, tenderness, erythema, and CNS changes. Teach female patient signs/symptoms of hypercalcemia (drowsiness, increased thirst, constipation, increased urine output) and to report this. Monitor Ca++ level in women with metastatic breast cancer closely during first few weeks of therapy.

II. ALTERATION IN NUTRITION, LESS THAN BODY REQUIREMENTS, related to NAUSEA AND VOMITING

Defining Characteristics: Occurs in 25% of patients; intensity is related to specific drug and dose. Tolerance occurs after a few weeks of therapy.

Nursing Implications: Inform patient that this may occur; teach self-administration of antiemetics prior to drug administration per physician order, and to take drug at bedtime to decrease nausea. Discuss with physician starting patient at low dose, with increase as tolerated.

III. ALTERATION IN MALE SEXUAL FUNCTION related to GYNECOMASTIA, LOSS OF LIBIDO, IMPOTENCE, AND VOICE CHANGE

Defining Characteristics: Gynecomastia may be prevented by pretreatment of breast with low dose of radiotherapy. Feminine characteristics disappear when therapy is stopped.

Nursing Implications: Explore with patient and partner reproductive and sexual patterns and impact that chemotherapy may have. Provide information, supportive counseling, and referral as indicated. Since alternative, superior hormonal manipulative drugs are available, discuss these with physician.

IV. POTENTIAL FOR FEMALE SEXUAL DYSFUNCTION related to BREAST TENDERNESS/ENGORGEMENT, UTERINE PROLAPSE, AND URINARY INCONTINENCE

Defining Characteristics: Breast engorgement may occur in postmenopausal women; uterine prolapse and exacerbation of preexisting uterine fibroids with possible uterine bleeding may occur, as may urinary incontinence.

Nursing Implications: Explore with patient sexual and reproductive patterns, and any impact the drug may have. Provide information, supportive counseling, and referral as needed. Discuss with physician alternative hormonal manipulative drugs as needed.

Drug: etoposide (VP-16, VePesid, Etopophos)

Class: Plant alkaloid, a derivative of the mandrake plant (mayapple plant).

Mechanism of Action: Inhibits DNA synthesis in S and G_2 so that cells do not enter mitosis. Causes single-strand breaks in DNA. Cell cycle specific for S and G_2 phases.

Metabolism: VP-16 is rapidly excreted in the urine and, to a lesser extent, in the bile. About 30% of drug is excreted unchanged. Binds to serum albumin (94%) and then becomes extensively tissue-bound.

Dosage/Range:
- 50–100 mg/m^2 IV qd × 5 days (testicular cancer) q3–4 weeks.
- 75–200 mg/m^2 IV qd × 3 days (small-cell lung cancer) q3–4 weeks.
- Many other doses based on tumor type being treated (e.g., lymphomas, ANLL, bladder, prostate, uterus, Kaposi's sarcoma).
- Oral dose is twice the intravenous dose, rounded to the nearest 50 mg.
- High dose (bone marrow transplantation): 750–2400 mg/m^2 IV, or 10–60 mg/kg over 1–4 hours to 24 hours, usually combined with other cytotoxic agents or total body irradiation.
- Dose modification if renal or hepatic dysfunction (see Special Considerations section).

Drug Preparation:
- Available in 5-cc (100-mg) vial as VePesid; the 100-mg Etopophos vial is reconstituted with 5 mL or 10 mL Normal Saline, D5W, sterile water, bacteriostatic sterile water, or bacteriostatic Normal Saline with benzyl alcohol to 20 mg/mL or 10 mg/mL, respectively. May be further diluted with NS or D5W to 0.1 mg/mL final concentration.
- Oral capsules are available in 50-mg and 100-mg capsules, and should be stored in the refrigerator.

Drug Administration:
- IV infusion: VePesid over 30–60 minutes to minimize risk of hypotension and bronchospasm (wheezing). In some instances, a test dose may be infused slowly (0.5 mL in 50 0.9% Sodium Chloride) and the remaining drug infused if no untoward reaction after 5 minutes. Etopophos: IVB over 5 minutes as drug is significantly less likely to cause hypotension.
- Stability: Drug must be diluted with either 5% Dextrose Injection USP or 0.9% Sodium Chloride solution and is stable 96 hours in glass and 48 hours in plastic containers at room temperature (25°C [77°F]) under normal fluorescent light at a concentration of 0.2 mg/mL.
- Inspect for clarity of solution prior to administration.
- Oral administration: may give as a single dose up to 400 mg; otherwise, divide dose into 2–4 doses.

Drug Interactions:

- Enhances warfarin action by increasing prothrombin time (PT); need to monitor closely.
- Increased toxicity of methotrexate when given concurrently.
- Cyclosporin: additive cytotoxicity when given concurrently.

Lab Effects/Interference:

- Increased PT with patients on warfarin.
- Increased LFTs, metabolic acidosis with higher doses.

Special Considerations:

- Nadir 7–14 days after treatment.
- Dose modifications: reduce drug dose by 50% if bili > 1.5 mg/dL, by 75% if bili > 3.0 mg/dL. Reduce drug 25% if creatinine clearance 10–50 mL/min; reduce by 50% if creatinine clearance < 10 mL/min.
- Synergistic drug effect in combination with cisplatin.
- Radiation recall may occur when combined therapies are used.
- Patients receiving high-dose therapy are at risk for the development of second malignancy or ethanol intoxication (injection contains polyethylene glycol with absolute alcohol).
- VePesid: drug stability is concentration-dependent, while Etopophos is prepared as a phosphate esther, which negates the need for concentration-dependent stability (equally stable for 24 hours at concentrations of 20 mg/mL to 0.1 mg/mL).

Table 1.9

Etoposide concentration (mg/mL)	5% Dextrose	0.9% Sodium Chloride
2	0.5 hour*	0.5 hour*
1	2 hours	2 hours
0.6	8 hours	8 hours
0.4	48 hours	48 hours
0.2	96 hours	96 hours

* Check for fine precipitate.

Source: Data from Dorr RT, Von Hoff DD (1994) *Cancer Chemotherapy Handbook* (2nd ed). Norwalk, CT: Appleton & Lange, p 462.

Potential Toxicities/Side Effects and the Nursing Process

I. POTENTIAL FOR INJURY related to ALLERGIC REACTION, HYPOTENSION, ANAPHYLAXIS DURING DRUG INFUSION

Defining Characteristics: Bronchospasm (wheezing) may occur, with or without fever, chills; hypotension may occur during rapid infusion. Anaphylaxis may occur, but is rare.

Nursing Implications: Infuse drug over at least 30–60 minutes in correct amount of IV solution (stability related to volume). Monitor temperature, vital signs prior to drug administration, and periodically during treatment. Remain with patient during first 15 minutes of infusion and assess for signs/symptoms of bronchospasm. Discontinue drug and notify physician if bronchospasm or signs/symptoms of anaphylacticlike reaction occur. Maintain patent IV, monitor VS, and have ready epinephrine, diphenhydramine, and hydrocortisone, as well as emergency equipment. Be familiar with institution's practice guidelines for management of anaphylaxis.

II. POTENTIAL FOR INFECTION AND BLEEDING related to BONE MARROW DEPRESSION

Defining Characteristics: Nadir 10–14 days after drug dose, with recovery on days 21–22. Neutropenia may be severe. Profound bone marrow suppression when given in high doses for bone marrow/stem cell rescue.

Nursing Implications: Monitor CBC, WBC, differential, and platelet count prior to chemotherapy and at expected nadir. Assess for signs/symptoms of infection or bleeding prior to drug administration; instruct patient in self-assessment and to report signs/symptoms immediately. Teach patient self-care measures to minimize risk of infection and bleeding, including avoidance of OTC aspirin-containing medications.

III. ALTERED NUTRITION, LESS THAN BODY REQUIREMENTS, related to NAUSEA AND VOMITING, ANOREXIA

Defining Characteristics: Nausea and vomiting are usually mild, occurring soon after infusion. Oral dosing has higher incidence of nausea/vomiting. Anorexia is mild but may be severe with oral dosing. Severe nausea and vomiting when given in high doses, requiring aggressive, maximal antiemesis. In addition, hepatitis, stomatitis, and metabolic acidosis may occur with high-dose therapy.

Nursing Implications: Premedicate with antiemetics and continue prophylactically for at least 4–6 hours after drug administration. Encourage small feedings of bland, cool foods and liquids; encourage spices as desired. Consult dietitian if anorexia is severe. Patients receiving high-dose therapy should have baseline and periodic assessment of laboratory parameters (e.g., LFTs and chemistries), as well as assessment of oral mucosa. Teach patients self-care, including oral assessment, use of oral hygiene regimen, and to report pain, burning, oral lesions.

IV. BODY IMAGE DISTURBANCE related to ALOPECIA

Defining Characteristics: Incidence is 20–90% and is dose-dependent; regrowth may occur between drug cycles.

Nursing Implications: Discuss with patient possible hair loss and potential coping strategies, including obtaining wig or cap. If hair loss is complete, instruct patient to wear cap or scarf at night to prevent loss of body heat in cold climates.

V. POTENTIAL SEXUAL DYSFUNCTION related to DRUG EFFECTS

Defining Characteristics: Drug is mutagenic and teratogenic.

Nursing Implications: Explore with patient and partner sexual patterns and reproductive goals. Teach about need for contraception as appropriate. Provide information, emotional support, and referral as needed.

VI. ALTERED SKIN INTEGRITY related to RADIATION RECALL, PERIVASCULAR IRRITATION IF DRUG INFILTRATES, AND SKIN LESIONS WITH HIGH DOSE THERAPY

Defining Characteristics: Drug is a radiosensitizer and an irritant. Patients receiving high-dose therapy may develop bullae on the skin (similar to Steven's Johnson syndrome).

Nursing Implications: Assess skin in area of prior radiation when combined therapies are given as well as mucous membranes. Drug may need to be withheld until skin healing occurs if radiation recall results in skin breakdown. Teach patient wound-management techniques. Use careful venipuncture and infuse drug through patent IV over 30–60 minutes, diluted according to manufacturer's specifications. Teach patients receiving high-dose therapy to report any skin changes.

VII. ALTERATION IN CARDIAC OUTPUT related to RARE MYOCARDIAL INFARCTION, ARRHYTHMIAS

Defining Characteristics: Rare myocardial infarction has been reported after prior mediastinal XRT in patients receiving etoposide-containing regimens. Arrhythmias are uncommon but may occur, especially in patients with preexisting coronary artery disease.

Nursing Implications: Monitor patient during infusion and instruct patient to report any unusual sensations. Discuss any abnormalities with physician.

VIII. SENSORY/PERCEPTUAL ALTERATION related to NEUROTOXICITY

Defining Characteristics: Peripheral neuropathies may occur but are uncommon and mild.

Nursing Implications: Assess motor and sensory function prior to drug administration. Instruct patient to report any changes in sensation or function. Discuss any abnormalities with physician. Encourage patient to verbalize feelings about discomfort and sensory loss, and discuss alternative coping strategies.

Drug: exemestane (Aromasin)

Class: Steroidal aromatase inactivator.

Mechanism of Action: Aromatase converts adrenal and ovarian androgens into estrogen, peripherally, in postmenopausal women. Exemestane acts as a false substrate (looks like androstenedione) and binds irreversibly to the aromatase enzyme, making it inactive ("suicide inhibition"). This results in a significant decrease (up to 95%) in circulating estrogen levels in postmenopausal women without affecting other adrenal enzymes. In the absence of estrogen, the stimulus for breast cancer growth is removed.

Metabolism: Oral drug is rapidly absorbed from the GI tract, with plasma levels increased by about 40% if taken after a high-fat breakfast. Drug is extensively distributed into the tissues, and is highly protein-bound (90%). Drug is extensively metabolized in the liver by the P450 3A4 (CYP 3A4) isoenzyme system, and excreted equally in urine and feces. After a single dose of 25 mg, maximal suppression of circulating estrogen occurs 2–3 days after the dose, and lasts for 4–5 days. In patients with either hepatic or renal insufficiency, the dose of exemestane was three times higher than in patients with normal liver or renal function. This does not require dosage adjustment, but studies looking at the safety of chronic dosing in these groups of patients have not been done.

Dosage/Range:
- 25 mg tab PO daily.

Drug Preparation:
- None. Store tablets at 77°F (25°C).

Drug Administration:
- Oral, once daily, after a meal.

Drug Interactions:
- Although metabolized by the P450 3A4 (CYP 3A4) isoenzyme system, it is unlikely that inhibitors of this system will significantly increase exemestane

serum levels; however, manufacturer cautions that known inducers of the enzyme system may decrease serum levels, and should be used together cautiously (see Chapter 15).

Lab Effects/Interference:
- Lymphopenia (20% incidence).
- Elevated LFTs (AST, ALT, alk phos, GGT) rarely.

Special Considerations:
- Drug is indicated for the 1) adjuvant treatment of post-menopausal women with ER positive early breast cancer who received 2–3 years of tamoxifen and who are switched to exemestane for completion of a total of five consecutive years of adjuvant hormonal therapy and 2) treatment of advanced breast cancer in postmenopausal women ONLY, whose disease has progressed following tamoxifen therapy. Drug should not be used for premenopausal women as the presence of estrogen may interfere with exemestane action.
- Drug should not be given to pregnant women.
- Drug is well tolerated, with mild to moderate side effects.
- Differs from other selective aromatase inhibitors in that drug irreversibly binds to aromatase, and androgens cannot displace drug from this enzyme. Body must synthesize new aromatase to start estrogen production again.
- Drug similar to or superior to megestrol acetate after tamoxifen failure in metastatic breast cancer (Kaufmann et al, 2000).

Potential Toxicities/Side Effects and the Nursing Process

I. ALTERATION IN ACTIVITY related to FATIGUE

Defining Characteristics: Overall incidence in studies is 22%, while incidence considered drug-related or of indeterminate cause is 8%.

Nursing Implications: Assess baseline activity tolerance, and self-care ability. Teach patient that fatigue may occur, but is usually mild to moderate. Teach patient to alternate rest and activity. Teach patient to manage activities of daily living using energy-saving strategies, e.g., shopping, cooking. Teach patient to accept assistance from friends and family as needed.

II. ALTERATION IN COMFORT related to HOT FLASHES, INCREASED SWEATING, PAIN

Defining Characteristics: Incidence of events attributable to exemestane were hot flashes, 13%, and increased sweating, 4%. In total evaluation of all adverse events, all patients, pain was reported in 13%.

Nursing Implications: Assess patient baseline comfort, and incidence and tolerance of hot flashes and increased sweating. Assess whether patient has any pain, and effectiveness of current pain-management regimen. Teach patient self-care strategies to maximize comfort, to keep cool (e.g., light, loose clothing, fans, cool drinks) and dry (e.g., use of corn starch after bathing, fan), and to minimize any painful discomfort (e.g., depending upon type and location of pain, OTC analgesics, application of heat, cold, Tiger Balm).

III. ALTERATION IN NUTRITION, POTENTIAL related to NAUSEA, INCREASED APPETITE

Defining Characteristics: Nausea appeared drug-related or of indeterminate cause in 9% of patients, and 3% of patients noted an increased appetite. 8% of patients receiving drug complained of weight gain (greater than 10% of baseline). These side effects are mild to moderate if they occur.

Nursing Implications: Assess baseline nutritional status, optimal and desired weight, and any changes. Teach patient to report nausea or weight gain. Teach patient strategies to minimize nausea (e.g., dietary modification, taking drug after meals) if it occurs, and discuss with physician antiemetic medication if dietary modification not effective. If patient experiences weight gain, discuss patient interest in gentle exercising, such as progressive muscle resistance, which would encourage weight gain as lean body mass rather than fat.

IV. SENSORY/PERCEPTION ALTERATIONS, POTENTIAL, related to DEPRESSION, INSOMNIA

Defining Characteristics: While not reported as side effects considered drugrelated or of indeterminate cause, depression and insomnia occurred in 13% and 11%, respectively, of patients participating in the clinical trials.

Nursing Implications: Assess baseline affect, use of effective coping strategies in dealing with disease and treatment, and usual sleep patterns. Teach patient to report changes in mood, such as depression, and difficulty falling asleep, or early awakening. If this occurs, further assess symptom, and suggest self-care strategies to minimize symptom. If nonpharmacologic measures are ineffective, discuss use of antidepressant or sleeping medication with physician, depending upon assessment.

Drug: floxuridine (FUDR, 2′-Deoxy-5-fluorouridine)

Class: Antimetabolite.

Mechanism of Action: Antimetabolite (fluorinated pyrimidine) that is metabolized to 5-FU when given by IV bolus, or metabolized to 5-FUDR-MP 5-fluoro-2′-deoxyuridine-5′-monophosphate when smaller doses are given, by continuous infusion intraarterially. FUDR-MP is four times more effective in inhibiting the enzyme thymidine synthetase than 5-FU. The inhibition prevents the synthesis of thymidine, an essential component of DNA, resulting in interruption of DNA synthesis and cell death. Other FUDR metabolites inhibit RNA synthesis. Drug is cell cycle specific, with activity during the S phase.

Metabolism: When given IV, drug is transformed to 5-FU; 70–90% of drug is extracted by liver on first pass. Metabolites are excreted by kidneys and lungs. Continuous infusion decreases metabolism of drug with more of the drug being converted to the active metabolite FUDR-MP.

Dosage/Range:
- Intraarterially by slow infusion pump: 0.3 mg/kg/day (range, 0.1–0.6 mg/kg/day), OR
- 5–20 mg/m^2/day every day × 14–21 days.
- IV: Investigational.

Drug Preparation:
- Reconstitute 500-mg vial of lyophilized powder with sterile water, then dilute with 0.9% Sodium Chloride.

Drug Administration:
- Usually administered by slow intraarterial infusion using a surgically placed catheter or percutaneous catheter in a major artery.
- H_2 antagonist antihistamine (i.e., ranitidine 150 mg PO bid) administered concurrently during intraarterial infusion to prevent development of peptic ulcer disease.

Drug Interactions:
- None significant.

Lab Effects/Interference:
- Decreased WBC, platelets.
- PT, total protein, sedimentation rate (abnormal values).
- Increased LFTs.

Special Considerations:
- Drug usually given for 14 days, then heparinized saline for 14 days to maintain line patency.
- Dose reductions or infusion breaks may be necessary depending on toxicity.
- FDA-approved for intrahepatic arterial infusion only.

Potential Toxicities/Side Effects and the Nursing Process

I. ALTERED NUTRITION, LESS THAN BODY REQUIREMENTS, related to NAUSEA/VOMITING, ANOREXIA, STOMATITIS/ ESOPHOPHARYNGITIS, DIARRHEA, GASTRITIS, HEPATIC DYSFUNCTION

Defining Characteristics: Nausea and vomiting occur infrequently and are mild; anorexia is common. Mucositis is milder than 5-FU when administered intrahepatically, but more severe when given via carotid artery. Diarrhea is mild to moderately severe. Gastritis may occur, with abdominal cramping and pain. Incidence is greater in patients receiving hepatic artery infusion. Duodenal ulcers may occur in 10% of patients, be painless, and lead to gastric outlet obstruction and vomiting. Chemical hepatitis may be severe, with increased alk phos in patients receiving drug via hepatic artery infusions.

Nursing Implications: Premedicate with antiemetics as ordered and teach patient in self-administration of prescribed antiemetics. Encourage small, frequent feedings of cool, bland foods. If intractable nausea and vomiting, severe diarrhea, or severe cramping occur, notify physician, stop drug, and infuse heparinized saline. Teach patient oral assessment and oral hygiene regimen, and instruct to report any signs/symptoms of stomatitis, esophopharyngitis. Instruct patient to report diarrhea. Teach self-care measures, including diet modification and self-administration of prescribed antidiarrheal medication. Assess for signs/symptoms of abdominal stress, cramping prior to and during infusion. Discuss with physician use of antacids and antisecretory medications. Catheter placement should be verified prior to each infusion cycle, and inadvertent drug infusion into gastric/duodenal-supplying arteries should be investigated. Monitor LFTs prior to drug initiation, during treatment, and at end of 14-day cycle. Discuss abnormalities and dose reductions with physician. Assess patient for signs/symptoms of liver dysfunction: lethargy, weakness, malaise, anorexia, fever, jaundice, icterus.

II. POTENTIAL FOR INJURY related to INTRAARTERIAL CATHETER PROBLEMS

Defining Characteristics: Catheter problems that may occur include leakage, arterial ischemia or aneurysm, bleeding at catheter site, catheter occlusion, thrombosis or embolism of artery, vessel perforation or dislodged catheter, infection, and biliary sclerosis.

Nursing Implications: Assess catheter carefully prior to each cycle of therapy for patency, signs/symptoms of infection. Ensure that catheter position and patency are determined prior to each cycle of therapy; do not force flushing solution—reaccess and try again. If still unsuccessful, notify physician.

III. SENSORY/PERCEPTUAL ALTERATIONS related to HAND-AND-FOOT SYNDROME AND OTHER CNS SYMPTOMS

Defining Characteristics: Hand-and-foot syndrome occurs in 30–40% of patients (numbness, sensory changes in hands and feet). Uncommonly, cerebellar ataxia, vertigo, nystagmus, seizures, depression, hemiplegia, hiccups, lethargy, and blurred vision may occur.

Nursing Implications: Assess baseline neurologic status prior to and during therapy. Teach patient that hand/foot syndrome may occur and instruct to report signs/symptoms. Discuss with physician use of pyridoxine 50 mg tid to prevent hand/foot syndrome. Assess ability to do activities of daily living and level of comfort.

IV. ALTERATION IN SKIN INTEGRITY related to LOCALIZED ERYTHEMA, DERMATITIS, NONSPECIFIC SKIN TOXICITY, OR RASH

Defining Characteristics: Erythema, dermatitis, pruritus, or rash may occur.

Nursing Implications: Assess for skin changes. Assess impact on comfort and body image. Teach patient self-care.

V. POTENTIAL FOR INFECTION AND BLEEDING related to BONE MARROW DEPRESSION

Defining Characteristics: Occurs rarely when FUDR is given as a single agent via continuous intraarterial infusion.

Nursing Implications: Assess baseline WBC, neutrophil count, and platelets, during treatment and at completion of 14-day infusion. Discontinue drug infusion if WBC < 3500/mm^3 or if platelet count < 100,000/mm^3, or per established physician orders; refill pump with heparinized saline.

Drug: fludarabine phosphate (Fludara)

Class: Antimetabolite.

Mechanism of Action: Inhibits DNA synthesis, probably by inhibiting DNA-polymerase-alpha, ribonucleotide reductase, and DNA primase.

Metabolism: Drug is rapidly converted to the active metabolite 2-fluoroara-A when given intravenously. The drug's half-life is about 10 hours. The major route of elimination is via the kidneys, and approximately 23% of the active drug is excreted unchanged in the urine.

Dosage/Range:

- 25 mg/m^2 IV over 30 minutes daily × 5 days, repeated every 28 days.

Drug Preparation:

- Aseptically add 2 mL sterile water for injection USP to the vial, resulting in a final concentration of 25 mg/mL. The drug may then be diluted further in 100 mL of 5% Dextrose or 0.9% Sodium Chloride. Once reconstituted, the drug should be used within 8 hours.

Drug Administration:

- IV infusion over 30 minutes.

Lab Effects/Interference:

- Decreased CBC.
- Tumor lysis syndrome.

Special Considerations:

- Indicated for the treatment of patients with B-cell chronic lymphocytic leukemia (CLL) who have not responded to treatment with at least one standard alkylating agent-containing regimen, or who have progressed on treatment.
- Dose-dependent toxicity: overdosage (four times recommended dose) has been associated with delayed blindness, coma, and death.
- Do not administer in combination with pentostatin, as fatal pulmonary toxicity can occur.
- Administer cautiously in patients with renal insufficiency.
- Drug is teratogenic.
- Drug may cause severe bone marrow depression.

Potential Toxicities/Side Effects and the Nursing Process

I. INFECTION AND BLEEDING related to BONE MARROW DEPRESSION

Defining Characteristics: Severe and cumulative bone marrow depression may occur; nadir, 13 days (range, 3–25 days).

Nursing Implications: Monitor CBC, platelet count prior to drug administration, as well as signs/symptoms of infection and bleeding. Instruct patient in self-assessment of signs/symptoms of infection and bleeding as well as self-care measures, including avoidance of OTC aspirin-containing medication.

II. POTENTIAL FOR ACTIVITY INTOLERANCE related to ANEMIA-INDUCED FATIGUE

Defining Characteristics: Bone marrow depression often includes red cell line.

Nursing Implications: Monitor Hgb, HCT; discuss transfusion with physician if HCT doesn't recover postchemotherapy. Teach patient high-iron diet as appropriate.

III. SENSORY/PERCEPTUAL ALTERATIONS related to CNS EFFECTS, PERIPHERAL NEUROPATHIES

Defining Characteristics: Agitation, confusion, visual disturbances, and coma have occurred. Objective weakness has been reported (9–65%), as have paresthesias (4–12%).

Nursing Implications: Assess baseline neurologic status; monitor neurologic vital signs. Teach patient signs/symptoms and instruct to report them if they occur. Evaluate these changes with physician and discuss continuation of therapy.

IV. POTENTIAL FOR IMPAIRED GAS EXCHANGE related to PULMONARY TOXICITY

Defining Characteristics: Pneumonia occurs in 16–22% of patients. Pulmonary hypersensitivity reaction characterized by dyspnea, cough, interstitial pulmonary infiltrate has been observed. Fatal pulmonary toxicity has occurred when drug is given in combination with pentostatin (Deoxycofomycin).

Nursing Implications: Instruct patient in possible side effects and to report dyspnea, cough, signs of breathlessness following exertion. Assess lung sounds prior to chemotherapy administration. DO NOT administer drug in combination with pentostatin.

V. POTENTIAL FOR SEXUAL DYSFUNCTION, related to TERATOGENICITY

Defining Characteristics: Drug is teratogenic; may cause testicular atrophy. It is unknown whether drug is excreted in breast milk.

Nursing Implications: As appropriate, explore with patient and partner issues of reproduction and sexuality patterns, and impact chemotherapy may have. Discuss strategies to preserve sexual and reproductive health (sperm banking, contraception). Mothers receiving drug should not breast-feed.

VI. ALTERED NUTRITION, LESS THAN BODY REQUIREMENTS, related to NAUSEA/VOMITING, DIARRHEA

Defining Characteristics: Nausea/vomiting occurs in about 30% of patients and can be prevented with standard antiemetics; diarrhea occurs in 15% of patients.

Nursing Implications: Premedicate with antiemetics; evaluate response to emetic protection. Encourage small, frequent meals of cool, bland foods and liquids. If vomiting occurs, assess for signs/symptoms of fluid/electrolyte imbalance; monitor I/O and daily weights, lab results. Encourage patient to report onset of diarrhea; teach patient to administer antidiarrheal medication as ordered.

Drug: 5-fluorouracil (Fluorouracil, Adrucil, 5-FU, Efudex [topical])

Class: Pyrimidine antimetabolite.

Mechanism of Action: Acts as a "false" pyrimidine, inhibiting the formation of an enzyme (thymidine synthetase) necessary for the synthesis of DNA. Also incorporates into RNA, causing abnormal synthesis. Methotrexate given prior to 5-FU results in synergism and enhanced efficacy.

Metabolism: Metabolized by the liver; most is excreted as respiratory CO_2, remainder is excreted by the kidneys. Plasma half-life is 20 minutes.

Dosage/Range:

- 12–15 mg/kg IV once per week, OR
- 12 mg/kg IV every day × 5 days every 4 weeks, OR
- 500 mg/m^2 every week or every week × 5 weeks.
- Hepatic infusion: 22 mg/kg in 100 mL 5% Dextrose infused into hepatic artery over 8 hours for 5–21 consecutive days.
- Head and neck: 1000 mg/m^2 day × 4–5 days as continuous infusion.
- Colon cancer: A variety of regimens, such as 500 mg/m^2 IVB 1 hour after start of leucovorin (500 mg/m^2 in a 2-hour IV infusion) every week × 6 weeks, or together with irinotecan and leucovorin as first line for metastatic colon cancer.

Drug Preparation:

- No dilution required. Can be added to 0.9% Sodium Chloride or 5% Dextrose.
- Store at room temperature; protect from light. Solution should be clear: if crystals do not disappear after holding vial under hot water, discard vial.

Drug Administration:

- Given via IV push or bolus (slow drip), or as continuous infusion.
- Topical: As cream.

Drug Interactions:

- When given with cimetidine, there are increased pharmacologic effects of fluorouracil.

- When given with thiazide diuretics, there is increased risk of myelosuppression.
- Leucovorin causes increased 5-fluorouracil cytotoxicity.

Lab Effects/Interference:
- Decreased CBC.

Special Considerations:
- Cutaneous side effects occur, e.g., skin sensitivity to sun, splitting of fingernails, dry flaky skin, and hyperpigmentation on face, palms of hands.
- Patients who have had adrenalectomy may need higher doses of prednisone while receiving 5-FU, or dose of 5-FU may be reduced in postadrenalectomy patients.
- Reduce dose in patients with compromised hepatic, renal, or bone marrow function and malnutrition.
- Inspect solution for precipitate prior to continuous infusion.

Potential Toxicities/Side Effects and the Nursing Process

I. POTENTIAL FOR INFECTION AND BLEEDING related to BONE MARROW DEPRESSION

Defining Characteristics: Nadir 10–14 days after drug dose; neutropenia, thrombocytopenia are dose-related. Toxicity is enhanced when combined with leucovorin calcium.

Nursing Implications: Assess baseline CBC, WBC, differential, and platelet count prior to chemotherapy, as well as for signs/symptoms of infection or bleeding. Teach patient signs/symptoms of infection or bleeding, and instruct to report these immediately; teach patient self-care measures to minimize risk of infection and bleeding. This includes avoidance of crowds, proximity to people with infections, and avoidance of OTC aspirin-containing medications.

II. ALTERED NUTRITION, LESS THAN BODY REQUIREMENTS, related to NAUSEA AND VOMITING, STOMATITIS, AND DIARRHEA

Defining Characteristics: Nausea and vomiting occur in 30–50% of patients and severity is dose-dependent. Stomatitis can be severe, with onset in 5–8 days; and may herald severe bone marrow depression. Diarrhea can be severe, and in combination with leucovorin calcium is the dose-limiting toxicity.

Nursing Implications: Premedicate patient with antiemetics (phenothiazines are usually effective), and continue for 24 hours, at least for the first cycle. Encourage small, frequent meals of cool, bland foods. Assess oral mucosa prior to drug administration and instruct patient to report changes. Teach patient oral hygiene measures and self-assessment. Instruct patient to report diarrhea, to self-administer prescribed antidiarrheal medications, and to drink adequate fluids. Moderate to severe stomatitis or diarrhea is an indication to interrupt therapy.

III. ALTERATION IN SKIN INTEGRITY related to ALOPECIA, CHANGES IN NAILS AND SKIN

Defining Characteristics: Alopecia is more common with five-day course and involves diffuse thinning of scalp hair, eyelashes, and eyebrows. Brittle nail cracking and loss may occur. Photosensitivity occurs. Chemical phlebitis may occur during continuous infusion with higher doses (pH > 8.0).

Nursing Implications: Teach patient about possible hair loss and skin changes; discuss possible impact on body image. Assess patient's risk for hair loss and skin changes during the therapy and discuss with patient strategies to minimize distress (wig, scarf, nail polish). Instruct patient to use sunblock when outdoors. Suggest implanted venous access device for continuous infusion of 5-FU, especially if patient will receive ongoing therapy.

IV. SENSORY/PERCEPTUAL ALTERATIONS related to PHOTOPHOBIA, CEREBELLAR ATAXIA, OCULAR CHANGES

Defining Characteristics: Photophobia may occur. Occasional cerebellar ataxia may occur and will disappear once drug is stopped. Drug is excreted in tears. Ocular changes that may occur are conjunctivitis, increased lacrimation, photophobia, oculomotor dysfunction, and blurred vision.

Nursing Implications: Assess baseline neurologic status, including vision. Instruct patient to report any changes. Teach patient safety precautions as needed.

Drug: flutamide (Eulexin)

Class: Antiandrogen.

Mechanism of Action: Inhibits androgen uptake or inhibits nuclear binding of androgen in target tissues or both.

Metabolism: Rapidly and completely absorbed. Excreted mainly via urine. Biologically active metabolite reaches maximum plasma levels in approximately 2 hours. Plasma half-life is 6 hours. Largely plasma-bound.

Dosage/Range:
- 250 mg every 8 hours.

Drug Preparation:
- None (provided in 125-mg tablets).

Drug Administration:
- Oral.

Drug Interactions:
- None reported.

Lab Effects/Interference:
- Increased LFTs.
- Increased BUN, creatinine.
- Monitor PSA for changes.

Special Considerations:
- None.

Potential Toxicities/Side Effects and the Nursing Process

I. POTENTIAL SEXUAL DYSFUNCTION related to DRUG EFFECTS

Defining Characteristics: Decreased libido and impotence can occur in 33% of patients; gynecomastia occurs in 10% of patients.

Nursing Implications: Assess patient's sexual pattern, any alterations, and patient response. Encourage patient to verbalize feelings; provide information, emotional support, and referral for counseling as available and appropriate.

II. ALTERATION IN COMFORT related to HOT FLASHES

Defining Characteristics: Hot flashes occur commonly.

Nursing Implications: Teach patient that this may occur, and encourage patient to report symptoms. Provide symptomatic support.

III. ALTERED NUTRITION, LESS THAN BODY REQUIREMENTS, related to DIARRHEA, NAUSEA AND VOMITING

Defining Characteristics: Diarrhea and nausea/vomiting occur in 10% of patients.

Nursing Implications: Teach patient that these may occur, and instruct to report them. Assess for occurrence; teach patient self-administration of prescribed antidiarrheal or antiemetic medications.

Agent: fulvestrant injection (Faslodex)

Class: Estrogen Downregulator.

Mechanism of Action: Fulvestrant is an estrogen receptor antagonist that binds to the estrogen receptor of cells that are dependent upon estrogen for growth, including breast cancer cells that are hormone positive. There is no agonist effect as with other antiestrogens, such as tamoxifen. In addition, the estrogen receptor is also degraded so that it is lost from the cell. Because of this, there is no chance that the hormone receptor can be stimulated by low concentrations of estrogen, as with other antiestrogens, and this theoretically reduces the development of resistance.

Metabolism: When given IM, it takes 7 days for the drug to reach maximal plasma levels, which are maintained for at least one month. Half-life is about 40 days, and after 3-6 monthly doses, steady-state plasma area under the curve levels are reached at 2.5 times that of a single-dose injection. Drug undergoes biotransformation similar to endogenous steroids (oxidation, aromatic hydroxylation, conjugation), and oxidative pathway is via cytochrome P-450 (CYP 3A4). Drug is metabolized by the liver and rapidly cleared from the plasma via the hepatobiliary route. 90% is excreted via the feces; renal excretion is < 1%. There were no pharmacokinetic differences found in the elderly and younger adults, men and women, different races, patients with renal impairment, and patients with mild hepatic impairment. However, patients with moderate to severe liver dysfunction have not been studied.

Dosage/Range:

- 250 mg given IM into the buttock monthly as either one 5 mL slow injection or 2 separate 2.5-mL slow injections into each buttock.

Drug Preparation:

- Drug available in refrigerated 5 ml/250 mg, and 2.5 ml/125 mg prefilled syringes; concentration is 50 mg/mL.
- Unopened vials should be stored in the refrigerator at 2°–8°C (36°–46°F), but do not freeze. Drug can be left at room temperature for a short period of time prior to injection to increase patient comfort.
- Remove glass syringe barrel from tray and ensure it is undamaged.
- Unopen Safety Glide needle and attach to luer lock end of the syringe.
- Expel any air.

Drug Administration:

- Administer slow IM in one buttock 5 mL (250 mg) or 2.5 mL (125 mg) into each buttock as solution is viscous.
- Z-track administration is recommended to prevent drug leakage into subcutaneous tissue.
- Following drug injection, activate needle protectin device when withdrawing needle from patient by pushing lever arm completely forward until needle tip is fully covered.
- If unable to activate, drop into sharps disposal container.

Drug Interactions:

- None significant as drug does not significantly inhibit the major CYP isoenzymes, including rifampin.

Lab Effects/Interference: None.

Special Considerations:

- Indicated for the treatment of hormone receptor positive metastatic breast cancer in postmenopausal women with disease progression following antiestrogen therapy.
- Contraindicated in pregnancy or in patients hypersensitive to the drug or its components.
- Drug should not be used by breastfeeding mothers.
- Injection site reactions more common when drug is given in two divided doses.

Potential Toxicities/Side Effects and the Nursing Process

I. ALTERATION IN COMFORT related to INJECTION SITE REACTION, ABDOMINAL PAIN, BACK PAIN

Defining Characteristics: Injection site reactions (pain and inflammation) occurred in 7% of patients receiving a single 5-mL injection (European Trial) as compared to 27% of patients (North American Trial) receiving two 2.5-mL injections, one in each buttock. Back and bone pain occurred in 15.8% of patients, while abdominal pain occurred in 11.8% of patients and often was associated with other gastrointestinal symptoms.

Nursing Implications: Teach patient this may occur and to report it. Consider using Z-track method, and if using 2 separate injection of 2.5 mL, try a single-dose injection to see if discomfort is reduced. Teach patient to report bone and/or back pain. Teach patient to use over-the-counter analgesics such as acetaminophen or nonsteroidal anti-inflammatory drugs as appropriate to bleeding history or risk factors. Discuss alternatives with physician if ineffective in symptom management.

II. ALTERATION IN NUTRITION, POTENTIAL related to NAUSEA, VOMITING, CONSTIPATION, DIARRHEA

Defining Characteristics: Nausea occurs in 26%, vomiting 13%, constipation 12.5%, diarrhea 12.3%, and anorexia 9%.

Nursing Implications: Assess baseline appetite, presence of nausea and/or vomiting, and bowel elimination pattern. Teach patient that these side effects may occur, self-care measures to minimize nausea and vomiting such as dietary modification, and to report these side effects. Discuss antiemetics with physician if dietary modification is ineffective. Teach patient to use dietary modification to relieve constipation or diarrhea and, if ineffective, to use over-the-counter laxatives or anti-diarrheal medicine. If ineffective, discuss pharmacologic management with physician.

III. ALTERATION IN SKIN INTEGRITY, POTENTIAL, related to HOT FLASHES AND PERIPHERAL EDEMA

Defining Characteristics: Vasodilation or hot flashes occurred in 17.7% of patients, and peripheral edema in 9% of patients.

Nursing Implications: Assess baseline skin integrity, history of hot flashes in post-menopausal patients, and presence of peripheral edema. Teach patient these side effects may occur and to report them. If hot flashes are severe, review common hot flash management including wearing loose, layered clothing that can be removed when the woman becomes hot, sipping cold beverages throughout the day, sleeping with light nightgown and window open, avoiding triggers such as caffeine or alcohol, and if ineffective, discuss use of venlaxafine (Effexor) or fluoxetine (Paxil) to reduce intensity and frequency of hot flashes (Loprinski et al, 2000). Teach patient self-assessment of peripheral edema, to wear loose stockings and shoes, to keep skin moisturized to prevent cracking, and comfort measures. Teach patient to report increasing edema or related problems.

Drug: gemcitabine (Gemzar, Difluorodeoxycitidine)

Class: Antimetabolite.

Mechanism of Action: Inhibits DNA synthesis by inhibiting DNA polymerase activity through a process called *masked chain termination*. It is a prodrug, structurally similar to ara-C, needing intracellular phosphorylation. It then inhibits DNA synthesis. Cell cycle specific for S phase, causing cells to accumulate at the G-S boundary.

Metabolism: Pharmacokinetics vary by age, gender, and infusion time. Half-life for short infusions ranges from 32–94 minutes, while that of long infusions ranges from 245–638 minutes. Following short infusions (< 70 minutes), the drug is not extensively tissue-bound; following long infusions (70–285 minutes), the drug slowly equilibrates within tissues. The terminal half-life of the parent drug, gemcitabine, is 17 minutes. There is negligible binding to serum proteins. Drug and metabolites are excreted in the urine, with 92–98% of the drug dose recovered in the urine within one week. Mean systemic clearance is 90 L/h/m^2. Clearance is about 30% lower in women than in men, and also reduced in the elderly, but this does not necessarily require a dose reduction.

Dosage/Range:

Adults:

- Breast cancer: 1250 mg/m^2 IV over 30 minutes d 1, 8 q 21 days, in combination with paclitaxel 175mg/m^2 IV over 3 hr administered prior to gemcitabine, day 1 repeated q 21 days.
- Pancreatic cancer: 1000 mg/m^2 IV infusion over 30 min every week for up to 7 weeks (or until toxicity necessitates dose reduction or delay), then followed by 1-week break. Treatment then continues weekly for 3 weeks, followed by 1 week off (i.e., treatment 3 weeks out of 4). See dose modifications for hematologic toxicity in Special Considerations. For patients who complete the initial 7 weeks, or a subsequent 3-week cycle at a dose of 1000 mg/m^2, the dose may be increased by 25% to 1250 mg/m^2 if the following conditions are met: the ANC NADIR is > 1500 × 10/L, platelet count NADIR is > 100,000 × 10/L, and nonhematologic toxicity has not been greater than WHO grade 1. If patient tolerates this course well, the dose for the next cycle can be increased an additional 20% if the above three criteria are met. (Source: Eli Lilly Co., Gemzar package insert.)
- Non-small-cell lung cancer (inoperable, locally advanced Stage IIIA and IIIB or metastatic) in combination with cisplatin: 4-week cycle: 1000 mg/m^2 IV over 30 minutes on day 1, 8, 15, repeat q28 days, with cisplatin 100 mg/m^2 IV on day 1 after the gemcitabine infusion; or as a 3-week cycle, with gemcitabine 1250 mg/m^2 IV over 30 minutes on day 1, 8; cisplatin 100 mg/m^2 IV is given following gemcitabine infusion on day 1, repeated q3 weeks.

Drug Preparation:

- Drug available in single-use vials of 200 mg/10 mL and 1 g/50 mL. Use 0.9% Sodium Chloride USP and reconstitute the 200-mg vial with 5 mL, and the 1-g vial with 25 mL. Shake to dissolve the powder. This results in a concentration of 38 mg/mL. Withdraw recommended dose and further dilute in 0.9% Sodium Chloride injection. Discard unused portion. Inspect solution for particulate matter or discoloration and do not use if these occur. Stable 24 hours at room temperature (20–25°C [68–77°F]). DO NOT refrigerate, as drug crystallization may occur.

Drug Administration:

- Administer IV over 30 minutes.

Drug Interactions:

- Administer cisplatin after gemcitabine to enhance renal drug clearance; paclitaxel should be administered before gemcitabine.

Lab Effects/Interference:

- Decreased CBC.
- Increased LFTs, RFTs.

Special Considerations:

- FDA-approved for first-line treatment of patients with unresectable non-small-cell lung cancer, in combination with cisplatin.
- FDA-approved for first-line treatment of patients with locally advanced (nonresectable Stage II or III), or metastatic (Stage IV) adenocarcinoma of the pancreas, in combination with paclitaxel, as first-line therapy for treatment of women with metastatic breast cancer who have failed prior anthracycline adjuvant chemotherapy, unless anthracyclines are contraindicated. Drug is also indicated for patients with pancreatic cancer previously treated with 5-FU.
- FDA-approved in combination with paclitaxel, as first-line therapy for treatment of patients with metastatic breast cancer who have failed prior anthracycline adjuvant chemotherapy, unless anthracyclines are contraindicated.
- Monitor liver and renal function at baseline and throughout therapy.
- Dose reduction or delay required for hematologic toxicity.

Table 1.10

ANC ($\times 10^6$/L)		Platelet Count ($\times 10^6$/L)	% of full dose
≥ 1000	and	≥ 100,000	100
500–999	or	50,000–99,000	75
< 500	or	< 50,000	hold

Source: Gemzar package insert (1998). Eli Lilly Company, Indianapolis, IN.

- Use with caution in patients with impaired renal function or hepatic dysfunction. (Studies have not been done to identify risks in this population.)
- Rarely, HUS (hemolytic uremic syndrome) has occurred. Discontinue drug if signs/symptoms occur (rapid decrease in hemoglobin and thrombocytopenia, together with elevated BUN/creatinine). Observe for elevation of serum bili or LDH.
- Drug can rarely cause severe pulmonary toxicity (interstitial pneumonitis, pulmonary fibrosis, pulmonary edema, adult respiratory distress syndrome), occurring up to 2 weeks following the last gemcitabine infusion. If patients develop dyspnea, with or without bronchospasm, stop gemcitabine until further pulmonary evaluation can proceed; discontinue drug if related to gemcitabine.
- Drug may cause sedation in 10% of patients; caution patient not to drive or operate heavy machinery until it is determined whether patient develops this side effect.
- Drug is embryotoxic; women of childbearing age should avoid pregnancy while receiving the drug.
- Drug may be irritating to the vein, requiring local heat; may require a central line for (long-term) administration.

Potential Toxicities/Side Effects and the Nursing Process

I. POTENTIAL FOR INFECTION AND BLEEDING related to BONE MARROW DEPRESSION

Defining Characteristics: Myelosuppression is dose-limiting toxicity. Incidence of leukopenia is 63%, thrombocytopenia 36%, and anemia 73%. Dose reductions required are shown in the Special Considerations section. Grades 3–4 thrombocytopenia are more common in the elderly, and grades 3–4 neutropenia and thrombocytopenia are more common in women (especially older women). Older women were less able to complete subsequent courses of therapy. Myelosuppression is usually short-lived with recovery within one week. Approximately 19% of patients require RBC transfusions.

Nursing Implications: Assess baseline CBC, WBC, differential, and platelet count prior to chemotherapy, as well as for signs/symptoms of infection or bleeding. Discuss dose reductions or delay based on neutrophil and platelet counts. Teach patient signs/symptoms of infection or bleeding, and instruct to report these immediately. Teach patient self-care measures to minimize risk of infection and bleeding. This includes avoidance of crowds, proximity to people with infections, and OTC aspirin-containing medications. Transfuse red blood cells and platelets as needed per physician order.

II. POTENTIAL ALTERATION IN NUTRITION, LESS THAN BODY REQUIREMENTS, related to NAUSEA AND VOMITING, DIARRHEA, STOMATITIS, AND ALTERATIONS IN LFTS

Defining Characteristics: Nausea and vomiting occur in 69% of patients, and of these, < 15% are severe. Nausea and vomiting are usually mild to moderate and are easily prevented or controlled by antiemetics. Diarrhea may occur (19% incidence), as may stomatitis (11% incidence). Abnormalities in liver transaminases occur in two-thirds of patients; rarely does this require drug discontinuance.

Nursing Implications: Premedicate patient with antiemetics (phenothiazides are usually effective). Encourage small, frequent meals of cool, bland foods. Teach patient self-administration of prescribed antiemetic medications, and to drink adequate fluids. Assess oral mucosa prior to drug administration, and instruct patient to report changes. Teach patient oral hygiene measures and self-assessment. Instruct patient to report diarrhea, to self-administer prescribed antidiarrheal medications, and to drink adequate fluids. Monitor LFTs baseline and periodically during therapy. Notify physician of any abnormalities and discuss implications. Drug should be used cautiously in any patient with hepatic dysfunction.

III. POTENTIAL ALTERATION IN COMFORT related to FLULIKE SYMPTOMS

Defining Characteristics: Flulike symptoms occur in 20% of patients with first treatment dose. Transient febrile episodes occur in 41% of patients.

Nursing Implications: Encourage patient to report flulike symptoms. Treat fevers with acetaminophen per physician. Assess for alterations in comfort, and discuss symptomatic measures. If severe, discuss drug discontinuance with physician.

IV. IMPAIRED SKIN INTEGRITY related to ALOPECIA, RASH, PRURITUS, EDEMA

Defining Characteristics: Skin rash occurs in about 30% of patients, often within 2–3 days of starting drug. The rash is erythematous, pruritic, and/or maculopapular, and may occur on the neck and extremities. Edema occurs in about 30% of patients, and is primarily peripheral but can rarely be facial or pulmonary. Edema is reversible after drug is discontinued, and appears unrelated to cardiac, renal, or hepatic impairment. Edema is usually mild to moderate. Minimal hair loss occurs in 15% of patients, and is reversible.

Nursing Implications: Assess skin integrity and presence of rash, pruritus, alopecia, and edema prior to dosing. Assess impact of these alterations on patient, and develop plan to manage symptom distress and promote skin integrity. Instruct patient to report rash, itching; discuss treatment of rash with topical corticosteroids. Teach patient self-assessment of signs/symptoms of edema, and instruct to notify health care provider if swelling occurs. If severe, discuss drug discontinuance with physician.

Drug: goserelin acetate (Zoladex)

Class: Synthetic analogue of luteinizing hormone-releasing hormone (LHRH).

Mechanism of Action: Inhibits pituitary gonadotropin, achieving a chemical orchiectomy in 2–4 weeks. Sustained-release medication provides continuous drug diffusion from the depot into subcutaneous tissue. This permits monthly injection instead of daily.

Metabolism: Absorbed slowly for first 8 days, then more rapid and constant absorption for remaining 28 days.

Dosage/Range:

Adults:

- Subcutaneous: 3.6-mg dose into upper abdominal wall, q28 days 10.8 mg q 3 months.

Drug Preparation/Administration:

- Inspect package for damage. Open package and inspect drug in translucent chamber.
- Select site on upper abdomen.
- Prepare site with alcohol swab, cleansing from center outward.
- Administer local anesthetic as ordered.
- Aseptically, stretch skin at site with nondominant hand, and insert needle into subcutaneous tissue with dominant hand at 45-degree angle.
- Redirect needle so it is parallel to the abdominal wall. Advance needle forward until hub touches skin. Withdraw needle 1 cm (approximately ½ inch).
- Depress plunger fully, expelling depot into prepared site.
- Withdraw needle carefully. Apply gentle pressure bandage to site. Confirm that tip of plunger is visible within needle tip.
- Document in chart.

Drug Interactions:

- None.

Lab Effects/Interference:

- Hypercalcemia in patients with bone metastases.
- Tests of pituitary/gonadal function may be inaccurate while on therapy due to suppression of pituitary/gonadal system.

Special Considerations:

- Compliance to 28-day injection schedule is important.
- Indicated for palliative treatment of advanced prostate cancer; treatment of Stage B2 (locally advanced) prostate cancer in combination with flutamide; palliative treatment of advanced breast cancer in pre- or peri-menopausal women; and for the treatment of endometriosis.
- Initially, there is transient increase in serum testosterone levels, with flare of symptoms.
- Well-tolerated treatment.

Potential Toxicities/Side Effects and the Nursing Process

I. SEXUAL DYSFUNCTION related to DECREASED TESTOSTERONE LEVELS

Defining Characteristics: Hot flashes, sexual dysfunction, and decreased erections can occur.

Nursing Implications: Assess normal sexual pattern. Refer as needed for sexual counseling.

II. POTENTIAL ALTERATION IN CARDIAC OUTPUT related to ARRYTHMIA, CARDIOVASCULAR DYSFUNCTION

Defining Characteristics: Arrhythmia, cerebrovascular accident (CVA), hypertension, myocardial infarction, peripheral vascular disease, chest pain may occur in 1–5% of patients.

Nursing Implications: Assess heart rate, blood pressure, peripheral pulses. Teach patient to report palpitations, shortness of breath, chest pain, or leg pain immediately. Evaluate abnormalities with physician.

III. SENSORY/PERCEPTUAL ALTERATION related to ANXIETY, DEPRESSION, HEADACHE

Defining Characteristics: Anxiety, depression, headache may occur (< 5%).

Nursing Implications: Assess baseline affect, comfort. Instruct patient to report mood disorder. Encourage patient to verbalize feelings, provide patient with emotional support. Assess efficacy of supportive care, and if needed, discuss pharmacologic management of symptoms with physician.

IV. ALTERATION IN NUTRITION, LESS THAN BODY REQUIREMENTS, related to VOMITING, HYPERGLYCEMIA

Defining Characteristics: Vomiting may occur (< 5%); also increased weight, ulcer, hyperglycemia.

Nursing Implications: Teach patient to report GI disturbances. Assess severity and discuss management with physician. Assess serum glucose, and if abnormal, discuss dietary or pharmacologic management, depending upon severity, with physician.

V. ALTERATION IN BOWEL ELIMINATION related to CONSTIPATION OR DIARRHEA

Defining Characteristics: Constipation or diarrhea may occur (< 5%).

Nursing Implications: Instruct patient to report problems in elimination. Teach symptomatic management.

VI. ALTERATION IN URINARY ELIMINATION related to OBSTRUCTION OR INFECTION

Defining Characteristics: Urinary obstruction, urinary tract infection, renal insufficiency may occur.

Nursing Implications: Monitor baseline urinary elimination pattern, baseline kidney function tests, and continue to monitor through therapy. Instruct patient to report signs/symptoms of urinary tract infection (UTI).

VII. ALTERATION IN COMFORT related to FEVER, CHILLS, TENDERNESS

Defining Characteristics: Chills, fever, breast swelling, and tenderness. Also, discomfort may result from injection, as a 16-gauge needle is used to inject depot.

Nursing Implications: Instruct patient to report discomfort. Discuss strategies to increase comfort. Administer local anesthetic prior to injection of medication (per physician's order).

Drug: histrelin implant (Vantas)

Class: Synthetic analogue of gonadotropin releasing factor (GnRH) or luteinizing hormone-releasing hormone (LHRH).

Mechanism of Action: Histrelin inhibits pituitary gonadotropin, achieving a chemical orchiectomy.

Metabolism: Implant delivers histrelin continuously for 12 months at 50–60 micrograms per day. Drug serum concentration 50% higher in patients with severe renal dysfunction, but this is not considered clinically significant.

Dosage/Range:
Adults:
- Histrelin implant (50 mg) is asceptically inserted subcutaneously under skin on upper, inner arm using implant tool; at 12 months, implant must be removed before new one is implanted.

Drug Preparation:
- Keep implant refrigerated until implant.
- Select site on upper inner arm, and follow guidelines in package insert using asceptic technique and implant tool.
- Implant is NOT radio-opaque so care must be given to carefully secure the implant as directed.

Drug Interactions:
- Unknown.

Lab Effects/Interference:
- Hypercalcemia in patients with bone metastases.
- Tests of pituitary/gonadal function may be inaccurate while on therapy due to suppression of pituitary/gonadal system.
- Decreased serum testosterone to below castrate levels (< ng/dL)

Special Considerations:
- Indicated for palliative treatment of advanced prostate cancer.

- Initially (1st week of treatment), there is transient increase in serum testosterone levels, with flare of symptoms or onset of new symptoms such as bone pain, neuropathy, hematuria, or ureteral/bladder outlet obstruction. If severe (rarely spinal cord compression, ureteral obstruction), these should be managed immediately.
- Patients with metastatic vertebral and/or urinary tract obstruction should be monitored very closely during the first few weeks of treatment.
- Generally well-tolerated treatment.
- Contraindicated in children and women.

Potential Toxicities/Side Effects and the Nursing Process

I. SEXUAL DYSFUNCTION related to DECREASED TESTOSTERONE LEVELS

Defining Characteristics: Hot flashes (66% with 2.3% severe), testicular atrophy (5.3%), gynecomastica (4.1%), decreased libido (2.3%) and erectile dysfunction (3.5%) can occur.

Nursing Implications: Assess normal sexual pattern. Encourage patient to verbalize feelings to assess impact of symptoms on sexual function; refer as needed for sexual counseling. Teach patient self-care strategies to reduce distress of hot flashes.

II. ALTERATION IN BOWEL ELIMINATION related to CONSTIPATION

Defining Characteristics: Constipation may occur (< 5%).

Nursing Implications: Instruct patient to report problems in elimination. Teach symptomatic management.

III. ALTERATION IN URINARY ELIMINATION related to OBSTRUCTION OR INFECTION

Defining Characteristics: Urinary obstruction, urinary tract infection, renal insufficiency may occur. Renal impairment occurs in 4.7% of patients.

Nursing Implications: Monitor baseline urinary elimination pattern, baseline kidney function tests, and continue to monitor through therapy. Instruct patient to report signs/symptoms of urinary tract infection (UTI).

IV. ALTERATION IN COMFORT related to IMPLANT SITE IRRITATION, ASTHENIA, AND INSOMNIA

Defining Characteristics: Implantation site reactions occur in at least 5.8% of patients: these include bruising, pain/soreness/tenderness after insertion or removal; rarely, erythema, and swelling may occur. Asthenia occurs in about 10% of patients, and insomnia 2.9% of patients.

Nursing Implications: Instruct patient to report discomfort. Discuss strategies to increase comfort. Teach patient to self-assess and reassure local effects will resolve. Teach patient to report any signs/symptoms of infection.

Drug: hydroxyurea (Hydrea, Droxia)

Class: Miscellaneous/antimetabolite.

Mechanism of Action: Prevents conversion of ribonucleotides to deoxyribonucleotides by inhibiting the converting enzyme ribonucleoside diphosphate reductase. DNA synthesis is thus inhibited. Cell cycle phase specific for S phase. May also sensitize cells to the effects of radiation therapy, although the process is not clearly understood.

Metabolism: Rapidly absorbed from GI tract. Peak plasma level reached in 2 hours, with plasma half-life of 3–4 hours. About half the drug is metabolized in the liver and half is excreted in urine as urea and unchanged drug. Some of the drug is eliminated as respiratory CO_2. Crosses BBB.

Dosage/Range:

- 500–3000 mg PO daily (dose reduced in renal dysfunction).
- 20–30 mg/kg/day PO as a continuous dose.
- 100 mg/kg IV daily × 3 days.
- Radiation sensitization: 80 mg/kg as a single dose every 3rd day starting at least 7 days before initiation of radiation.
- Sickle cell disease: To prevent painful crises, initial 15 mg/kg/day, increased by 5 mg/kg every 12 weeks to a maximum dose of 35 mg/kg/day as tolerated.

Drug Preparation:

- None. Hydrea available in 500-mg capsules or Droxia in 200-mg, 300-mg, and 400-mg tablets.

Drug Administration:

- Oral.
- High-dose IV continuous infusions are being studied with doses of 0.5–1 g/m^2/day × 5–12 weeks (investigational).

Drug Interactions:

- None significant.

Lab Effects/Interference:

- Decreased CBC.
- Increased BUN, creatinine, uric acid.

- Increased hepatic enzymes.

Special Considerations:

- Hydroxyurea has a side effect of dramatically lowering the WBC in a relatively short period of time (24–48 hours). In leukemia patients endangered by the potential complication of leukostasis, this is the desired effect.
- May need to pretreat with allopurinol to protect patient from tumor lysis syndrome.
- Dermatologic radiation recall phenomena may occur.
- In combination with radiation therapy, mucosal reactions in the radiation field may be severe.
- Drug used in the treatment of chronic myelogenous leukemia (CML) in chronic phase, as a radiosensitizer (primary brain tumors, head and neck cancer, cancer of the cervix or uterus, non-small-cell lung cancer), and in sickle cell anemia.
- Drug should not be used during pregnancy, or by breast-feeding mothers as drug is excreted in breast milk.
- Dose modification in renal dysfunction: Reduce dose by 50% if creatinine clearance 10–50 mL/min; reduce dose 80% (give only 20% of dose) if creatinine clearance < 10 mL/min.

Potential Toxicities/Side Effects and the Nursing Process

I. INFECTION AND BLEEDING related to BONE MARROW DEPRESSION

Defining Characteristics: WBC begins to decrease 24–48 hours after beginning therapy, with nadir in 10 days and recovery within 10–30 days. Leukopenia more common than thrombocytopenia and anemia, and is dose-related.

Nursing Implications: Assess CBC, WBC with differential, and platelet count prior to drug administration, as well as for signs/symptoms of infection or bleeding. Doses may need to be reduced if patient has undergone prior radiotherapy or chemotherapy. Dose must be reduced if patient has renal dysfunction. Discuss any abnormalities with physician prior to drug administration. Teach patient signs/symptoms of infection and bleeding, and instruct to report them immediately. Teach self-care measures to minimize risk of infection and bleeding, including avoidance of OTC aspirin-containing medications.

II. ALTERED NUTRITION, LESS THAN BODY REQUIREMENTS, related to NAUSEA AND VOMITING, DIARRHEA, STOMATITIS, ANOREXIA, HEPATIC DYSFUNCTION

Defining Characteristics: Nausea and vomiting are uncommon, anorexia is mild to moderate, stomatitis is uncommon, diarrhea is uncommon, and hepatic dysfunction is rare, although abnormal LFTs may occur.

Nursing Implications: Premedicate with antiemetics as needed. Teach self-administration of prescribed medications. Instruct patient to report nausea/vomiting, diarrhea, anorexia, and stomatitis. Teach patient oral hygiene regimen and assess baseline oral mucosa. Monitor baseline LFTs, and monitor them periodically during therapy.

III. POTENTIAL ALTERATION IN FLUID/ELECTROLYTES/RENAL ELIMINATION STATUS related to TUMOR LYSIS SYNDROME

Defining Characteristics: When drug is first started in patients with high tumor burden, e.g., CML with high WBC, this often results in rapid death of a large number of malignant cells. The lysis or breakdown of these cells results in the release of intracellular contents into the systemic circulation. The resulting metabolic abnormalities are hyperkalemia, hyperphosphatemia, hypocalcemia, and hyperuricemia. If these persist, renal failure with oliguria can result.

Nursing Implications: Assess baseline chemistries, including metabolic panel, renal function. Expect that if the patient is at risk for the development of tumor lysis syndrome, the patient will begin allopurinol 200–300 mg/m^2/day prior to therapy, and receive hydration with alkalination (e.g., 50–100 mEq bicarbonate added per liter) to deliver 3 liters/m^2/day. Assess serum potassium, phosphate, calcium, uric acid, and BUN and creatinine at least daily, and discuss any abnormalities with physician to revise current regimen. Monitor I/O, weights, and total body balance carefully, and at least daily.

IV. SENSORY/PERCEPTUAL ALTERATIONS related to DROWSINESS, HALLUCINATIONS, OTHER CNS EFFECTS

Defining Characteristics: Drug crosses the BBB, so CNS effects may occur, such as drowsiness, confusion, disorientation, headache, vertigo; symptoms last < 24 hours.

Nursing Implications: Assess baseline mental status and neurologic functioning. Instruct patient to report signs/symptoms, and reassure that they will resolve. If symptoms persist, discuss interrupting drug with physician.

V. POTENTIAL SEXUAL/REPRODUCTIVE DYSFUNCTION related to DRUG EFFECTS

Defining Characteristics: Drug is mutagenic and teratogenic. Drug is excreted in breast milk.

Nursing Implications: Assess patient's sexual patterns and reproductive goals. Discuss with patient and partner potential toxicity and impact on sexuality. Provide information, emotional support, and referral as needed. Patient should use contraceptive measures; a mother receiving the drug should not breast-feed.

Drug: idarubicin (Idamycin, 4-Demethoxydaunorubicin)

Class: Antitumor antibiotic.

Mechanism of Action: Cell cycle phase specific for S phase. Analogue of daunorubicin. Has a marked inhibitory effect on RNA synthesis.

Metabolism: Excreted primarily in the bile and urine, with approximately 25% of the intravenous dose accounted for over 5 days. The half-life is 6–9.4 hours.

Dosage/Range:
- 12 mg/m^2 qd × 3 days in combination with ara-C 100 mg/m^2 continuous infusion × 7 days, OR
- In combination with ara-C, 25 mg/m^2 IVP followed by ara-C 200 mg/m^2 continuous infusion daily × 5 days.
- 8–15 mg/m^2 IV every 3 weeks has been studied.

Drug Preparation:
- Available as a red powder.
- The drug is reconstituted with 0.9% Sodium Chloride injection to give a final concentration of 1 mg/1 mL.

Drug Administration:
- Drug is a vesicant. Administer IV over 10 to 15 minutes into the sidearm of a freely running IV.

Drug Interactions:
- Other myelosuppressive drugs: additive bone marrow suppression; monitor patient closely.
- Incompatible with heparin—causes precipitant.

Lab Effects/Interference:
- Decreased CBC.
- Increased LFTs, RFTs.

Special Considerations:
- Vesicant.
- Discolored urine (pink to red) may occur up to 48 hours after administration.
- Cardiomyopathy is less common and less severe than with doxorubicin and daunorubicin.
- Drug is light-sensitive.
- Dose-reduce for renal dysfunction.

- Dose-reduce for hepatic dysfunction: give 50% of dose if serum bili is 2.5 mg/dL; do not give dose if serum bili is > 5 mg/dL.

Potential Toxicities/Side Effects and the Nursing Process

I. INFECTION AND BLEEDING related to BONE MARROW DEPRESSION

Defining Characteristics: Hematologic toxicity is dose limiting. Leukopenia nadir 10–20 days with recovery in 1–2 weeks. Thrombocytopenia usually follows leukopenia and is mild. Bone marrow toxicity is not cumulative.

Nursing Implications: Evaluate WBC, neutrophil, and platelet count and discuss any abnormalities with physician prior to drug administration. Assess for signs/symptoms of infection or bleeding and instruct patient in signs/symptoms of infection and bleeding and to report them immediately. Suggest strategies to minimize risk of infection and bleeding, including avoidance of OTC aspirin-containing medications.

II. ALTERATION IN CARDIAC OUTPUT related to CUMULATIVE DOSES OF IDARUBICIN

Defining Characteristics: Cardiac toxicity is similar characteristically but less severe than that seen with daunorubicin and doxorubicin; CHF due to cardiomyopathy seen after large cumulative doses.

Nursing Implications: Assess cardiac status prior to chemotherapy administration: signs/symptoms of CHF, quality/regularity and rate of heartbeat, results of prior GBPS or other test of LVEF. Teach patient to report dyspnea, palpitations, swelling in extremities. Maintain accurate records of total dose; expect GBPS to be repeated periodically during treatment and the drug to be discontinued if there is a significant drop in heart function.

III. ALTERED NUTRITION, LESS THAN BODY REQUIREMENTS, related to NAUSEA/VOMITING, ANOREXIA, STOMATITIS, DIARRHEA, AND HEPATIC DYSFUNCTION

Defining Characteristics: Nausea/vomiting is usually mild to moderate, although it is seen to some degree in most patients; anorexia commonly occurs; stomatitis is mild; diarrhea is infrequent and mild; hepatitis is rare but may occur, and there are also disturbances in LFTs.

Nursing Implications: Premedicate with combination antiemetics and continue protection for 24 hours. If patient has a central line, slower infusion of drug over 1 hour decreases nausea/vomiting. Encourage small, frequent meals of bland foods. Anorexia occurs frequently: teach patient or caregiver to make foods ahead of time and use spices; encourage weekly weights. Stomatitis and esophagitis may occur in patients who have received prior radiation and during posttreatment visits. Teach patient oral hygiene regimen and self-assessment techniques. Encourage patient to report onset of diarrhea; administer or teach patient to self-administer antidiarrheal medications. Monitor SGOT, SGPT, LDH, alk phos, and bili periodically during treatment. Notify physician of any elevations.

IV. ALTERATION IN SKIN INTEGRITY related to ALOPECIA, SKIN CHANGES

Defining Characteristics: Alopecia occurs in about 30% of patients after oral drug and can be partial after IV drug; begins after 3+ weeks and hair may grow back while on therapy; may be slight to diffuse thinning. Skin changes include darkening of nail beds, skin ulcer/necrosis, sensitivity to sunlight, skin itching at irradiated areas, radiation recall, and potential necrosis with extravasation.

Nursing Implications: Discuss with patient hair loss, anticipated impact, and strategies to decrease distress, e.g., obtaining wig prior to hair loss. Assess disturbance of body image from hyperpigmentation and discuss strategies to minimize this, e.g., nail polish. Drug must be administered via patent IV. Assess need for venous access device early. If drug administered as continuous infusion, IT MUST BE GIVEN VIA A CENTRAL LINE.

V. POTENTIAL SEXUAL/REPRODUCTIVE DYSFUNCTION related to DRUG EFFECTS

Defining Characteristics: Gonadal function and fertility may be affected (may be permanent or transient). Reported to be excreted in breast milk.

Nursing Implications: As appropriate, explore with patient and partner issues of reproductive and sexuality patterns and impact chemotherapy will have; discuss strategies to preserve sexuality and reproductive health (e.g., contraception, sperm banking).

Drug: idoxifene (investigational)

Class: Synthetic tamoxifen analogue, nonsteroidal antiestrogen.

Mechanism of Action: Overcomes tamoxifen limitations, such as the estrogenic effects that tamoxifen possesses, and maximizes antiestrogen activity. (Only about 50% of estrogen-positive women with breast cancer respond to tamoxifen, acquired resistance to tamoxifen eventually develops, and it is probable that the estrogen agonist activity of tamoxifen accounts for the increased risk of developing endometrial cancer after tamoxifen therapy.) Drug has 2.5–5-fold higher affinity for estrogen receptors than tamoxifen. It is 1.5-fold more effective in inhibiting estrogen-induced growth in tumor cells, and potently inhibits calmodulin activity (important in breast cancer cell growth) (Coombes et al, 1995).

Metabolism: Peak plasma levels at 2–8 hours after a single dose, achieving steady-state levels with daily dosing in 6–12 weeks, as compared to tamoxifen's 2–6 weeks, and possessing a very long elimination phase (terminal half-life is 23.3 ± 5 days, about three times longer than tamoxifen).

Dosage/Range:
- Doses studied include 10- to 60-mg daily dosing for 2 weeks, and then 20-mg maintenance doses.
- Refer to study protocol.

Drug Preparation:
- None.

Drug Administration:
- Oral.

Drug Interactions:
- Unknown, but probably similar to tamoxifen.

Lab Effects/Interference:
- None known.

Special Considerations:
- Possesses ability to reverse multi-anticancer drug resistance mediated by P-glycoprotein (at least as effective as tamoxifen and verapamil).
- Probably has partial cross-resistance with tamoxifen, so may be effective in tamoxifen-resistant patients.

Potential Toxicities/Side Effects and the Nursing Process

I. ALTERATION IN NUTRITION, LESS THAN BODY REQUIREMENTS, related to NAUSEA AND VOMITING

Defining Characteristics: Nausea and vomiting may occur and are transient.

Nursing Implications: Inform patient of possibility of nausea, vomiting, and anorexia. Encourage small, frequent feedings of high-calorie, high-protein foods. Assess need for antiemetic medications, and discuss with physician. Teach patient self-administration as needed.

II. ACTIVITY INTOLERANCE related to TIREDNESS, LETHARGY, WEAKNESS

Defining Characteristics: Tiredness, lethargy, weakness may occur, but do not appear to be dose-related.

Nursing Implications: Assess baseline activity level and changes that occur with drug. Discuss with patient impact of activity intolerance or symptoms on quality of life.

Drug: ifosfamide (Ifex)

Class: Alkylating agent.

Mechanism of Action: Destroys DNA throughout the cell cycle by binding to protein and by DNA crosslinking and causing chain scission as well as inhibition of DNA synthesis. Analogue of cyclophosphamide and is cell cycle phase nonspecific. Ifosfamide has been shown to be effective in tumors previously resistant to cyclophosphamide. Activated by microsomes in the liver.

Metabolism: Only about 50% of the drug is metabolized, with much of the drug excreted in the urine almost completely unchanged. Half-life is 13.8 hours for high dose vs 3–10 hours for lower doses.

Dosage/Range:
- IV bolus/push: 50 mg/kg/day, OR.
- 700 mg–2 grams/m^2/day × 5 days, OR.
- 2400 mg/m^2/day × 3 days.
- Continuous infusion: 1200 mg/m^2/day × 5 days.
- Single dose: 5000 mg/m^2 q3–4 weeks.
- Dose-reduce by 25–50% if serum creatinine is 2.1–3.0 mg/dL and hold if creatinine > 3.0 mg/dL.
- High dose (bone marrow transplant/stem cell rescue): 7.5–16 grams/m^2 IV in divided doses over several days.

Drug Preparation:
- Available as a powder and should be reconstituted with sterile water for injection.
- Solution is chemically stable for 7 days, but discard after 8 hours due to lack of bacteriostatic preservative in the solution.
- May be diluted further in either 5% Dextrose or 0.9% Sodium Chloride.

Drug Administration:
- IV bolus: Administer over 30 minutes. Mesna (20% of ifosfamide dose) should be administered with ifosfamide: mesna is begun 15 minutes prior to ifosfamide and repeated at 4 and 8 hours after the ifosfamide (see drug sheet on mesna). Mesna, ascorbic acid, and mucomycin have been used to protect the bladder. Pre- and posthydration (1500–2000 mL/day) or continuous bladder irrigations are recommended to prevent hemorrhagic cystitis.
- Continuous infusion: Administer intravenously for 5 days. Mesna is mixed with ifosfamide in equal amounts (1:1 mix). Prior to initiating continuous

infusion, mesna is given IVB (10% of total ifosfamide dose). Following completion of the infusion, mesna alone should be infused for 12–24 hours to protect from delayed drug excretion activity against the bladder.

Drug Interactions:
- Activity/toxicity affected by allopurinol, chloroquine, phenothiazides, potassium iodide, chloramphenicol, imipramine, vitamin A, corticosteroids, succinylcholine.
- Mesna binds to and inactivates ifosfamide metabolite, thus preventing bladder toxicity.

Lab Effects/Interference:
- Decreased CBC.
- Increased RFTs.

Special Considerations:
- Metabolic toxicity is increased by simultaneous administration of barbiturates.
- Renal function: BUN, serum creatinine, and creatinine clearance must be determined prior to treatment.
- Therapy requires the concomitant administration of a uroprotector such as mesna and pre- and posthydration; may also require catheterization and constant bladder irrigation, and/or ascorbic acid.
- Test urine for occult blood.
- Dose-limiting toxicity has been renal and bladder dysfunction.
- Increased risk for toxicity in patients who have received prior or concurrent radiotherapy or other antineoplastic agents.
- Drug active in cancers of lung, breast, ovary, pancreas, and stomach; Hodgkin's and NHL, acute and chronic lymphocytic leukemias.

Potential Toxicities/Side Effects and the Nursing Process

I. ALTERED URINARY ELIMINATION related to HEMORRHAGIC CYSTITIS AND RENAL TOXICITY

Defining Characteristics: Symptoms of bladder irritation; hemorrhagic cystitis with hematuria, dysuria, urinary frequency; preventable with uroprotection and hydration. Symptoms of renal toxicity; increased BUN and serum creatinine, decreased urine creatinine clearance (usually reversible); acute tubular necrosis, pyelonephritis, glomerular dysfunction; metabolic acidosis.

Nursing Implications: Assess presence of RBC in urine prior to successive doses, especially if symptoms are present, as well as BUN and creatinine. Administer drug with concomitant uroprotector (e.g., mesna). Encourage prehydration: oral intake of 2–3 L/day prior to chemotherapy; posthydration: increase oral fluids to 2–3 L for 2 days after chemotherapy. If possible, administer drug in morning to minimize drug accumulation in bladder during sleep. Instruct patient to empty bladder every 2–3 hours, before bedtime, and during night when awake. Monitor urinary output and total body balance. Assess urinary elimination pattern prior to each drug dose. If rigorous regimen is adhered to, minimal renal toxicity will result. Monitor BUN and creatinine.

II. ALTERED NUTRITION, LESS THAN BODY REQUIREMENTS, related to NAUSEA AND VOMITING, HEPATOTOXICITY

Defining Characteristics: Nausea and vomiting occur in 58% of patients; dose and schedule-dependent, with increased severity with higher dose and rapid injection. Occurs within a few hours of drug administration and may last 3 days. Elevations of serum transaminase and alk phos may occur; usually transient and resolve spontaneously without apparent sequelae.

Nursing Implications: Premedicate with antiemetics and continue prophylactically to prevent nausea and vomiting for 24 hours at least for the first treatment. Encourage small, frequent feedings of cool, bland foods and liquids. Refer to section on nausea and vomiting. Monitor LFTs during treatment.

III. INFECTION AND BLEEDING related to BONE MARROW DEPRESSION

Defining Characteristics: Leukopenia is mild to moderate. Thrombocytopenia and anemia are rare. Dosage adjustment may be necessary when ifosfamide is combined with other chemotherapy agents. Patients at risk for bone marrow depression include patients with impaired renal function and decreased bone marrow reserve (bone marrow metastases, prior XRT).

Nursing Implications: Evaluate WBC, with neutrophil, and platelet count and discuss any abnormalities with physician prior to drug administration. Assess for signs/symptoms of infection or bleeding and instruct patient in signs/symptoms of infection and bleeding, and to report them immediately; discuss strategies to minimize risk of infection and bleeding, including avoidance of OTC aspirin-containing medications. Assess patient's Hgb/HCT and signs/symptoms of fatigue; teach patient self-assessment and to alternate rest and activity as needed.

IV. ALTERATION IN SKIN INTEGRITY related to ALOPECIA, STERILE PHLEBITIS, SKIN CHANGES

Defining Characteristics: The incidence of alopecia is 83%, with 50% experiencing severe hair loss in 2–4 weeks. Sterile phlebitis may occur at injection site; irritation occurs with extravasation. Hyperpigmentation, dermatitis, and nail ridging may occur.

Nursing Implications: Discuss with patient anticipated impact of hair loss; suggest wig, as appropriate, prior to actual hair loss. Explore with patient response to hair loss and alternative strategies to minimize distress. Carefully monitor injection site during drug administration for signs/symptoms of phlebitis, irritation, vein patency. Assess skin integrity. Assess impact of skin changes on body image. Discuss strategies to minimize distress.

V. POTENTIAL SEXUAL/REPRODUCTIVE DYSFUNCTION related to DRUG EFFECTS

Defining Characteristics: Drug is carcinogenic, mutagenic, and teratogenic. Drug is excreted in breast milk.

Nursing Implications: As appropriate, explore with patient and partner issues of reproductive and sexual patterns, and impact chemotherapy will have. Discuss strategies to preserve sexuality and reproductive health (e.g., sperm banking, contraception).

VI. SENSORY/PERCEPTUAL ALTERATIONS related to CONFUSION, ACTIVITY INTOLERANCE, FATIGUE

Defining Characteristics: Intact drug passes easily into CNS; however, active metabolites do not. Lethargy and confusion may be seen with high doses, lasting 1–8 hours, usually spontaneously reversible. CNS side effects occur in about 12% of patients treated, including somnolence, confusion, depressive psychosis, hallucinations. Less frequent side effects: dizziness, disorientation, cranial nerve dysfunction, seizures. Incidence of CNS side effects may be higher in patients with compromised renal function, as well as in patients receiving high doses.

Nursing Implications: Identify patients at risk (decreased renal function) and observe closely. Assess neurologic and mental status prior to and during drug administration and on follow-up. Instruct patient to report any alterations in behavior, sensation, perception. Develop a plan of care with patient and family if side effects develop to manage distress and promote safety.

Drug: irinotecan (Camptosar, Camptothecan-11, CPT-11)

Class: Topoisomerase I inhibitor.

Mechanism of Action: Induces protein-linked DNA single-strand breaks and blocks DNA and RNA synthesis in dividing cells, thus preventing cells from entering mitosis. The active metabolite, SN-38, prevents repair (religation) of previous, reversible single-strand breaks in DNA by binding to topoisomerase I. Topoisomerase I is an enzyme that relaxes tension in the DNA helix torsion by initially causing this single-strand break in DNA so that DNA replication can occur. Topoisomerases I and II then work together to bring about replication, transcription, and recombination of DNA material. Topoisomerase I is found in higher-than-normal concentrations in certain malignant cells, such as colon adenocarcinoma cells and non-Hodgkin's lymphoma cells.

Metabolism: Metabolized to its active metabolite SN-38 in the liver; 11–20% of the drug is excreted in the urine, and 5–39% in the bile over a 48-hour period. Mean terminal half-life is 6 hours, while that of SN-38 is 10 hours. Drug is moderately protein-bound (30–68%), while SN-38 is highly protein-bound (95%).

Dosage/Range:

IFL (Saltz) regimen:

- Metastatic colorectal cancer (in combination with 5-FU and leukovorin): Irinotecan 125 mg/m^2 IV over 90 minutes (day 1, 8, 15, 22); leukovorin 20 mg/m^2 IVB immediately after irinotecan (day 1, 8, 15, 22); 5-FU 500 mg/m^2 IVB immediately after leukovorin (day 1, 8, 15, 22), followed by 2-week rest period (total, 6-week cycle). Requires *very* close monitoring and supportive care.
- Colon and rectal cancers that have recurred following 5-FU-based therapy: Starting dose is 125 mg/m^2 IV over 90 minutes weekly × 4 weeks, followed by a 2-week rest period. This 6-week cycle is then repeated.
- Dose increase up to 150 mg/m^2 as tolerated.
- 350 mg/m^2 IV day 1 repeated every 21 days (300 mg/m^2 for patients > 70 years old, those who have received prior pelvic/abdominal radiotherapy, or those with a performance status of 2).
- Dose modifications based on tolerance of prior cycle of therapy (see Tables 1.9a–d).

Douillard

- Metastatic colorectal cancers: Day 1: Irinotecan 180 mg/m^2 IV over 90 min, at the same time as Leucovorin 200 mg/m^2 IV over 2hr through separate arms of a Y-tubing, followed by 5-FU 400 mg/m^2 IVB, then 22 hr 5-FU 600 mg/m^2 IV continuous infusion (CI). Day 2: leucovorin 200 mg/m^2 IV over 2 hr, then 5-FU 400 mg/m^2 IVB, then 22 hr 5-FU 600 mg/m^2 IV continuous infusion (CI). Repeat q 2 weeks.

Drug Preparation:

- Store unopened vials at room temperature and protect from light.
- Dilute and mix drug in 5% Dextrose (preferred) or 0.9% Sodium Chloride to a final concentration of 0.12–1.1 mg/mL. Commonly, the drug is diluted in 500 mL 5% Dextrose.

- Diluted drug is stable 24 hours at room temperature. If diluted in 5% Dextrose, the drug is stable for 48 hours if refrigerated (2–8°C [36–46°F]) and protected from light.

Drug Administration:
- Administer IV bolus over 90 minutes.

Lab Effects/Interference:
- Decreased CBC.

Special Considerations:
- IFL (Saltz) regimen may result in increased deaths. Use cautiously and monitor patients closely, especially patients with ↓ Performance Status (2), elderly, or patients with prior pelvic/abdominal radiation, or with hepatic dysfunction. Assess for s/s dehydration, febrile neutropenia, diarrhea. Modify dose per manufacturer's guidelines.
- Independent expert panel reviewed clinical trial data and did not recommend changes in starting doses; potential life-threatening toxicity was highlighted, especially severe myelosuppression, and both *early* and late diarrhea.
- Patient must have weekly assessment for toxicity.
- Patient must have dose reduction as recommended; drug should not be administered if the patient is neutropenic or has diarrhea.
- Patient must be taught to notify provider if toxicity develops, and how to manage diarrhea, nausea, vomiting, potential infection. (www.asco.org/people/nr/html/jco-early.htm.)
- Drug is indicated for first-line treatment of metastatic colon or rectal cancer in combination with 5-FU and leukovorin, and as a single agent for colorectal cancer recurring or progressing after treatment with 5-FU.
- Dose-limiting toxicities are diarrhea and severe myelosuppression.
- Drug is teratogenic and thus contraindicated in pregnant women; women of childbearing age should be taught and encouraged to use birth control.
- Drug is an irritant. If extravasation occurs, the manufacturer recommends flushing the IV site with sterile water, and then applying ice.
- All patients should receive self-care instructions on management of diarrhea, self-administration of loperamide for delayed diarrhea, and assessment of the patient's ability to purchase loperamide, and ability to comply with instructions.
- Patient response to treatment is usually apparent within two courses of therapy (12 weeks).
- Flushing (vasodilation) may occur during drug infusion, and usually does not require intervention.
- Patient educational material is available from Pharmacia/Upjohn Co.

- Rarely, patients may lack an enzyme necessary for drug metabolism, resulting in increased toxicity (Gilbert's syndrome, abnormal gucouronidation of bilirubin).
- Dose reductions must be made for neutropenia and severe diarrhea, and are different for combination therapy (irinotecan/5-FU/leukovorin) and irinotecan as a single agent.
- Contraindications: serum BR > 2.0 mg/dL although no studies done, grades ¾ neutropenia occurred in patients with BR 1–2 mg/dL.

Potential Toxicities/Side Effects and the Nursing Process

I. ALTERATION IN ELIMINATION related to DIARRHEA

Defining Characteristics: Diarrhea may be early or late. Early diarrhea is characterized by onset within 24 hours of drug dose and is mediated by cholinergic pathway(s), as the metabolite SN-38 inhibits acetylcholinesterase; diaphoresis and abdominal cramping may precede diarrhea, and may be prevented by atropine. Other cholinergic effects that may appear are salivation, lacrimation, visual disturbances, piloerection, and bradycardia. This can be managed effectively with atropine 0.25–1.0 mg IV or scopalomine. Late diarrhea occurs > 24 hours after the drug dose, can be severe, prolonged, and lead to dehydration and electrolyte imbalance; the etiology appears related to changes in intestinal mucosal epithelium that prevent the reabsorption of water and electrolytes, which are then lost during diarrhea. 88% of patients may experience late diarrhea, and 31% have severe, or grade ¾ diarrhea. Loperamide is effective in halting late diarrhea. Irinotecan should be held for grade 3 diarrhea (7–9 stools/day, incontinence, or severe cramping) and grade 4 (> 10 stools/day, grossly bloody stool, or need for parenteral support). Once recovered, decrease drug dose at next treatment per manufacturer's guidelines and per physician order.

Nursing Implications: Acute diarrhea: teach patient to report diarrhea, sweating, and abdominal cramping during or after drug administration. Administer atropine 0.25–1 mg IVP per physician order, unless contraindicated, to prevent diarrhea. Delayed diarrhea: teach patient self-management of diarrhea (diet, fluids, avoidance of laxatives), and to notify nurse or physician of vomiting, fever, or if signs/symptoms of dehydration occur (fainting, light-headedness, dizziness). Teaching about diet should include drinking 8–10 large glasses of fluid/day, including soup/broth, soda, Gatorade; avoiding dairy products; eating small meals often; using BRAT diet (bananas, rice, applesauce, toast); and adding other foods as tolerated, such as bland, low-fiber foods, white chicken meat without skin, scrambled eggs, crackers, or pasta without sauce. Also teach patient to avoid foods that worsen diarrhea (fatty, fried, or greasy foods, high-fiber foods with bran, raw fruits and vegetables, popcorn, beans, nuts, chocolate). Review patient's medication profile, including over-the-counter medicines, and teach patient to stop taking any laxatives. Teach patient to avoid cigarette smoking to promote comfort. Instruct patient to record stools, and to take loperamide, not as indicated on the medication package, but as instructed: At the first episode of late-onset diarrhea, take 4 mg (2 [2-mg] capsules) of loperamide, then 2 mg (1 capsule) every 2 hours until free of diarrhea for at least 12 hours. Take a 4-mg dose (2 [2-mg] capsules) at bedtime (Camptosar recommendations). Patient should notify doctor or nurse if diarrhea is unrelieved by loperamide taken as instructed. Assess patient's ability to purchase loperamide if impoverished, and identify other sources that can provide the medication prior to patient's discharge from clinic after drug therapy. Review patient's medication profile to ensure that the patient is not taking any cathartics. Diarrhea must be monitored closely and managed aggressively to prevent morbidity and mortality.

II. POTENTIAL FOR INFECTION, ANEMIA related to BONE MARROW DEPRESSION

Defining Characteristics: Leukopenia has been noted in 63% of patients on single-dose schedules, with an overall neutropenia incidence of 54%, and grade ¾ neutropenia occurring in 26% of patients. Thrombocytopenia is uncommon, occurring in about 3% of patients. Anemia is common (61%). Nadir is commonly on day 6–9.

Nursing Implications: Evaluate WBC, with neutrophil, and platelet count, and discuss any abnormalities with physician prior to drug administration. Refer to Special Considerations section for dosage modifications based on hematologic toxicity. Assess patient tolerance of chemotherapy and nadir blood counts, especially Cycle 1. Assess for signs/symptoms of infection or bleeding; instruct patient in signs/symptoms of infection and bleeding, and to report them immediately. If febrile neutropenia develops, assess and begin antibiotic therapy ASAP. Instruct in measures to minimize risk of infection and bleeding, including avoidance of OTC aspirin-containing medications. Assess patient's Hgb/HCT and signs/symptoms of fatigue; teach patient self-assessment and to alternate rest and activity as needed.

III. POTENTIAL ALTERATION IN NUTRITION, LESS THAN BODY REQUIREMENTS, related to NAUSEA AND VOMITING, DEHYDRATION

Defining Characteristics: Moderate to severe nausea and vomiting occur in 35–60% of patients, with 17% experiencing NCI grade ¾ nausea and 13% experiencing NCI grade ¾ vomiting. Aggressive combination antiemetics are effective in preventing nausea/vomiting.

Nursing Implications: Premedicate with aggressive combination antiemetics such as serotonin antagonist (dolestron, granisetron, or ondansetron) plus dexamethasone 10 mg IV 30 minutes prior to chemotherapy to prevent nausea and vomiting. Encourage small, frequent meals of cool, bland foods and liquids. Teach patients to monitor their fluid intake, and take daily weights if nausea/vomiting occurs. Assess for signs/symptoms of fluid and electrolyte imbalance. Teach patients self-assessment, and instruct to notify doctor or nurse if these occur. Late-onset nausea and vomiting may occur, and dopamine antagonists such as prochlorperazine are then recommended. If dehydration develops, replace fluid and electrolytes to prevent worsening dehydration and cardiovascular complications.

IV. POTENTIAL FOR IMPAIRED GAS EXCHANGE, POTENTIAL related to DYSPNEA, PULMONARY INFILTRATES, FEVER

Defining Characteristics: Pulmonary effects may occur in up to 22% of patients, ranging from transient dyspnea to pulmonary infiltrates, fever, increased cough, and decreased DLCO in a small number of patients.

Nursing Implications: Assess baseline pulmonary status, and teach patient to report any changes. Assess pulmonary status prior to each treatment and at visits between treatment. If patient develops dyspnea, discuss patient having PFTs with physician, and evaluating whether related to drug. Teach patient to manage dyspnea if it occurs, including alternating activity and rest periods.

Drug: ketoconazole (investigational as an anticancer agent)

Class: Azole antifungal, antiadrenal.

Mechanism of Action: High-dose therapy interferes with conversion of lanosterol to cholesterol, a major precursor of several hormones. Drug has inhibitory effect on gonadal and adrenal steroid synthesis, thus lowering serum testosterone concentrations and suppressing corticosteroid secretion. Both hormones return to baseline levels when ketoconazole therapy is discontinued.

Metabolism: Rapidly absorbed from GI tract in acid environment. Decreased absorption in patients with gastric hypochlorhydria (25% of all AIDS patients) or in patients taking medications that raise pH (antacids, H_2 antagonists). Distributed widely but cerebrospinal penetration is unpredictable. Drug is ~90% protein-bound. Partially metabolized in liver, and mostly excreted in the feces via bile.

Dosage/Range:
- For lymphoma: 200 mg/day PO.

- For metastatic prostate cancer: 400 mg PO 3 times per day with hydrocortisone 20 mg PO q A.M. and 10 mg PO q P.M.

Drug Preparation:
- Store in tightly closed container at < 40°C (104°F).

Drug Administration:
- Orally in single dose.
- May take with meals to decrease GI side effects (unclear whether food increases absorption).
- In patients with gastric achlorhydria, patient may be instructed to dissolve ketoconazole in 4 mL aqueous solution of 0.2 N hydrochloric acid and drink through a straw; follow with 4 oz (120 mL) water.

Drug Interactions:
- Drugs that increase gastric pH: Antacids, cimetidine, rantidine, famotidine, sucralfate decrease ketoconazole absorption; give these drugs at least 2 hours after ketoconazole.
- Other hepatotoxic drugs: Use cautiously, and monitor liver function studies closely.
- Rifampin or rifampin plus isoniazid: Decreased ketoconazole levels, especially if isoniazid is taken as well. Increase ketoconazole dose.
- Acyclovir: Synergism and increased antiviral action against herpes simplex virus.
- Norfloxacin: Theoretically increases antifungal action of ketoconazole, but studies are inconsistent.
- Coumarin anticoagulants: Increased PT; monitor patient closely and decrease anticoagulant dose accordingly.
- Cyclosporine: Increased cyclosporine serum level; monitor serum level and decrease cyclosporine dose accordingly.
- Phenytoin: May have altered serum levels of phenytoin or ketoconazole; monitor serum levels of each and adjust dosages accordingly.
- Theophylline: May decrease theophylline serum concentrations; monitor serum levels and increase dosage accordingly.
- Terfenadine (Seldane): May increase terfenadine serum level with possible prolongation of QT interval on EKG, and/or ventricular tachycardia. Do not administer concomitantly.
- Corticosteroids: May increase corticosteroid serum level; may need to decrease dosage.

Lab Effects/Interference:

Major clinical significance:
- ALT, alk phos, AST, serum bili values may be elevated.
- ACTH-induced serum corticosteroid concentrations and serum testosterone concentrations may be decreased by doses of 800 mg/day of ketoconazole;

serum testosterone concentrations are abolished by values of 1.6 g/day of ketoconzole but return to baseline values when ketoconazole is discontinued.

Special Considerations:

- Monitor liver function studies.
- High failure rate in HIV-infected patients due to achlorhydria.
- Addisonian crisis may occur if ketoconazole not given with hydrocortisone.

Potential Toxicities/Side Effects and the Nursing Process

I. ALTERATION IN MALE SEXUAL FUNCTION related to GYNECOMASTIA, BREAST TENDERNESS, OLIGOSPERMIA, DECREASED LIBIDO, AND IMPOTENCE

Defining Characteristics: Breast enlargement and tenderness may occur in some men, lasting weeks to duration of therapy. Oligospermia, azoospermia, decreased libido, and impotence may also occur.

Nursing Implications: Inform patient that these side effects may occur. Explore with patient and partner reproductive and sexual patterns, and impact that therapy may have. Provide information and supportive counseling, and referral as appropriate. Assess for presence of side effects on follow-up, as well as comfort level, breast tenderness, and impact on body image and sexual relationships.

II. ALTERATION IN NUTRITION, LESS THAN BODY REQUIREMENTS, related to GI SIDE EFFECTS

Defining Characteristics: Nausea, vomiting is seen in 3–10% of patients; anorexia affects about 10% as well. Diarrhea, abdominal pain, flatulence, constipation may occur less frequently. Increased LFTs may occur: AST, ALT, alk phos. Hepatotoxicity is less common, is usually reversible, and is rarely fatal.

Nursing Implications: Assess baseline nutritional and elimination status. Instruct patient to report GI disturbances. Administer and teach patient to self-administer antiemetics and antidiarrheals as needed and as ordered. Although an acidic environment enhances absorption, taking ketoconazole with milk or food reduces nausea. Alternatively, starting patient at lower dose and gradually increasing dose will also reduce nausea. Teach patient importance of nutritious diet, and suggest small, frequent, high-calorie, high-protein meals as appropriate. Assess baseline LFTs and monitor periodically during treatment. Discuss abnormalities and drug interruption with physician. Assess whether taking other hepatotoxic drugs (see Special Considerations section). Assess for increased fatigue, jaundice, dark urine, pale stools (signs of hepatotoxicity) and discuss drug discontinuance immediately with physician.

III. ALTERATION IN COMFORT related to GYNECOMASTIA AND BREAST TENDERNESS

Defining Characteristics: Breast enlargement and tenderness may occur in some men, lasting weeks to duration of therapy.

Nursing Implications: Assess for occurrence in male patients. Assess comfort level, degree of tenderness, and self-care measures used to increase comfort. Assess impact on body image.

IV. ALTERATION IN SKIN INTEGRITY related to ALLERGIC REACTION

Defining Characteristics: Rash, dermatitis, purpura, urticaria occur in 1% of patients; rarely, anaphylaxis may occur.

Nursing Implications: Assess baseline skin condition and integrity. Teach patient to report itch, rash, other skin changes. Teach patient skin care and symptomatic measures. If rash or dermatitis progresses, discuss drug discontinuance with physician. Assess for signs/symptoms of anaphylaxis.

V. ALTERATIONS IN SENSORY/PERCEPTUAL PATTERNS related to CNS EFFECTS

Defining Characteristics: Dizziness, headache, nervousness, insomnia, lethargy, somnolence, and paresthesia have occurred in ~1% of patients.

Nursing Implications: Assess baseline neurologic function and comfort, and monitor during treatment. Instruct patient to report any changes. Discuss any abnormalities with physician.

Drug: letrozole (Femara)

Class: Nonsteroidal aromatase inhibitor.

Mechanism of Action: Highly selective, potent agent that significantly suppresses (90%) serum estradiol levels within 14 days, without interfering with other steroid hormone synthesis. Binds to the heme group of aromatase, a cytochrome P-450 enzyme necessary for the conversion of androgens to estrogens. Aromatase is thus inhibited, leading to a significant reduction in plasma estradiol, estrone, and estrone sulfate. After six weeks of therapy, there is 97% suppression of estradiol.

Metabolism: Rapidly and completely absorbed after oral administration, with a terminal half-life of 2 days. Metabolized in the liver and excreted in the urine.

Dosage/Range:
- 2.5 mg PO qd.
- Dose reduction recommended in patients with cirrhosis and severe hepatic dysfunction.

Drug Preparation/Administration:
- Oral.

Drug Interactions:
- Tamoxifen: coadministration with tamoxifen decreased letrozole plasma levels by 38%.

Lab Effects/Interference:
- Liver transaminases may be transiently elevated.
- Increase in total cholesterol (non-fasting, adjuvant studies).

Special Considerations:
- Indicated for 1) adjuvant treatment of postmenopausal women with hormone receptor positive early breast cancer, 2) the extended adjuvant treatment of early breast cancer in postmenopausal women who have received 5 years of adjuvant tamoxifen therapy; 3) the first-line treatment of postmenopausal women with hormone receptor positive or unknown, locally advanced or metastatic breast cancer; 4) treatment of advanced breast cancer in postmenopausal women with disease progression following antiestrogen therapy.
- Letrozole was compared to tamoxifen in postmenopausal women and found to be superior in terms of response (30% vs 20%), time to disease progression (41 weeks vs 25 weeks), and rate of clinical benefit (49% vs 38%) (Mouridsen et al, 2001).
- Potent aromatase inhibitor with response rate of 20%.
- Drug has not been evaluated in premenopausal women.
- About 200 times more potent than aminoglutethamide.
- Letrozole may cause fetal harm when administered to pregnant women as drug is embryotoxic and fetotoxic in lab animals. If there is exposure to letrozole during pregnancy, the patient should be apprised of the potential hazard to the fetus and potential risk for loss of the pregnancy.

Potential Toxicities/Side Effects and the Nursing Process

I. ALTERATION IN COMFORT related to PAIN, FATIGUE, AND HOT FLASHES

Defining Characteristics: Most common side effects were musculoskeletal pain (21%: muscle, skeletal, back, arm, leg), arthralgia (8%), headache (9%), fatigue (8%), and chest pain (6%). Hot flashes occur in approximately 6% of patients.

Nursing Considerations: Assess baseline comfort levels, and teach patient that this discomfort may occur. Teach patient symptomatic measures, and instruct to report if symptoms are unrelieved.

II. ALTERATION IN NUTRITION, LESS THAN BODY REQUIREMENTS, related to NAUSEA/VOMITING, ANOREXIA

Defining Characteristics: Nausea occurs in 13% of patients, with less frequent vomiting and anorexia.

Nursing Implications: Determine baseline weight, and monitor at each visit. Teach patient that these side effects may occur, and instruct to report this. Discuss strategies to minimize nausea, including diet and dosing time.

III. ALTERATION IN BOWEL ELIMINATION related to DIARRHEA AND CONSTIPATION

Defining Characteristics: Diarrhea or constipation occurs in about 6% of patients.

Nursing Implications: Assess for change in bowel patterns, and instruct patient to report diarrhea or constipation. Teach patient that diarrhea or constipation are usually relieved by nonprescription medications such as Kaolin pectate combinations (Kaopectate) for diarrhea, and stool softeners or Psyllium for constipation. Instruct patient to report unrelieved diarrhea or constipation.

Drug: leuprolide acetate (Lupron, Viadur)

Class: Antihormone.

Mechanism of Action: It is a luteinizing hormone-releasing hormone (LHRH) analogue that suppresses the secretion of follicle-stimulating hormone (FSH) and luteinizing hormone (LH) from the pituitary gland. The decrease in LH causes the Leydig cells to reduce testosterone production to castrate levels.

Metabolism: 95% of the drug is absorbed after SQ injection, and 85–100% of the drug is absorbed after IM or SQ injection. Drug is slightly protein bound (7–15%).

Dosage/Range:

- For palliative treatment of prostate cancer: Depot suspension 7.5 mg IM q month, OR 22.5 mg IM q 3 months, OR 30 mg IM q 4 months, OR Viadur implant 65 mg q 12 months, OR 1 mg/day SQ injection.

Drug Preparation:
- Use syringes, diluent, kit provided by manufacturer.
- Injection: 5 mg/mL; kit 5 mg/mL for 7.5-mg, 22.5-mg doses.
- Powder for injection: 7.5 mg.
- Viadur implant kit contains implant, implanter, and sterile field/supplies. Sterile gloves must be added. Procedure is sterile, and uses a special implant technology.

Drug Administration:
- Depot is administered IM or SQ.
- Daily solution is given SQ.
- Viadur: Kit contains specific directions for insertion of implant, removal, and reinsertion of subsequent dose after 1 year.

Drug Interactions:
- None reported.

Lab Effects/Interference:
- Decreased PSA, testosterone levels; increased calcium, decreased WBC, decreased serum total protein.
- Injection: Increased BUN and creatinine.
- Depot: Increased LDH, alk phos, AST, uric acid, cholesterol, LDL, triglycerides, glucose, WBC, phosphate; decreased potassium, platelets.

Special Considerations:
- Patient should be instructed in proper administration techniques, and in signs/symptoms of infection at site. Sites should be rotated. For Viadur, patient has implant inserted by MD/RN once yearly.
- Initially, drug causes increased LH secretion, resulting in increased testosterone secretion and tumor flare. Usually disappears after 2 weeks.
- Drug has been studied in the treatment of breast and islet cell cancers.
- Studies on Viadur show that implant delivers 120 micrograms of leuprolide acetate per day over 12 months, reducing testosterone levels to castration levels within 2–4 weeks after insertion.

Potential Toxicities/Side Effects and the Nursing Process

I. ALTERATION IN COMFORT related to HOT FLASHES, TUMOR FLARE, EDEMA

Defining Characteristics: Headache, dizziness, and hot flashes may occur. Vasodilation most common, with 67.9% incidence. Sweating may affect 5% of patients. Tumor flare may also occur initially (bone and tumor pain, transient increase in tumor size due to transient increase in testosterone levels). Breast tenderness has been reported. Peripheral edema may occur in 8% of patients.

Nursing Implications: Inform patient that symptoms may occur, that flare reaction will subside after the initial two weeks of therapy. Encourage patient to report symptoms early. Develop symptom management plan with patient and physician.

II. POTENTIAL SEXUAL DYSFUNCTION related to LIBIDO, IMPOTENCE

Defining Characteristics: Frequently causes decreased libido and erectile impotence in men. Gynecomastia occurs in 3–6.9% of patients. In women, amenorrhea occurs after ten weeks of therapy.

Nursing Implications: As appropriate, explore with patient and significant other issues of reproductive and sexual patterns and the impact chemotherapy may have on them. Discuss strategies to preserve sexuality and reproductive health.

III. DEPRESSION, POTENTIAL related to DRUG EFFECT

Defining Characteristics: Depression may affect up to 5.3% of patients, and less commonly, patients may develop emotional lability, insomnia, nervousness, anxiety.

Nursing Implications: Assess baseline affect and usual coping strategies. Teach patient to report change in affect. Assess effectiveness of coping strategies, encourage patient to verbalize feelings, and provide emotional support. Assess need for referral to psychiatric nurse specialist or social worker if supportive efforts ineffective.

IV. ALTERED NUTRITION, LESS THAN BODY REQUIREMENTS, related to GI SIDE EFFECTS

Defining Characteristics: Anorexia, nausea, and vomiting may occur rarely, with an incidence of $< 5\%$.

Nursing Implications: If patients experience symptoms, encourage small, frequent feedings of favorite foods, especially high-calorie, high-protein foods. Monitor weight weekly. Assess incidence and pattern of nausea, vomiting, or anorexia if they occur. Discuss need for antiemetic with physician and patient.

V. ALTERATION IN SKIN INTEGRITY, POTENTIAL related to INSERTION, REMOVAL OF 12-MONTH IMPLANT

Defining Characteristics: Insertion and removal of implant caused local site bruising (34.8%) and burning (5.6%). In general, the reactions lasted two weeks, and then resolved completely. In about 10% of patients, reactions lasted longer than two weeks, or reactions didn't develop until after two weeks.

Nursing Implications: Assess baseline skin integrity after implant insertion, or removal. Teach patient that these reactions may occur, and will resolve, usually within two weeks. Teach patients to use local measures to minimize feeling of burning.

Drug: lomustine (CCNU, CeeNU)

Class: Alkylating agent (nitrosourea).

Mechanism of Action: Nitrosourea alkylates DNA with a reactive chloroethyl carbonium ion, producing strand breaks and crosslinks that inhibit RNA and DNA synthesis. Interferes with enzymes and histadine utilization. Is cell cycle phase nonspecific.

Metabolism: Completely absorbed from GI tract. Metabolized rapidly, partly protein-bound. Undergoes hepatic recirculation. Lipid soluble: crosses BBB; 75% excreted in urine within 4 days.

Dosage/Range:
- 130 mg/m^2 PO every 6 weeks.
- 100 mg/m^2 if given with other myelosuppressive drugs.

Drug Preparation:
- Oral: Available in 10-mg, 30-mg, and 100-mg capsules.

Drug Administration:
- Administer on an empty stomach at bedtime.

Drug Interactions:
- Myelosuppressive drugs increase hematologic toxicity; reduce dose.

Lab Effects/Interference:
- Decreased CBC.
- Increased LFTs, RFTs.

Special Considerations:
- Give orally on an empty stomach.
- Consumption of alcohol should be avoided for a short period after taking CCNU.
- Absorbed 30–60 minutes after administration; consequently, vomiting does not usually affect efficacy.

Potential Toxicities/Side Effects and the Nursing Process

I. INFECTION AND BLEEDING related to MYELOSUPPRESSION

Defining Characteristics: Nadir of platelets: 26–34 days, lasting 6–10 days; nadir of WBC: 41–46 days, lasting 9–14 days. Delayed and cumulative bone marrow depression with successive dosing: recovery takes 6–8 weeks. Bone marrow depression is dose-limiting toxicity.

Nursing Implications: Drug should be administered every 6–8 weeks due to delayed nadir and recovery. Monitor CBC, platelets prior to drug administration (WBC > $4000/mm^3$ and platelets > $100{,}000/mm^3$). Dispense only one dose at a time.

II. ALTERATION IN NUTRITION, LESS THAN BODY REQUIREMENTS related to NAUSEA/VOMITING, ANOREXIA, DIARRHEA

Defining Characteristics: Onset of nausea/vomiting occurs 2–6 hours after taking dose; may be severe. Anorexia may last for several days. Diarrhea is uncommon.

Nursing Implications: Administer drug on an empty stomach at bedtime. Premedicate with antiemetic and sedative or hypnotic to promote sleep. Discourage food or fluid intake for two hours after drug administration. Encourage small, frequent feedings of favorite foods. Encourage high-calorie, high-protein foods; monitor weekly weights. Encourage patient to report onset of diarrhea. Administer or teach patient to self-administer antidiarrheal medication.

III. ALTERATION IN URINARY ELIMINATION related to RENAL COMPROMISE

Defining Characteristics: After prolonged therapy with high cumulative doses, tubular atrophy, glomerular sclerosis, and interstitial nephritis have occurred, leading to renal failure.

Nursing Implications: Monitor BUN, creatinine prior to dosing, especially in patients receiving prolonged or high cumulative dose therapy. If abnormalities are noted, a creatinine clearance should be determined.

IV. POTENTIAL FOR SEXUAL DYSFUNCTION related to MUTAGENIC AND TERATOGENIC QUALITIES OF CCNU

Defining Characteristics: Drug is teratogenic, mutagenic, and carcinogenic.

Nursing Implications: As appropriate, discuss birth control measures.

V. ACTIVITY INTOLERANCE related to LETHARGY, CONFUSION

Defining Characteristics: Neurologic dysfunction may occur rarely: confusion, lethargy, disorientation, ataxia.

Nursing Implications: Perform neurologic assessment as part of prechemotherapy assessment. Assess orientation and level of consciousness, gait, activity tolerance.

VI. POTENTIAL SENSORY/PERCEPTUAL ALTERATIONS (VISUAL) related to OCULAR DAMAGE

Defining Characteristics: Ocular damage may occur rarely: optic neuritis, retinopathy, blurred vision.

Nursing Implications: Assess vision during prechemotherapy assessment. Encourage patient to report any visual changes.

Drug: mechlorethamine hydrochloride (Mustargen, Nitrogen Mustard, HN_2)

Class: Alkylating agent.

Mechanism of Action: Produces interstrand and intrastrand cross-linkages in DNA, causing miscoding, breakage, and failures of replication. Cell cycle phase nonspecific.

Metabolism: Undergoes chemical transformation after injection with less than 0.01% excreted unchanged in urine. Drug is rapidly inactivated by body fluids. 50% of the inactive metabolites are excreted in the urine within 24 hours.

Dosage/Range:
- IV: 0.4 mg/kg, or 12–16 mg/m^2 IV as single agent; 6 mg/m^2 IV days 1 and 8 of 28-day cycle with MOPP regimen.
- Topical: Dilute 10 mg in 60 mL sterile water; apply with rubber gloves.
- Intracavitary: Pleural, peritoneal, pericardial: 0.2–0.4 mg/kg.

Drug Preparation:
- Add sterile water or 0.9% Sodium Chloride to each vial. Wear eye and hand protection when mixing.
- Administer via sidearm or rapidly running IV.
- Drug must be used within 15 minutes of reconstitution.

Drug Administration:
- Intravenous: This drug is a potent vesicant. Give through a freely running IV to avoid extravasation, which can lead to ulceration, pain, and necrosis. Check hospital's policy and procedure for administration of a vesicant.

Drug Interactions:
- Myelosuppressive drugs: Additive hematologic toxicity; dose reduce or monitor patient closely.

Lab Effects/Interference:
- Decreased CBC.
- Increased uric acid, RFTs.

Special Considerations:

- Drug is a vesicant. Give through a running IV to avoid extravasation. Antidote is sodium thiosulfate: dilute 4 mL sodium thiosulfate injection USP (10%) with 6 mL sterile water for injection, USP and inject SQ in area of infiltration.
- Nadir is 6–8 days after treatment.
- Side effects occur in the reproductive system, such as amenorrhea and azoospermia.
- Severe nausea and vomiting.
- Systemic toxic effects may occur with intracavitary drug administration.

Potential Toxicities/Side Effects and the Nursing Process

I. ALTERATION IN NUTRITION, LESS THAN BODY REQUIREMENTS related to NAUSEA AND VOMITING, ANOREXIA, DIARRHEA

Defining Characteristics: Nausea and vomiting occur in ~100% of patients, within 30 minutes to 2 hours of drug administration, and up to 8 hours afterward. Nausea and vomiting can be severe, but can be prevented by the use of combination antiemetics such as serotonin antagonist (granisetron or ondansetron) and dexamethasone. Anorexia and taste distortion (metallic taste) occur commonly. Diarrhea may occur up to several days after drug administration.

Nursing Implications: Premedicate with combination antiemetics such as serotonin antagonist (granisetron or ondansetron) and dexamethasone. Continue prophylactically. Antiemetic and sedative may need to be started the evening before if patient develops anticipatory nausea and vomiting. Encourage small, frequent feedings of cool, bland foods, dry toast, crackers. Monitor I/O to detect fluid volume deficit. Notify physician of the need for more aggressive antiemetic if vomitus > 750 mL. Encourage small, frequent feedings of high-calorie, high-protein foods. Encourage use of spices for anorexia, weekly weights. Encourage patient to report onset of diarrhea. Administer or teach patient to self-administer antidiarrheal medication and teach diet modifications (low residue) as appropriate.

II. INFECTION AND BLEEDING related to BONE MARROW DEPRESSION

Defining Characteristics: Potent myelosuppressant with nadir 6–8 days, recovery in 4 weeks. Patients at risk for profound bone marrow depression are those with previous extensive XRT, previous chemotherapy, or compromised bone marrow function. Lymphocyte depression occurs within 24 hours of drug dose.

Nursing Implications: Evaluate WBC, with neutrophil, and platelet count, and discuss any abnormalities with physician prior to drug administration. Assess for signs/symptoms of infection or bleeding; instruct patient in signs/symptoms of infection and bleeding, and to notify nurse or physician if they arise. Teach patient self-care measures to minimize risk of infection and bleeding, including avoidance of OTC aspirin-containing medications. Assess patient's Hgb/HCT and signs/symptoms of fatigue; teach patient self-assessment and to alternate rest and activity as needed. Transfuse red blood cells and platelets per physician order.

III. IMPAIRED SKIN INTEGRITY related to ALOPECIA, DRUG EXTRAVASATION

Defining Characteristics: Alopecia usually occurs as diffuse thinning. Drug is a potent vesicant, causing tissue necrosis and sloughing if extravasation occurs. Thrombosis or thrombophlebitis may occur despite all precautions, and venous access device may be required. Delayed cutaneous hypersensitivity is seen with topical application.

Nursing Implications: Discuss with patient hair loss, anticipated impact, and strategies to decrease distress, e.g., obtaining wig prior to hair loss. Assess body disturbance from hyperpigmentation and discuss strategies to minimize this, e.g., nail polish. Drug must be administered via patent IV. Assess need for venous access device early. Delayed cutaneous hypersensitivity (topical application) is not an indication to stop the drug. Discuss symptomatic management with physician. If extravasation is suspected, stop drug; aspirate any residual drug and blood from IV tubing, IV catheter/needle, and IV site if possible; instill antidote, sodium thiosulfate (1–6 molar), into area of apparent infiltration as per physician orders and institutional policy and procedure; apply cold or topical medication as per physician orders and institutional policy and procedure. Assess site regularly for pain, progression of erythema, induration, and for evidence of necrosis. When in doubt about whether drug is infiltrating, TREAT AS AN INFILTRATION. Teach patient to assess site, and instruct to notify physician if condition worsens. Arrange next clinic visit for assessment of site depending on drug, amount infiltrated, extent of potential injury, and patient variables. Document in patient's record as per institutional policy. Warm packs may decrease discomfort of phlebitis. Have standing orders and sodium thiosulfate injection USP (10%) close by in the event of actual infiltration of drug; dilute sodium thiosulfate with sterile water for injection and inject SQ in area of infiltration.

IV. ALTERATION IN COMFORT related to CHILLS, FEVER, DIARRHEA

Defining Characteristics: Chills, fever, diarrhea may occur after drug administration. Also weakness, drowsiness, headache may occur.

Nursing Implications: Assess patient for these symptoms during hour following treatment. Instruct patient to report these symptoms and teach self-management at home if outpatient. Provide symptomatic management per physician with acetaminophen, antidiarrheal medication.

V. POTENTIAL SEXUAL DYSFUNCTION related to DRUG EFFECTS

Defining Characteristics: Drug is teratogenic, carcinogenic. Amenorrhea occurs in females. Impaired spermatogenesis occurs in males. If administered to pregnant patients, spontaneous abortion or fetal abnormalities may occur.

Nursing Implications: As appropriate, explore with patient and partner issues of reproductive and sexual patterns, and anticipated impact chemotherapy will have. Discuss strategies to preserve sexuality and reproductive health (sperm banking, contraception).

VI. POTENTIAL FOR SENSORY/PERCEPTUAL ALTERATIONS related to CRANIAL NERVE INJURY

Defining Characteristics: Tinnitus, deafness, and other signs of eighth cranial nerve damage occur rarely, with high drug doses or regional perfusion techniques. Temporary aphasia and paresis occurs very rarely.

Nursing Implications: Assess hearing ability, presence of tinnitus prior to drug doses. If high doses of drug are given, or regional perfusion used, schedule patient for periodic audiometry. Instruct patient to report signs/symptoms of hearing loss.

Drug: melphalan hydrochloride (Alkeran, L-Phenylalanine Mustard, L-PAM, L-Sarcolysin)

Class: Alkylating agent.

Mechanism of Action: Prevents cell replication by causing breaks and cross-linkages in DNA strands with subsequent miscoding and breakage. Cell cycle phase nonspecific. Drug is derivative of nitrogen mustard.

Metabolism: Variable bioavailability after oral administration, especially if taken with food. Therefore, dose is titrated to WBC count; 20–50% of drug is excreted in feces over 6 days, 50% excreted in urine within 24 hours. After IV administration, parent compound disappears from plasma, with a half-life of about 2 hours.

Dosage/Range:

- Multiple myeloma: Several regimens, including 0.25 mg/kg/day × 4 days, in combination with prednisone 2 mg/kg/day, repeated every 6 weeks; OR 6

mg/m² orally daily × 5 days every 6 weeks for myeloma; OR 0.1 mg/kg PO × 2–3 weeks, then maintenance of 2–4 mg daily when bone marrow has recovered.
- 8 mg/m² IV daily × 5 days (investigational).
- Bone marrow transplantation: 50–60 mg/m² IV, but may be as high as 140–200 mg/m² (investigational).

Drug Preparation:
- Oral: Available in 2-mg tablets. Take on empty stomach.
- IV: Reconstitute 50-mg vial with 10 mL of provided diluent resulting in concentration of 5 mg/mL. Further dilute in 100–150 mL to produce a final concentration ≤ 2 mg/mL in 0.9% Sodium Chloride. Use provided 0.45-μm filter. Administer over 30–45 minutes. Stable for 1 hour at room temperature.

Drug Administration:
- Serious hypersensitivity reactions reported with IV administration.
- IV drug can cause anaphylaxis.
- IV drug is an irritant—avoid extravasation.

Drug Interactions:
- Myelosuppressive chemotherapy: Increases hematologic toxicity; dose-reduce or monitor patient very carefully.
- Cyclosporine: Increases nephrotoxicity.
- Drug activity is enhanced with concurrent administration of misonidazol (investigational).

Lab Effects/Interference:
- Decreased CBC.

Special Considerations:
- Nadir is 14–21 days after treatment.
- Increased risk of nephrotoxicity when given with cyclosporine.
- Drug dose reductions are recommended in patients with renal compromise.
- Drug is used in regional perfusion.

Potential Toxicities/Side Effects and the Nursing Process

I. INFECTION AND BLEEDING related to BONE MARROW DEPRESSION

Defining Characteristics: Bone marrow depression may be pronounced; leukopenia and thrombocytopenia occur 14–21 days after intermittent dosing schedules. May be delayed in onset, and cumulative with nadir extended to 5–6 weeks. Combined immunosuppression from disease (e.g., multiple myeloma) and drug may prolong vulnerability to infection. Thrombocytopenia may be persistent.

Nursing Implications: Evaluate WBC, with neutrophil, and platelet count and discuss any abnormalities with physician prior to drug administration. Assess for signs/symptoms of infection or bleeding; instruct patient in signs/symptoms of infection and bleeding, and to notify nurse or physician if they arise. Teach patient self-care measures to minimize risk of infection and bleeding, including avoidance of OTC aspirin-containing medications. Assess patient for Hgb/HCT and signs/symptoms of fatigue; teach patient self-assessment and to alternate rest and activity as needed. Transfuse packed red blood cells and platelets per physician order.

II. ALTERATION IN NUTRITION, LESS THAN BODY REQUIREMENTS, related to NAUSEA AND VOMITING, ANOREXIA

Defining Characteristics: Nausea and vomiting are mild at low, continuous dosing; severe following high doses. Anorexia occurs rarely.

Nursing Implications: Administer drug (oral) on empty stomach. Premedicate with antiemetic (oral) one hour before oral dose. Use aggressive antiemetic regimen for IV Alkeran. Encourage small, frequent feedings of favorite foods, especially high-calorie, high-protein foods. Encourage use of spices; weekly weights.

III. ALTERATION IN CARDIAC OUTPUT, PERFUSION related to ANAPHYLAXIS

Defining Characteristics: Severe hypersensitivity reactions can occur with IV administration, including diaphoresis, hypotension, and cardiac arrest.

Nursing Implications: Review standing orders for management of patient in anaphylaxis and identify location of anaphylaxis kit containing epinephrine 1:1000, hydrocortisone sodium succinate (Solucortef), diphenhydramine HCl (Benadryl), aminophylline, and others. Prior to drug administration, obtain baseline vital signs and record mental status. Administer drug slowly, diluted as per physician's order. Observe for following signs/symptoms, usually occurring within first 15 minutes of infusion. Subjective signs are generalized itching, nausea, chest tightness, crampy abdominal pain, difficulty speaking, anxiety, agitation, sense of impending doom, uneasiness, desire to urinate/defecate, dizziness, chills. Objective signs are flushed appearance (angioedema of face, neck, eyelids, hands, feet), localized or generalized urticaria, respiratory distress ± wheezing, hypotension, cyanosis. For generalized allergic reaction, stop infusion and notify physician. Place patient in supine position to promote perfusion of visceral organs. Monitor VS. Provide emotional reassurance to patient and family. Maintain patent airway and have CPR equipment ready if needed. Document incident. Discuss with physician desensitization for further dosing vs drug discontinuance.

IV. POTENTIAL SEXUAL DYSFUNCTION related to DRUG EFFECTS

Defining Characteristics: Potentially mutagenic and teratogenic.

Nursing Implications: Encourage patient to verbalize goals about family; discuss options, such as sperm banking. As appropriate, discuss or refer for counseling about birth control measures during therapy.

V. POTENTIAL FOR INJURY related to SECOND MALIGNANCY

Defining Characteristics: Acute myelogenous and myelomonocytic leukemias may occur after continuous long-term dosing, especially in patients with ovarian cancer and multiple myeloma. Heralded by preleukemic pancytopenia of several weeks' duration. Chromosomal abnormalities characteristic of acute leukemia.

Nursing Implications: Patients receiving prolonged continuous therapy should be closely followed during and after treatment.

VI. POTENTIAL FOR IMPAIRED GAS EXCHANGE related to PULMONARY TOXICITY

Defining Characteristics: Rare, but may occur, especially with continued chronic dosing. Bronchopulmonary dysplasia and pulmonary fibrosis.

Nursing Implications: Assess pulmonary status for signs/symptoms of pulmonary dysfunction. Assess lung sounds prior to dosing. Instruct patient to report cough or dyspnea. Discuss PFTs to be performed periodically with physician. Long-term follow-up is important.

VII. IMPAIRED SKIN INTEGRITY related to ALOPECIA, MACULOPAPULAR RASH, URTICARIA

Defining Characteristics: Alopecia is minimal if it occurs at all. Maculopapular rash and urticaria are infrequent.

Nursing Implications: Assess skin integrity and presence of rash, urticaria, alopecia prior to dosing. Assess impact of these alterations on patient and develop plan to manage symptom distress.

Drug: menogaril (Menogarol) (investigational)

Class: Antitumor (anthracycline) antibiotic.

Mechanism of Action: Appears to have a mechanism different from other anthracyclines in that the drug does not appear to bind too strongly to DNA for its cytotoxicity; drug also appears to act in the cytoplasm of the cell rather than in the cell nucleus.

Metabolism: Metabolized in the liver to its metabolite(s) following IV administration. Limited oral bioavailability; 5% elimination via either the bile or kidneys. Drug elimination half-life of 30 hours, and of its metabolite 58 hours.

Dosage/Range:
- 140–200 mg/m^2 IV over 2 hours every 3–4 weeks (investigational).
- 50 mg/m^2/day × 5 days every 3–4 weeks (investigational).

Drug Preparation:
- Vial is kept refrigerated and protected from light.
- Reconstitute 50-mg vial with 10 mL sterile water and shake well for 2 minutes; solution is stable for 14 days at room temperature and 6 weeks refrigerated.
- Withdraw dose and further dilute in 5% Dextrose ONLY to a final concentration of 0.1 mg/mL. Commonly, drug is mixed in 500 mL of 5% Dextrose.

Drug Administration:
- Administer by slow IV infusion over 1–2 hours by central line if possible to avoid phlebitis.
- Oral administration has been studied: drug is mixed in grape juice.

Drug Interactions:
- Drug becomes a gel when mixed in sodium-containing solutions.
- Incompatible with heparin and sodium bicarbonate.

Lab Effects/Interference:
- Decreased CBC.
- Increased LFTs.

Special Considerations:
- Drug is being studied in a number of malignancies.

Potential Toxicities/Side Effects and the Nursing Process

I. POTENTIAL FOR INFECTION AND BLEEDING related to BONE MARROW DEPRESSION

Defining Characteristics: Neutropenia is dose-limiting toxicity, with nadir occurring 2–3 weeks after treatment, and recovery by week 4. Thrombocytopenia and anemia are less common, with 10–12% incidence.

Nursing Implications: Evaluate WBC, ANC, and platelet count, and discuss any abnormalities with physician prior to drug administration. Assess for signs/symptoms of infection or bleeding, and teach patient to notify nurse or physician if they arise. Teach patient self-care measures to minimize risk of infection and bleeding, including avoidance of OTC aspirin-containing medications. Assess patient for Hgb/HCT and signs/symptoms of fatigue; teach patient self-assessment and to alternate rest and activity as needed. HIGH DOSE: Bone marrow aplasia expected; refer to investigational protocol.

II. ALTERATION IN NUTRITION, LESS THAN BODY REQUIREMENTS, related to NAUSEA, DIARRHEA, STOMATITIS, ANOREXIA, HEPATIC ENZYME ELEVATIONS

Defining Characteristics: Nausea/vomiting is mild if it occurs. Stomatitis is dose-limiting in leukemic patients. Anorexia has an incidence of 25%, and diarrhea has been reported. SGOT and SGPT may become mildly elevated.

Nursing Implications: Teach patient to report GI side effects, and teach self-care measures as appropriate. Monitor SGOT, SGPT, LDH, alk phos, and bili baseline and monitor SGPT and SGOT periodically during treatment. Notify physician of any elevations.

III. POTENTIAL FOR IMPAIRED SKIN INTEGRITY related to ALOPECIA, PHLEBITIS, URTICARIA

Defining Characteristics: Drug is irritating to vein. Phlebitis, inflammation, and pain at the IV injection site are common. Erythema may occur along the vein path during administration in 10% of patients. Urticaria may be severe, is dose-related, and may result in blister formation. Alopecia occurs and is mild.

Nursing Implications: Consider central line, especially if higher dose is given. Assess patient for signs/symptoms of hair loss. Discuss with patient impact of hair loss, and strategies to minimize distress. Teach patient that skin reactions may occur, and instruct to report them. Develop management strategies to maintain skin integrity and comfort.

IV. POTENTIAL ALTERATION IN OXYGENATION related to CARDIOTOXICITY

Defining Characteristics: Drug is less cardiotoxic than doxorubicin. However, atrial fibrillation, sinus bradycardia, myocardial infarction, ventricular arythmias, and decreased LVEF may occur. Incidence of the last abnormality is 10%.

Nursing Implications: Assess patient risk (history of prior anthracycline chemotherapy, history of cardiovascular disease). Assess cardiac status prior to chemotherapy administration: signs/symptoms of CHF, quality/regularity and rate of heart beat, results of prior GBPS or other test of LVEF. Instruct patient to report dyspnea, palpitations, swelling in extremities. Maintain accurate records of total dose, and expect GBPS to be repeated periodically during treatment, and the drug to be discontinued if there is a significant drop in heart function.

Drug: mercaptopurine (Purinethol, 6-MP)

Class: Antimetabolite.

Mechanism of Action: One of two thiopurine antimetabolites (with 6-TG) that are converted to monophosphate nucleotides and inhibit de novo purine synthesis. The nucleotides are also incorporated into DNA. Cell cycle phase specific for S phase.

Metabolism: Metabolized by the enzyme xanthine oxidase in the kidney and liver; 50% of the drug is excreted in the urine. Plasma half-life is 20–40 minutes.

Dosage/Range:
- 100 mg/m^2 PO daily × 5 days.
- Children: 70 mg/m^2 daily for induction, then 40 mg/m^2 daily for maintenance.
- IV: 500–1000 mg/m^2/day × 2–3 days (investigational).

Drug Preparation:
- Oral: none; available in 50-mg tablets.
- IV: reconstitute 500-mg vial with sterile water for concentration of 10 mg/mL; store IV solution at room temperature; discard after 8 hours.
- Further dilute to a final concentration of 1–2 mg/mL in 5% Dextrose or 0.9% Sodium Chloride. Stable 3 days either refrigerated or at room temperature.

Drug Administration:
- Oral.
- IV: Infuse over 1 hour or longer per protocol.

Drug Interactions:
- Allopurinol: increased mercaptopurine levels; reduce dose to 25–35% of normal.
- Hepatotoxic drugs: additive hepatotoxicity; monitor LFTs closely.
- Warfarin: decreases or increases PT; monitor PT closely.
- Nonpolarizing muscle relaxants: decreased neuromuscular blockage; use together cautiously.

Lab Effects/Interference:
- Decreased CBC.
- Increased LFTs.
- Increased RFTs: tumor lysis.

Special Considerations:
- Elevated serum glucose levels and elevated serum uric acid levels could be related to the effects of medication.
- Reduce dose in cases of hepatic or renal dysfunction.
- Because xanthine oxidase is inhibited by allopurinol, concurrent use of the latter necessitates a dose reduction of 6-MP to ¼ the normal dose.

Potential Toxicities/Side Effects and the Nursing Process

I. POTENTIAL FOR INFECTION AND BLEEDING related to BONE MARROW DEPRESSION

Defining Characteristics: Nadir varies from 5 days to 6 weeks after treatment. Leukopenia more prominent than thrombocytopenia. Blood counts may continue to fall after therapy is stopped.

Nursing Implications: Evaluate WBC, with neutrophil, and platelet count, and discuss any abnormalities with physician prior to drug administration. Assess for signs/symptoms of infection or bleeding; instruct patient to notify nurse or physician if they arise. Teach patient self-care measures to minimize risk of infection and bleeding, including avoidance of OTC aspirin-containing medications. Assess patient's Hgb/HCT and signs/symptoms of fatigue; teach patient self-assessment and to alternate rest and activity as needed.

II. ALTERATION IN NUTRITION, LESS THAN BODY REQUIREMENTS related to HEPATOTOXICITY, GI SYMPTOMS

Defining Characteristics: Reversible cholestatic jaundice may develop after 2–5 months of treatment. Hepatic necrosis may develop. Nausea, vomiting, anorexia, diarrhea are infrequent. Stomatitis uncommon, but appears as white patchy areas similar to thrush.

Nursing Implications: Monitor SGOT, SGPT, LDH, alk phos, and bili periodically during treatment. Notify physician of any elevations. Hepatic toxicity may be an indication for discontinuing treatment. Instruct patient to report GI side effects and to perform self-care measures as appropriate.

III. POTENTIAL FOR IMPAIRED SKIN INTEGRITY related to RASH

Defining Characteristics: Skin eruptions; rash may occur.

Nursing Implications: Advise patient these changes may occur. Instruct patient in symptomatic care if distress related to skin reactions occurs.

Drug: methotrexate (Amethopterin, Mexate, Folex)

Class: Antimetabolite, folic acid antagonist.

Mechanism of Action: Blocks the enzyme dihydrofolate reductase (DHFR), which inhibits the conversion of folic acid to tetrahydrofolic acid, resulting in an inhibition of the key precursors of DNA, RNA, and cellular proteins. May synchronize malignant cells in the S phase: at high plasma levels, passive entry of the drug into tumor cells can potentially overcome drug resistance.

Metabolism: Bound to serum albumin; concurrent use of drugs that displace methotrexate from serum albumin should be avoided. Salicylates, sulfonamides, dilantin, some antibacterials—including tetracycline, chloramphenicol, paraminobenzoic acid—and alcohol should be avoided, as they will delay excretion. Drug is absorbed from GI tract and peaks in 1 hour. Plasma half-life is 2 hours; 50–100% of dose is excreted into the systemic circulation, with peak concentration 3–12 hours after administration.

Dosage/Range:
- IV: Low: 10–50 mg/m^2; med: 100–500 mg/m^2; high: 500 mg/m^2 and above with leucovorin rescue.
- IT: 10–15 mg/m^2.
- IM: 25 mg/m^2.

Drug Preparation:
- 5-, 50-, 100-, and 200-mg vials are available already reconstituted.
- Powder is available in vials without preservative for IT and high-dose administration (reconstitute with preservative-free 0.9% Sodium Chloride).

Drug Administration:
- 5–149 mg: slow IVP.
- 150–499 mg: IV drip over 20 minutes.
- 500–1500 mg: infusion, per protocol, with leucovorin rescue.

Drug Interactions:
- Protein-bound drugs (aspirin, sulfonamides, sulfonylureas, phenytoin, tetracycline, chloramphenicol) increase toxicity; give together cautiously and monitor patient closely.
- NSAIDs (nonsteroidal anti-inflammatory drugs, e.g., indomethacin, ketoprofen) increased and prolonged methotrexate levels; DO NOT administer concurrently with high doses of methotrexate; monitor patients closely who are receiving moderate or low-dose methotrexate.

- Cotrimoxazole increased methotrexate serum level; DO NOT use concurrently.
- Pyrimethamine increased methotrexate serum level; DO NOT use concurrently.

Lab Effects/Interference:
- Decreased CBC.
- Increased LFTs, RFTs.

Special Considerations:
- High doses cross the BBB; reconstitute with preservative-free 0.9% Sodium Chloride.
- With high doses (1–7.5 gm/m^2), urine should be alkalinized both before and after administration, as the drug is a weak acid and can crystallize in the kidneys at an acid pH. Alkalinize with bicarbonate; add to pre- and posthydration. High doses should only be given under the direction of a qualified oncologist at an institution that can provide rapid serum methotrexate level readings.
- Leucovorin rescue must be given on time per orders to prevent excessive toxicity and to achieve maximum therapeutic response (see Leucovorin Calcium).
- Avoid folic acid and its derivatives during methotrexate therapy. Kidney function must be adequate to excrete drug and avoid excessive toxicity. Check BUN and creatinine before each dose.

Potential Toxicities/Side Effects and the Nursing Process

I. ALTERATION IN NUTRITION, LESS THAN BODY REQUIREMENTS, related to GI SIDE EFFECTS

Defining Characteristics: Nausea and vomiting are uncommon with low dose; more common (39%) with high dose; may occur during drug administration and last 24–72 hours. Anorexia is mild. Stomatitis is a common indication for interruption of therapy: occurs in 3–5 days with high dose, 3–4 weeks with low dose; appears initially at corners of mouth. Diarrhea is common and is an indication for interruption of therapy, as enteritis and intestinal perforation may occur; melena, hematemesis may occur. Hepatotoxicity is usually subclinical and reversible, but can lead to cirrhosis; increased risk of hepatotoxicity when given with other agents, like alcohol; transient increase in LFTs with high dose 1–10 days after treatment—may cause jaundice.

Nursing Implications: Premedicate with antiemetics if giving high-dose methotrexate; continue prophylactically for 24 hours (at least) to prevent nausea and vomiting. Encourage small, frequent feedings of cool, bland foods and liquids. Assess for symptoms of fluid and electrolyte imbalance: monitor I/O, daily weights if administered to inpatient. Assess oral cavity every day. Teach patient oral assessment and mouth care regimens. Encourage patient to report early stomatitis. Provide pain relief measures, if indicated. Explore patient compliance to rescue; discuss increase in rescue dose if moderate GI toxicity. Assess patient for diarrhea: guaiac all stools; encourage patient to report onset of diarrhea. Administer or teach patient to self-administer antidiarrheal medications. Monitor LFTs prior to drug dose, especially with high-dose methotrexate. Assess patient prior to and during treatment for signs/symptoms of hepatotoxicity.

II. POTENTIAL FOR INFECTION AND BLEEDING related to BONE MARROW DEPRESSION

Defining Characteristics: Nadir is seen 7–9 days after drug administration. Bone marrow depression occurs in about 10% of patients.

Nursing Implications: Monitor CBC and platelet count prior to drug administration, as well as signs/symptoms of infection or bleeding. Instruct patient in self-assessment of signs/symptoms of infection or bleeding measures to decrease risk. Administer leucovorin calcium as ordered.

III. POTENTIAL FOR ALTERATION IN URINARY ELIMINATION related to RENAL TOXICITY

Defining Characteristics: As an organic acid, methotrexate is insoluble in acid urine. At doses greater than 1 gm/m^2 (i.e., high dose), drug may precipitate in renal tubules, causing acute renal tubular necrosis (ATN).

Nursing Implications: Prehydrate patient with alkaline solution for several hours prior to drug administration. Maintain high urine output with a urine pH greater than 7.0 (hydration fluid may need further alkalinization); dipstick each void. Record I/O. Monitor BUN and serum creatinine before, during, and after drug administration. Increases in these values may require methotrexate dose reductions or leucovorin dose increases.

IV. POTENTIAL FOR IMPAIRED GAS EXCHANGE related to PULMONARY TOXICITY

Defining Characteristics: Pneumothorax (high dose): rare, occurs within first 48 hours after drug administration in patients with pulmonary metastasis. Allergic pneumonitis (high dose): rare but accompanied by eosinophilia, patchy pulmonary infiltrates, fever, cough, shortness of breath. Occurs 1–5 months after initiation of treatment. Pneumonitis (low dose) symptoms usually disappear within a week, with or without use of steroids; interstitial pneumonitis may be a fatal complication.

Nursing Implications: Assess for signs/symptoms of pulmonary dysfunction before each dose and between doses (see Defining Characteristics section). Discuss PFTs to be performed periodically with physician. Assess lung sounds prior to drug administration. Instruct patient to report cough or dyspnea.

V. POTENTIAL FOR ALTERATION IN SKIN INTEGRITY related to ALOPECIA, DERMATITIS

Defining Characteristics: Alopecia and dermatitis are uncommon. Pruritus, urticaria may occur. Photosensitivity, sunburnlike rash 1–5 days after treatment; also, patient can develop radiation recall reaction.

Nursing Implications: Assess patient for signs/symptoms of hair loss. Discuss with patient impact of hair loss and strategies to minimize distress. Instruct patient to avoid sun if possible and to stay covered or wear sunblock if sun exposure is unavoidable.

VI. POTENTIAL FOR SENSORY AND PERCEPTUAL ALTERATIONS related to CNS CHANGES

Defining Characteristics: CNS effects: dizziness, malaise, blurred vision. IT administration may increase CSF pressure. Brain XRT followed by IV methotrexate may also cause neurologic changes.

Nursing Implications: Monitor for CNS effects of drug: dizziness, blurred vision, malaise. Monitor for symptoms of increased CSF pressure: seizures, paresis, headache, nausea and vomiting, brain atrophy, fever. If IV methotrexate follows brain XRT, monitor for symptoms of increased CSF pressure.

VII. POTENTIAL FOR ALTERATIONS IN COMFORT related to PAIN

Defining Characteristics: Sometimes causes back pain during administration.

Nursing Implications: Monitor patient for back and flank pain. Slow down infusion rate if it occurs. Administer analgesics if pain occurs (must avoid aspirin-containing products, as they displace methotrexate from serum albumin).

Drug: methyl-CCNU (Semustine, MeCCNU) (investigational)

Class: Alkylating agent (nitrosourea); investigational agent.

Mechanism of Action: Alkylation and carbamoylation by semustine metabolites interfere with the synthesis and function of DNA, RNA, and proteins. Also inhibits DNA repair. Semustine is lipid-soluble and easily enters the brain. Cell cycle phase nonspecific.

Metabolism: 10–20% of the drug is excreted in the urine.

Dosage/Range:

- 150–200 mg/m^2 PO once every 6–12 weeks.

Drug Preparation:

- Oral: Available in 10-, 50-, and 100-mg capsules.

Drug Administration:

- Administer at bedtime on an empty stomach or 3–4 hours after a meal to minimize nausea and vomiting.

Drug Interactions:

- Myelosuppressive drugs: Additive toxicity if similar nadir; use cautiously at decreased dose.

Lab Effects/Interference:

- Decreased WBC and platelets.
- Increased BUN, creatinine.
- Increased SGOT, alk phos, bili.

Special Considerations:

- Dose reduction necessary if patient has liver impairment.
- Dispense one dose of semustine at a time.
- Bone marrow recovery should occur prior to administration: WBC > 4000/mm^3 and platelets > 100,000/mm^3.

Potential Toxicities/Side Effects and the Nursing Process

I. POTENTIAL FOR INFECTION AND BLEEDING related to MYELOSUPPRESSION

Defining Characteristics: Nadir of platelets: 4 weeks, but may be delayed to 8 weeks, with recovery 4–10 weeks later; nadir of WBC: occurs later than platelets. Cumulative bone marrow suppression with subsequent dosing may occur: Second or third drug dose may need to be reduced 25–50%. Persistent thrombocytopenia may occur.

Nursing Implications: Monitor WBC and platelets prior to drug administration (see Special Considerations section). WBC should be > 4000/mm^3 and platelets > 100,000/mm^3. Dispense only one drug dose at a time. Do not administer more often than once every 6 weeks. Dose-reduce with bone marrow or liver impairment.

II. ALTERED NUTRITION, LESS THAN BODY REQUIREMENTS, related to GI SIDE EFFECTS

Defining Characteristics: Onset of nausea and vomiting occurs 4–6 hours after drug dosing and may be severe. Stomatitis, hepatic dysfunction are rare.

Nursing Implications: Premedicate with antiemetic and sedative or hypnotic. Administer at night on empty stomach. Discourage food or fluid for 6 hours after drug dose. Encourage favorite foods, especially those that are high-calorie, high-protein. Encourage small, frequent meals. Inspect oral mucosa prior to dosing. Teach patient oral exam, mouth care after meals and at bedtime. Monitor SGOT, LDH, alk phos, bili. Notify physician of elevations and discuss prior to administering subsequent dose.

III. ALTERATION IN URINARY ELIMINATION related to RENAL DYSFUNCTION

Defining Characteristics: Renal dysfunction infrequent but may occur late in treatment. Tubular atrophy and glomerular sclerosis; ultimately, renal failure.

Nursing Implications: Monitor BUN, creatinine prior to dosing, especially in patients receiving prolonged or high cumulative doses. If abnormalities are noted, determine renal creatinine clearance.

IV. POTENTIAL SEXUAL DYSFUNCTION related to DRUG EFFECT

Defining Characteristics: Drug is teratogenic and mutagenic.

Nursing Implications: Assess patient's risk of becoming pregnant. Give information about adverse effects on fetus. As appropriate, discuss birth control measures.

V. ACTIVITY INTOLERANCE related to NEUROLOGIC DYSFUNCTION

Defining Characteristics: Neurologic dysfunction may occur rarely, including disorientation, lethargy, ataxia.

Nursing Implications: Perform neurologic assessment as part of prechemotherapy assessment. Assess orientation and level of consciousness, gait, activity tolerance.

VI. SENSORY/PERCEPTUAL ALTERATIONS (VISUAL) related to OCULAR DAMAGE

Defining Characteristics: Ocular damage may occur rarely, including optic neuritis, retinopathy, blurred vision.

Nursing Implications: Assess vision during prechemotherapy assessment. Encourage patient to report any visual changes.

VII. IMPAIRED GAS EXCHANGE related to PULMONARY FIBROSIS

Defining Characteristics: Pulmonary fibrosis occurs rarely.

Nursing Implications: Assess patients at risk, particularly those with (1) preexisting lung disease and (2) high cumulative doses. Monitor PFTs periodically for pulmonary dysfunction.

Drug: mitomycin (Mitomycin C, Mutamycin, 3 Mitozytrex)

Class: Antitumor antibiotic.

Mechanism of Action: Drug acts as alkylating agent and inhibits DNA synthesis by crosslinking of DNA. Alkylating and crosslinking mitomycin metabolites interfere with structure and function of DNA.

Metabolism: Drug is rapidly cleared by the liver. May need to modify dose in presence of liver abnormalities; 10% of drug is excreted unchanged.

Dosage/Range:
- 2 mg/m^2 IV every day × 5 days.
- 5–20 mg/m^2 IV every 6–8 weeks.
- Bladder instillations 20–60 mg (1 mg/mL).
- May be used at different dosages for autologous bone marrow transplant.

Drug Preparation:
- Depending on vial size, dilute with sterile water to obtain concentration of 0.5 mg/mL.

Drug Administration:
- IV: Drug is potent vesicant.
- Give through the sidearm of a running IV to avoid extravasation, which can lead to ulceration, pain, and necrosis. Check individual hospital policy for administration of a vesicant.

Drug Interactions:
- Myelosuppressive agents: Additive toxicity if overlapping nadirs; use cautiously.

Lab Effects/Interference:
- Decreased CBC, especially WBC and platelets.
- Hemolytic uremic syndrome (rare): Decreased hemoglobin, platelets, and increased creatinine.

Special Considerations:
- Indicated for treatment of disseminated adenocarcinoma of the stomach or pancreas in proven combinations with other approved chemotherapeutic agents and as palliative treatment when other modalities have failed.
- May cause interstitial pneumonitis.

- Rarely, hemolytic uremic syndrome can occur (characterized by rapid fall in hemoglobin, renal failure, severe thrombocytopenia) and progress to pulmonary edema and hypotension.
- Drug may be given intraarterially.
- Manufacturer's recommendations on dosage modification based on hematologic toxicity (NADIR AFTER PRIOR DOSE).

Potential Toxicities/Side Effects and the Nursing Process

I. POTENTIAL FOR INFECTION related to MYELOSUPPRESSION

Defining Characteristics: Myelosuppression is the dose-limiting toxicity. Toxicity is delayed and cumulative. Initial nadir occurs at approximately 4–6 weeks. Usually by the third course, 50% drug modifications are necessary.

Nursing Implications: Monitor WBC, HCT, platelets prior to drug administration. Monitor patients for signs/symptoms of infection. Teach patient self-assessment. Drug dosage should be reduced or held for lower-than-normal blood values.

II. ALTERATION IN NUTRITION, LESS THAN BODY REQUIREMENTS, related to NAUSEA, VOMITING, ANOREXIA, STOMATITIS

Defining Characteristics: Mild-to-moderate nausea and vomiting occur within 1–2 hours, lasting up to 3 days, but may be prevented by adequate premedication. Anorexia occurs commonly, and stomatitis may occur.

Nursing Implications: Premedicate with aggressive antiemetics, i.e., serotonin antagonist to prevent nausea and vomiting at least for the first treatment. Encourage small, frequent feedings of cool, bland foods and liquids. Teach patient and family member preparation of meals in advance, and encourage the use of spices when patient has little appetite. Teach patient oral assessment and oral hygiene regimen, and encourage patient to report early stomatitis.

III. POTENTIAL FOR ACTIVITY INTOLERANCE related to FATIGUE

Defining Characteristics: Fatigue is common.

Nursing Implications: Assess baseline activity level. Teach patient to report fatigue and activity intolerance. Teach self-management strategies, including alternating rest and activity periods, as well as stress reduction.

IV. POTENTIAL FOR IMPAIRED SKIN INTEGRITY related to DRUG EXTRAVASATION, ALOPECIA

Defining Characteristics: Extravasation of drug can cause severe tissue necrosis, erythema, burning, tissue sloughing. Delayed erythema or ulceration has been reported weeks to months after drug dose, at the injection site or distant from it, and despite the fact that there was no evidence of extravasation. Alopecia occurs frequently.

Nursing Implications: Use scrupulous IV technique to prevent extravasation of the drug. If there is doubt as to whether drug has infiltrated, treat as an infiltration, aspirate any drug in the tubing, and discontinue IV. IV line must be patent. Assess for need of venous access device early. Refer to hospital policy for management of extravasation. (If unclear what best strategy is, application of 1–2 mL 99% DMSO to the site every 6 hours × 14 days may offer some benefit [Alberts and Dorr, 1991].) Assess site regularly for pain, progression of erythema, induration, and evidence of necrosis. Discuss with patient hair loss, anticipated impact, and strategies to decrease distress, e.g., obtaining wig prior to hair loss.

V. POTENTIAL FOR INJURY related to HEMOLYTIC UREMIC SYNDROME

Defining Characteristics: 2% of patients may experience significant increase in creatinine unrelated to total dose or duration of therapy. Hold drug if creatinine is > 1.7 mg/dL. Thrombotic microangiopathy may occur with anemia, thrombocytopenia. Blood transfusions may exacerbate condition. Can often be fatal.

Nursing Implications: Monitor renal function, HCT, and platelets prior to each drug dose; hold dose if serum creatinine is > 1.7 mg/dL. If renal failure occurs, hemofiltration or dialysis may be necessary. Discuss risks and benefits with physician and patient if renal insufficiency is present and blood transfusion(s) is required.

VI. POTENTIAL ALTERATION IN OXYGENATION related to INTERSTITIAL PNEUMONITIS

Defining Characteristics: Rarely, interstitial pneumonitis occurs and can be quite severe (ARDS). signs/symptoms include nonproductive cough, dyspnea, hemoptysis, pneumonia, pulmonary infiltrates on X-ray. Incidence may be reduced by dexamethasone 20 mg IV prior to dose (Chang et al, 1986).

Nursing Implications: Assess baseline pulmonary status, and monitor prior to each drug dose. Teach patient to report dyspnea, new onset cough, or any respiratory symptoms. Discuss abnormalities with physician, and plan for further diagnostic workup.

VII. POTENTIAL FOR INJURY related to VENO-OCCLUSIVE DISEASE OF THE LIVER AFTER BONE MARROW TRANSPLANT

Defining Characteristics: Hepatic veno-occlusive disease has been reported in patients who have received mitomycin C and autologous bone marrow transplant. signs/symptoms are abdominal pain, hepatomegaly, and liver failure.

Nursing Implications: Assess baseline LFTs, and monitor periodically during therapy. Notify physician of any abnormalities, and discuss further diagnostic workup and management. Refer to autologous bone marrow transplant protocol.

Drug: mitotane (o, p′-DDD, Lysodren)

Class: Antihormone.

Mechanism of Action: Adrenocortical suppressant with direct cytotoxic effect on mitochondria of adrenal cortical cells. Forces a drop in steroid secretion and alters the peripheral metabolism of steroids.

Metabolism: 34–45% of oral dose is absorbed from the GI tract. Metabolized partly in the liver and kidneys to a water-soluble metabolite that is then excreted in the bile and urine. Small amount of drug passes into the CSF.

Dosage/Range:
- Dose ranges from 2–16 g/day PO.
- Usual doses 2–10 g/day.
- Treatment usually begins with low doses (2 g/day) and gradually increases.
- Daily dose is divided into 3–4 doses.

Drug Preparation:
- None.

Drug Administration:
- Oral.

Drug Interactions:
- Neurotoxic drugs may have additive toxicity; use cautiously.

Lab Effects/Interference:
- None.

Special Considerations:
- Hypersensitivity reactions are rare but have occurred.

Potential Toxicities/Side Effects and the Nursing Process

I. ALTERATION IN NUTRITION, LESS THAN BODY REQUIREMENTS, related to GI SIDE EFFECTS

Defining Characteristics: Nausea and vomiting occur in 75% of patients and may be dose-limiting toxicity. Anorexia may also occur. Diarrhea occurs in 20% of patients.

Nursing Implications: Nausea and vomiting may be reduced by beginning therapy with a low dose and increasing it as tolerated. Premedicate with antiemetics to prevent nausea and vomiting; continue as needed. Encourage small, frequent meals of cool, bland foods and liquids. Inform patient that nausea and vomiting can occur; encourage patient to report onset. Encourage patient to report onset of diarrhea. Administer or teach administration of antidiarrheal medication. If diarrhea is protracted, ensure adequate hydration, monitor I/O and electrolytes, teach perineal hygiene.

II. POTENTIAL FOR INJURY related to NEUROLOGIC TOXICITY

Defining Characteristics: Lethargy and somnolence are most common; resolve with discontinuation of therapy. Dizziness, vertigo occur in about 15% of patients. Other CNS manifestations are depression, muscle tremors, confusion, headache.

Nursing Implications: Teach the patient and family about possible neurologic toxicity; assess safety of planned activities (e.g., patient should avoid activities that require alertness). Encourage patient and family to report onset of symptoms, as they may necessitate discontinuing therapy.

III. POTENTIAL FOR IMPAIRED SKIN INTEGRITY related to RASH

Defining Characteristics: Skin irritation or rash occurs in about 15% of patients. Sometimes resolves during treatment.

Nursing Implications: Inform patient that rash is expected and will resolve when treatment is finished. Assess skin for integrity; recommend measures to decrease irritation, if indicated.

Drug: mitoxantrone (Novantrone)

Class: New class of antineoplastics—anthracenediones. Antitumor antibiotic.

Mechanism of Action: Inhibits both DNA and RNA synthesis regardless of the phase of cell division. Intercalates between base pairs, thus distorting DNA structure. DNA-dependent RNA synthesis and protein synthesis are also inhibited.

Metabolism: Excreted in both the bile and urine for 24–36 hours as virtually unchanged drug. Mean half-life is 5.8 hours. Peak levels achieved immediately. FDA-approved for acute nonlymphocytic leukemia in adults.

Dosage/Range:
- 12 mg/m^2 IV daily for 3 days, in combination with cytosine arabinoside 100 mg/m^2/day × 7 days continuous infusion for induction therapy of ANLL.
- 10–14 mg/m^2 IV every 3–4 weeks (refer to protocol).

Drug Preparation:
- Available as dark blue solution.
- May be diluted in 5% Dextrose, 0.9% Sodium Chloride, or 5% Dextrose in 0.9% Sodium Chloride.
- Solution is chemically stable at room temperature for at least 48 hours.
- Intact vials should be stored at room temperature. If refrigerated, a precipitate may form. This precipitate can be redissolved when vial is warmed to room temperature.

Drug Administration:
- IV push over 3 minutes through the sidearm of a freely running infusion.
- IV bolus over 5–30 minutes.

Drug Interactions:
- Myelosuppressive agents: Increased hematologic toxicity if nadir overlaps; use together cautiously.

Lab Effects/Interference:
- Decreased CBC.
- Decreased electrolytes.
- Increased LFTs, uric acid.

Special Considerations:
- Nonvesicant. There have been rare reports of tissue necrosis after drug infiltration.
- Incompatible with admixtures containing heparin.
- Patient may experience blue-green urine for 24 hours after drug administration.
- Cardiotoxicity is less than that of doxorubicin or daunorubicin.

Potential Toxicities/Side Effects and the Nursing Process

I. POTENTIAL FOR INJURY related to BONE MARROW DEPRESSION

Defining Characteristics: Potent bone marrow depression; nadir 9–10 days. Granulocytopenia is usually the dose-limiting toxicity, and toxicity may be cumulative. Thrombocytopenia uncommon, but can be severe when it occurs. Hypersensitivity has been reported occasionally with hypotension, urticaria, dyspnea, rashes.

Nursing Implications: Monitor WBC, HCT, platelets prior to drug administration. Instruct patient in self-assessment for signs/symptoms of infection. Drug dosage should be reduced or held for lower-than-normal blood values. Instruct patient in self-assessment of signs/symptoms of bleeding. Prior to drug administration, obtain baseline vital signs. Observe for signs/symptoms of allergic reaction. Subjective signs/symptoms: generalized itching, dizziness. Objective signs/symptoms: flushed appearance (angioedema of face, neck, eyelids, hands, feet), localized or generalized urticaria. Document incident. Discuss with physician desensitization for future dose vs drug discontinuance.

II. POTENTIAL FOR ALTERATION IN CARDIAC OUTPUT related to CARDIOTOXICITY

Defining Characteristics: CHF with decreased LVEF occurs in about 3% of patients. Increased cardiotoxicity with cumulative dose greater than 180 mg/m^2; cumulative lifetime dose must be reduced if patient has had previous anthracycline therapy.

Nursing Implications: Assess for signs/symptoms of cardiomyopathy. Assess quality and regularity of heartbeat. Baseline EKG. Instruct patient to report dyspnea, shortness of breath, swelling of extremities, orthopnea. Discuss frequency of GBPS with physician.

III. ALTERATION IN NUTRITION, LESS THAN BODY REQUIREMENTS, related to NAUSEA/VOMITING AND MUCOSITIS

Defining Characteristics: Nausea and vomiting are typically not severe and occur in 30% of patients. Mucositis is more common with prolonged dosing; occurs in 5% of patients, usually within one week of therapy.

Nursing Implications: Premedicate with antiemetic and continue prophylactically for 24 hours to prevent nausea and vomiting, at least for the first treatment. Encourage small, frequent feedings of cool, bland foods and liquids. Teach patient oral assessment and oral hygiene regimen. Encourage patient to report early stomatitis.

IV. POTENTIAL FOR IMPAIRED SKIN INTEGRITY related to ALOPECIA AND EXTRAVASATION

Defining Characteristics: Alopecia is mild to moderate; occurs in 20% of patients. Drug is not a vesicant. Stains skin blue without ulcers. There have been rare reports of tissue necrosis following extravasation.

Nursing Implications: Discuss with patient impact of hair loss. Suggest wig as appropriate prior to actual hair loss. Explore with patient response to actual hair loss and plan strategies to minimize distress, e.g., wig, scarf, cap. Use careful technique during venipuncture and IV administration. Administer drug through freely flowing IV, constantly monitoring IV site and patient response.

V. POTENTIAL FOR ANXIETY related to ABNORMAL COLOR OF URINE SCLERA

Defining Characteristics: Urine will be green-blue for 24 hours. Sclera may become discolored blue.

Nursing Implications: Explain to patient changes that may occur with therapy and that they are only temporary.

VI. POTENTIAL SEXUAL DYSFUNCTION related to DRUG EFFECT

Defining Characteristics: Drug is mutagenic and teratogenic.

Nursing Implications: As appropriate, explore with patient and partner issues of reproductive and sexuality patterns and impact chemotherapy may have. Discuss strategies to preserve sexual and reproductive health (e.g., sperm banking, contraception).

Drug: nilutamide (Nilandron)

Class: Antiandrogen.

Mechanism of Action: Irreversibly binds to androgen receptors and inhibits androgen binding. Unlike steroidal antiandrogens, nilutamide binds specifically to adrenal androgen receptor and does not interact with progestin or glucocorticoid receptors.

Metabolism: Following oral administration, nilutamide is rapidly and completely absorbed. Steady-state levels are achieved after about two weeks. Though the drug is extensively metabolized, it appears that the parent drug is the active compound. The drug is excreted in the urine as metabolite. Renal impairment does not alter the properties of the drug.

Dosage/Range:
- 300 mg/day for 30 days, then 150 mg/day.

Drug Preparation/Administration:
- Oral.

Drug Interactions:
- Has been shown to inhibit the liver cytochrome P-450 isoenzymes and may decrease the metabolism of compounds requiring these systems.
- Drugs with a low therapeutic margin, such as vitamin K antagonists, phenytoin, and theophylline, could delay elimination. Dose reduction of these drugs may be necessary.

Contraindications:
- In patients with severe hepatic impairment (baseline hepatic enzymes should be evaluated prior to treatment).
- In patients with severe respiratory insufficiency.
- In patients with hypersensitivity to nilutamide or any component of this preparation.

Lab Effects/Interference:
- Causes increased liver enzymes (see below); may cause increased serum glucose.

Special Considerations:
- Treatment should begin the day of or the day after surgical castration.
- If transaminases rise to greater than 2–3 times the upper limit of normal, therapy should be discontinued.

Potential Toxicities/Side Effects and the Nursing Process

I. ALTERATION IN NUTRITION, LESS THAN BODY REQUIREMENTS, related to NAUSEA, ANOREXIA

Defining Characteristics: Nausea, anorexia occur infrequently.

Nursing Implications: Teach patient to report occurrence of loss of appetite or nausea. Encourage small, frequent feedings and consider antiemetic if necessary.

II. ALTERATION IN CARDIAC OUTPUT related to HYPERTENSION, ANGINA

Defining Characteristics: Angina occurs in 2% of patients; unclear whether increased incidence of hypertension (9%) due to drug alone.

Nursing Implications: Instruct patient in signs and symptoms of angina, and to report to physician if they occur. Monitor BP on follow-up visits.

III. ALTERATION IN COMFORT related to DIZZINESS, HOT FLASHES, DYSPNEA, VISUAL CHANGES

Defining Characteristics: Hot flashes occur in 28% of patients and are the most common side effect. Dyspnea is rare but is related to interstitial pneumonitis, a serious side effect of the drug. Many patients experience impaired adaptation to light.

Nursing Implications: Inform patient that side effects may occur and to report dyspnea immediately to physician, as therapy must be discontinued if it occurs. Baseline chest X-ray should be done prior to treatment. Patients should be discouraged from driving at night because of visual changes and may find it helpful to wear tinted glasses during the day.

Drug: oxaliplatin (Eloxatin)

Class: Alkylating agent (3rd-generation platinum analogue).

Mechanism of Action: Blocks DNA replication and transcription into RNA by causing intrastrand and interstrand crosslinks in DNA strands.

Metabolism: Heavily bound (90%) to plasma proteins; following 2-hour drug infusion, 15% of drug is found in plasma and 85% in tissue or excreted in the urine. Binds irreversibly in red blood cells. The drug concentrates in the kidney and spleen, and is excreted as platinum-containing metabolites.

Dosage/Range:

- FOLFOX 4: *Day 1*: Oxaliplatin 85 mg/m^2 IV infusion in 250–500 ml 5% Dextrose in water and leucovorin 200 mg IV infusion in 5% dextrose in water, each over 2 hours simultaneously in different bags connected by a Y-line, followed by 5-FU 400 mg/m^2 IVB over 2–4 minutes, followed by 5-FU 600 mg/m^2 in 250–500 mL D5W as a 22-hour continuous infusion. *Day 2*: Leucovorin 200 mg/m^2 IVB over 2 hours, followed by 5-FU 400 mg/m^2 IVB over 2–4 minutes, followed by 5-FU 600 mg/m^2 in 250–500 mL D5W as a 22-hour continuous infusion.

Dose Reductions:

- Persistent grade 2 neurotoxicity: Reduce oxaliplatin to 65 mg/m^2.
- Grade 3 neurotoxicity: Discontinue oxaliplatin.
- Grades 3–4 gastrointestinal toxicity: Decrease oxaliplatin dose to 65 mg/m^2 and 5-FU by 20% (300mg/m^2 IVB and 500 mg/m^2 CI).
- Grades 3–4 hematological toxicity (ANC < 1500/l, platelets < 100,000/l): Decrease oxaliplatin dose to 65 mg/m^2 and 5-FU by 20% (300 mg/m^2 IVB and 500 mg/m^2 CI).

- Nausea, vomiting or other acute symptoms: Infuse oxaliplatin over a period of up to 6 hours as this lowers peak serum levels by 32%, revise antiemetic regime.

Drug Preparation:
- Add 10 mL bacteriostatic water for injection or 5% dextrose injection to the 50-mg vial of lyophilized powder and 20 mL to the 100-mg vial. Further dilute in 250–500 mL of 5% dextrose injection.
- DO NOT use chloride-containing solutions.
- DO NOT use aluminum needles or infusion sets containing aluminum.

Drug Administration:
- Administer IV infusion over 2 or more hours through central line, preferably.
- Drug classified as an irritant, but extravasations have resulted in induration and formation of nodule lasting 9 months or more.
- If given peripherally, it may cause infusion site pain; relieve this by further diluting the drug in 500 mL 5% Dextrose in water.

Drug Interactions:
- Incompatible with 5-FU and other highly alkaline solutions.
- Incompatible with chloride-containing solutions (forms precipitate).
- Physically incompatible with diazepam (forms precipitate).
- Nephrotoxic drugs: renal excretion of oxaliplatin could be reduced with increased serum levels of oxaliplatin.
- At high doses (130 mg/m^2), increases plasma levels of 5-FU by 20%.

Lab Effects/Interference:
- Decreased CBC, especially WBC and platelets.

Special Considerations:
- Indicated for the (1) adjuvant treatment of patients with Stage III colon cancer, and (2) first-line treatment of metastatic colon and rectal cancers in combination with infusional 5-fluorouracil (5-FU) and leucovorin (LV) for the treatment of patients with metastatic carcinoma of the colon or rectum. In the MOSAIC study of 2246 patients receiving adjuvant chemotherapy for colon cancer, Stage III patients receiving FOLFOX 4 had a superior survival compared to patients receiving 5FU/LV alone (24% risk reduction for recurrence) 4 years out (de Gramont, 2005). In addition, 99% of patients with grade 3 neurotoxicity had resolved or decreased by 1-year post treatment (deGramont et al, 2003).
- Peripheral neuropathy (sensory) is dose-limiting toxicity. Two distinct neurotoxicity syndromes: acute, lasting less than 14 days, and chronic persistent peripheral neuropathy (PN) similar to cisplatin.
- Rare pulmonary fibrosis and veno-occlusive disease of the liver.

Potential Toxicities/Side Effects and the Nursing Process

I. SENSORY/PERCEPTUAL ALTERATIONS related to ACUTE SENSORY NEUROPATHY

Defining Characteristics: Acute neurotoxicity appears related to ion channelopathy. It is common, affecting up to 56% of patients. It is temporary, and occurs during, within hours of, or up to 14 days following oxaliplatin administration. Often precipitated by exposure to cold and characterized by dysesthesias, transient paresthesias, or hypothesias of the hands, feet, perioral area, and throat. Acute events can be minimized by slower infusion of oxaliplatin, increasing the infusion time from 2 to 6 hours, as this lowers peak serum levels. Studies are ongoing to determine whether glutamine can prevent these, and also studies exploring 1 gm calcium/1 gm magnesium IVB prior to and after the oxaliplatin infusion. Most frightening for patients is pharyngolaryngeal dysesthesia characterized by a sensation of discomfort or tightness in the back of the throat and inability to breathe. It may be accompanied by jaw pain, and is often precipitated by exposure to cold. Cramping of muscles, such as fisted hand, occurs due to prolonged action potential. Rarely, dysarthria (difficulty articulating words), eye pain, and a feeling of chest pressure can occur.

Nursing Implications: Teach patient that acute neurotoxicity can occur but is not dangerous. Teach patient to minimize occurrence by avoiding exposure to cold during and for 3–5 days after drug administration, such as wearing scarves over the face in the winter, warm gloves if going outside or reaching into the refrigerator or freezer. Teach patient to avoid exposure to cold and cold liquids, if lip paresthesias present. Teach patient to use straw if drinking cool liquids. Teach patient to avoid cold air conditioning in the car or home during the summer. Teach patient how to reassure themselves they are breathing if pharyngolaryngeal dysesthesia occurs (cup hands in front of mouth or hold mirror so that breath can be felt or seen on the mirror). Teach patient to warm area, such as fingers or toes, if they become cold, such as running warm water over affected area, as this may help resolve the feeling.

II. SENSORY/PERCEPTUAL ALTERATIONS related to PERSISTENT, CHRONIC SENSORY NEUROPATHY

Defining Characteristics: Peripheral neurotoxicity affects about 48% of patients, and usually occurs when a cumulative dose of 800 mg/m^2 is reached. Symptoms include paresthesias, dysesthesias, hypoesthesias, in a stocking and glove distribution, and altered proprioception (knowing where body parts are in relation to the whole). This can become manifest in difficulty writing, walking, swallowing, and buttoning buttons. IF allowed to progress, motor pathways will become involved. When drug is stopped, symptoms resolve in 4–6 months in many patients. Ongoing studies are looking at temporarily stopping the drug when grade 2 or 3 neurotoxicity occurs, and resuming when the patient has grade 0 or 1 toxicity (OPTIMOX trial). In the MOSAIC trial, an adjuvant trial, although 23% of patients developed grade 3 neurotoxicity after 6 months, all patients except 1% had complete resolution of toxicity (de Gramont, 2003).

Nursing Implications: Assess baseline neurologic status (sensory and motor); instruct patient to report signs/symptoms. Identify patients at risk: those with preexisting neuropathies (e.g., ethanol- and diabetes mellitus-related). Assess motor function, and monitor over time prior to each treatment, such as picking up a dime from a smooth/flat surface, buttoning shirt, and writing name. Specifically, assess whether function impaired, as this necessitates a dose reduction, or if ability to perform activities of daily living impaired, as this necessitates drug cessation. In either case, discuss with physician as complete neurological exam should be performed prior to treatment decision. Assess impact on patient and quality of life. Drug holiday or discontinuance based on grade of neurotoxicity.

III. POTENTIAL FOR INFECTION, BLEEDING, and FATIGUE related to BONE MARROW DEPRESSION

Defining Characteristics: Mild leukopenia, and mild to moderate thrombocytopenia occur. Anemia common.

Nursing Implications: Assess baseline CBC, WBC, differential, and platelet count prior to chemotherapy as well as signs/symptoms of infection, bleeding, or fatigue. Teach patient signs/symptoms of infection or bleeding, and to report these immediately. Teach patient self-care measures to minimize risk of infection and bleeding. This includes avoidance of crowds, proximity to people with infections, and OTC aspirin-containing medications. Teach energy-conserving techniques and ways to minimize fatigue, such as gentle exercise as tolerated.

IV. ALTERATION IN NUTRITION, LESS THAN BODY REQUIREMENTS, related to NAUSEA AND VOMITING

Defining Characteristics: Nausea and vomiting occur commonly and are severe if patient does not receive aggressive antiemesis.

Nursing Implications: Premedicate patient with aggressive combination antiemetics: serotonin antagonist (granisetron or ondansetron) and dexamethasone. Encourage small, frequent feedings of cool, bland foods. Instruct patient to report nausea, and teach self-administration of antiemetics if patient is receiving drug as an outpatient.

V. POTENTIAL FOR INJURY related to DELAYED HYPERSENSITIVITY OR ANAPHYLAXIS REACTIONS (often after 10–12 cycles of therapy)

Defining Characteristics: Delayed hypersensitivity may occur after 10–12 cycles of therapy with symptoms ranging from local rash or vague symptoms such as new onset of vomiting, to anaphylaxis and severe hypersensitivity (characterized by dyspnea, hypotension requiring treatment, angioedema, and generalized urticaria). Anecdotal reports show successful desensitization using carboplatin desensitization regimens.

Nursing Implications: Assess baseline VS and mental status prior to drug administration. If patient has symptoms, discuss premedication using corticosteroid, antihistamine, and H2 antagonist as ordered. Monitor VS every 15 minutes, and remain with patient during first 15 minutes of drug infusion. Stop drug if signs/symptoms of hypersensitivity or anaphylaxis occur, and notify physician. *Subjective symptoms*: generalized itching, nausea, chest tightness, crampy abdominal pain, difficulty speaking, anxiety, agitation, sense of impending doom, uneasiness, desire to urinate/defecate, dizziness, chills. *Objective signs*: flushed appearance; angioedema of face, neck, eyelids, hands, feet; localized or generalized urticaria; respiratory distress with or without wheezing; hypotension; cyanosis. Provide fluid resuscitation for hypotension per MD order, and maintain a patent airway.

Drug: paclitaxel (Taxol)

Class: Taxoid, mitotic inhibitor.

Mechanism of Action: Promotes early microtubule assembly and prevents depolymerization, resulting in cell death.

Metabolism: Extensively protein-bound, resulting in an initial sharp decline in serum level. Metabolized primarily by hepatic hydroxylation using the P-450 enzyme system. Metabolites are excreted in the bile. Less than 10% of the intact drug is excreted in the urine.

Dosage/Range:

- Previously untreated ovarian cancer: 135 mg/m^2 IV over 24 hours, followed by cisplatin 75 mg/m^2 every 3 weeks or paclitaxel 175 mg IV over 3 hours followed by cisplatin 75 mg/m^2 q 3 weeks.
- Previously treated ovarian cancer: 135mg or 175 mg/m^2 IV over 3 hours every 3 weeks.
- Adjuvant node positive breast cancer: 175 mg/m^2 IV over 3 hours, every 3 weeks, for 4 courses, administered sequentially to doxorubicin-containing combination chemotherapy.

- Metastatic breast cancer, after failure of initial therapy or relapse within 6 months of adjuvant therapy: 175 mg/m^2 IV over 3 hours every 3 weeks.
- Metastatic breast cancer, weekly paclitaxel 80 mg/m^2 IV over 1 hour q wk.
- Non-small-cell lung cancer (NSCLC): 135 mg/m^2 IV over 24 hours, followed by cisplatin 75 mg/m^2 repeated every 3 weeks.
- AIDS-related Kaposi's sarcoma: 135 mg/m^2 IV over 3 hours, repeated every 3 weeks, or 100 mg/m^2 IV over 3 hours, repeated every 2 weeks (dose intensity of 45–50 mg/m^2 per week.
- Less myelosuppression with 3-hour vs 24-hour infusion.

Other regimens used/being studied/reported:

- Metastatic breast cancer overexpressing *HER*-2 protein: 175 mg/m^2 IV over 3 hours, every 3 weeks in combination with trastuzumab.
- Advanced or metastatic NSCLC: Weekly paclitaxel 50 mg/m^2 IV over 1 hour in combination with carboplatin AUC 2 with concurrent XRT, and after completion of XRT, paclitaxel 200 mg/m^2 and carboplatin AUC 6 q3 weeks × 2 cycles.
- Activity in other tumor types (bladder, small-cell lung, head and neck cancers).

Drug Preparation:

- Drug is poorly soluble in water, so is formulated using polyoxyethylated castor oil (Cremaphor EL) and dehydrated alcohol.
- Further dilute in 5% Dextrose or 0.9% Sodium Chloride.

Drug Administration:

- Glass or polyolefin containers MUST BE USED, and polyethylene-lined administration sets must be used. DO NOT USE polyvinylchloride containers or tubing since the polyoxyethlated caster oil (Cremaphor EL) causes leaching of plasticizer diethylhexlphthalate (DEHP) from polyvinylchloride plastic into the infusion fluid. Do not use Chemo Dispensing Pin device or similar devices since the device may cause the stopper to collapse, sacrificing sterility of the paclitaxel solution.
- Inline filter of < 0.22 microns MUST be used.
- Assess vital signs baseline, and remain with patient during first 15 minutes of infusion. Monitor vital signs every 15 minutes or per hospital policy.
- Assess CBC: Patients with solid tumors: absolute neutrophil count (ANC) must be at least 1500 cells/mm^3 and platelet count at least 100,000/mm^3; patients with AIDS-related Kaposi's sarcoma: ANC at least 1,000 cells/mm^3.

Premedication with corticosteroids:

- Solid Tumors: Dexamethasone 20 mg PO 12 and 6 hours prior to treatment. Administer diphenydramine 50 mg and H2 antagonist (cimetidine 300 mg, famotidine 20 mg, or ranitidine 50 mg) IV 30–60 minutes prior to treatment.

- AIDS-related Kaposi's sarcoma: Dexamethasone 10 mg PO 12 and 6 hours prior to treatment; administer diphenydramine 50 mg and H2 antagonist (cimetidine 300 mg, famotidine 20 mg, or ranitidine 50 mg) IV 30–60 minutes prior to treatment.
- Administer paclitaxel IV over 3 hours via infusion controller.
- DO NOT give drug as a bolus, as this may cause bronchospasm and hypotension.
- Assess for hypersensitivity reaction (most often occurs during first 10 minutes of infusion) and for cardiovascular effects (arrhythmia, hypotension).
- Keep resuscitation equipment nearby.
- Administer paclitaxel first when given in combination with cisplatin or carboplatin. There is increased cytotoxic activity when given in this sequence.
- Paclitaxel is being studied as a radiosensitizer, given weekly doses 80–100 mg/m^2 as a 1-hour infusion.
- Intraperitoneal infusion (investigational): Dilute dose into 1–2 liters of 0.9% NS, or as ordered; warm to 37°C and infuse as rapidly as tolerated into peritoneal cavity; assist patient to change position every 15 minutes per protocol × 2 hours to maximize distribution in peritoneal cavity.

Drug Interactions:

- Cisplatin: Myelosuppression is more severe when cisplatin is administered prior to paclitaxel (due to 33% reduction in paclitaxel clearance from the plasma). Therefore, paclitaxel must be given prior to cisplatin when drugs are administered sequentially.
- Ketoconazole, other azole antifungal agents: May inhibit metabolism of paclitaxel. Use together cautiously, and closely monitor for paclitaxel toxicity.
- Carboplatin: Possible increased cytotoxicity when given *after* taxol. Also, combination of paclitaxel and carboplatin results in less thrombocytopenia than would be expected from dose of carboplatin alone (etiology of plateletsparing effect unknown).
- Paclitaxel is metabolized by P450 cytochrome isoenzymes CYP2C8 and CYP3A4. Potential interactions may occur, including antiretroviral protease inhibitors. Use together cautiously with other drugs metabolized by this system (substrates or inhibitors).
- Doxorubicin and liposomal doxorubicin: Increased incidence of neutropenia and stomatitis when paclitaxel is administered prior to doxorubicin (due to significant decrease in doxorubicin clearance, possibly due to competition for biliary excretion of both agents). Therefore, doxorubicin should be given prior to paclitaxel.
- Doxorubicin: Increased risk of cardiotoxicity when given in combination with paclitaxel, with sharp increase in risk of congestive heart failure once cumulative dose of doxorubicin is > 380 mg/m^2. Consider stopping combination therapy when cumulative doxorubicin dose is 340–380 mg/m^2 and

continuing paclitaxel as a single agent, as this does not increase risk of CHF (Gianni et al, 1998).
- Beta-blockers, calcium-channel blockers, digoxin: Additive bradycardia may occur; assess/monitor patients closely.
- Immunosuppressive agents, other antineoplastic agents: Additive immunosuppression may occur; assess toxicity and patient response closely.

Lab Effects/Interference:
- Decreased CBC.
- Increased LFTs.

Special Considerations:
- Reversal of multidrug resistance has been studied with quinidine, cyclosporine, quinine, verapamil.
- Drug has radiosensitizing effects.
- Drug is embryotoxic; avoid use in pregnancy. Women of childbearing age should use effective contraception.
- Drug may be excreted in breast milk, so breast-feeding should be avoided during drug therapy.
- ANC should be $\geq 1500/mm^3$ prior to initial or subsequent doses of paclitaxel.
- Dose reductions: 20% dose reduction if severe neuropathy or severe neutropenia (ANC $< 500/mm^3$ for 7+ days) develop and/or consider addition of colony-stimulating factor support with next cycle; 25–50% dose reduction if hepatic dysfunction (hepatic metastasis > 2 cm) occurs (Chabner and Longo, 2001); 50% or more dose reduction for moderate or severe hyperbilirubinemia or significantly increased serum transferase levels, with dose of paclitaxel not exceeding 50–75 mg/m^2 IV over 24 hours, or 75–100 mg/m^2 IV over 3 hours; if AST > 2 times upper limit of normal, patient dose should not exceed 50 mg/m^2 IV over 24 hours (Venook et al, 1998).
- One-hour infusion of paclitaxel as well as weekly dosing regimens are being studied/used. Lower doses, e.g., 80–100 mg/m^2 IV over 1 hour weekly × 3 with 1 week off per cycle, weekly × 6 with 2 weeks off per cycle, or weekly > 12 weeks, appear to inhibit angiogenesis, and allow for increased dose density.

Potential Toxicities/Side Effects and the Nursing Process

I. POTENTIAL FOR INJURY related to HYPERSENSITIVITY OR ANAPHYLAXIS REACTIONS

Defining Characteristics: Hypersensitivity occurs in 10% of patients, with anaphylaxis and severe hypersensitivity reactions in 2–4% (characterized by dyspnea, hypotension requiring treatment, angioedema, and generalized urticaria). Reaction is to cremaphor in paclitaxel preparation. Signs/symptoms include tachycardia, wheezing, hypotension, facial edema; incidence of supraventricular tachycardia with hypotension and chest pain occurs in 1–2%. Patients who have severe hypersensitivity reaction should not be rechallenged with drug. Those who have less severe reactions have received 24 hours of corticosteroid prophylaxis, and have been successfully rechallenged with drug infused at a slower rate.

Nursing Implications: Assess baseline VS and mental status prior to drug administration. Ensure that patient has taken dexamethasone premedication, and administer diphenhydramine and H2 antagonist as ordered. Monitor VS every 15 minutes, and remain with patient during first 15 minutes of drug infusion as most reactions occur during the first 10 minutes. Stop drug if cardiac arrhythmia (irregular apical pulse), hypotension, or hypertension occur, and discuss continuance of infusion with physician. Recall signs/symptoms of anaphylaxis, and if these occur, stop drug immediately and notify physician. *Subjective symptoms*: generalized itching, nausea, chest tightness, crampy abdominal pain, difficulty speaking, anxiety, agitation, sense of impending doom, uneasiness, desire to urinate/defecate, dizziness, chills. *Objective signs*: flushed appearance; angioedema of face, neck, eyelids, hands, feet; localized or generalized urticaria; respiratory distress with or without wheezing; hypotension; cyanosis. Review standing orders or nursing procedure for patient management of anaphylaxis, and be prepared to stop drug immediately if signs/symptoms occur, keep IV line open with 0.9% Sodium Chloride, notify physician, monitor VS, and administer ordered medications, which may include epinephrine 1:1000, hydrocortisone sodium succinate, and diphenhydramine. Teach patient the potential of a hypersensitivity or anaphylactic reaction and to immediately report any unusual symptoms.

II. POTENTIAL FOR INFECTION AND BLEEDING related to BONE MARROW DEPRESSION

Defining Characteristics: Neutropenia may be severe, especially when drug is administered via 24-hour infusion. Neutropenia is also more severe when cisplatin precedes paclitaxel in sequential administration, as it reduces paclitaxel clearance by 33%. Neutropenia is also more pronounced in patients who have received prior radiotherapy. Nadir is 7–10 days after dose with recovery in one week. Neutropenia is dose-dependent, with severe neutropenia (ANC $< 500/mm^3$) occurring in 47–67% of patients. Anemia occurs frequently, but thrombocytopenia is uncommon.

Nursing Implications: Assess baseline CBC, WBC, differential, and platelet count prior to chemotherapy, as well as signs/symptoms of infection or bleeding. Teach patient the signs/symptoms of infection or bleeding, and to report these immediately, and teach patient self-care measures to minimize risk of infection and bleeding. This includes avoidance of crowds, proximity to people with infections, and OTC aspirin-containing medications. Administer paclitaxel PRIOR to cisplatin or carboplatin when either is given in combination with paclitaxel. Teach patient self-administration of G-CSF as ordered to prevent severe neutropenia. Transfuse red blood cells and platelets per physician order.

III. SENSORY/PERCEPTUAL ALTERATIONS related to SENSORY NEUROPATHY

Defining Characteristics: Frequency and incidence is dose-dependent but appears not to be influenced by infusion duration. Overall incidence is 60%, with 3% severe neuropathy in women with breast or ovarian cancer treated with single-agent paclitaxel, but severe neuropathy occurred in 8–13% of patients with NSCLC who also received cisplatin. Onset related to cumulative dose, with incidence after first course 27% and remainder occurring after 2–10 courses. Sensory symptoms usually resolve after two or more months following paclitaxel discontinuance. Sensory alterations are paresthesias in a glove-and-stocking distribution, and numbness. There may be a loss of sensation, symmetrically, vibration, proprioception, temperature, and pinprick. Sensory and motor neuropathy may occur in patients receiving both paclitaxel and cisplatin. There is an increased risk for motor and autonomic dysfunction in patients with neuropathy from diabetes mellitus or alcohol ingestion prior to treatment with paclitaxel. Arthralgias and myalgias affect 60% of patients, begin 2–3 days after treatment, then resolve in a few days; may be ameliorated by low-dose dexamethasone.

Nursing Implications: Assess baseline neurologic status. Instruct patient to report signs/symptoms of pins and needle sensation, numbness, pain, increased discomfort with certain sensations, especially in the extremities, or motor weakness. Identify patients at risk: prior cisplatin, or having preexisting neuropathies (ethanol- and diabetes mellitus-related). Assess sensory and motor function prior to each treatment, and if abnormality found, assess impact on patient function, safety, independence, and quality of life. Test patient's ability to button a shirt, or pick up a dime from a flat surface. If severely impacting safety or quality of life, discuss with patient and physician drug reduction (20%) or discontinuance or use of cytoprotective agent. Teach self-care strategies, including maintaining safety when walking, getting up, taking bath or washing dishes and unable to sense temperature, and the need to keep extremities warm in cold weather. See NCI Common Toxicity Criteria, Appendix II: grade 3 motor = objective weakness, interfering with ADLs; grade 3 sensory = sensory loss or paresthesia interfering with ADLs; grade 4 motor = paralysis; grade 4 sensory = permanent sensory loss that interferes with function.

IV. ALTERATION IN SKIN INTEGRITY related to ALOPECIA

Defining Characteristics: Complete alopecia occurs in most patients and is reversible.

Nursing Implications: Discuss potential impact of hair loss prior to drug administration. Discuss coping strategies and plan to minimize body image distortion (e.g., wig, scarf, cap). Assess patient for signs/symptoms of hair loss. Assess patient's response and use of coping strategies, and help patient to build on effective strategies.

V. ALTERATION IN NUTRITION, LESS THAN BODY REQUIREMENTS, related to NAUSEA AND VOMITING, DIARRHEA, STOMATITIS, HEPATOTOXICITY

Defining Characteristics: Nausea and vomiting occur commonly in 52% of patients and are mild and preventable with antiemetics. Diarrhea occurs in 38% of patients and is mild. Stomatitis occurs in 31% and is mild, appears to be dose- and schedule-dependent, and is more common with 24-hour infusions than 3-hour infusions. Mild increase in LFTs may occur (7% bilirubin, 22% alk phos, 19% AST). Rarely, hepatic necrosis and hepatic encephalopathy leading to death have been reported. If severe hepatic dysfunction occurs, paclitaxel dose should be reduced (see Special Considerations section).

Nursing Implications: Premedicate patient with antiemetic (either serotonin antagonist or dopamine antagonist). Encourage small, frequent meals of cool, bland foods. Instruct patient to report nausea, and teach self-administration of antiemetics if receiving drug as an outpatient. If nausea/vomiting occur and is severe, assess for signs/symptoms of fluid/electrolyte imbalance. Encourage patient to report onset of diarrhea and to self-administer antidiarrheal medications. Assess baseline oral mucous membranes. Teach patient oral assessment and to report any alterations. Assess LFTs prior to drug administration and periodically during treatment.

VI. POTENTIAL ALTERATION IN CIRCULATION related to HYPOTENSION, ARRYTHMIA

Defining Characteristics: Hypotension during first three hours of infusion in 12% of patients, and bradycardia in 3% of patients have been reported; most often patients were asymptomatic, and patients did not require intervention. Significant cardiovascular events (syncope, rhythm abnormalities, hypertension, and venous thrombosis) occurred in 1% of patients receiving single-agent paclitaxel, but the incidence was 12–13% in patients with NSCLC receiving cisplatin as well. Of those patients with normal baseline EKGs at the beginning of paclitaxel therapy, 14% of patients developed an abnormal EKG tracing (nonspecific repolarization abnormalities, sinus bradycardia, sinus tachycardia, premature beats). Whether or not the patient received prior anthracycline therapy did not influence these events. Prior anthracycline therapy did influence the rare incidence of CHF. Rarely, patients developed myocardial infarction, atrial fibrillation, and supraventricular tachycardia. For patients receiving doxorubicin in combination with paclitaxel, there is increased risk of CHF once the cumulative dose of doxorubicin is > 380 mg/m^2. (Gianni et al, 1998). Severe conduction abnormalities have been described in $< 1\%$ of patients, and required pacemaker insertion in some patients.

Nursing Implications: Assess baseline cardiac status, history, and risk for development of CHF. Closely monitor patient during paclitaxel infusion, especially if patient has history of hypertension, or is on cardiac medications (see Drug Interactions section). Teach patient to report any dyspnea, SOB, chest pain, or heart palpitations, or any unusual feeling. If any abnormalities occur, stop infusion as appropriate and discuss further management with physician. If patient is receiving doxorubicin and paclitaxel, discuss with physician stopping combination therapy when cumulative doxorubicin dose is 340–380 mg/m^2, and continuing paclitaxel as a single agent, as this does not increase risk of CHF (Gianni et al, 1998). If the patient develops significant conduction abnormalities, discuss medical management with physician, and expect that patient will have cardiac monitoring during subsequent paclitaxel therapy.

VII. ALTERATION IN COMFORT related to FATIGUE, ARTHRALGIAS AND MYALGIAS

Defining Characteristics: Fatigue occurs commonly, and arthalgias and myalgias affect about 44% of all patients, with 8% experiencing severe symptoms. Arthralgias and myalgias commonly occurred 2–3 days after the drug was given, and resolved within a few days.

Nursing Implications: Teach patient that fatigue may occur, and ways to minimize exertion and energy expenditure by alternating rest and activity, and organizing chores so that they are done as efficiently as possible. Arthalgias and myalgias may be troublesome, and can be managed with NSAIDs, application of warmth, and other comfort measures. Some patients report that swimming is helpful in minimizing discomfort. Studies of gabapentin, glutamine, and steroids have been disappointing. Opioids may be needed if severe.

Drug: paclitaxel protein bound particles for injectable suspension, albumin-bound (Abraxane, nab paclitaxel.

Class: Taxane, Nanoparticle albumin-bound paclitaxel, mitotic inhibitor.

Mechanism of Action: Promotes early microtubule assembly and prevents depolymerization, resulting in cell death; drug is combined with human albumin in a nanoparticle state, resulting in increased intra-tumoral concentrations of paclitaxel, lower drug concentrations in normal tissue, and potentially greater anti-tumor activity as higher doses can be given compared to cremaphor-dissolved paclitaxel.

Metabolism: Lower AUC, slower metabolism of paclitaxel nanoparticles, more rapid and extensive distribution into tissues; and longer half-life than paclitaxel.

Dosage/Range:

- 260 mg/m^2 q 21 day cycle, IV over 30 min; ANC must be > 1500 cells/mm^3;
- Dose reduce to 220 mg/m^2 if nadir ANC < 500/mm^3 for 1+ weeks or severe neuropathy; further reduce to 180 mg/m^2 if severe neutropenia or neuropathy recur; resume chemotherapy only when neuropathy resolves to grades 1–2, and ANC > 1500 cells/mm^3.
- Also being studied: 100 g/m^2 IV weekly.

Drug Preparation/Administration:

- Available in single use 100 mg vials. Gently dilute in Normal Saline, place in IV bag, and administer IV over 30 minutes. If not used immediately after mixing, may be stored in refrigerator for 8 hours. See package insert.

Drug Interactions:

- Metabolism of paclitaxel is catalyzed by the P450 micro-enzyme system: CYP2C8 and CYP3A4, but studies have not been done to determine extent of interaction; use together cautiously with protease inhibitors, e.g., retonivir.
- Cisplatin: Myelosuppression is more severe when cisplatin is administered prior to paclitaxel (due to 33% reduction in paclitaxel clearance from the plasma). Therefore, paclitaxel must be given prior to cisplatin when drugs are administered sequentially.
- Ketoconazole, other azole antifungal agents: May inhibit metabolism of paclitaxel. Use together cautiously, and closely monitor for paclitaxel toxicity.
- Carboplatin: Possible increased cytotoxicity when given *after* paclitaxel. Also, combination of paclitaxel and carboplatin results in less thrombocytopenia than would be expected from dose of carboplatin alone (etiology of plateletsparing effect unknown).

- Doxorubicin and liposomal doxorubicin: Increased incidence of neutropenia and stomatitis when paclitaxel is administered prior to doxorubicin (due to significant decrease in doxorubicin clearance, possibly due to competition for biliary excretion of both agents). Therefore, doxorubicin should be given prior to paclitaxel.
- Doxorubicin: Increased risk of cardiotoxicity when given in combination with paclitaxel, with sharp increase in risk of congestive heart failure once cumulative dose of doxorubicin is > 380 mg/m^2. Consider stopping combination therapy when cumulative doxorubicin dose is 340–380 mg/m^2 and continuing paclitaxel as a single agent, as this does not increase risk of CHF (Gianni et al, 1998).
- Beta-blockers, calcium-channel blockers, digoxin: Additive bradycardia may occur; assess/monitor patients closely.

Lab Effects/Interference:

- Decreased white blood cell count, neutrophil count, platelet count, decreased red blood cell count; 1/3 of patients had elevated alkaline phosphatase, AST.

Special Considerations:

- Indicated for the treatment of breast cancer after failure of combination chemotherapy for metastatic disease or relapse within six months of adjuvant chemotherapy. Prior therapy should have included an anthracycline unless clinically contraindicated.
- Drug is a Cremaphor-free, protein-engineered nanotransporter of paclitaxel. No pre-medication for hypersensitivity is required.
- Drug needs no special tubing, filter.
- Rarely, pneumothorax, interstitial pneumonia, lung fibrosis, pulmonary embolism have been reported.

Potential Toxicities/Side Effects and the Nursing Process

I. POTENTIAL FOR INFECTION AND BLEEDING related to BONE MARROW DEPRESSION

Defining Characteristics: Neutropenia is dose dependent and reversible, with grade 4 reported as 9% at doses of 260 mg/m^2, without growth factor support. Febrile neutropenia occurred in 2% of patients, compared to 1% in the paclitaxel arm. Neutropenia may be more pronounced in patients who have received prior radiotherapy. Infectious complications occurred in 24% of patients, with oral candidiasis, respiratory tract infection, and pneumonia the mose commonly reported. Thrombocytopenia is uncommon, with bleeding reported in 2% of patients. Anemia occurred in 33% of patients, and was severe in 1% of patients (hgb < 8 g/dL).

Nursing Implications: Assess baseline CBC, WBC, differential, and platelet count prior to chemotherapy, as well as signs/symptoms of infection or bleeding. Teach patient the signs/symptoms of infection or bleeding, and to report these immediately, and teach patient self-care measures to minimize risk of infection and bleeding. This includes avoidance of crowds, proximity to people with infections, and OTC aspirin-containing medications. Administer paclitaxel PRIOR to cisplatin or carboplatin when either is given in combination with paclitaxel.

II. SENSORY/PERCEPTUAL ALTERATIONS related to SENSORY NEUROPATHY

Defining Characteristics: Sensory neuropathy is dose related, and common, occurring in 71% of patients in clinical studies (10% severe), compared to 56% in patients receiving paclitaxel. Grade 3 neuropathy reversible in many patients, within a mean 22 days. No grade 4 severity have been reported in clinical trials. Rare motor or autonomic neuropathy (e.g., ileus). Ocular/visual disturbances may occur rarely, especially at higher doses, and in the literature, persistent optic nerve damage related to paclitaxel has been reported.

Nursing Implications: Assess baseline neurologic status. Instruct patient to report signs/symptoms of pins and needle sensation, numbness, pain, increased discomfort with certain sensations, especially in the extremities, or motor weakness. Identify patients at risk: prior cisplatin, or having pre-existing neuropathies (ethanol- and diabetes mellitus-related). Assess sensory and motor function prior to each treatment, and if abnormality found, assess impact on patient function, safety, independence, and quality of life. Test patient's ability to button a shirt, or pick up a dime from a flat surface. Teach self-care strategies as needed, including maintaining safety when walking, getting up, taking bath or washing dishes and unable to sense temperature, and the need to keep extremities warm in cold weather (see NCI Common Toxicity Criteria, Appendix).

III. POTENTIAL ALTERATION IN CIRCULATION related to HYPOTENSION, ARRYTHMIA

Defining Characteristics: Hypotension during first three hours of infusion in 5% of patients, and bradycardia in < 1% of patients have been reported; most often patients were asymptomatic, and patients did not require intervention. Significant cardiovascular events (chest pain, cardiac arrest, supraventricular tachycardia, edema, thombosis, pulmonary embolism, hypertension, cerebral vascular accident) occurred in 3% of patients receiving single-agent paclitaxel albumin-bound particles for injection. Of those patients with normal baseline EKGs at the beginning of single-agent paclitaxel albumin-bound particles for injection therapy, 35% of patients developed an abnormal EKG tracing (non-specific repolarization abnormalities, sinus bradycardia, sinus tachycardia).

Nursing Implications: Assess baseline cardiac status, history, and risk for development of CHF. Closely monitor patient during paclitaxel infusion, especially if patient has history of hypertension, or is on cardiac medications (see Drug Interactions section). Teach patient to report any dyspnea, SOB, chest pain, or heart palpitations, or any unusual feeling. If any abnormalities occur, stop infusion as appropriate and discuss further management with physician.

IV. ALTERATION IN SKIN INTEGRITY related to ALOPECIA

Defining Characteristics: Alopecia occurs commonly (90% of patients studied).

Nursing Implications: Discuss potential impact of hair loss prior to drug administration. Discuss coping strategies and plan to minimize body image distortion (e.g., wig, scarf, cap). Assess patient for signs/symptoms of hair loss. Assess patient's response and use of coping strategies, and help patient to build on effective strategies.

V. ALTERATION IN NUTRITION, LESS THAN BODY REQUIREMENTS, related to NAUSEAVOMITING, DIARRHEA, MUCOSITIS, AND HEPATOTOXICITY

Defining Characteristics: Nausea, vomiting, diarrhea and mucositis were reported in 30%, 18%, 26%, and 7% of patients respectively. Rarely, hepatic necrosis, hepatic encephalopathy, intestinal obstruction, intestinal perforation, pancreatitis, and ischemic colitis have been reported in patients receiving paclitaxel albumin-bound injection.

Nursing Implications: Premedicate patient with antiemetic (either serotonin antagonist or dopamine antagonist). Encourage small, frequent meals of cool, bland foods. Instruct patient to report nausea, and teach self-administration of antiemetics. If nausea/vomiting occur and is severe, assess for signs/symptoms of fluid/electrolyte imbalance. Assess bowel elimination pattern and oral mucosa baseline and prior to each treatment. Teach patient to report diarrhea unrelieved with self-administered anti-diarrheal medications and adequate fluid replacement. Teach patient to assess oral mucosa and to use systematic oral cleansing after meals and at bedtime. Teach patient to report difficulty drinking fluids or ingesting food.

VI. ALTERATION IN COMFORT related to FATIGUE, ARTHRALGIAS AND MYALGIAS

Defining Characteristics: Fatigue occurs commonly, and arthalgias and myalgias affect about 44% of all patients, with 8% experiencing severe symptoms. Arthralgias and myalgias commonly occurred 2–3 days after the drug was given, and resolved within a few days.

Nursing Implications: Teach patient that fatigue may occur, and ways to minimize exertion and energy expenditure by alternating rest and activity, and organizing chores so that they are done as efficiently as possible.

Drug: pamidronate disodium (Aredia)

Class: Biphosphonate; hypocalcemic agent.

Mechanism of Action: Probably inhibits osteoclast activity in bone (which causes bone breakdown and lytic bone lesions) and may also block dissolution of minerals (hydroxyapatite) in bone, thus preventing calcium release from bone. Indicated for skeletal metastasis of breast cancer and multiple myeloma.

Metabolism: Not metabolized, renally excreted.

Dosage/Range:
- For bone metastases from breast cancer: 90 mg in 250 mL NS or D5W IV over 2 hours every 3–4 weeks.
- For bone metastases from multiple myeloma: 90 mg in 500 mL NS or D5W IV over 4 hours every 4 weeks.

Drug Preparation/Administration:
- Reconstitute by adding 10 mL sterile water for injection to 30-mg vial. Further dilute in 1 L 0.95 Sodium Chloride or 5% Dextrose Injection as per manufacturer's directions.
- Infuse over 2–24 hours via infusion pump or rate controller.

Drug Interactions:
- None.

Lab Effects/Interference:
- Decreased Ca.
- Decreased K+, decreased Mg, decreased P (phosphate).

Special Considerations:
- Saline hydration to maintain urinary output of 2 L/day should be maintained during treatment.
- Clinical studies show 64% of patients have corrected serum calcium levels by 24 hours after beginning therapy, and after 7 days 100% of the 90-mg

group had normal corrected levels. For some (33–53%), normal or partially corrected calciums in the 60-mg and 90-mg groups persisted × 14 days.
- Has been shown to reduce bony metastasis in patients with multiple myeloma and to reduce pain.
- Patients with preexisting anemia, leukopenia, or thrombocytopenia should be monitored closely for 2 weeks after pamidronate disodium treatment.

Potential Toxicities/Side Effects and the Nursing Process

I. ALTERATIONS IN NUTRITION, LESS THAN BODY REQUIREMENTS, related to GI SIDE EFFECTS

Defining Characteristics: Rarely, nausea, vomiting, abdominal discomfort, constipation, and anorexia may occur.

Nursing Implications: Assess baseline nutritional and elimination status and monitor during treatment. Ensure adequate hydration and urinary output of 2 L/day. Administer ordered antiemetics. Administer oral phosphates as cathartics if ordered. Assess food differences and offer small, frequent feedings.

II. ALTERATION IN ELECTROLYTES related to HYPOCALCEMIA, HYPERCALCEMIA

Defining Characteristics: Rarely, if drug is very effective, hypocalcemia may occur; conversely, if drug is ineffective, hypercalcemia may occur. Hypokalemia, hypomagnesemia, hypophosphatemia may occur.

Nursing Implications: Monitor serum Ca+ closely. Assess for signs/symptoms of hypocalcemia (muscle twitching, spasm tetany, seizures) and hypercalcemia (bone pain, nausea, vomiting, polyuria, polydipsia, constipation, bradycardia, lethargy, muscle weakness, psychosis). Notify physician, recheck serum calcium immediately, and institute corrective measures as ordered. Monitor serum potassium, magnesium, phosphate levels, and notify physician of abnormalities.

III. ALTERATIONS IN COMFORT related to LOCAL VEIN IRRITATION

Defining Characteristics: Transient fever (1°C or 3°F elevation) may occur 24–48 hours after drug administration (27% of patients); local reactions (pain, irritation, phlebitis) are common with 90-mg dose.

Nursing Implications: Assess baseline temperature, and monitor during and after infusion. Administer antipyretics as ordered. Assess IV site and restart new IV as needed for 90-mg dose in large vein where drug can be rapidly diluted. Apply warm packs as needed to site.

IV. ALTERATIONS IN FLUID BALANCE related to AGGRESSIVE HYDRATION

Defining Characteristics: Patients receive aggressive saline hydration to ensure urinary output of 2 L/day. Hypertension may occur. Patients with history of heart disease or renal insufficiency are at risk for fluid overload.

Nursing Implications: Assess baseline hydration status, total body fluid balance; monitor q4h. Discuss with physician need for diuretics once hydrated to keep body fluid balance equal (I = O). Monitor VS q4h during hydration, and notify physician of changes.

Drug: pegasparaginase

Class: Miscellaneous agent (enzyme).

Mechanism of Action: Pegasparaginase is a modified form of L-asparaginase, wherein units of monomethoxypolethylene glycol (PEG) are covalently conjugated to L-asparaginase, forming the active ingredient PEG-L-asparaginase. The enzyme hydrolyzes serum asparagine, a nonessential amino acid for both normal and leukemic cells. Unlike normal cells, leukemic cells are unable to synthesize their own asparagine, resulting in cell death.

Metabolism: Unclear.

Dosage/Range:
- Adults under 21 and adolescents: 2500 IU/m^2 every 14 days.
- Children with BSA ≥ 0.6 m^2: 2500 IU/m^2 every 14 days.
- Children with BSA ≤ 0.6 m^2: 82.5 IU/kg body weight every 14 days.
- NOTE: Safety and efficacy have been established only in patients from 1–21 years of age.

Drug Preparation/Administration:
- For intravenous use, reconstitute with sterile water for injection, and dilute further in 100 cc NS or D5W. If giving IM, reconstitute in no more than 2 cc NS for injection. If more than 2 cc of NS is used, more than one injection site must be used.
- IM is the preferred route of administration, because of the lower incidence of hepatotoxicity, coagulopathy, and gastrointestinal and renal disorders as compared with the intravenous route.

Drug Interactions:
- Nonsteroidal anti-inflammatory drugs (NSAIDs), aspirin, dipyridamole, heparin, warfarin, and blood-dyscrasia-causing medications: Pegasparaginase causes imbalances in coagulation factors, predisposing patients to bleeding and/or thrombosis.

- Hepatotoxic medications (increased risk of toxicity).
- Methotrexate: Drug antagonizes antifolate effects of MTX if given before MTX administration. If given 24 hours after MTX, its antifolate activity will be terminated at that point.
- Vaccines, both live and killed virus: Patient's antibody response to the killed vaccine may be reduced for up to one year by the immunosuppression brought on by pegasparaginase. Such immunosuppression may also potentiate the replication of live-virus vaccines, increase the side effects of the vaccine virus, and/or may decrease the patient's antibody response to the vaccine.

Lab Effects/Interference:
- Increased LFTs, serum glucose, BUN, and uric acid.
- Prolonged PT.

Special Considerations:
- Drug should NOT be given in patients with:
  - —Pegasparaginase allergy
  - —Bleeding disorders associated with prior asparaginase therapy
  - —Pancreatitis, or history of
- Hypersensitivity reactions occur more frequently with pegasparaginase than with the vast majority of chemotherapeutic agents. Patients must be closely monitored for signs of allergic/anaphylactic reactions. Ensure immediate access to adverse-reaction kit.

Potential Toxicities/Side Effects and the Nursing Process

I. POTENTIAL FOR INJURY related to HYPERSENSITIVITY OR ANAPHYLACTIC REACTIONS

Defining Characteristics: Occurs less often with IM route of administration. May be life-threatening reaction, but is usually mild.

Nursing Implications: Discuss with physician use of test dose prior to drug administration. Assess baseline VS and mental status prior to drug administration. Review standing orders or nursing procedure for management of anaphylaxis and be prepared to stop drug immediately if signs/symptoms occur; keep IV line open with 0.9% Sodium Chloride, notify physician, monitor vital signs, and administer ordered medications, which may include epinephrine 1:1000, hydrocortisone sodium succinate, and diphenhydramine. Teach patient the potential of a hypersensitivity or anaphylactic reaction and to immediately report any unusual symptoms. *Escherichia coli* preparation of L-asparaginase and *Erwinia carotovora* preparation are non-cross-resistant, so if an anaphylactic reaction occurs with one, the other preparation may be used.

II. POTENTIAL FOR INJURY related to HEPATIC DYSFUNCTION OR THROMBOEMBOLISM

Defining Characteristics: Most patients have elevated LFTs starting within first two weeks of treatment, e.g., SGOT, bili, and alk phos. Hepatically derived clotting factors may be depressed, resulting in excessive bleeding or blood clotting. Relatively uncommon.

Nursing Implications: Monitor SGOT, bili, alk phos, albumin, and clotting factors CPT, PTT, fibrinogen. Teach patient of the potential for excessive bleeding or blood clotting, and instruct to report any unusual symptoms. Assess patient for signs/symptoms of bleeding.

III. ALTERED NUTRITION, LESS THAN BODY REQUIREMENTS, related to NAUSEA/VOMITING, ANOREXIA, HYPERGLYCEMIA

Defining Characteristics: Many patients experience mild-to-moderate nausea and vomiting. Anorexia commonly occurs. Hyperglycemia is a transient reaction caused by effects on the pancreas with decreased insulin synthesis. Pancreatitis occurs in some patients.

Nursing Implications: Premedicate with antiemetics and continue prophylactically for 24 hours to prevent nausea and vomiting. Encourage small, frequent meals of cool, bland foods and liquids, as well as favorite foods, especially high-calorie, high-protein foods. Encourage use of spices and do weekly weights. Teach patient about the potential of hyperglycemia and pancreatitis, and instruct to report any unusual symptoms: e.g., increased thirst, urination, and appetite (hyperglycemia) and abdominal or stomach pain, constipation, or nausea and vomiting (pancreatitis). Monitor serum glucose, amylase, and lipase levels periodically during treatment. Report any laboratory elevations to physician. Treat hyperglycemia issues with diet or insulin as ordered by physician. Treat pancreatitis per physician orders.

IV. SENSORY/PERCEPTUAL ALTERATIONS related to NEUROTOXICITY

Defining Characteristics: Neurotoxicity may occur in some patients—commonly, lethargy, drowsiness, and somnolence; rarely coma. Seen more frequently in adults.

Nursing Implications: Teach patient about the potential of CNS toxicity, and instruct to report any unusual symptoms. Obtain baseline neurologic and mental function. Assess patient for any neurologic abnormalities and report changes to physician. Discuss with patient the impact of malaise on his/her general sense of well-being and strategies to minimize the distress.

V. INFECTION, BLEEDING, AND FATIGUE related to BONE MARROW DEPRESSION

Defining Characteristics: Bone marrow depression is not common. Mild anemia may occur. Serious leukopenia and thrombocytopenia are rare.

Nursing Implications: Monitor CBC, platelet count prior to drug administration, as well as signs/symptoms of infection, bleeding, or anemia. Instruct patient in self-assessment of signs/symptoms of infection, bleeding, or anemia and to report immediately.

Drug: pemetrexed (Alimta)

Class: Multi-targeted antifolate (antimetabolite).

Mechanism of Action: Inhibits key metabolic enzymatic steps (Thymidylate synthase [TS], dihydrofolate reductase [DHFR], and glycinamide ribonucleotide formyl-transferase [GARFT]) critical to pyrimidine and purine synthesis, thus preventing DNA synthesis and cell division. Drug is carried into tumor cells via reduced folate carriers, metabolized intracellularly to polyglutamated form of pemetrexed that potently inhibits purine and pyrimidine synthesis. Antitumor effect dependent upon size of cellular folate pools, so folic acid must be co-administered to increase drug efficacy and minimize toxicity. Polyglutamates accumulate in the cell, with a long cellular half-life, and increased cytotoxicity.

Metabolism: Following IV administration, peak plasma levels are achieved within 30 minutes. Drug is widely distributed in body tissues, especially liver, kidneys, small intestines and colon. Excreted by kidneys (glomerular and tubular) into the urine, with up to 90% of the drug excreted unchanged during the first 24 hours after administration. Plasma half-life is about 3 hours, with prolonged terminal half-life of 20 hours.

Dosage/Range:

- Malignant-pleural mesothelioma: 500 mg/m^2 IV over 10 minutes q 21 days together with cisplatin 75 mg/m^2 IV over 2 hours, beginning 30 minutes after the end of the pemetrexed dose.
- Non-Small Cell Lung Cancer: 500 mg/m^2 IV over 10 minutes q 21 days

Drug Preparation/Administration:

- Reconstitute pemetrexed 500 mg vial by adding 20 mL 0.9% sodium chloride for injection, resulting in a concentration of 25 mg/mL.
- Asceptically remove dose and add to 100 mL 0.9% sodium chloride for injection.
- Administer as a 10-minute IV infusion.

- Patient should take dexamethasone 4 mg PO twice daily on the day before, day of, and day after treatment to help prevent skin rash.
- Patient must take daily folic acid supplement (350 to 1000 μg) po beginning 1 week prior to treatment, and continuing throughout treatment and post-treatment.
- Patient must receive vitamin B_{12} (1000 μg) IM injections every 3 cycles, beginning 1 week prior to treatment, and continuing throughout treatment every 3 cycles thereafter
- Full dose if ANC > 1500 cells/mm^3, platelets > 100,000 cells/mm^3, AND creatinine clearance > 45 mL/min.

Dose Reductions:

- Hematologic: Nadir ANC < 500 cells/mm^3 and platelet count > 50,000 cells/mm^3 DOSE REDUCE both drugs to 75% of previous doses.
- Hematologic: Nadir platelets < 50,000 cells/mm^3 regardless of ANC nadir DOSE REDUCE both drugs to 50% of previous doses.
- Pemetrexed should be discontinued for any grade 3 or 4 hematologic or non-hematologic toxicity after 2 dose reductions, or immediately if grade 3 or 4 neurologic toxicity.
- If grade 1 neurotoxicity, no dose modifications of either drug. If grade 2 neurotoxicity, 100% pemetrexed dose, but cisplatin is 50% of previous dose.

Drug Interactions:

- Nephrotoxic drugs: Potentially delayed pemetrexed excretion.
- Drugs secreted by renal tubules (e.g., probenecid): potential delayed pemetrexed excretion.
- Ibuprofen in people with normal renal function: 20% increase in AUC of pemetrexed, due to 20% reduction in pemetrexed clearance.
- NSAIDs (short half-lives, e.g., ibuprofen): AVOID if renal compromise (creatinine clearance < 80 mL/min), stop NSAIDs 2 days prior to pemetrexed administration, the day of administration, and for 2 days following pemetrexed administration.
- NSAIDs (long half-lives): stop NSAID 5 days before, the day of, and for 2 days following pemetrexed administration.

Lab Effects/Interference: None known.

Special Considerations:

- FDA indicated in combination with cisplatin for the treatment of patients with malignant pleural mesothelioma whose disease is unresectable or who are otherwise not candidates for curative surgery.
- FDA indicated as a single agent for the treatment of patients with locally advanced or metastatic nonsmall cell lung cancer after prior chemotherapy.

- Do not administer drug if creatinine clearance is < 45 mL/min using Cockcroft and Gault formula (estimated creatinine clearance).
  $$\text{Males} = \frac{[140 - \text{age in years}] \times \text{actual body weight (kg)}}{72 \times \text{Serum creatinine (mg/dL)}} = \text{mL/min}$$
  Females = Estimated creatinine clearance for males × 0.85
- Pemetrexed is fetotoxic and teratogenic. Women of child-bearing age should use effective birth control measures. Women should not breast feed an infant while receiving pemetrexed.

Potential Toxicities/Side Effects and the Nursing Process

I. POTENTIAL INFECTION, BLEEDING, AND FATIGUE related to BONE MARROW DEPRESSION

Defining Characteristics: Bone marrow depression is dose-limiting toxicity. Nadir is day 8 with recovery by day 15 of each cycle. Neutropenia occurred in 58% of patients, with grade 3 (19%), and grade 4 (5%). For grades 3 and 4 neutropenia, the incidence in between patients who were fully supplemented was 24%, in contrast to patients who were never supplemented (38%). The overall incidence of thrombocytopenia is 27%, with grades 3 and 4 (4%/1%, respectively). Anemia occurred in 33% of patients overall.

Nursing Implications: Assess baseline CBC, WBC, differential and ANC, and platelet count prior to chemotherapy as well as for signs and symptoms of infection, bleeding, or anemia. Ensure labs ANC > 1500 cells/mm^3, platelets $> 100{,}000$ cells/mm^3, AND creatinine clearance > 45 mL/min prior to drug administration. Ensure that patient has taken vitamin supplements prior to drug administration: low dose oral folic acid or multivitamin with folic acid q d (at least 5 daily doses of folic acid must be taken during the 7-day period prior to the first dose of pemetrexed, and dosing should continue during the full course of therapy, and for 21 days after the last drug dose; Vitamin B_{12} 100 μg IM during the week prior to cycle 1, then every 3 cycles. Subsequent doses can be given on same day as pemetrexed treatment). Discuss dose reductions based on nadir counts with physician as needed. Teach patient signs/symptoms of infection, and bleeding, and instruct to report them right away. Teach measures to minimize infection and bleeding, such as avoidance of crowds, proximity to people with infection, and to avoid aspirin or NSAID-containing medications. Teach patient strategies to minimize fatigue, such as alternating rest with activity, and ways to organize shopping to minimize energy expenditure.

II. POTENTIAL ALTERATION IN NUTRITION, LESS THAN BODY REQUIREMENTS, related to NAUSEA, CONSTIPATION, ANOREXIA, DIARRHEA, STOMATITIS

Defining Characteristics: Nausea occurs in 84% of patients, vomiting 58%, constipation 44%, anorexia 35%, stomatitis/pharyngitis 28%, and diarrhea 26%, in combination with cisplatin.

Nursing Implications: Premedicate with antiemetics, and ensure patient has antiemetics to take to prevent delayed emesis from cisplatin. Teach patient and family delayed emesis regime. Encourage small, frequent meals of cool, bland foods, and to increase fluid intake. Assess oral mucosa prior to drug administration and instruct patient to report changes. Teach patient oral hygiene measures and self-assessment. Instruct patient to report diarrhea, to self-administer prescribed antidiarrheal medications and to drink adequate fluids. Monitor LFTs baseline and periodically during therapy. Notify physician of any abnormalities and discuss implications as drug studied only in patients with elevated LFTs related to liver metastases.

III. ALTERATION IN SKIN INTEGRITY related to RASH

Defining Characteristics: Incidence of rash with or without desquamation was 22%.

Nursing Implications: Assess baseline skin integrity. Teach patient that this may occur, and to take recommended dexamethasone premedication 4 mg po bid the day before, the day of, and the day after pemetrexed administration. Teach patient potential side effects of corticosteroid administration, including difficulty sleeping, mood alterations, and depression.

IV. POTENTIAL FOR IMPAIRED GAS EXCHANGE related to DYSPNEA

Defining Characteristics: Dyspnea was reported in 66% of patients receiving pemetrexed and cisplatin therapy; 10% had grade 3 dyspnea, and 1% had grade 4 toxicity.

Nursing Implications: Teach patient that this may occur, and to report it right away if severe or worsening. Assess baseline pulmonary status, at rest, and with activity. Assess oxygen saturation with vital signs. Discuss severe or worsening dyspnea with physician.

Drug: plicamycin (Mithramycin, Mithracin)

Class: Antibiotic isolated from *Streptomyces plicatus.*

Mechanism of Action: In the presence of magnesium ions the drug binds with guanine bases of DNA and inhibits DNA-directed RNA synthesis. Cell cycle specific for S phase.

Metabolism: Metabolism is not clearly understood. About half of the drug is excreted within 18–24 hours. Crosses BBB. Concentrations of drug in CSF equal blood concentration 4–6 hours after elimination.

Dosage/Range:

- Dose for testicular cancer: 25–30 μg/kg IV, alternating days until toxicity occurs.
- Hypercalcemia: 25 μg/kg IV for one dose.

Drug Preparation:

- For each 2.5-mg vial, add sterile water to obtain concentration of 500 μg/mL.

Drug Administration:

- IV drug is an irritant; avoid extravasation. Administer over 4–6 hours to minimize nausea and vomiting.

Drug Interactions:

- Myelosuppressive agents: Increased hematologic toxicity if overlapping nadirs; use cautiously and monitor patient closely or reduce drug dose.

Lab Effects/Interference:

- Decreased CBC (especially platelets).
- Decreased electrolytes, especially Ca, K, P.
- Increased LFTs, RFTs.
- Increased PT, bleeding time.

Special Considerations:

- Alternate-day therapy greatly reduces the incidence and severity of stomatitis, hemorrhage, and facial flushing and swelling.
- Do not administer to patient with a coagulation disorder or impaired bone marrow function because of the risk of hemorrhagic diathesis.
- Crosses the BBB.
- Metallic taste with administration.

Potential Toxicities/Side Effects and the Nursing Process

I. ALTERATION IN NUTRITION, LESS THAN BODY REQUIREMENTS, related to NAUSEA/VOMITING, ANOREXIA, AND STOMATITIS

Defining Characteristics: Severe nausea and vomiting begin 6+ hours after dose and may last 24 hours (at therapeutic doses); anorexia commonly occurs; alternate-day therapy greatly reduces the incidence and severity of stomatitis; taste alterations can occur.

Nursing Implications: Premedicate with antiemetics and continue prophylactically to prevent nausea and vomiting, at least for the first treatment. Encourage small, frequent meals of cool, bland foods and liquids. Encourage small, frequent feedings of favorite foods, especially high-calorie, high-protein foods. Encourage use of spices; weekly weights. Teach patient oral assessment and oral hygiene regimens. Encourage patient to report early stomatitis. Administer pain relief measures, e.g., diclone, viscous xylocaine oral gargles if needed. Suggest increased use of spices as tolerated. Help patient and partner develop menu based on past favorite foods. Dietary consultation as needed. Discuss dietary supplements of zinc and selenium.

II. POTENTIAL FOR IMPAIRED SKIN INTEGRITY related to ALOPECIA

Defining Characteristics: Occurs in 30–50% of patients, especially with IV dosing. Some degree of hair loss is expected in all patients. Begins after 3+ weeks, and hair may grow back in therapy. May be slight to diffuse thinning.

Nursing Implications: Assess patient for signs/symptoms of hair loss. Discuss with patient impact of hair loss and strategies to minimize distress (e.g., wig, scarf, cap); begin before therapy initiated. Assess patient for changes in skin, nails. Discuss with patient impact of changes and strategies to minimize distress; e.g., wearing nail polish, long-sleeved tops. Hyperpigmentation of nails and skin, transverse ridging of nails ("banding") may occur.

III. POTENTIAL FOR INFECTION AND BLEEDING related to BONE MARROW DEPRESSION

Defining Characteristics: Leukopenia nadir 7–14 days with recovery by 1–2 weeks. Less frequent thrombocytopenia, but one-third of patients develop a coagulopathy. Alternate-day instead of daily dosing reduces bleeding complications. Mild anemia. Potent immunosuppressant.

Nursing Implications: Monitor CBC, platelet count prior to drug administration, as well as signs/symptoms of infection or bleeding. Instruct patient in self-assessment of signs/symptoms of infection or bleeding and risk reduction. Dose reduction often necessary (35–50%) if there is compromised bone marrow function.

IV. POTENTIAL SEXUAL DYSFUNCTION related to DRUG EFFECTS

Defining Characteristics: Drug is mutagenic and teratogenic. Testicular atrophy sometimes occurs with reversible oligo- and azoospermia. Amenorrhea often occurs in females. Drug is excreted in breast milk.

Nursing Implications: As appropriate, explore with patient and partner issues of reproductive and sexuality patterns and the impact chemotherapy will have. Discuss strategies to preserve sexual and reproductive health (e.g., sperm banking, contraception).

V. ALTERATION IN METABOLISM related to HYPOCALCEMIA

Defining Characteristics: Drug may decrease calcium and lead to hypocalcemia. Monitor for muscle stiffness, twitching. In some cases when calcium is abnormally high (as in hypercalcemia from breast cancer), this drug may be used to decrease calcium level.

Nursing Implications: Monitor blood calcium levels. Instruct patient about signs/symptoms of neuromuscular involvement such as muscle stiffness, weakness, or twitching. Instruct patient about CNS manifestations of hypocalcemia: weakness, drowsiness, lethargy, irritability, headache, confusion, depression.

Drug: polifeprosan 20 with carmustine (BCNU) implant (Gliadel®)

Class: Alkylating agent.

Mechanism of Action: Wafer (copolymer) containing carmustine is implanted in the surgical cavity created when brain tumor is resected. In water, the anhydride bonds of the wafer are hydrolyzed, releasing the carmustine into the surgical cavity. The carmustine diffuses into the surrounding brain tissue, reaching any residual tumor cells, and causing cell death by alkyating DNA and RNA.

Metabolism: Unknown. Dime-sized wafer is biodegradable in brain tissue, with a variable rate. More than 70% of the copolymer degrades by three weeks, slowly releasing 7.7 mg of carmustine in concentrations. In some patients, wafer fragments remained up to 232 days after implantation, with almost all drug gone.

Dosage/Range:

- Each wafer contains 7.7 mg of carmustine, and the recommended dose is 8 wafers, or a total dose of 61.6 mg of carmustine.

Drug Preparation:

- Drug must be stored at or below 20°C (−4°F) until time of use.

- Unopened foil packages can stay at room temperature for a maximum of 6 hours at a time. The manufacturer recommends that the treatment box be removed from the freezer and taken to the operating room just prior to surgery.
- The box and pouches should be opened just before the surgeon is ready to implant the wafers. Open the sealed treatment box and remove double foil packages, handling the unsterile outer foil packet by the crimped edge VERY CAREFULLY to prevent damage to the wafers. See product information for opening the inner foil pouch and removing the wafer with sterile technique.
- Chemotherapy precautions should be used to limit exposure to the chemotherapy: surgical instruments used to remove and implant the wafers should be kept separate from other instruments and sterile fields, and should be cleaned after the procedure according to hospital chemotherapy procedure; all personnel handling the wafers of the inner foil pouches containing the wafers should wear double gloves, which, along with unused wafers or fragments, inner foil packages, and opened outer foil package, should be disposed of as chemotherapeutic waste.

Drug Administration:
- Neurosurgeon places 8 wafers into surgical resection cavity if size and shape appropriate; wafers are placed contiguously or with slight overlapping.
- Wafer may be broken into 2 pieces *only* if needed.

Drug Interactions:
- Unknown but unlikely as drug is probably not systemically absorbed.

Lab Effects/Interference:
- Unknown, but unlikely.

Special Considerations:
- Indicated for the treatment of newly diagnosed patients with high-grade malignant glioma as an adjunct to surgery and radiation.
- Indicated for use as an adjunct to surgery to prolong survival in patients with recurrent glioblastoma multiforme for whom surgical resection is indicated.
- Manufacturer reports that in a study of 222 patients with recurrent glioma who failed initial surgery and radiotherapy, the six-month survival rate after surgery increased from 47% (placebo) to 60%, and in patients with glioblastoma multiforme, the six-month survival for patients receiving placebo was 36% vs 56% for patients receiving polifeprosan 20 with camustine implant.
- Patients require close monitoring for complications of craniotomy, as intracerebral mass effect has occurred that does not respond to corticosteroid treatment; in one case, this resulted in brain herniation.

- Studies have not been conducted during pregnancy or in nursing mothers. Carmustine is a known teratogen, and is embryotoxic. Use during pregnancy should be avoided, and mothers should stop nursing during use of the drug.

Potential Toxicities/Side Effects and the Nursing Process

I. POTENTIAL SENSORY/PERCEPTUAL ALTERATIONS related to SEIZURES, BRAIN EDEMA, MENTAL STATUS CHANGES

Defining Characteristics: In clinical testing, the incidence of new or worsened seizures was 19% in both the group receiving the implant and those receiving the placebo. Seizures were mild to moderate in severity. In patients with new or worsened seizures postoperatively, the group receiving the implant had a 56% incidence, with median time to first new or worsened seizure of 3.5 days, versus placebo incidence of 9%, and median time to first new or worsened seizure of 61 days. Incidence of brain edema was 4%, and there were cases of intracerebral mass effect that did not respond to corticosteroids. Other nervous system effects were hydrocephalus (3%), depression (3%), abnormal thinking (2%), ataxia (2%), dizziness (2%), insomnia (2%), visual field defect (2%), monoplegia (2%), eye pain (1%), coma (1%), amnesia (1%), diplopia (1%), and paranoid reaction (1%). Rarely (< 1%), cerebral infarct or hemorrhage may occur.

Nursing Implications: Monitor neurovital signs closely postoperatively, and notify physician of any abnormalities. If intracranial pressure increases, a mass effect is suspected, and if it is nonresponsive to corticosteroids, expect the patient to be taken to surgery, with possible removal of wafer or remnants. Assess baseline mental status and regularly during postoperative care. Validate changes with family members. Discuss abnormalities with physician immediately and continue to monitor closely.

II. POTENTIAL FOR INFECTION related to HEALING ABNORMALITIES

Defining Characteristics: Most abnormalities were mild to moderate, occurred in 14% of patients, and included cerebrospinal leaks, subdural fluid collections, subgaleal or wound effusions, and breakdown. The incidence of intracranial infection (e.g., meningitis or abscess) was 4%. Incidence of deep wound infection was 6% (same as placebo) and included infection of subgaleal space, bone, meninges, and brain tissue.

Nursing Implications: Using aseptic technique, assess postoperative wound/dressing immediately postoperatively, and regularly thereafter. Assess systematically for signs/symptoms of infection or wound breakdown. Notify physician immediately and discuss antimicrobial therapy.

III. ALTERATION IN NUTRITION, LESS THAN BODY REQUIREMENTS, related to GI SIDE EFFECTS, ELECTROLYTE ABNORMALITIES

Defining Characteristics: Rarely, GI disturbances occurred: diarrhea (2%), constipation (2%), dysphagia (1%), gastrointestinal hemorrhage (1%), fecal incontinence (1%). Hyponatremia (3%), hyperglycemia (3%), and hypokalemia (1%) also occurred.

Nursing Implications: Assess baseline nutritional status, including electrolytes. Assess bowel elimination status and monitor nutritional and bowel elimination status closely during postoperative time. Discuss interventions for abnormalities with physician.

IV. ALTERATION IN CIRCULATION, POTENTIAL, related to CHANGES IN BLOOD PRESSURE

Defining Characteristics: Hypertension occurred in 3% of patients, and hypotension in 1%.

Nursing Implications: Assess baseline VS and monitor closely during postoperative phase. Discuss abnormalities with physician.

V. ALTERATION IN COMFORT related to EDEMA, PAIN, ASTHENIA

Defining Characteristics: The following occur rarely: peripheral edema (2%), neck pain (2%), rash (2%), back pain (1%), asthenia (1%), chest pain (1%).

Nursing Implications: Assess baseline comfort level and monitor closely during postoperative phase. Provide comfort measures. If ineffective, discuss symptom-management strategies with physician.

Drug: procarbazine hydrochloride (Matulane)

Class: Miscellaneous agent.

Mechanism of Action: Uncertain but appears to affect preformed DNA, RNA, and protein. It is a methylhydrazine derivative.

Metabolism: Most of the drug is excreted in the urine. Procarbazine crosses the BBB. Rapidly absorbed from the GI tract; metabolized by the liver.

Dosage/Range:
- 100 mg/m^2 PO daily from 7–14 days every 4 weeks.
- Given in combination with other drugs.

Drug Preparation:
- None.

Drug Administration:
- Oral.
- Available in 50-mg capsules.

Drug Interactions:
- Procarbazine is synergistic with CNS depressants. Barbiturate, antihistamine, narcotic, and hypotensive agents or phenothiazine antiemetics should be used with caution.
- Disulfirim (Antabuse)-like reaction may result if the patient consumes alcohol. Symptoms include headache, respiratory difficulties, nausea and vomiting, chest pain, hypotension, and mental status changes.
- Exhibits weak MAO(monoamine oxidase) inhibitor activity. Foods containing high amounts of tyramine should be avoided: substances such as beer, wine, cheese, brewer's yeast, chicken livers, and bananas. Consumption of foods high in tyramine in combination with procarbazine may lead to intracranial hemorrhage or hypertensive crisis.
- When taken in combination with digoxin, there is a decreased bioavailability of digoxin.

Lab Effects/Interference:
- Decreased CBC.
- Increased LFTs, RFTs.

Special Considerations:
- Discontinue if CNS signs/symptoms (paresthesia, neuropathy, confusion), stomatitis, diarrhea, or hypersensitivity reaction occur.

Potential Toxicities/Side Effects and the Nursing Process

I. POTENTIAL FOR INFECTION AND BLEEDING related to BONE MARROW DEPRESSION

Defining Characteristics: Major dose-limiting toxicity. Thrombocytopenia occurs in 50% of patients, evidenced by a delayed onset (28 days after treatment) and lasting 2–3 weeks. Leukopenia seen in two-thirds of patients, with nadirs occurring after initial thrombocytopenia. Anemias may be due to bone marrow depression or hemolysis.

Nursing Implications: Monitor CBC, platelet count prior to drug administration, as well as signs/symptoms of infection, bleeding, and anemia. Instruct patient in self-assessment of signs/symptoms of infection, bleeding, and anemia and to report this immediately. Dose reduction often necessary (35–50%) if compromised bone marrow function. Platelet and red cell transfusions per physician order.

II. ALTERATION IN NUTRITION, LESS THAN BODY REQUIREMENTS, related to GI SIDE EFFECTS

Defining Characteristics: Nausea and vomiting occur in 70% of patients and may be a dose-limiting toxicity. Diarrhea is uncommon, but rarely may be protracted and thus would be an indication for dose reduction.

Nursing Implications: Premedicate with antiemetics and continue prophylactically for 24 hours to prevent nausea and vomiting. Encourage small, frequent meals of cool, bland foods and liquids. Minimize nausea and vomiting by dividing the total daily dosage into 3–4 doses. Also, taking the pills at bedtime may decrease the sense of nausea. May administer nonphenothiazine antiemetics. Encourage patients to report onset of diarrhea. Administer, or teach patient to self-administer, antidiarrheal medications.

III. POTENTIAL FOR SENSORY/PERCEPTUAL ALTERATIONS

Defining Characteristics: Symptoms occur in 10–30% of patients and are seen as lethargy, depression, frequent nightmares, insomnia, nervousness, or hallucinations. Tremors, coma, convulsions are less common. Symptoms usually disappear when drug is discontinued. Crosses into CSF.

Nursing Implications: Teach patient the potential for neurotoxicity and provide early counseling about these effects. Assess patients for any symptoms of neurotoxicity. Discuss strategies with patient to preserve general sense of well-being. Obtain baseline neurologic and motor function. CNS toxicity may be manifested as reactions to other drugs, e.g., barbiturates, narcotics, and phenothiazine antiemetics.

IV. ACTIVITY INTOLERANCE related to PERIPHERAL NEUROPATHY

Defining Characteristics: 10% of patients exhibit paresthesias, decrease in deep tendon reflexes. Foot drop and ataxia occasionally reported. Reversible when drug is discontinued.

Nursing Implications: Obtain baseline neurologic and motor function. Assess patient for any changes in motor function, e.g., ability to pick up pencil, button buttons.

V. ALTERATION IN COMFORT related to FLULIKE SYNDROME

Defining Characteristics: Fever, chills, sweating, lethargy, myalgias, and arthralgias commonly occur.

Nursing Implications: Teach patient the potential for flulike syndromes and how to distinguish from actual infection. Instruct patient to report any changes in condition.

VI. POTENTIAL FOR IMPAIRED SKIN INTEGRITY related to RARE DERMATITIS REACTIONS

Defining Characteristics: Rarely occurs as alopecia, pruritus, rash, hyperpigmentation.

Nursing Implications: Assess patient for changes in skin, nails, and hair loss. Discuss with patient impact of changes and strategies to minimize distress, e.g., wearing nail polish, long-sleeved tops, wigs, scarfs, caps.

VII. POTENTIAL SEXUAL DYSFUNCTION related to DRUG EFFECTS

Defining Characteristics: Drug is teratogenic. Causes azoospermia. Causes cessation of menses, although may be reversible.

Nursing Implications: As appropriate, explore with patient and partner issues of reproductive and sexuality patterns and the impact chemotherapy may have. Discuss strategies to preserve sexual and reproductive health (e.g., sperm banking, contraception).

Drug: progestational agents: medroxyprogesterone acetate (Provera, Depo-Provera), megestrol acetate (Megace)

Class: Hormone.

Mechanism of Action: Unclear, but progestational agents compete for androgen and progestational receptor sites on the cell. Has potent antiestrogenic properties that disturb estrogen receptor cycle. Also increases synthesis of RNA by interacting with DNA.

Metabolism: Rapidly absorbed from GI tract. Metabolized in the liver. Excreted in the urine. Peak plasma levels reached in 1–3 hours; biological half-life, 3.5 days.

Dosage/Range:

Medroxyprogesterone acetate:

- Provera: 20–80 mg PO daily.

Depo-Provera:

- —400–800 mg IM every month
- —100 mg IM three times weekly
- —1000–1500 mg daily (high dose)

Megestrol acetate:

- Megace, mg PO qid (breast cancer): 80 mg PO qid (endometrial cancer).

Drug Preparation:

- IM preparation is ready to use; shake vial well before drawing up medication.

Drug Administration:
- Give via deep IM injection.

Drug Interactions:
- None.

Lab Effects/Interference:
- Increased LFTs.
- Changes in TFTs.

Special Considerations:
- Patients may become sensitive to oil carrier (oil in which drug is mixed).
- Small risk of hypersensitivity reaction.

Potential Toxicities/Side Effects and the Nursing Process

I. POTENTIAL FOR INJURY related to FLUID RETENTION, THROMBOEMBOLISM

Defining Characteristics: Fluid retention. Thromboembolic complications may occur. Sterile abscess may occur with IM injection.

Nursing Implications: Inform patient of potential for fluid retention and of signs/symptoms to watch for and to report to nurse or physician. Assess for signs/symptoms of fluid overload. Teach patient and family signs/symptoms of thromboembolic events: positive Homan's sign, localized pain, tenderness, erythema, sudden CNS changes, shortness of breath. Instruct patient to notify nurse or physician if any of the above occur. Give drug via deep IM injection: apply pressure to injection site after administering. Inspect used sites; rotate sites systematically.

II. ALTERED NUTRITION, LESS THAN BODY REQUIREMENTS, related to NAUSEA

Defining Characteristics: Nausea is rare.

Nursing Implications: Inform patient that nausea can occur; encourage patient to report nausea. Encourage small, frequent meals of cool, bland foods and liquids.

Drug: raloxifene hydrochloride (Evista®)

Class: Selective estrogen receptor modulator (SERM).

Mechanism of Action: Selectively modulates estrogen receptors by binding to estrogen receptors. This binding causes expression of multiple estrogen-regulated genes in different tissues. Acts as antagonist by inhibiting breast epithelial and uterine/endometrial proliferation; acts as an agonist (like estrogen) in bone to preserve bone mineral density, and on lipid metabolism to lower low-density lipids and total cholesterol, while not affecting high-density lipids or triglycerides.

Metabolism: Primarily metabolized in the liver, with rapid systemic clearance.

Dosage/Range:
- 60 mg PO qd.

Drug Preparation:
- Oral, available in 60-mg tablets.

Drug Administration:
- Take orally without regard to food or meals.

Drug Interactions:
- Cholestyramine: Causes 60% reduction in absorption of raloxifene. DO NOT GIVE CONCURRENTLY.
- Warfarin: 10% decrease in PT has been noted; monitor prothrombin closely if drugs are given concurrently.
- Highly protein-bound drugs: Raloxifene is >95% protein-bound. Use together with the following drugs cautiously, and monitor for underdosing or toxicity: clofibrate, indomethacin, naproxen, ibuprofen, diazepam, diazoxide.

Lab Effects/Interference:
- Unknown.

Special Considerations:
- Indicated for the prevention of osteoporosis in postmenopausal women, at doses of 30 mg–150 mg/day, together with calcium replacement.
- Recent evidence shows that raloxifene used to treat osteoporosis in postmenopausal women reduces risk of invasive breast cancer by 76% (*Multiple Outcomes of Raloxifene Evaluation*, 1999). Raloxifene decreased estrogen receptor-positive breast cancer by 90% but did not decrease estrogen receptor-negative breast cancer risk; benefit seems to be for postmenopausal women who commonly have receptor-positive receptor status.
- As compared to tamoxifen, raloxifene has 3 times the risk of causing thromboembolic disease but does significantly increase the risk of endometrial cancer (tamoxifen increases the risk 4 times).
- Currently being tested against tamoxifen in preventing breast cancer [National Surgical Adjuvant Breast and Bowel Project—PT (Prevention Trial) 2, sometimes referred to as the STAR (Study of Tamoxifen and Raloxifene)].

- Contraindicated in individuals who are hypersensitive to the drug, have or have had thromboembolic disorders, pregnant women, women who may become pregnant.
- Use cautiously in patients with cardiovascular disease, uterine cancer, or renal or hepatic dysfunction.
- When used to preserve bone density in postmenopausal women, drug should be combined with supplemental calcium and vitamin D, weight-bearing exercises, lifestyle changes such as cessation of smoking and reduced alcohol consumption.

Potential Toxicities/Side Effects and the Nursing Process

I. ALTERATION IN CIRCULATION, POTENTIAL, related to THROMBOEMBOLIC EVENT

Defining Characteristics: Drug can cause thromboembolic events, including deep vein thrombosis, pulmonary embolism, and retinal vein thrombosis. Greatest risk is during first four months of treatment. Rarely, patients may experience chest pain. Drug is contraindicated for individuals who have had or currently have thromboembolic events.

Nursing Implications: Assess baseline risk (e.g., history of CHF, malignancy). Teach patient to report pain in the legs, especially the calves, any redness or swelling of the legs, sudden-onset shortness of breath with chest pain. If leg pain, assess Homan's sign, and if positive, discuss with physician and anticipate sending patient to radiology for a duplex ultrasound to rule out thromboembolism or thrombophlebitis. If pulmonary embolism suspected, assess pulmonary status, discuss VQ scan with physician. Drug should be discontinued at least 72 hours prior to and during prolonged bed rest (e.g., postoperative care) resumed when the patient is fully ambulatory. Teach patient to move around while traveling to avoid prolonged time in one position.

II. ALTERATION IN NUTRITION related to GASTROINTESTINAL SYMPTOMS

Defining Characteristics: Nausea, vomiting, dyspepsia, flatulence, gastroenteritis, and weight gain have all been reported as occurring > 2% of the time.

Nursing Implications: Assess baseline nutritional status. Teach patient that these symptoms may occur and to report them. Teach patient symptomatic management. If problems persist or are severe, discuss pharmacologic symptom management and possible drug discontinuance.

III. SENSORY/PERCEPTUAL ALTERATIONS related to CNS CHANGES

Defining Characteristics: Migraine headaches, depression, insomnia, and fever have all been reported as occurring in > 2% of patients.

Nursing Implications: Assess baseline neurological status, including affect and sleeping pattern. Teach patient that these symptoms may occur and to report them. Teach symptomatic management. If symptoms do not resolve or become severe, discuss with physician pharmacologic symptom management and possible discontinuance of drug.

IV. ALTERATION IN COMFORT related to HOT FLASHES, ARTHRALGIAS, MYALGIAS, COUGH, RASH

Defining Characteristics: Hot flashes (25%), arthralgias (11%), myalgias (8%), leg cramps (6%), arthritis (4%), rash (6%), and flulike syndrome (15%) have all been described. Hot flashes usually occur during first six months of treatment.

Nursing Implications: Assess baseline comfort level and history of muscle and joint aches or pains. Assess skin integrity and respiratory status. Teach patient that these symptoms may occur and to report them, especially rash. Teach symptomatic management. If symptoms persist or become severe, discuss drug discontinuance with physician.

V. ALTERATION IN SEXUALITY related to VAGINITIS, LEUKORRHEA

Defining Characteristics: Vaginitis, urinary tract infections (UTIs), cystitis, and leukorrhea have been reported to occur in at least 2% of patients.

Nursing Implications: Assess baseline gynecologic status and history of UTIs and cystitis. Teach patient that these problems may occur and to report them. Teach patient symptomatic management and, if these are ineffective, discuss other strategies with physician.

Drug: raltitrexed (Tomudex, NSC-639186, ZD 1694, ICI-D1694) (investigational)

Class: Antimetabolite folate antagonist.

Mechanism of Action: Quinazoline-based folic acid analogue that acts as a folic acid antagonist; by selectively inhibiting the enzyme thymidylate synthase, it blocks purine synthesis. This causes breaks in DNA strands, and thus, DNA, RNA, and protein synthesis cannot proceed and the cell dies.

Metabolism: Drug has triphasic kinetics when administered intravenously over 15 minutes. The drug is rapidly distributed into tissue, with peak plasma levels occurring during or immediately after drug infusion. Cells actively take up drug, which is metabolized intracellularly into polyglutamates (more potent inhibitors of thymidylate synthase than parent drug). Polyglutamates have a long half-life in the cell, simulating continuous infusion therapy, with a terminal elimination half-life 8.2–105^{+} hours. Except for cellular metabolism, drug is excreted unchanged in the urine and is actively excreted by the renal tubules.

Dosage/Range:
- Per protocol.
- Colorectal cancer: 3 mg/m^2 IV q3 weeks.

Drug Preparation:
- Available in 2-mg vials, which should be protected from light, and refrigerated at 2–8°C (36–46°F).
- Reconstitute with 4 mL sterile water for injection, producing a concentration of 0.5 mg/mL.
- Withdraw dose, and further dilute in 50–250 mL 0.9% Normal Saline or 5% Dextrose.
- Reconstituted and diluted solutions are stable refrigerated for 24 hours.

Drug Administration:
- IV infusion over 15 minutes.
- Hold if urine creatinine clearance is $<$ 25 mL/min.
- Contraindicated in patients with uncontrolled diarrhea, or hypersensitivity.

Drug Interactions:
- Potential interaction with other drugs that compete for excretion in the renal tubules: penicillin, indomethacin, methotrexate (Taylor, 2000).
- Folate, folic acid: Interferes, decreases cytotoxicity.

Lab Effects/Interference:
- Decreased WBC, neutrophil count, platelet count, Hgb/HCT.
- Increased bili and/or alk phos, liver transaminases (ALT, AST).

Special Considerations:
- Has been used for a long time in Europe; is being studied in the United States in the following tumor types: colorectal, with and without 5-FU/leucovorin and/or irinotecan, oxaliplatin; breast; NSCLC; ovary; pancreas.
- Some U.S. clinical studies in colorectal cancer have shown conflicting results and higher mortality, possibly because dose was not adjusted in renal dysfunction.
- Use cautiously, and monitor closely patients who have previously been heavily pretreated with chemotherapy or radiotherapy, especially if persistent stomatitis, bone marrow depression, hepatic or renal dysfunction; pa-

tients with history of gastrointestinal problems (e.g., diarrhea); and patients with hepatic or renal dysfunction.

- Patients should NOT take folate or folate-containing vitamins during therapy, as this interferes with cytotoxicity of drug.
- Drug should not be used during pregnancy or by breast-feeding mothers.
- Dose reduce for myelosuppression, gastrointestinal toxicity, renal dysfunction per protocol; reduced dose should be given only when toxicity resolved.
- Allergic responses (e.g., stridor and wheezing) following first dose are rare, but have been reported.

Potential Toxicities/Side Effects and the Nursing Process

I. POTENTIAL FOR INFECTION, BLEEDING, AND FATIGUE related to BONE MARROW DEPRESSION

Defining Characteristics: Bone marrow depression is one of dose-limiting toxicity. 60% incidence of leukopenia, and severe in 10–22% of patients. Nadir is day 8, but may be delayed to day 21; recovery begins day 10. Thrombocytopenia is less common, occurring in 25% of patients, and is severe in 2%.

Nursing Implications: Assess baseline WBC, differential, platelet and Hgb/HCT prior to chemotherapy, as well as for signs/symptoms of infection or bleeding. Teach patient signs/symptoms of infection and bleeding and to report these immediately; teach patient self-care measures to minimize risk of infection and bleeding. This includes avoidance of crowds, proximity to people with infections, and OTC aspirin-containing medications. Teach patient to report fatigue and teach measures to conserve energy, such as alternating rest and activity periods. Discuss transfusion of red blood cells as needed. Consult protocol for dose reductions if patient has severe bone marrow suppression, renal dysfunction, or severe hepatic dysfunction.

II. ALTERATION IN NUTRITION, LESS THAN BODY REQUIREMENTS, related to DIARRHEA, NAUSEA, VOMITING, STOMATITIS

Defining Characteristics: Diarrhea may be dose-limiting in some studies. Incidence is 11–26%, and drug is contraindicated in patients with uncontrollable diarrhea. Nausea and vomiting are mild to moderate if they occur, with an incidence of 11–19%, and are preventable with antiemetics. Stomatitis may occur, and in some studies had an incidence of 48%. Rarely, patients may experience anorexia or constipation (1–10% incidence).

Nursing Implications: Teach patient that these side-effects may occur and to report them. Assess baseline weight and nutritional status, bowel elimination pattern, and oral mucosal integrity, and monitor before each treatment and throughout treatment. Administer premedication to prevent nausea/vomiting. Teach patient to self-administer antiemetics at home, and to report unrelieved or persistent nausea/vomiting. Teach patient to notify provider if diarrhea occurs, to take OTC antidiarrheal medications if diarrhea develops, and to call nurse/physician if diarrhea persists or recurs. Teach patient self-care of oral mucosa, including assessment, when to notify provider, and oral hygiene regimen. Refer to protocol for dose reductions for gastrointestinal toxicity.

III. ALTERATION IN ACTIVITY related to ASTHENIA, FATIGUE

Defining Characteristics: Asthenia is very common, and may be severe. Appears to be dose-related. Anemia is very common, affecting up to 70% of patients.

Nursing Implications: Assess baseline activity tolerance, and level of fatigue. Teach patient that these side-effects may occur and to report them. Teach patient to alternate rest and activity periods. Teach fatigue self-care measures, such as strategies to maximize energy use and conservation while shopping, interacting with friends, and other activities.

IV. POTENTIAL FOR ALTERATION IN COMFORT related to FEVER, RASH, PAIN

Defining Characteristics: Fever occurs in 20% of patients, usually 1–3 days after drug administration. Rash may occur (35% incidence), is papular and pruritic, and commonly affects head and upper trunk. Alopecia and cellulitis have been reported rarely (1–10%). Pain may occur.

Nursing Implications: Assess baseline skin texture, presence of rashes, general comfort level, and also, whether patient commonly has fevers. Teach patient to report fever, pain, or rash. Teach patient to take acetaminophen or other agent to relieve fever or pain. Teach patient to use skin emollient or cream if rash appears to reduce itching. If itching and/or rash persist or are severe, discuss further management with physician.

Drug: rebeccamycin analogue (NSC 655649) (investigational)

Class: Antitumor antibiotic.

Mechanism of Action: Rebeccamycin is isolated from an actinomycete strain, but is not water soluble. It causes breaks in DNA. Its analogue, NSC 655649, has a tartrate salt (glycosyl-dichloro-indolecarbazole) that is water soluble and that appears to bind to or intercalate into the base pairs of DNA. It causes unwinding of the supercoiled DNA double helix. It also inhibits topoisomerase II.

Metabolism: Long terminal half-life of drug, and large volume of distribution, leading to marked bone marrow suppression. Appears to be exclusively metabolized in the liver and excreted in the bile. Five-day treatment provides therapeutic plasma concentrations for 7–8 days versus 2–3 days with one-day treatment q 21 days.

Dosage/Range:

- Per protocol, in studies, given as a 30–60 minute IV infusion q 21 days at MTD of 500 mg/m^2 (heavily pretreated patients) or 572 mg/m^2 (minimal pretreatment), or IV qd × 5, repeated q 21 days at 141 mg/m^2/d (heavily pretreated) or 165 mg/m^2/d (minimal pretreatment).

Drug Preparation/Administration:

- Drug available from NCI in 20 mL vials containing 10 mg/mL with one equivalent (2.24 mg/mL) of l-tartaric acid in sterile water for injection. Desired drug dose is further diluted in 0.9% Normal Saline and infused over 1 hour via a central line.

Drug Interactions:

- Unknown.

Lab Effects/Interference:

- Transient elevation of hepatic transaminases peaking on day 8 or 15 of each cycle.

Special Considerations:

- Bone marrow suppression is dose-limiting toxicity (Dowlati et al, 2001).
- Phlebitis related to dose necessitates use of central venous catheter for MTD infusions.
- One patient developed acute myeloid leukemia 13 months after completing therapy (described with topoisomerase II inhibitor therapy).
- Appears marked activity in hepatobiliary cancers in chemotherapy-naïve patients (2 PRs, 2 minor responses, and 6 prolonged (> 6 month); stable disease in 3 patients with gallbladder cancer and 1 patient cholangiocarcinoma.

Potential Toxicities/Side Effects and the Nursing Process

I. POTENTIAL FOR INFECTION, BLEEDING, FATIGUE related to NEUTROPENIA, THROMBOCYTOPENIA, ANEMIA

Defining Characteristics: Neutropenia and thrombocytopenia may occur at MTD. Anemia is uncommon but may occur at highest dose level. Many patients required dose delays due to neutropenia, but neutropenic fever is rare.

Nursing Implications: Evaluate WBC, ANC, platelet count, hemoglobin/hematocrit baseline and monitor regularly during therapy per protocol. Discuss abnormalities with physician prior to drug administration. Assess for signs/symptoms of infection or bleeding, and teach patient to notify nurse or physician if they arise. Teach patient self-care measures to minimize risk of infection and bleeding, including avoidance of OTC aspirin-containing medications. Assess patient Hgb/Hct and signs/symptoms of fatigue. Teach patient self-assessment and energy conservation strategies, such as alternating rest and activity periods.

II. ALTERATION IN NUTRITION, LESS THAN BODY REQUIREMENTS related to NAUSEA, VOMITING, MUCOSITIS, AND TRANSIENT INCREASED TRANSAMINASES

Defining Characteristics: Nausea and vomiting is mild and easily prevented by serotonin antagonists. Mild stomatitis may occur. Hepatic transaminases often increase, usually between days 8–15 of each cycle.

Nursing Implications: Assess nutritional status and weight baseline and monitor regularly at each visit. Premedicate with antiemetic prior to each treatment. Assess efficacy of plan, and revise as needed. Assess oral mucosa and dentition baseline and prior to each treatment. Teach patient systematic oral hygiene, self-assessment, and to report development of stomatitis. Teach patient dietary modifications if following symptoms develop: nausea, vomiting, stomatitis, and weight loss. Assess LFTs baseline and prior to each treatment per protocol. Discuss elevated transaminases with physician.

Drug: rubitecan (9-Nitro-20(S)-Camptothecin, 9NC, RFS 2000) (investigational)

Class: Topoisomerase I inhibitor.

Mechanism of Action: Induces protein-linked DNA single-strand breaks and blocks DNA and RNA synthesis in dividing cells, thus preventing cells from entering mitosis. Prevents repair (religation) of previous, reversible single-strand breaks in DNA by binding to topoisomerase I. Topoisomerase I is an enzyme that relaxes tension in the DNA helix torsion by initially causing this single-strand break in DNA so that DNA replication can occur. Topoisomerases I and II then work together to bring about replication, transcription, and recombination of DNA material. Topoisomerase I is found in higher-than-normal concentrations in certain malignant cells, such as colon adenocarcinoma cells and non-Hodgkin's lymphoma cells.

Metabolism: Drug is well absorbed after oral administration, with maximal serum levels in 2–4 hours after the first dose, and is converted to 9-aminocamptothecin and other metabolites. Drug is water insoluble, unlike other topoisomerase inhibitors (e.g., irinotecan, topotecan), which are water soluble.

Drug is metabolized in the liver, and slowly excreted in the urine, with a terminal half-life of 10.6 hours.

Dosage/Range:
- Studies in solid tumors: 1.5 $mg/m^2/d$ PO on days 1–5, with no therapy on days 6–7, repeated q week.
- Studies in hematologic malignancies: 2 $mg/m^2/d$ on days 1–5, with no therapy on days 6–7, repeated q week.

Drug Preparation:
- Per protocol.

Drug Administration:
- Oral, available in 1.25-mg and 0.5-mg capsules.

Drug Interactions:
- Unknown.

Lab Effects/Interference:
- Unknown.

Special Considerations:
- Drug is a radiosensitizer.
- Being studied in the following cancers: pancreatic (phase III), myelodysplastic syndrome (phase II), refractory ovarian (phase II), advanced colorectal (phase II), metastatic melanoma (phase II), previously treated NSCLC (phase II), sarcoma (phase II), relapsed metastatic breast cancer (phase II), refractory prostate cancer (phase II), recurrent glioma (phase II), chronic phase CML (phase II), refractory/relapsed AML (phase II), refractory lymphoma (phase II).
- Patients should drink 3 L of fluid daily to prevent hemorrhagic cystitis.
- Drug is contraindicated in patients with hypersensitivity to the drug, or to 9-amino-camptothecin.

Potential Toxicities/Side Effects and the Nursing Process

I. POTENTIAL FOR INFECTION, BLEEDING, AND FATIGUE related to BONE MARROW DEPRESSION

Defining Characteristics: Bone marrow depression is the dose-limiting toxicity. 30% of patients in pancreatic clinical trials experienced neutropenia, 11% severe (grades 3/4). Thrombocytopenia in these studies affected 35%, with 21% graded severe (grades 3/4). Finally, anemia was common, with an incidence of 53%, with 16% severe (grades 3/4).

Nursing Implications: Assess baseline WBC, differential, platelet, and Hgb/HCT prior to chemotherapy as well as for signs/symptoms of infection or bleeding. Teach patient signs/symptoms of infection and bleeding and to report these immediately; teach patient self-care measures to minimize risk of infection and bleeding. This includes avoidance of crowds, proximity to people with infections, and OTC aspirin-containing medications. Teach patient to report fatigue and teach measures to conserve energy, such as alternating rest and activity periods. Discuss transfusion of red blood cells as needed.

II. ALTERATION IN NUTRITION, LESS THAN BODY REQUIREMENTS, related to NAUSEA, VOMITING, AND DIARRHEA

Defining Characteristics: Nausea and vomiting are common, but preventable with antiemetics. Incidence in pancreatic studies was 50%, with only 5% having severe (grades 3/4). The incidence of diarrhea in these studies was 28%, with 5% severe (grades 3/4).

Nursing Implications: Teach patient that these side-effects may occur and to report them. Teach patients to take ordered antiemetic medications one hour prior to their dose, and to notify provider right away if nausea and/or vomiting persist, or if unable to drink/keep down fluids. Teach patient to take antidiarrheal medications if diarrhea develops, and to notify provider if diarrhea persists or recurs.

III. POTENTIAL FOR ALTERATION IN COMFORT related to FEVER

Defining Characteristics: In the pancreatic studies, 13% of patients reported fever.

Nursing Implications: Teach patient to report fever. Teach patient to take acetaminophen or other agent to relieve fever if it occurs.

IV. ALTERATION IN URINE ELIMINATION, related to CYSTITIS

Defining Characteristics: Interstitial cystitis may occur and be hemorrhagic; in clinical studies, cystoscopy revealed punctate mucosal ulcerations. Histopathologic exam revealed interstitial cystitis, coagulative mucosal necrosis, and little inflammatory infiltrate (Natelson et al, 1996). This is preventable by maintaining hydration. Incidence in patients described in pancreatic studies was 3%.

Nursing Implications: Teach patient that it is imperative to drink 3 L of fluid a day, and to avoid alcoholic beverages, as they may cause diuresis. Teach patient that if nausea and/or vomiting develop, and unable to drink this amount, to notify provider immediately.

Drug: streptozocin (Zanosar)

Class: Alkylating agent (nitrosourea).

Mechanism of Action: A weak alkylating agent (nitrosourea) that causes interstrand cross-linking in DNA and is cell cycle phase nonspecific. Appears to have some specificity for neoplastic pancreatic endocrine cells. Glucose attached to nitrosourea appears to diminish myelotoxicity.

Metabolism: 60–70% of total dose and 10–20% of parent drug appear in urine. Drug is rapidly eliminated from serum in 4 hours, with major concentrations occurring in liver and kidneys.

Dosage/Range:
- 500 mg/m^2 IV qd × 5 days. Repeat every 3–4 weeks; OR
- 1500 mg/m^2 IV every week.

Drug Preparation:
- Add sterile water or 0.9% Sodium Chloride to vial.
- If powder or solution contacts skin, wash immediately with soap and water.
- Solution is stable 48 hours at room temperature, 96 hours if refrigerated.

Drug Administration:
- Administer via pump over 1 hour.
- Has also been given as continuous infusion or continuous arterial infusion into the hepatic artery.
- If local pain or burning occurs, slow infusion and apply cool packs above injection site.
- Irritant; avoid extravasation.
- Administer with 1–2 L of hydration to prevent nephrotoxicity.

Drug Interactions:
- Nephrotoxic drugs: additive nephrotoxicity; avoid concurrent use.

Lab Effects/Interference:
- Decreased CBC.
- Increased RFTs (especially BUN).
- Increased LFTs.
- Changes in glucose, phosphorus.

Special Considerations:
- Renal function must be monitored closely.
- Drug is an irritant; give through the sidearm of a running IV over 15 minutes to 6 hours.

Potential Toxicities/Side Effects and the Nursing Process

I. POTENTIAL FOR ALTERATION IN URINARY ELIMINATION related to RENAL DYSFUNCTION

Defining Characteristics: 60% of patients experience renal dysfunction. Usually transient proteinuria and azotemia, but this may progress to permanent renal failure, especially if other nephrotoxic drugs are given concurrently. Signs/symptoms include proteinuria, increased BUN, hypophosphatemia, glycosuria, renal tubular acidosis, decreased creatinine clearance. Hypophosphatemia is probably earliest sign of renal dysfunction.

Nursing Implications: Closely monitor BUN, creatinine, phosphorus, urine protein, and 24-hour creatinine clearance prior to each treatment. Monitor BUN, creatinine, pH of urine, glucose/protein of urine every shift during therapy. If creatinine clearance is < 25 mL/min, dose should be reduced by 50–75%. Strictly monitor I/O during therapy. Hydration per physician, but usually 2–3 L/day.

II. ALTERATION IN NUTRITION, LESS THAN BODY REQUIREMENTS, related to GI SIDE EFFECTS

Defining Characteristics: Nausea and vomiting occur in up to 90% of patients, beginning 1–4 hours after drug dose, and can be significantly reduced when drug is given as continuous infusion. Nausea and vomiting may worsen during 5-consecutive-day therapy; increased severity with doses > 500 mg/m^2. 10% of patients experience diarrhea with abdominal cramping. LFTs may be elevated but normalize with time. Hepatotoxicity occurs in ~50% of patients. Liver enzymes increase 2–3 weeks after therapy. Albumin decreases. Symptoms rarely occur. Painless jaundice.

Nursing Implications: Premedicate with antiemetics and continue prophylactically for 24 hours; use aggressive antiemetics when drug is given IV over 1 hour (serotonin antagonists effective). Encourage small, frequent feedings of cool, bland foods and liquids. If patient has emesis > 250 mL or vomiting > 2 times in 8 hours, discuss with physician more aggressive antiemetics. Monitor I/O closely and replace fluids. Encourage patient to report onset of diarrhea. Administer or teach patient to self-administer antidiarrheal medications. Teach patient diet modifications. Monitor LFTs prior to each treatment (alk phos, SGOT, SGPT, albumin). Assess for signs/symptoms of hepatic dysfunction: jaundice, yellowing of skin, sclera; orange-colored urine; white or clay-colored stools; itchy skin.

III. ALTERATIONS IN GLUCOSE METABOLISM related to HYPOGLYCEMIA

Defining Characteristics: Appears that damage to pancreatic beta cells causes sudden release of insulin, with resulting hypoglycemia in about 20% of patients. Hyperglycemia may occur in patients with insulinomas and decreased glucose tolerance. Increased fasting or postprandial blood levels may occur.

Nursing Implications: Monitor serum glucose levels every day or more frequently as needed; check urine glucose. Assess for, and instruct patient to report, the following signs/symptoms of hypoglycemia: muscle weakness and lethargy, perspiration, flushed feeling, restlessness, headache, confusion, trembling, epigastric hunger pains. If signs/symptoms are found, encourage patient to eat or drink high-glucose food and juice and notify physician. Hypoglycemia can be prevented with nicotinamide. Assess for signs/symptoms of hyperglycemia in patient with insulinomas and instruct patient in self-assessment.

IV. POTENTIAL FOR INFECTION AND BLEEDING related to BONE MARROW DEPRESSION

Defining Characteristics: Bone marrow depression occurs in about 9–20% of patients. Nadir 1–2 weeks after administration. Occasionally, severe leukopenia and thrombocytopenia occur. Mild anemia may occur.

Nursing Implications: Monitor CBC, platelets prior to drug administration, as well as assess for signs/symptoms of infection or bleeding. Instruct patient in self-assessment of signs/symptoms of infection or bleeding.

V. POTENTIAL FOR INJURY related to SECONDARY MALIGNANCIES

Defining Characteristics: Drug is carcinogenic; secondary malignancies are well described.

Nursing Implications: Patients receiving prolonged therapy should be screened periodically.

Drug: tamoxifen citrate (Nolvadex)

Class: Antiestrogen.

Mechanism of Action: Nonsteroidal antiestrogen that binds to estrogen receptors, forming an abnormal complex that migrates to the cell nucleus and inhibits DNA synthesis.

Metabolism: Well absorbed from GI tract and metabolized by liver. Undergoes enterohepatic circulation, prolonging blood levels. Excreted in feces. Elimination half-life is 7 days.

Dosage/Range:
- 20–80 mg PO daily (most often, 10 mg bid).

Drug Preparation:
- Available in 10-mg tablets.

Drug Administration:
- Oral.

Drug Interactions:
- Anticoagulants: increased PT; monitor PT closely and reduce anticoagulant dose.

Lab Effects/Interference:
- Decreased CBC.
- Increased LFTs.
- Increased Ca.
- Interference in lab tests such as TFTs and hyperlipidemia.

Special Considerations:
- Measurement of estrogen receptors in tumor may be important in predicting tumor response and should be performed at same time as biopsy and before antiestrogen treatment is started.
- Avoid antacids within 2 hours of taking enteric-coated tablets.
- A flare reaction with bony pain and hypercalcemia may occur. Such reactions are short-lived and usually result in a tumor response if therapy is continued.
- No evidence exists that doses > 20 mg/day are more efficacious.
- FDA-approved to reduce the incidence of breast cancer in high-risk women.
- FDA-indicated also for reducing the risk of contralateral breast cancer.
- FDA-approved for use to reduce the risk of invasive breast cancer in women with ductal carcinoma.
- Tamoxifen resulted in a significant decrease in development of invasive breast cancer in woman with atypical hyperplasia (88%).
- Rare side effects include uterine sarcoma, stroke, uterine cancer, blood clot formation.
- Tamoxifen is being studied as an adjunct to in vitro fertilization (IVF) for women with breast cancer who wish to have a child, given with FSH. The addition of either tamoxifen or letrozole with FSH increased the number of ovarian follicles, more mature eggs, and more embryos (Oktay et al, 2005).

Potential Toxicities/Side Effects and the Nursing Process

I. POTENTIAL FOR SEXUAL DYSFUNCTION related to CHANGES IN MENSES, HOT FLASHES

Defining Characteristics: May cause menstrual irregularity, hot flashes, milk production in breasts, vaginal discharge, and bleeding. Symptoms occur in about 10% of patients and are usually not severe enough to discontinue therapy.

Nursing Implications: As appropriate, explore with patient and partner issues of reproductive and sexuality patterns and the impact drug may have on them. Discuss strategies to preserve sexual and reproductive health.

II. POTENTIAL FOR ALTERATION IN COMFORT related to FLARE REACTION

Defining Characteristics: May cause flare reaction initially (bone and tumor pain, transient increase in tumor size). Nausea, vomiting, and anorexia may occur.

Nursing Implications: Inform patient of possibility of flare reaction, signs/symptoms to be aware of, and encourage patient to report any signs/symptoms. Inform patient of possibility of nausea, vomiting, and anorexia. Encourage small, frequent meals of high-calorie, high-protein foods.

III. POTENTIAL FOR SENSORY/PERCEPTUAL ALTERATION related to VISUAL CHANGES

Defining Characteristics: Retinopathy has been reported with high doses. Corneal changes (infrequent), decreased visual acuity, and blurred vision have occurred. Headache, dizziness, and light-headedness are rare.

Nursing Implications: Obtain visual assessment prior to starting therapy. Encourage patient to report any visual changes. Instruct patient to report headache, dizziness, light-headedness.

IV. POTENTIAL FOR INFECTION AND BLEEDING related to BONE MARROW DEPRESSION

Defining Characteristics: Mild, transient leukopenia and thrombocytopenia occur rarely.

Nursing Implications: Monitor CBC, platelets prior to drug administration and after therapy has begun. Instruct patient in self-assessment of signs/symptoms of infection or bleeding.

V. POTENTIAL FOR SKIN INTEGRITY IMPAIRMENT related to RASH, ALOPECIA

Defining Characteristics: Skin rash, alopecia, peripheral edema are rare.

Nursing Implications: Assess patient for signs/symptoms of hair loss, edema, and skin rash. Instruct patient to report any of these symptoms. Discuss with patient the impact of skin changes.

VI. POTENTIAL FOR INJURY related to HYPERCALCEMIA

Defining Characteristics: Hypercalcemia uncommon.

Nursing Implications: Obtain serum calcium levels prior to therapy and at regular intervals during therapy. Instruct patient in signs/symptoms of hypercalcemia: nausea, vomiting, weakness, constipation, loss of muscle tone, malaise, decreased urine output.

Drug: temozolamide (Temodar®)

Class: Alkylating agent.

Mechanism of Action: Drug is a member of the imidazotetrazine class and related to dacarbazine. Drug is a pro-drug, forming the metabolite monomethyl triazenoimidazole carboxamide (MTIC) when chemically degraded, and is further metabolized to 5-aminoimidazole-4-carboxamide (AIC), the active cytotoxic metabolite. Drug can pass through the BBB, where it has been shown to be effective against some brain tumors, possibly because of the alkyline pH. MTIC causes alkylation of DNA and RNA strands.

Metabolism: Well absorbed from the GI tract following oral dose (100% bioavailability), with peak concentrations in 1 hour when taken on empty stomach. The elimination half-life is 1.8 hours. The drug is degraded into MTIC in plasma and tissues. 15% of drug is excreted unchanged in the urine. Differs from dacarbazine in that formation of MTIC does not require liver metabolism. Food decreases the rate and extent of drug absorption.

Dosage/Range:

Refractory anaplastic astrocytoma that has failed prior chemotherapy:

- 150 mg/m^2/day × 5 days if patient has received prior chemotherapy, repeated q28 days.
- Dose should be adjusted to keep ANC 1000–1500/mm^3 and platelet count 50,000–100,000/mm^3.

Newly diagnosed glioblastoma multiforme (GBM) concomitantly with (at the same time as) radiotherapy and then as maintenance treatment.

- 75 mg/m^2 qd starting the first day of RT through the last day of RT, for 42 days (maximum 49 days) as long as ANC > 1500 cells/mm^3, platelet count > 100,000 cells/mm^3, and other toxicity (except alopecia, nausea, vomiting) are less than grade 1 (CTC),
- Prophylaxis for Pneumocystis carinii pneumonia while receiving concomitant RT and temozolamide, then 4 weeks after completion of RT.
- Maintenance dose (temozolamide PO qd × 5, then 23 days without treatment, repeated × 6):
- Cycle 1: Temozolamide 150 mg/m^2 PO qd × 5, then 23 days without treatment (as long as ANC > 1500 cells/mm^3, platelet count >100,000 cells/mm^3, and other toxicity (except alopecia, nausea, vomiting) are less than grade 1 (CTC),
- Cycle 2-6: Temozolamide 200 mg/m^2 PO qd × 5 then 23 days without treatment, repeated for 5 more cycles (as long as ANC > 1500 cells/mm^3, platelet count > 100,000 cells/mm^3, and other toxicity (except alopecia, nausea, vomiting) are <, grade 1 (CTC),
- Monitor CDC on day 22 then weekly until ANC > 1500 cells/mm^3, and platelets > 100,000 cells/mm^3; see package insert for dose reductions based on nadir counts and worst CTC toxicity.

Drug Preparation:
- None.
- Available in 250-mg, 100-mg, 20-mg, and 5-mg strengths.
- Drug is stored at room temperature, protected from light and moisture.

Drug Administration:
- Give orally with full glass of water on an empty stomach. Patient should take medicine at around the same time of day each day, e.g., bedtime.
- Do not crush or dissolve capsule.

Drug Interactions:
- Valproic acid: reduces temozolomide clearance by 5% but may not be clinically significant; monitor drug effect closely if used together.

Lab Effects/Interference:
- Elevated liver function tests (e.g., ALT, AST; occur in up to 40% of patients), increase in alk phos; decreased WBC, Hgb and platelet count; hyperglycemia; elevated renal function tests.

Special Considerations:
- Drug is indicated for the treatment of adults with 1) refractory anaplastic astrocytoma who have experienced disease progression on a nitrosurea and procarbazine (after first relapse), and 2) with newly diagnosed glioblastoma multiforme (GBM) concomitantly with (at the same time as) radiotherapy and then as maintenance treatment.

- Drug has also been used for treatment of glioma after first relapse and advanced metastatic malignant melanoma, and is being studied in a variety of solid tumors.
- Drug causes severe myelosuppression, and thrombocytopenia is the dose-limiting factor.
- Active in high-grade malignant glioma (gioblalstoma multiforme, anaplastic astrocytoma) and metastatic melanoma.
- Use with caution, if at all, in the following patients: hypersensitive to dacarbazine; myelosuppressed; have bacterial or viral infection; have renal dysfunction; have received prior chemotherapy or radiation; and women who are pregnant or who are breast-feeding.
- Rarely (1% of patients), hypercalcemia may occur with the 5-day regimen.
- PET (positive emission tomography) scanning showed reduced uptake of fluorodeoxyglucose (FDG) in patients who responded, in 7–14 days following a 5-day course of treatment, as opposed to those patients who did not respond, and who showed increased FDG uptake (Newlands et al, 1997).
- Overall response rate in some studies of patients with malignant glioma that had recurred or progressed after surgery and radiation therapy was 15–25% and 30% in newly diagnosed patients prior to XRT (Bower et al, 1997).

Potential Toxicities/Side Effects and the Nursing Process

I. POTENTIAL FOR INFECTION, BLEEDING, AND FATIGUE related to BONE MARROW DEPRESSION

Defining Characteristics: Thrombocytopenia and leukopenia are dose-limiting factors and occur in grade 2 or higher 40% of the time. This does not usually require administration of G-CSF. Nadir at 21–22 days, unless using 5-day treatment schedule, where nadir is day 28–29. Recovery for platelets is 7–42 days and in shorter time for WBC. Anemia may also occur, but is infrequent and less severe. Severity of bone marrow depression depends on dose and schedule, as well as disease process. In one trial, patients with malignant glioma had severe lymphopenia (41% grade 3 and 15% grade 4).

Nursing Implications: Assess baseline WBC, differential, platelet and Hgb/HCT prior to chemotherapy, as well as for signs/symptoms of infection or bleeding. Teach patient signs/symptoms of infection and bleeding and to report these immediately; teach patient self-care measures to minimize risk of infection and bleeding. This includes avoidance of crowds, proximity to people with infections, and OTC aspirin-containing medications. Teach patient to report fatigue and teach measures to conserve energy, such as alternating rest and activity periods. Discuss transfusion of red blood cells as needed.

II. ALTERED NUTRITION, LESS THAN BODY REQUIREMENTS, related to NAUSEA AND VOMITING, STOMATITIS, AND DIARRHEA

Defining Characteristics: Nausea and vomiting occur in 75% of patients, usually grade 1 or 2, and usually occurring on day 1. In one trial, using a 5-day treatment regimen, 21% had grade 3 nausea, and 23% had grade 4. Stomatitis may occur in up to 20% of patients. Diarrhea, constipation, and/or anorexia may affect up to 40% of patients.

Nursing Implications: Teach patient to self-medicate with antiemetics (serotonin antagonist effective) one hour prior to dose and suggest evening dosing to minimize nausea/vomiting. Encourage small, frequent feedings of cool, bland foods. Teach patient to notify provider right away if nausea/vomiting persists. Assess oral mucosa prior to drug administration and teach patient to report changes. Teach patient oral hygiene measures and self-assessment. Teach patient to report diarrhea, to self-administer prescribed antidiarrheal medications, and to drink adequate fluids. Teach patient to report constipation, and manage with stool softeners or laxatives. If patient has anorexia, teach patient to select acceptable foods and to eat small portions q2 hours and at bedtime.

III. ALTERATION IN SKIN INTEGRITY/COMFORT related to RASH, PRURITUS, ALOPECIA

Defining Characteristics: Skin rash, itching, and mild alopecia may occur, and are mild.

Nursing Implications: Teach patient about the possibility of these side effects and to notify the nurse if any develop. Discuss rash with physician if moderate or severe. Teach patient local symptom-management strategies for itch. Reassure patient that hair loss is usually thinning with mild hair loss and will grow back.

IV. ACTIVITY INTOLERANCE POTENTIAL, related to CENTRAL NERVOUS SYSTEM EFFECTS

Defining Characteristics: Lethargy (up to 40% in patients with malignant glioma), fatigue, headache, ataxia, and dizziness may occur, and in clinical testing, it was unclear whether this was due to neurological disease (i.e., malignant glioma), concurrent other drug therapy, or temozolomide.

Nursing Implications: Assess baseline energy and activity level. Teach patients that these side effects may occur, especially if the primary diagnosis is malignant glioma. Teach patient to report them. Teach patient to alternate rest and activity periods, to use supportive device such as a cane if ataxia or dizziness occurs, and other measures to maximize activity tolerance and to prevent injury.

Drug: teniposide (Vumon, VM-26)

Class: Plant alkaloid, a derivative of the mandrake plant (*Mandragora officinarum*).

Mechanism of Action: Cell cycle specific in late S phase, early G_2 phase, causing arrest of cell division in mitosis. Inhibits uptake of thymidine into DNA so DNA synthesis is impaired.

Metabolism: Drug binds extensively to serum protein. Metabolized by the liver and excreted in bile and urine.

Dosage/Range:
- 100 mg/m^2 weekly for 6–8 weeks.
- 50 mg/m^2 twice weekly × 4 weeks.

Drug Preparation:
- Available in 50-mg/5-mL glass ampules.
- Add desired 0.9% Sodium Chloride for injection or 5% Dextrose in water to reach final concentration of 0.1 mg/mL–0.4 mg/mL (stable 24 hours) or 1.0 mg/mL (stable 4 hours).
- USE ONLY non-DEHP containers such as glass or polyolefin plastic bags or containers.
- DO NOT USE polyvinylchloride IV bags, as the plasticizer DEHP will leach into the solution.

Drug Administration:
- Assess for presence of precipitate and do not administer solution if precipitate is seen.
- Administer over at least 30–60 minutes.

Drug Interactions:
- Doses of tolbutamide, sodium salicylate, and sulfamethizole will need to be reduced.
- Heparin causes a precipitate.

Lab Effects/Interference:
- Increased LFTs, RFTs.
- Decreased CBC.

Special Considerations:
- Rapid infusion may cause hypotension and sudden death.
- Chemical phlebitis may occur if drug is not properly diluted, or infused too rapidly.

- Severe myelosuppression may occur.
- Hypersensitivity reactions, including anaphylaxis-like symptoms, may occur with initial or repeated doses.

Potential Toxicities/Side Effects and the Nursing Process

I. POTENTIAL FOR INJURY DURING DRUG ADMINISTRATION related to HYPOTENSION AND HYPERSENSITIVITY REACTION

Defining Characteristics: Hypotension may occur during rapid IV infusion. Hypersensitivity reactions occur in 5% of patients, characterized by fever, chills, tachycardia, dyspnea, flushing, lumbar pain, bronchospasm, and progressive hypotension or hypertension. It is thought that hypersensitivity may be to the drug suspension of castor oil and denatured alcohol, which is used because the drug is poorly water-soluble.

Nursing Implications: Assess baseline temperature (T), VS prior to drug administration, and periodically during infusion. Ensure that drug is properly diluted, and infuse over at least 30–60 minutes. Instruct patient to report untoward signs/symptoms immediately. Have emergency equipment and medications, including epinephrine, diphenhydramine, hydrocortisone nearby. If signs/symptoms develop, stop infusion, keep IV line open, notify physician, monitor VS, and support patient. Be familiar with institution's standing orders or practice guidelines on management of anaphylaxis.

II. POTENTIAL FOR INFECTION AND BLEEDING related to BONE MARROW DEPRESSION

Defining Characteristics: Leukopenia is dose-limiting toxicity but thrombocytopenia may occur; nadir day 7 (3–14 days). Dose reductions need to be made if patient previously received chemotherapy or radiotherapy.

Nursing Implications: Assess CBC, WBC, differential, and platelet count prior to drug administration, as well as for signs/symptoms of infection and bleeding. Teach patient signs/symptoms of infection and bleeding, and instruct to report them immediately. Teach patient self-care measures to minimize infection and bleeding, including avoidance of OTC aspirin-containing medications.

III. ALTERATION IN NUTRITION, LESS THAN BODY REQUIREMENTS, related to NAUSEA AND VOMITING, HEPATIC DYSFUNCTION, MUCOSITIS

Defining Characteristics: Nausea and vomiting occur in 29% of patients but are usually mild; mucositis occurs at high drug doses. Mild elevation of LFTs may occur.

Nursing Implications: Premedicate with antiemetics prior to drug administration, and continue prophylactically for 24 hours, at least for the first cycle. Assess oral mucosa at baseline prior to drug administration; teach patient self-assessment and self-care measures. Monitor LFTs prior to drug administration; discuss dose reduction with physician if results abnormal.

IV. POTENTIAL FOR IMPAIRED SKIN INTEGRITY related to ALOPECIA AND PHLEBITIS

Defining Characteristics: Alopecia is uncommon (9–30% of patients) and is reversible. Phlebitis can occur if drug is improperly diluted or administered too rapidly.

Nursing Implications: If patient develops hair loss, discuss impact of loss and suggest coping strategies, such as wig or cap. Encourage patient to verbalize feelings and provide emotional support. Administer drug only through patent IV, properly diluted, and over at least 30–60 minutes.

V. POTENTIAL FOR SENSORY/PERCEPTUAL ALTERATIONS related to NEUROLOGIC TOXICITY

Defining Characteristics: Peripheral neuropathies may occur and are mild.

Nursing Implications: Assess baseline neurologic status. Teach patient to report any changes in motor or sensory functioning. Encourage patient to verbalize feelings regarding discomfort and sensory loss if these occur.

VI. POTENTIAL FOR ALTERATION IN CARDIAC OUTPUT related to HYPOTENSION AND PALPITATIONS

Defining Characteristics: Hypotension is related to rapid infusion of drug. Palpitations may occur during drug infusion.

Nursing Implications: Assess baseline cardiac status, noting heart rate, rhythm, and monitor heart rate and BP periodically during infusion. Infuse drug over at least 30–60 minutes.

VII. POTENTIAL SEXUAL DYSFUNCTION related to DRUG EFFECT

Defining Characteristics: Drug is carcinogenic, mutagenic, and teratogenic. It is not known if drug is excreted in breast milk.

Nursing Implications: Assess patient's and partner's sexual patterns and reproductive goals. Provide information, supportive counseling, and referral as needed and appropriate. Teach importance of contraception and discuss coping strategies for alterations in fertility (e.g., sperm banking). Mothers receiving drug should not breastfeed.

Drug: thioguanine (Tabloid, 6-Thioguanine, 6-TG)

Class: Thiopurine antimetabolite.

Mechanism of Action: Converts to monophosphate nucleotides and inhibits *de novo* purine synthesis. The nucleotides are also incorporated into DNA. Cell cycle phase specific for S phase. Thioguanine interferes with nucleic acid biosynthesis, resulting in sequential blockage of the synthesis and utilization of the purine nucleotides.

Metabolism: Absorption is incomplete and variable orally. Is metabolized in the liver by deamination and methylation. Metabolites are excreted in the urine and feces. Plasma half-life is 80–90 minutes.

Dosage/Range:
- Children and adults: 100 mg/m^2 PO q12h for 5–10 days, usually in combination with cytarabine.
- 100 mg/m^2 IV daily × 5 days (investigational).
- 1–3 mg/kg PO daily.

Drug Preparation:
- Available in 40-mg tablets.
- Dilute 75-mg vial with 5 mL 0.9% Sodium Chloride USP (15 mg/mL).
- Further dilute drug in 5% Dextrose or 0.9% Sodium Chloride (stable for 24 hours at room temperature or under refrigeration).

Drug Administration:
- Given orally between meals; can be given as a single dose.
- Given via IV bolus over 5–30 minutes (investigational).

Drug Interactions:
- Busulfan: increased hepatotoxicity; use caution when used together; monitor patient closely during long-term therapy.

Lab Effects/Interference:
- Decreased CBC.
- Increased LFTs.
- Increased uric acid.

Special Considerations:
- Oral dose is to be given on empty stomach to facilitate complete absorption.
- Dose is titrated to avoid excessive stomatitis and diarrhea.
- Thioguanine can be used in full doses with allopurinol.

Potential Toxicities/Side Effects and the Nursing Process

I. ALTERATION IN NUTRITION, LESS THAN BODY REQUIREMENTS, related to GI SIDE EFFECTS

Defining Characteristics: Nausea and vomiting occur commonly, especially in children, but are dose-related; anorexia is rare; stomatitis is rare, but most common with high doses; hepatotoxicity is rare, but may be associated with hepatic veno-occlusive disease or jaundice.

Nursing Implications: Treat symptomatically with antiemetics. Encourage small, frequent feedings of cool, bland foods and liquids. If vomiting occurs, assess for fluid and electrolyte imbalance. Monitor I/O and daily weights if patient is hospitalized. Encourage small, frequent meals of favorite foods, especially high-calorie, high-protein foods. Encourage use of spices; weekly weights. Teach oral assessment and oral hygiene regimen. Encourage patient to report early stomatitis. Provide pain relief measures, if indicated. Monitor LFTs prior to drug dose. Assess patient prior to and during treatment for signs/symptoms of hepatotoxicity.

II. POTENTIAL FOR INFECTION AND BLEEDING related to BONE MARROW DEPRESSION

Defining Characteristics: Bone marrow depression occurs 1–4 weeks after treatment. Leukopenia and thrombocytopenia are most common. Drug may have prolonged or delayed nadir.

Nursing Implications: Monitor CBC, platelet count prior to drug administration as well as for signs/symptoms of infection or bleeding. Instruct patient in self-assessment of signs/symptoms of infection or bleeding. Administer platelet, red cell transfusions per physician's order.

III. POTENTIAL FOR SENSORY/PERCEPTUAL ALTERATION related to LOSS OF VIBRATORY SENSE

Defining Characteristics: Loss of vibratory sensation; unsteady gait may occur.

Nursing Implications: Assess vibratory sensation, gait before each dose and between treatments. Report changes to physician. Encourage patient to report any changes.

Drug: thiotepa (Thioplex, Triethylenethiophosphoramide)

Class: Alkylating agent.

Mechanism of Action: Selectively reacts with DNA phosphate groups to produce chromosome cross-linkage with blocking of nucleoprotein synthesis. Acts as a polyfunctional alkylating agent. Cell cycle phase nonspecific agent. Mimics radiation-induced injury.

Metabolism: Rapidly cleared following IV administration; 60% of dose is eliminated in urine within 24–72 hours. Slow onset of action, slowly bound to tissues, extensively metabolized.

Dosage/Range:

Intravenous:
- 8 mg/m² (0.2 mg/kg) IV every day × 5 days, repeated every 3–4 weeks, OR
- 0.3–0.4 mg/kg IV, q 1–4 weeks.

Intracavitary:
- Bladder: 60 mg in 60 mL sterile water once a week for 3–4 weeks.

Drug Preparation:
- Add sterile water to vial of lyophilized powder.
- Further dilute with 0.9% Sodium Chloride or 5% Dextrose.
- Do not use solution unless it is clear.
- Refrigerate vial until use (reconstituted solution is stable for 5 days).

Drug Administration:
- IV, IM; intracavitary, intratumor, intraarterial.

Drug Interactions:
- Myelosuppressive drugs: additive hematologic toxicity.

Lab Effects/Interference:
- Decreased CBC (especially WBC and platelets).
- Increased LFTs and RFTs.

Special Considerations:
- Hypersensitivity reactions have occurred with this drug.
- Is an irritant; should be given IVP via a sidearm of a running IV.
- Increased neuromuscular blockage when given with nondepolarizing muscle relaxants.

Potential Toxicities/Side Effects and the Nursing Process

I. POTENTIAL FOR INFECTION AND BLEEDING related to BONE MARROW DEPRESSION

Defining Characteristics: Nadir is 5–30 days after drug administration. Thrombocytopenia and leukopenia may occur. Anemia may occur with prolonged use. May be cumulative toxicity with recovery of bone marrow in 40–50 days. Thrombocytopenia is dose-limiting.

Nursing Implications: Monitor CBC, platelet count prior to drug administration; monitor for signs/symptoms of infection or bleeding. Instruct patient in self-assessment of signs/symptoms of infection or bleeding and to report them immediately. Administer red cells and platelet transfusions per physician's orders.

II. ALTERATION IN NUTRITION, LESS THAN BODY REQUIREMENTS, related to GI SIDE EFFECTS

Defining Characteristics: Nausea and vomiting occur in 10–15% of patients; dose-dependent; occurs 6–12 hours after drug dose; anorexia occurs occasionally.

Nursing Implications: Premedicate with antiemetics especially with parenteral dosing of high dose. Continue antiemetics at least 12 hours after drug is given. Encourage small, frequent meals of cool, bland, dry foods, and favorite foods, especially high-calorie, high-protein foods. Encourage use of spices; assess weight weekly.

III. POTENTIAL SEXUAL DYSFUNCTION related to DRUG EFFECT

Defining Characteristics: Drug is mutagenic. Sterility may be reversible and incomplete. Amenorrhea often reverses in 6–8 months.

Nursing Implications: As appropriate, explore with patient and partner issues of reproductive and sexuality patterns and the anticipated impact chemotherapy may have. Discuss strategies to preserve sexuality and reproductive health (e.g., sperm banking).

IV. POTENTIAL FOR INJURY related to ALLERGIC REACTION

Defining Characteristics: Allergic responses occur rarely: hives, bronchospasm, skin rash (dermatitis). Secondary malignancies may occur with prolonged therapy.

Nursing Implications: Assess for signs/symptoms of allergic response during drug administration. Stop drug if bronchospasm occurs and notify physician. Discuss symptomatic treatment with physician. Instruct patient receiving prolonged therapy about importance of regular health maintenance examinations during and after therapy by primary care provider and oncologist.

V. ALTERATION IN COMFORT related to DIZZINESS, FEVER, PAIN

Defining Characteristics: Dizziness, headache, fever, and local pain may occur.

Nursing Implications: Assess for alterations in comfort. Treat symptomatically.

Drug: TLK 286 (Telcyta, investigational)

Class: Cell activated chemotherapeutic agent.

Mechanism of Action: Drug is a prodrug, and is activated when split into its two component parts—glutathione analogue and cytotoxic fragment, by the enzyme glutathione S-transferase P1-1(GST P1-1). This enzyme is overexpressed in many cancers, and confers a poor prognosis, and resistance to many chemo agents. The cytotoxic fragment then interacts with DNA, RNA and proteins to bring about cell death. The glutathione fragment may bind to GST P1-1 and reduce its ability to inactivate other chemotherapeutic agents, thus reducing drug resistance.

Metabolism: Unknown.

Dosage/Range:
Per protocol, phase II study 75 mg/m^2.

Drug Interactions: Unknown.

Lab Effects/Interference: Decreased neutrophil and platelet counts.

Special Considerations:

- Drug appears synergistic with platinums, taxanes, and anthracyclines.
- Drug is being studied in breast, ovarian, NSCLC, colorectal cancers.
- Drug has activity in patients with NSCLC resistant to cisplatin.

Potential Toxicities/Side Effects and the Nursing Process

I. INFECTION AND BLEEDING, POTENTIAL, related to BONE MARROW DEPRESSION

Defining Characteristics: Neutropenia is the dose-limiting toxicity. Grade 3 neutropenia occurred in 28% of NSCLC study patients, and grade 3 thrombocytopenia in 5%.

Nursing Implications: Monitor CBC and platelet count prior to drug administration as well as signs/symptoms of infection or bleeding. Instruct patient in self-assessment of signs/symptoms of infection or bleeding.

II. ALTERATION IN NUTRITION, LESS THAN BODY REQUIREMENTS, related to NAUSEA AND VOMITING,

Defining Characteristics: Nausea and vomiting in patients with NSCLC who received drug with cisplatin.

Nursing Implications: Premedicate with anti-emetics per protocol, and teach patient self-administration of anti-emetics at home if needed. Encourage small, frequent feedings of cool, bland, dry foods. Assess for symptoms of fluid and electrolyte imbalance: monitor I/O and daily weights if administered to an inpatient.. Ensure adequate hydration, nutrition, and monitor I/O.

Drug: topotecan hydrochloride for injection (Hycamtin)

Class: Topoisomerase I inhibitor.

Mechanism of Action: Causes single-strand breaks in DNA to permit relaxation of DNA helix prior to DNA replication. Topotecan binds to the topoisomerase I-DNA complex thus preventing repair (religation) of the strand breaks. This leads to double-strand DNA breaks that cannot be repaired; thus, drug prevents DNA synthesis and replication and leads to cell death.

Metabolism: 30% of dose is excreted in the urine. Patients with moderate renal impairment have a 34% decrease in plasma clearance and require a dosage adjustment. Minor metabolism by the liver, so patients with liver dysfunction do not require dose modification.

Dosage/Range:
- Metastatic carcinoma of the ovary after failure of initial or subsequent chemo: 1.5 mg/m^2 IV infusion over 30 minutes for 5 consecutive days every 21 days, but many oncologists use dose of 1.25 mg/m^2, which the manufacturer says has equal efficacy.
- Small-cell lung cancer after failure of first-line chemotherapy: same.

Drug Preparation:
- Available as a 4 mg vial.
- Reconstitute vial with 4 mL sterile water for injection.
- Further dilute in 0.9% Sodium Chloride or 5% Dextrose.
- Use immediately.

Drug Administration:
- Administer IV over 30 minutes × 5 days.
- Baseline ANC for initial course must be $\geq 1500/mm^3$ and platelets $\geq 100{,}000/mm^3$, and for subsequent courses, ANC $\geq 1000/mm^3$, platelets $\geq 100{,}000/mm^3$, and hemogloblin ≥ 9mg/dL.
- G-CSF may be required if neutropenia develops.

Drug Interactions:
- None known.

Lab Effects/Interference:
- Decreased CBC.
- Increased LFTs, RFTs.

Special Considerations:
Dosage Modifications:
- Renal impairment: MILD (creatinine clearance 40–60 mL/minute): use reduced dose of 0.75 mg/m²; MODERATE (creatinine clearance 29–39 mL/minute): manufacturer makes no recommendation, but physician may discontinue drug.
- Hematologic toxicity: SEVERE NEUTROPENIA: reduce dose by 0.25 mg/m² for subsequent doses, or may use G-CSF instead to prevent neutropenia beginning on day 6 of the course (24 hours after last day of topotecan infusion).
- Minimum of 4 courses needed, as clinical responses occur 9–12 weeks after beginning of therapy.
- Indicated for the treatment of relapsed or refractory metastatic ovarian cancer and small-cell lung cancer sensitive disease after first relapse.
- Currently, an oral formulation of the drug is being studied in clinical trials.
- Drug appears to cross BBB.

Potential Toxicities/Side Effects and the Nursing Process

I. INFECTION AND BLEEDING related to BONE MARROW DEPRESSION

Defining Characteristics: Myelosuppression is the dose-limiting toxicity. Severe grade 4 neutropenia is seen during the first course of therapy in 60% of patients. Febrile neutropenia or sepsis may occur in up to 26% of patients. Nadir occurs on day 11. Prophylactic G-CSF is needed in 27% of courses after the first cycle. Thrombocytopenia (grade 4 with platelet count $< 25{,}000/mm^3$) occurs in 26% of patients. Platelet nadir occurs on day 15. Severe anemia (Hgb < 8 gm/dL) occurs in 40% of patients, and transfusions were needed for 56% of patients.

Nursing Implications: Monitor CBC and platelet count prior to drug administration as well as signs/symptoms of infection or bleeding. Assess renal function baseline and prior to each treatment. Discuss dose reductions with physician (see Special Considerations section). Instruct patient in self-assessment of signs/symptoms of infection or bleeding. Administer RBCs and platelet transfusions per physician's orders. Teach patient self-administration of G-CSF as ordered.

II. ALTERATION IN NUTRITION, LESS THAN BODY REQUIREMENTS, related to NAUSEA AND VOMITING, DIARRHEA, ELEVATED LFTS

Defining Characteristics: Nausea occurs in 77% of patients, and vomiting in 58% without premedication with antiemetics. Diarrhea occurs in 42% of patients, while constipation occurs in 39%. Abdominal pain may occur in 33% of patients. Asparate aminotransferase (AST, previously SGOT) and alanine aminotransferase (ALT, previously SGPT) elevations occur in 5% of patients.

Nursing Implications: Premedicate with a serotonin antagonist or dopamine antagonist antiemetic, and continue prophylactically for 24 hours to prevent nausea and vomiting, at least for the first treatment. Encourage small, frequent feedings of cool, bland, dry foods. Assess for symptoms of fluid and electrolyte imbalance: monitor I/O and daily weights if administered to an inpatient. Teach patient oral assessment and oral hygiene regimen. Encourage patient to report early stomatitis. Provide pain relief measures if indicated (e.g., topical anesthetics). Encourage patient to report onset of diarrhea. Administer or teach patient to self-administer antidiarrheal medication. Ensure adequate hydration, monitor I/O. Monitor LFTs baseline and periodically during treatment.

III. POTENTIAL FOR HEPATOTOXICITY related to HYPOALBUMINEMIA, PREEXISTING HEPATIC INSUFFICIENCY

Defining Characteristics: Evidence of increased drug toxicity in patients with low protein and hepatic dysfunction. Dose reductions may be necessary.

Nursing Implications: Monitor LFTs prior to drug dose. Assess patient prior to administering drug and during treatment for signs/symptoms of hepatotoxicity.

Drug: toremifene citrate (Fareston)

Class: Synthetic tamoxifen analogue.

Mechanism of Action: Estrogen antagonist.

Metabolism: Extensively metabolized in the liver by the P-450 enzyme system. Peak serum level after single dose is 3 hours, with terminal half-life of 6.2 days. Increased terminal half-life (decreased clearance) in patients with hepatic dysfunction to 10.9 days and 21 days for the principal metabolite. Only slightly protein-bound (0.3%). Clearance not significantly changed with renal impairment.

Dosage/Range:

- 60 mg PO qd.

Drug Preparation:

- None.

Drug Administration:

- Oral.

Drug Interactions:

- Metabolism is inhibited by testosterone and cyclosporin.
- Appears to enhance inhibition of multidrug-resistant cell lines by vinblastine.
- Appears to be cross-resistant with tamoxifen.

Lab Effects/Interference:

- Decreased WBC and platelets (mild).

Special Considerations:

- Activity, side effects, toxicity in postmenopausal women or women with unknown receptor status appear similar.

Potential Toxicities/Side Effects and the Nursing Process

I. POTENTIAL FOR SEXUAL DYSFUNCTION related to MENSTRUAL IRREGULARITIES, HOT FLASHES

Defining Characteristics: Similar to tamoxifen toxicity profile. May cause menstrual irregularity, hot flashes (most common), milk production in breasts, and vaginal discharge and bleeding.

Nursing Implications: As appropriate, explore with patient and partner issues of reproductive and sexuality patterns and the impact drug may have on them. Discuss strategies to preserve sexual and reproductive health.

II. POTENTIAL FOR ALTERATION IN COMFORT related to FLARE REACTION

Defining Characteristics: May cause flare reaction initially (bone and tumor pain, transient increase in tumor size). Nausea, vomiting, and anorexia may occur. Tremor may occur and be significant in some patients.

Nursing Implications: Inform patient of flare reaction, signs/symptoms to be aware of, and encourage patient to report any signs/symptoms. Inform patient of possibility of nausea, vomiting, and anorexia. Encourage small, frequent feedings of high-calorie, high-protein foods. Teach patients to report tremor, and discuss impact on self-care ability and comfort.

III. POTENTIAL FOR INFECTION AND BLEEDING related to BONE MARROW DEPRESSION

Defining Characteristics: Mild, transient leukopenia and thrombocytopenia occur rarely. Lowest WBC count in clinical trials was 2500/mm^3.

Nursing Implications: Monitor CBC and platelet count prior to drug administration and after therapy has begun. Instruct patient in self-assessment of signs/symptoms of infection or bleeding.

IV. POTENTIAL FOR SKIN INTEGRITY IMPAIRMENT related to RASH, ALOPECIA

Defining Characteristics: Skin rash, alopecia, and peripheral edema are rare.

Nursing Implications: Assess patient for signs/symptoms of hair loss, edema, and skin rash. Instruct patient to report any of these symptoms. Discuss with patient the impact of skin changes.

Drug: trimetrexate (Neutrexin)

Class: Antimetabolite.

Mechanism of Action: Nonclassical folate antagonist; potent inhibitor of dihydrofolate reductase. May be able to overcome mechanism(s) of methotrexate resistance as drug reaches higher concentration within tumor cells. Also, inhibits growth of parasitic infective agents (causing *Pneumocystis carinii* pneumonia [PCP], toxoplasmosis) in patients with immunodeficiency or myelodysplastic disorders.

Metabolism: Significant percentage of drug is protein-bound. Metabolized by liver; 10–20% of dose is excreted by kidneys in 24 hours.

Dosage/Range:

For PCP indication:

- 45 mg/m^2 qd IV infusion over 60–90 minutes × 21 days.
- Leucovorin 20 mg/m^2 IV over 5–10 minutes q6 hours (80 mg/m^2 24-hour total dose), or 20 mg/m^2 PO qid for days of trimetrexate treatment, extending 72 hours past the last dose of trimetrexate, for a total of 24 days.

Drug Preparation:

- Reconstitute with 2 mL 5% Dextrose USP or sterile water for injection (12.5 mg of trimetrexate/mL).
- Filter with 0.22-μm filter prior to further dilution; observe for cloudiness or precipitate.
- Further dilute in 5% Dextrose to a final concentration of 0.25–2.00 mg/mL.
- Stable 24 hours at room temperature or refrigerated.

Drug Administration:

- IV infusion over 60 minutes.
- Incompatible with chloride solutions, as precipitate forms immediately, and leucovorin.
- Leucovorin can be started either before or after first trimetrexate dose, but ensure that IV line is flushed with at least 10 mL of 5% Dextrose between drugs.

Drug Interactions:

- Drug is metabolized by P-450 enzyme system, so interactions are possible with erythromycin, fluconazole, ketoconazole, rifabutin, rifampin, protease inhibitors.

Lab Effects/Interference:

- Decreased CBC.
- Increased LFTs, RFTs (especially creatinine).
- Decreased Ca, Na.

Special Considerations:

- Indicated for alternative treatment of moderate-to-severe PCP in patients with immunodeficiency, including AIDS patients who are intolerant or refractory to trimethoprim-sulfamethoxazole (TMP-SMX), or for whom TMP-SMX is contraindicated.
- Increased toxicity is seen in patients with low protein (drug is highly proteinbound) and hepatic dysfunction. Dose reduction is indicated.
- Leukopenia is dose-limiting toxicity.
- Other side effects are nausea and vomiting, rash, mucositis, AST elevations, thrombocytopenia.
- Drug is fetotoxic and embryotoxic. Women of childbearing age should use contraceptive measures to prevent pregnancy while receiving the drug.
- Zidovudine (AZT) therapy should be interrupted while receiving trimetrexate.
- Use cautiously in patients with renal, hepatic, or hematologic impairment.
- Transaminase levels or alk phos > 5 times upper limit of normal: HOLD DOSE.
- Serum creatinine ≥ 2.5 mg/dL due to trimetrexate: HOLD DOSE.
- Severe mucosal toxicity (unable to eat): HOLD DOSE, and continue leucovorin.
- Temperature ≥ 40.5°C (105°F) uncontrolled by antipyretics: HOLD DOSE.
- Hematologic toxicity: HOLD DOSE and consult package insert.

Potential Toxicities/Side Effects and the Nursing Process

I. INFECTION AND BLEEDING related to BONE MARROW DEPRESSION

Defining Characteristics: Leukopenia is a dose-limiting toxicity. Thrombocytopenia also occurs commonly.

Nursing Implications: Monitor CBC, platelet count prior to drug administration, as well as for signs/symptoms of infection or bleeding. Instruct patient in self-assessment of signs/symptoms of infection or bleeding. Administer red cells and platelet transfusions per physician's orders.

II. ALTERATION IN NUTRITION, LESS THAN BODY REQUIREMENTS, related to GI SIDE EFFECTS

Defining Characteristics: Nausea and vomiting have been reported in clinical trials; drug has been reported to cause stomatitis; diarrhea may occur also.

Nursing Implications: Premedicate with antiemetics and continue prophylactically for 24 hours to prevent nausea and vomiting, at least for the first treatment. Encourage small, frequent feedings of cool, bland, dry foods. Assess for symptoms of fluid and electrolyte imbalance: monitor I/O, daily weights if administered to an inpatient. Teach patient oral assessment and oral hygiene regimen. Encourage patient to report early stomatitis. Provide pain relief measures if indicated (e.g., topical anesthetics). Encourage patient to report onset of diarrhea. Administer or teach patient to self-administer antidiarrheal medication. Guaiac all stools. Ensure adequate hydration; monitor I/O.

III. POTENTIAL FOR IMPAIRED SKIN INTEGRITY related to ALOPECIA

Defining Characteristics: Alopecia is total in 42% of patients.

Nursing Implications: Discuss with patient the impact of hair loss. As appropriate, suggest wig prior to actual hair loss. Explore patient's response to actual hair loss and plan strategies to minimize distress (e.g., wig, scarf, cap).

IV. ALTERATION IN COMFORT related to HEADACHE

Defining Characteristics: Headache occurs in 21% of patients. Paresthesias may affect 9% of patients.

Nursing Implications: Teach patient that headache may occur and is usually relieved by acetaminophen. Instruct patient to report headache that is not relieved by usual methods.

V. ALTERATION IN OXYGEN POTENTIAL related to DYSPNEA

Defining Characteristics: Dyspnea may occur in 20% of patients, and is severe in 4% of patients.

Nursing Implications: Assess baseline pulmonary status, including presence of dyspnea, and history since last treatment prior to successive drug administrations. Instruct patient to report new onset or worsening of dyspnea. Discuss occurrences with physician to determine further diagnostic evaluation.

Drug: UFT (Ftorafur [Tegafur] and Uracil) (investigational)

Class: Dihydropyrimidine dehydrogenase inhibitory fluoropyrimidines.

Mechanism of Action: Tegafur is a fluorouracil pro-drug, which then acts as a "false" pyrimidine, inhibiting the formation of an enzyme (thymidine synthetase) necessary for the synthesis of DNA. Also incorporates into RNA, causing abnormal synthesis and resultant suppression of tumor cell multiplication. Uracil competitively inhibits the degradation of 5-FU (see Metabolism section). Tegafur appears to directly increase apoptosis in cancer cells, but may also decrease intratumoral angiogenesis.

Metabolism: Quickly absorbed by the GI tract. Tegafur is metabolized by the liver into 5-FU; most is excreted as respiratory CO_2 and a small amount is excreted by the kidneys. Uracil is rapidly metabolized and excreted but enhances the cytotoxic effect of 5-FU by increasing its concentration in tumors and inhibiting its degradation.

Dosage/Range:

Check protocol, but these are examples:

- 200 mg/m^2/day and may be combined with with 5 or 50 mg leucovorin × 28 days per cycle.
- 300–350 mg/m^2/day in three divided doses (8 h apart) × 28 days.

Drug Preparation:

- Oral.

Drug Administration:

- Oral.

Drug Interactions:

- Unknown.

Lab Effects/Interference:

- Decreased CBC.
- Decreased K, Mg.
- Increased or decreased Ca.

- Increased PT.
- Increased LFTs.

Special Considerations:
- Cutaneous side effects occur, e.g., pigmentation changes.
- Can cause asthenia, paresthesias, and headaches.
- Uracil may increase 5-FU concentrations within tumor more than within normal tissues.

Potential Toxicities/Side Effects and the Nursing Process

I. POTENTIAL FOR INFECTION AND BLEEDING related to BONE MARROW DEPRESSION

Defining Characteristics: Usually mild, reversible.

Nursing Implications: Assess baseline CBC, WBC, differential, and platelet count prior to chemotherapy, as well as for signs/symptoms of infection or bleeding. Teach patient signs/symptoms of infection or bleeding, and instruct to report these immediately. Teach patient self-care measures to minimize risk of infection and bleeding, including avoidance of crowds, proximity to people with infections, and OTC aspirin-containing medications.

II. ALTERATION IN NUTRITION, LESS THAN BODY REQUIREMENTS, related to NAUSEA AND VOMITING, STOMATITIS, AND DIARRHEA

Defining Characteristics: Nausea and vomiting, anorexia, and diarrhea can be severe, and are the dose-limiting toxicities. Dehydration may result. Mucositis and stomatitis also occur.

Nursing Implications: Premedicate patient with antiemetics, and continue for 24 hours, at least for the first cycle. Encourage small, frequent meals of cool, bland foods. Assess oral mucosa prior to drug administration and instruct patient to report changes. Teach patient oral hygiene measures and self-assessment. Instruct patient to report diarrhea, to self-administer prescribed antidiarrheal medications, and to drink adequate fluids.

Drug: UFT (Ftorafur [Tegafur] and Uracil) plus leucovorin (Orzel) (investigational)

Class: Dihydropyrimidine dehydrogenase inhibitory fluoropyrimidines.

Mechanism of Action: Tegafur is a fluorouracil pro-drug, which then acts as a “false” pyrimidine, inhibiting the formation of an enzyme (thymidine synthetase) necessary for the synthesis of DNA. Also incorporates into RNA, causing abnormal synthesis and resultant suppression of tumor cell multiplication. Uracil competitively inhibits the dihydropyrimidine dehydrogenase (DPD), which is the primary enzyme degrading 5-FU into its metabolites. This results in sustained levels of 5-FU in plasma and tumor (see Metabolism section). Leucovorin potentiates the activity of 5-fluorouracil (5-FU). Tegafur appears to directly increase apoptosis in cancer cells, but may also decrease intratumoral angiogenesis.

Metabolism: Quickly absorbed by the GI tract. Tegafur is metabolized by the liver into 5-FU (via hepatic microsomal cytochrome P-450 system as well as by thymidine phosphorylase, which exists in tumor and body tissues); most is excreted as respiratory CO_2; small amount is excreted by the kidneys. Uracil is rapidly metabolized and excreted but enhances the cytotoxic effect of 5-FU by increasing its concentration in tumors and inhibiting its degradation.

Dosage/Range:
- Metastatic colorectal cancer: UFT 300 mg/m^2/day PO in 3 divided doses × 28 days with 1-week rest period. Leucovorin 75–90 mg/da PO in 3 divided doses.

Drug Preparation:
- Oral. Capsules contain uracil (224 mg) and tegafur (100 mg) in a 4:1 molar ratio.

Drug Administration:
- Oral.

Drug Interactions:
- Unknown.

Lab Effects/Interference:
- Decreased CBC.
- Decreased K, Mg.
- Increased or decreased Ca.
- Increased PT.
- Increased bili.

Special Considerations:
- Combination gives double modulation of 5-FU.
- Cutaneous side effects occur, e.g., pigmentation changes.
- Can cause asthenia, paresthesias, and headaches.
- Single daily dose causes more myelosuppression and diarrhea than if drug dose is given in three divided doses.
- Does NOT cause hand-foot syndrome seen with 5-FU or 5-FU analogues.
- Drug may have usefulness in breast, head and neck, and other gastrointestinal cancers.

- Appears to have efficacy comparable to IV fluorouracil and leucovorin with less toxicity.
- 5-FU is excreted in human tears, so increased lacrimation, conjunctivitis may occur.

Potential Toxicities/Side Effects and the Nursing Process

I. POTENTIAL FOR INFECTION AND BLEEDING related to BONE MARROW DEPRESSION

Defining Characteristics: Usually mild, reversible.

Nursing Implications: Assess baseline CBC, WBC, differential, and platelet count prior to chemotherapy, as well as for signs/symptoms of infection or bleeding. Teach patient signs/symptoms of infection or bleeding, and instruct to report these immediately; teach patient self-care measures to minimize risk of infection and bleeding, including avoidance of crowds, proximity to people with infections, and OTC aspirin-containing medications.

II. ALTERATION IN NUTRITION, LESS THAN BODY REQUIREMENTS, related to NAUSEA AND VOMITING, STOMATITIS, AND DIARRHEA

Defining Characteristics: Nausea and vomiting, and diarrhea may occur; diarrhea is the dose-limiting toxicity. Dehydration may result. Mucositis and stomatitis also occur.

Nursing Implications: Premedicate patient with antiemetics, and continue for 24 hours, at least for the first cycle. Teach patient to report nausea and/or vomiting so that antiemetic regimen can be revised, and patient can be compliant with oral regimen. If nausea, vomiting occur, encourage small, frequent meals of cool, bland foods. Assess oral mucosa prior to drug administration, and instruct patient to report changes. Teach patient oral hygiene measures and self-assessment. Instruct patient to report diarrhea, to self-administer prescribed antidiarrheal medications, to drink adequate fluids, and to call provider right away if diarrhea does not resolve. Consult protocol re dose modifications for diarrhea and other gastrointestinal toxicity.

Drug: valrubicin (Valstar)

Class: Anthracycline antitumor antibiotic.

Mechanism of Action: Semisynthetic analogue of doxorubicin; drug is highly lipophilic and is made soluble in Cremophor EL. Apparently, the drug does not interact with negatively charged molecules, and thus is less irritating to bladder mucosa. Drug metabolites appear to inhibit topoisomerase II so that cellular DNA cannot replicate, thus inhibiting DNA synthesis and causing chromosomal damage and cell death.

Metabolism: Drug is well absorbed by bladder mucosa with little if any systemic absorption unless bladder is injured/perforated. Used for bladder instillation, and excreted unchanged in the urine (98.6%).

Dosage/Range:
- Intravesicular therapy of BCG-refractory carcinoma in situ of the urinary bladder: 800 mg q week × 6 weeks.
- High incidence of metastases in patients receiving drug in clinical trials, probably due to delayed cystectomy. Therefore, therapy should be discontinued in patients not responding to treatment after three months.

Drug Preparation:
- Available as injection form, 200 mg in 5-mL vial, which should be stored in the refrigerator 2–8°C (36–46°F).
- Remove vials from refrigerator and allow to warm to room temperature without heating; dilute by adding 800 mg (20 mL) to 55 mL of 0.9% Normal Saline Injection, USP.

Drug Administration:
- Bladder lavage by intravesicular administration of drug (total volume of 75 mL when diluted as above), allowed to dwell for 2 hours, and then voided out.
- Non-PVC tubing and non-DEHP containers and administration sets should be used to prevent leaching of PVC into drug volume (due to Cremophor EL).

Drug Interactions:
- None known due to limited, if any, systemic absorption.

Lab Effects/Interference:
- Hyperglycemia.

Special Considerations:
- Contraindicated in patients with hypersensitivity to anthracycline antibiotics, Cremophor EL, or any drug components, during pregnancy, in breastfeeding mothers, or in patients with urinary tract infection at time treatment is planned or with small bladder unable to hold 75 mL.
- Drug should NOT be given if bladder is injured, inflamed, or perforated, as systemic absorption will occur via loss of mucosal integrity.
- Use with caution in patients with severe irritable bladder symptoms, as drug may cause symptoms of irritable bladder (during instillation and dwell time).
- Teach patients that urine will be red- or pink-tinged for 24 hours.

- Patients with diabetes need to check blood glucose levels, as hyperglycemia may occur with treatment (1% incidence).

Potential Toxicities/Side Effects and the Nursing Process

I. ALTERATION IN URINE ELIMINATION related to DRUG EFFECTS

Defining Characteristics: Intravesicular administration of drug is associated with signs/symptoms of bladder irritation: frequency (61% of patients), dysuria (56%), urgency (57%), bladder spasm (31%), hematuria (29%), pain in bladder (28%), incontinence (22%), cystitis (15%), and urinary tract infection (15%). Less commonly, nocturia (7%), burning on urination (5%), urinary retention (4%), pain in the urethra (3%), pelvic pain (1%).

Nursing Implications: Assess baseline urinary elimination pattern, history of signs/symptoms of bladder irritation. Teach patient that these side effects may occur and to report them. Teach patient to drink 3 L of fluid for at least 2–3 days beginning day of treatment to flush bladder. Reassure patient that signs/symptoms will resolve and to report any persistent symptoms.

II. ALTERATION IN OXYGENATION, POTENTIAL, related to RARE CARDIAC EFFECTS

Defining Characteristics: Rarely, chest pain may occur (2%) as may vasodilation (2%) or peripheral edema (1%).

Nursing Implications: Assess patient's baseline cardiac status, and history of chest pain, peripheral edema. Teach patient to report any pain, or swelling in hands or feet. If this occurs, discuss management with physician. If possible, do EKG while patient is having chest pain to see if ischemia exists. Systemic absorption is possible only if bladder mucosal surfaces are injured, so this should be considered.

III. ALTERATION IN COMFORT, POTENTIAL, related to PAIN, RASH, WEAKNESS, MYALGIA

Defining Characteristics: The following discomfort may occur: headache (4%), malaise (4%), dizziness (3%), fever (2%), rash (3%), abdominal pain (5%), weakness (4%), back pain (3%), myalgia (1%).

Nursing Implications: Assess baseline comfort level, and any pain and the usual pain relief plan. Teach patient that these problems may occur rarely and to report them if they do. Teach patient these symptoms should resolve, and to use local measures to minimize discomfort. Teach patient to report any symptoms that do not resolve or that become worse.

IV. ALTERATION IN NUTRITION, POTENTIAL, related to NAUSEA, DIARRHEA, VOMITING

Defining Characteristics: Rarely, gastrointestinal symptoms may occur: nausea affects approximately 5% of patients, diarrhea 3% of patients, and vomiting 2% of patients.

Nursing Implications: Assess baseline nutritional status, history of nausea, vomiting, or diarrhea. Teach patient that these may occur rarely and to report them if they do. If patient does develop symptoms, teach patient to take antiemetic medication as ordered, and OTC antidiarrheal medicine. Teach patient to call right away if symptoms do not resolve.

Drug: vinblastine (Velban)

Class: Plant alkaloid extracted from the periwinkle plant (*Vinca rosea*).

Mechanism of Action: Drug binds to microtubular proteins, thus arresting mitosis during metaphase; may inhibit RNA, DNA, and protein synthesis. Cell cycle phase specific for M phase and active in S phase.

Metabolism: About 10% of drug is excreted in feces. Vinblastine is partially metabolized by the liver. Minimal amount of the drug is excreted in urine and bile. Dose modification may be necessary in the presence of hepatic failure.

Dosage/Range:
- 0.1 mg/kg; 6 mg/m^2 IV weekly: continuous infusion 1.5–2.0 mg/m^2/d in 1L D_5W or NS × 5 days.

Drug Preparation:
- Available in 10-mg vials. Store in refrigerator until use.

Drug Administration:
- IV: This drug is a vesicant. Give slow IVP over 1–2 min through the sidearm of a running IV so as to avoid extravasation, which can lead to ulceration, pain, and necrosis. Refer to individual hospital policy and procedure for administration of a vesicant.

Drug Interactions:
- Decreased pharmacologic effects of phenytoin when given with this drug.
- Increases cellular uptake of methotrexate by certain malignant cells when administered sequentially, but less so than vincristine.

Lab Effects/Interference:
- Decreased WBC.

Special Considerations:
- Drug is a vesicant; give through a running IV to avoid extravasation.

- Dose modification may be necessary in the presence of hepatic failure.

Potential Toxicities/Side Effects and the Nursing Process

I. POTENTIAL FOR INFECTION AND BLEEDING related to BONE MARROW DEPRESSION

Defining Characteristics: May cause severe bone marrow depression; nadir 4–10 days. Neutrophils greatly affected. In patients with prior XRT or chemotherapy, thrombocytopenia may be severe.

Nursing Implications: Monitor CBC, platelet count prior to drug administration. Assess for signs/symptoms of infection or bleeding. Instruct patient in self-assessment of signs/symptoms of infection or bleeding. Dose reduction if hepatic dysfunction: 50% if bili > 1.5 mg/dL; 75% if bili > 3.0 mg/dL. Administer red blood cell and platelet transfusions per physician's orders.

II. POTENTIAL FOR SENSORY/PERCEPTUAL ALTERATIONS related to PERIPHERAL OR CENTRAL NEUROPATHY

Defining Characteristics: Occur less frequently than with vincristine. Occur in patients receiving prolonged or high-dose therapy. Symptoms: paresthesias, peripheral neuropathy, depression, headache, malaise, jaw pain, urinary retention, tachycardia, orthostatic hypotension, seizures. Rare ocular changes: diplopia, ptosis, photophobia, oculomotor dysfunction, optic neuropathy.

Nursing Implications: Assess sensory/perceptual changes prior to each drug dose, especially if dose is high (> 10 mg) or patient is receiving prolonged therapy. Notify physician of alterations. Discuss with patient the impact changes have had, as well as strategies to minimize dysfunction and decrease distress.

III. ALTERATION IN BOWEL ELIMINATION related to CONSTIPATION

Defining Characteristics: Constipation results from neurotoxicity (central) and is less common than with vincristine. Risk factor: high dose (> 20 mg). May lead to adynamic ileus, abdominal pain.

Nursing Implications: Assess bowel elimination pattern with each drug dose, especially if dose > 20 mg. Teach patient to promote bowel elimination with fluids (3 L/day), high-fiber, bulky foods, exercise, stool softeners. Suggest laxative if unable to move bowels at least once a day. Instruct patient to report abdominal pain.

IV. ALTERATION IN NUTRITION, LESS THAN BODY REQUIREMENTS, related to GI SIDE EFFECTS

Defining Characteristics: Nausea and vomiting rarely occur. Stomatitis is uncommon but can be severe.

Nursing Implications: Premedicate with antiemetics and continue prophylactically for 24 hours to prevent nausea and vomiting, at least for the first treatment. Encourage small, frequent feedings of cool, bland foods and liquids. Assess for symptoms of fluid and electrolyte imbalance: monitor I/O, daily weights if administered to an inpatient. Teach patient oral assessment. Teach, reinforce teaching, regarding oral hygiene regimen. Encourage patient to report early stomatitis. Provide pain relief measures if indicated (e.g., topical anesthetics).

V. POTENTIAL FOR IMPAIRED SKIN INTEGRITY related to ALOPECIA

Defining Characteristics: Alopecia is reversible and mild and occurs in 45–50% of patients receiving drug. Drug is a potent vesicant and can cause irritation and necrosis if infiltrated.

Nursing Implications: Discuss with patient the impact of hair loss. Suggest wig as appropriate prior to actual hair loss. Explore with patient response to actual hair loss and plan strategies to minimize distress (e.g., wig, scarf, cap). Careful technique is used during venipuncture and intravenous administration. Administer vesicant through freely flowing IV, constantly monitoring IV site and patient response. Nurse should be THOROUGHLY familiar with institutional policy and procedure for administration of a vesicant agent. If vesicant drug is administered as a continuous infusion, drug must be given through a PATENT CENTRAL LINE. If extravasation is suspected, stop drug administration and aspirate any residual drug and blood from IV tubing, IV catheter/needle, and IV site if possible. If drug infiltration is suspected, manufacturer suggests the following after withdrawing any remaining drug from IV: local installation of hyaluronidase; application of moderate heat. Assess site regularly for pain, progression of erythema, induration, and for evidence of necrosis. When in doubt about whether drug is infiltrating, TREAT AS AN INFILTRATION. Teach patient to assess site, and instruct to notify physician if condition worsens. Arrange next clinic visit for assessment of site depending on drug, amount infiltrated, extent of potential injury, and patient variables. Document in patient's record as per institutional policy and procedure.

VI. POTENTIAL FOR SEXUAL DYSFUNCTION related to REPRODUCTIVE HAZARD

Defining Characteristics: Drug is possibly teratogenic. Likely to cause azoospermia in men.

Nursing Implications: As appropriate, explore with patient and partner issues of reproductive and sexuality patterns and the anticipated impact chemotherapy may have. Discuss strategies to preserve sexual health (e.g., sperm banking).

Drug: vincristine (Oncovin)

Class: Plant alkaloid extracted from the periwinkle plant (*Vinca rosea*).

Mechanism of Action: Drug binds to microtubular proteins, thus arresting mitosis during metaphase. Cell cycle phase specific for M phase and active in S phase.

Metabolism: The primary route for excretion is via the liver with about 70% of the drug being excreted in feces and bile. These metabolites are a result of hepatic metabolism and biliary excretion. A small amount is excreted in the urine. Dose modification may be necessary in the presence of hepatic failure.

Dosage/Range:
- 0.4–1.4 mg/m^2 weekly (initially limited to 2 mg per dose).

Drug Preparation:
- Supplied in 1-mg, 2-mg, and 5-mg vials. Refrigerate vials until use.

Drug Administration:
- IV: This drug is a vesicant. Give IVP through sidearm of a running IV to avoid extravasation, which can lead to ulceration, pain, and necrosis. Refer to hospital's policy and procedure for administration of a vesicant.

Drug Interactions:
- Neurotoxic drugs: additive neurotoxicity can occur; use cautiously.
- Decreased bioavailability of digoxin when given with this drug.
- Increased cellular uptake of methotrexate by some malignant cells when given sequentially.

Lab Effects/Interference:
- Decreased WBC, platelets.
- Increased uric acid.

Special Considerations:
- Dose is a vesicant; give through a running IV to avoid extravasation.
- Dose modifications may be necessary in the presence of hepatic failure.

Potential Toxicities/Side Effects and the Nursing Process

I. POTENTIAL FOR SENSORY/PERCEPTUAL ALTERATIONS related to PERIPHERAL CENTRAL NEUROPATHY

Defining Characteristics: Peripheral neuropathies occur as a result of toxicity to nerve fibers: absent deep tendon reflexes, numbness, weakness, myalgias, cramping, and late severe motor difficulties. Reversal or discontinuance of therapy is necessary. Increased risk exists in elderly. Cranial nerve dysfunction may occur (rare), as well as jaw pain (trigeminal neuralgia), diplopia, vocal cord paresis, mental depression, and metallic taste.

Nursing Implications: Assess sensory/perceptual changes prior to each drug dose, e.g., presence of numbness or tingling of fingertips or toes. Assess for loss of tendon reflexes: foot drop, slapping gait. Assess for motor difficulties: clumsiness of hands, difficulty climbing stairs, buttoning shirt, walking on heels. Notify physician of alterations; discuss holding drug if loss of deep tendon reflexes occurs. Discuss with patient the impact alterations have had, and strategies to minimize dysfunction and decrease distress. Discuss with patient type of alteration: memory and sensory/perceptual changes are temporary and reversible when drug is stopped. Assess patient for signs/symptoms of nerve dysfunction before each dose. Notify physician of any changes.

II. ALTERATION IN BOWEL ELIMINATION related to CONSTIPATION

Defining Characteristics: Autonomic neuropathy may lead to constipation and paralytic ileus. A concurrent use of vincristine, narcotic analgesics, or cholinergic medication may increase risk of constipation.

Nursing Implications: Assess bowel elimination pattern prior to each chemotherapy administration. Teach patient to include bulky and high-fiber foods in diet, increase fluids to 3 L/day, and exercise moderately to promote elimination. Suggest stool softeners if needed. Teach patient to use laxative if unable to move bowels at least once every two days. Instruct patient to report abdominal pain.

III. POTENTIAL FOR IMPAIRED SKIN INTEGRITY related to ALOPECIA

Defining Characteristics: Complete hair loss occurs in 12–45% of patients. Both men and women are at risk for body image disturbance. Hair will grow back. Dermatitis is uncommon. Drug is potent vesicant causing irritation and necrosis if infiltrated.

Nursing Implications: Discuss with patient anticipated impact of hair loss. Suggest wig or toupee as appropriate prior to actual hair loss. Explore with patient response to actual hair loss and plan strategies to minimize distress (e.g., wig, scarf, cap). Assess impact on patient: body image, comfort. Careful technique is used during venipuncture and intravenous administration. Administer vesicant through freely flowing IV, constantly monitoring IV site and patient response. Nurse should be THOROUGHLY familiar with institutional policy and procedure for administration of a vesicant agent. If vesicant drug is administered as a continuous infusion, drug must be given THROUGH A PATENT CENTRAL LINE. If extravasation is suspected, stop drug administration and aspirate any residual drug and blood from IV tubing, IV catheter/needle, and IV site if possible. If drug infiltration is suspected, manufacturer suggests the following after withdrawing any remaining drug from IV: local installation of hyaluronidase, application of moderate heat. Assess site regularly for pain, progression of erythema, induration, and evidence of necrosis. When in doubt about whether drug is infiltrating, TREAT AS AN INFILTRATION. Teach patient to assess site and notify physician if condition worsens. Arrange next clinic visit for assessment of site depending on drug, amount infiltrated, extent of potential injury, and patient variables. Document in patient's record as per institutional policy and procedure.

IV. POTENTIAL FOR INFECTION AND BLEEDING related to BONE MARROW DEPRESSION

Defining Characteristics: Rare myelosuppression, mild when it occurs. Nadir 10–14 days after treatment begins.

Nursing Implications: Monitor CBC, HCT, platelet count prior to drug administration. Dose reduction if hepatic dysfunction: 50% reduction if bili > 1.5 mg/dL; 75% reduction if bili > 3.0 mg/dL.

V. POTENTIAL SEXUAL DYSFUNCTION related to IMPOTENCE

Defining Characteristics: Impotence may occur related to neurotoxicity.

Nursing Implications: As appropriate, explore with patient and partner issues of reproductive and sexuality patterns, and impact chemotherapy may have. Discuss strategies to preserve sexual health, e.g., alternative expressions of sexuality. Reassure patient that impotency, if it occurs, is usually temporary, and reversible after drug discontinuance.

Drug: vindesine (Eldisine, Desacetylvinblastine) (investigational)

Class: Synthetic derivative of vinblastine; synthetic vinca alkyloid.

Mechanism of Action: Inhibits microtubule formation, causing metaphase arrest during M phase. Causes some cell death during S phase. Cell cycle phase specific.

Metabolism: Short plasma half-life (probably binds to tissue). Prolonged elimination suggesting drug may accumulate with repeated dosing. Excreted primarily by bile.

Dosage/Range:
- 3–4 mg/m^2 every 1–2 weeks.
- 1.0–1.3 mg/m^2/day × 5–7 days, repeated every 3 weeks.
- 1.5–2.0 mg/m^2 twice weekly.

Drug Preparation:
- 10-mg vial of lyophilized powder, reconstituted with provided diluent or 0.9% Sodium Chloride. Solution is stable for two weeks if refrigerated.

Drug Administration:
- Vesicant precautions: administer slowly as intravenous push through sidearm of freely running IV; also may be given as continuous infusion.

Drug Interactions:
- Do not give with other vinca alkaloids, such as vincristine or vinblastine, as there is potential for cumulative neurotoxicity.

Lab Effects/Interference:
- Decreased CBC, especially WBC.

Special Considerations:
- Dose reduction may be necessary in patients with abnormal liver function or if patient has received maximal doses of other vinca alkaloids.

Potential Toxicities/Side Effects and the Nursing Process

I. POTENTIAL FOR INFECTION AND BLEEDING related to BONE MARROW DEPRESSION

Defining Characteristics: Dose-limiting side effect. Nadir 5–10 days. Neutropenia is mild to moderate. Thrombocytopenia is mild, rare (may increase on treatment).

Nursing Implications: Monitor CBC, HCT, platelet count prior to drug administration as well as for signs/symptoms of infection or bleeding. Instruct patient in self-assessment of signs/symptoms of infection or bleeding. Dose reduction is often necessary (35–50%) if compromised bone marrow function exists.

II. POTENTIAL FOR SENSORY/PERCEPTUAL ALTERATIONS related to PERIPHERAL, CENTRAL NEUROPATHIES

Defining Characteristics: Neurotoxicity is similar to vincristine. Cumulative toxicity, mild. Begins with distal paresthesias, proximal muscle weakness, loss of deep tendon reflexes. Abdominal cramping is common; constipation and paralytic ileus are less common. Hoarseness, jaw pain (severe and transient) may occur.

Nursing Implications: Obtain visual assessment prior to starting therapy. Encourage patient to report any visual changes. Instruct patient to report headache, dizziness, light-headedness.

III. POTENTIAL FOR IMPAIRED SKIN INTEGRITY related to ALOPECIA

Defining Characteristics: Alopecia affects 80–90%, with 25–50% experiencing complete hair loss. Alopecia may be progressive. Both men and women are at risk for body image disturbance. Hair will grow back. Drug is a vesicant. Inapparent or obvious infiltrations can occur. Presentation is delayed; pain, phlebitis, blister formation occur; may progress to ulceration and necrosis. Management similar to vincristine extravasation.

Nursing Implications: Discuss with patient anticipated impact of hair loss. Suggest wig or toupee as appropriate prior to actual hair loss. Explore with patient response to actual hair loss and plan strategies to minimize distress (e.g., wig, scarf, cap). Assess impact on patient: body image, comfort. Careful technique is used during venipuncture and intravenous administration. Administer vesicant through freely flowing IV, constantly monitoring IV site and patient response. Nurse should be THOROUGHLY familiar with institutional policy and procedure for administration of a vesicant agent. If vesicant drug is administered as a continuous infusion, drug must be given THROUGH A PATENT CENTRAL LINE. If extravasation is suspected, stop drug administration and aspirate any residual drug and blood from IV tubing, IV catheter/needle, and IV site if possible. If drug infiltration is suspected, manufacturer suggests the following after withdrawing any remaining drug from IV: local installation of hyaluronidase, application of moderate heat. Assess site regularly for pain, progression of erythema, induration, and for evidence of necrosis. When in doubt about whether drug is infiltrating, TREAT AS AN INFILTRATION. Teach patient to assess site and instruct to notify physician if condition worsens. Arrange next clinic visit for assessment of site depending on drug, amount infiltrated, extent of potential injury, and patient variables. Document in patient's record as per institutional policy and procedure.

IV. ALTERATION IN BOWEL ELIMINATION related to CONSTIPATION

Defining Characteristics: Autonomic neuropathy may lead to constipation and paralytic ileus.

Nursing Implications: Assess bowel elimination pattern prior to each chemotherapy administration. Teach patient to include bulky and high-fiber foods in diet, increase fluids to 3 L/day, and exercise moderately to promote elimination. Suggest stool softeners if needed. Teach patient to use laxative if unable to move bowels at least once every two days. Instruct patient to report abdominal pain.

V. ALTERATION IN NUTRITION, LESS THAN BODY REQUIREMENTS, related to GI SIDE EFFECTS

Defining Characteristics: Nausea and vomiting typically not severe; occur in 30% of patients. Diarrhea is uncommon but rarely may be protracted and thus would be an indication for dose reduction.

Nursing Implications: Premedicate with antiemetic and continue prophylactically for 24 hours to prevent nausea and vomiting, at least for the first treatment. Encourage small, frequent feedings of cool, bland food and liquids. Encourage patient to report onset of diarrhea. Administer, or teach patient to self-administer, antidiarrheal medications.

Drug: vinorelbine tartrate (Navelbine)

Class: Semisynthetic vinca alkaloid derived from vinblastine.

Mechanism of Action: Inhibits mitosis at metaphase by interfering with microtubule assembly. Also appears to interfere with some aspects of cellular metabolism, including cellular respiration and nucleic acid biosynthesis. Cell cycle specific.

Metabolism: Slow elimination; extensive tissue binding (80% bound to plasma proteins); metabolized by the liver. Terminal half-life is 27–43 hours. Excreted in feces (46%) and urine (18%).

Dosage/Range:
- 30 mg/m^2 IV weekly or in combination with cisplatin.

Drug Preparation:
- Drug is available as 10 mg/mL in 1- or 5-mL vials.
- Further dilute drug in syringe or IV bag in 0.9% Sodium Chloride or 5% Dextrose to a final concentration of 1.5–3.0 mg/mL in a syringe, or 0.5–2.0 mg/mL in an IV bag.
- Stable for 24 hours if refrigerated.
- Also available as a 40-mg gelatin capsule.

Drug Administration:
- Infuse diluted drug IV over 6–10 minutes into sidearm port of freely flowing IV infusion, either peripherally or via central line. Use port CLOSEST TO THE IV BAG, not the patient.

- Flush vein with at least 75–125 mL of IV fluid after drug infusion.
- Use vesicant precautions.
- Oral capsule should be taken on an empty stomach at bedtime.

Drug Interactions:

- Increased granulocytopenia occurs when given in combination with cisplatin.
- Possible pulmonary reactions occur when given in combination with mitomycin C, characterized by dyspnea and severe bronchospasm. May require management with bronchodilators, corticosteroids, and/or supplemental oxygen.

Lab Effects/Interference:

- Decreased CBC (especially WBC).
- Increased LFTs.

Special Considerations:

- Drug indicated as single agent or in combination with cisplatin for the first-line treatment of advanced, unresectable, non-small-cell lung cancer (Stage III, combination therapy; Stage IV, single agent, or in combination with cisplatin).
- Increased nausea, vomiting, and diarrhea with oral administration.
- Drug is embryotoxic and mutagenic, so female patients of childbearing age should use contraception.
- Administer cautiously to patients with hepatic insufficiency. Contraindicated in patients with ANC $< 1000/mm^3$.

Dosage modifications:

- Hematologic toxicity: if ANC on day of treatment is $1000–1499/mm^3$, use 50% dose (i.e., 15 mg/m^2); drug should be held if ANC $< 1000/mm^3$. If drug is held for 3 consecutive weeks due to ANC $< 1000/mm^3$, discontinue drug. If patient develops neutropenic fever or sepsis, or drug is held for neutropenia for 2 consecutive doses, dose should be reduced 25% (i.e., 22.5 mg/m^2) if ANC $< 1500/mm^3$; if ANC is $1000–1499/mm^3$, drug should be decreased to 11.25 mg/m^2 as per package insert.
- Hepatic dysfunction: if total bili is 2.1–3.0 mg/dL, use 50% dose reduction (i.e., 15 mg/m^2); if total bili is > 3.0 mg/dL, use 75% dose reduction (i.e., 7.5 mg/m^2).

Potential Toxicities/Side Effects and the Nursing Process

I. INFECTION AND BLEEDING related to BONE MARROW DEPRESSION

Defining Characteristics: Leukopenia is dose-limiting toxicity; bone marrow depression noncumulative and short-lived (< 7 days), with nadir at 7–10 days.

Use with caution in patients with history of prior radiotherapy or chemotherapy. Severe thrombocytopenia and anemia are uncommon.

Nursing Implications: Monitor CBC, ANC, HCT, and platelet count prior to drug administration, as well as for signs/symptoms of infection or bleeding. Instruct patient in self-assessment of signs/symptoms of infection or bleeding. Teach patient self-care measures, including avoidance of OTC aspirin-containing medications. Dose reduction necessary for hematologic toxicity (see Special Considerations section).

II. POTENTIAL FOR SENSORY/PERCEPTUAL ALTERATIONS related to NEUROLOGIC TOXICITY

Defining Characteristics: Incidence of mild-to-moderate neuropathy is 25%. Paresthesias occur in 2–10% of patients, but incidence is increased if patient has received prior chemotherapy with vinca alkaloids or abdominal XRT. Decreased deep tendon reflexes occur in 6–29% of patients. Constipation may occur in 29% of patients. Neuropathy is reversible.

Nursing Implications: Assess baseline neuromuscular function, and reassess prior to drug infusion, especially in the presence of paresthesias; risk is increased if drug is given concurrently with cisplatin. Teach patient to report any changes in sensation or function. Identify strategies to promote comfort and safety.

III. ALTERATION IN NUTRITION, LESS THAN BODY REQUIREMENTS, related to NAUSEA/VOMITING, DIARRHEA, STOMATITIS, HEPATOTOXICITY

Defining Characteristics: Incidence of nausea/vomiting increases with oral dosing; mild in IV dosing, with an incidence of 44%. Vomiting occurs in 20% of patients. Diarrhea increases with oral dosing (17% incidence). Stomatitis is mild to moderate with < 20% incidence. Transient increases in LFTs (AST) occur in 67% of patients, and are without clinical significance.

Nursing Implications: Premedicate with antiemetic, such as a serotonin antagonist, prior to drug administration. Encourage small, frequent meals of cool, bland foods and liquids. Assess for symptoms of fluid/electrolyte imbalance if patient has severe nausea and vomiting. Monitor I/O, daily weights, and lab electrolyte values. Encourage patient to report onset of diarrhea. Administer, or teach patient to self-administer, antidiarrheal medications. Teach patient oral assessment. Teach and reinforce teaching of systemic oral hygiene regimen. Instruct patient to report early stomatitis, and provide pain relief measures as needed. Assess LFTs prior to drug administration baseline and periodically during treatment. Dose modifications may be necessary for hepatic dysfunction (see Special Considerations section).

IV. POTENTIAL FOR ALTERATION IN SKIN INTEGRITY related to ALOPECIA, EXTRAVASATION

Defining Characteristics: Gradual alopecia occurs in 10% of patients, rarely progressing to complete hair loss or requiring a wig. Severity is related to treatment duration. Drug is a moderate vesicant, primarily causing venous irritation and phlebitis; 30% of patients experience injection-site reactions commonly characterized by erythema, vein discoloration, tenderness; rarely, pain and venous irritation at sites proximal to injection site.

Nursing Implications: Discuss potential impact of hair loss prior to drug administration, coping strategies, and plans to minimize body-image distortion (e.g., wig, scarf, cap). Assess patient for signs/symptoms of hair loss. Assess patient's response and use of coping strategies. Scrupulous venipuncture technique is used during venipuncture. Administer vesicant through freely flowing IV via IV port closest to IV fluid bag, not patient, and administer maximally diluted drug over 6–10 minutes (not longer). If extravasation is suspected, TREAT AS AN INFILTRATION and aspirate any remaining drug from IV tubing, locally instill hyaluronidase in area of suspected infiltration, and apply moderate heat. Assess site regularly for pain, progression of erythema, and evidence of necrosis. Document in patient's record. Schedule next clinic visit for assessment of site depending on drug, amount infiltrated, extent of potential injury, and other patient variables.

V. POTENTIAL FOR SEXUAL/REPRODUCTIVE DYSFUNCTION related to TERATOGENICITY

Defining Characteristics: Drug is teratogenic and fetotoxic.

Nursing Implications: As appropriate, explore with patient and partner issues of reproductive and sexuality patterns and the anticipated impact chemotherapy may have. Counsel female patients of childbearing age in contraceptive options.

Chapter 2

Biologic Response Modifier Therapy

Surgery, chemotherapy, and radiation therapy are the three most commonly used treatments against cancer. Biotherapy, or the use of biologic response modifiers (BRMs), comprises the fourth traditional treatment modality for cancer management. BRMs work in a variety of ways to modify the immune response so that cancer cells are injured or killed. This category includes antibodies, cytokines, and other substances that stimulate the immune system. It has recently been greatly expanded to include gene therapy and immunomodulating agents, such as vaccines. In this book, Chapter 5 addresses new agents that target specific abnormal molecular events that promote malignant transformation, such as over-expression of cell surface growth factors like Epidermal Growth Factor receptor. Inhibitors that target abnormal signal transduction and transcription factors are also included. Monoclonal antibodies are classically targeted against molecular flaws, such as the angiogenesis inhibitor, bevaacizumab (Avastin) and epidermal growth factor receptor inhibitor cetuximab (Erbitux). Even though they are technically biological agents, for this edition, they appear in Chapter 5, Molecular Targeted Therapies. Biological response modifiers can

- Have direct antitumor activity or help cancer cells become recognizable as foreign so that the host immune system can kill the cancer cells.
- Restore, augment, or modulate the host's immune system, such as inhibiting viral infection, and activating natural killer (NK) and lymphocyte-activated killer (LAK) cells.
- Help the host's normal ability to repair or replace damaged cells (e.g., damaged by chemotherapy or radiotherapy).
- Interfere with tumor cell differentiation, transformation, or metastasis.

Cytokines are substances released from activated lymphocytes and include the interferons (IFNs), interleukins (ILs), tumor necrosis factor (TNF), and colony stimulating factors (CSFs). Other BRMs are the monoclonal antibodies (MoAbs or MAbs), and vaccine.

Interferons occur naturally in the body and were the first cytokine to be studied. IFN-alfa (α) is stimulated by viruses and tumor cells; its antiviral activity is greater than its antiproliferative activity, which is greater than its immunomodulatory effects. There are twenty subtypes of IFN-α. IFN-beta (β) is also stimulated by viruses; it has equal antiviral, antiproliferative, and immunomodulatory effects. There are two subtypes of IFN-β. IFN-gamma (γ) is stimulated by cell-mediated immune response and IL-2; it is released by activated T lymphocytes and natural killer cells. Its immunomodulatory action is greater than its antiproliferative effect, which is greater than its antiviral effect. There is only one type of this interferon. IFN-alfa 2a is used in the treatment of hairy-cell leukemia, acquired immunodeficiency syndrome (AIDS)-related Kaposi's sarcoma, chronic myelogenous leukemia (CML), chronic hepatitis C, and adjuvant therapy of malignant melanoma. IFN-alpha 2b is used for condyloma acuminata, hepatitis B and C, hairy-cell leukemia, high-risk malignant melanoma, and AIDS-related Kaposi's sarcoma. IFN-beta 1a is being studied as to its usefulness in treating AIDS-related Kaposi's sarcoma, metastatic renal cell cancer, malignant melanoma, and cutaneous T-cell lymphoma. IFN-gamma is used for B-cell malignancies, chronic myelogenous leukemia, renal cell cancer, and is being studied in ovarian cancer. Common side effects of interferons include flulike symptoms, anorexia, and fatigue.

Colony stimulating factors include hematopoietic growth factors. They too occur naturally in the body and help immature blood cell elements develop into mature, effective white blood cells, red blood cells, and platelets. Recombinant DNA techniques have permitted the manufacture of large quantities of these substances. An "r" prefix (e.g., r-IL-2) indicates that it was produced using recombinant technology. The use of these cytokines has permitted increased doses of chemotherapy to be safely given. Filgrastim, or granulocyte-colony stimulating factor (G-CSF), is approved to prevent febrile neutropenia following bone marrow suppressive chemotherapy, as well as for other uses, and a sustained-duration pegylated formulation requiring less frequent dosing is available (pegfilgrastim or Neulasta). Sargramostim, or granulocyte-macrophage colony stimulating factor (GM-CSF), is approved for myeloid reconstitution after autologous bone marrow transplantation and for other uses. It is now being studied in use with dendritic cell vaccines. Both G-CSF and GM-CSF can be used to mobilize stem cells that will be used to rescue the bone marrow after high-dose chemotherapy. EPO or rHuEPO (erythropoietin) has become standard therapy in many situations, especially in radiation therapy, as it has become clear that cytotoxic damage from radiation is enhanced if the hemoglobin is > 12–14g/dL (hypoxic cells require almost three times the dose of radiation therapy to kill the cell than normally oxygenated cells [Kumar, 1999]). In addition, EPO helps prevent the need for red blood cell transfusions during chemotherapy and helps to minimize the fatigue associated with anemia. Efforts to produce an erythropoietin growth factor requiring less frequent dosing has resulted in the drug darbapoietin, now available.

Platelet growth factor, oprelvekin (Neumega), or interleukin-11 can be used to prevent and treat thrombocytopenia following myelosuppressive chemotherapy, and results in a modest increase in platelets. Research continues on thrombopoietin (TPO), which has a peak effect in twelve days, which often is when the nadir effect of chemotherapy occurs. In addition, new technology permits fused growth factors, such as GM-CSF fused together with interleukin-3 (IL-3) in the molecule PIXY-321. Common side effects of colony stimulating factors may include bone pain, fatigue, anorexia, and fever. In order to provide guidance and recommendations for evidence-based practice, the American Society of Clinical Oncology (ASCO) published guidelines for the use of colony stimulating factors. Together with American Society of Hematology colleagues, both organizations said there is strong evidence to use epoetin as a treatment option for patients with chemotherapy-associated anemia with a hemoglobin concentration below 10g/dL (Rizzo et al, 2002).

IL-2 is another naturally occurring cytokine that is made using recombinant technology. It is indicated for the treatment of adults with metastatic renal cell carcinoma and adults with metastatic malignant melanoma; recently, an inhaled high-dose form given together with dacarbazine has been shown to reduce lung metastases from malignant melanoma (Enk et al, 2000). IL-12 is gaining much attention due to its ability to stimulate natural killer (NK) activity and antitumor potential, as well as its synergistic action with IL-2, GM-CSF, and calcium ionophore to enhance dendritic cell function (Bedrosian et al, 2000). IL-12 is being studied in gene therapy (Divino et al, 2000). Side effects of interleukins include flulike symptoms, fatigue, and anorexia, as well as substance-specific side effects; for example, IL-2 can cause serious side effects, depending upon dose, such as capillary leak syndrome.

While many BRMs are still investigational (i.e., being studied in clinical research trials to determine their effectiveness, optimal dose, and method of administration), many are quickly being approved for use. Expected side effects vary according to agent, dose, and patient characteristics. In general, flulike symptoms (fever, chills, rigor, malaise, arthralgias, headache, myalgias, and anorexia) may occur. Routes of administration include intravenous (IV), intramuscular (IM), intraperitoneal (IP), subcutaneous (SQ), intralesional, inhaled and topical.

Currently, palifermin or recombinant human keratinocyte growth factor has shown remarkable success in decreasing the oral mueositis associated with bone marrow transplant, and is being considered for approval by the FDA.

Monoclonal antibodies are produced to target a single foreign antigen, and are designed to attach to specific cancer antigens. Monoclonal antibodies can become targeted therapies and have demonstrated an active role in molecularly targeted therapies. Therefore, further discussion of monoclonal antibodies and specific agents can be found in Chapter 5, Molecular Targeted Therapies.

References

Amgen. Prescribing Package Insert: Neulasta. Thousand Oaks, CA: Amgen, Inc. 2002

Bedrosian I, Roras JG, Xu S, et al. Granulocyte-Macrophage Colony-Stimulating Factor, Interleukin-2a and Interleukin-12 Synergize with Calcium Ionophore to Enhance Dendritic Cell Function. *J Immunother* 2000;23(3):311–320

Benstein K. Future of Basic/Clinical Hematopoiesis: Research in the Era of Hematopoietic Growth Factor Availability. *Semin Oncol* 1992;19(4):441–448

Bronchud MH, Scarffe JH, Thatcher N, et al. Phase I/II Study of Recombinant Human Granulocyte Colony-Stimulating Factor in Patients Receiving Intensive Chemotherapy for SCLC. *Br J Cancer* 1987;56:809–813

Chabner BA, Longo DL. *Cancer Chemotherapy and Biotherapy,* 2nd ed. Philadelphia: Lippincott-Raven; 1996

Clark JW, Longo DL. Biologic Response Modifiers. *Mediguide Oncology* 1986;6:1–10

Dorr RT, Von Hoff DD. *Cancer Chemotherapy Handbook,* 2nd ed. Norwalk, CT: Appleton & Lange; 1994

Egrie JC, Dwyer E, Lykos M, et al. Novel Erythropoiesis Stimulating Protein (NESP) Has a Longer Serum Half-life and Greater in vivo Biological Activity than Recombinant Human Erythropoietin (rHuEPO). *Blood* 1997;90(10): abstract 243 (Suppl 1)

Enk AH, Nashan D, Rubben A, Knop J. High Dose Inhalation Interleukin-2 Therapy for Lung Metastases in Patients with Malignant Melanoma. *Cancer* 2000;88(9): 2042–2046

Farese AM, Roskos L, Cheung E, et al. A Single Administration of r-met-HuGCSF-SD/01 (SD/01) Significantly Improves Neutrophil Recovery Following Autologous Bone Marrow Transplantation. *Blood* 1998;92 (suppl):112A (abstract 455)

Gabrilove JL, Cleeland CS, Livingston RB. Clinical Evaluation of Once Weekly Dosing of Epoetin Alfa in Chemotherapy Patients: Improvements in Hemoglobin and Quality of Life are Similar to Three Times Weekly Dosing. *J Clin Oncol* 2001;19 (11):2875–2882

Genentech. Herceptin Package Insert S. San Francisco,, Genentech BioOncology 1998

Glaspy JA, Glode DW. Clinical Applications of the Myeloid Growth Factors. *Semin Hematol* 1989;26 (Suppl 2):14–17

Hahn MB, Jassak PF. Nursing Management of Patients Receiving Interferon. *Semin Oncol Nurs* 1988;4:120–125

Irwin MM. Patients Receiving Biologic Response Modifiers: Overview of Nursing Care. *Oncol Nurs Forum* 1987;14 (Suppl):32–37

Jassak PF. Biotherapy. In Groenwald SL, Frogge MH, Goodman M, Yarbro CH, (eds), *Cancer Nursing Principles and Practice,* 2nd ed. Sudbury, MA: Jones and Bartlett;1990;284–306

Kammula US, White D, Rosenberg SA. Trends in the Safety of High Dose Bolus Interleukin-2 Administration in Patients with Metastatic Cancer. *Cancer* 1998;83(4): 797–805

Kumar P. Tumor Hypoxia and Anemia: Impact upon the Efficacy of Radiation Therapy. *Anemia YK Symposium* New Orleans, LA 3 December 1999

MacDougall IC, Gray SJ, Orlaith E, et al. Pharmacokinetics of Novel Erythropoiesis Stimulating Protein Compared with Epoetin Alfa in Dialysis Patients. *J Am Soc of Nephrology* 1999;10(11):2411–2419

Moldawer NP, Figlin RA. Tumor Necrosis Factor: Current Clinical Status and Implications for Nursing Management. *Semin Oncol Nurs* 1988;4:95–101

Neumega Prescribing Information. Cambridge, MA: Genetics Institute, Inc.; 1998

Rizzo JD, Lichtin AE, Woolf SH, et al. Use of Epoetin in patients with Cancer: Evidence-based Clinical Practice Guidelines of the American Society of Clinical Oncology and the American Society of Hematology. *Blood* 2002;100(7):2303–2320

Simpson C, Seipp CA, Rosenbery SA. The Current Status and Future Applications of Interleukin-2 and Adoptive Immunotherapy in Cancer Treatment. *Semin Oncol Nurs* 1988;4:132–141

Solimando DA, Bressler LR, Kintzel PE, Geraci MC. *Drug Information Handbook for Oncology,* 2nd ed. Cleveland, OH: Lexi-Comp Inc.; 2000

Spielberger R, Emmanouilides C, Stiff P, et al. Use of recombinant human keratinocyte growth factor (rHuKGF) can reduce severe oral mucositis in patients with hematologic malignancies undergoing autologous peripheral blood progenitor cell transplantation (auto-PBPCT) after radiation-based conditioning—results of a phase 3 trial. *Proc Am Soc Clin Oncol* 2003;22:122, abstract 3642

Swanson G, Bergstrom K, Stump E, et al. Growth Factor Usage Patterns and Outcomes in the Community Setting: Collection through a Practice-based Computerized Clinical Information System. *J Clin Oncol* 2000;18(8):1764–1770

Yasko JM, Dudjak LA, eds. *Biological Response Modifier Therapy: Symptom Management.* New York: Park Row Publishers; 1990

Agent: darbepoetin alfa (Aranesp)

Class: Cytokine, CSF.

Mechanism of Action: Recombinant DNA protein that is an erythropoiesis-stimulating protein, closely resembling erythropoietin. Drug is produced in the Chinese hamster ovary. Drug stimulates erythropoiesis in the same way that endogenous erythropoietin does in response to hypoxia. Darbepoetin alfa interacts with progenitor stem cells to stimulate red blood cell production.

Metabolism: Drug is slowly absorbed after subcutaneous injection, with bioavailabilty of 37%, a peak serum level 34 hours after administration (24–72 hour range), and half-life of 49 hours (27–89 hour range) in patients with Chronic Renal Failure. In patients with cancer, the peak serum concentration occurs at 90 hours with a range of 71–123 hours. When given IV, the drug has a biphasic profile, with a distribution half-life of 1.4 hours, and terminal half-life of 21 hours, which is about 3 times longer than Epoetin alfa.

Dosage/Range:

- Cancer Patients Receiving Chemotherapy: 2.25 mcg/kg SQ q week as starting dose
  - —If less than 1.0 g/dL increase in hgb after 6 weeks of therapy, increase dose to 4.5 mcg/kg.

— If hgb increases by > 1.0 g/dL in 2-week period or exceeds 12 g/dL, reduce dose by 25%.
— If hgb > 13 g/dL, hold dose until hgb falls to 12g/dL and restart at 75% of prior dose.

- Chronic Renal Failure Patients: 0.45 mcg/kg IV or SC q week as starting dose
  — Titrate to achieve/maintain hemoglobin at 12 g/dL, increasing dose q month.
  — If increase in hgb is < 1.0 g/dL over 4 weeks and iron stores are adequate, increase dose by 25% of the previous dose; dose may be increased at 4-week intervals until target hemoglobin reached.
  — If hgb increases by > 1 g/dL in 2-week period, decrease dose by 25%.
  — Convert from Epoetin alfa to darbepoetin alfa (Special Considerations).
  — May be able to give drug every 2 weeks.

Drug Preparation:

- Drug available in single-dose vials containing 25, 40, 60, 100, 150, 200, 300, or 500 mcg of darbepoetin alfa; contains no preservative so should not be pooled.
- Do not shake drug as it may denature it; do not dilute; visually inspect drug for discoloration or particulate matter prior to parenteral administration, and discard if found.
- Drug available with either polysorbate or albumin solution.
- Store at 2° to 8°C (36° to 46°F). Do not freeze or shake, and protect from light.

Drug Administration:

- Administer SQ or IV weekly to start, and may be able to give every 2 weeks depending upon response to drug.

Drug Interactions:

- No studies have been performed.

Lab Effects/Interference:

- Increased hemoglobin and hematocrit.

Special Considerations:

- Contraindicated in patients with uncontrolled hypertension, or known hypersensitivity to any of the active substance or excipients (albumin or polysorbate).
- Drug may increase the risk of cardiovascular events in patients with Chronic Renal Failure (CRF) due to high hemoglobin and risk increased in patients who had a rise of 1 g/dL or more in a 2-week period.
- Once starting drug, weekly hemoglobin should be monitored until stabilized and maintenance dose has been established; once dose has been adjusted, the hemoglobin should be monitored weekly for at least 4 weeks until stabi-

lization occurs; once maintenance established, hemoglobin should be monitored at regular intervals.

- Rarely, patients may develop antibodies that neutralize the effect, and rarely can lead to red cell aplasia. If a patient loses response to darbepoetin alfa, evaluation should be done to find cause, including presence of binding and neutralizing antibodies to darbepoetin alfa, native erythropoietin, and any other recombinant erythropoietin administered to the patient.
- Overall incidence of thrombotic events 6.2% compared to 4.1% for placebo, characterized by pulmonary embolism, thromboembolism, thrombosis, and thrombophlebitis (deep and/or superficial).
- Edema occurred in 21% of patients as compared to 10% with placebo.
- The possibility that darbepoetin alfa can stimulate tumor growth, especially as a growth factor of myeloid malignancies, has not been studied.
- Iron status should be assessed before and during treatment to ensure effective erythropoiesis; supplemental iron is recommended for patients with serum ferritin < 100 mcg/L or whose serum transferring saturation is < 20%. If patient does not respond to darbepoetin alfa, folic acid and vitamin B_{12} levels should also be assessed and deficiencies corrected.
- No studies have been performed on use of the drug in pregnant women. Drug should be used only if potential benefit outweighs risk to the fetus; it is unknown if the drug is excreted in human milk, so caution should be used if used in a nursing mother.
- Rarely, allergic reactions can be severe, including skin rash and urticaria. Drug should be discontinued if serious allergic or anaphylactic reactions occur.
- Patients who have controlled hypertension should have regular assessment of blood pressure. Patients should be encouraged to be compliant with their anti-hypertensive medication regime.
- Dosing in Chronic Renal Faillure: Estimated Darbepoetin alfa starting doses (mcg/week) based on Prior Epoetin alfa dose (units/week):

Previous Weekly Epoetin alfa dose (units/wk)	**Weekly Darbepoetin alfa dose (mcg/week)**
< 2500	6.25
2500–4999	12.5
5000–10,999	25

Previous Weekly Epoetin alfa dose (units/wk)	Weekly Darbepoetin alfa dose (mcg/week)
11,000–17,999	40
18,000–33,999	60
34,000–89,999	100
≥ 90,000	200

Potential Toxicities/Side Effects and the Nursing Process

I. ACTIVITY INTOLERANCE related to FATIGUE

Defining Characteristics: 33% of cancer patients reported fatigue compared to 30% in the placebo group. Patients had advanced disease, which may explain the high incidence.

Nursing Implications: Assess baseline activity and energy levels. Assess baseline fluid.

II. ALTERATION IN SKIN INTEGRITY, POTENTIAL related to PERIPHERAL EDEMA, RASH

Defining Characteristics: Peripheral edema occurred in 21% of cancer patients in clinical trials as compared to 10% in the placebo group; rash occurred in 7% of patients receiving darbepoietin alfa compared to 3% in the placebo group.

Nursing Implications: Perform baseline skin assessment, assess baseline weight and presence of edema. Teach patient to report development of peripheral edema. Teach patient self-assessment of skin, weight, and peripheral edema, and to report rash right away. Assess degree of peripheral edema if it develops, and discuss significant edema with physician to determine etiology and management. Teach patient local skin care, including avoidance of tight clothing and shoes, keeping skin moisturized to prevent cracking, and local comfort measures. If rash develops, assess extent, presence of urticaria, and implications regarding allergic reaction and drug discontinuance.

III. ALTERATION IN COMFORT related to HEADACHE, DIZZINESS, FEVER, MYALGIA, ARTHRALGIA

Defining Characteristics: Headache occurred in 12% of cancer patients in the clinical trials compared to 8% in the placebo group; dizziness 14% compared to 8% in placebo group; fever 19% compared to 16% in placebo group; myalgias 13% compared to 6% in placebo group, and myalgias 8% compared to 5% in the placebo group, probably due to bone marrow expansion.

Nursing Implications: Teach patient bone pain may occur and discuss use of nonsteroidal anti-inflammatory drugs with patient and physician for symptom management. Teach patient to remain seated or lying down if feeling dizzy, and when dizziness has resolved, to change position gradually. Monitor hemoglobin weekly during dose determination period, and weekly for at least 4 weeks after each dose adjustment. Teach patient headache, fever, dizziness, myalgia, and arthralgia may occur and to report them if they do not respond to usual management strategies.

IV. ALTERATION IN ELIMINATION related to DIARRHEA

Defining Characteristics: Diarrhea occurred in 22% of cancer patients receiving the drug in clinical trials compared to 12% of placebo group; 18% experienced constipation compared to 17% in the placebo group.

Nursing Implications: Assess baseline patient bowel elimination pattern. Teach patient to report these side effects so that they can be evaluated. Teach patient self-care measures, including dietary modification, local comfort measures, and over-the-counter anti-diarrheal medication. Teach patient to report symptoms that persist, and discuss with physician possible other etiologies and management plan.

V. KNOWLEDGE DEFICIT related to SELF-ADMINISTRATION TECHNIQUE

Defining Characteristics: Drug is administered once weekly or if response is adequate, may be given once every 2 weeks.

Nursing Implications: Assess baseline psychomotor ability, knowledge, and willingness to learn technique of self-injection. Teach how to refrigerate drug, self-administer using pre-filled syringes, how to activate needle guard, and safely collect used syringes for proper disposal. Drug insert has "Information for Patients and Caregivers." Use written and video supplements to teaching process and have patient correctly demonstrate technique prior to performing at home. Make referral to visiting-nurse agency to reinforce teaching if needed. Teach patient telephone number and who to call if questions or problems arise, and ensure patient can correctly repeat information.

Agent: epoetin alfa (Epogen, Erythropoietin, Procrit)

Class: Cytokine, colony stimulating factor (CSF).

Mechanism of Action: Stimulates the division and differentiation of erythrocyte stem cells in the bone marrow and is a hormone produced by recombinant DNA techniques. Has a naturally occurring counterpart, erythropoietin. Results in the release of reticulocytes into the bloodstream in 7–10 days, where they mature into erythrocytes, taking 2–6 weeks to increase hemoglobin.

Metabolism: Following SC injection, 21–31% of drug is bioavailable, with rapid distribution to tissues. Drug is taken up in the liver, kidneys, and bone marrow. Onset of action in a few days to 2 weeks; peak effect in 2–3 weeks. Half-life is 4–13 h. Eliminated via the liver and urine (10% unchanged drug).

Dosage/Range:

I. 50–150 units/kg TIW; if no increase in HCT within 8 weeks, increase dose by 25–50 units/kg/dose up to 300 units/kg TIW.

II. 40,000 U as a single dose once a week SQ; if HCT does not rise 5–6% in 8 weeks, increase dose to 60,000 units/week; if no response, increase dose to 80,000 units/week (maximum).

- Interrupt therapy if HCT > 40%, and resume at 75% of dose when HCT is 36%.
- Usual target range 30–36% HCT.
- IV doses must be 40–50% higher than subcutaneous doses to achieve same effect.

Drug Preparation:

- DO NOT SHAKE vial as it may denature the glycoprotein.
- Available as preservative-free injection in 2000-U/mL, 3000-U/mL, 4000-U/mL, 10,000-U/mL, and 40,000-U/mL vials. These must be refrigerated and unused portions should be discarded.
- Injection, preserved with benzyl alcohol: available as 10,000–U/mL (2 mL multidose) and 20,000-U/mL vials.

Drug Administration:

- SQ or IV injection.

Drug Interactions:

- None reported.

Lab Effects/Interference:

- Expect increase in Hgb/HCT in 2–6 weeks.

Special Considerations:

- Drug is contraindicated in patients with uncontrolled hypertension.
- Iron stores need to be checked, and replaced to maximize response to therapy.
- Used for management of chemotherapy-related anemia and anemia of chronic disease.

Potential Toxicities/Side Effects (Dose- and Schedule-Dependent) and the Nursing Process

I. ALTERATION IN COMFORT related to PYREXIA, FATIGUE, HEADACHE

Defining Characteristics: May be due to HIV disease, rather than drug, and occurs in 20–25% of patients. Allergic reactions including urticaria may occur. Anaphylaxis has not been reported.

Nursing Implications: Assess baseline temperature (T) and energy level. Instruct patient to report signs/symptoms, and discuss measures to increase comfort.

II. POTENTIAL ALTERATION IN OXYGENATION related to POLYCYTHEMIA

Defining Characteristics: Polycythemia may result if target range is exceeded (HCT of 40%).

Nursing Implications: Monitor weekly HCT: dose should be interrupted if HCT > 40%, then resumed at 75% dose once HCT is 36%. When HCT is stabilized, discuss monitoring HCT with physician (e.g., testing).

III. KNOWLEDGE DEFICIT related to SELF-ADMINISTRATION TECHNIQUE

Defining Characteristics: Most often drug is administered SQ three times per week.

Nursing Implications: Assess baseline psychomotor ability, knowledge, and willingness to learn technique of self-injection. Teach how to prepare drug, self-administer, and safely collect used syringes for proper disposal. Use written and video materials as supplements to teaching process and have patient correctly demonstrate technique prior to performing at home. Make referral to visiting-nurse agency to reinforce teaching.

Agent: filgrastim (Neupogen, G-CSF)

Class: Cytokine, CSF.

Mechanism of Action: Recombinant DNA protein (G-CSF) that regulates the production of neutrophils in the bone marrow (proliferation, differentiation, activation of mature neutrophils). Drug is produced by the insertion of the human G-CSF gene into *Escherichia coli* bacteria.

Metabolism: Elimination half-life is 3.5 hours.

Dosage/Range:

- Starting dose 5 μg/kg/day SQ or IV; dose increase by 5 μg/kg for each chemotherapy cycle, based on duration and severity of neutropenia at nadir.
- BMT: After BMT, 10 μg/kg/day as IV infusion of 4 or 24 hours, or as a continuous subcutaneous, 24-hour infusion, and then titrated based on ANC.
- Mobilization of peripheral blood progenitor cells (PBPC) is 10 mcg/kg/day SQ × at least 4 days until the first leukapheresis procedure, and continued until the last leukapheresis. Modify dose if WBC > 100,000/mm^3.
- Patients with acute myeloid leukemia receiving induction or consolidation: 5 mcg/kg/da SQ beginning 24 hrs after last dose of chemotherapy until ANC > 1000/mm^3 for 3 consecutive days.

Drug Preparation:

- Drug available in refrigerated vials of 300 μg/mL; discard unused portions.
- Unopened vials should be stored in the refrigerator at 2–8°C (36–46°F).
- Avoid shaking.
- Remove from refrigerator 30 minutes prior to injection. Discard if left out > 6 hours.

Drug Administration:

- SQ or IV, daily, beginning at least 24 hr postadministration of chemotherapy, continuing up to 2 weeks or until ANC > 10,000/mm^3.

Drug Interactions:

- None significant.

Lab Effects/Interference:

- Increased WBC and neutrophil counts.

Special Considerations:

- PEGylated form of filgrastim (sustained duration) is available and is given once a treatment cycle; it is equivalent to daily injections of filgrastim (see p.364, pegfilgrastim).
- Indicated for accelerating the recovery of neutrophil counts after myelosuppressive chemotherapy, including BMT and prevention of febrile neutropenia.
- Indicated for the mobilization of hematopoietic progenitor cells into the periphery for collection by leukopheresis, and reinfusion for stem cell rescue.
- Studies showed no statistical difference between Neupogen or placebo group in complete remission rate, disease-free survival, time to disease progression, or overall survival when used in patients with acute myeloid leukemia after induction or consolidation therapy.

Potential Toxicities/Side Effects (Dose- and Schedule-Dependent) and the Nursing Process

I. ALTERATION IN COMFORT related to SKELETAL PAIN

Defining Characteristics: Patients (22%) may report transient skeletal pain, believed due to the expansion of cells in the bone marrow in response to G-CSF.

Nursing Implications: Teach patient this may occur and discuss use of nonsteroidal anti-inflammatory drugs (NSAIDs) with patient and physician for symptom management. Monitor WBC and ANC twice weekly during therapy; dose should be discontinued when ANC > 10,000/mm^3.

II. KNOWLEDGE DEFICIT related to SELF-ADMINISTRATION TECHNIQUE

Defining Characteristics: Drug is administered daily for up to two weeks by SQ injection (outpatients).

Nursing Implications: Assess baseline psychomotor ability, knowledge, and willingness to learn technique of self-injection. Teach how to prepare drug, self-administer, and safely collect used syringes for proper disposal. Use written and video supplements to teaching process and have patient correctly demonstrate technique prior to performing at home. Make referral to visiting-nurse agency to reinforce teaching. Patient instructions in English are on package insert. Video and more detailed patient education are available from Amgen (Thousand Oaks, CA) representative.

Agent: Imiquimod 5% topical cream (Aldara®)

Class: Immune response modifier.

Mechanism of Action: Stimulates the immune system to release cytokines, including interferon, which stimulate Langerhans cells to kill skin cancer cells. Has been shown to reduce the expression of Bcl-2 (a protein that causes the cell to avoid apoptosis, or programmed cell death, by preventing the activation of the proapoptotic proteins called capases) and increase apoptosis of basal skin cancer cells.

Metabolism: Unknown.

Dosage/Range:
Imiquimod 5% topical cream is applied to the superficial basal cell carcinoma (sBCC) lesion (must be 2 cm or less in diameter), including a 1cm margin around the lesion as shown in the table below.

Target tumor diameter	Size of cream droplet to be used (diameter)	Amount of Imiquimod cream used
0.5cm—< 1.0 cm	4 mm	10 mg
> 1.0 cm—< 1.5 cm	5 mm	25 mg
> 1.5 cm—2.0cm	7 mm	40 mg

Available in single use packets, supplied 12 per box.

Drug Preparation/Administration: Wash hands before and after application of cream, and wear gloves. Wash skin area(s) with mild soap and water, then dry thoroughly before application, and again, after 8 hours application. Apply cream to lesion with an additional 1 cm surrounding the lesion(s), at bedtime leaving the cream on at least 8 hours, 5 nights a week, × 6 weeks.

Drug Interactions: Unknown.

Lab Effects/Interference: None known.

Special Considerations:

- Indicated for the treatment of sBCC on the body, neck, arms or legs (not the face, hands or feet) when surgical removal is not an option.
- Drug is also used for the treatment of external genital and non-genital warts, molluscum contagiosum, solar keratoses.

Potential Toxicities/Side Effects (More Severe with Higher Dosing) and the Nursing Process

I. POTENTIAL ALTERATION IN SKIN INTEGRITY AND COMFORT related to SKIN IRRITATION

Defining Characteristics: Redness, swelling, development of a sore or blister, peeling, itching, and burning are common application site reactions. Response to therapy cannot be determined until the skin reaction resolves, sometimes up to 12 weeks.

Nursing Implications: Explain to the patient that these side effects may occur. Teach patient to wash skin prior to application, and again after 8 hours. Teach patient to assess skin reactions, and to report any symptoms that interfere with activities of daily living as a rest period of a few days may be necessary if symptoms are severe. In addition, instruct patient to stop cream and report infection in the application area right away.

II. KNOWLEDGE DEFICIT related to SELF-ADMINISTRATION OF CREAM

Defining Characteristics: Treatment is for 6 weeks and must be applied properly for adequate tumor exposure.

Nursing Implcations: Teach patient self-administration of the cream, and to keep a diary to keep track of the application schedule. Teach patient to wash hands before and after application. Teach patient verbally and through demonstration to wash treatment area with mild soap and water, then to dry prior to application. Cream should be applied to extend 1 cm beyond the lesion borders, and rubbed into the treatment area until no longer visible. Keep cream away from eyes. Cream should be on for at least 8 hours, and then removed using mild soap and water.

Agent: interferon alfa (α) (Alpha interferon, IFN, Interferon alpha-2a, rIFN-A, Roferon A)

Class: Cytokine.

Mechanism of Action: Antiviral, antiproliferative, and immunomodulatory effects. Activates prenatural killer cells, increases cytotoxicity of NK cells, and enhances immune response.

Metabolism: Well absorbed following SQ or IM injection with 90% bioavailability after SQ injection. Drug peaks at 6–8 hours, and has an elimination half-life of 2 hours (IM/IV) and 3 hours (SQ). Renal filtration and tubular reabsorption as catabolites; minor hepatic metabolism and biliary excretion.

Dosage/Range:

- Hairy-cell leukemia: IFN-α_{2a}: Induction 3 mIU qd for 16–24 weeks (IM, SQ); maintenance 3 mIU three times per week for 6–24 months.
- CML: 9mIU qd SQ × up to 18 months.
- AIDS-related Kaposi's sarcoma: IFN-α_{2a}: Induction 3 mIU qd for 10–12 weeks (IM, SQ); can escalate dose from 3 mIU → 9 mIU → 18 mIU over 3 days to 36 mIU; maintenance 36 mIU three times per week.
- Malignant melanoma: 3mIU qd × 8–48 weeks.

Drug Preparation:

- IFN-α_{2a} available as injection solution (3–mIU vial or 18–mIU multidose vial) or powder for injection (3 mIU/0.5 mL in 18–mIU vial). Do not shake or freeze. Store in refrigerator and use reconstituted solution within 30 days.

Drug Administration:

- IM, SQ, or IV.

Drug Interactions:

- May decrease elimination of aminophylline by 33–81% via inhibition of cytochrome P-450 enzyme system.
- Increased effects of CNS depressants.
- Increased bone marrow suppressant effects with zidovudine (AZT).

- Cimetidine may increase antitumor effect in melanoma.
- Vinblastine: may increase incidence of peripheral neuropathy.

Lab Effects/Interference:

- Dose-dependent; leukopenia; elevated liver serum transaminases.

Potential Toxicities/Side Effects (More Severe with Higher Dosing) and the Nursing Process

I. ALTERATION IN COMFORT related to FLULIKE SYNDROME

Defining Characteristics: Chills 3–6 hours after dose in 40–60% of patients; fever (74–98% of patients) with onset 30–90 minutes after chill, lasting up to 24 hours. Temperature 39–40°C (102–104°F), tachyphylaxis (decrease in severity/occurrence after successive treatments) common. Fatigue (89–95% of patients) and malaise are cumulative and dose-limiting. Headache, myalgias occur in 60–70% of patients, as well as arthralgias (5–24% of patients).

Nursing Implications: Assess baseline T, vital signs (VS), neurologic status, and comfort level; monitor every 4–6 hours if patient is in hospital. Discuss with physician premedication and regular dosing of antipyretic (e.g., acetaminophen ± diphenhydramine, NSAID). Teach patient self-care measures, including monitoring T, comfort level, self-administration of prescribed medications prior to dose and regularly postdose, as well as the use of heat or cold for myalgias, arthralgias. Encourage patient to increase oral fluids and alternate rest and activity periods. If patient is in hospital and experiences rigor, discuss with physician IV meperidine (25 mg IVq15min to maximum 100 mg in 1 hour) and monitor BP for hypotension. Teach patient to alternate rest and activity periods.

II. POTENTIAL FOR INFECTION AND BLEEDING related to NEUTROPENIA AND THROMBOCYTOPENIA

Defining Characteristics: Although uncommon, increased risk with increased dose; dose-limiting thrombocytopenia; reversible. Onset usually in 7–10 days, nadir at day 14, but may be delayed in hairy-cell leukemia (20–40 days); recovery in 21 days.

Nursing Implications: Assess baseline CBC, WBC, differential, and platelet count, and signs/symptoms of infection or bleeding. Discuss any abnormalities with physician before drug administration. Teach patient signs/symptoms of infection and bleeding, and to report them immediately. Teach patient self-care measures to minimize infection and bleeding, including avoidance of OTC aspirin-containing medications, and oral hygiene regimen.

III. ALTERATION IN NUTRITION, LESS THAN BODY REQUIREMENTS, related to NAUSEA, DIARRHEA, ANOREXIA

Defining Characteristics: Anorexia occurs (46–65% of patients) and is cumulative and dose-limiting. Nausea (32–51% of patients) is mild with tachyphylaxis after one week. Diarrhea (29–42% of patients) is mild, and vomiting is rare (10–17% of patients). Taste alterations and xerostomia may occur.

Nursing Implications: Assess baseline nutritional status. Teach patient potential side effects and self-care measures, including oral hygiene. Encourage patient to prepare favorite high-calorie, high-protein foods ahead of time so can snack when hungry. Teach self-administration of prescribed antiemetics and antidiarrheals as needed. Refer to dietitian as appropriate.

IV. SENSORY/PERCEPTUAL ALTERATION related to CNS EFFECTS

Defining Characteristics: Dizziness (21–41% of patients), confusion (8–10% of patients), decreased mental status (17% of patients), and depression (16% of patients). Somnolence, irritability, poor concentration, seizures, paranoia, hallucinations, psychoses may occur in 70% of patients but are reversible. Use drug cautiously in patients with history of seizures or CNS dysfunction.

Nursing Implications: Assess baseline mental status and neurologic status prior to drug administration. Assess patient for changes (impaired memory/attention, disorientation, slow/vague responses to questions, increased lethargy) during treatment. Instruct patient to report signs/symptoms; provide information and emotional support, as well as interventions to ensure safety if signs/symptoms occur.

V. POTENTIAL ALTERATION IN CARDIAC OUTPUT related to TACHYCARDIA, CHEST PAIN, DYSRHYTHMIAS

Defining Characteristics: Uncommon but dose-related with increased risk in elderly and patients with preexisting cardiac dysfunction: tachycardia, pallor, cyanosis, chest pain, orthostatic hypotension or hypertension arrhythmias, CHF, syncope.

Nursing Implications: Assess baseline cardiopulmonary status and risk (elderly, preexisting cardiac dysfunction). EKG testing is done baseline and during treatment for high-risk individuals. Monitor VS and I/O, every four hours while receiving drug in hospital. Teach patient to report signs/symptoms of dyspnea, chest pain, edema, or other abnormalities immediately.

VI. POTENTIAL ALTERATION IN ELIMINATION related to RENAL AND HEPATIC DYSFUNCTION

Defining Characteristics: Dose-related increased BUN, creatinine, LFTs (increased AST 42–46%) may occur, as well as proteinuria. Patient may develop interstitial nephritis.

Nursing Implications: Assess baseline renal and hepatic function studies and urinalysis prior to drug initiation, and periodically during therapy. Discuss abnormalities with physician.

VII. POTENTIAL FOR SEXUAL DYSFUNCTION related to IMPOTENCE, MENSTRUAL IRREGULARITIES

Defining Characteristics: Impotence and decreased libido, menstrual irregularities, and increased spontaneous abortions have occurred. Drug is excreted in breast milk.

Nursing Implications: Assess patient's baseline sexual patterns and discuss potential alterations. Provide information, emotional support, and referral as appropriate and needed. Encourage patient to use contraceptive measures; mothers receiving the drug should not breast feed.

VIII. POTENTIAL ALTERATION IN SKIN INTEGRITY related to RASH, PARTIAL ALOPECIA, DRYNESS

Defining Characteristics: Partial alopecia (8–22% of patients), rash (11–18% of patients), throat dryness (15% of patients), as well as skin dryness, flushing, pruritus, and irritation at injection site may occur.

Nursing Implications: Assess baseline skin integrity. Instruct patient to report signs/symptoms. Discuss/teach symptomatic management, including the use of mild soaps and rinsing skin thoroughly after bathing. Encourage patient to use alcohol-free, oil-based moisturizers on skin.

IX. KNOWLEDGE DEFICIT related to SELF-ADMINISTRATION TECHNIQUE

Defining Characteristics: Often patients must receive daily dosing or thrice weekly dosing in the home setting by SQ injection, and they are unfamiliar with technique.

Nursing Implications: Assess baseline psychomotor ability, knowledge, and willingness to learn technique of self-injection. Teach how to prepare drug, self-administer, and safely collect used syringes for proper disposal. Use written and video materials as supplements to teaching process and have patient correctly demonstrate technique prior to performing at home. Make referral to visiting-nurse agency to reinforce teaching.

Agent: interferon alfa-2b (Intron A, IFN-alpha-2b Recombinant, α-2–Interferon, rIFN-α-2)

Class: Cytokine.

Mechanism of Action: Antiviral, antiproliferative, and immunomodulatory effects. Activates prenatural killer cells, increases cytotoxicity of NK cells, and enhances immune response.

Metabolism: Well absorbed following SQ or IM injection with 90% bioavailability after SQ injection. Drug peaks at 6–8 hours, and has an elimination half-life of 2 hours (IM/IV) and 3 hours (SQ). Renal filtration and tubular reabsorption as catabolites; minor hepatic metabolism and biliary excretion.

Dosage/Range:
- Hairy-cell leukemia: IFN-α_{2b}: 2 mIU/m^2 IM or SQ three times per week × 2–6 months.
- AIDS-related Kaposi's sarcoma: IFN-α_{2b}: 30 mIU/m^2 SQ or IM three times per week.
- Malignant melanoma: Induction: 20 mIU/m^2 IV days 1–5/week for 4 weeks; maintenance: 10 mIU/m^2 SQ three times per week for 48 weeks.
- NHL: 5 mIU TIW.

Drug Preparation:
- IFN-α_{2b} (Intron A): Available in powder for injection (3-, 5-, 10-, 25-, 50-mIU vials).
- Albumin free: in 3-, 5-, 10-, 18-, and 25-mIU vials.
- Powder for injection (lyophilized): 3-, 5-, 10-, 18-, 25-, and 50-mIU vials.
- Multidose pens with 6 doses of 3 mIU (18 mIU) or 5 mIU (30 mIU) or 10 mIU (60 mIU).

Drug Administration:
- IM, SQ, or IV (IVB, intermittent or continuous infusion).

Drug Interactions:
- May decrease elimination of aminophylline by 33–81% via inhibition of cytochrome P-450 enzyme system.
- Increased effects of CNS depressants.
- Increased bone marrow suppressant effects with zidovudine (AZT).
- Increased risk of peripheral neuropathy when combined with vinblastine.

Lab Effects/Interference:
- Dose-dependent; leukopenia; elevated liver serum transaminases.

Potential Toxicities/Side Effects (More Severe with Higher Dosing) and the Nursing Process

I. ALTERATION IN COMFORT related to FLULIKE SYNDROME

Defining Characteristics: Chills 3–6 hours after dose in 40–60% of patients; fever (74–98% of patients) with onset 30–90 minutes after chill, lasting up to 24 hours. Temperature 39–40°C (102–104°F); tachyphylaxis (decrease in severity/occurrence after successive treatments) common. Fatigue (89–95% of patients) and malaise are cumulative and dose-limiting. Headache, myalgias occur in 60–70% of patients, as well as arthralgias (5–24% of patients).

Nursing Implications: Assess baseline T, vital signs (VS), neurologic status, and comfort level; monitor every 4–6 hours if patient is in hospital. Discuss with physician premedication and regular dosing of antipyretic (e.g., acetaminophen ± diphenhydramine, NSAID). Teach patient self-care measures, including monitoring T, comfort level, self-administration of prescribed medications prior to dose and regularly postdose, as well as the use of heat or cold for myalgias, arthralgias. Encourage patient to increase oral fluids and alternate rest and activity periods. If patient is in hospital and experiences rigor, discuss with physician IV meperidine (25 mg IV q15min to maximum 100 mg in 1 hour) and monitor BP for hypotension. Teach patient to alternate rest and activity.

II. POTENTIAL FOR INFECTION AND BLEEDING related to NEUTROPENIA AND THROMBOCYTOPENIA

Defining Characteristics: Although uncommon, increased risk with increased dose; dose-limiting thrombocytopenia, reversible. Onset in 7–10 days, nadir in 14 days (may be delayed 20–40 days in patients with hairy-cell leukemia), and recovery at day 21.

Nursing Implications: Assess baseline CBC, WBC, differential, and platelet count, and signs/symptoms of infection or bleeding. Discuss any abnormalities with physician before drug administration. Teach patient signs/symptoms of infection and bleeding, and to report them immediately. Teach patient self-care measures to minimize infection and bleeding, including avoidance of OTC aspirin-containing medications, and oral hygiene regimen.

III. ALTERATION IN NUTRITION, LESS THAN BODY REQUIREMENTS, related to NAUSEA, DIARRHEA, ANOREXIA

Defining Characteristics: Anorexia occurs (46–65% of patients) and is cumulative and dose-limiting. Nausea (32–51% of patients) is mild with tachyphylaxis after one week. Diarrhea (29–42% of patients) is mild, and vomiting is rare (10–17% of patients). Taste alterations and xerostomia may occur.

Nursing Implications: Assess baseline nutritional status. Teach patient potential side effects and self-care measures including oral hygiene. Encourage patient to prepare favorite high-calorie, high-protein foods ahead of time so can snack when hungry. Teach self-administration of prescribed antiemetics and antidiarrheals as needed. Refer to dietitian as appropriate.

IV. SENSORY/PERCEPTUAL ALTERATION related to CNS EFFECTS

Defining Characteristics: Dizziness (21–41% of patients), confusion (8–10% of patients), decreased mental status (17% of patients), and depression (16% of patients). Somnolence, irritability, poor concentration, seizures, paranoia, hallucinations, psychoses may occur in 70% of patients but are reversible. Use drug cautiously in patients with history of seizures or CNS dysfunction.

Nursing Implications: Assess baseline mental status and neurologic status prior to drug administration. Assess patient for changes (impaired memory/attention, disorientation, slow/vague responses to questions, increased lethargy) during treatment. Instruct patient to report signs/symptoms; provide information and emotional support, as well as interventions to ensure safety if signs/symptoms occur.

V. POTENTIAL ALTERATION IN CARDIAC OUTPUT related to TACHYCARDIA, CHEST PAIN, DYSRHYTHMIAS

Defining Characteristics: Uncommon but dose-related with increased risk in elderly and patients with preexisting cardiac dysfunction: tachycardia, pallor, cyanosis, chest pain, orthostatic hypotension or hypertension arrhythmias, CHF, syncope.

Nursing Implications: Assess baseline cardiopulmonary status and risk (elderly, preexisting cardiac dysfunction). EKG testing is done baseline and during treatment for high-risk individuals. Monitor VS and I/O, every four hours while receiving drug in hospital. Teach patient to report signs/symptoms of dyspnea, chest pain, edema, or other abnormalities immediately.

VI. POTENTIAL ALTERATION IN ELIMINATION related to RENAL AND HEPATIC DYSFUNCTION

Defining Characteristics: Dose-related increased BUN, creatinine, LFTs (increased AST in 42–46%) may occur, as well as proteinuria. Patient may develop interstitial nephritis.

Nursing Implications: Assess baseline renal and hepatic function studies and urinalysis prior to drug initiation, and periodically during therapy. Discuss abnormalities with physician.

VII. POTENTIAL FOR SEXUAL DYSFUNCTION related to IMPOTENCE, MENSTRUAL IRREGULARITIES

Defining Characteristics: Impotence and decreased libido, menstrual irregularities, and increased spontaneous abortions have occurred. Drug is excreted in breast milk.

Nursing Implications: Assess patient's baseline sexual patterns and discuss potential alterations. Provide information, emotional support, and referral as appropriate and needed. Encourage patient to use contraceptive measures; mothers receiving the drug should not breast feed.

VIII. POTENTIAL ALTERATION IN SKIN INTEGRITY related to RASH, PARTIAL ALOPECIA, DRYNESS

Defining Characteristics: Partial alopecia (8–22% of patients), rash (11–18% of patients), throat dryness (15% of patients), as well as skin dryness, flushing, pruritus, and irritation at injection site may occur.

Nursing Implications: Assess baseline skin integrity. Instruct patient to report signs/symptoms. Discuss/teach symptomatic management, including the use of mild soaps and rinsing skin thoroughly after bathing. Encourage patient to use alcohol-free, oil-based moisturizers on skin.

IX. KNOWLEDGE DEFICIT related to SELF-ADMINISTRATION TECHNIQUE

Defining Characteristics: Often patients must receive daily dosing or thrice weekly dosing in the home setting by SQ injection, and they are unfamiliar with technique.

Nursing Implications: Assess baseline psychomotor ability, knowledge, and willingness to learn technique of self-injection. Teach how to prepare drug, self-administer, and safely collect used syringes for proper disposal. Use written and video materials as supplements to teaching process and have patient correctly demonstrate technique prior to performing at home. Make referral to visiting-nurse agency to reinforce teaching.

Agent: interferon gamma (Actimmune, IFN-gamma (γ), rIFN-gamma)

Class: Cytokine.

Mechanism of Action: Antiviral, antiproliferative, and immunomodulatory effects. Activates phagocytes and appears to generate toxic oxidative metabolites in phagocytes; interacts with interleukins to orchestrate immune effect, and enhances antibody-dependent cellular cytotoxicity, NK activity, and mounting of antigen on monocytes (Fc expression).

Metabolism: Slowly absorbed following SQ or IM injection, with 89% bioavailability. Peaks in 4–13 hours following IM injection, and 6–7 hours after SQ injection. Elimination half-lives for IV injection is 30–60 minutes, and 2–8 hours for IM or SC injection. Renal filtration and tubular reabsorption as catabolites; minor hepatic metabolism and biliary excretion.

Dosage/Range:
- Per protocol.
- CML: 0.5–1.5 mg/m^2 IV TIW OR 0.75–1.5 mg/m^2 IV 5 times/week OR 1.5 mg/m^2 IV qd.
- Renal cell carcinoma: 100 micrograms SQ q week OR 0.25 mg IM qd × 8 days q21–28 days.

Drug Preparation:
- Available in 100-μg (3 million units) vials, which should be refrigerated at 2–8°C (36–46°F); do not freeze. Vials stable at room temperature for up to 12 hours.

Drug Administration:
- IM, SQ, or IV.

Drug Interactions:
- May decrease elimination of aminophylline by 33–81% via inhibition of cytochrome P-450 enzyme system.
- Increased effects of CNS depressants.
- Increased bone marrow suppressant effects with zidovudine (AZT).

Lab Effects/Interference:
- Dose-dependent, leukopenia; elevated liver serum transaminases.
- Increased serum creatinine, BUN, proteinuria.

Potential Toxicities/Side Effects (More Severe with Higher Dosing) and the Nursing Process

I. ALTERATION IN COMFORT related to FLULIKE SYNDROME

Defining Characteristics: Chills 3–6 hours after dose in 20% of patients; fever (80% of patients), with onset 30–90 minutes after chill. Tachyphylaxis (decrease in severity/occurrence after successive treatments) common. Fatigue (20% of patients) and myalgia (10%) can occur. Headache occurs in 50% of patients.

Nursing Implications: Assess baseline T, vital signs (VS), neurologic status, and comfort level; monitor every 4–6 hours if patient is in hospital. Discuss with physician premedication and regular dosing of antipyretic (e.g., acetaminophen ± diphenhydramine, NSAID). Teach patient self-care measures, including monitoring T, comfort level, self-administration of prescribed medications prior to dose and regularly postdose, as well as the use of heat or cold for myalgias, arthralgias. Encourage patient to increase oral fluids and alternate rest and activity periods. If patient is in hospital and experiences rigor, discuss with physician IV meperidine (25 mg IV q15min to maximum 100 mg in 1 hour) and monitor BP for hypotension. Teach patient to alternate rest and activity.

II. POTENTIAL FOR INFECTION AND BLEEDING related to NEUTROPENIA AND THROMBOCYTOPENIA

Defining Characteristics: Although uncommon, increased risk with increased dose; dose-limiting thrombocytopenia; reversible.

Nursing Implications: Assess baseline CBC, WBC, differential, and platelet count, and signs/symptoms of infection or bleeding. Discuss any abnormalities with physician before drug administration. Teach patient signs/symptoms of infection and bleeding, and to report them immediately. Teach patient self-care measures to minimize infection and bleeding, including avoidance of OTC aspirin-containing medications, and oral hygiene regimen.

III. ALTERATION IN NUTRITION, LESS THAN BODY REQUIREMENTS, related to NAUSEA, DIARRHEA, ANOREXIA

Defining Characteristics: Anorexia occurs (46–65% of patients) and is cumulative and dose-limiting. Nausea (32–51% of patients) is mild with tachyphylaxis after one week. Diarrhea (29–42% of patients) is mild, and vomiting is rare (10–17% of patients). Taste alterations and xerostomia may occur.

Nursing Implications: Assess baseline nutritional status. Teach patient potential side effects and self-care measures, including oral hygiene. Encourage patient to prepare favorite high-calorie, high-protein foods ahead of time so can snack when hungry. Teach self-administration of prescribed antiemetics and antidiarrheals as needed. Refer to dietitian as appropriate.

IV. SENSORY/PERCEPTUAL ALTERATION related to CNS EFFECTS

Defining Characteristics: Incidence 1–10%: dizziness, confusion, seizures, gait instability, and depression (3% of patients). Use drug cautiously in patients with history of seizures or CNS dysfunction.

Nursing Implications: Assess baseline mental status and neurologic status prior to drug administration. Assess patient for changes (impaired memory/attention, disorientation, slow/vague responses to questions, increased lethargy) during treatment. Instruct patient to report signs/symptoms; provide information and emotional support, as well as interventions to ensure safety if signs/symptoms occur.

V. POTENTIAL ALTERATION IN CARDIAC OUTPUT related to TACHYCARDIA, CHEST PAIN, DYSRHYTHMIAS

Defining Characteristics: Uncommon but dose-related with increased risk in elderly and patients with preexisting cardiac dysfunction: tachycardia, pallor, cyanosis, chest pain, orthostatic hypotension or hypertension arrhythmias, CHF, syncope.

Nursing Implications: Assess baseline cardiopulmonary status and risk (elderly, preexisting cardiac dysfunction). EKG testing is done baseline and during treatment for high-risk individuals. Monitor VS and I/O, every four hours while receiving drug in hospital. Teach patient to report signs/symptoms of dyspnea, chest pain, edema, or other abnormalities immediately.

VI. POTENTIAL ALTERATION IN ELIMINATION related to RENAL AND HEPATIC DYSFUNCTION

Defining Characteristics: Dose-related increased BUN, creatinine, LFTs (increased AST in 42–46%) may occur, as well as proteinuria. Patient may develop interstitial nephritis.

Nursing Implications: Assess baseline renal and hepatic function studies and urinalysis prior to drug initiation, and periodically during therapy. Discuss abnormalities with physician.

VII. POTENTIAL FOR SEXUAL DYSFUNCTION related to IMPOTENCE, MENSTRUAL IRREGULARITIES

Defining Characteristics: Impotence and decreased libido, menstrual irregularities, and increased spontaneous abortions have occurred. It is unknown whether drug is excreted in breast milk.

Nursing Implications: Assess patient's baseline sexual patterns and discuss potential alterations. Provide information, emotional support, and referral as appropriate and needed. Encourage patient to use contraceptive measures; mothers receiving the drug should not breast feed.

VIII. KNOWLEDGE DEFICIT related to SELF-ADMINISTRATION TECHNIQUE

Defining Characteristics: Often patients must receive daily dosing or thrice weekly dosing in the home setting by SQ injection, and they are unfamiliar with technique.

Nursing Implications: Assess baseline psychomotor ability, knowledge, and willingness to learn technique of self-injection. Teach how to prepare drug, self-administer, and safely collect used syringes for proper disposal. Use written and video materials as supplements to teaching process and have patient correctly demonstrate technique prior to performing at home. Make referral to visiting-nurse agency to reinforce teaching.

Agent: interleukin-2 (Aldesleuken, Proleukin)

Class: Cytokine.

Mechanism of Action: IL-2, previously called T-cell growth factor, is produced by helper T cells following antibody-antigen reaction (processed antigen is mounted on macrophage) and IL-1. IL-2 amplifies the immune response to an antigen by immunomodulation and immunorestoration. IL-2 stimulates T-lymphocyte proliferation, enhances killer T-cell activity, increases antibody production (secondary to increased B-cell proliferation), helps to increase synthesis of other cytokines (IFNs, IL-1, -3, -4, -5, -6, CSFs), and stimulates production and activation of natural killer (NK) cells and other cytotoxic cells (LAK and TIL).

Metabolism: Half-life is 3–10 minutes when given by IV bolus, but 30–120 minutes when given by continuous infusion.

Dosage/Range:

Metastic renal cell carcinoma and metastatic malignant melanoma:

- 600,000 IU/kg (0.037 mg/kg) IVB over 15 minutes every 8 hours for a maximum of 14 doses over 5 days, then a 9-day rest, followed by 14 additional doses every 8 hours, for a maximum of 28 doses per course as tolerated. Evaluate for response 4 weeks after completion of a course and prior to next treatment course. Tumor shrinkage should be seen before retreatment. 7-week rest period should separate discharge from the hospital and retreatment. Delay and drug holiday should be used rather than drug dose reduction to manage toxicity.

Contraindications (based on toxicity) to retreatment:

- Sustained ventricular tachycardia (5 beats), uncontrolled cardiac rhythm disturbances, ECG changes showing angina or MI, cardiac tamponade.
- Intubation > 72 hours.
- Renal failure requiring dialysis > 72 hrs.
- Coma or toxic psychosis lasting > 48 hrs; difficult to control seizures.
- Bowel ischemia or perforation, GI bleeding requiring surgery.

Delay with resumption of dose after resolution of symptoms and condition resolved or ruled out.

- Persistent atrial fibrillation, supraventricular tachycardia or bradycardia.
- Hypotension (SBP < 90 mmHg with need for pressors).
- ECG change showing MI, ischemia, myocarditis.
- O2 sat < 90%.
- Mental status changes (confusion, agitation).
- Sepsis.
- Serum creatinine > 4.5 mg/dL or ≥ with severe volume overload, acidosis, or hyperkalemia; persistent oliguria, urine output < 10 mL/hr for 16–24 hours with increasing serum creatinine.
- Signs of hepatic failure (encephalopathy, increasing ascites, liver pain, hypoglycemia): stop this course of treatment, and reinitiate new course after at least 7 weeks of rest.
- Stool guaiac repeatedly > 3–4+.
- Bullous dermatitis or marked worsening of pre-existing skin condition (don't use topical steroid therapy).

Drug Preparation:
- Vial containing 22 mIU (1.3 mg) should be reconstituted with 1.2 mL of sterile water for injection, USP so each mL contains 18 IU of drug. DO NOT SHAKE. Further dilute in 50 mL of 5% Dextrose injection, USP. If patient weight < 40 kg, use smaller volume. Refrigerate and use within 48 hrs of preparation. Bring to room temperature prior to administration.

Drug Administration:
- IV (IVB or 24–hour continuous infusion); SQ; intraperitoneal (IP).
- Administer IV over 15 minutes.

Drug Interactions:
- Potentiation of CNS effects when given in combination with psychotropic drugs.
- Combination with nephrotoxic, myelotoxic, cardiotoxic, or hepatotoxic will increase toxicity of aldesleukin in these organ systems.
- Increased risk of hypersensitivity reactions when sequential high dose aldesleukin combined with dacarbazine, cisplatin, tamoxifen, and interferon-alpha.
- Interferon alpha and aldesleukin concurrently: increased risk of myocardial injury (MI, myocarditis, severe rhabdomyolysis).
- Glucocorticoid steroids: decreased antitumor effectiveness, do not use together.
- Beta-blockers, antihypertensives: potentiate hypotension of aldesleukin.
- Iodinated contrast medium: increased risk of atypical adverse reaction (12.6% incidence) characterized by fever, chills, nausea, vomiting, pruritus, rash, diarrhea, hypotension, edema, and oliguria, and can happen when contrast is given within 4 weeks of aldesleukin dosing.

Lab Effects/Interference:

- Anemia, leukopenia, thrombocytopenia.
- Elevated LFTs.

Special Considerations:

- FDA-indicated for treatment patients with metastatic renal cell cancer or metastatic malignant melanoma.
- Patient must have NORMAL cardiac, pulmonary, hepatic, renal (serum creatinine $\leq$ 1.5 mg/dL) and CNS function prior to treatment, and be free of any known infection.
- Drug may worsen symptoms of patients with unknown/untreated CNS metastases. Thorough evaluation and treatment of CNS metastases should precede treatment so patient has a negative scan before starting aldesleukin.
- Use caution when patient receiving other drugs that are hepatic or renally toxic.
- Drug may increase rejection in allogeneic transplant patients, exacerbation of autoimmune disease and inflammatory disorders.
- Contraindicated in male or female patients of child-bearing age/intention not using effective contraception; nursing mothers should not nurse while taking the drug unless benefit outweighs unknown risk.
- Pegylated interleukin-2 with a longer drug half-life is being studied but still has the same cardiopulmonary toxicity; inhaled interleukin-2 for patients with pulmonary metastases continues to be studied, and offers few systemic side effects.

Potential Toxicities/Side Effects (Dose-1 and Schedule-Dependent) and the Nursing Process

I. ALTERATION IN COMFORT related to FLULIKE SYNDROME

Defining Characteristics: Chills may occur 2–4 hours after dose; rigors are possible; fever to 39–40°C (102–104°F); and headache. Myalgia and arthralgias may occur at high doses due to accumulation of cytokine deposits/lymphocytes in joint spaces. Incidence of chills 52%, fever 29%, malaise 27%, asthenia 23%, anorexia 20%.

Nursing Implications: Assess baseline T, VS, neurologic status, and comfort level, and monitor every 4–6 hours if patient in hospital. Discuss with physician premedication and regular dosing of antipyretic (e.g., acetaminophen ± diphenhydramine, NSAID). Teach patient self-care measures, including monitoring T, comfort level, self-administration of prescribed medications prior to dose and regularly postdose, as well as the use of heat or cold for myalgias, arthralgias. Encourage patient to increase oral fluids and alternate rest and activity periods. If patient is in hospital and experiences rigor, discuss with physician IV meperidine (25 mg IV every 15 minutes to maximum 100 mg in 1 hour), and monitor BP for hypotension.

II. SENSORY/PERCEPTUAL ALTERATION related to CNS EFFECTS

Defining Characteristics: Confusion, irritability, disorientation, impaired memory, expressive aphasia, sleep disturbances, depression, hallucinations, and psychoses may occur, resolving within 24–48 hours after last drug dose. Mental status abnormalities exaggerated by anxiety and sleep deprivation.

Nursing Implications: Assess baseline mental status and neurologic status prior to drug administration. Assess patient for changes (impaired memory/attention, disorientation, slow/vague responses to questions, increased lethargy) during treatment. Teach patient to report signs/symptoms. Provide information, emotional support, and interventions to ensure safety if signs/symptoms occur.

III. ALTERATION IN CARDIAC OUTPUT related to HYPOTENSION (HIGH-DOSE THERAPY)

Defining Characteristics: Increased risk with doses > 100,000 IU/kg. Capillary leak syndrome (peripheral edema, CHF, pleural effusions, and pericardial effusions) may occur and is reversible once treatment is stopped. Atrial arrhythmias may occur; occasionally, supraventricular tachycardia, myocarditis, chest pain; and rarely, myocardial infarction. IL-2 causes peripheral vasodilation, decreased systemic vascular resistance, and hypotension that may lead to decreased renal perfusion. A decrease in SBP occurs 2–12 hours after start of therapy, and typically will progress to significant hypotension (SBP < 90 mmHg or a 20 mmHg drop from baseline SBP) with hypoperfusion. In addition, protein and fluids will extravasate into the extravascular space forming edema and new effusions.

Nursing Implications: Assess baseline cardiopulmonary status and patients at risk (the elderly, those with preexisting cardiac dysfunction). Monitor VS and pulse oximetry frequently, at least q 4 hour (if hypotensive, q 1 hr), noting rate, rhythm of heartbeat, blood pressure, urinary output, fluid status, I/O q 4 hours or more frequent, and daily weights during therapy. Discuss any abnormalities with physician and revise plan as needed (e.g., diuretics, plasma expanders, ICU transfer). Instruct patient to report signs/symptoms of dyspnea, chest pain, edema, or other abnormalities immediately. Hypotension requires fluid replacement, and patient should be monitored with continuous cardiac monitoring if SBP < 90 mmHg. Any ectopy should be documented on EKG. Manufacturer states that early administration of dopamine (1–5 μg/kg/min) to patients with capillary leak syndrome before the onset of hypotension can improve organ perfusion and preserve urinary output. Increased dopamine doses (6–10 μg/kg/min) or the addition of phenylephrine hydrochloride (1–5 μg/kg/min) to low dose dopamine have been described. Once blood pressure stabilized, use of diuretics often effective in relieving edema and pulmonary congestion.

IV. POTENTIAL ALTERATION IN OXYGENATION

Defining Characteristics: Pulmonary symptoms are dose-related, such as dyspnea and tachypnea. Pulmonary edema may occur with hypoxia, due to fluid shifts.

Nursing Implications: Assess baseline cardiopulmonary status every four hours during therapy, noting rate, rhythm, depth of respirations, presence of dyspnea, and breath sounds (presence of wheezes, crackles, rhonchi). Identify patients at risk: those with preexisting cardiac or pulmonary disease, prior treatment with cardio- or pulmonary-toxic drugs or radiation, and smoking history. Instruct patient to report cough, dyspnea, or change in respiratory status. Strictly monitor I/O, total fluid balance, and daily weight. Discuss abnormalities with physician, as well as the need for oxygen, diuretics, or transfer to ICU.

V. POTENTIAL ALTERATION IN NUTRITION, LESS THAN BODY REQUIREMENTS, related to NAUSEA/VOMITING, DIARRHEA, MUCOSITIS, ANOREXIA

Defining Characteristics: Nausea and vomiting are mild and are effectively controlled by antiemetics. Diarrhea is common, can be severe, and may require bicarbonate replacement. Stomatitis is common but mild.

Nursing Implications: Assess patient's baseline nutritional status. Administer antiemetics as ordered. Teach patient potential side effects and self-care measures, including oral hygiene, and encourage patient to eat favorite high-calorie, high-protein foods. Teach self-administration of prescribed antiemetics and antidiarrheals as needed. Refer to dietitian as appropriate.

VI. POTENTIAL ALTERATION IN ELIMINATION related to RENAL DYSFUNCTION, HEPATOTOXICITY

Defining Characteristics: IL-2 causes direct tubular cell injury and decreased renal blood flow with cumulative doses. Oliguria, proteinuria, increased serum creatinine and BUN, increased LFTs (bili, AST, ALT, LDH, alk phos). Anuria (i.e., 10 mL of urine/hour for 8 hours) occurs in 38% of patients; renal dysfunction is reversible after drug discontinuance. Hepatomegaly and hypoalbuminemia may occur.

Nursing Implications: Assess baseline renal and hepatic functions and monitor during treatment. Assess fluid and electrolyte balance, urine output hourly, and total body balance. Dipstick urine for protein. Discuss abnormalities with physician and revise plan.

VII. POTENTIAL FOR FATIGUE AND BLEEDING related to ANEMIA, THROMBOCYTOPENIA

Defining Characteristics: Severe anemia occurs in 70% of patients, requiring RBC transfusion. Thrombocytopenia occurs commonly but rarely requires transfusion.

Nursing Implications: Assess baseline CBC and platelet count, and signs/symptoms of fatigue, severe anemia, bleeding. Instruct patient to report signs/symptoms immediately and to manage self-care (alternate rest/activity, minimize bleeding by avoidance of OTC aspirin-containing medicines). Transfuse red cells and platelets as ordered.

VIII. POTENTIAL ALTERATION IN SKIN INTEGRITY related to DIFFUSE RASH

Defining Characteristics: All patients develop diffuse erythematous rash, which may desquamate (soles of feet, palms of hands, between fingers). Pruritus may occur with or without rash.

Nursing Implications: Assess baseline skin integrity. Teach patient to report signs/symptoms. Discuss/teach symptomatic management, including the use of mild soaps and rinsing skin thoroughly after bathing. Encourage the use of alcohol-free, oil-based moisturizers on skin and the protection of desquamated areas.

Agent: interleukin-3 (investigational)

Class: Cytokine.

Mechanism of Action: Binds to early progenitor cells. Species-specific stimulator of bone marrow progenitor cells (CFU-GEMM [colony forming unit-granulocyte, erythrocyte, megakaryocyte, and macrophage]). Production of immature neutrophils is enhanced when drug is administered after GM-CSF.

Metabolism: IL-3 is produced by activated T lymphocytes. Other cytokines released after administration of IL-3 include IL-6 (B-lymphocyte growth factor). Short half-life of 4–8 minutes.

Dosage/Range:
- Per investigational protocol, but effective doses have been found to be 60 $\mu g/m^2$/day to 500 $\mu g/m^2$/day for 15 days.

Drug Preparation:
- Per protocol.

Drug Administration:
- SQ qd for 15 days (no difference between IV or SQ injection, and less toxicity; best delivery may be via depot injection or prolonged infusions).

Drug Interactions:
- None reported, but data is being accumulated in clinical trials.

Lab Effects/Interference:
- Expect increase in neutrophils, platelets.

Special Considerations:
- Bone marrow depression/bone marrow failure after chemotherapy: dose-dependent increases in neutrophils in 15 days, and in platelets.
- Myelodysplastic syndrome: respond more slowly, with neutrophil production peak at 19 days, and peak platelet count at 15–25 days.

Potential Toxicities/Side Effects (Dose-1 and Schedule-Dependent) and the Nursing Process

I. ALTERATION IN COMFORT related to FLULIKE SYNDROME

Defining Characteristics: Fever occurs, especially on first day of therapy, and lasts 2–16 hours after administration. Headache and stiff neck also affect comfort but are not severe. Facial flushing, erythema at the injection site, mild bone pain, and edema may occur. When given IV, flulike symptoms, hypotension, rash, headache, and purpura occur (Dorr and Von Hoff, 1994).

Nursing Implications: Assess baseline T, VS, neurologic status, and comfort level, and monitor every 2–16 hours if patient is in hospital. Discuss with physician premedication and regular dosing of antipyretic (e.g., acetaminophen ± diphenhydramine, NSAID). Teach patient self-care measures, including monitoring T, comfort level, self-administration of prescribed medications prior to dose and regularly postdose, and use of heat or cold for myalgias and arthralgias. Encourage patient to increase oral fluids and alternate periods of rest and activity.

Agent: interleukin-6 (investigational)

Class: Cytokine.

Mechanism of Action: Acts primarily as a cofactor in the differentiation and proliferation of cytotoxic T cells (Dorr and Von Hoff, 1994) but has some antitumor activity. Also stimulates differentiation of megakaryocytes, resulting in increased peripheral platelets (thrombopoiesis). Mediates increased osteoclast activity and bone absorption. Probably augments IL-3 activity. IL-6 is produced by T lymphocytes, monocytes, endothelial cells, and fibroblasts.

Metabolism: Probably triphasic elimination, with peak serum levels five hours after administration.

Dosage/Range:
- Per investigational protocol, but effective doses have been found to be 2.5 μg/kg/day administered by SQ injection.

Drug Preparation:
- Per protocol.

Drug Administration:
- SQ.

Drug Interactions:
- None reported, but data is being accumulated in clinical trials.

Lab Effects/Interference:
- Anemia.
- Increased LFTs.

Special Considerations:
- Not recommended therapy for patients with history of cardiac disease, as atrial fibrillation has occurred.
- Contraindicated in patients with diabetes, T- or B-cell malignancy, and multiple myeloma.
- Clinical studies in patients with melanoma, ovarian cancer, and post-BMT in Hodgkin's disease.

Potential Toxicities/Side Effects (Dose- and Schedule-Dependent) and the Nursing Process

I. ALTERATION IN COMFORT related to FLULIKE SYNDROME

Defining Characteristics: Fever and chills commonly occur, along with headaches, which can be severe. These occur 1–4 hours after drug administration. Anorexia and arthralgias can occur. Symptoms can be ameliorated or prevented by prophylactic antipyretics and anti-inflammatory agents.

Nursing Implications: Assess baseline T, VS, neurologic status, and comfort level, and monitor if patient is in hospital. Discuss with physician premedication and regular dosing of antipyretic (e.g., acetaminophen ± diphenhydramine, NSAID). Teach patient self-care measures, including monitoring T, comfort level, self-administration of prescribed medications prior to dose and regularly postdose, and use of heat or cold for myalgias and arthralgias. Encourage patient to increase oral fluids and alternate rest and activity periods.

II. POTENTIAL ALTERATION IN NUTRITION, LESS THAN BODY REQUIREMENTS, related to ALTERATIONS IN HEPATIC FUNCTION STUDIES AND GLUCOSE

Defining Characteristics: Transient alterations in serum alk phos, transaminases, and fasting blood glucose can occur. Development of significant alteration in alk phos in one patient who developed hepatic necrosis has been reported at higher doses (30 μg/kg/day).

Nursing Implications: Assess patient's baseline LFTs and blood glucose. Monitor during therapy. Discuss any alterations with physician.

III. POTENTIAL FOR ACTIVITY INTOLERANCE related to ANEMIA

Defining Characteristics: Anemia appears a few days after beginning therapy. Recovery occurs within one week of cessation of IL-2. Platelet counts rise and neutrophil counts are unchanged.

Nursing Implications: Assess baseline WBC, Hgb/HCT hematocrit, and platelet counts, and monitor during therapy. Assess impact of anemia on patient, and reassure that Hgb/HCT will rise once treatment has stopped.

Agent: interleukin-12 (investigational)

Class: Cytokine.

Mechanism of Action: Stimulates strong natural-killer (NK) cell-mediated antitumor response and enhances cytotoxic lymphocytes (called *cytotoxic lymphocyte maturation factor* and *NK stimulatory factor*). Synergistic with GMCSF, IL-2, and calcium ionophore to enhance maturation of dendritic cell function (Bedrosian et al, 2000); being studied in gene therapy.

Metabolism: Unknown.

Dosage/Range:
- Per investigational protocol.

Drug Preparation:
- Per protocol.

Drug Administration:
- Per protocol.

Drug Interactions:
- Unknown.

Lab Effects/Interference:
- Increased triglycerides and LFTs.
- Hyperglycemia.

- Decreased white and red blood cell counts, platelet count.

Special Considerations:

- Interleukin-12 gene therapy being studied in patients with unresectable/recurrent or refractory squamous cell cancer of the head and neck, and AIDS-related Kaposi's sarcoma.

Potential Toxicities/Side Effects (Dose- and Schedule-Dependent) and the Nursing Process

I. ALTERATION IN COMFORT related to FLULIKE SYNDROME

Defining Characteristics: Flulike symptoms and delayed fever commonly occur.

Nursing Implications: Assess baseline T, VS, neurologic status, and comfort level, and monitor if patient is in hospital. Discuss with physician pre-medication and regular dosing of antipyretic (e.g., acetaminophen ± diphenhydramine, NSAID) and per protocol. Teach patient self-care measures, including monitoring T, comfort level, self-administration of prescribed medications prior to dose and regularly post-dose, and use of heat or cold for myalgias and arthralgias. Encourage patient to increase oral fluids and alternate rest and activity periods.

II. POTENTIAL ALTERATION IN NUTRITION, LESS THAN BODY REQUIREMENTS, related to STOMATITIS, ALTERATIONS IN HEPATIC FUNCTION STUDIES AND GLUCOSE

Defining Characteristics: Stomatitis occurs, as do transient alterations in LFTs, triglycerides, and fasting blood glucose. Hyperglycemia, elevated triglycerides, and LFTs common.

Nursing Implications: Assess oral mucosa baseline and regularly during therapy. Teach patient self-care strategies, including self-assessment, self-administration of oral hygiene regimen, and to report alterations. Assess patient's baseline LFTs, triglycerides, and blood glucose. Monitor during therapy. Discuss any alterations with physician.

III. POTENTIAL FOR INFECTION, BLEEDING, FATIGUE related to BONE MARROW SUPPRESSION

Defining Characteristics: Bone marrow suppression can occur.

Nursing Implications: Assess baseline CBC, WBC, differential, and platelet count, and signs/symptoms of infection or bleeding. Discuss any abnormalities with physician before drug administration. Teach patient signs/symptoms of infection and bleeding, and to report them immediately. Teach patient self-care measures to minimize infection and bleeding, including avoidance of OTC aspirin-containing medications. Teach patient to alternate rest and activity periods and strategies to conserve energy.

Nursing Implications: Assess baseline WBC, Hgb/HCT, and platelet counts, and monitor during therapy. Assess impact of anemia on patient, and reassure that Hgb/HCT will rise once treatment has stopped.

Agent: levamisole hydrochloride (Ergamisol)

Class: Anthelmintic.

Mechanism of Action: Stimulate immunorestoration in deficient host. Nonspecific immunomodulating agent has antiproliferating action against tumor metastases (with small tumor burdens) rather than primary tumor. Thus, drug is combined with chemotherapy (e.g., 5-FU) and/or surgery (e.g., colon resection).

Metabolism: Rapidly absorbed from GI tract, with elimination half-life of 3–4 hours. Extensively metabolized by liver, and metabolites excreted by kidneys (70% over three days). Unchanged drug is excreted in urine (< 5%) and feces (< 0.2%).

Dosage/Range:

Adjuvant chemotherapy with 5-FU for Duke's Stage C colon cancer:

- Initial therapy: 50 mg PO q8h × 3 days (starting day 7–30 postsurgery); 5-FU 450 mg/m²/day IV × 5 days (concomitant with levamisole, starting 21–34 days postsurgery).
- Maintenance: 50 mg PO q8h × 3 days every 2 weeks for 1 year; 5-FU 450 mg/m²/day every week beginning 28 days after initiation of 5-day course.
- See package insert for 5-FU dose reductions for stomatitis, diarrhea, leukopenia.

Drug Preparation:

- Available as 50-mg tablets in 36-tablet blister pack.

Drug Administration:

- Oral.

Drug Interactions:

- Alcohol may produce disulfiram-like effect (flushing, throbbing in head and neck, throbbing headaches, respiratory difficulty, nausea and vomiting, sweating, chest pain, dyspnea, hypotension, weakness, blurred vision, confusion, coma, and death).
- Increased phenytoin levels occur when coadministered with levamisole and 5-FU: phenytoin dose may need to be decreased.

Lab Effects/Interference:

- Leukopenia, increased bili when given together with 5-FU.

Special Considerations:

- Indicated for adjuvant treatment in combination with 5-FU after surgical resection of Duke's Stage C colon cancer.
- May be used investigationally with other protocols.

Potential Toxicities/Side Effects (in Combination with 5-fluorouracil) and the Nursing Process

I. ALTERATION IN NUTRITION, LESS THAN BODY REQUIREMENTS, related to NAUSEA/VOMITING, DIARRHEA, STOMATITIS, ANOREXIA

Defining Characteristics: Stomatitis or diarrhea (i.e., 5 stools/day) is an indication to interrupt 5-day course and weekly 5-FU injection; if stomatitis or diarrhea develops during weekly 5-FU, dose-reduce subsequent 5-FU doses. Nausea may occur more commonly than vomiting.

Nursing Implications: Assess baseline oral mucosa, elimination pattern. Inform patient of potential side effects and need to report them if they develop. Premedicate with antiemetic, at least for the first cycle. Assess oral mucosa; ask about incidence of diarrhea during and prior to each course of therapy. Teach patient self-care measures, including diet modifications, self-medication with prescribed antiemetic, and oral hygiene regimen. If stomatitis or diarrhea develops, discuss modification of therapy with physician.

II. POTENTIAL FOR INFECTION AND BLEEDING related to BONE MARROW DEPRESSION

Defining Characteristics: Agranulocytosis may occur and may be preceded by flulike syndrome (fever, chills). Neutropenia is usually reversible on discontinuance of therapy.

Nursing Implications: Monitor CBC, WBC, differential, platelet count prior to initial drug treatment and then weekly prior to each 5-FU dose. Discuss with physician if abnormalities occur. Manufacturer recommends holding 5-FU dose until WBC $> 3500/mm^3$, and holding both 5-FU and levamisole if platelets $< 100{,}000/mm^3$. If 5-FU nadir $< 2500/mm^3$, next 5-FU dose should be reduced by 20%. Teach patient signs/symptoms of infection and bleeding, and instruct to report these immediately. Teach patient self-care measures to minimize infection and bleeding, including avoidance of OTC aspirin-containing medications.

III. POTENTIAL ALTERATION IN SKIN INTEGRITY related to DERMATITIS, SKIN CHANGES

Defining Characteristics: Dermatitis (23% of patients), alopecia (22% of patients), and pruritus may occur.

Nursing Implications: Assess skin and teach patient about potential side effects. Discuss potential impact hair loss will have, as well as coping strategies (e.g., wig, scarf). Discuss/teach symptom management depending on character of dermatitis.

IV. SENSORY/PERCEPTUAL ALTERATIONS related to NEUROLOGIC CHANGES

Defining Characteristics: Dizziness, headaches, paresthesia, ataxia, taste perversion, and altered sense of smell may occur (4–8% of patients). Less commonly, somnolence, depression, nervousness, insomnia, and anxiety may occur (2% of patients).

Nursing Implications: Assess baseline mental status and neurologic status. Instruct patient to report any abnormalities. Notify physician of any abnormalities and discuss therapy modification depending on severity of side effects.

V. ALTERATION IN COMFORT related to FLULIKE SYMPTOMS

Defining Characteristics: Fever, chills, fatigue, chest pain may occur, although they are rare. Fever and chills may precede agranulocytosis.

Nursing Implications: Teach patient that these may occur, and instruct to report fever and chills. Assess CBC, WBC, differential if fever and chills occur. Discuss symptom management with patient, self-administration of prescribed NSAIDs or acetaminophen, and alternation of rest/activity periods.

Agent: megakaryocyte growth and development factor (MGDF) (investigational)

Class: Cytokine.

Mechanism of Action: Growth-factor-specific for megakaryocyte precursor lineage.

Metabolism: Unknown.

Dosage/Range:
- Per protocol.

Drug Preparation/Administration:
- SQ daily for 5 days, or per protocol.

Drug Interactions:
- None known.

Lab Effects/Interference:
- Expect increase in platelet count.

Special Considerations:
- Minimal toxicity.
- Current studies are exploring platelet recovery after induction therapy for acute myelogenous leukemia (AML), and activity of MGDF as a mobilizing agent for peripheral blood stem cells.
- For further information, contact Amgen (Thousand Oaks, CA).

Potential Toxicities/Side Effects and the Nursing Process

I. POTENTIAL FOR KNOWLEDGE DEFICIT related to INVESTIGATIONAL AGENT

Nursing Diagnosis: Knowledge deficit related to drug's status as an investigational agent.

Defining Characteristics: Clinical studies are defining a toxicity profile, but no toxicity has been reported as yet.

Nursing Interventions: Reinforce teaching about cytokine, including indication, expected benefit, and administration. Instruct patient to report any side effects or unusual occurrences.

Drug: novel erythropoiesis stimulating protein (darbepoietin, NESP) (investigational)

Class: Cytokine, colony simulating factor (CSF).

Mechanism of Action: NESP is a hyperglycosylated analogue of recombinant human erythropoietin (EPO, r-HuEPO), which has a terminal half-life 3 times longer than EPO (r-HuEPO). Stimulates the division and differentiation of erythrocyte stem cells in the bone marrow and is a hormone produced by recombinant DNA techniques. Has a naturally occurring counterpart, erythropoietin. When administered once weekly, drug is 20 times more efficacious than rHuEPO (Egrie et al, 1997). NESP has five N-linked carbohydrate chains as compared to endogenous hormone and rHuEPO, which each have only three.

Metabolism: When given IV, terminal half-life is 25.3 hours (compared to 8.5 for rHuEPO), with significantly increased serum concentration-time curve and lower clearance as compared to rHuEPO. When given SQ, mean terminal half-life was 48.8 hours, with peak concentration 10% of the level achieved when given IV, with 37% bioavailability.

Dosage/Range:

- Per protocol; in renal failure patients, optimal dose appeared to be 0.45 μg/kg SQ or IV once weekly, although in some studies every-2-week dosing showed effectiveness.

Drug Preparation:

- Per protocol.

Drug Administration:

- SQ or IV.

Special Considerations:

- Studies have shown NESP to be equally effective when given weekly as compared to rHuEPO given TIW in patients with renal dysfunction (MacDougall et al, 1999).

Potential Toxicities/Side Effects and the Nursing Process

I. POTENTIAL ALTERATION IN OXYGENATION related to POLYCYTHEMIA

Defining Characteristics: Polycythemia may result if target range is exceeded (HCT of 40%).

Nursing Implications: Monitor weekly HCT: dose should be interrupted if HCT > 40%, then resumed at 75% dose once hematocrit is 36%. When HCT is stabilized, discuss monitoring HCT with physician (e.g., testing).

II. KNOWLEDGE DEFICIT related to SELF-ADMINISTRATION TECHNIQUE

Defining Characteristics: Drug is administered IV or SQ once a week to once every two weeks. If the drug is to be given SQ, patient must be instructed in self-injection technique.

Nursing Implications: Assess baseline psychomotor ability, knowledge, and willingness to learn technique of self-injection. Teach how to prepare drug, self-administer, and safely collect used syringes for proper disposal. Use written and video materials as supplements to teaching process and have patient correctly demonstrate technique prior to performing at home. Make referral to visiting-nurse agency to reinforce teaching.

Drug: oprelvekin (Neumega)

Class: Biological (interleukin).

Mechanism of Action: IL-11 is a thrombopoietin growth factor that stimulates directly the bone marrow stem cells and megakaryocyte progenitor cells so that the production of platelets is increased. Produced by recombinant DNA technology. Results in higher platelet nadir and accelerates time to platelet recovery postchemotherapy.

Metabolism: Peak serum concentrations reached in approximately 3 ± 2 hours, with a terminal half-life of approximately 7 ± 1 hours. Bioavailability is < 80%. Clearance decreases with age, and drug is rapidly cleared from the serum, is distributed to organs with high perfusion, metabolized, and excreted by the kidneys. Little intact drug is found in the urine.

Dosage/Range:
- Adults: 50 μg/kg SQ qd.

Drug Preparation/Administration:
- Available as single-use vial containing 5 mg of oprelvekin as a lyophilized, preservative-free powder. This is reconstituted with 1 mL sterile water for injection, USP, gently swirled to mix, and results in a concentration of 5 mg/1 mL in a single-use vial. NOTE: 5 mL of diluent is supplied, but only 1 mL should be withdrawn to reconstitute drug. Drug should be used within 3 hours of reconstitution. If not used immediately, store reconstitued solution in refrigerator or at room temperature, but DO NOT FREEZE OR SHAKE.
- The drug should be administered SQ every day (abdomen, thigh or hip, or upper arm). Begin daily administration 6–24 hours after the completion of chemotherapy, and continue until the postnadir platelet count is equal to or greater than 50,000 cells/mL. Do not give for more than 21 days, and stop at least 2 days before starting the next planned cycle of chemotherapy. Drug has *not* been evaluated in patients receiving chemotherapy regimens longer than 5 days, nor has it been shown to cause delayed myelosuppression (e.g., Mitomycin C, nitrosoureas).

Drug Interactions:
- Unknown.

Lab Effects/Interference:
- Increase in platelet count.
- Anemia associated with increased circulating plasma volume.

Special Considerations:
- Indicated for the prevention of severe thrombocytopenia and to decrease the need for platelet transfusion in patients with nonmyeloid malignancies receiving myelosuppressive chemotherapy.

- Causes fluid retention, so must be used with caution in patients with CHF or in patients receiving chronic diuretic therapy (sudden deaths reported in patients receiving ifosfamide and chronic diuretic therapy due to severe hypokalemia).
- Monitor platelet count frequently during oprelvekin therapy, and at the time of the expected nadir to identify when recovery will begin.
- Contraindicated in pregnant females and nursing mothers.

Potential Toxicities/Side Effects and the Nursing Process

I. ALTERATIONS IN FLUID AND ELECTROLYTE BALANCE related to FLUID RETENTION

Defining Characteristics: Most patients develop mild to moderate fluid retention (peripheral edema, dyspnea on exertion) but without weight gain. Fluid retention is reversible in a few days after drug is stopped. Patients with preexisting pleural effusions, pericardial effusions, or ascites may develop increased fluid, and may require drainage. Patients receiving chronic administration of potassium-excreting diuretics should be monitored extremely closely, as there are reports of sudden death due to severe hypokalemia in patients receiving ifosfamide and chronic diuretic therapy. Capillary leak syndrome has *not* been reported.

Nursing Implications: Assess baseline fluid and electrolyte balance, and weight prior to beginning drug. Assess presence of history of cardiac problems, or CHF, and risk of developing fluid volume overload. If diuretic therapy is ordered, monitor fluid and electrolyte balance very carefully, and replete electrolytes as indicated and ordered. Teach patients that mild-to-moderate peripheral edema and shortness of breath on exertion are likely to occur during the first week of treatment and will disappear after treatment ends. If the patient has CHF or pleural effusions, instruct to report worsening dyspnea to their nurse or physician.

II. ALTERATION IN CIRCULATION related to ATRIAL FIBRILLATION

Defining Characteristics: 10% of patients experience transient arrhythmias, including atrial fibrillation or flutter, after treatment with oprelvekin; it is believed to be due to increased plasma volume rather than the drug itself. Arrhythmias may be symptomatic, are usually brief in duration, and are not clinically significant. Some patients have spontaneous conversion to a normal sinus rhythm, while others require rate-controlling drug therapy. Most patients can receive drug without recurrence of the atrial arrhythmia. Risk factors for developing atrial arrhythmias are: (1) advancing age, (2) use of cardiac medications, (3) history of doxorubicin exposure, (4) history of atrial arrhythmia.

Other cardiovascular events include tachycardia, vasodilatation, palpitations, and syncope.

Nursing Implications: Assess baseline risk. If patient has history or presence of atrial arrhythmias, discuss with the physician potential benefit versus risk, and monitor very closely. Monitor baseline heart rate and other VS at each visit. Instruct patient to report immediately palpitations, lightheadedness, dizziness, or any other change in condition, especially if patient has any risk factors.

III. ALTERATION IN SENSORY PERCEPTION related to VISUAL BLURRING

Defining Characteristics: Transient, mild visual blurring has been reported, as has papilledema in 1.5% of patients. Dizziness (38%), insomnia (33%), and injection of conjunctiva (19%) may also occur.

Nursing Implications: Assess risk for papilledema (existing papilledema, CNS tumors); assess for changes in pupillary response in these patients. Teach patients that dizziness and insomnia may occur, and to change positions slowly and to hold onto supportive structures. If insomnia is severe, discuss sleep medications with physician.

IV. ALTERATION IN NUTRITION, LESS THAN FULL BODY REQUIREMENTS, related to GI SYMPTOMS

Defining Characteristics: Nausea, vomiting, mucositis, and diarrhea may occur, although percentage was not significantly greater than placebo control. Oral candidiasis occurred in 14% of patients, and this was significantly greater than control.

Nursing Implications: Instruct patient to report changes, and assess impact on nutrition. Inspect oral mucosa and teach patient to as well. Since patient is receiving myelosuppressive chemotherapy, teaching should include oral hygiene regimen, and frequent self-assessment by patient.

V. ALTERATIONS IN BREATHING PATTERN, INEFFECTIVE, POTENTIAL, related to DYSPNEA, COUGH

Defining Characteristics: Dyspnea (48% of patients), rhinitis (42%), increased cough (29%), pharyngitis (25%), and pleural effusions (10%) may occur.

Nursing Implications: Assess baseline pulmonary status and presence of pleural effusions. Instruct patient to report dyspnea and any other changes. Discuss significant changes with physician.

Drug: palifermin (Kepivance)

Class: Keratinocyte Growth Factor.

Mechanism of Action: Palifermin is a keratinocyte growth factor (KGF) produced by recombinant DNA technology, similar to the naturally occurring, endogenous KGF. Once EGF binds to its receptor found on epithelial cells including those of the tongue, buccal mucosa, mammary gland, skin (hair follicles and sebaceous gland), lung, liver, and the lens of the eye, it stimulates proliferation, differentiation, and migration of epithelial cells. KGF decreases the incidence and duration of severe stomatitis in patients with hematologic malignancies who undergo high dose chemotherapy and radiation therapy with stem cell rescue.

Metabolism: Palifermin has an elimination half-life of 4.5 hour (average).

Dosage/Range:

- 60 mcg/kg/day IV bolus for 3 consecutive days before and 3 consecutive days after myelotoxic therapy for a total of 6 doses.

Drug Preparation:

- Reconstitute Kepivance lyophilized powder with Sterile Water for Injection USP, asceptically, by slowly injecting 1.2 mL Sterile Water for Injection USP to yield final volume of 5 mg/mL. Do not shake or agitate the vial.
- Protect from light.
- Reconstituted solution may be refrigerated in its carton for up to 24 hours at 2°–8° C (36°–46° F); prior to injection, may leave at room temperature for up to 1 hour protected from light. Inspect for discoloration or particulates, and if found, do not use.
- Do not filter drug during reconstitution or administration.

Drug Administration:

- Pre-myelotoxic therapy: the 3rd dose should be 24–48 hours before myelotoxic chemotherapy is administered.
- Post-myelotoxic therapy: the first of the 3 doses should be given after, but on the same day of the hematopoietic stem cell infusion, and at least 4 days after the most recent administration of palifermin.

Drug Interactions:

- Heparin: palifermin binds to heparin, so drugs should not be used concomitantly; flush central line well with saline prior to administration of palifermin.
- Myelotoxic chemotherapy: if given with chemotherapy, KGF increases the severity and duration of oral mucositis. Palifermin should NOT be administered within 24 hours before, during infusion of, or after the administration of myelotoxic chemotherapy.

Lab Effects/Interference:

- Increase in serum amylase and lipase.

Special Considerations:

- Palifermin is FDA-approved to decrease the incidence and duration of severe oral mucositis in patients with hematologic malignancies receiving myelotoxic therapy requiring hermatopoietic stem cell support.
- Drug is being studied in the treatment of patients with solid tumors, but the safety and efficacy has not been established at this time. KFG in laboratory studies can enhance malignant cell growth in tissues with KFG receptors.
- Drug is contraindicated in patients with known hypersensitivity to *E. coli* derived proteins.
- Drug is embryotoxic to lab animals when given in higher doses; drug should be used in pregnant women only when the potential benefit to the mother exceeds the risk to the fetus.

Potential Toxicities/Side Effects and the Nursing Process

I. POTENTIAL ALTERATION IN SKIN INTEGRITY related to SKIN RASH

Defining Characteristics: Skin rash was the most common serious adverse reaction, and occurred in 62% of patients in clinical studies. Skin toxicity was manifested by rash, erythema (32%), edema (28%), pruritis (35%). Median time to onset was 6 days after the first of 3 doses, and lasted a median of 5 days.

Nursing Implications: Teach patient that skin changes may occur and to report them. Teach patient self-care strategies to promote comfort and reduce the risk of infection.

II. ALTERATION IN NUTRITION AND COMFORT, related to ORAL TOXICITIES

Defining Characteristics: Dysesthesia, tongue discoloration, tongue thickening, alterations in taste occur related to the increased keratin layer on the lining of the oral cavity.

Nursing Implications: Inform patient that these side effects may occur. Teach patient systematic oral cleansing after meals and at hs. Inform patient to report discomfort or inability to chew or swallow, and develop plan with measures to promote comfort and nutrition. Many patients are already receiving TPN. If taste alterations are bothersome, suggest dietitian referral for measures to stimulate taste.

III. ALTERATION IN COMFORT related to PAIN, ARTHRALGIAS, AND DYSESTHESIAS

Defining Characteristics: Dysesthesia, pain, and arthralgias may occur and affect about 12% of patients.

Nursing Implications: Assess baseline comfort, as well as existing arthralgias and dysesthesias. Perform a basic neurologic assessment. Inform patient these side effects may occur and to report them if they occur. Develop a plan of care that includes self-care activities to promote comfort, such as the use of heat or cold for arthralgias. If pain related to stomatitis is severe, then patient-controlled analgesia may be necessary. Teach patient to report any dysesthesias, hyperesthesias, hypoesthesia, or paresthesias that occur. Develop a plan to minimize discomfort, such as keeping sheets off feet if patient has hyperesthesias.

Agent: pegfilgrastim (Neulasta)

Class: Cytokine, CSF.

Mechanism of Action: Recombinant DNA protein (G-CSF) that regulates the production of neutrophils in the bone marrow (proliferation, differentiation, activation of mature neutrophils). Drug is produced by the insertion of the human G-CSF gene into Escherichia coli bacteria. Drug has longer half-life and different excretion pattern as compared to the parent drug, filgrastim.

Metabolism: Clearance of drug decreases with increased dose, body weight, and is directly related to the number of neutrophils so that as neutrophil recovery begins after myelosuppressive chemotherapy, serum concentration of pegfilgrastim declines rapidly. In patients with increased body weight, systemic exposure to the drug was higher despite dose normalized for body weight. Pharmacokinetics variable, with a half-life of 15–80 hours after SQ injection. Pharmacokinetics did not vary with age (elderly) or gender.

Dosage/Range:
- 6 mg SQ once per chemotherapy cycle.

Drug Preparation:
- Drug available in refrigerated 6 mg (0.6mL) prefilled syringes with UltraSafe needle guards.
- Unopened vials should be stored in the refrigerator at 2–8°C (36–46°F) in the original carton to protect from light.
- Avoid shaking. Screen for visible particulate matter or discoloration and do not use if found.

- Remove from refrigerator 30 minutes prior to injection, but drug may be left at room temperature for up to 48 hours.
- If drug accidently freezes, allow to thaw in the refrigerator prior to administration; if frozen a second time, discard.

Drug Administration:
- SQ × 1 *at least 14 days prior to or more than 24 hours after* chemotherapy administration.
- Following injection, activate UltraSafe Needle Guard holding hands behind the needle, and sliding the guard forward until the needle is completely covered and guard clicks into place. If no click is heard, drop entire syringe/needle into sharps disposal container.

Drug Interactions:
- Lithium: may potentiate the release of neutrophils from the bone marrow: monitor neutrophil count more frequently.

Lab Effects/Interference:
- Increased white blood cell count and neutrophil count.
- Elevated LDH, alkaline phosphatase, uric acid may occur but is reversible and less frequent than with filgrastim.

Special Considerations:
- Indicated to decrease the incidence of infection (febrile neutropenia) in patients with non-myeloid malignancies receiving myelosuppressive anti-cancer therapy associated with a significant incidence of febrile neutropenia.
- Contraindicated in patients with known hypersensitivity to *E. coli* derived proteins, pegfilgrastim, filgrastim, or any product component; contraindicated in peripheral blood progenitor cell (PBPC) mobilization as the drug has not been studied in this population.
- Splenic rupture has been reported in patients receiving the parent drug, filgrastim, for PBPC. If a patient receiving pegfilgrastim complains of left upper abdominal or shoulder tip pain, s/he should be evaluated immediately for an enlarged spleen or splenic rupture.
- Adult Respiratory Distress Syndrome (ARDS) has been reported in neutropenic patients with sepsis receiving the parent drug filgrastim, probably related to the influx of neutrophils to inflammed pulmonary sites. Neutropenic patient receiving pegfilgrastim who develop fever, lung infiltrates, or respiratory distress should be immediately evaluated for ARDS. If ARDS is suspected, pegfilgrastim should be stopped until ARDS resolves with appropriate medical care.
- Severe sickle cell crisis, rarely fatal, has been reported in patients with sickle cell disease (homozygous sickle cell anemia, sickle/hemoglobin C disease, sickle/α-thalassemia) who received filgrastim, the parent drug. Pegfilgrastim should be used in this population only when the potential ben-

efit outweighs the risk, and patients should be well hydrated and closely monitored for sickle cell crisis, with immediate intervention.

- Pegfilgrastim should not be administered within *14 days prior to* and *for 24 hours after chemotherapy administration* as this will increase the sensitivity of rapidly dividing myeloid cells to the chemotherapy.
- G-CSF receptor to which drug binds is also found in tumor cell lines (some myeloid, T-lymphoid, lung, head and neck, and bladder cancer) and the potential for the drug to be a tumor growth factor exists.
- Drug should be used in pregnant women only when the potential benefit outweighs risk of fetal harm as there are no adequate controlled studies in pregnant women, and laboratory animals had increased number of abortions and wavy ribs in fetuses.
- Do not use in infants, children, and smaller adolescents whose weight is < 45 kg.

Potential Toxicities/Side Effects (dose and schedule-dependent) and the Nursing Process

I. ALTERATION IN COMFORT related to SKELETAL PAIN, HEADACHE, MYALGIA, ABDOMINAL PAIN, ARTHRALGIA

Defining Characteristics: Patients (26%) may report transient mild to moderate skeletal pain believed due to the expansion of cells in the bone marrow in response to G-CSF. About 12% used non-opioid analgesics and less than 6% required opioid analgesics. Leukocytosis of more than 100–109/L occurred in < 1% of patients. Other pain related to headache, myalgia and arthralgia, and abdominal pain may occur less commonly, but is easily managed.

Nursing Implications: Teach patient bone pain may occur and discuss use of nonsteroidal anti-inflammatory drugs with patient and physician for symptom management. Monitor white blood cell count (WBC), hematocrit and platelet count as appropriate prior to each cycle of chemotherapy. Teach patient headache, myalgia, arthralgia, abdominal pain may occur and to report them if they do not respond to usual management strategies.

II. ALTERATION IN NUTRITION, POTENTIAL, related to NAUSEA, VOMITING, CONSTIPATION, DIARRHEA, ANOREXIA, STOMATITIS, MUCOSITIS

Defining Characteristics: Nutritional symptoms are rarely reported and may be related to the underlying malignancy.

Nursing Implications: Perform baseline patient nutritional assessment, history of nausea and vomiting, bowel elimination pattern, oral assessment, and usual appetite. Teach patient to report these sideeffects so that they can be evaluated. Teach patient self-care measures, including dietary modification, local comfort measures as well as pharmacologic management as determined by the nurse/physician team. Teach patient to report symptoms that persist and do not respond to the planned therapy.

III. ALTERATION IN SKIN INTEGRITY, POTENTIAL related to PERIPHERAL EDEMA, ALOPECIA

Defining Characteristics: Peripheral edema and alopecia are rarely reported, and may be related to other factors, such as the chemotherapy agents administered.

Nursing Implications: Perform baseline skin and scalp assessment. Teach patient to report development of peripheral edema, hair loss. Discuss with patient acceptable management strategies depending upon impact of hair loss, if it occurs. Assess degree of peripheral edema if it develops, and discuss significant edema with physician to determine etiology and management. Teach patient local skin care, including avoidance of tight clothing and shoes, keeping skin moisturized to prevent cracking, and local comfort measures.

IV. KNOWLEDGE DEFICIT related to SELF-ADMINISTRATION TECHNIQUE

Defining Characteristics: Drug is administered once per chemotherapy cycle, more than 14 days prior to chemotherapy administration or more than 24 hours after chemotherapy is given.

Nursing Implications: Assess baseline psychomotor ability, knowledge, and willingness to learn technique of self-injection. Teach how to refrigerate drug, self-administer using pre-filled syringes, how to activate needle guard, and safely collect used syringes for proper disposal. Drug insert has "Information for Patients and Caregivers." Use written and video supplements in teaching process and have patient correctly demonstrate technique prior to performing at home. Make referral to visiting-nurse agency to reinforce teaching if needed. Teach patient telephone number and whom to call if questions or problems arise, and ensure that patient can correctly repeat information.

Drug: PIXY-321 (GM-CSF/IL-3 fusion protein)

Class: Fusion protein.

Mechanism of Action: Synergism of IL-3 together with GM-CSF causes a rapid rise in neutrophils due to GM-CSF and a slower rise in platelets due to IL-3.

Metabolism: Unknown in humans.

Dosage/Range:

- 750–1000 μg/m^2 SQ or IV 24 hours after chemotherapy per protocol.

Drug Preparation/Administration:

- SQ or IV (per protocol).

Drug Interactions:

- Under investigation.

Lab Effects/Interference:

- Increase in neutrophils, with slower increase in platelets.

Special Considerations:

- Has been studied in patients with breast or ovarian cancers, and patients undergoing BMT. In patients with breast cancer receiving PIXY-321, there was decreased incidence and duration of severe (grades 3 and 4) neutropenia, with more rapid recovery of neutrophils than those patients not receiving it; however, patients had more pronounced systemic toxicity and thrombocytopenia in later cycles of therapy.
- Limited data as to toxicity profile in humans, but it is expected that toxicity from each component (i.e., flulike symptoms), did not occur at doses > 500 μg/m^2.

Potential Toxicities/Side Effects (Dose- and Schedule-Dependent) and the Nursing Process

I. POTENTIAL ALTERATION IN SKIN INTEGRITY related to ERYTHEMA AT INJECTION SITE

Defining Characteristics: This is the most common toxicity at doses up to 500 μg/m^2. More toxicity may be seen with higher doses.

Nursing Implications: Select and rotate sites, assess and monitor skin for reaction and skin integrity. Implement strategies to maintain intact skin.

II. ALTERATION IN COMFORT related to FEVER

Defining Characteristics: Fever is mild if it occurs. Flulike symptoms do not occur at doses < 500 μg/m^2, but toxicity may be more pronounced at higher doses. Toxicity is being studied in humans at higher doses.

Nursing Implications: Monitor T at baseline and during therapy. Teach patient to take own T and to report elevations. If severe, discuss premedication with physician.

Drug: recombinant human keratinocyte growth factor (Palifermin, rHuKGF) (investigational)

Class: Cytokine.

Mechanism of Action: Selectively stimuates the growth and differentiation of epithelial cells. Reduces duration and incidence of severe oral mucositis in patients undergoing high-dose chemotherapy, radiotherapy, and total body irradiation (TBI) followed by stem cell support, such as peripheral blood progenitor cell transplantation (PBPCT).

Metabolism: Unknown.

Dosage/Range:
Per protocol, but in one study 60 μg/kg/day for 3 consecutive days before TBI and 3 consecutive days after PBPCT.

Drug Preparation/Administration: Per protocol.

Drug Interactions: Unknown.

Lab Effects/Interference: Transient, asymptomatic increases in serum amylase and lipase.

Special Considerations:
- Preliminary studies show drug significantly reduces duration and incidence of severe oral mucositis of patients with hematologic malignancies undergoing PBPCT after TBI and chemotherapy conditioning (Spielberger et al, 2003).
- Keratinocytes stimulate the growth and development of epithelial cells, such as those lining the oral mucosa; keratinocyte growth factor occurs naturally, and stimulates the growth of keratinocytes.

Potential Toxicities/Side Effects and the Nursing Process

I. POTENTIAL ALTERATION IN SKIN INTEGRITY related to SKIN AND ORAL ERYTHEMA

Defining Characteristics: Mild to moderate skin and oral erythema may occur, with or without edema.

Nursing Implications: Assess oral mucosa and skin baseline, and during treatment. Teach patient to self-assess, and use systematic cleansing pc and hs.

Agent: sargramostim (Leukine, GM-CSF) (investigational)

Class: Cytokine.

Mechanism of Action: Granulocyte-macrophage colony-stimulating factor that regulates growth of all levels of granulocytes and stimulates production of monocytes and macrophages; GM-CSF induces synthesis of other cytokines and enhances cytotoxic action. Manufactured using recombinant DNA technology.

Metabolism: Peak serum levels 2–3 hours after injection. Initial half-life 12–17 min, with a terminal half-life of 1.6–2.6 hours.

Dosage/Range:

- 250 μg/m²/day as a 2–hour infusion for 21 days, beginning 2–4 hours after autologous marrow infusion, > 24 hours after last chemotherapy dose, and > 12 hours after last radiation treatment; administer for 14 days when used for BMT failure.
- Neutrophil recovery after chemotherapy for AML: 250 μg/m²/day IV over 4 hours beginning on day 11 (4 days after completion of induction chemotherapy if day 10 bone marrow biopsy shows hypoplasia with < 5% blasts).
- Mobilization of peripheral blood progenitor cells (PBPCs): 250 μg/m²/day IV over 24 hours or SQ daily; continue through PBPC collection.

Drug Preparation:

- Reconstitute per manufacturer's directions. Do *not* filter.
- Further dilute in 0.9% Sodium Chloride.
- If final concentration is < 10 μg/mL, human albumin (dilute to final concentration of 0.1% human albumin in 0.9% Sodium Chloride) should be added before adding GM-CSF to prevent absorption of drug in IV container and tubing.

Drug Administration:

- Administer IV over 2 hours, or according to research protocol.

Drug Interactions:

- Corticosteroids, lithium: may ↑ myeloproliferation.
- Sargramostim effect may be ↓ in patients who have received chemotherapy containing alkylating agents, anthracyclines, antibiotics, antimetabolites.

Lab Effects/Interference:

- Increased stem cell, granulocyte, macrophage production.
- Serum glucose, BUN, cholesterol, bili, creatinine, ALT, alk phos; ↓ serum albumin, Ca.
- Leukocytosis, eosinophilia.

Special Considerations:
- Indicated for acceleration of bone marrow recovery (myeloid cells) after autologous or allogeneic BMT; following induction chemotherapy in acute myelogenous leukemia; mobilization and following transplant of autologous PBPCs; and in BMT failure or engraftment delay.
- Produces fever more commonly than G-CSF, and fluid retention.
- Stop drug when WBC > 50,000 cells/mm^3, or ANC > 20,000 cells/mm^3.
- Administer > 24 hours after last chemotherapy, or > 12 hours after radiotherapy.

Potential Toxicities/Side Effects (Dose- and Schedule-Dependent) and the Nursing Process

I. ALTERATION IN COMFORT related to FLULIKE SYNDROME

Defining Characteristics: Fever, myalgias, chills, rigors, fatigue, and headache may occur.

Nursing Implications: Assess baseline T, VS, neurologic status, and comfort level, and monitor q4–6h if patient in hospital. Discuss with physician premedication and regular dosing of antipyretic (e.g., acetaminophen ± diphenhydramine, NSAID). Teach patient self-care measures, including monitoring T, comfort level, self-administration of prescribed medications prior to dose and regularly postdose, as well as the use of heat or cold for myalgias, arthralgias. Encourage patient to increase oral fluids and alternate rest and activity periods. If patient is in hospital and experiences rigor, discuss with physician IV meperidine (25 mg IV every 15 minutes to maximum 100 mg in 1 hour) and monitor BP for hypotension.

II. ALTERATION IN COMFORT related to SKELETAL PAIN

Defining Characteristics: Transient skeletal pain may occur and is believed to be due to bone marrow expansion in response to GM-CSF.

Nursing Implications: Teach patient this may occur and discuss use of NSAIDS with patient and physician for symptom management. Monitor WBC, ANC twice weekly during therapy; dose reduction or discontinuation depends on purpose of drug.

III. POTENTIAL ALTERATION IN SKIN INTEGRITY related to RASH, FLUSHING, INJECTION SITE REACTION

Defining Characteristics: Facial flushing, generalized rash, and inflammation at injection site may occur.

Nursing Implications: Teach patient that these may occur, and instruct to report rash, inflammation. Teach patient to rotate injection sites. Assess rash, and teach symptomatic management.

IV. POTENTIAL ALTERATION IN OXYGENATION related to DYSPNEA AND FLUID RETENTION

Defining Characteristics: Some patients developed dyspnea during initial 2–6 hours of continuous infusion GM-CSF, thought to be due to migration of neutrophils in the lung. Fluid retention may also occur.

Nursing Implications: Assess baseline pulmonary and fluid status. Teach patient to weigh self daily and instruct to report any changes in weight, breathing (e.g., dyspnea).

Agent: tumor necrosis factor (TNF) (investigational)

Class: Cytokine.

Mechanism of Action: Binds to target cell membranes. TNF (cachectin) is produced by activated macrophages. It appears to halt cell growth in G_2 phase of cell cycle (cytostatic), is cytotoxic, and may cause vascular endothelial injury in tumor capillaries, leading to hemorrhage and necrosis of tumor cells. It also activates immune elements: increased NK cytotoxic activity, increased production of NK cells, B cells, and neutrophils.

Metabolism: Half-life is 20 minutes when given as IV bolus but varies with dose and route of administration.

Dosage/Range:
- Per individual protocol.

Drug Preparation:
- Per individual protocol.

Drug Administration:
- IVB or continuous infusion SQ and IM. Refer to protocol for guidelines. When given IV, agent must be administered using a solution of 0.9% Sodium Chloride containing human serum albumin at a concentration of 2 mg/mL. This albumin prevents TNF from adhering to bag or tubing; prime tubing with solution before adding TNF to bag.

Drug Interactions:
- None reported, but data is being accumulated in clinical trials.

Lab Effects/Interference:
- Granulocytopenia, thrombocytopenia.

Potential Toxicities/Side Effects (Dose- and Schedule-Dependent) and the Nursing Process

I. ALTERATION IN COMFORT related to FLULIKE SYMPTOMS

Defining Characteristics: Fever to 39–40°C (102–104°F) and chills occur within 1–6 hours of dose, dependent on administration route; rigor, fatigue, myalgia, arthralgia, headache (dull, aching), and back pain may occur. Gradual disappearance of symptoms with repeated dosing (tachyphylaxis).

Nursing Implications: Assess baseline T, VS, neurologic status, and comfort level, and monitor every 4–6 hours if patient in hospital. Discuss with physician premedication and regular dosing of antipyretic (e.g., acetaminophen ± diphenhydramine, NSAID). Teach patient self-care measures, including monitoring T, comfort level, self-administration of prescribed medications prior to dose and regularly postdose, as well as the use of heat or cold for myalgias, arthralgias. Encourage patient to increase oral fluids and alternate rest and activity periods. If patient is in hospital and experiences rigor, discuss with physician IV meperidine (25 mg IV every 15 minutes to maximum 100 mg in 1 hour) and monitor BP for hypotension.

II. POTENTIAL ALTERATION IN NUTRITION, LESS THAN BODY REQUIREMENTS, related to ANOREXIA, NAUSEA, VOMITING, DIARRHEA

Defining Characteristics: Do not appear dose-dependent. Weight loss is not significant, and nausea/vomiting can be effectively managed.

Nursing Implications: Assess baseline nutritional status. Teach patient potential side effects, and self-care measures, including oral hygiene and preparing favorite high-calorie, high-protein foods ahead of time so patient can snack when hungry. Teach self-administration of prescribed antiemetics and antidiarrheals as needed. Refer to dietitian as appropriate.

III. ALTERATION IN CARDIAC OUTPUT related to ORTHOSTATIC HYPOTENSION

Defining Characteristics: Transient orthostatic hypotension (SBP < 90 mm Hg) may occur after IV or SQ injection and resolve with IV saline infusion. Hypertension may occur secondary to rigors.

Nursing Implications: Assess baseline cardiovascular status and orthostatic BP. Teach patient to change position slowly, to report light-headedness, and to increase oral fluids to 3 L/day.

IV. POTENTIAL FOR INFECTION AND BLEEDING related to GRANULOCYTOPENIA, THROMBOCYTOPENIA

Defining Characteristics: Dose-related, especially if > 100 mg/m^2 day, with normalization when treatment terminated.

Nursing Implications: Assess baseline CBC, WBC, differential, and platelet count, and signs/symptoms of infection or bleeding. Discuss any abnormalities with physician before drug administration. Teach patient signs/symptoms of infection, bleeding, and instruct to report them immediately. Teach patient self-care measures to minimize infection and bleeding, including avoidance of OTC aspirin-containing medications, and oral hygiene regimen.

V. POTENTIAL SENSORY/PERCEPTUAL ALTERATIONS related to NEUROLOGIC TOXICITY

Defining Characteristics: Seizures, confusion, aphasia may occur transiently and rarely.

Nursing Implications: Assess baseline mental status and history of seizures. Instruct patient to report any changes and ensure patient safety.

VI. POTENTIAL ALTERATION IN OXYGENATION related to DYSPNEA

Defining Characteristics: Dyspnea may occur, possibly related to alveolar endothelial damage.

Nursing Implications: Assess patient's risk (preexisting pulmonary dysfunction) and baseline pulmonary status. Instruct patient to report any changes.

Chapter 3

Antineoplastic Treatment Agonists: Radiosensitizers, Chemosensitizers, and Chemical Adjuncts

Radiation is the third major cancer treatment modality. Ionizing radiation causes cell damage and death to frequently dividing cells within the radiation port (site being radiated). Damage to DNA in malignant cells depends on the oxygenation of the tumor—cells that are well supplied with oxygen are sensitive to radiation effects, while those that are hypoxic (i.e., large, necrotic tumors) are radioresistant. Oxygen appears to be necessary at the time of radiation because it promotes formation of free radicals, causing DNA damage and preventing DNA repair (Noll, 1992).

Certain drugs called *radiosensitizers* may be administered concurrently with radiation therapy to increase the radiation damage to sensitive cells, thus increasing the tumor response (i.e., tumor reduction) to radiation therapy. Radiosensitizers are classified into three broad groups based on ability to sensitize hypoxic tumor cells and mechanism of action (Noll, 1992).

Hypoxic cell sensitizers mimic oxygen in chemical reactions that occur after ionizing radiotherapy, thus making the hypoxic cells sensitive to radiation damage. Examples are etanidazole, Fluosol DA with 100% oxygen breathing, and buthionine, which depletes sulfhydryl-containing compounds from damaged cells so they are unable to repair their DNA.

Nonhypoxic cell sensitizers include the halogenated pyrimidines, which, because they are analogues of the DNA pyrimidine thymidine, are actively taken up by dividing cells and incorporated into DNA. This enhances radiosensitivity of the tumor cells and theoretically increases tumor response to radiotherapy. Drugs undergoing clinical testing include bromodeoxyuridine (BUdR) and iododeoxyuridine (IUdR).

A third group is composed of *chemotherapy agents* that are capable of radiosensitization. They are administered either prior to radiotherapy as part of combined modality therapy or concurrently in low doses to enhance radiosensitivity of tumor cells. These drugs include cisplatin, 5-fluorouracil, gemcitabine, carboplatin, paclitaxel, gemcitabine, bleomycin, and mitomycin. Recent research on gemcitabine showed that the radiosensitization mechanism of action is different than when the drug is used as a chemotherapy agent (cytotoxic): When the cancer cells start to move through the Synthesis phase of the cell cycle and the DNA strands are damaged by radiation, the cell undergoes programmed cell death (apoptosis) [Symon Z et al, 2002].

Finally, a fourth group called *molecular targeted agents* can also produce radiosensitization, thus increasing the therapeutic index (so cancer cells are killed rather than normal cells). These include epidermal growth factor receptor (EGFR) tyrosine kinase inhibitors cetuximab (Erbitux), the EGFR tyrosine kinase inhibitor gefitinib (Iressa), and farnesyl transferase inhibitors [Lawrence TS and Nyati MK, 2002].

This is a promising frontier in cancer treatment, and the next decade will bring greater understanding and options in radiotherapy, chemosensitization, and new adjuncts.

References

Brown JM. Therapeutic Targets In Radiotherapy. *Int J Radiat Oncol Biol Phys* 2001; 49(2):319–326

Bunn PA. Triplet Combination Chemotherapy and Targeted Therapy Regimens. *Oncology* 2001;15(3 Suppl 6):26–32

Coleman CN. Radiation and Chemotherapy Sensitizers and Protectors. Chabner Band, Longo DL, (eds), *Cancer Chemotherapy and Biotherapy,* 2nd ed. Philadelphia: Lippincott Raven;1996;553–584

Coleman CN, Bump EA, Kramer RA. Chemical Modifiers of Cancer Treatment. *J Clin Oncol* 1989;6:709–733

Craighead PS, Pearcey R, Stuart G. A Phase I/II Evaluation of Tirapazamine Administered Intravenously Concurrent with Cisplatin and Radiotherapy in Women with Locally Advanced Cervical Cancer. *Int J Radiat Oncol Biol Phys* 2000;48(3):791–795

Denny WA, Wilson WR. Tirapazamine: A Bioreductive Anticancer Drug that Exploits Tumour Hypoxia. *Expert Opin Investig Drugs* 2000;9(12):2889–2901

Dische S. Chemical Sensitizers for Hypoxic Cells: A Decade of Experience in Clinical Radiotherapy. *Radiother Oncol* 1985;3:97–111

Fowler JF. Chemical Modifiers of Radiosensitivity: Theory and Reality: A Review. *Int J Radiat Oncol Biol Phys* 1985;11:665–674

Goldberg Z, Evans J, Birrell G, Brown JM. An Investigation of the Molecular Basis for the Synergistic Interaction of Tirapazamine and Cisplatin. *Int J Radiat Oncol Biol Phys* 2001;49(1):175–182

Kinsella TJ, Mitchell JB, Russo A, et al. The Use of Halogenated Thymidine Analogues as Clinical Radiosensitizers: Rationale, Current Status, and Future Prospects. *Int J of Radiat Oncol Biol Phys* 1984;10:1399–1406

Lawrence TS, Nyati MK. Small-molecule Tyrosine Kinase Inhibitors as Radiosensitizers. *Semin Radiat Oncol* 2002;12 (suppl 2):33–36

Mallinkckrodt, Phosphocol P32 Package Insert. St. Louis: Mallinkckrodt Inc. 1997

Noll L. Chemical Modifiers of Radiation Therapy. In Hassey-Dow K, Hilderly LJ, (eds), *Nursing Care in Radiation Oncology* Philadelphia: WB Saunders; 1992
Novartis Pharmaceuticals Corp (2005) Exjade. East Hanover, NJ: Novartis Pharmaceuticals Corporation
Rischin D, Peters L, Hicks R, et al. Phase I Trial of Concurrent Tirapazamine, Cisplatin, and Radiotherapy in Patients with Advanced Head and Neck Cancer. *J Clin Oncol* 2000;19(2):535–545
Symon Z, Davis M, McGinn CJ, et al. Concurrent Chemoradiotherapy with Gemcitabine and Cisplatin for Pancreatic Cancer: From Laboratory to the Clinic. *Int J Radiat Oncol Biol Phys* 2002;53:140–145

Drug: chromic phosphate P32 suspension (Phosphocol™ P32)

Class: Radiopharmaceutical agent.

Mechanism of Action: Provides local irradiation by beta emission and is administered into cavities for the treatment of peritoneal or pleural effusions due to metastatic cancer; it may also be given interstitially to treat cancer.

Metabolism: Phosphorus P32 decays by beta emission with a physical half-life of 14.3 days, with a residence time of 495 hours. The mean energy of the beta particle is 695 keV. Distribution in the pleural or peritoneal space is nonuniform, with extremes of local dosage.

Dosage/Range:
- Intraperitoneal: 370–740 megabecquerels (10–20 millicuries).
- Intrapleural: 222–444 megabecquerels (6–12 millicuries).
- Interstitial (e.g., prostate): based on estimated gram weight of tumor, about 3.7–18.5 megabecquerels/gm (0.2–0.5 millicuries/gm).
- 37 kilobecquerels = 1 millicurie (mCi) = 7.3 grays = 730 rads.

Drug Preparation:
- None.
- Available as chromic phosphate P32 suspension in 10–mL vials containing 555 megabecquerels (15 mCi) with a concentration of up to 185 megabecquerels (5 mCi)/mL.

Drug Administration:
- Always given into pleural or peritoneal cavity, or may be given interstitially (e.g., prostate), but NEVER intravenously.
- For pleural effusions:

Interventional radiologist visualizes pleural space with ultrasound to ensure that it is open without adhesions.
Interventional radiologist places a thoracentesis catheter in the pleural space, having a three-way stopcock, and verifies position by ultrasound; removes pleural fluid by opening ports 1 and 2.

Port 2 is closed and port 3 is opened for a qualified M.D. to administer chromic phosphate P32 suspension (injecting 6–12 mCi into the port, then rinses with 10 mL 0.9% NS).
Close ports and ensure that they are closed to prevent leakage of radionucleotide and radiation contamination. The catheter is then removed. If there is leakage or contamination, refer to institutional policy/procedure for radiation spill.
Reposition patient from supine to prone, onto the right side, and onto the left side, and lastly, have the patient stand and bend over.
CXR is done to make certain there is no pneumothorax.
Patient is given one-month follow-up appointment for a CXR, and is asked to return if shortness of breath occurs, as this may signify reaccumulation of effusion.

Drug Interactions:
- Unknown.

Lab Effects/Interference:
- Unknown.

Special Considerations:
Eligible candidates for treatment of pleural effusion:
- History of prior pleurodesis with talc.
- Evidence of pleural plaques.
- Prior treatment using a chest tube.
- Emphysema.
- History of pleural asbestos exposure.

Contraindications:
- Presence of ulcerative tumors.
- Pregnant or nursing mothers, unless benefit outweighs risks.
- Presence of large tumor masses.
- Risk of improper placement: intestinal fibrosis or necrosis, and chronic fibrosis of body wall have been described.
- Radiation damage may occur if injected interstitially or into a loculation.
- Treatment may be less effective if effusion bloody.

Potential Toxicities/Side Effects and the Nursing Process

I. POTENTIAL FOR INFECTION, BLEEDING, AND FATIGUE related to BONE MARROW DEPRESSION

Defining Characteristics: Bone marrow suppression, if it occurs, is transitory.

Nursing Implications: Assess baseline WBC, differential, platelet and Hgb/HCT prior to treatment, as well as for signs/symptoms of infection or bleeding. Teach patient signs/symptoms of infection and bleeding and to report these immediately; teach patient self-care measures to minimize risk of infection and bleeding. This includes avoidance of crowds, proximity to people with infections, and avoidance of OTC aspirin-containing medications. Teach patient to report fatigue, and teach measures to conserve energy, such as alternating rest and activity periods. Discuss transfusion of red blood cells as needed.

II. PAIN related to PLEURITIS, PERITONITIS, AND ABDOMINAL CRAMPING

Defining Characteristics: Symptoms depend upon area treated, with pleuritis arising from treatment of pleural effusion, and peritonitis, abdominal cramping, and nausea arising from treatment of peritoneal effusion.

Nursing Implications: Assess baseline pain level. Teach patient of potential side effects and to report them. Teach patient symptom-management techniques and discuss with physician medications for analgesia and nausea. Teach patient to report if symptoms do not subside or improve.

III. ALTERATION IN COMFORT related to RADIATION SICKNESS

Defining Characteristics: Exposure to ionizing radiation causes symptoms, the severity of which are dependent upon the volume of radiation, the length of time of exposure, and the area of the body affected. Moderate symptoms may occur from treatment with chromic phosphate P32 suspension, and these include headache, nausea, vomiting, anorexia, and diarrhea. Long-term exposure may result in sterility, malformation of the fetus in a pregnant woman, and cancer.

Nursing Implications: Assess baseline comfort level. Teach patient that moderate symptoms may arise. Teach patient to report symptoms as soon as possible, and discuss management strategies. Discuss pharmacologic management of nausea/vomiting and diarrhea with physician and give patient prescriptions for antiemetic and antidiarrheal medications for PRN use.

Drug: deferasirox tablets for oral suspension (Exjade)

Class: Iron chelating agent.

Mechanism of Action: Orally active chelator that binds iron, thus preventing iron overload resulting from multiple red blood cell transfusions (transfusional hemosiderosis).

Metabolism: Drug is absorbed after oral ingestion with 70% bioavailability (compared to an IV dose), achieving maximum plasma concentrations at a median of 1.5–4 hours. Area Under the Curve (AUC) was increased when drug is taken with food. Drug is highly (~99%) protein bound, primarily to serum albumin. Deferasirox is metabolized via the glucuronidation pathway, and excreted in the bile. Although UGT1A1 and to a lesser extent, UGT1A3, are involved, there is no apparent induction or inhibition of metabolic enzymes. Drug and metabolites are primarily excreted in the feces (84%), and to a lesser extent via the kidneys (8%). Mean elimination half-life is 8–16 hours. In children < 6 years of age, systemic exposure was 50% lower than adults.

Dosage/Range:

- Therapy is recommended when a patient has evidence of chronic iron overload (transfusion of ~100 mL/kg of packed red blood cells or 20 units for a 40 kg patient, and a serum ferritin consistently > 1000 mcg/L).
- Initial daily dose: 20 mg/kg qd.
- Maintenance: Adjust dose of deferasirox tablets for oral suspension every 3–6 months, based on trends of monthly serum ferritin levels. Dose adjustments should be made in increments of 5–10 mg/kg based on response and therapeutic goals (e.g., maintenance or reduction of iron burden). Dose should not exceed 30 mg/kg per day. Dose should be interrupted if serum ferritin falls consistently < 500 mcg/L.

Dose Adjustments

- Increased serum creatinine (reduction, interruption, or discontinuation): in clinical trials, dose was reduced by 10 mg/kg if serum creatinine increase on 2 consecutive measures was > 33% in patients > 15 years old, or > 33% and greater than the age-appropriate upper limit of normal in patients < 15 years old.
- Increased liver function tests (LFTs): dose reduction, interruption or discontinuation if increase in LFTs severe or persistent.
- Severe rash: drug may be interrupted, and reintroduced at a lower dose with escalation in combination with a short period of oral steroids.
- Auditory or ocular disturbances: dose reduction or interruption.

Drug Preparation/Administration:

- Drug is available in 125 mg, 250 mg, and 500 mg tablets for oral suspension.
- Teach patient
  - Patient should have the following tests prior to starting drug, and then regularly during therapy:
    - Auditory and ophthalmic testing baseline and every 12 months.
    - Serum creatinine and liver function tests baseline and monthly; urine protein baseline and regularly.
  - Take drug as follows on an empty stomach, 30 minutes before eating.
    - Disperse tablet for oral suspension in water, orange juice, or apple juice until a fine suspension results. Dose should be calculated to the nearest whole tablet size. If dose is < 1 g, use 3.5 oz of liquid, and if > 1 g, use 7 oz of liquid.

  - Once the suspension is swallowed, ensure all the dose is ingested by filling the glass again with a small amount of liquid to resuspend the residue, and swallow this as well.
- DO NOT chew or swallow tablets whole.
- DO NOT take with aluminum-containing antacid products.
- DO NOT drive or operate machinery if patient experiences dizziness.

Drug Interactions:
- Aluminun-containing antacids: potential interaction; deferasirox should not be taken with aluminum-containing antacids.
- Other iron chelating agents: safety has not been determined; do not take in combination.

Lab Effects/Interference:
- Serum ferritin: decrease in serum ferritin. Monitor baseline and monthly.
- Serum creatinine: increased (dose-dependent) in 38% of patients. Monitor serum creatinine baseline, and at least monthly.
- Urine protein: intermittent proteinuria occurred in 18.6% patients on clinical trials. Assess baseline and monitor closely.
- Liver function studies: increased in some patients. Monitor baseline and monthly.
- Liver iron concentration (LIC): decreased; however, correlation coefficient between serum ferritin and LIC is 0.63 so serum ferritin levels may not always reflect changes in LIC.

Special Considerations:
- Drug is indicated for the treatment of chronic iron overload due to blood transfusions in patients aged 2 and older.
- Drug is contraindicated in patients with hypersensitivity to deferasirox or to any other drug component.
- In clinical trials, 4 patients discontinued drug due to hepatic abnormalities: chemical hepatitis, or increased serum transaminases.
- Patients should have baseline serum ferritin, creatinine, liver function tests, urine protein, and auditory and ophthalmic (slit lamp and dilated fundoscopy) testing. Serum lab tests should be repeated monthly, urine protein regularly, and auditory and ocular testing yearly during treatment.
- Drug is not carcinogenic, mutagenic, and has no adverse effects on fertility or reproductive performance in laboratory animals.
- Although drug was not teratogenic in lab animals, drug should be used in pregnancy only if clearly needed (Pregnancy Category B).
- Drug is excreted in breast milk of lab animals, so caution should be exercised when drug is administered to a nursing woman.
- During the 1 year clinical trial, safety and efficacy of pediatric patients was similar to that of adults so recommended starting dose and dosing modifica-

tions are the same. During this time, the growth and development of the children were within normal limits.

- Use drug cautiously in elderly patients due to the greater frequency of decreased hepatic, renal, or cardiac function, and polypharmacy.

Potential Toxicities/Side Effects and the Nursing Process

I. POTENTIAL FOR SENSORY/PERCEPTUAL ALTERATIONS related to AUDITORY AND OCULAR DISTURBANCES

Defining Characteristics: Auditory disturbances (high frequency hearing loss, decreased hearing), and ocular disturbances (lens opacities, cataracts, elevated intraocular pressure, retinal disorders) were reported rarely (< 1%).

Nursing Implications: Ensure that patient has had baseline auditory and ophthalmic (slit lamp and full fundoscopy examinations). Teach patient to report any changes in hearing or vision right away. Ensure that patient has 12 month follow up auditory and ophthalmic examinations during therapy.

II. ALTERATION IN URINARY ELIMINATION, POTENTIAL, related to INCREASED SERUM CREATININE

Defining Characteristics: Increased serum creatinine occurred in 11.1% of patients, and appeared to be dose-related.

Nursing Implications: Assess baseline serum creatinine, and monitor monthly during treatment. If increased, discuss dose adjustment (interruption, reduction, or discontinuance) with physician.

III. ALTERATION IN NUTRITION, LESS THAN BODY REQUIREMENTS related to NAUSEA/VOMITING, DIARRHEA

Defining Characteristics: Nausea occurred in 10.5%, vomiting 10%, and diarrhea in 11.8% of patients. Gastrointestinal side effects appear dose related.

Nursing Implications: Reinforce teaching to administer drug on an empty stomach 30 minutes before a meal. Teach patient to report nausea, vomiting, and/or diarrhea. If nausea and/or vomiting occur, discuss premedication with an antiemetic with physician. Encourage small, frequent feedings of favorite foods. If diarrhea occurs, teach patient to self-administer antidiarrheal medication.

IV. ALTERATION IN SKIN INTEGRITY related to RASH

Defining Characteristics: Rash affected 8.4% of patients and appears dose-related. Rash can be mild to moderate or severe, and often resolves spontaneously.

Nursing Implications: Assess skin integrity and presence of rash baseline and periodically during treatment. Teach patient to report skin rash, and explain that rash often resolves spontaneously. If rash is severe, discuss dose interruption with physician. Teach patient that once rash resolves, drug can be reintroduced at lower dose with escalation in combination with a short course of oral steroids.

V. ALTERATION IN COMFORT related to ABDOMINAL PAIN, ARTHRALGIA, FATIGUE

Defining Characteristics: Abdominal pain occurred in about 14% of patients in 1 study, compared to about 10% in the comparator group who received deferoxamine IV. Arthralgia occurred in 7.4% of patients and fatigue in 6.1%.

Nursing Implications: Teach patient that abdominal pain may occur, and to report it. Teach local measures to improve comfort. If abdominal pain persists or worsens, discuss further testing and drug interruption with physician. Liver function tests should be monitored baseline and monthly; chemical hepatitis occurred in 2 patients, and should be ruled out. Teach patient that fatigue and arthralgias are uncommon, but may occur. Teach local comfort measures, and teach patient to report symptoms that worsen.

Drug: etanidazole (investigational)

Class: Nitrolmidazole, hypoxic radiosensitizer.

Mechanism of Action: Sensitizes hypoxic tumor cells to the effects of ionizing radiotherapy by mimicking oxygen. This enhances formation of free radicals, which damage cellular DNA and prevent DNA repair so that tumor cell kill is enhanced.

Metabolism: Metabolized by liver.

Dosage/Range:
- Per protocol.

Drug Preparation/Administration:
- Per protocol, but may be administered as a rapid intravenous infusion three times per week, immediately prior to radiotherapy.

Drug Interactions:
- Unknown.

Special Considerations:
- Peripheral neuropathy is dose-limiting toxicity.
- Less toxic than nitrolmidazole, with less nerve tissue penetration.

Potential Toxicities/Side Effects and the Nursing Process

I. SENSORY PERCEPTUAL ALTERATION related to PERIPHERAL NEUROPATHY

Defining Characteristics: Peripheral neuropathy occurs, with sensory loss and paresthesias of feet, toes, hands. May have decreased sensitivity to pinprick, decreased vibratory sense. May resolve over days, while severe neuropathies may be permanent. Related to cumulative drug exposure.

Nursing Implications: Assess baseline neurologic status. Assess for numbness, tingling, burning, loss of temperature sensation, and ache at each visit. Instruct patient to report these or other changes immediately. Discuss drug discontinuance with physician as appropriate to prevent permanent severe neuropathy.

II. ALTERATION IN NUTRITION, LESS THAN BODY REQUIREMENTS, related to GI SIDE EFFECTS

Defining Characteristics: Nausea and vomiting may occur.

Nursing Implications: Assess baseline nutritional status and signs/symptoms of nausea, vomiting. Instruct patient to report occurrence of nausea, vomiting. Discuss premedication with physician and administer prescribed antiemetic prior to drug. Teach patient to self-administer prescribed antiemetic at home.

III. ALTERATION IN COMFORT related to RASH, ARTHRALGIAS

Defining Characteristics: Rash, transient arthralgias may occur.

Nursing Implications: Assess baseline comfort level. Assess for rash, arthralgias, and instruct patient to report these side effects. If they occur, provide and teach patient symptomatic measures to reduce discomfort.

Drug: fluosol DA (20%) (investigational)

Class: Perfluorocarbon emulsion, hypoxic radiosensitizer.

Mechanism of Action: Hydrocarbon with hydrogen atom replaced by fluorine, so acts as artifical oxygen carrier. Thus, it decreases cell hypoxia and enhances formation of free radicals, which damage tumor cell DNA and prevent DNA repair.

Metabolism: By liver.

Dosage/Range:
- Per protocol.

Drug Preparation/Administration:
- Per protocol.

Drug Interactions:
- None known.

Special Considerations:
- Administer prior to radiation with patient breathing 100% oxygen before and during radiation.
- Increases solid tumor response to radiotherapy without increased damage to normal cells.
- Mild myelosuppression may be due to radiotherapy rather than drug.

Potential Toxicities/Side Effects and the Nursing Process

I. ALTERATION IN COMFORT related to DRUG ALLERGY

Defining Characteristics: Allergic-type reaction may occur with first dose, characterized by facial flushing, chest pressure, and/or chills and fever. Premedication with antihistamines and corticosteroids prevents further episodes.

Nursing Implications: Assess baseline drug allergies, temperature, VS. Teach patient to report sensation of warmth, chest pressure, chills, facial flushing. Discuss with physician premedication with antihistamines and corticosteroids.

II. ALTERATION IN NUTRITION, LESS THAN BODY REQUIREMENTS, related to HEPATOTOXICITY

Defining Characteristics: Transient, self-limited increases in LFTs may occur (AST, ALT, alk phos).

Nursing Implications: Assess baseline LFTs and monitor throughout treatment. Discuss abnormalities with physician.

Drug: leucovorin calcium (Folinic Acid, Citrovorum Factor)

Class: Water-soluble vitamin in the folate group (folinic acid).

Mechanism of Action: Potentiates antitumor activity of 5-FU when given prior to or concurrently with 5-FU, ± XRT. Acts as an antidote for methotrexate and other folic acid antagonists. Circumvents the biochemical block of the enzyme inhibitors (e.g., dihydrofolate reductase [DHFR]) to permit DNA and RNA synthesis.

Metabolism: Leucovorin is metabolized to polyglutamates that are more effective in potentiating 5-FU tumor cell kill. Metabolized primarily in the liver;

50% of the single dose is excreted in 6 hours in the urine (80–90% of the dose) and stool (8% of the dose).

Dosage/Range:

Antidote for methotrexate:

- Dose of drug and duration of rescue is dependent on serum methotrexate levels:

Methotrexate Level	Leucovorin
$< 5.0\ (10)^{-7}$M	10 mg/m^2 q6h
$5\ (10)^{-7}$M$(10)^{-6}$M	30–40 mg/m^2 q6h
$> 5\ (10)^{-6}$M	100 mg/m^2 q3–6h

- Potentiation of 5-FU ± XRT: dose varies leucovorin 20 mg/m^2/d–2.5 g/m^2 CI.

Drug Preparation:

- Drug is supplied in ampules or vials.
- Reconstitute vials with sterile water for injection.
- Dilute reconstituted vials or ampules further with 5% Dextrose or 0.9% Sodium Chloride.

Drug Administration:

- With 5-FU, in a variety of combinations; e.g., leucovorin: 500 mg/m^2/week for 6 weeks as a 2-hour infusion; 5-FU: 500–600 mg/m^2/week for 6 weeks, IVB midway through leucovorin infusion, then 2-week rest, then repeat 6-week cycle.
- Administered 24 hours after first methotrexate dose is begun. Dose every 6 hours for up to 12 doses.
- First dose is given IV; others can be given IM or PO when given as methotrexate "rescue."
- IV doses are given via bolus over 15 minutes unless otherwise specified.
- When given as a rescue dose, must be given exactly on time in order to rescue normal cells from methotrexate toxicity.

Drug Interactions:

- 5-FU: potentiation.
- Folic acid: provides folinic acid so cells can make DNA (antagonizes drug effect).
- Phenobarbital, phenytoin, primidone: decreases anticonvulsant action (when leucovorin given in large doses); monitor patient closely and increase anticonvulsant as needed.

Lab Effects/Interference:

- None.

Special Considerations:

- It is imperative that the patient receive the leucovorin on schedule to avoid fatal methotrexate toxicity. Notify the physician if the patient is unable to take the dose orally, as it must then be given IV.
- Usually free of side effects, but allergic reaction and local pain may occur.

Potential Toxicities/Side Effects and the Nursing Process

I. POTENTIAL FOR INJURY related to HYPERSENSITIVITY, DRUG INTERACTIONS

Defining Characteristics: Allergic sensitization has been reported: facial flushing, itching. Leucovorin in large amounts may counteract the antiepileptic effects of phenobarbital, phenytoin, and primidone.

Nursing Implications: Monitor patient for signs/symptoms of allergic reaction. Diphenhydramine is effective for relieving symptoms of allergic reaction. Monitor patient for symptoms of increased seizure activity (if on antiepileptic drugs); monitor antiepileptic drug levels.

II. ALTERED NUTRITION, LESS THAN BODY REQUIREMENTS, related to NAUSEA, VOMITING

Defining Characteristics: Oral leucovorin rarely causes nausea or vomiting.

Nursing Implications: Administer oral leucovorin with antacids, milk, or juice.

Drug: porfirmer (Photofrin)

Class: Photosensitizing agent.

Mechanism of Action: Porfirmer is selectively distributed and maintained in tumor tissue. When exposed to 630 nanometer laser light, porfirmer is activated and a chain reaction ensues, resulting in damage to tumor cell mitochondria and intracellular membranes. The therapy also causes the release of thromboxane A, resulting in vasoconstriction, activation and aggregation of platelets, and increased clotting. Ischemic necrosis ensues, causing tissue and tumor death.

Metabolism: Distributed through a variety of tissues, but is selectively retained by tumors, skin, and organs of the reticuloendothelial system (liver, spleen). Drug is not dialysable.

Dosage/Range:

- 2 mg/kg body weight, injected over 3–5 minutes.

- May be given for a total of 3 courses of therapy, each separated by at least 30 days.

Drug Preparation/Administration:
- Add 31.8 mL D5W or NS to the 75-mg vial, producing a concentration of 2.5 mg/ml.
- Protect reconstituted solution from bright light and use immediately.

Drug Interactions:
- The following drugs may decrease the effectiveness of profirmer therapy: allopurinol, corticosteroids (glucocorticoid), calcium channel blockers, prostaglandin synthesis inhibitors, Thromboxane A inhibitors, beta carotene, DMSO, ethanol, formate, and mannitol.
- Some drugs may increase photosensitivity, including griseofulvin, phenothiazines, sulfonamides, sulfonylurea hypoglycemia agents, tetracyclines, and thiazide diuretics.

Lab Effects/Interference:
- None.

Special Considerations:
- Drug is for use in esophageal and non-small-cell lung carcinoma (NSCLC).
- Photodynamic therapy should NOT be used in patients with:
  porphyria
  tumor erosion into a major blood vessel
  bronchoesophageal fistula
  tracheoesophageal fistula
  tumor erosion into the trachea or bronchial tree
- Extreme caution should be exercised when deciding candidacy for therapy, as it can cause an initial inflammation at the site and can cause fistulas as tumors shrink.
- When photodynamic therapy is preceded or followed by local radiation therapy, sufficient time should be allowed between treatments for inflammation to subside (e.g., radiation therapy should not be given to the site until at least 2–4 weeks after photodynamic therapy).
- If extravasation occurs during IV administration, the area should be protected from light for 30 days.

Potential Toxicities/Side Effects and the Nursing Process

I. POTENTIAL FOR INJURY related to ANEMIA, INFLAMMATION AT SITE OF THERAPY

Defining Characteristics: Photodynamic therapy can cause significant tumor bleeding at the site of treatment, sometimes resulting in anemia. Inflammation at the site can cause narrowing and/or obstruction of vital structures and pulmonary and cardiovascular changes (pleural effusion or edema, atrial fibrillation and angina), particularly since much of this therapy occurs in the mediastinal area.

Nursing Implications: Monitor respiratory, cardiovascular systems during treatment. Instruct patient to contact physician immediately for dyspnea, excessive coughing, abdominal pain, fever, dysphagia, bleeding/hemoptysis, chest pain, etc. Substernal chest pain in esophageal cancer patients can be treated with opioids.

II. POTENTIAL FOR INJURY related to PHOTOSENSITIVITY

Defining Characteristics: May cause photosensitivity reactions for 30 days after administration, both to sunlight and bright indoor light. Skin around the eyes may be particularly sensitive. Sunscreens are not protective, as phototherapy causes sensitivity to visible light. Porfirmer is slowly inactivated by ambient light.

Nursing Implications: Patients should test skin (do not use facial skin) by exposing a small area to sunlight for 10 minutes. If area is free of erythema, blistering, and edema 24 hours later, patient may gradually increase exposure. Patients should wear dark glasses that transmit less than 4% of white light for 30 days after treatment.

Drug: tirapazamine (investigational)

Class: Hypoxic cell cytoxin (benzotriazine bioreductive compound).

Mechanism of Action: When given concurrently with radiotherapy, increases damage to aerobic malignant cells throughout different oxygen levels, probably due to the fact that in hypoxic conditions, tirapazamine is reduced to a free radical form, which produces DNA strand breaks. Drug also shows marked potentiation of cisplatin, probably by preventing repair of cisplatin-induced DNA cross-linkages in hypoxic cells. Additive effect when given with cisplatin, and synergy when given before cisplatin. It is possible that under hypoxic conditions, tirapazamine may act as a topoisomerase II inhibitor.

Metabolism: Is metabolized by reductases to form a transient oxidizing radical, which is scavenged by molecular oxygen. In hypoxic conditions, the oxidizing radical removes a proton from DNA to form DNA radicals (at the C4' position on the ribose ring). The radicals are then oxidized, forming DNA strand breaks, preventing cell division, and causing cell death.

Dosage/Range:
Maximum tolerated dose is 290 mg/m² IV on days 1, 15, and 29, and 220 mg/m² on days 8, 10, 12, 22, 24, and 26 concurrent with cisplatin and radiotherapy (Craighead PS et al, 2000).

Drug Preparation/Administration: Administer IV over 2 hours followed 1 hour later by cisplatin IV given over 1 hour, followed immediately by radiotherapy. When given without cisplatin, radiotherapy follows 30–120 minutes after tirapazamine infusion.

Drug Interactions:
- Additive cytotoxicity when given concurrently with cisplatin.
- Synergy with increased cell kill when given prior to cisplatin.

Lab Effects/Interference:
- Unknown.

Special Considerations:
- Administer prior to cisplatin chemotherapy.
- Is being studied in treatment of head and neck, advanced cervical and ovarian cancers.

Potential Toxicities/Side Effects and the Nursing Process

I. ALTERATION IN NUTRITION, LESS THAN BODY REQUIREMENTS, related to NAUSEA, VOMITING, DIARRHEA

Defining Characteristics: Nausea and vomiting can be severe, especially when drug is given in combination with cisplatin. Diarrhea can also occur, but is usually mild.

Nursing Implications: Ensure aggressive antiemesis, with serotonin antagonists and dexamethasone recommended to prevent nausea and vomiting. Assess efficacy of regime, and modify as needed. Explain to patient that this may occur, and teach dietary modifications, including the avoidance of greasy, spicy foods.

II. POTENTIAL FOR INFECTION AND BLEEDING related to NEUTROPENIA AND THROMBOCYTOPENIA

Defining Characteristics: In one study, febrile neutropenia necessitated decreasing the dose and frequency of tirapazamine. Thrombocytopenia was uncommon.

Nursing Implications: Assess baseline CBC and differential prior to therapy, and at least weekly during therapy. Teach patient to report signs and symptoms of infection and bleeding right away. Teach patient to check temperature during treatment, and to report T > 100.5°F. If infection occurs, discuss antibiotic treatment, and teach patient self-care strategies.

III. ALTERATION IN COMFORT related to MUSCLE CRAMPS

Defining Characteristics: Muscle cramps can occur, especially during the first 2 weeks of treatment, generally resolving by the 3rd week of treatment.

Nursing Implications: Teach patient that muscle cramps may occur, and to report them. Teach patient self-care measures to minimize discomfort. Discuss alternative approaches with physician if plan is ineffective. Refer to protocol for other management strategies.

IV. POTENTIAL ALTERATION IN SKIN INTEGRITY related to RASH

Defining Characteristics: Rash that is transient may occur.

Nursing Implications: Teach patient that rash may occur, and to report it. Discuss local management with physician.

Chapter 4

Cytoprotective Agents

Advances in the development of effective, new chemotherapeutic agents have been slow, although a number of excellent agents have recently been approved for use. All traditional chemotherapeutic agents work by interfering with DNA and RNA replication, and protein synthesis, causing cell death or stasis. Unfortunately, the chemotherapy, unless attached to a targeted vehicle, such as a monoclonal antibody, is nonselective, and normal cells are damaged by the chemotherapy. Often, the dose-limiting toxicity is myelosuppression, but organ toxicity specific to the chemotherapy agent may limit the drug's usefulness. Specific organ toxicity that can occur includes neurotoxicity (e.g., cisplatin, oxaliplatin, the taxanes), cardiotoxicity (e.g., anthracyclines, alone or together with trastuzumab), bladder toxicity (e.g., high-dose cyclophosphamide, ifosfamide), and nephrotoxicity (e.g., cisplatin). Thus, both doses and duration of therapy of treatment are often limited by these organ toxicities. This can compromise optimal treatment, as well as compromise quality of life. Similarly, radiation therapy causes cell damage (e.g., ionization causes the formation of free radicals, which, in the presence of oxygen, cause damage to DNA, leading to cell death when the cell tries to replicate). Again, normal tissue in the radiation port also are damaged, such as the bone marrow in the skull, sternum, and heads of long bones, and can lead to side effects such as bone marrow depression, which results in the need for treatment breaks and less-than-optimal radiotherapy.

In an effort to protect normal cells from treatment toxicity and to limit organ toxicities, a number of agents have been developed that offer cyto (cell) or organ protection, and even more are being studied (investigational agents). Agents that are currently approved for use are amifostine (Ethyol), Mesna, and dexrazoxane (Zinecard, a chelating agent). Amifostine has shown "broad spectrum" activity in protecting multiple organ systems, such as the kidneys, bone marrow, and nerves. In addition, it protects the parotid glands from radiation damage. Amifostine is indicated for the reduction of cumulative nephrotoxicity from cisplatin in patients with advanced ovarian and NSCLC, as well as for reducing the incidence of moderate-to-severe xerostomia in patients with head and neck cancer whose radiation port covers the parotid glands. Mesna is included in this chapter because it provides bladder protection from the toxic effects of high-dose cyclophosphamide and ifosfamide. Leucovorin is also a classic cytoprotectant in that it "rescues" normal cells from methotrexate toxicity (bone marrow and mucosal cells). This drug appears in Chapter 3. In an effort to help establish a practice standard for the use of currently available cytoprotectants in patients not enrolled on clinical trials, the American Society of Clinical Oncology (ASCO) has developed guidelines (ASCO, 1999).

One organ toxicity that is receiving increased attention is neurotoxicity. Many highly effective agents are limited in both dose and duration of treatment by the development of peripheral neuropathy, such as the taxanes (paclitaxel causes axonal degeneration and demyelination), oxaliplatin, and cisplatin (segmental demyelination). This side effect can be one of the most clinically challenging problems for oncology nurses. See Table 4.1 for a list of antitumor agents that cause neurotoxicity. Peripheral neuropathy is defined as the injury, inflammation, or degeneration of any nerve outside the central nervous system. Chemotherapy may cause damage to the sensory and motor axons. Symptoms of sensory damage include tingling, pricking or numbness of the extremities, a sensation of wearing an invisible glove or sock and thus the term *glove and stocking distribution*; burning or freezing pain; sharp, stabbing, or electric shock-like pain; and extreme sensitivity to touch. Patients, in some cases, will be reluctant to admit to these symptoms because they believe that if they do, their chemotherapy drug will be stopped. If the motor neurons are affected, then symptoms include muscle weakness and loss of balance or coordination. If myelinated nerves are injured, then there is a reduction in conduction velocity of the nerve impulse, and on examination, the patient has depressed or absent deep tendon reflexes (Wilkes, 2004). Although in many instances, peripheral neuropathy may be reversible, it may take many months for this to occur. Unfortunately, damage to peripheral nerves can have long-term effects on quality of life, and cause much discomfort, injury, and distress. In addition, while the exact percentage of patients with cancer who experience peripheral neuropathy is unknown, the economic impact is considerable. It has been estimated that it costs $5,507 per patient to treat neuropathy (both medical and indirect costs) (Calhoun et al, 1999). Nurses have been pivotal in performing assessments of sensory and motor function, and assessing the impact of peripheral neuropathy on the patient's safety and quality of life, making them strong advocates for patients. Nurses monitor patients' neurological status prior to each treatment and between treatment cycles. A simple six-step neurosensory exam should be performed throughout the course of chemotherapy to identify any potential deficits. The exam should include a history, such as the questionnaire developed by Berghorn and shown in Figure 4.1, as well as a physicial exam of gait, motor and sensory systems, and testing of reflexes. Grading of neurotoxicity is based on a neurosensory exam that includes assessment of gait, motor and sensory system, functional ability, and reflexes, and is scored from 0–4 according to the National Cancer Institute (NCI) Common Toxicity Criteria (see Appendix II). In obtaining the history, since it is imperative to involve patients in the assessment of function and ability to perform activities of daily living, an excellent patient neurotoxicity questionnaire has been developed by Berghorn et al (2000) and incorporated in one clinical trial evaluating neuroprotectants. (see Figure 4.1.) Patients are asked if they have difficulties in performing their normal activities of daily living, such as buttoning a shirt or holding a fork to eat (fine motor movement), mobility in terms of difficulty going up or down stairs, and communicating. Currently, in clinical practice, the offending drug is usually stopped if the patient develops grade 3 or 4 toxicity. Fortunately, clinical studies are being conducted to find effective neuroprotectants that have little or no toxicity. Agents being studied include amifostine, BNP7787, and glutamine. These agents are included in this chapter.

Table 4.1 Chemotherapy Agents Likely to Cause Neurotoxicity

High Incidence (very common > 80% incidence)	
Cisplatin	Interferon (especially at HD)
Interleukin-2 (if patient develops capillary leak syndrome)	
Moderate Incidence (common, 20–80% incidence)	
Arsenic trioxide	Methotrexate (IT, HD)
Carmustine (intra-arterial)	Oxaliplatin, ormaplatin
Cytosine arabinoside (HD)	Paclitaxel
Docetaxel	Procarbazine
Hexamethylmelamine	Suramin
Ifosfamide	Tretinoin
l-asparaginase	Vincristine, vinblastine, vinorelbine
Uncommon (< 20% incidence)	
Busulfan	Fludarabine
Capecitabine	5-fluorouracil
Cladrabine	Pentostatin
Etoposide	Teniposide

IT = intrathecal; HD = high dose
Data from: Armstrong T, Rust D, and Kohtz JR (1997); Cheson BD, Vena DA, Foss FM, and Sorensen JM (1994); Furlong TG (1993); Weiss RB (2001).

References

Armstrong T, Rust D, Kohtz JR. Neurologic, Pulmonary, and Cutaneous Toxicities of High-Dose Chemotherapy. *Oncology Nursing Forum* 1997;24(Suppl 1):23–33

Berghorn E, Hausheer F. Bionumerik Patient Neurotoxicity Questionnaire. San Antonio, TX: Bionumerick Pharmaceuticals, Inc.; 2000

For each of the following 2 items, please indicate by placing a check in the box that best describes how you have felt over the past 4 weeks.

1. □ I have no numbness, pain, or tingling in my hands or feet.
   □ I have mild tingling, pain, or numbness in my hands or feet. This does not interfere with my activities.
   □ I have moderate tingling, pain, or numbness in my hands or feet. This interferes with some of my activities.
   □ I have moderate to severe tingling, pain, or numbness in my hands or feet. This interferes with my activities of daily living.
   □ I have severe tingling or numbness in my hands or feet. It completely prevents me from doing most activities.
2. □ I have no weakness in my arms or legs.
   □ I have a mild weakness in my arms or legs. This does not interfere with my activities.
   □ I have moderate weakness in my arms or legs. This interferes with some of my actities.
   □ I have moderate to severe weakness in my arms or legs. This interferes with my activities of daily living.
   □ I have severe weakness in my arms or legs. It completely prevents me from doing most activities.

To help you complete this form, listed below are some examples of activities of daily living:

Dressing:	ability to button blouse/shirt, put on earrings, tying shoes, put in contact lenses
Eating:	ability to use knife, fork, and spoon or chopsticks
Mobility:	ability to walk, climb stairs
Communication:	writing, typing on a keyboard
Other:	interference with sleep, driving, operation of remote controls

Figure 4.1 Patient Neurotoxicity Questionnaire
Source: Berghorn E and Hausheer F (2000) Bionumerik Patient Neurotoxicity Questionnaire. San Antonio, TX, Bionumerik Pharmaceuticals, Inc.

Boyle FM, Wheeler HR, Shenfield GM. Glutamine Ameliorates Experimental Vincristine Neuropathy. *J Pharmacol Exp Ther* 1996;279(1):410–415

Boyle FM, Wheeler HR, Shenfield GM. Amelioration of Experimental Cisplatin and Paclitaxel Neuropathy with Glutamate. *J Neuro-Oncol* 1999;41:107–116

Calhoun EA, Fishman DA, Roland PY, Lurain JR, Bennett CL. Total Cost of Chemotherapy-induced Hematologic and Neurologic Toxicity. *Proc Am Soc Clin Oncol* 1999;18A:1606

Cheson BD, Vena DA, Foss FM, Sorensen JM. Neurotoxicity of Purine Analogues: A Review. *J Clin Oncology* 1994;12(10):2216–2228

Furlong TG. Neurologic Complications of Immunosuppressive Cancer Therapy. *Oncology Nursing Forum* 1993;20(9):1337–1352

Hensley ML, Schuchter LM, Lindley C, et al. American Society of Clinical Oncology Clinical Practice Guidelines for the Use of Chemotherapy and Radiotherapy Protectants. *J Clin Oncol* 1999;17(10):3333–3355
Liu T, Liu Y, He S, et al. Use of Radiation with or without WR-2721 in Advanced Rectal Cancer. *Cancer* 1992;69(11):2820–2825
Savarese D, Boucher J, Corey B. Glutamine Treatment of Paclitaxel-induced Myalgias and Arthralgias [letter]. *J Clin Oncol* 1998;16(12):3918–3939
Schuchter LM, Luginbuhl WE, Meropol NJ. The Current Status of Toxicity Protectants in Cancer Therapy. *Semin Oncol* 1992;19(6):742–751
Viele CS, Holmes BC. Amifostine: Drug Profile and Nursing Implications of the First Pancytoprotectant. *Oncol Nurs Forum* 1998;25(3):515–523
Weiss RB. Miscellaneous Toxicities. In DeVita VT Jr, Hellman S, Rosenberg SA, (eds), *Principles and Practice of Oncology,* 5th ed. New York, NY: Lippincott-Raven Publishers;1997;2802
Weiss RB. Miscellaneous Toxicities, Adverse Effects of Treatment. DeVita VT Jr, Hellman S, Rosenberg SA, (eds), *Principles and Practice of Oncology,* 6th ed. New York, NY: Lippincott-Raven Publishers; 2001: Chapter 55
Wilkes GM. Peripheral Neuropathy. In Yarbro CH, Frogge MH, Goodman M, (eds), *Cancer Symptom Management,* 3rd ed. Sudbury, MA: Jones and Bartlett Publishers;2004;362–367

Drug: allopurinol sodium (Aloprim, Zyloprim, Zurinol)

Class: Xanthine oxidase inhibitor.

Mechanism of Action: Drug inhibits xanthine oxidase, the enzyme necessary for conversion of hypoxanthine (natural purine base) to xanthine, and then xanthine to uric acid, without affecting biosynthesis of purines. This lowers serum and urinary uric acid levels.

Metabolism: Well absorbed orally and IV with comparable oxypurinol (major pharmacologic component) serum levels with the relative bioavailability of oxypurinol 100%. Time to peak serum concentration is 30–120 minutes, with half-life of allopurinol 1–3 hours, and of oxypurinol 18–30 hours. Drug metabolized in liver to active metabolite oxypurinol, and excreted by kidneys and enterohepatic circulation.

Dosage/Range:

- Oral: 600 mg–800 mg/day for 2–3 days with hydration (dose-reduce if creatinine clearance is < 60 mg/mL.
- IV: in management of patients with leukemia, lymphoma, and solid tumors receiving cancer therapy expected to cause elevated serum and urinary uric acid levels and who cannot tolerate oral therapy:

Adults: 200–400 mg/m²/day, maximum 600 mg/day as a single dose or in divided doses every 6, 8, or 12 hours; optimally begin allopurinol 24–48 hours prior to chemotherapy.
Dose-reduce for renal dysfunction based on creatinine clearance (10–20 mL/min = 200 mg/day; 3–10 mL/min = 100 mg/day).

Drug Preparation:

- Oral: available in 100-mg and 300-mg tablets.
- IV: available as 30-mL vial containing 500 mg allopurinol lyophilized powder, which is stable at room temperature (25°C, 77°F).
- Reconstitute by adding 25 mL Sterile Water for Injection.
- The ordered dose should be withdrawn, and further diluted in 0.9% NS Injection or 5% Dextrose for Injection to achieve a final concentration of no greater than 6 mg/mL.
- Store at 20–25°C (68–77°F) for up to 10 hours after reconstitution.
- Do not refrigerate reconstituted or diluted product.

Drug Administration:

- Oral: give with food or immediately after meals to decrease gastric irritation.
- IV: administer over appropriate period of time given volume of diluted drug.

Drug Interactions:

- Dicoumarol: PT may be prolonged due to prolonged half-life; monitor PT closely and adjust dose as needed.
- Mercaptopurine/azathioprine: allopurinol decreased drug metabolism so dose of mercaptopurine or azathioprine must be reduced to 1/3 or 1/4 the usual dose, and then subsequent dose adjusted based on clinical response.
- Uricosuric agents: decreases the inhibition of xanthine oxidase by oxypurinol and increases the urinary excretion of uric acid. Avoid concomitant use.
- Ampicillin/amoxicillin: increased frequency of skin rash; use together cautiously.
- Chlorpropamide: allopurinol may prolong half-life of drug as both drugs compete for excretion in renal tubule; monitor closely for hypoglycemia if drugs used concomitantly in a patient with renal dysfunction.
- Cyclosporin: cyclosporine levels may be increased, so drug levels should be monitored closely, and dose of cyclosporine adjusted accordingly.
- Theophylline: prolonged half-life when used together; monitor theophylline levels closely and adjust dose accordingly.

Physical incompatibilities with IV allopurinol:

- Amikacin sulfate, amphotericin B, carmustine, cefotaxime sodium, chlorpromazine HCl, cimetidine HCl, clindamycin phosphate, cyarabine, dacarbazine, daunorubicin HCl, diphenhydramine HCl, doxorubicin HCl, doxycycline hyclate, droperidol, floxuridine, gentamycin sulfate, haloperidol lactate, hydroxyzine HCl, idarubicin HCl, imipenem-cilastin sodium, mechlorethamine HCl, meperidine HCl, metoclopramide HCl, methylprednisolone sodium succinate, minocycline HCl, nalbuphine HCl, netimicin sulfate, ondansetron HCl, prochlor perazine edisylate, promethazine HCl, sodium bicarbonate, streptozocin, tobramycin sulfate, vinorelbine tartrate.

Lab Effects/Interference:

- Increased alk phos, AST, ALT, bili.

Special Considerations:

- Dose reduction necessary in renal dysfunction.
- Contraindicated in patients hypersensitive to drug (even mild allergic reaction).
- Discontinue at first sign of a rash.
- Use cautiously with patients on diuretics, as may decrease renal function and increase serum levels of allopurinol.
- Allopurinol hypersensitivity syndrome may occur rarely and is characterized by fever, chills, leukopenia or leukocytosis, eosinophilia, arthralgias, rash, pruritus, nausea, vomiting, renal and hepatic compromise.
- Drug MUST be discontinued immediately if rash develops.
- To prevent tumor lysis syndrome, patient should receive aggressive IV hydration and alkalinization of urine, together with allopurinol.

Potential Toxicities/Side Effects and the Nursing Process

I. POTENTIAL SENSORY/PERCEPTUAL ALTERATIONS related to CNS EFFECTS

Defining Characteristics: Drowsiness, chills, and fever have been reported in > 10% of patients. Headaches, and somnolence occur in 1–10% of patients. Rarely, seizure, myoclonus, twitching, agitation, mental status changes, cerebral infarction, coma, paralysis, and tremor can occur. If fever and chills are associated with rash, eosinophilia, nausea, vomiting, they are most likely related to rare allopurinol hypersensitivity reaction.

Nursing Implications: Assess baseline neurological status, including mental status, and periodically during treatment. If any abnormalities, discuss with physician right away. Teach patient to report chills, fever, drowsiness, or any changes, if they occur. If they do, teach patient self-management strategies, and to report if they are ineffective. If so, discuss management strategies with physician. If fever and chills are associated with rash, eosinophilia, nausea, vomiting, they are most likely related to rare allopurinol hypersensitivity reaction and should be discussed with the physician immediately, and drug discontinued.

II. ALTERATION IN SKIN INTEGRITY, POTENTIAL, related to RASH, STEVENS-JOHNSON SYNDROME

Defining Characteristics: More than 10% of patients develop maculopapular rash, often associated with urticaria and pruritus; may be exfoliative. Less common but more severe, 1–10% of patients develop Stevens-Johnson syndrome or toxic epidermal necrolysis, which may be fatal. For IV administration, local injection site reactions may occur. Alopecia has been reported in 1–10% of patients.

Nursing Implications: Assess baseline skin integrity and intactness of scalp hair. Teach patient that rash may occur, and to report it right away, as drug must be discontinued. Teach patient self-care strategies, including skin cream to moisturize the skin and to prevent itching. Discuss drug discontinuance and management with physician. Teach patient to report any hair loss. If it occurs, discuss impact on patient, self-care strategies, and if severe, discuss drug discontinuance with physician.

Drug: amifostine for injection (Ethyol, WR-2721)

Class: Cytoprotectant; free-radical scavenger, metabolized to a free thiol.

Mechanism of Action: Drug is phosphorylated by alkaline phosphatase bound in tissue membranes, producing free thiol. Inside the cell, free thiol binds to and detoxifies reactive metabolites of cisplatin and other chemotherapeutic agents, thus neutralizing the chemotherapy drug in normal tissues so that cellular DNA and RNA are not damaged. Normal cells are protected because of differences in cell physiology (higher alkaline phosphatase concentrations and tissue pH, as well as more effective vascularity in normal cells as compared to malignant cells) and transport mechanisms that promote the preferential uptake of free thiol into normal tissues. Free thiol may also scavenge reactive free-radical reactive oxygen molecules resulting from chemotherapy or radiotherapy. Free thiol may also upregulate p53 expression, so that cells accumulate in the G_1-S cell cyle phase, enabling DNA repair.

Metabolism: Drug is rapidly metabolized to an active free-thiol metabolite and cleared from the plasma, so the drug should be administered 30 minutes prior to drug dose.

Dosage/Range:

- Chemoprotectant: 740 mg/m^2 in 50 mL 0.9% NS administered intravenously (IV) over 5 minutes, 30 minutes prior to beginning chemotherapy.
- Radioprotectant: 200 mg/m^2/day IVP over 3 minutes, 15–30 minutes prior to standard fraction radiation therapy (1.8–2.0 Gy).

- Clinical studies: myelodysplastic syndrome: 200 mg/m^2 IV 3d/week × 3 weeks, then 2 weeks off, q5 weeks; evaluate response after 2 cycles (10 weeks).
- Clinical studies: reversal of neurotoxicity: 500 mg/m^2 IV qd × 5q 21 days × 3 cycles (evaluate response after 2 cycles).

Drug Preparation:

- Available in 10-mL vials containing 500 mg of drug; store at room temperature.
- Use only 0.9% Sodium Chloride.
- Reconstitute vial with 9.7 mL of sterile 0.9% Sodium Chloride.
- Further dilute with sterile 0.9% Sodium Chloride to total 50 mL.
- Stable at 5 mg/mL to 40 mg/mL for 5 hours at room temperature, and for 24 hours if refrigerated.

Drug Administration:

- Hypertension medicines should be stopped 24 hours prior to drug administration.
- Place patient in supine position.
- Administer combination antiemetics.
- Infuse amifostine IV over 15 minutes, beginning 30 minutes prior to chemotherapy or IVP 15–30 minutes prior to radiotherapy.
- Administer IV antiemetic medication 1 hour prior, and oral antiemetic 2 hours prior to amifostine administration.
- Generally, patients should be hydrated with 1 L 0.9% NS prior to amifostine when used as a chemoprotectant.
- Monitor BP baseline, immediately after amifostine infusion and as needed until BP returns to baseline.
- Resume diuretic(s) and/or antihypertensive medications 30 minutes after amifostine infusion is complete as long as patient is normotensive.

Drug Interactions:

- Antihypertensive and diuretic medications may potentiate hypotension.

Lab Effects/Interference:

- May cause hypocalcemia.

Special Considerations:

- Patients unable to tolerate cessation of antihypertensive medications are not candidates for the drug.
- Drug is indicated to reduce the cumulative renal toxicity from cisplatin in patients with advanced ovarian cancer or non-small-cell lung cancer.
- Studies have shown no decrease in drug efficacy when given with first-line therapy in ovarian cancer.
- No evidence exists that drug interferes with tumor response from chemotherapy in other cancers, but research is ongoing.

- Offers significant protection of kidneys.
- Offers protection of bone marrow and nerves.
- Drug has been shown to protect skin, mucous membranes, and bladder and pelvic structures against late moderate-to-severe radiation reactions.

Potential Toxicities/Side Effects and the Nursing Process

I. ALTERATION IN NUTRITION, LESS THAN BODY REQUIREMENTS, related to NAUSEA AND VOMITING, HYPOCALCEMIA

Defining Characteristics: Incidence is frequent, and nausea and vomiting may be severe. These are preventable by using serotonin antagonist and dexamethasone. Hypocalcemia noted in trials using higher doses.

Nursing Implications: Administer serotonin antagonist (e.g., granisetron, ondansetron, or dolasetron) and dexamethasone 20 mg IV prior to amifostine. Encourage small, frequent meals of cool, bland foods and liquids. Teach patient self-management tips and to avoid greasy or heavy foods. Instruct patient to report nausea and/or vomiting that is not resolved by antiemetics. Teach patient to maintain oral hydration as tolerated. Identify patients at risk for hypocalcemia, i.e., nephrotic syndrome and depletion from many courses of cisplatin. Check baseline calcium and albumin, and monitor during therapy. Assess for signs/symptoms of hypocalcemia. Patients may receive calcium supplements as needed.

II. ALTERATION IN OXYGENATION related to HYPOTENSION, POTENTIAL

Defining Characteristics: Drug causes transient, reversible hypotension in 62% of patients at a dose of 910 mg/m^2. Hypotension is usually manifested by a 5- to 15-minute transient decrease in systolic BP of $\geq$ 20 mm Hg. Incidence is less when dose is 740 mg/m^2, and infused over 5 minutes.

Nursing Implications: Assess patient's medication profile. Antihypertensives should be stopped 24 hours prior to drug administration. Assess baseline BP, heart rate, and hydration status. Ensure that patient is well hydrated, and per physician, administer 1 L of 0.9% NS IV prior to amifostine if needed to assure euhydration; if dehydrated, patient may require 2 L. Place patient in supine position during administration of drug, and monitor BP q5min during administration, immediately after administration, and as needed postinfusion. If the BP falls below threshold (see tabulation below), interrupt infusion and give an IVB of 0.9% NS per physician order. If BP comes back above threshold (returns to threshold within 5 minutes and patient is asymptomatic), then resume infusion and give full dose. If BP does not return to threshold within 5 minutes, infusion should be terminated and IV hydration fluids administered per physician, and patient placed in Trendelenburg position, if symptomatic. If

BP does not return to normal in 5 minutes, dose should be reduced in next cycle. Manufacturer recommends the following thresholds for supine BP:

Systolic BP (SBP)	Threshold SBP in mm Hg
< 100	< 80
100–119	75–94
120–139	90–109
140–179	100–139
≥180	≥130

III. ALTERATION IN COMFORT related to FLUSHING, CHILLS, DIZZINESS, SOMNOLENCE, HICCUPS, AND SNEEZING

Defining Characteristics: These effects may occur during or after drug infusion and are mild. Allergic reactions are rare, ranging from skin rash to rigors, but anaphylaxis has not been reported.

Nursing Implications: Assess comfort level, and ask patient to report these symptoms. Discuss with patient comfort measures.

Drug: dexrazoxane for injection (Zinecard)

Class: Cardioprotector.

Mechanism of Action: Enters easily through cell membranes, but the exact mechanism of cardiac cell protection is unclear. A possible mechanism is that the drug becomes a chelating agent within the cell and interferes with ironmediated free-radical formation that otherwise would cause cardiotoxicity from anthracyclines. Drug is a derivative of edetic acid (EDTA).

Metabolism: 42% of the dose is excreted in the urine. No plasma protein binding of drug.

Dosage/Range:
- 10:1 ratio of dexrazoxane to doxorubicin (i.e., 500 mg/m^2 of dexrazoxane to 50 mg/m^2 of doxorubicin).

Drug Preparation:
- Available in 250- or 500-mg vials.
- Reconstitute drug with provided diluent.
- Drug may be further diluted in 0.9% Sodium Choride or 5% Dextrose to a concentration of 1.3–5 mg/mL.
- Stable 6 hours at room temperature or refrigerated.
- USE SAFE CHEMOTHERAPEUTIC AGENT HANDLING PRECAUTIONS!

Drug Administration:

- Give slow IV push or IVB < 30 minutes prior to beginning doxorubicin.

Drug Interactions:

- None known.

Lab Effects/Interference:

- May increase myelosuppression of concomitant doxorubicin, with leukopenia, neutropenia, and thrombocytopenia.

Special Considerations:

- Drug is indicated for reduction of the incidence and severity of cardiomyopathy associated with doxorubicin in women with metastatic breast cancer who have received a cumulative doxorubicin dose of 300 mg/m^2 and who would benefit from continuing doxorubicin.
- Drug may reduce the response from 5–FU, doxorubicin, and cyclophosphamide (FAC) chemotherapy when given concurrently on the first cycle of therapy (48% response rate vs. 63% without the drug, and shorter time to disease progression).
- Drug requires SAFE CHEMOTHERAPEUTIC AGENT HANDLING PRECAUTIONS!

Potential Toxicities/Side Effects and the Nursing Process

I. POTENTIAL FOR INJURY related to ENHANCED BONE MARROW DEPRESSION

Defining Characteristics: Drug may increase doxorubicin-induced bone marrow depression.

Nursing Implications: Monitor WBC, HCT/Hgb, and platelets baseline and prior to each dose. Instruct patient in self-assessment for signs/symptoms of infection and bleeding, and how to report them. Teach patient self-care measures to minimize risk.

II. POTENTIAL ALTERATION IN METABOLISM related to HEPATIC AND RENAL ALTERATIONS

Defining Characteristics: Possible elevations in liver and renal function studies may occur. Incidence did not differ from patients who received same chemotherapy (FAC) without the protector.

Nursing Implications: Assess hepatic and renal function tests (bili, BUN, creatinine, and alk phos), baseline and prior to each treatment. Notify physician of any abnormalities.

III. ALTERATION IN COMFORT related to PAIN AT INJECTION SITE

Defining Characteristics: Pain at the injection site may occur.

Nursing Implications: Assess site during and after infusion. Instruct patient to notify nurse if discomfort arises. Apply local measures to reduce discomfort.

Drug: glutamine (investigational)

Class: Nutrient (amino acid).

Mechanism of Action: Glutamine is the most abundant amino acid in blood and human tissues. It is a precursor of neurotransmitters and necessary in nucleic acid and nucleotide synthesis. Deficiency can occur during metabolic stress or catabolic periods. It is unclear how glutamine may protect or reduce neurotoxicity related to taxanes, or how it may reduce the arthralgias and myalgias related to paclitaxel administration.

Metabolism: Unknown.

Dosage/Range:
- Per research protocol.
- Neuroprotectant: glutamine 10 g PO tid beginning 24 hours after HD paclitaxel × 3–4 days prior to autologous BM.
- Prevention of arthralgias and myalgias: paclitaxel dose > 135 mg/m^2: glutamine 10 g tid starting on day 2 × 4 days; paclitaxel plus radiotherapy: glutamine 10 g tid 24 hours after paclitaxel × 3 days.

Drug Preparation:
- Oral, available in packets of 10 g per envelope; mix powder with water or preferred beverage.

Drug Administration:
- Per research protocol; drink immediately after mixing tid.

Drug Interactions:
- None known.

Lab Effects/Interference:
- None known.

Special Considerations:
- In laboratory animals, glutamine was shown to improve neuropathy associated with vincristine, cisplatin and paclitaxel.
- Anecdotal reports have shown prevention of arthralgias and myalgias in patients receiving paclitaxel who were their own controls.
- Numerous clinical research studies are ongoing to determine effectiveness, mechanism of action, pharmacokinetics.

- Glutamine available from health food stores.

Potential Toxicities/Side Effects and the Nursing Process

I. LACK OF KNOWLEDGE RE DRUG, SELF-ADMINISTRATION related to NEW PRODUCT

Defining Characteristics: Unclear how nutrient may work, but there are published reports suggesting its effectiveness. Randomized clinical trials are being undertaken to determine effectiveness, pharmacokinetics, and mechanism of action. There are no known side effects.

Nursing Implications: Assess baseline knowledge of nutrient, and its use. Teach patient dosing and self-administration per protocol.

Drug: mesna for injection (Mesnex)

Class: Sulfhydryl.

Mechanism of Action: Used to prevent ifosfamide-induced hemorrhagic cystitis. Drug is rapidly metabolized to the metabolite dimesna. In the kidney, dimesna is reduced to mesna, which binds to the urotoxic ifosfamide and cyclophosphamide metabolites acrolein and 4-hydroxyfosfamide, resulting in their detoxification.

Metabolism: Rapidly metabolized, remains in the intravascular compartment, and is rapidly eliminated by the kidneys. The drug is eliminated in 24 hours as mesna (32%) and dimesna (33%). Majority of the dose is eliminated within 4 hours. Oral mesna has 50% bioavailability of IV dose.

Dosage/Range: Initial dose should be given IV; subsequent doses can be given PO or IV

- Recommended IV-IV-IV: clinical dose 20% of the Mesna dose IV bolus 15 minutes before (or at the same time as the Ifosfamide), 4 hours and 8 hours after ifosfamide or cyclophosphamide dose. Mesna dose is 20% of ifosfamide or cyclophosphamide dose, with total daily dose 60% of the ifosphamide or cyclophosphamide dose.
- IV-oral-oral: Mesna is given as an IV bolus injection in a dosage equal to 20% of the ifosfamide dosage at the time of ifosfamide administration. Mesna tablets are given orally in a dosage equal to 40% of the ifosfamide dose at 2 and 6 hours after each dose of ifosfamide. The total daily dose of mesna is 100% of the ifosfamide dose.
- Patients who vomit within two hours of taking oral mesna should repeat the dose or receive IV mesna. The efficacy and safety of this ratio of IV-oral-

oral mesna has not been established as being effective for daily doses of ifosfamide higher than 2.0 gm/m^2 for 3–5 days.

- For continuous ifosfamide infusions, mesna is mixed with ifosfamide in equal amounts (1:1 mix). Prior to initiating continuous infusion, mesna is given IVB (10% of total ifosfamide dose). Following completion of the infusion, mesna alone should be infused for 12–24 hours to protect against delayed drug excretion activity against the bladder.
- Oral mesna: dose is 40% of ifosfamide or cyclophosphamide dose (not recommended for initial dose if the patient experiences nausea and vomiting).

Drug Preparation:

- Dilute mesna with 5% Dextrose, 5% Dextrose/0.9% Sodium Chloride, or 0.9% Sodium Chloride to create a designated fluid concentration.
- For continuous ifosfamide infusion, mesna should be mixed together with the ifosfamide.

Drug Administration:

- Diluted solution is stable for 24 hours at room temperature.
- Refrigerate and use reconstituted solution within 6 hours.
- Oral preparation can be diluted from 1:1–1:10 in cola, chilled fruit juice, or plain or chocolate milk (if patient vomits within 1 hour, patient should receive repeated IV dose).

Drug Interactions:

- Ifosfamide: mesna binds to drug metabolites; is given concurrently for bladder protection.

Lab Effects/Interference:

- None.

Special Considerations:

- At clinical doses, mild nausea, vomiting, and diarrhea are the only side effects expected.
- Can cause false-positive result on urinalysis for ketones.

Potential Toxicities/Side Effects and the Nursing Process

I. POTENTIAL FOR INJURY related to MAINTENANCE OF BLADDER MUCOSAL INTEGRITY

Defining Characteristics: Mesna uniquely concentrates in the bladder and has a very low degree of toxicity, making it the uroprotector of choice against ifosfamide-related urotoxicity.

Nursing Implications: Assess daily urinalysis. Assess for hematuria per hospital policy and procedure. Hydrate vigorously.

II. ALTERATION IN NUTRITION, LESS THAN BODY REQUIREMENTS, related to NAUSEA/VOMITING, DIARRHEA

Defining Characteristics: Nausea and vomiting are minor in incidence and severity. Diarrhea is mild if it occurs.

Nursing Implications: Assess baseline nutritional status. Usual antiemetics for ifosfamide or cyclophosphamide-induced nausea/vomiting protect against mesna contribution. Encourage small, frequent meals and liquids. Teach patient to avoid greasy, fried, or fatty foods. Encourage patient to report onset of nausea/vomiting or diarrhea.

Chapter 5

Molecularly Targeted Therapies

The new millennium has brought exciting promise to patients with cancer and to their nurses. As a better understanding of the process of carcinogenesis and metastases has emerged, with it has come identified molecular flaws that can be therapeutically targeted. For the past decades, systemic and local therapies have provided cure, disease stabilization, and palliation for many patients with cancer. However, the physical cost of these benefits was often significant, and included bone marrow depression with increased risk of infection and bleeding, nausea, and vomiting. The "magic bullet" was always sought so that benefit could be achieved with minimal toxicity. Today, a number of molecularly targeted agents have been FDA approved and thousands more are undergoing clinical testing. This chapter lays the groundwork for a sound understanding of the molecular basis of cancer, the identified and potential molecular flaws and targets, and the agents that target them. The presentation is simplified, and if the reader wishes more in-depth discussion of the material covered, please consult the references for more advanced readings.

Dr. Andrew von Eschenbach MD, NCI Director, describes our knowledge of the process of cancer (http://cancer.gov/BenchMarks/archives/2003_04/feature_article.html#q3):

"Today we understand cancer as both a genetic disease and a cell signaling failure. Genes that control orderly replication become damaged, allowing the cells to reproduce without restraint. A single cell's progress from normal, to malignant, to metastatic, appears to involve a series of interactive processes, each controlled by a different gene or set of genes. These altered genes produce defective protein signals, which are, in turn, mishandled by the cell. This understanding of the biology of cancer is enabling us to design interventions to preempt the cancer's progression to uncontrolled growth."

In order to better understand the molecular basis of cancer, it is important to recall early courses in biology and genetics. The following will be reviewed: basic cell biology, genetic mutations, malignant transformation, communication within the cell (signal transduction), over-expression of growth factor genes and their receptors, cell cycle regulation, loss of apoptosis, loss of telomerase activity, invasion, angiogenesis, and metastases.

BASIC CELL BIOLOGY

Cancer is a disease of the cell. The nucleus of the cell is where the genetic material, or Deoxyribonucleic Acid (DNA), is located. DNA is the building block of life, an incredibly simple yet complex double helix in which each strand is made up of millions of chemical bases, and each chemical base attaches to its complementary pair in a specific way (cytosine with guanine, thymine with adenosine). See Figure 5.1.

Genes are a subunit of DNA, and each gene contains a code for a specific product, such as a protein or enzyme. Scientists have now identified all the 35,000 or so genes in the human genome. Genes carry the blueprint of who we are. All cells have the genetic blueprint, but only the genes we need are "turned on," such as blue eyes. The genes we don't need at the moment are turned off. In early fetal growth, many genes are turned on, and then when the embryo develops into a baby, the unnecessary genes are "turned off." Genes code for specific proteins and are contained in a chromosome. Humans have 46 chromosomes: 22 autosomal pairs and 1 pair of sex chromosomes. When the body needs to make a specific protein or enzyme, or to make more cells, this requirement message comes to the cell, attaches to a receptor, such as a growth receptor, on the outside of the cell membrane. Once complexed at the growth factor receptor site, there is dimerization or pairing of receptors, or the receptor can be autostimulated; this begins the message, which is now sent through the membrane to tyrosine kinase molecules, which exchange the currency of a phosphate (phosphorylation) to send the message from one molecule to another (signal transduction). The information goes to the cell nucleus, the DNA strands separate exposing the gene that codes for that enzyme or protein, and information from the gene is copied.

The sequence of chemical bases in the gene are copied base by base onto a new strand of messenger ribonucleic acid (m-RNA) so that the complementary base is shown on the m-RNA. This piece of m-RNA then travels out of the nucleus into the cytoplasm of the cell to the ribosomes, which are the cell's "protein factory." Here the gene copy is transferred by transfer RNA (t-RNA) to the ribosome, and the copy is now identical to the original gene, telling the ribosome to make the specific protein or enzyme. Amino acids are then assembled into a completed protein molecule. See Figure 5.2

When a cell needs to divide, such as a cell lining the gastrointestinal tract, the cell's nucleus receives a message from a growth factor to divide. Recall the process of cell division in terms of the cell cycle, as discussed in Chapter 1. When each cell prepares to divide, the DNA is copied during the Synthesis (S) Phase to make a duplicate set of DNA for the daughter cell. Millions of coded genes are copied during cell division, or when the necessary proteins or enzymes are being made. Occasionally a mistake is made, such as when one

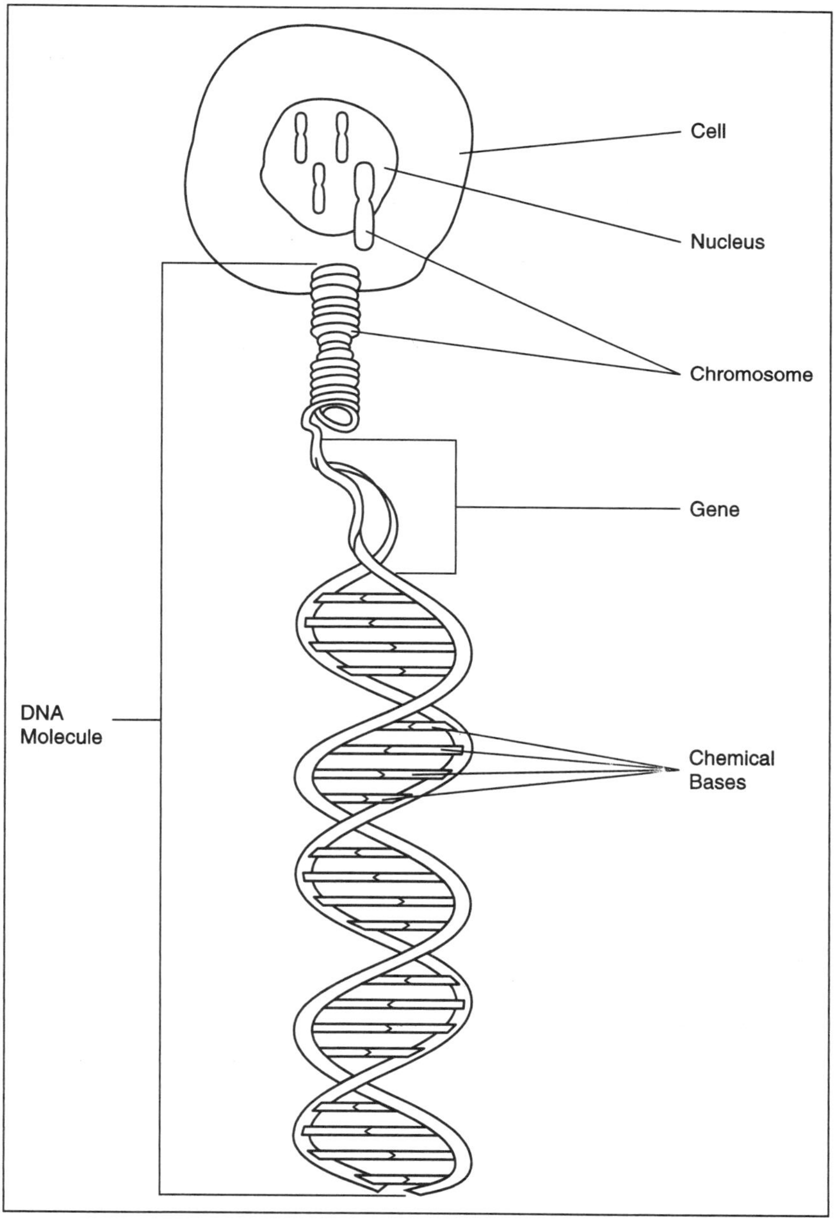

Figure 5.1 DNA: base pairs and double helix (NCI, Understanding Gene Testing, p ii, 1997)

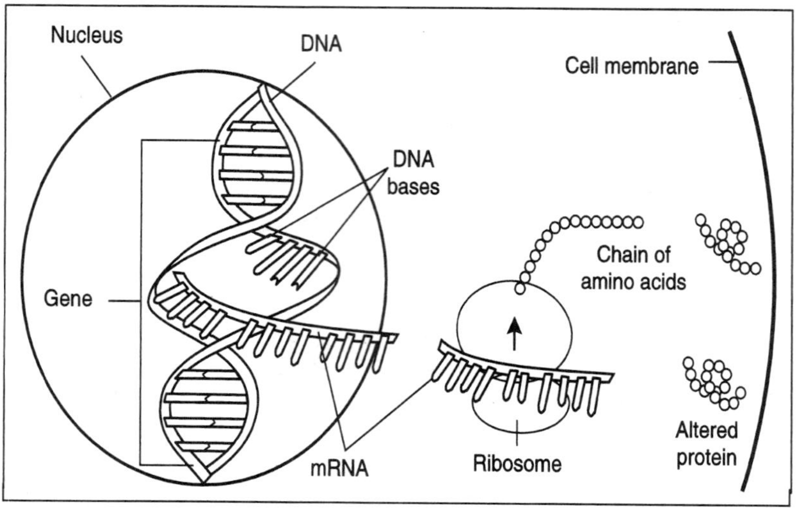

Figure 5.2 Protein synthesis (NCI, Understanding Gene Testing p 2, 1995)

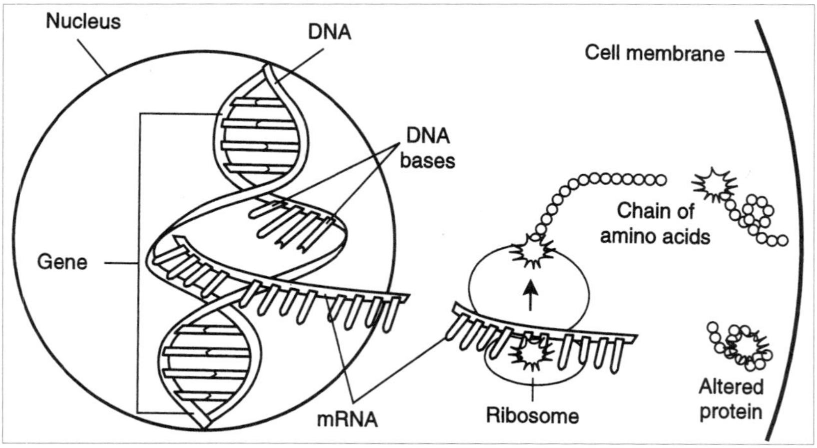

Figure 5.3 Mutation Leading to Abnormal Protein Production (NCI, Understanding Gene Testing p 4, 1995)

chemical base is not correctly copied. Often this is quickly fixed, but sometimes a mutation can result in the production of an abnormal protein, enzyme, or product. Figure 5.3 shows how a mutation can lead to the production of an abnormal protein. Different types of mutations are shown in Figure 5.4.

One example of a serious mutation is the reciprocal translocation between chromosome 9 and 22, forming an extra-long chromosome 9. The other chro-

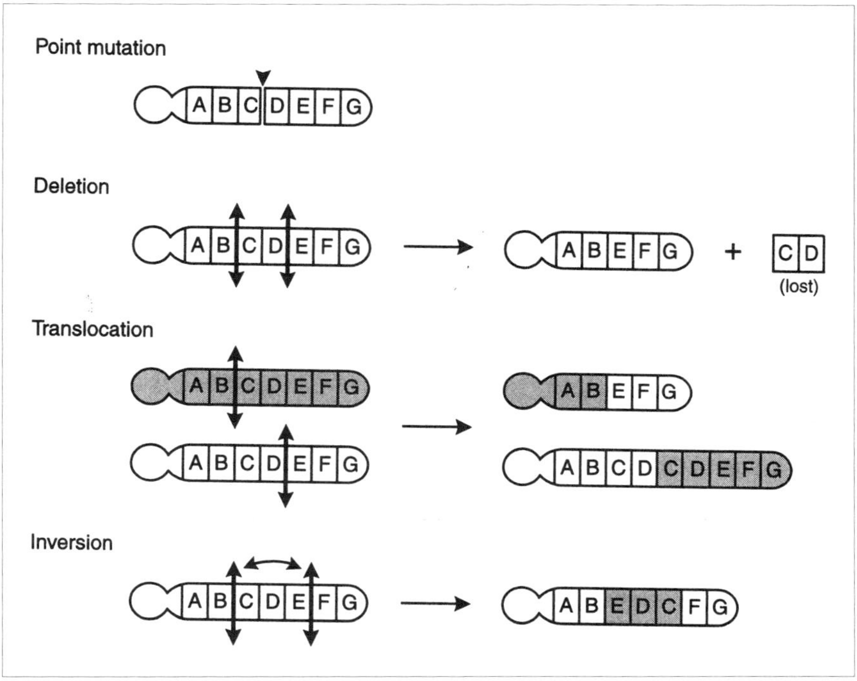

Figure 5.4 Types of Chromosomal Mutations

mosome is short, called the Philadelphia chromosome (Ph[1]) which contains the fused ABL-BCR gene, and is shown in Figure 5.5. This genetic abnormality occurs in 90% of patients with Chronic Myelogenous Leukemia (CML), and results in the formation of an abnormal receptor tyrosine kinase. Imatinib mesylate (Gleevec), a receptor tyrosine kinase inhibitor that selectively targets this flaw, has been FDA approved due to its extraordinary ability to block this mutation.

It appears that all malignancies are caused by mutations in cellular DNA. However, it usually takes at least four mutations to cause malignant transformation. This is shown in Figure 5.6.

Approximately 10% of these mutations are inherited or carried in the DNA of reproductive cells in individuals with parents carrying the gene, while 90% of mutations are acquired and considered sporadic. These develop during the course of one's life, due to exposure to carcinogens and are related to relationships among and between genes and the environment. Most cancers are not inherited, although two examples of inherited vulnerability to cancer are:

- Women who carry the BRCA-1 gene, who represent 5% or so of women who develop breast cancer, and

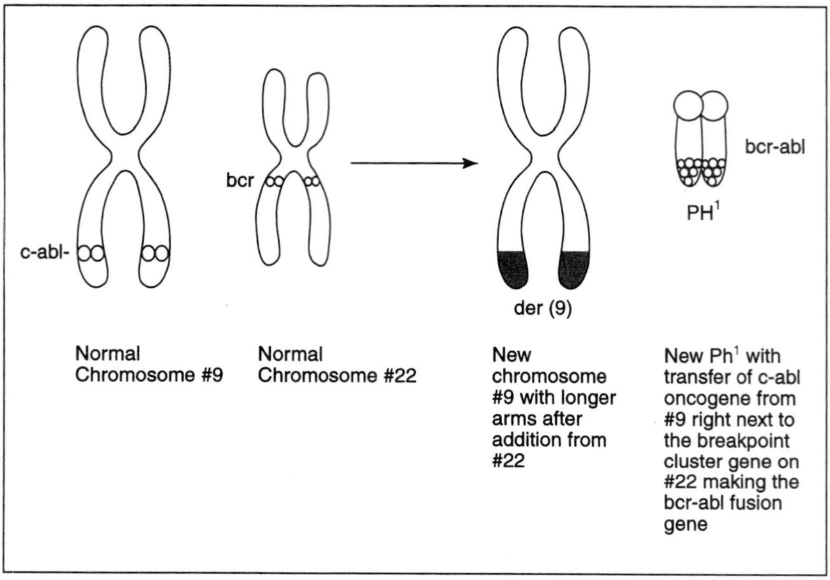

Figure 5.5 Philadelphia Chromosome

- Individuals with hereditary polyposis in which one allele of the APC tumor suppressor gene is silenced. This gene is located in the intraepithelial cells of the intestines. When the second allele becomes mutated, the gene no longer functions as a tumor suppressor gene. Thousands of polyps are formed, and many can progress to malignancy. Fortunately, COX-2 inhibitors appear to prevent many polyps from forming. This also suggests that cyclo-oxygenase 2 (COX-2) is an important mediator of not only inflammation, but also of malignant transformation. COX-2 is overexpressed in many premalignant and malignant tumors, in addition to colorectal adenomas and cancer, such as pancreatic cancer, oral leucoplakia and head and neck cancer, prostate intraepithelial neoplasia and prostate cancer, ductal carcinoma in situ, and breast cancer. Specifically, it appears that COX-2 plays a role in angiogenesis, apoptosis, inflammation, immunosuppression, and invasiveness (Dannenberg AJ et al, 2001).

Thus, people who have a genetic mutation start with one mutation. Most cancers, however, are related to acquired mutations, occurring when the genes become damaged during one's lifetime by factors in the environment or chemicals made in the cells. Genetic errors may be added during cell division when enzymes are copying DNA so that the mutation is copied into permanent DNA. Usually the body's DNA repair mechanism catches the mistake, and if unable to repair it, causes the cell to die (programmed cell death or apoptosis).

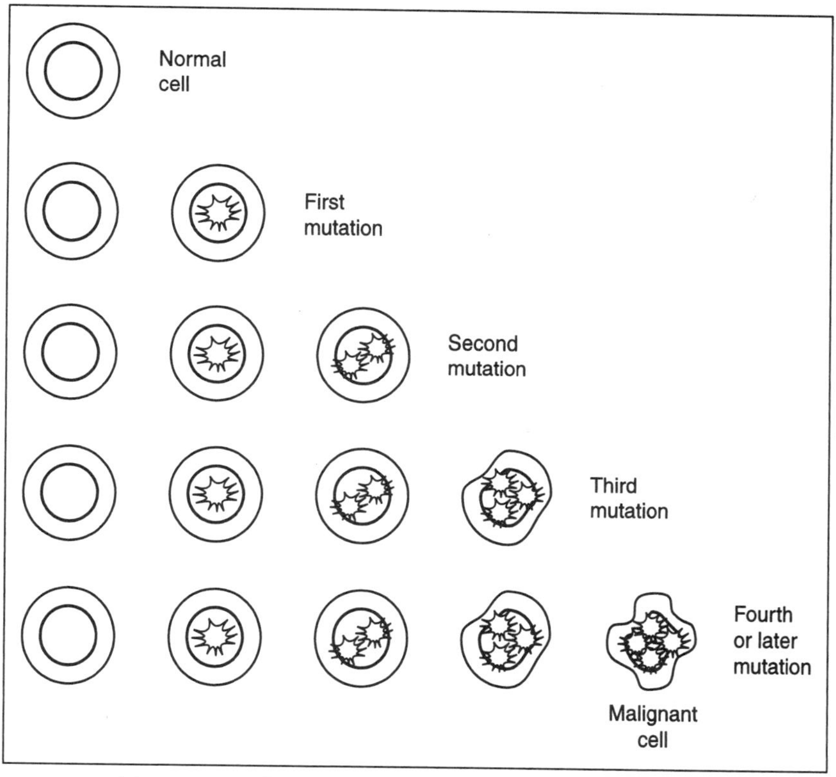

Figure 5.6 Mutations and Malignant Transformation (NCI, Understanding Gene Testing, p 13, 1995)

Sometimes, the system fails, and the error becomes permanent, and are passed on to successive generations of cells.

According to Lippman (2000) mutations in DNA can result from:

- **Gain of function:** The mutation activates one or more genes that lead to malignant transformation, such as with the *Ras, Myc, Epidermal Growth Factor Receptor* family. This results in the speeding up of cell growth and division, which makes more cells than the body needs.
- **Loss of function:** The mutation(s) inactivate genes that control cell growth, such as the tumor suppressor gene p53. In this case, the genetic mutation is not caught, the DNA is not repaired or destroyed, and the genetic flaw is perpetuated with each further cell division.

CELL COMMUNICATION (SIGNAL TRANSDUCTION)

How does a cell know when it needs to divide or make proteins or other cellular products? Signal transduction is the communication link between and among cells. It depends on signals that often originate on the cell surface, such as the growth factors or hormones that attach to cell surface receptors. These are called *ligands.* Once the growth factor attaches to the receptor, the receptor dimerizes with another receptor, and a message is generated. The receptor has three domains: one that sticks outside the cell (external), one that is transmembrane, and one that is internal. The message from a growth factor telling the cell to divide starts when it attaches to the receptor's external domain or "docking station." The message passes through the transmembrane domain into the internal domain, which changes in shape to allow it to interact with the receptor tyrosine kinases or "information-relaying molecules" in the cytoplasm (Scott and Pawson, 2000). Receptor tyrosine kinases pick the message up from the internal end of the receptor and pass it along from one molecule to another until it gets to the cell nucleus. The name *kinase* means enzyme, and this group adds a specific phosphate group to the amino acid tyrosine, called phosphorylation. This transfer of chemical energy activates the tyrosine kinase and it passes the message along from one molecule to another, like a "bucket brigade" or "signal cascade" (Weinberg, 1996). This way, the message is relayed "downstream" to the cell nucleus or down specific signaling pathways to get the desired effect, such as normal cell growth, cell division, differentiation (specialization), or cell death (apoptosis). It is a precise system and has many redundant parallel pathways. As the understanding of the complexity of cell signal transduction has grown, the many potential targets for anticancer therapy have skyrocketed! Figures 5.7 and 5.8 show schemas of cell signals resulting in important cell functions.

Important growth factors are the epidermal growth factor family (EGF or erb-1, erb-2 or HER-2-neu, erb-3, and erb-4), platelet derived growth factor (PDGF), vascular endothelial growth factor (VEGF), transforming growth factor α (TGF-α), and fibroblast growth factor (FGF). The EGF receptor family is very important for cell growth, differentiation, and survival. Many cancers overexpress this receptor resulting in a more aggressive tumor with increased tendency for invasion and metastases and shorter survival. HER-2-neu has become well known because it is overexpressed in about 20% of breast cancer cases, again conferring a poor prognosis. A number of monoclonal antibodies have been developed to block the external domain of the EGF-1 receptor (cetuximab or Erbitux), and the EGF-2 receptor (trastuzumab or Herceptin), and the internal domain [receptor tyrosine kinase inhibitors such as imatinib mesylate (Gleevec).

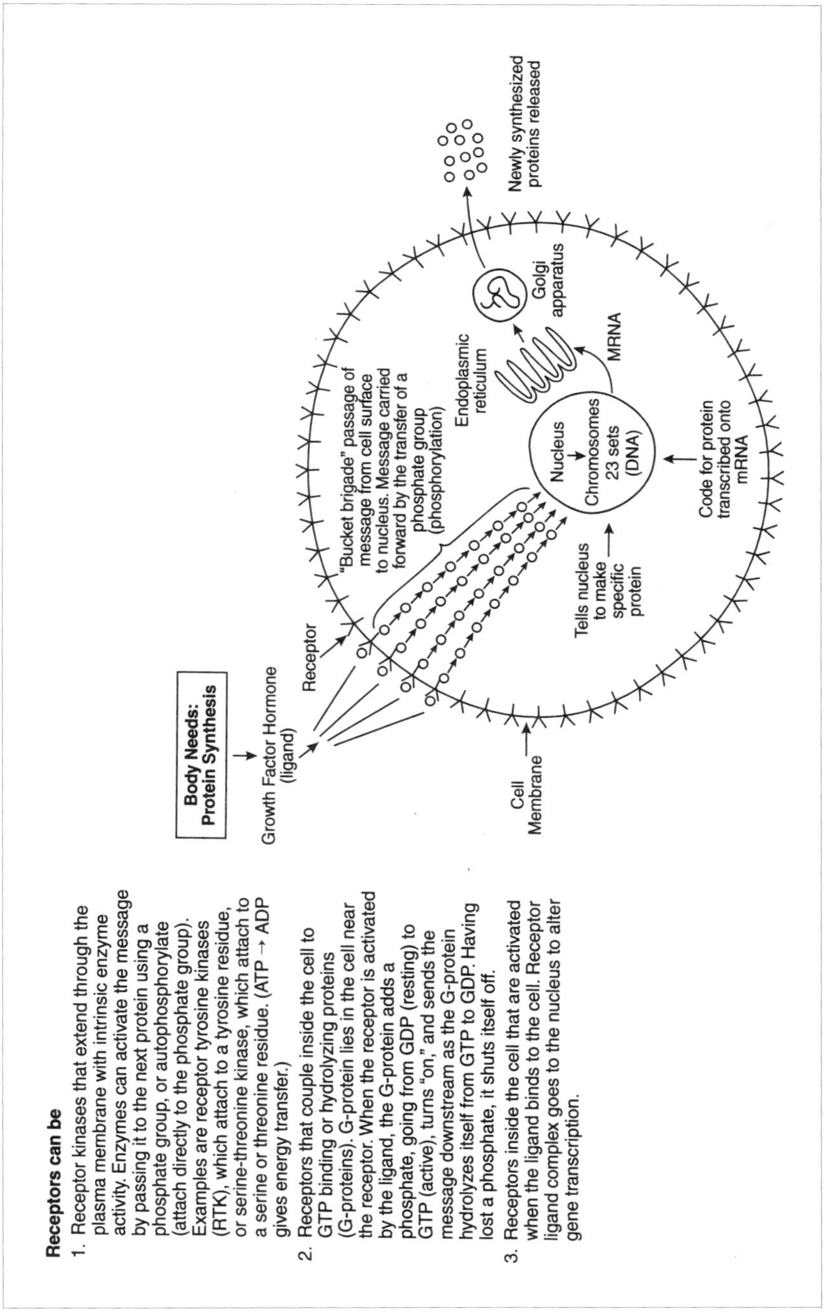

Figure 5.7 Cell Communication: The Inside Story (Scott JD and Pawson T. Scientific American, June 2000)

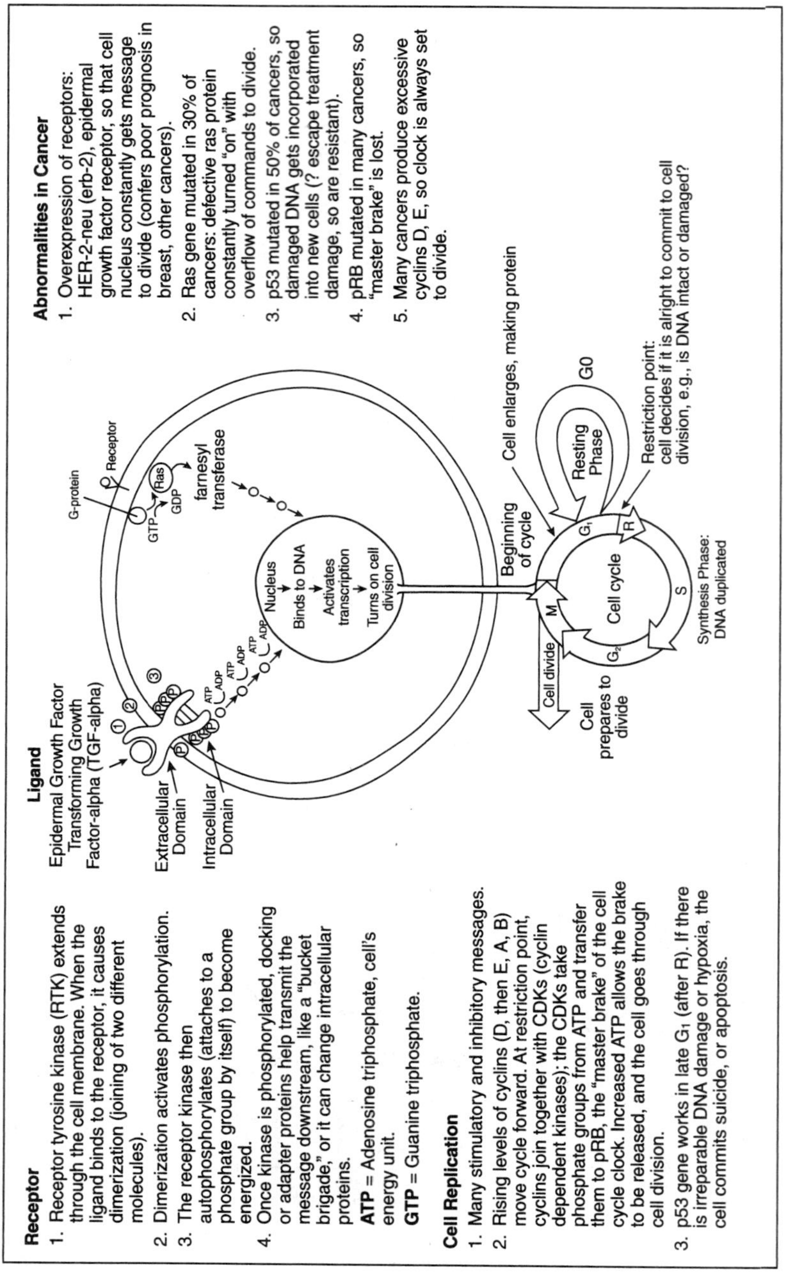

Figure 5.8 Epidermal Growth Factor Receptor and Its Role in Signal Transduction and Tumor Progression (Harari and Huang, 2000)

MALIGNANT TRANSFORMATION

How exactly does the malignant transformation occur? Normally, cell division occurs only when the tissue needs to replace lost or dead cells. Proto-oncogenes are normal cells that encourage cell growth. They are balanced by tumor suppressor genes that not only tell the cell nucleus not to divide if cells are not needed, but they also prevent injured or mutated cells from going through cell division and passing on genetic errors. Mutations must occur in both oncogenes and suppressor genes to get malignant transformation.

For example, a mutation in a proto-oncogene can start the process. This is because proto-oncogenes often produce the protein molecules in the bucket brigade. As a result, the mutates oncogene keeps sending the message to the nucleus for the cell to divide over and over again, leading to uncontrolled cell division. Other mutated oncogenes can also lead to the overproduction of growth factors. PDGF or TGF-α can repeatedly tell the cell to divide, while HER-2-neu overexpression causes proliferation of cell surface receptors that flood the cell with signals to divide, again leading to uncontrolled cell division.

Other proto-oncogenes code for other molecules in the signal cascade, such as the *ras* family of proto-oncogenes which are the H-ras gene, the K-ras-gene, and the N-ras gene (Weinberg, 1996). Normally, the *ras* gene, a proto-oncogene, codes for proteins that bring the message from the cell surface growth factor receptors to other protein messengers further down the signal cascade as part of the bucket brigade, activating downstream effectors such as the Raf-1/mitogen-activating protein kinase (MAPK) pathway, and the Rac/Rho pathway (Rowinsky et al, 1999). Once the message is sent to the nucleus, the ras protein is turned "off," and remains off until recruited again to the cell membrane to bring another message from the extracellular growth factor to inside the cell, and down to the cell nucleus. If the ras proto-oncogene is mutated and then activated, it becomes locked in an "on" position, and keeps sending the message to divide even when there is no growth factor binding to the surface receptor, and no message was actually generated. In order to become activated and to attach to the inner surface of the cell membrane, ras has a molecule added called farnesyl isoprenoid; it depends upon an enzyme called farnesytansferase (FTase) to catalyze this addition. If the enzyme is inhibited, then the ras protein is blocked, and in many tumors, causes cells to undergo dysregulation of the cell cycle and programmed cell death (apoptosis). Tipifarnib (R115777, Zarnestra) is a farnesyltransferase inhibitor (FTI) that has shown exciting results in phase III clinical trials. If farnesylation is not blocked, and the ras protein goes to the cell membrane, then Raf-1 kinase is activated and phosphorylates two MAPK kinases (MEK_1 and MEK_2 that are also known as extracellular signal-regulated kinases 1 and 2). Once activated, (phosphorylated), the MAPKs move to the nucleus, where they start a chain reaction leading to cell proliferation (Rowinsky et al, 1999). Sorafenib (BAY 43-9006) is a multi-targeted protein kinase inhibitor that inhibits Raf-kinase, as well as two kinases involved in angiogenesis (VEGF-2, PDGF-β, which is being studied in Phase III trials. It is estimated that 33% of all cancers have a mutated *ras* oncogene, especially cancers Sorof the colon, pancreas, and lungs (Weinberg, 1996). These oncogenes, or their products, are therapeutic targets being studied in clinical trials to block their function so that, for example, the abnormal *ras* proteins are not produced.

Another key pathway that appears to play an important role in cancer is the STAT (Signal Transducers and Activators of Transcription) pathway. This pathway is made up of proteins in the cytoplasm of the cell that join together (dimerize) when activated by tyrosine phosphorylation (Haura et al, 2005). This causes the activated STAT proteins to move into the cell nucleus, then into the DNA where they bind to gene promoters and regulate the expression of certain genes involved in malignancy. The STAT proteins that are activated by themselves without normal growth regulation (constitutive) during malignant transformation regulate pathways such as cell-cycle progression, programmed cell death (apoptosis), angiogenesis, invasion, metastases, and evasion of the immune system by tumor (Haura et al, 2005). Many tumors have dysregulation of Stat 3, Stat 4, and loss of Stat 1 function. Agents are being studied to target the flaws in the STAT signaling pathway.

Via an analogous bucket brigade of inhibitory signals from the cell surface to the nucleus, the normal cell nucleus also receives messages from tumor suppressor genes telling it not to divide unless the body tissues need more cells. This normally prevents the mutated oncogene from causing uncontrolled cell growth, and can be thought of as "putting brakes on" the cell division process. However, tumor suppressor genes also become mutated, and this must occur in order for the malignant transformation to happen. The most famous of these tumor suppressor genes is p53; it appears to be mutated in over 50% of human cancers.

Once there are mutations in both the proto-oncogene and tumor suppressor genes, then there is no longer balance between cell growth and division. Instead, there is uncontrolled cell growth. How does this happen? Again, recall the cell cycle as shown in Figures 5.8 and 5.9. Normally, the nucleus activates the cell cycle by putting the cell into cell division mode only when the stimulatory signals are greater than the inhibitory signals. When this happens, levels of cyclins rise (cyclin D, followed by E, A, and B) as the cell moves through the phases of the cell cycle. This starts the cell to cycle, initiating in the G_1 phase. During this phase, the cell produces new proteins that make RNA in preparation for cell division. The cell enlarges, and the time spent in this phase is highly variable. If division is not needed, then the cell goes into a resting phase called G_0. Near the end of G_1, the cell decides whether to proceed into cell division that is called the *Restriction point.* Weinberg (1996) describes this as a time when the molecular switch needs to be moved from the "off" mode to "on mode," as follows: Cyclins D then E combine/activate cyclin-dependent kinases, enzymes which then transfer phosphate groups from adenosine triphosphate (ATP), the energy molecule, to the retinoblastoma protein (pRB) which is the "master brake" of the cell cycle. If no phosphate groups are added to pRB, the brake stays in the "off" position; however, the brake is lifted when sufficient phosphate groups are added. When the brake is lifted, transcription factors are released which interact with genes so that proteins are actively synthesized for progression through the cell cycle. Mutations can also occur in important inhibitory proteins that would otherwise stop the cell cycle from progressing forward, specifically p53, pRB, p16, and p15. This is important because the cell's DNA is examined to see whether there are any mutations or mistakes, and, if so, the cell tries to repair them. If the DNA cannot be repaired, p53 causes the cell to go into "programmed cell death," or apoptosis. This normally eliminates any abnormal cells from the body. Unfortunately, in over 50% of cancers this protein is inactive. In some cancers, such as cervical cancer, both p53 and pRB are both inactivated (Weinberg, 1996), and in small cell lung cancer and retinoblastoma, pRB is lost. Other proteins such as the cyclins or cyclin-dependent kinases (CDK), which can be synthesized in greater number, or loss of CDK inhibitors, can move the cell through the cell cycle relentlessly. Unfortunately, most cancers have some abnormalities in the cell cycle machinery, and each of these becomes a molecular flaw that can be targeted.

The genes for p53 and pRB are also active in regulating normal cell senescence, leading to programmed cell death. All somatic cells have a finite life of 50–60 doublings after which the cell dies. At the end of the chromosomes, caps called *telomeres* count each of the cell divisions, and snip off a piece of the chromosome with each division. After 50–60 divisions, the chromosome is too short to divide again. In a developing embryo, where there is rapid cell division, the chromosome is protected from being snipped off with each division by the enzyme telomerase, which replaces each snipped piece. This enzyme is not found in normal cells after the embryo develops into a fetus but is found in all tumor cells. If there is a mutation that inactivates either of these genes, the cells can use telomerase to replace each of the snipped off pieces of chromosome, to become immortal. Again, telomerase becomes a molecular target.

2003 saw the arrival of a unique class of antineoplastic targeted therapy: proteasome inhibitors. Bortezomib (Velcade) is the first of this class that is FDA approved for cancer therapy, specifically multiple myeloma as it interferes with the interaction of the myeloma cells with the bone marrow microenvironment. Proteasomes are enzyme complexes that are the housekeeping enzymes which degrade or breakdown proteins in the cell nucleus so that the

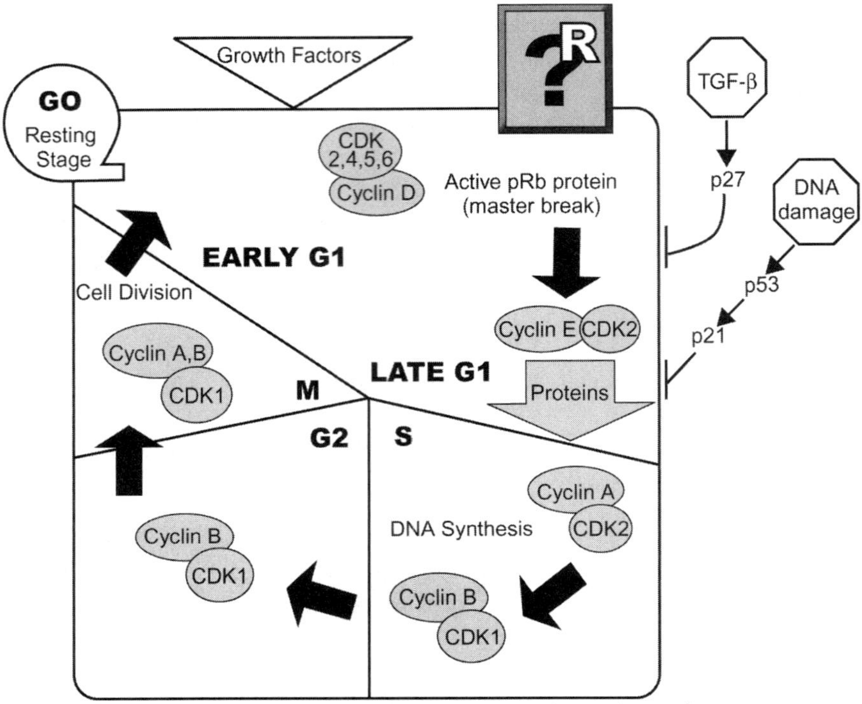

Figure 5.9 The Cell Cycle (Merkle CJ, Loescher LJ. The Biology of Cancer. In Yarbro CH, Frogge MH and Goodman M, (eds). *Cancer Nursing: Principles and Practice*, 6th ed. Sudbury, MA: Jones and Bartlett Inc; 2005;15)

proteins can be recycled and used again. They are found in every cell of the body. The proteasomes know which proteins to degrade because they are tagged with ubiquitin. The ubiquitin-proteasome pathway regulates protein homeostasis within the cell (Kemple, 2003). Proteasome inhibitors block this process from occurring, so the cell gets conflicting signals about cell regulation. The high volume of the conflicting messages the cell nucleus receives causes malignant cells to go into apoptosis or programmed cell death, while normal cells are less sensitive to this overload and can recover. Specifically, 3 pathways are affected by proteasome inhibition: the cell cycle (proteins active in the cell cycle such as cyclins, cyclin-dependent kinase inhibitors, tumor suppressor p53), apoptosis (proteins which inhibit apoptosis like XIAP, cIAP, and Bcl-2 proteins), and Nuclear Factor-kappa B dependent signaling (inhibitor of this pathway is I kappa B-alpha) [Glickman and Ciechanover, 2002]. Nuclear Factor (NF)-kappa B is a transcription factor that has been found to regulate a number of genes that control malignant transformation and metastases. Inactive proteins p50, p65, I kappa B- alpha, and NF-kappa B are found in the cytoplasm of the cell (outside the nucleus). When NF-kappa B is activated by carcinogens, tumor promoter factors, inflammatory cytokines, and some chemotherapy agents, I kappa B-alpha is broken down and the other two proteins move into the nucleus. They attach to DNA in the nucleus at a promoter region and activate the gene. Once NF-kappa B is activated, it can stop apoptosis, which leads to tumor formation and resistance to chemotherapy. There is much excitement about using chemoprevention strategies to block activation of the NF-kappa B by inhibiting its signaling pathway, such as the proteasome does. In addition, it theoretically increases tumor sensitivity to chemotherapy (Bharti and Aggarwal, 2002).

A number of agents are being investigated that target Bcl-2 or other proteins that may suppress apoptosis. Since Bcl-2 protein inhibits apoptosis and makes the cells resistant to treatment with standard chemotherapy, drugs such as anti-sense oligonucleotides theoretically can disable Bcl-2 and restore responsiveness to chemotherapy. Oblimersen sodium is an anti-sense oligonucleotide that binds to Bcl-2 messenger RNA (mRNA), leading to the degradation of Bcl-2 mRNA, which then results in decreased Bcl-2 protein translation or downregulation of Bcl-2 (Klaska et al, 2002).

Another exciting group of agents being explored is the histone deacetylase (HDAC) inhibitors. HDACs complex with cell regulatory proteins to regulate gene transcription, and are key components of cell proliferation, angiogenesis, apoptosis, and cell differentiation. HDAC inhibitors are intended to help malignant cells become normal again, since they target and accumulate in malignant cells. An example of one such agent is suberoylanilide hydroxamic acid (SAHA), which has demonstrated activity in cutaneous T-cell lymphoma, diffuse large B-cell lymphoma, and mesothelioma. SAHA is synergistic with radiation, tyrosine kinase inhibitors, and cytotoxic agents (NCI, 2004).

INVASION AND METASTASES

Once a mutation of an epithelial cell occurs, for example, further development and transformation into malignancy occurs in stages. In this case, the first mutation causes hyperplasia or increased proliferation of normal-appearing cells, and the second leads to dysplasia. The cells now appear abnormal. A third mutation may cause a change to carcinoma in situ, in which the cells remain within normal tissue boundaries. If allowed to continue, the cells may again mutate and develop invasiveness, allowing them to invade underlying tissue and enter blood and lymphatic vessels. As cells are shed, they travel via the blood or lymph system to distant sites. This is called *metastases.* It initially seemed that metastases begins after the development of a detectable tumor, but it is now clear that, in some tumors, metastases can begin even before the primary tumor is detectable. In general, a tumor cannot grow beyond a size of 2 mm (the head of a pin) unless it forms new blood vessels (angiogenesis).

However, not all cancers are invasive or metastasize. The explosion of scientific discovery about cell function and the molecular processes of metastases has led to the clinical trials of numerous molecularly targeted therapies, including agents that interrupt different steps in the metastases process. Fortunately, it appears that the metastatic process is highly inefficient, especially in late disease, and, in addition, each of the steps is "rate limiting," so that if one step is not achieved, the process can't move forward (Stetler-Stevenson and Kleiner, 2001).

Stetler-Stevenson and Kleiner (2001) identify eight steps in the "metastatic cascade," each controlled by a number of gene products in the malignant cell. Some aggressively permit invasion and others subvert the normal body's defenses against metastases. These steps include the detachment of cells from the primary tumor, invasion of the underlying basement membrane and extracellular tissue, movement of cells into blood vessels, and survival in the venous or lymphatic circulation until reaching a capillary bed. There the malignant cell must attach to the basement membrane of the blood vessel, enter the tissue of the organ fed by the capillary bed, respond to local growth factors, begin cell division to form a small tumor, and begin the formation of local blood vessels to support growth beyond 2 mm.

1. As seen, a cell undergoes multiple mutations during malignant transformation. A single cell (clone) that goes through multiple mutations usually results in cells that are not all alike (heterogenous). Some of the cells are more likely to metastasize than others. Activation of the *ras* oncogene turns a malignant cell into one that invades and metastasizes, and there appears to be a survival advantage for more aggressive cells that respond to local growth factors. The new, tiny tumor gets nourishment by simple diffusion. However, once the tumor reaches 2 mm, it can grow no bigger until it gets its own blood supply to increase the delivery of nutrients.
2. As the tumor grows, the cells on the outside get nourishment (e.g., oxygen), but the cells in the inside (core) become hypoxic. This causes the activation of an "angiogenic switch," involving secretion of angiogenic growth factors (e.g., Vascular Endothelial Growth Factor, VEGF) and suppressing normal inhibitors of angiogenesis (e.g., angiostatin). The blood vessels that form are leaky but have an invasiveness not seen in normal new blood vessels. If the tumor grows near an existing vessel, it may invade and use existing vessels before making its own. Unfortunately, studies have shown that turning on the angiogenic switch is associated with increased frequency of metastases, disease recurrence, and shorter survival (Weidner, 1998).

3. Cells continue to mutate in the primary tumor, and a clone of cells emerges that is superior in growth and is highly invasive. This clone of cells turns down (down regulates) the activity of substances that keep normal cells sticking to their neighboring cells (cell-cell adhesion molecules called *cadherins*, and in epithelial cells, *E-cadherin*) and to the extracellular matrix (integrins). Thus, the tumor cells become mobile and can separate from the rest of the primary tumor. Stromolysin-1 is a matrix metalloproteinase (MMP) that can degrade E-cadherin, and is associated with tumor progression. The tumor cell then uses enzymes (e.g., MMPs) to destroy the integrity of the basement membrane that the tumor lies on, as well as the extracellular matrix. Imagine it like a tank destroying the area ahead so that the invading army can move forward. Now the malignant cells can invade neighboring normal tissue and the newly made leaky blood vessels or nearby thin-walled lymph vessels. Normal cells must remain attached to the extracellular matrix or they die. It is unclear how malignant cells can overcome this. Integrins are critical molecules in the extracellular matrix and also have a role in cell signal transduction and cell growth. Changes in integrin-mediated signaling allow the malignant cell to become invasive and to migrate. Integrin attached to the extracellular matrix gives the malignant cell adhesive traction. As the actin filaments in the cell's cytoskeleton contract, the cell body is propelled forward. Proportionate to the age and size of the primary tumor, huge numbers and clumps of malignant cells can be shed into the bloodstream. The clinical effect depends on whether the embolized cells reach a favorable environment and can achieve the steps in metastases.
4. Individual cells or clumps of cells are carried in the blood or lymph circulation, and many do not survive. The cells need to survive the turbulence of blood flow as well as the circulating cell-mediated and humoral immune cell elements (e.g., cytotoxic and killer lymphocytes). Most die.
5. Cells that survive the ride to distant organs or lymph nodes either get stuck in the microcirculation or attach to specific endothelial cells in capillaries or lymph vessels. In addition, they may attach to an exposed basement membrane of the organ or lymph node.
6. The cells "extravasate" from the blood or lymph vessel into the extracellular tissue and either grow in response to growth factors or stay dormant in this secondary site. Malignant cells migrate to find a "favorable" site. Many die.
7. If successful in finding an hospitable local environment, after some growth to 2 mm, the tumor cells release angiogenic growth factors to build blood vessels in this secondary site. This increases the ability of the metastastic cells to metastasize again.

8. How the metastatic cells evade the body's host immune responses is not well known.

ANGIOGENESIS

Many similarities exist between angiogenesis and tumor invasion and, as a result, they may have similar molecular targets. The body normally needs the ability to make new blood vessels for processes such as wound healing, female menstruation, rebuilding the endometrial lining, or making the placenta during pregnancy. The body maintains a fine balance between turning angiogenesis on and turning it off. When there are more factors favoring angiogenesis than opposing it (inhibitors), angiogenesis occurs. Factors that are angiogenic growth factors are shown in Table 5.1. When cells are hypoxic or lacking oxygen, they release vascular endothelial growth factor (VEGF), also known as vascular permeability factor. VEGF initiates new blood vessel growth and casuses the release of nitric oxide (NO) from the endothelial cells lining the blood vessel, which causes them to dilate. There are a number of VEGF receptors on the endothelial cells, and the most important appears to be VEGF-R2. Others are VEGF-R1, VEGF-R3 (Flt-4), which when stimulated send the message for proliferation and migration of endothelial cells via a tyrosine kinase system, and neuropilin, which is a non-tyrosine kinase receptor. Neuropilin is hypothesized to be a survival factor for tumors (Parikh et al, 2004). Bevacizumab prevents VEGF (the ligand) from binding to VEGF-R2. Numerous agents are being developed and tested to block the VEGF-R2 receptor (monoclonal anti-

Table 5.1 Natural Factors that Stimulate or Inhibit Angiogenesis

Factors Stimulating Angiogenesis	Factors Inhibiting Angiogenesis
• Angiopoietin-1	• Cartilage derived inhibitor (CDI)
• Fibroblast growth factor	• Herparinases
• Interleukin-8	• Human chorionic gonadotropin (hCG)
• Tumor Necrosis Factor (TNF) alpha	• Interferon (alpha, beta, gamma)
• Transforming Growth Factor (TGF) alpha and beta	• Interleukin-12
• Plasminogen activator inhibitor retinoids	• Plasminogen activator inhibitor retinoids
• Platelet derived growth factor (PDGF) BB	• Tissue inhibitors of metaloproteinases called TIMPs
• Granulocyte-Colony Stimulating Factor (G-CSF)	• Thrombospondin-1
• VEGF, also known as vascular permeability factor (VPF)	• Vasculostatin
	• Platelet factor-4

bodies with longer half-lives), and tyrosine kinases (TKIs, which are given orally and have short-half-lives). Of interest, clinical trials with bevacizumab showed not only the cessation of tumor angiogenesis and growth, but also tumor regression suggesting that when combined with chemotherapy, anti-angiogenesis agents alter the tumor blood flow so that the chemotherapy is more effective in killing tumor cells. In addition, it is now believed that there are VEGF- receptors are on tumor cells which are involved in tumor cell migration and invasion; thus, anti-angiogenesis agents appear to directly affect tumor cells (Fan et al, 2005). New agents with ability to target multiple receptors are being developed.

Platelet derived growth factor is necessary for the pericytes outside the newly formed blood vessel to give it stability. Sorafenib (BAY 43-9006), a multiple targeted protein tyrosine kinase inhibitor as well as an anti-angiogenesis agent, appears to block the Raf kinase step in the ras pathway, as well as VEGF-2 and PDGF-β.

Drugs such as bevacizumab (Avastin) neutralize Vascular Endothelial Growth Factor (VEGF), which is released by tumors to start the process of angiogenesis. This drug has shown a significant delay in disease recurrence and increased overall survival in patients with metastatic colon and rectal cancers when combined with chemotherapy. The drug is being studied in the adjuvant setting and it is hoped that it may prevent metatases in patients with Stage III colon cancer. It has also been shown to increase overall survival when combined with carboplatin and paclitaxel in patients with non-squamous NSCLC.

Some substances in the extracellular matrix components undergo proteolysis and release angiogenesis inhibitors such as endostatin and others (Stetler-Stevenson and Kleiner, 2001). On their Web site, http://www.angio.org/providers/oncology/oncology.html, the Angiogenesis Foundation describes the process of angiogenesis (see also Figure 5.10) as follows:

- Angiogenic growth factors are released, normally by injured tissue, and in the case of malignancy, by tumor cells that require blood vessels to grow beyond their current size. The growth factors diffuse into the neighboring tissue.
- The growth factors bind to receptors on the endothelial cells of a nearby blood vessel, activating the endothelial cells.
- Once activated, the endothelial cells send a signal from the cell membrane into the cell nucleus telling the nucleus (genes) to make new molecules, including enzymes.
- The enzymes dissolve tiny holes in the basement membrane of the blood vessels in the area.
- The endothelial cells are stimulated to divide, making more endothelial cells that migrate through the holes in the basement membrane and move toward

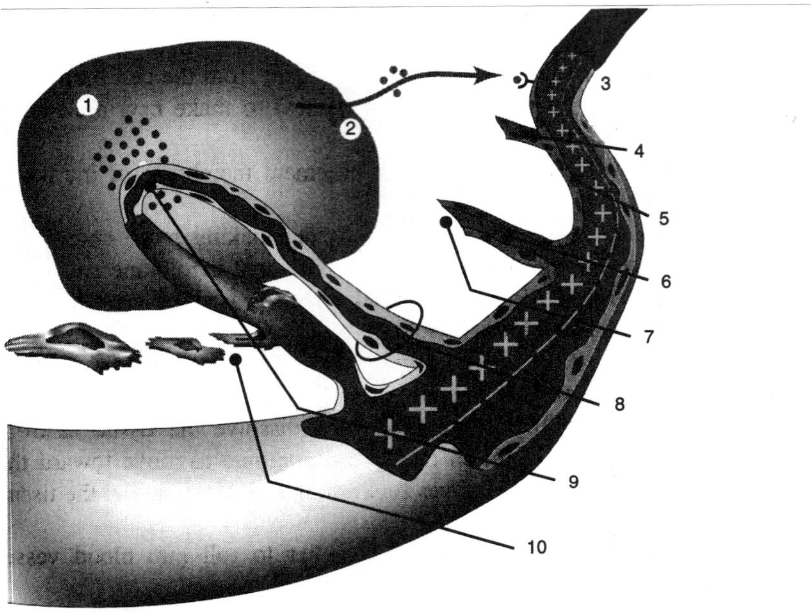

1. Hypoxic or injured tissues produce and release angiogenic growth factors (proteins) that diffuse into the nearby tissues.
2. The angiogenic growth factors bind to endothelial receptors located on the endothelial cells (EC) of nearby preexisting blood vessels.
3. Once growth factors bind to their receptors, the endothelial cells become activated. Signals are sent from the cell's surface to the nucleus. The endothelial cell's machinery begins to produce new molecules, including enzymes
4. Enzymes dissolve tiny holes in the sheath-like covering (basement membrane) surrounding all existing blood vessels.
5. The endothelial cells begin to divide (proliferate), and they migrate out through the dissolved holes of the existing vessels towards the diseased tissue (tumor),
6. Specialized molecules called adhesion molecules, or integrins (avb3, avb5), serve as grappling hooks to help pull the sprouting new blood vessel forward.
7. Additional enzymes (matrix metalloproteinases, or MMP) are produced to dissolve the tissue in front of the sprouting vessel tip in order to accommodate it. As the vessel extends, the tissue is remolded around the vessel.
8. Sprouting endothelial cells roll up to form a blood vessel tube.
9. Individual blood vessel tubes connect to form blood vessel loops that can circulate blood.
10. Finally, newly formed blood vessel tubes are stabilized by specialized muscle cells (smooth muscle cells, pericytes) that provide structural support. Blood flow then begins.

Figure 5.10 The Angiogenesis Cascade (Modified from the Angiogenesis Foundation, 2000, Angiogenesis Cascade) the injured tissue or malignant cells that released the growth factor, like tiny sprouting new blood vessels.

- Adhesion molecules (integrins) act like little grappling hooks and pull the sprouting new blood vessels forward toward the tumor.
- Additional enzymes (MMPs) are made and dissolve the tissue in front of the sprouting blood vessel so that it can continue to move toward the tumor. After the blood vessel moves forward, the MMPs remodel the tissue to anchor the blood vessel.
- The sprouting endothelial cells come together to roll into blood vessel tubes.
- The individual blood vessel tubes connect to form blood vessel loops.
- Smooth muscle cells stabilize the blood vessels, and blood begins to flow from the parent blood vessel to the new blood vessel loops.

Table 5.2 lists agents currently being tested to inhibit angiogenesis. These are only some of the many agents undergoing clinical testing. In addition, altering the dose and administration schedule of some standard chemotherapy agents appears to change the mechanism of action. As illustrated in the complex steps of metatastases, there are innumerable opportunities for interruption, causing the arrest of the metastatic cascade.

FINDING AND ESTABLISHING A METASTATIC SITE

Ruoslahti (1996) describes the "area code" hyposthesis first developed by Dreyer and Sperry in the late 1960s. The theory helps to explain how certain malignancies develop metastases in preferential areas given that, as we have seen, metastatic cells are blindly embolized into the bloodstream.

First, in order to be embolized, malignant epithelial cells must overcome two types of adhesion, which keep normal cells adhering to one another and attached to the protein meshwork (extracellular matrix), especially in epithelial tissue. This is important because most cancers are epithelial, arising from the epithelial covering of the outer layer of skin and outer layer and lining of many organs, such as the gut and lungs.

Cell-to-cell adhesion molecules keep normal cells orderly. One molecule is especially important, E-cadherin, which ensures intercellular adhesion. Early studies show that when this molecule is manipulated in cancer cells, it changes a cell from a non-invasive cell to an invasive cell capable of forming tumors. When functional E-cadherin is restored, this tendency can be reversed. Malignant cells are able to inactivate E-cadherin and are released from this requirement of cell-to-cell adhesion.

Table 5.2 Agents Currently Being Tested to Inhibit Angiogenesis

MMP Inhibitors	Growth Factor Inhibitors	Small Molecule Inhibitors
• COL-3 (synthetic, tetracycline derivative) • BMS-275291 (synthetic) • Marimastat (synthetic) • AG3340 (synthetic) • Neovastat (natural)	• SU 6668 (blocks vascular endothelial growth factor (VEGF), fibroblast growth factor (FGF), and epidermal growth factor (EGF) signaling from the receptor to the cell nucleus) • Anti-VEGF Ab (monoclonal antibody to VEGF) • Interferon alfa (inhibits bFGF) • Thalidomide (recently found to inhibit VEGF, others) • SU5416 (blocks VEGF signaling from the receptor to cell nucleus)	• Angiostatin (inhibits proliferation of endothelial cells) • Endostatin (inhibits proliferation of endothelial cells) • EMD 121974 (blocks endothelial integrin) • TNP-470 (inhibits proliferation of endothelial cells) • Combretastatin (causes programmed cell death of proliferating endothelial cells) • IM862 (inhibits endothelial cells.

Source: From Folkman (2001), others

In addition, for cell survival and reproduction, normal cells must adhere to the extracellular matrix. In laboratory tests, cells in culture cannot grow unless they attach to a surface, or achieve *anchorage dependence* (Ruoslahti and Reed, 1994). The molecules on the cell surface that actually do the attachment are *integrins.* Integrins must be intact for cell growth and cell division. It appears that integrins influence a protein in the cell nucleus called cyclin E-CDK2 complex (cyclin dependent kinase [CDK]), which is necessary for the cell cycle (division) clock to move toward cell growth and division. When cells do not adhere to the extracellular matrix, the lack of integrin adherence causes inhibition of cyclin E-CDK2 in the cell nucleus; the cell cycle clock stops; and the cell commits suicide (programmed cell death, or apoptosis). Unfortunately, cancer cells are able to circumvent this process, to become *anchorage independent* so cyclin E-CDK2 stays active whether or not the cell is attached, and cells keep growing and dividing, thus avoiding programmed death. In addition, with only a few exceptions (e.g., neutrophils), normal cells cannot penetrate through the underlying basement membrane on which they rest, or through basement membranes of blood vessels (endothelial lining). Like neutrophils, malignant cells release the enzymes called *matrix metalloproteinases (MMPs)* that dissolve parts of the basement membrane as well as the extracellular matrix, like a military tank, so that the cells can migrate away from the primary tumor and into the blood vessels for the process of metastases.

Once in the blood vessel, it is estimated that only one cell in 10,000 is successful in setting up a new metastatic site distant from the primary tumor. As stated, it must attach to the inner lining of capillaries and dissolve holes in the blood vessel basement membrane to escape into the extravascular tissue. It appears that most cells get trapped in the nearest capillary bed they encounter after leaving the primary tumor. Metastatic cells tend to be large and easily trapped, and many secrete clotting factors that cause platelets to aggregate around them. The primary destination for venous blood from most organs is the lungs, thus this is the most common metastatic site. Venous blood leaves the gut and goes to the liver first; the liver is the most common metastatic site for intestinal tumors. While this is true, it appears that, in addition, the cell surface adhesion molecules are directed to specific organ locations, via a code much like telephone area codes, so that malignant cells migrate to specific areas, such as prostate cancer to bone. This was further defined by Muller et al (2001). It also appears that there is "metastatic inefficiency"; some cells go to places without "area codes," or cells from a primary tumor that lacks metastatic qualities undergo apoptosis (Wong et al, 2001).

By studying neutrophils, normal cells that migrate where needed to fight infection, Muller et al (2001) were able to demonstrate that chemokines, soluble substances that carry messages between cells, are responsible for directing breast cancer cells to the primary organs where breast cancer metastasizes: lymph nodes, bone marrow, lung, and liver. Chemokines are small molecules that resemble cytokines and that connect with specific receptors on the cell surface causing rearrangement of the cell's cytoskeleton. This allows cells to adhere firmly to endothelial cells (lining blood vessels) and migrate in a specific direction. Chemokines work with integrins and other proteins on the surface of the cell to direct the breast cancer cells to specific organs. The authors found that breast cancer cells have functionally active chemokine receptors. When these receptors are activated by binding with a ligand (a substance that binds to a receptor on the cell surface and that turns on signal transduction within a cell), the cell starts active actin (which gives structure to a cell) polymerization and formation of pseudopods (fake feet) that allow the cell to migrate and invade tissue. The tissues in which these ligands are overexpressed are the primary metastatic sites in breast cancer. Further, by neutralyzing interactions between the chemokines and their receptors, there is a significant inhibition of metastases to lymph nodes and lung. As more is learned about the process of metastases, new agents can be developed to inhibit each of the critical steps, thus preventing the process.

Thus, as the twenty-first century moves forward, there is tremendous momentum in transforming cancer care. The human genome project and other molecular research have given great insight into the process of carcinogenesis, metastases, and molecular flaws that can be targeted to provide cytostatic and cytocidal effects. This chapter presents investigational as well as FDA approved agents in which the mechanism of action is taking advantage of the molecular flaw, and interrupting the malignant process. As targets are identified, often they can be directly attacked, as with the fusion protein denileukin diftitox (Ontak) which carries the diphtheria toxin directly to high-affinity IL-2 receptors containing a CD25 component, such as activated T- and B-cell lymphocytes. The drug is indicated in the treatment of persistent or recurrent cutaneous T-cell lymphoma (CTCL or mycoses fungoides). The uses of monoclonal antibodies include:

- blocking a receptor, such as the Erb-B1 (EGFR) or Erb-B2 (HER-2-neu) which prevents over-expressed growth factor receptors from sending the signal for cell division
- targeting the internal ptotein receptor kinases, such as gefitinib (Iressa) or erlotinib (OSI-774, Tarceva) which are tyrosine kinase inhibitors.
- carrying chemotherapy or radioisotopes which, when internalized into the cell, cause cell death, such as gemtuzumab ozogamicin (Mylotarg) and ^{90}Y ibritumomab (Zevalin).

Figure 5.11 shows mechanisms of monoclonal antibody therapy.

Tables 5.3 and 5.4 show current agents in clinical trials that target molecular flaws.

Matrix metalloproteases (*MMPs*) have been shown to be overexpressed in breast, lung, and prostate cancers, and it appears that certain MMPs are necessary for the formation of new capillaries (angiogenesis), movement of the cancer cells into neighboring tissue (invasion), and metastases. Normally, the extracellular matrix provides structure between cells, with basement membranes that separate subdivisions within tissues. This matrix prevents aberrant cells from invading other tissues or moving into the bloodstream to go elsewhere in the body. MMPs are zinc-dependent enzymes that maintain the extracellular matrix of tissues by breaking down different parts of the matrix as needed for ongoing remodeling (synthesis and breakdown of these proteins) over time. There are five main subcategories, based on their site of action: collagenases (MMP-1, MMP-8, MMP-13); gelatinases (MMP-2, MMP-9); stromelysins (MMP-3, MMP-7, MMP-10); membrane-type MMPs or MT-MMPs (MMP-14, MMP-15, MMP-16, MMP-17); and others (MMP-11, MMP-12, MMP-18) (Agouron Pharmaceuticals, 1999; Chambers and Matrisian, 1997). The principal MMPs that appear to be involved in tumor angiogenesis, invasion, and metastases are gelatinase A (MMP-2), gelatinase B (MMP-9), and MT-MMP-1 (MMP-14). It is known that tumors larger than 2 mm require new blood vessels to nourish the tumor cells and support tumor growth. As the tu-

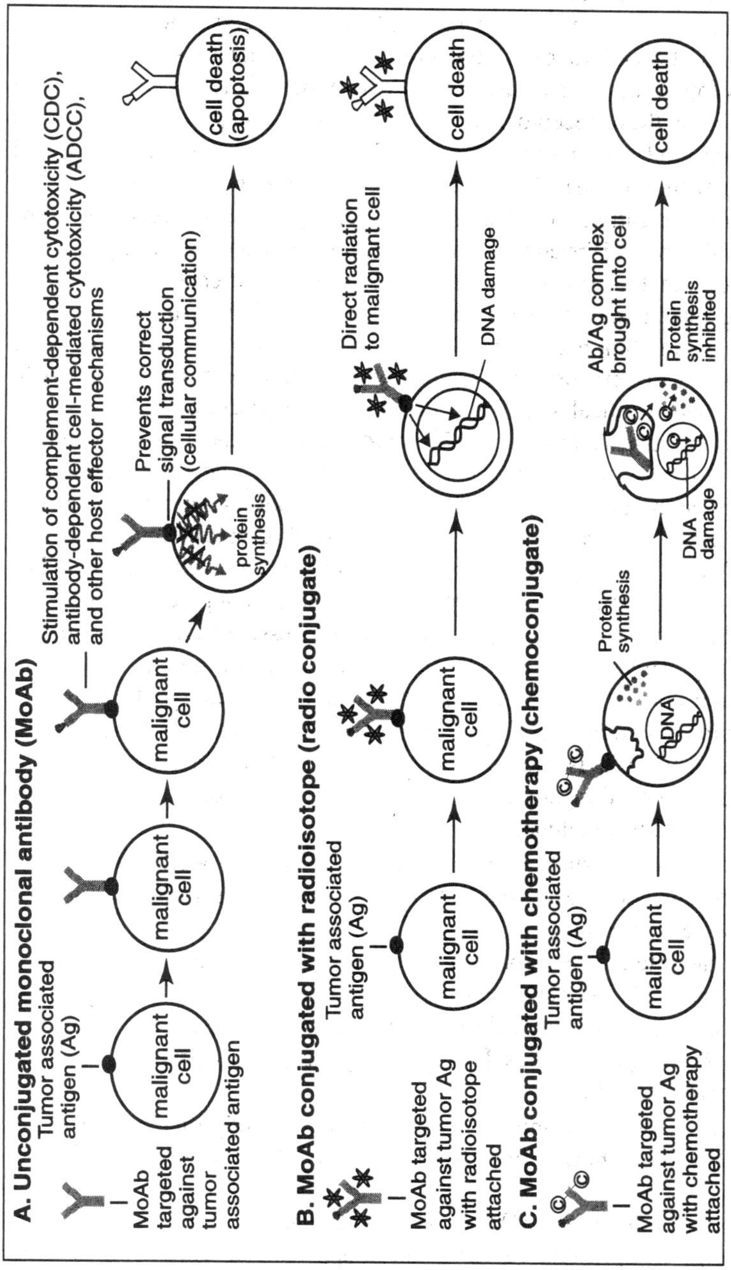

Figure 5.11 Mechanisms of Monoclonal Antibody Therapy

Source: Modified from Wyeth-Ayerest Laboratories (1999) *Antibody-Targeted Chemotherapy.* Philadelphia, PA: Wyeth-Ayerest Laboratories, p. 3

Table 5.3 Molecular Targeted Therapy: Selected Agents Undergoing Clinical Testing

Agent	Mechanism of Action
Cetuximab (Erbitux)	Monoclonal Antibody (MoAb) against EGF receptor
Erlotinib	Small molecule directed against EGF receptor tyrosine kinase
(Tarceva)	MoAb against VEGF Oral immunomodulatory analogue of thalidomide which as
Bevacizumab (Avastin)	
Lenalidomide (Revimid)	Oral iMID (immunomodulatory) analogue of thalidomide which has VEGF antagonist activity
Arasentan (ABT-627)	Endothelin-A receptor antagonist
SCH 44342, BMS-186511, others	Farnesyl Transferase Inhibitors

Table 5.4 Quick Tips on Understanding Monoclonal Antibody Names

1st syllable	Name unique to the product	Tras
2nd syllable	Target, tumor = tu	Tu
3rd syllable	Identifies the source, where 0 = mouse u = human I = chimeric (mouse and human)	U
4th syllable	mab = monoclonal antibody	Mab
X and z	Consonants to link syllables	Tras tu z u mab

mor grows, it releases MMPs to enable cells to break from the tumor and attach to pieces of the extracellular matrix, then to break down the extracellular matrix so the cells can move through the tissue compartments, and, finally, to move through the created openings to invade blood and lymphatic vessels and travel to distant sites. It is hoped that through inhibiting the MMPs, new blood vessel growth (angiogenesis), invasion, and metastases can be prevented. Currently, MMP inhibitors (MMPIs) can be specific, such as inhibiting MMP-2 and MMP-9, or broad spectrum, and are being clinically tested either alone as a single agent, or together with chemotherapy, and then continued as a maintenance agent. Clinical studies with MMPIs have been disappointing, and this book will be updated as more promising agents appear.

Retinoids appear to function by interfering with tumor differentiation. They are believed to have a role in cancer prevention as well as therapy. There are receptors in the cell nucleus that are retinoid-dependent and function in the transcription of proteins. When retinoids bind to the receptors, it is believed that they dimerize nuclear proteins, the complex then binds to DNA, and then there is transcription of a number of target genes. Thus, these activated retinoid receptors regulate the expression of genes responsible for differentiation and replication of cells. Retinoids have been effective in treating superficial Kaposi's sarcoma lesions (alitretinoin) and acute promyelocytic leukemia (tretinoin). In acute promyelocytic leukemia (APL), there is a translocation of a gene called retinoic-receptor alpha (RAR-alpha) on chromosome 17 that is switched with a gene called PML on chromosome 15. It appears that this translocation of RAR-alpha is part of the etiology of APL. Treatment with all-trans retinoic acid induces the primitive leukemic blast cells to differentiate, with replacement by normal myelocyte cells. This drug is now indicated for induction remission in patients with APL with subtype 3, including the M3 variant of AML. Other cancers that appear sensitive to 13-*cis* retinoic acid in combination with interferon alpha are squamous cell cancers of the skin and cervix. Alitretinoin (9-*cis*-retinoic acid) occurs naturally in the body and is able to bind and activate intracellular retinoid receptors. It has been shown to inhibit the growth of Kaposi's sarcoma when used topically and is now indicated for topical treatment of cutaneous lesions in patients with AIDS-related Kaposi's sarcoma who do not require systemic therapy.

It is an exciting time in cancer care. Genetic arrays are being perfected, thus improving diagnosis and treatment and promising to pave the way for individualized multidimensional therapy. It may be possible in the near future to prevent tumors from enlarging beyond 2 mm, and to prevent metastases. Given world politics and individual lifestyle choices, it is probably not possible to eliminate environmental carcinogens. However, the future looks promising that cancer, if not cured, will soon be a chronic, not terminal, disease.

References

Agus DB, Gordon MS, Taylor C, et al. Phase I clinical study of pertuzumab, a novel HER dimerization inhibitor, in patients with advanced cancer. *J Clin Oncol* 2005;23(11):2534–2543

Agus DB, Sweeny CJ, Morris M, et al. Efficacy and safety of single agent pertuzumab (rhuMAb 2C4), a HER dimerization inhibitor, in hormone refractory prostate cancer after failure of taxane-based therapy. *J Clin Oncol* 2005;23(16s):408s, abstact 4624

Bartlett JB, Dredge K, Dalgleish AG. The evolution of thalidomide and its IMiD derivatives as anticancer agents *Nat Rev Cancer* 2004;4(4):314–322

Bharti AC, Aggarwal BB. Nuclear Factor-kappa B and Cancer:Its Role in Prevention and Therapy. *Biochem Pharmacol* Sept 2002;64(5-6):883–888

Blankenberg F, Chang JT, Tidmarsh G, et al. Independent Review of Response to Iodine-131 Anti-B1 Antibodies in Low Grade or Transformed Low Grade NHL. *Proc Am Soc Clin Oncol* 1998;17:20, abstract 77

Browder T, Butterfield CE, Kraling BM, et al. Antiangiogenic Scheduling of Chemotherapy Improves Efficacy Against Experimental Drug-Resistant Cancer. *Cancer Res* 2000;60:1878–1886

Carducci MA, Nelson JB, Padley RJ, et al. The Endothelin-A Receptor Antagonist Atrasentan (ABT-627) Delays Clinical Progression in Hormone Refractory Prostate Cancer: A Multinational, Randomized Double-Blind, Placebo-Controlled Trial. *Proc Am Soc Clin Oncol* 2001;20(Part 1):174a Abstract 694. 37th Annual Meeting: San Francisco, CA

Chan S, Scheulen ME, Johnston S. et al. Phase II study of temsirolimus (CCI-779), a novel inhibitor of mTOR, in heavily pretreated patients with locally advanced or metastatic breast cancer. *J Clin Oncol* 2005;23:1–9

Connor KM. Understanding Vaccine Therapy. 1998; www.oncolink.upenn.edu/specialty/med onc/vaccine therapy.html

Cortes J, Baselga J, Kellokumpu-Lehtinen P, et al. Open label, randomized phase II study of pertuzumab (P) in patients (pat) with metastatic breast cancer with low expression of HER-2. *Proc Am Soc Clin Oncol* 2005; abstract 3068

Cunningham D, Humblet Y, Siena S, et al. Cetuximab (C225) alone or in combination with irinotecan (CPT-11) in patients with epidermal growth factor receptor (EGFR)-positive, irinotecan refractory metastatic colorectal cancer (MCRC). *Proc Am Soc Clin Oncol* 2003;22:252, abstract 1012

Dannenberg AJ, Altorki NK, Boyle JO, et al. Cyclo-oxygenase 2: A pharmacological target for the Prevention of Cancer. *Lancet Oncology* 2001;2(9):544–551

Demetri GD, Desai J, Fletcher JA, et al. SU11248: a multi-targeted tyrosine kinase inhibitor, can overcome imatinib (IM) resistance caused by diverse genomic mechanisms in patients with metastatic gastrointestinal stromal tumor (GIST). *Proc Am Soc Clin Oncol* 2004;23:195, abstract 3001

Dimopoulous M, Weber D, Chen C, et al. Evaluating oral lenalidomide (revlimid) and dexamethasone versus placebo and dexamethasone in patients with relapsed or refractory multiple myeloma. *European Hematology Assoc 10th Conference* June 2–5 2005, Stockholm, Sweden, abstract 0402

Divino CM, Chen SH, Yang W, et al. Anti-tumor Immunity Induced by Interleukin-12 Gene Therapy in a Metastatic Model of Breast Cancer Is Mediated by Natural Killer Cells. *Breast Cancer Res Treat* 2000;60(2):129–134

Fan F, Wey JS, McCarty MF, et al. Expression and function of vascular endothelial growth factor receptor 1 on human colorectal cancer cancer cells. *Oncogene* 2005; 24:2647–2653

Ferrara N, Alitalo K. Clinical Applications of Angiogenic Growth Factors and Their Inhibitors. *Nature Medicine* 1999;5:1359–1364

Folkman J. Pharmacology of Cancer Biotherapeutics: Antiangiogenesis Agents. In DeVita VT, Hellman S, Rosenberg SA, (eds), *Principles and Practice of Oncology*, 6th ed. Philadelphia, PA: Lippincott, Williams and Wilkins 2001;509–521

Fonseca R, Anderson KC, Weber D. Scientific Symposium: IMiDs: Results of Phase III Studies in Relapsed/Refractory Myeloma (SS10). Program of the 41st Annual Meeting of the American Society of Clinical Oncology. May 13–17, 2005; Orlando, FL

Francois B, Jourdes P, Benabid A. AE-941 (Neovastat) Induces the Expression of Angiostatin in Experimental Glioma. *Proc Am Soc Clin Oncol* 2001;20(Part 1):100a. Abstract 395. 37th Annual Meeting: San Francisco

Galanis E, Buckner JC, Maurer MJ, et al. N997B: Phase II trial of CCI-779 in recurrent glioblastoma multiforme (GBM): Updated results and correlative laboratory analysis. *Proc Am Soc Clin Oncol* 2005;Abstract 1505. 41st Annual Meeting: Orlando, FL

Gasparini G. Prognostic Value of Vascular Endothelial Growth Factor in Breast Cancer. *The Oncologist* 2000;5(suppl 1):37–44

Genentech, Avastin package insert. South San Francisco, CA: Genetech, Inc. 2004

Glickman MH, Ciechanover A. The Ubiquitin-Proteasome Proteolytic Pathway: Destruction for the Sake of Construction. *Physiology Review* 2002;82:373–428

Gorre ME, Mohammed M, Ellwood K, et al. Clinical Resistance to STI-571 Cancer Therapy Caused by Bcr-Abl Gene Mutation or Amplification. *Science* 2001; 293(5531):876–880

Hanahan D, Folkman J. Patterns and Emerging Mechanisms of the Angiogenic Switch During Tumorigenesis. *Cell* 1996;86:353–358

Harari PM, Huang SM. Modulation of Molecular Targets to Enhance Radiation. *Clin Cancer Res* 2000;6:323–325

Harris AL, Zhang H, Moghaddam A, et al. Breast Cancer Angiogenesis. New Approaches to Therapy Via Antiangiogenesis, Hypoxic Activated Drugs, and Vascular Targeting. *Breast Cancer Research Treatment* 1996;38:97–108

Haura EB, Turkson J, Jove R. Mechanisms of Disease: Insights into the Emerging Role of Signal Transducers and Activators of Transcription in Cancer. *Nature Clinical Practice Oncology* 2(6):315–324

Hidalgo M, Siu LL, Neumanitis J, et al. Phase I and Pharmacologic Study of OSI-774, an Epidermal Growth Factor Receptor Tyrosine Kinase Inhibitor, in Patients with Advanced Solid Malignancies. *J Clin Oncol* 2001;19(13):3267–3279

Hurwitz H, Fehrenbacher L, Novotny W, et al. Bevacizumab plus irinotecan, fluorouracil, and leucovorin for metastatic colorectal cancer. *N Engl J Med* 2004;350(23): 2335–2342

Imclone Systems, Erbitux package insert. NY.Imclone Systems, Inc. 2004

Keating M, Byrd J, Rai K, et al. Multicenter Study of Campath-1H in Patients with CLL Refractory to Fludarabine. *Blood* 1999;94:3118 (abstract)

Keefe DL. Trasuzumab-associated Cardiotoxicity. *Cancer* 2002;95(7):1592–1600

Kemple SN. *The proteasome: A novel target in multiple myeloma.* Cambridge, MA: Millennium Pharma 2003

Kern FG, Lippman ME. The Role of Angiogenic Growth Factors in Breast Cancer Progression. *Cancer Metastatasis Rev* 1996;15:213–219

Lancet JE, Gotlib J, Gojo I, et al. Tipifarnib (ZARNESTRA™ in Previously Untreated Poor-Risk AML of the Elderly: Updated Results of a Multicenter Phase 2 Trial. *Blood* (ASH Annual Meeting Abstracts), November 2004;104:874

Li F. Angiogenesis. The Angiogenesis Foundation. 2000; (http://www.angio.org)

Liekens S, DeClercq E, Neyts J. Angiogenesis: Regulators and Clinical Applications. *Biochem Pharmacol* 2001;61(3):253–270

Linderholm B, Grankvist K, Wilking N, et al. Correlation of Vascular Endothelial Growth Factor Content with Recurrences, Survival, and First Relapse Site in Primary Node-postiive Breast Carcinoma after Adjuvant Treatment. *J Clin Oncology* 2000;18:1423–1431

List A, Kurtin S, Roe DJ, et al. Efficacy of lenalidomide in myelodysplastic syndromes. *N Eng J Med* 2005;352:549–557

Lippman ME. New Approaches to the Treatment of Breast Cancer in the Next Century. *Clinical Dialogues in Oncology,* Kingston, NJ: Medicom; 2000

Liu ET. Tumor Suppressor Genes: Changing Concepts. ASCO Educational Book. 35th Annual Meeting, Atlanta, GA: 1999

Maloney DG, Grillo-Lopez AJ, White CA, et al. IDEC-C2B8 (Rituximab) Anti-CD_{20} Monoclonal Antibody Therapy in Patients with Relapsed Low-Grade Non-Hodgkin's Lymphoma. *Blood* 1997;90(6):2188–2195

Lynch TJ, Bell DW, Sordella R, et al. Activating Mutations in the Epidermal Growth Factor Receptor Underlying Responsiveness of Non-Small-Cell Lung Cancer to Gefitinib. *N Eng J Med* 2004;350(21):2129–2139

Malik I, Hecht J, Patnaik A, et al. Safety and efficacy of panitumumab monotherapy in patients with metastatic colorectal cancer (mCRC). Poster presented at the 41st Annual American Society of Clinical Oncologists (ASCO). Orlando, FL;May 2005, abstract K4, 3520

McMahon G. VEGF Receptor Signaling in Tumor Angiogenesis. *The Oncologist* 2000; 5(suppl 1):3–10

Merkle CJ , Loescher LJ. The Biology of Cancer. In Yarbro CH, Frogge MH, Goodman M, (eds), *Cancer Nursing: Principles and Practice,* 6th ed. Sudbury, MA:Jones and Bartlett Publishers, Inc.;2005;15

Meyerson M. Role of Telomerase in Normal and Cancer Cells. *J Clin Oncol* 2000; 18(13):2626–2634

Muller A, Homey B, Soto H, et al. Involvement of Chemokine Receptors in Breast Cancer Metastases. *Nature* 2001;410:50–56

Motzer RJ, Rini BL, Michaelson MD, et al. SU 11248, a novel tyrosine kinase inhibitor, shows antitumor activity in second-line therapy for patients with metastatic renal cell carcinoma. Results of a Phase II trial. *Proc Am Soc Clin Oncol* 2004;23:381, abstract 4500

Murray JL, Witzig TE, Wiseman GA, et al. Zevalin Therapy Can Convert Peripheral Blood bcl-2 Status from Positive to Negative in Patients with Low-grade, Follicular or Transformed Non-Hodgkin's Lymphoma (NHL). *Proc ASCO* 2000;19:22a (77) New Orleans, LA: May 20–23, 2000

National Cancer Institute, *Histone Deacetylase Inhibitors.* 2004; Available at http://cancer.gov/clinicaltrials. Accessed June 13, 2004

Nelson JB, Carducci MA. The Role of Endothelin-1 and Endothelin Receptor Antagonists in Prostate Cancer. *BJU Int* 2000;85(Suppl 2):45–48

Nelson JB, Carducci MA, Padley RJ, et al. The Endothelial-A Receptor Antagonist Atrasentan (ABT-627) Reduces Skeletal Remodeling Activity in Men with Advanced, Hormone Refractory Prostate Cancer. *Proc Am Soc Clin Oncol* 2001; 20(Part 1):4a. Abstract 12. 37th Annual Meeting: San Francisco, CA

Novartis. Gleevec Package Insert. New Jersey: Novartis Pharma AG; May 2001

Onyx Pharmaceuticals . Sorafenib. http://www.onyx-pharma.com/wt/page/bay 43 9006. Accessed June 22, 2005

Parikh AA, Fan F, Liu WB, et al. Neuropilin-1 in human colon cancer: Expression, regulation, and role in induction of angiogenesis. *Am J Pathology* 2004;164(6): 2139–2151

Perez EA, et al. Interim cardiac safety analysis of NCCTG N9831. *Proc Am Soc Clin Oncol* 2005; Scientific Session presented May 16, 2005, 41st Am Soc Clin Oncol Meeting, Orlando, FL

Piccart-Gebhart MJ. First results of the HERA trial. *Proc Am Soc Clin Oncol* 2005; Scientific Session presented May 16, 2005, 41st Am Soc Clin Oncol Meeting, Orlando, FL

Punt CJ, Nagy A, Douillard JY, et al. Edrecolomab alone or in combination with fluorouracil and folinic acid in the adjuvant treatment of Stage III colon cancer: A randomized study. *Lancet* 2002;360:671–677

Raponi M, Lowenberg R, Lancet JE, et al. Identification of Molecular Predictors of Response to ZARNESTRA™ (Tipifarnib, R115777) in Relapsed and Refractory Acute Myeloid Leukemia. *Blood* (ASH Annual Meeting Abstracts) November, 2004;104: 861

Riethmuller G, Schneider-Gadicke E, Schlimok G, et al. Randomised trial of monoclonal antibody for adjuvant therapy of resected Dukes' C colorectal carcinoma. *Lancet* 1994;343:1177–1183

Rituximab Prescribing Information. San Francisco/San Diego,, IDEC Pharmaceuticals and Genentech, Inc 1997

Robert F, Ezekiel MP, Spencer SA, et al. Phase I Study of Anti-epidermal Growth Factor Receptor Antibody Cetuximab in Combination with Radiation Therapy in Patients with Advanced Head and Neck Cancer. *J Clin Oncol* 2001;19(13):3234–3243

Romond EH, et al. Doxorubicin and cyclophosphamide followed by paclitaxel with or without trastuzumab as adjuvant therapy for patients with HER-2 positive operable breast cancer: Combined analysis of NSABP-B31/NCCTG-N9831. *Proc Am Soc Clin Oncol* 2005; Scientific Session presented May 16, 2005, 41st Am Soc Clin Oncol Meeting, Orlando, FL

Rosenberg SA. Molecular Targets and Early Clinical Trials of New Therapeutics and Prevention. ASCO 2000 Educational Book 36th Annual Meeting, New Orleans. 2000

Rowinsky EK, Schwartz GH, Gollob JA, et al. Safety, pharmakinetics, and activity of ABX-EGF, a fully human anti-epidermal growth factor receptor monoclonal antibody in patients with metastatic renal cell cancer. *J Clin Onco* 2004;22(15): 3003–3015

Rowinsky EK, Windle JJ, Von Hoff DD. Ras protein farnesyltransferase: A strategic target for anticancer therapeutic development. *J Clin Oncol* 1999;17(11):3631–3652

Ruoslahti E. How Cancer Spreads. Scientific American (Sept 1996). 1996; http://www.sciam.com/0996issue/0996ruoslahti.html

Ruoslahti E, Reed JC. Anchorage Dependence, Integrins, and Apoptosis. *Cell* 1994; 77(4):477–478

Sandler AB, Blumenschein GR, Henderson T, et al. Phase I/II trial evaluating the anti-VEGF MAb bevacizumab in combination with erlotinib, a HER1/EGFR-TK inhibitor, for patients with recurrent non-small cell lung cancer. 2004 ASCO Annual Meeting Proceedings, Post Meeting Edition. *J Clin Oncol* 2004;22(14S):2000

Sandler AB, Gray R, Bhramer J, et al. Randomized phase II/III trial of paclitaxel (P) plus carboplatin © with or without bevacizumab (NSC 704865) in patients with advanced non-squamous non-small cell lung cancer: An Eastern Cooperative Oncology Group (ECOG) trial-E4599. *Proc Am Soc Clin Oncol* 2005; abstract LBA4

Sausville EA. Cyclin Dependent Kinases: Novel Targets for Cancer Development. ASCO 1999 Educational Book 35th Annual Meeting, Atlanta: 1999

Shi N, Pardridge WM. Noninvasive Gene Targeting to the Brain. *Proc Natl Acad Sci USA* 2000;97(13):7567–7572

Siegel JA. Revised Nuclear Regulatory Commission Regulation for Release of Patients Administered Radioactive Materials: Outpatient Iodine-131 Anti-B1 Therapy. *J Nucl Med* 1998;39(8):285–335

Siemeister G, Martiny-Baron G, Marme D. The Pivotal Role of VEGF in Tumor Angiogenesis: Molecular Facts and Therapeutic Opportunities. *Cancer Metastases Rev* 1998;17:241–245

Singh A, Padley RJ, Ashraf T. The Selective Endothelin-A Receptor Antagonist Atrasentan Improves Quality of Life Adjusted Time to Progression (QATTP) in Hormone Refractory Prostate Cancer Patients. *Proc Am Soc Clin Oncol* 2001;20(Part 2): 393a. Abstract 1567. 37th Annual Meeting: San Francisco

Sledge G, Milelr K, Novotny W, et al. A Phase II Trial of Single-Agent rhuMAb VEGF (Recombinant Humanized Monoclonal Antibody to Vascular Endothelial Cell Growth Factor) in Patients with Relapsed Metastatic Breast Cancer. *Proc Am Soc Oncol* 2000;19:3a, abstract 5C

Stetler-Stevenson WG, Kleiner DE. Molecular Biology of Cancer: Invasion and Metastases. In DeVita VT, Hellman S, Rosenberg SA, (eds), *Principles and Practice of Oncology,* 6th ed. Philadelphia, PA: Lippincott Williams and Wilkins;2001:123–137

U.S. Department of Health and Human Services. Understanding Gene Testing. Washington, DC, National Cancer Institute, NIH Publication,1995;96–3905

Vose J, Saleh M, Lister A, et al. Iodine-131 Anti-B1 Antibody for Non-Hodgkin's Lymphoma (NHL): Overall Clinical Trial Experience. *Proc Am Soc Clin Oncol* 1998;17:38, abstract 38

Wahl RL, Tidmarsh G, Krolls , et al. Successful Retreatment of Non-Hodgkin's Lymphoma (NHL) with Iodine-131 Anti-B1 Antibody. *Proc Am Soc Clin Oncol* 1998; 17:40, abstract 156

Weidner N. Tumoural Vascularity as a Prognostic Factor in Cancer Patients: The Evidence Continues to Grow. *J Pathol* 1998;184:119–120

Weinberg RA. Fundamental Understandings: How Cancer Arises. Scientific American. Sept 1996; http://www.sciam.com/0996

Weiner LM. Phase 1 Open-Label Dose Escalation Trial, poster presented at the 41st Annual American Society of Clinical Oncologists (ASCO), Orlando, FL, May 2005, abstract K4, 3509

Wilkes GM, Ingwersen K, Barton-Burke M. Oncology Nursing Drug Reference. Sudbury, MA: Jones and Bartlett; 2001

Wiseman GA, Leigh BR, Gordon LI, et al. Zevalin Radioimmunotherapy (RIT) for B-Cell Non-Hodgkin's Lymphoma (NHL): Biodistribution and Dosimetry Result. *Proc ASCO* 2000;19:10a (29) New Orleans, LA: May 20–23, 2000

Witzig TE, White CA, Wiseman GA, et al. Phase I/II trial of IDEC-Y2B8 Radioimmunotherapy for Treatment of Relapsed or Refractory CD_{20} + B-Cell Non-Hodgkin's Lymphoma. *J Clin Oncol* 1999;17:3793–3803

Wong CW, Lee A, Shientag L, et al. Apoptosis: An Early Event in Metastatic Inefficiency. *Cancer Res* 2001;61(1):333–338

Wyeth-Ayerst Laboratories. Antibody-Targeted Chemotherapy: Coming of Age. Philadelphia, PA: Wyeth-Ayerest Laboratories; 1999

Drug: alemtuzumab (campath-1H anti-CD52 Monoclonal Antibody, Humanized IgG1 MoAb)

Class: Monoclonal antibody.

Mechanism of Action: Humanized monoclonal antibody, which targets the CD52 antigen present on the surface of most normal human lymphocyte cells, as well as malignant T cell and B-cell malignant lymphocytes (lymphomas). Once the monoclonal antibody binds with the CD52 antigen, it initiates antibodydependent cellular toxicity and complement binding, which then lead to apoptosis, or programmed cell death, and activation of normal T-cell cytotoxicity against the malignant cells.

Metabolism: When given subcutaneously or intravenously, bioavailability appears similar. Host antibodies may develop 14–21 days after the first dose and theoretically can decrease lymphocyte killing. Drug half-life 12 days.

Drug Preparation:

- Available in single use vials containing 30 mg alemtuzumab in 1 mL of diluent. Draw up ordered dose, and dilute in 100 mL sterile 0.9% sodium chloride USP or 5% dextrose in water. Gently invert IV bag to mix. Use within 8 hours. Store at room temperature or refrigerated.

Drug Administration:

- TIW dose initially is 3 mg, then dose escalated to 10 mg, then 30 mg if well tolerated during the first week (tolerance usually achieved within 3–7 days) as IV infusion over 2 hours.
- Stop drug if reaction during infusion.
- Premedicate with acetaminophen 650 mg and diphenhydramine 50 mg 30 min prior to beginning infusion. Severe reactions may require hydrocortisone 200 mg.
- Subsequent dosing: 30 mg IV over 2 h 3-times-a-week, for a minimum of 4 weeks, but may continue up to 12 weeks. Give on Mon, Wed, Fri.
- If dose held more than 7 days, reinstitute gradually with dose escalation.

- Anti-infective prophylaxis recommended, starting on day 8 and continuing for 2 months after treatment completed or stopped, or CD4 count ≥ 200 cells/μL, e.g., with trimethoprim and sulfamethoxazole (Bactrim) DS/bid.
- Dose Reduce ANC < 250/μL and/or platelet count ≤ 25,000/μL. See package insert.

Drug Interactions:

- Unknown.

Lab Effects/Interference:

- An immune e response to the drug may interfere with subsequent serum laboratory tests using antibodies.

Special Considerations:

- Indicated for the treatment of B-cell chronic lymphocytic leukemia (B-CLL) in patients who have received alkylating agents and failed fludarabine.
- Patients who have received multiple courses of chemotherapy prior to campath-1H are at increased risk for bacterial, viral, and other opportunistic infections.
- Immunosuppression related to drug may reactivate herpes simplex infections, septicemia.
- Subcutaneous and intravenous have similar efficacy and effect.
- Following 3-times-a-week therapy, destruction of CLL cells takes about 14 days before being removed from the blood, with no cells detectable at 5 weeks (Solimandro et al, 2000).
- Is being studied in the treatment of chronic lymphocytic leukemia, lowgrade lymphoma, graft-versus-host disease, multiple sclerosis, and rheumatoid arthritis.

Potential Toxicities/Side Effects (Dose- and Schedule-Dependent) and the Nursing Process

I. POTENTIAL FOR INJURY related to HYPERSENSITIVITY REACTION DURING INFUSION

Defining Characteristics: Infusion reactions are common and require premedication to prevent them. Hypotension occurs in 16%, rash in 50%, nausea in 62% of patients, and fever and rigors in 80% of patients. Infusion reactions usually resolve after one week of therapy.

Nursing Implications: Assess vital signs baseline and frequently during infusion, especially during dose escalation. Teach patient that reactions may occur and to tell nurse or physician immediately. Administer premedication as ordered, usually acetaminophen and diphenhydramine. Dose is begun low at 3 mg, then gradually increased based on patient tolerance to 10-mg dose, then to a 30-mg dose. If the patient has a treatment break of seven days or more, then it is necessary to reintroduce drug at the lower dose and gradually escalate dose. If reaction happens, stop infusion but keep main IV line open, notify physician, and, if rigors, give meperidine and any other medications ordered by physician. Expect reaction to resolve in 20 minutes or so, and gradually resume infusion per physician order. Assess skin for integrity and presence of rash. Teach patient to report this, and discuss management with physician. Teach patient that nausea may develop, and to report it right away. Discuss antiemetic agent with physician, and administer as ordered.

II. POTENTIAL FOR INFECTION AND BLEEDING related to BONE MARROW DEPRESSION

Defining Characteristics: All patients develop leukopenia, with approximately 28% of patients developing neutropenia. There is a dramatic fall in WBC during the first week. As both T and B cell lymphocytes are injured, patients are at an increased risk for bacterial, viral, and other opportunistic infections. Most patients require prophylactic antibiotic with/without antiviral therapy, especially heavily pretreated patients. Most common pulmonary infections are opportunistic: *Pneumocystis carinii* pneumonia, cytomegalus virus (CMV) pneumonia, and pulmonary aspergillosis. Commonly, there is reactivation of herpes simplex infections and development of oral candidiasis. Thrombocytopenia affects 22%, with platelet recovery weeks 7 to 12. Incidence of anemia is 36%.

Nursing Implications: Assess baseline leukocyte, platelet, and Hgb/HCT and monitor before each treatment, during therapy, and more often as needed. Hold drug for ANC $< 250/\mu L$ or platelets $\leq 25{,}000/\mu L$. See package insert for dose modifications. Assess risk for infection and integrity of skin and mucous membranes, pulmonary status, and ability to clear secretions, as well as history of past infections, baseline and prior to each treatment. Teach patient to self-administer prophylactic antibiotics and antiviral agents as ordered by physician. Teach patient to self-administer oral antifungal agent if oral candidiasis develops. Teach patient to self-assess for signs/symptoms of infection, and to call provider immediately or come to the emergency room if temperature $> 100.5°F$, shaking chills, or rash, productive cough, burning on urination, or any signs/symptoms of infection or bleeding. Teach self-care strategies to minimize risk of infection and bleeding, including avoidance of OTC aspirin-containing medications.

III. ALTERATION IN COMFORT related to PAIN, ASTHENIA, PERIPHERAL EDEMA, HEADACHE, DYSTHESIAS, DIZZINESS

Defining Characteristics: Pain is common, and in clinical studies 24% of patients experienced skeletal pain, 13% asthenia, 13% peripheral edema, 10%

back or chest pain, 9% malaise, 24% headache, 15% dysthesias, and 12% dizziness.

Nursing Implications: Assess comfort and presence of peripheral edema, baseline and prior to each treatment. Teach patient that these side effects may occur and to report them. Teach patient local comfort measures, and discuss management plan with physician if ineffective.

IV. ALTERATION IN OXYGENATION, POTENTIAL, related to HYPOTENSION, HYPERTENSION, TACHYCARDIA

Defining Characteristics: Hypotension is common, affecting 32% of patients in clinical studies, while 11% had hypertension. 11% of patients also had sinus or supraventricular tachycardia.

Nursing Implications: Assess baseline cardiac status, including blood pressure and heart rate, noting rhythm and rate. Assess past medical history for arrhythmia, hypertension. If heart rate irregular, document rhythm on EKG, monitor blood pressure for evidence of decompensation, and discuss management with physician. If hypertension noted, discuss management with physician. If hypotension noted, assess patient tolerance and need for intervention; discuss management with physician.

Drug: alitretinoin gel 0.1% (Panretin®)

Class: Retinoid.

Mechanism of Action: A9-*cis*-retinoic acid, alitretinoin is a naturally occurring, endogenous retinoid necessary for regulation of gene expression responsible for cell differentiation and replication. 9-*cis*-retinoic acid binds to and activates intracellular retinoid receptors that enable transcription of these genes. Alitretinoin has been found to inhibit the growth of Kaposi's sarcoma (KS) cells directly.

Metabolism: Drug is used topically, without any detectable plasma concentrations or metabolites.

Dosage/Range:
- Sufficient gel applied to cover the lesion with "generous" coating.
- Available in 60-gram tube.

Drug Preparation:
- None.
- Gel tube should be stored at room temperature.

Drug Administration:

- Use glove to apply generous coating of gel to lesions bid, avoiding surrounding skin.
- DO NOT APPLY on or near mucosal surfaces.
- Allow to dry for 3–5 minutes before covering with clothing.
- Gradually increase applications to 3–4 per day.
- If severe skin irritation develops, stop application for a few days until irritation resolves.
- DO NOT USE an occlusive dressing over gel.

Drug Interactions:

- DEET (*N*, *N*-diethyl-*m*-toluamide) insect repellent or products containing DEET, as gel increases DEET toxicity.
- No testing has been done to assess possible interactions between systemic antiretroviral agents, or other agents used in the systemic management of HIV infection.

Lab Effects/Interference:

- None known.

Special Considerations:

- Responses may be seen in 2 weeks, but most often take longer, rarely 14 weeks. Gel should be used as long as there is clinical benefit.
- Indicated for TOPICAL treatment of cutaneous KS lesions in patients with AIDS. It should not be used when systemic therapy for KS is necessary (> 10 KS lesions in prior month, or symptomatic lymphedema, pulmonary KS, or visceral involvement).
- Contraindicated in patients having hypersensitivity to retinoids.
- Women of childbearing age should use contraception to prevent pregnancy, as it is unknown whether topical gel can modulate endogenous 9-*cis*-retinoic levels. 9-*Cis*-retinoic acid is teratogenic.
- Drug SHOULD NOT BE USED by nursing mothers; mothers must discontinue nursing prior to using the drug.
- Drug may increase photosensitivity, so patients should be taught to AVOID sunlamps and to minimize sunlight exposure.
- Safety testing has not been done in pediatric or geriatric (> 65 yr) populations.
- Toxicity almost exclusively related to skin reactions at the application site.

Potential Toxicities/Side Effects and the Nursing Process

I. ALTERATION IN COMFORT AND SKIN INTEGRITY, POTENTIAL, related to APPLICATION SITE REACTIONS

Defining Characteristics: Toxicity begins as erythema. This may increase, and edema may develop with continued application. Most of reactions are mild to moderate, but in some patients (10%), severe reactions may occur with intense erythema, edema, and formation of vesicles. Other skin reactions occurring in >5% of patients are rash, pain, pruritus, exfoliative dermatitis, cracking, crusting, drainage, oozing, stinging, or tingling.

Nursing Implications: Assess baseline skin integrity and condition of KS cutaneous lesions. Teach patient to apply gel only to lesions and AVOID surrounding skin, as irritation will occur. Teach patient to assess and report any changes in the lesions, such as erythema, and edema. Teach patient to reduce frequency of application if skin reaction occurs, to stop use of the gel if severe reactions occur, and to report this as soon as possible.

Drug: arasentan (ABT-627) (investigational)

Class: Endothelin-A receptor antagonist.

Mechanism of Action: Cytostatic. Blocks the endothelin-A (ET-A) receptor, which, when stimulated, would inhibit apoptosis (programmed cell death) resulting in malignant cell proliferation (prostate cancer cells and osteoblasts).

Endothelin-1 is important in inducing osteoblastic changes (G-protein couples with RT-A receptor).

Dosage/Range:
- Per protocol. Doses studied are 2.5-mg and 10-mg tablets.

Drug Preparation/Administration:
- Administer orally, once daily.

Drug Interactions:
- Unknown.

Lab Effects/Interference:
- Unknown.

Special Considerations:
- Drug showed improved quality of life (37% higher) in patients using 10 mg dose (Singh et al, 2001).
- Drug appears to inhibit progression of skeletal metastases in hormone-refractory prostate cancer (Nelson et al, 2001).
- Significant increase in median time to clinical progression for men with hormone-refractory prostate cancer (196 days at 10 mg dose) compared to placebo (129 days) and time to PSA progression (155 days at 10 mg dose) compared to placebo (71 days) (Carducci et al, 2001).
- Toxicity profile mild and drug is well tolerated.

Potential Toxicities/Side Effects and the Nursing Process

I. ALTERATION IN COMFORT related to PERIPHERAL EDEMA, RHINITIS, AND HEADACHE

Defining Characteristics: Peripheral edema developed in 35% of patients receiving the drug as compared to 14% receiving placebo. Edema was mild and easily managed. Rhinitis affected 28% in the treatment group and 13% receiving placebo, while 20% receiving the drug had headache as compared to 10% in the placebo group.

Nursing Implications: Assess comfort and presence of edema baseline and at each visit, and teach patient these side effects may occur and to report them. Assess degree of peripheral edema if it develops, and discuss need for diuretics if permitted by protocol with physician. Discuss symptomatic treatment of rhinitis if it develops with physician based on protocol.

Drug: bevacizumab (Avastin)

Class: Recombinant humanized Monoclonal Antibody targeted against Vascular Endothelial Growth Factor (VEGF); Angiogenesis inhibitor.

Mechanism of Action: VEGF binds to receptors on endothelial cells, turning on the cell surface receptors KDR and Flt-1, which then function as tyrosine kinases sending the message to the cells to proliferate and migrate. This leads to the establishment of new blood vessels (neovascularization) in tumors. Studies show that tumors that express VEGF tend to be more aggressive, more invasive, and more likely to metastasize. Bevacizumab binds to all human forms of VEGF, thus preventing it from binding to its receptors on the endothelial cells. This theoretically prevents one step in the process of angiogenesis from occurring.

Metabolism: Humanized via recombinant technologies resulting in a 93% human monoclonal antibody. It is widely distributed throughout the body and has a terminal half-life of approximately 20 days (range 11–50 days). It appears to reach steady state in 100 days. Drug clearance varies by body weight, gender, and tumor burden: men and patients with a large tumor burden have higher clearances than females, but this does not appear to decrease drug efficiency. Drug clearance has not been studied in patients with either renal or hepatic impairment. Concurrent administration of 5-fluourouracil, carboplatin, doxorubicin, cisplatin, or paclitaxel does not affect pharmacokinetics of the drug.

Dosage/Range:
5 mg/kg IV q 2 weeks

Drug Preparation/Administration:

- Single use vials contain 4 mL to deliver 100 mg, and 16 mL to deliver 400 mg per vial. Use within 8 hours of opening. Store at 2–8°C (36–46°F). Protect from light. Do not freeze or shake.
- Further dilute in 100 mL 0.9% Normal Saline for injection.
- Administer IV over 90 minutes as an infusion. If tolerated well without fever and/or chills, may give second dose over 60 minutes; if this is well tolerated, administer all subsequent doses as a 30 minute infusion.

Drug Interactions:

- SN-38 (the active metabolite of irinotecan) concentration is 33% higher when bevacuzimab is given concurrently
- Incompatible with dextrose solutions

Lab Effects/Interference:

- Thrombocytopenia
- Proteinuria
- Leukopenia
- Hypokalemia
- Bilirubinemia

Special Considerations:

- FDA approved for first-line treatment of patients with metastatic colon or rectal cancer in combination with a fluorouracil-based regimen. Is being studied in adjuvant treatment of patients with Stage III colon cancer. Bevacuzimab has been shown to increase the overall survival of patients with metastatic colorectal cancer when given with IFL (irinotecan, 5-fluorouracil or 5-FU, leucovorin or LV) chemotherapy by 4.7 months as compared to IFL alone, and by 4.1 months in combination with 5-FU/LV as compared to 5-FU/LV alone (Hurwitz et al, 2004).
- Interim analysis of a phase III study showed that patients receiving bevacizumab together with paclitaxel and carboplatin had a 30% improvement in overall survival compared to patients receiving paclitaxel and carboplatin alone (Sandler et al, 2005).
- Black box warnings include risk of 1) gastrointestinal perforations/complications of wound healing, and 2) hemorrhage (fatal hemoptysis occurred in 5 patients with NSCLC- squamous cell and adenocarcinoma histologies); Postmarketing: UP to 5% incidence of arterial thrombi with risk of stroke, myocardial infarction, transient ischemic attacks, angina. Risk factors for development of arterial thromboembolic events: history of arterial thromboembolism and age > 65.
- Discontinue drug in patients who develop gastrointestinal perforation, wound dehiscence requiring medical intervention, serious bleeding, nephrotic syndrome, hypertensive crisis.

- Temporarily suspend drug in patients with moderate to severe hypertension uncontrolled with medical management, and for patients who require elective surgery, at least several weeks prior to surgery.
- Bevacuzimab may increase the incidence and severity of hypertension, and severe hypertensive crisis may rarely occur.
- Proteinuria may occur, and rarely, nephrotic syndrome.
- Contraindicated in patients with hemoptysis.
- Drug may impair fertility, and is teratogenic. Women of child bearing age taking drug should use contraceptive measures during treatment, and for the expected time of drug elimination from the body (half-life is 20 days, with a range of 11–50 days) after the drug is stopped. Nursing mothers should discontinue nursing during treatment with bevacuzimab and for the expected time of drug elimination after the drug is stopped.
- Drug toxicities that occur more commonly in the elderly (> 2%) were asthenia, sepsis, deep thrombophlebitis, hypertension, hypotension, myocardial infarction, congestive heart failure, diarrhea, constipation, anorexia, leukopenia, anemia, dehydration, hypokalemia, and hyponatremia. In those aged 75 or older, in addition, dyspepsia, gastrointestinal hemorrhage, edema, epistaxis, increased cough, and voice alteration occurred more commonly than those under age 65.

Potential Toxicities/Side Effects and the Nursing Process

I. ALTERATION IN INTESTINAL AND SKIN INTEGRITY related to GASTROINTESTINAL PERFORMATION AND WOUND DEHISCENCE

Defining Characteristics: Rarely, patients may develop gastrointestinal perforation, sometimes fatal. It may be associated with intra-abdominal abcesses, and occur at variable times during the treatment. Incidence in pre-approval studies was 2–4%, as compared to 0.3% in the bolus IFL-only arm. Presenting symptoms were abdominal pain associated with nausea and constipation. Colonoscopy has a similar risk of GI perforation, so drug should be stopped 28 days before a planned colonoscopy. Also in clinical testing, 1% of patients receiving bevacuzimab plus either IFL or 5-FU/LV developed wound dehiscence, compared to 0.5% in the IFL arm alone. It is unknown how long the interval between surgery and treatment with bevacuzimab should be, but it may be greater than 2 months; similarly, it is not known how long the interval should be between treatment with bevacuzimab and elective surgery, but it certainly should be longer than the elimination time of the drug (half life 20 days). In one small clinical study, 15% of patients who had surgery following bevacuzimab treatment had wound healing or bleeding complications (Genentech, 2004). Exfoliative dermatitis occurred in 19% of patients receiving 5-FU/LV plus bevacuzimab.

Nursing Implications: Assess baseline bowel, skin integrity, and healing of any wounds or incisions; assess for dehiscence, and presence of rash at each visit. Teach patient that very rarely GI perforation or wound dehiscence may occur, to report abdominal pain associated with nausea, constipation, or other symptoms; or problems with wound healing right away for immediate evaluation. Bevacuzimab should be discontinued if perforation or wound dehiscence occur. Bevacuzimab should not be started until at least 28 days before or after major surgery, and the surgical incision is fully healed. Drug should be stopped at least 28 days (drug half-life is 20 days, with a range of 10–50 days) before elective surgery. Teach patient to self-assess skin for rash, and to report it right away.

II. ALTERATION IN HEMOSTASIS related to BLEEDING and THROMBOSIS

Defining Characteristics: Two patterns of bleeding may rarely occur: minor hemorrhage such as mild epistaxis, and serious hemorrhage. Of note, hemorrhage (pulmonary) occurred when drug was being studied in patients with lung cancer, with a higher incidence (31% in a small study) in patients with squamous cell histology. Many of these patients bled from a cavitation or area of necrosis in the pulmonary tumor. CNS bleeding has not been evaluated at this time, as patients with brain metastases were excluded from clinical trials following CNS hemorrhage in a patient with brain metastases. Rarely, the following other events were described in clinical trials: gastrointestinal hemorrhage (24% compared to 6% In IFL alone patients), subarachnoid hemorrhage, hemorrhagic stroke, thrombosis (grade 3/4 incidence 3% compared to 1% in IFL only group), embolism, epistaxis, hematemesis, hemoptysis, and bleeding at tumor sites. Epistaxis occurred in 35% of patients receiving bevacizumab + IFL, compared to 10% in IFL-alone arm. Epistaxis is easily controlled with pressure application.Thrombocytopenia may occur in 5% of patients. Deep vein thrombosis may occur in 6–9%, and epistaxis in 32–35% of patients. Patients on low-dose coumadin for implanted port patency had no increased risk of bleeding. There was no increased venous thromboembolism in a review of clinical studies when bevacizumab was added to chemotherapy, although there may be a small increase in arterial thromboembolic events (Novotny et al, 2004).

Nursing Implications: Assess baseline hematologic parameters and monitor during therapy. Teach patient that bleeding may occur and is most commonly epistaxis; but may also rarely occur as bleeding in the gastrointestinal tract, vagina in women, or elsewhere, and to report signs/symptoms of bleeding, changes in mental status, mobility, vision, weakness, or any new sign or symptom right away. Teach patient to assess for and report right away signs/symptoms of thrombosis: new swelling, pain, skin warmth and/or change in color (e.g., erythema, mottling) on the legs or thighs; new onset pain in the abdomen; dysnpnea or shortness of breath, rapid heartbeat, chest pain, or pressure that may signal a pulmonary embolism; and any changes in vision, new onset of severe headache, lightheadedness, or dizziness. Assess baseline mental status and neurological signs and monitor during therapy, especially in patients with brain metastases. Teach patients to apply pressure if epistaxis occurs. Discuss any abnormalities with physician. Bevacuzimab should be discontinued if the patient develops serious hemorrhage, and is contraindicated in patients with recent hemoptysis.

III. POTENTIAL ALTERATION IN CIRCULATION related to HYPERTENSION and CONGESTIVE HEART FAILURE

Defining Characteristics: Bevacuzimab may increase the incidence and severity of hypertension. Incidence of hypertension (> 150/100 mm Hg) was 60% in the clinical study arm IFL+ bevacuzimab and 67% in the arm 5-FU/LV + bevacuzimab arm, compared to 43% in the IFL arm. Severe hypertension defined as > 200/110 mm Hg occurred in 7% of patients in the clinical study arm IFL+ bevacuzimab and 10% in the arm 5-FU/LV+bevacuzimab arm, compared to 2% in the IFL-only arm. Hypertension may persist following drug cessation, as shown in clinical studies: 69% in patients receiving IFL+bevacuzimab, and 80% in the IFL-only arm. Grade 3/4 hypertension occurred in 12% of patients in clinical trials, compared to 2% in the IFL group. Severe hypertension necessitated hospitalization or drug discontinuation, and was complicated by hypertensive encepthalopathy or subarachnoid hemorrhage in some patients. Overall incidence of hypertension is 23–34%, with 12% grade 3/4. Rarely, 2% of patients may develop grade 2–4 congestive heart failure (CHF). Incidence is higher in combination with, or if a past history of, receiving anthracycline chemotherapy with or without left chest wall irradiation.

Nursing Implications: Assess baseline BP prior to and during treatment, at least for the first treatment, then prior to each drug administration. If the patient has a history of hypertension, monitor BP more closely, although hypertension develops over time rather than during the drug infusion. Blood pressure should continue to be monitored after patient has stopped the drug. Teach patient drug administration, potential side-effects, and self care measures if prescribed antihypertensive medication, such as angiotensin-converting enzyme inhibitors, beta blockers, diuretics, and calcium channel blockers. Drug should be permanently discontinued if the patient develops hypertensive crisis (diastolic blood pressure > 120 mm Hg). Drug can be temporarily suspended in patients with severe hypertension until BP can be controlled with medical management.

IV. POTENTIAL FOR INJURY related to HYPERSENSITIVITY REACTION DURING INFUSION

Defining Characteristics: Although the recombinant DNA product is 93% humanized, allergic reactions are still possible. Incidence is <3%, and slower infusion time greatly reduces the incidence. Infusion syndrome is characterized by fever, rigors, chills, or myalgias. Premedication is not necessary unless the patient experiences an infusion reaction in prior treatments. However, stridor and wheezing may occur. Rash with desquamation may also occur.

Nursing Implications: Assess vital signs baseline and as needed. Teach patient that reactions may occur and to tell nurse or physician immediately. First dose is MENT administered over 90 minutes, 2nd infusion over 60 minutes if previously well tolerated, and then subsequent infusions can be given over 30 minutes if tolerated well. If a reaction occurs, stop infusion but keep main IV line open, notify physician, and if rigors, give meperidine and any other medications ordered by physician. Expect reaction to resolve over 20 minutes or so, and gradually resume infusion per physician order. Monitor blood pressure, and implement ordered medical management plan. Stop drug if severe infusion reactions occur, such as stridor or wheezing, and be prepared to administer oxygen, fluids, and/or antihistamines. Monitor baseline skin integrity, and teach patient to report rash or skin changes. Develop local management plan, and discuss plan revision with physician if ineffective. Fever is treated symptomatically.

V. ALTERATION IN RENAL FUNCTION related to NEPHROTIC SYNDROME

Defining Characteristics: Nephrotic syndrome and proteinuria may occur. 17–28% of patients receiving bevacuzimab in combination with IFL or 5-FU/LV had 2+ proteinuria compared to 14% of patients on IFL alone. 2–4% had grade 3 proteinuria (>3.5 g protein/24 h), as compared to 0% in the IFL arm. Nephrotic syndrome is rare, occuring in 0.5% of patients, but 1 of the 5 affected patients required dialysis and 1 patient died. Although there may be an improvement in renal function, no patient had normalization following drug discontinuation.

Nursing Implications: Assess baseline renal function and presence of protein in urine (1+ or greater by dipstick), and monitor prior to and between treatments. Discuss any abnormalities with the physician. Patients with 2+ or higher proteinuria by urine dipstick should be asked to collect a 24 hour urine sample for protein. Drug should be held for proteinuria >2 g/24 h, and resume when proteinuria <2 g/24 h. Monitor patients closely if moderate to severe proteinuria until improved or resolved.

VI. ALTERATION IN NUTRITION, LESS THAN BODY REQUIREMENTS related to DIARRHEA, STOMATITIS, VOMITING, CONSTIPATION, and TASTE DISORDER

Defining Characteristics: Patients on clinical studies developed the following symptoms compared to patients receiving IFL-only: stomatitis (30–32% vs 18%), dyspepsia (17–24% vs 15%), flatulence (11–19% vs 10%), and vomiting (47–52% vs 47%). Grade 3/4 diarrhea occurred in 34% of patients, compared to 25% receiving IFL-only. Grade 3/4 constipation occurred in 4% of patients, compared to 2% receiving IFL-only. GI hemorrhage occurred in 19–24% vs 6% in the IFL group. Taste disorder occurred in 14–21% of patients compared to 9% in the IFL-alone arm.

Nursing Implications: Assess baseline weight, nutritional status, taste distortion and monitor prior to each treatment. Teach patient that these side effects may occur and to report them. Develop symptom management plan with physician. Make referral to dietitian as appropriate.

VII. ALTERATION IN COMFORT related to ARTHRALGIA, ASTHENIA, PAIN, HEADACHE, COUGH, DYSPNEA, EXCESS LACRIMATION

Defining Characteristics: Discomfort may occur, with symptoms occuring with the following frequency: arthralgias, asthenia (73–74%), myalgia (8–15%), pain (61–62%), headache (26%), cough, or dyspnea (25–26%). Pain and asthenia were common grade 3/4 toxicities in clinical studies. Voice alterations occurred in 6–9% of patients. Underlying disease process may account for many of these symptoms rather than drug, but it was unclear in clinical studies. Excess lacrimation occurred in 18% of patients receiving 5-FU/LV+bevacuzimab, compared to 2–6% in IFL alone or with bevacuzimab arm.

Nursing Implications: Assess baseline comfort, pulmonary status, and eye tearing, and teach patient to report any changes. Discuss further evaluation of symptoms with physician. Develop symptom management plan with physician and implement. Revise plan as appropriate.

VIII. POTENTIAL FOR INFECTION related to LEUKOPENIA

Defining Characteristics: Infection may occur without neutropenia. The incidence of Grade 3/4 leukopenia was 37% in patients receiving the combination, compared to 31% in patients receiving IFL alone. Grade 3/4 neutropenia was 21% in the combination arm, compared to 14% in the IFL arm. Thrombocytopenia occurs in 5% of patients.

Nursing Implications: Assess baseline white blood cell count, differential, and absolute neutrophil count, and monitor closely prior to each treatment when given in combination with irinotecan. Teach patient to avoid opportunities for infection (crowds, people with colds), and to report signs/symptoms of infection right away. Ensure that patient has a thermometer and knows how to use it; alternatively, a family member can monitor patient's temperature at home. Teach patient to monitor temperature, and report temperature > 100.5°F. If patient develops febrile neutropenia, discuss immediate antibiotics and hospitalization as needed.

Drug: bexarotene (Targretin oral capsules and topical gel)

Class: Retinoid

Mechanism of Action: Retinoid that selectively binds to and activates retinoid × receptors, which have biologic activity distinct from retinoic acid receptors. The activated receptors can partner with receptor partners (e.g., retinoic acid receptors), and then function as transcription factors that regulate the expression of genes which control cellular differentiation and proliferation. The exact mechanism of action in cutaneous T-cell lymphoma is unknown.

Metabolism: Drug is well absorbed after oral administration, especially after a fat-containing meal, with a terminal half-life of seven hours. Drug is highly protein-bound (> 99%). Drug appears to be metabolized by the cytochrome P4503A4 isoenzyme system in the liver, forming glucuronidated oxidative metabolites. Four metabolites are formed and are active, but it is unclear which metabolites or whether the parent drug are responsible for the efficacy of the drug. Probably excreted via the hepatobiliary system.

Dosage/Range:
Oral capsules:
- Indicated for the treatment of cutaneous manifestations of cutaneous T-cell lymphoma in patients who are refractory to at least one prior systemic therapy.
- Initial dose of 300 mg/m^2 PO per day for up to 97 weeks (maximum in clinical trials).
- Dose-reduce for toxicity to 200 mg/m^2 PO qd, then down to 100 mg/m^2 PO qd, or stop temporarily until toxicity resolves. After resolution, gradually titrate dose upward.
- Evaluate treatment efficacy at 8 weeks, and if no tumor response but the drug is well tolerated, increase dose to 400 mg/m^2 PO qd and monitor closely.

Topical gel:

- 1% gel indicated for the topical treatment of skin lesions in patients with early stage cutaneous T-cell lymphoma who have failed other therapies.

Drug Preparation:
- Available as 75-mg gelatin capsules in bottles of 100 capsules. The contents of the bottle should be protected from light, high temperatures, and humidity once opened.
- Store at 2–25°C (36–77°F).
- 1% gel available in tube.

Drug Administration:
- Oral: single daily oral dose with a meal.
- Topical gel: apply to affected areas only (NOT entire body) as needed.

Drug Interactions: *Oral capsules:*
- Presumed to be related to P4503A4 isoenzyme system metabolism.
- Inhibitors of cytochrome P4503A4 enzyme system (e.g., ketoconazole, itraconazole, erythromycin, gemfibrozil, grapefruit juice) theoretically can increase serum levels of bexarotene; DO NOT GIVE GEMFIBROZIL concomitantly with bexarotene.
- Inducers of cytochrome P4503A4 enzyme system (e.g., rifampin, phenytoin, Phenobarbital) may cause a decrease in serum bexarotene concentrations. If used concomitantly, assess response, and increase bexarotene accordingly.
- Theoretically, as drug is highly protein bound, it is possible that baxarotene can displace drugs or be displaced by drugs which bind to plasma proteins; use together cautiously.
- Insulin, sulfonylureas, or insulin-sensitizers: may increase action with resultant hypoglycemia; use together cautiously.

Lab Effects/Interference: *Oral capsules:*
- CA 125 assay values in patients with ovarian cancer may be increased.
- Significantly increased serum triglycerides, total cholesterol, and decreased HDL.
- Increased LFTs.
- Decreased TSH and total T4.
- Leukopenia and neutropenia.
- Increased LDH.

Special Considerations:

Oral capsules:
- Baseline serum lipid levels must be assessed prior to initiation of therapy, and any abnormalities treated so that fasting triglycerides are normal before starting therapy.
- Drug is contraindicated during pregnancy as it is teratogenic. Women of childbearing age should use effective contraception — optimally, two forms

unless abstinence is chosen. This should continue during therapy and for one month after the completion of therapy. A pregnancy test should be done one week prior to beginning therapy, and repeated monthly during therapy. If pregnancy occurs, the drug must be stopped immediately and the woman counseled.

- Male patients with sexual partners who are pregnant, possibly pregnant, or who could become pregnant, should use condoms during therapy, and for one month after therapy is ended.
- Most patients have major lipid abnormalities, and one patient died of pancreatitis. In general, patients with risk factors for pancreatitis should not take the drug (e.g., history of pancreatitis, uncontrolled hyperlipidemia, uncontrolled diabetes mellitus, biliary tract disease, or medications known to increase triglyceride levels or to be associated with pancreatic toxicity).
- Drug is contraindicated in nursing mothers.
- Drug should be used cautiously in patients who have hypersensitivity to other retinoids.
- Drug may cause cataracts; patients who experience visual difficulties should have an opthamologic exam.
- Baseline laboratory assessment prior to starting drug should include WBC with differential, thyroid function tests, fasting blood lipid profile, and liver function tests.
- Patients should limit vitamin A intake to ≤ 15,000 IU/day to avoid possible additive toxicity.
- Patients should avoid direct sunlight and artificial ultraviolet light while taking bexarotene as severe sunburn and skin sensitivity reactions may occur due to photosensitization.
- No studies have been done with patients having hepatic dysfunction, but theoretically, hepatic dysfunction would greatly reduce metabolism/excretion and increase serum drug levels. Use cautiously if at all in this setting.
- Response rate in patients with cutaneous T-cell lymphoma who were refractory to one prior systemic therapy was 32%.
- Drug being studied in clinical trials of patients with advanced breast cancer or moderate/severe psoriasis.

1% gel:

- Main side effects are rash, itching, and pain at application site.

Potential Toxicities/Side Effects and the Nursing Process

I. ALTERATION IN NUTRITION, POTENTIAL, related to ABNORMAL LIPID LEVELS, PANCREATITIS, ELEVATED LFTs, AND NAUSEA (oral capsules)

Defining Characteristics: Almost all patients experience major lipid abnormalities, including elevated fasting triglycerides (70% receiving doses of ≥ 300 mg/m²/day had elevations of more than 2.5 times upper limits of normal (ULN), and 55% had values over 800 mg/dL with a median of 1200 mg/dL), elevated cholesterol (60% of patients receiving 300 mg/m²/day, and 75% of patients receiving doses of ≥ 300 mg/m²/day), and decreased levels of the protective high-density lipoproteins (HDL) to < 25 mg/dL (55% of patients receiving a dose of 300 mg/m²/day, and 90% of patients receiving a dose of > 300 mg/m²/day). These values normalize after bexarotene is stopped. In most patients, either antilipemic medication or dose reduction of bexarotene allowed contol over elevated levels. Rarely, patients with markedly elevated triglycerides (lowest level 770 mg/dL) can develop pancreatitis, which can be fatal. Patients with risk factors for pancreatitis should not receive the drug (e.g., history of pancreatitis, uncontrolled hyperlipidemia, uncontrolled diabetes mellitus, biliary tract disease, or medications known to increase triglyceride levels or to be associated with pancreatic toxicity). Uncommonly, patients may have elevated LFTs (5% of patients receiving an initial dose of 300 mg/m²/day and 7% when doses of > 300 mg/m²/day were used), but one patient developed cholestasis and died of liver failure in clinical trials. Nausea/vomiting occurs in 15%/3% of patients receiving a dose of 300 mg/m²/day and 7%/13% of patients receiving doses of > 300 mg/m²/day. Anorexia affects 2% of patients receiving a dose of 300 mg/m²/day, and 22% of patients receiving higher doses.

Nursing Implications: Assess baseline triglyceride, cholesterol, and HDL levels. If abnormal, discuss pharmacological management plan, e.g., atorvastatin, as fasting triglyceride level should be normal before patient begins therapy. Gemfibrozzil should NOT be used. Fasting triglyceride level should then be monitored weekly until the lipid response to bexarotene is known (2–4 weeks), then at 8-week intervals. Goal is to keep fasting triglyceride level < 400 mg/dL to prevent pancreatitis. If fasting triglyceride level becomes elevated during treatment, discuss with physician antilipemic medication, e.g., atorvastatin, and if no response, discuss with physician bexarotene dose reduction or drug holiday. Teach patient about importance of testing fasting triglycerides, and monitoring level throughout treatment. LFTs should be assessed baseline, and after 1, 2, and 4 weeks of starting treatment; if stable, then assess every 8 weeks during treatment. Monitor serum LFTs, HDL, and discuss any abnormalitites with physician (manufacturer recommends suspension or discontinuance of bexarotene if LFTs (SGOT/AST, SGPT/ALT, and bilirubin) > 3x ULN). Assess baseline nutritional status, teach patient that nausea, vomiting, and anorexia may occur and to report them. If these occur, teach strategies to minimize occurrence, and if ineffective or symptoms are severe, discuss pharmacologic management with physician.

II. ALTERATION IN ACTIVITY, POTENTIAL, related to HYPOTHYROIDISM (oral capsules)

Defining Characteristics: Bexarotene binds and activates retinoid × receptors, and can partner with thyroid receptor; once activated, the receptor functions as a transcription factor that regulates gene expression controlling cellular differentiation and proliferation. Drug induces reversible clinical hypothyroidism in about 50% of patients (decrease in TSH in 60% of patients, and total T4 in 45% of patients at a dose of 300 mg/m^2/day), and hypothyroidism was reported in 29% of patients. Asthenia occurs in 29.8% of patients at a dose of 300 mg/m^2/day and in 45% of patients at higher doses.

Nursing Implications: Assess baseline thyroid function tests (TFTs), and discuss pharmacologic replacement of thyroid hormone with physician if values indicate hypothyroidism. Monitor TFTs during treatment. Teach patient that this may occur, importance of laboratory testing, fact that hypothyroidism induced by drug is reversible following discontinuance of drug, and to report signs/symptoms of hypothyroidism (e.g., weight gain, lethargy, slowed thinking, skin dryness, constipation, joint pain/stiffness). Teach patient to alternate rest and activity periods, and other measures to conserve energy.

III. POTENTIAL FOR INFECTION related to LEUKOPENIA (oral capsules)

Defining Characteristics: Reversible leukopenia (WBC/mm^3 1000–3000) occurred in 18% of patients receiving dose of 300 mg/m^2/day, and in 43% of patients receiving higher doses. Patients receiving 300 mg/m^2/day had grade 3 (12%) and grade 4 (4%) neutropenia. Incidence of bacterial infection was 1.2% in patients receiving dose of 300 mg/m^2/day (overall body infection was 13%), and bacterial infection was 13% (overall infections 22%) in patients receiving higher doses. Onset of leukopenia was 4–8 weeks. Resolution of leukopenia/neutropenia occurred in 30 days with drug dose reduction or discontinuance in most patients (82–93%). There were rare serious adverse events associated with leukopenia/neutropenia.

Nursing Implications: Assess baseline WBC, ANC and periodically during therapy. Teach patient that leukopenia may occur, and teach self-care measures, including self-assessment for infection, minimizing risk of infection, and when to notify provider. Teach patient/family signs/symptoms of infection, and how to take temperature if this is not known.

IV. ALTERATION IN BOWEL ELIMINATION related to DIARRHEA (oral capsules)

Defining Characteristics: Diarrhea is uncommon in patients receiving dose of 300 mg/m^2/day, but is more common (41%) when dose is increased.

Nursing Implications: Assess baseline elimination status, and monitor throughout treatment. Teach patient that diarrhea may occur, especially if dose is > 300 $mg/m^2/day$, and to report it. Teach patient self-care measures, including dietary modification (decreased insoluble fiber, increased soluble fiber, and increased fluid) and self-administration of OTC medicines to manage diarrhea. Teach patient to report diarrhea that does not resolve in 24 hours, or is severe, and discuss management with physician.

V. ALTERATION IN COMFORT related to HEADACHE, ABDOMINAL PAIN, CHILLS, FEVER, FLU SYNDROME, BACK PAIN, INSOMNIA (oral capsules)

Defining Characteristics: Symptoms occur with the following incidence (300 $mg/m^2/day$ dose vs higher dose): headache (30% vs 42%), abdominal pain (11% vs 4%), chills (9% vs 13%), fever (5% vs 17%), insomnia (5% vs 11%), flulike symptoms (3% vs 13%), back pain (2% vs 11%).

Nursing Implications: Assess baseline comfort status. Teach patient that these symptoms may occur and teach self-management measures. Teach patient to report fever > 100.5°F, chills, or symptoms that persist or are severe. Discuss management with physician if these occur.

VI. POTENTIAL ALTERATION IN SKIN INTEGRITY related to RASH, DRY SKIN, ALOPECIA, PERIPHERAL EDEMA (oral capsules), and RASH, PRURITUS, PAIN AT GEL APPLICATION SITE (topical gel)

Defining Characteristics: Oral capsules: Symptoms occur with the following incidence (300 $mg/m^2/day$ vs higher dose): rash (17% vs 23%), exfoliative dermatitis (10.7% vs 9%), alopecia (3.6% vs 11%), and peripheral edema (13% vs 11%). Topical gel: Commonly, rash, pruritus, and pain at application site occur.

Nursing Implications: Oral capsules: Assess baseline skin integrity and extent of cutaneous lesions, and teach patient to report rash right away after taking capsules, especially if peeling. Discuss drug continuance with physician if this occurs. Teach patient to use skin cream to keep skin moist, to prevent cracking and peeling, and to prevent itching as directed by the physician. Teach patient to report any hair thinning, and if it occurs, assess impact on patient's body image. Discuss measures to enhance coping, such as use of scarf, measures to protect hair follicles (e.g., gentle shampoo, avoidance of hair perms or use of curling iron), encourage patient to verbalize feelings, and provide emotional support. Teach patient to report swelling of feet or hands, to keep skin moisturized to prevent cracking or dryness, and to report skin changes that persist or are severe. Discuss management with physician. Topical gel: Assess integrity/extent of cutaneous lesions prior to patient starting therapy. Teach patient application of topical gel on areas of lesions only. Teach patient to report rash, persistent itching, or pain at application site. Teach patient self-care measures to manage itching, or pain at application site if they occur. Discuss with physician management of rash, and if severe, discontinuance of gel.

Drug: bortezomib (Velcade)

Class: Proteasome inhibitor.

Mechanism of Action: A reversible inhibitor of the 26S proteasome; inhibits the breakdown of ubiquiniated intracellular proteins and disrupts the ubiquitin-proeasome pathway. This pathway normally regulates the intracellular concentration of specific proteins, thus controlling homeostasis. When disrupted, multiple signaling pathways within the cell are disrupted, encouraging the cell to undergo apoptosis. In addition, cell cycle movement (cell division) stops, cells are unable to migrate, and sensitivity to chemotherapy is increased. In multiple myeloma, it interferes with cellular adhesion molecules so that tumor cells cannot bind to the bone marrow.

Metabolism: Following IV administration, mean elimination half-life is 9–15 hours following the first dose. Drug undergoes oxidative metabolism via cytochrome P450 enzymes 3A4, 2D6, 2C19, 2C9, and 1A2. Drug is deboronated into 2 metabolites that are then hydroxylated into several metabolites. Unknown elimination path.

Dosage/Range:
- 1.3 mg/m^2 per dose IVB twice weekly × 2 weeks (days 1, 4, 8, 11) followed by a 10-day rest period (d 12–21). Cycle repeated q 21 days. Doses should be separated by at least 72 hours (to give normal cells a chance to recover).

Dose Reductions:
- Hold drug at onset any grade 3 non-hematologic toxicity or grade 4 hematologic toxicity.
- Once signs/symptoms resolved, reinitiate drug at 25% dose reduction (1.3 mg/m^2 reduced to 1.0 mg/m^2/dose.
- Neuropathic pain and/or sensory neuropathy: see dose reduction in Nursing section.
- Recalculate dose if weight loss of > 8% between cycles.

Drug Preparation:
- Available in 10 mL vials containing 3.5 mg of bortezomib powder; store unopened vials at room temperature 25°C (77°F), and protect from light.
- Reconstitute each vial with 3.5 mL 0.9% Sodium chloride Injection USP, forming a colorless and clear solution (stable for 8 hours at controlled room temperature).

- Draw up prescribed amount (stable in syringe for 3 hours).

Drug Administration:

- Administer IVP over 3–5 seconds, followed by saline flush.
- Ensure serum sodium > 130 mg/dL prior to drug administration.

Drug Interactions:

- Unknown but theoretically may increase/decrease serum level of other drugs metabolized via the P450 microenzyme system, and serum level of bortezomib can be increased or decreased by drugs metabolized by microenzyme system (depending upon whether inducers or inhibitors of CYP 3A4, 2C19, 1A2).
- In clinical trials, the additional of dexamethasone 20 mg PO given the day of and day after bortezomib resulted in increased response rate in patients with stable disease or progressive disease on bortezomib alone.

Lab Effects/Interference:

- Decreased neutrophil, platelet and red blood cell counts.
- Hyponatremia and hypokalemia; rarely, hypercalcemia and hypomagnesemia.

Special Considerations:

- Indicated for the treatment of multiple myeloma patients who have disease progression after at least one prior therapy. Drug is being studied in other malignancies with promising results, such as NSCLC.
- Contraindicated in patients with hypersensitivity to bortezomib, boron, or mannitol; avoid if pregnant and do not breastfeed while receiving the drug.
- Additive/synergistic antitumor effect when given with chemotherapy.
- No studies have been conducted with patients having hepatic dysfunction, renal dysfunction, pediatric patients, or to determine whether age, gender, or race affect the drug pharmacokinetics.
- Clinical studies conducted in patients with creatinine clearances ranging from 13.8 to 220 mL/min.
- Most patients in clinical trials had received prior therapy, including high-dose chemotherapy with stem cell rescue or transplant.
- Studies showed 28% response to bortezomib, with median response 1 year.

Potential Toxicities/Side Effects and the Nursing Process

I. POTENTIAL SENSORY/PERCEPTUAL ALTERATIONS related to SENSORY PERIPHERAL NEUROPATHY

Defining Characteristics: 80% of patients on clinical trials had a preexisting baseline peripheral neuropathy. 37% of patients had new onset or aggravation of existing peripheral neuropathy (PN). 14% developed grade 3 PN overall, with 5% occurring in patients without baseline PN symptoms. There were no grade 4 PN. Symptoms often improved off therapy, but this has not been characterized.

Nursing Implications: Teach patient to report new onset or worsening of PN symptoms (paresthesias, dysesthesias), any changes in sensory function (temperature sensation, knowing where body parts are in relation to the whole, etc.), functional ability (e.g., especially senses of smell and taste), and ability to carry out activities of daily living (ADLs). Assess severity of symptom(s) if they arise and potential for injury. If moderate, consult protocol and discuss medical intervention with physician. Teach patient measures to minimize symptoms and ensure safety. Discuss coadministered medication profile with physician as concomitant administration of the following drugs increases risk of PN: amiodarone, antivirals, isoniazid, nitrofurantoin, or statins. Discuss adding agents that may decrease development or worsening of PN, such as glutamine.

Dose Reductions:

- Grade 1 (paresthesias +/or loss of reflexes) without pain or loss of function: no action.
- Grade 1 with pain or Grade 2 (interfering with function but not ADLs): ↓ dose to 1.0 mg/m^2/dose.
- Grade 2 with pain or Grade 3 (interfering with ADLs): hold drug until toxicity resolves, then reinitiate with dose reduced to 0.7 mg/m^2 and change treatment schedule to once a week.
- Grade 4 (permanent sensory loss that interferes with function): discontinue drug.

II. POTENTIAL FOR INFECTION AND BLEEDING related to BONE MARROW DEPRESSION

Defining Characteristics Thrombocytopenia occurred in 43% of patients (27% gr 3, 3% gr 4) and neutropenia in 24% of patients (13% gr 3 and 3% gr 4). Febrile neutropenia occurred in < 1% of patients. Thrombocytopenia was dose related and occurred on days 1–11, returning to baseline during rest period (days 12–21). Anemia incidence was 32%.

Nursing Implications: Assess baseline leukocyte, platelet, and Hgb/HCT and monitor before each treatment, during therapy, and more often as needed. Hold drug for Grade 4 hematologic toxicity (NCI, see Appendix 1) and dose reduce 25%. Assess risk for infection and integrity of skin and mucous membranes, pulmonary status, and ability to clear secretions, as well as history of past infections, baseline and prior to each treatment. Teach patient to self-assess for signs/symptoms of infection, and to call provider immediately or come to the emergency room if temperature < 100.5°F, shaking chills, or rash, productive cough, burning on urination, or any signs/symptoms of infection or bleeding.

Teach self-care strategies to minimize risk of infection and bleeding, including avoidance of OTC aspirin-containing medications.

III. ALTERATION IN NUTRITION, LESS THAN BODY REQUIREMENTS, related to NAUSEA, DIARRHEA, DECREASED APPETITE, CONSTIPATION, VOMITING, AND DEHYDRATION

Defining Characteristics: Patients on clinical studies developed these symptoms with the following incidence: nausea (64%), diarrhea (51%), decreased appetite (43%), constipation (43%), vomiting (36%), dehydration (18%). Diarrhea, nausea, and vomiting occur 6–24 hours after infusion. Diarrhea and constipation may occur during cycles 1 and 2, and then disappear.

Nursing Implications: Assess baseline weight and nutritional status, and monitor prior to each treatment. Assess electrolytes prior to each treatment to weekly, especially serum sodium and potassium; replete as necessary and teach diet high in sodium and potassium. Teach patient that serum electrolytes may be decreased and to assess for s/s: hyponatremia (confusion, weakness, seizures), hypokalemia (muscle weakness, confusion, irregular heart beats), hypercalcemia (constipation, thirst, confusion, muscle cramps, sleepiness), and hypomagnesemia (muscle cramps, headache, weakness). Teach patient that side effects may occur, self-care strategies, and to report them if symptoms do not resolve. Use aggressive antiemetics to prevent nausea and vomiting: serotonin antagonist IV prior to bortezomib dose, and for 36 hours after each drug dose. If diarrhea develops after 1st treatment, teach patient to take loperamide prior to next dose of bortezomib and after every loose stool × 36 hours (not to exceed 8 tablets a day), as well as to use the BRAT diet (bananas, rice, applesauce, toast). If patient develops constipation, teach preventative self-care (stool softener, flax seed oil, MOM, prunes or prune juice q am to ensure BM at least q o day). Teach patient to drink 2 quarts of fluid daily, drinking 1 glass an hour while awake to prevent dehydration. Teach patient to report dizziness, lightheadedness, or fainting spells, and to avoid operating heavy machinery or driving a car if these occur. Develop symptom management plan with physician. Make referral to dietitian as appropriate.

IV. ALTERATION IN OXYGENATION, POTENTIAL, related to HYPOTENSION

Defining Characteristics: Orthostatic hypotension/postural hypotension can affect up to 12% of patients throughout therapy.

Nursing Implications: Identify patients at risk: patients with history of syncope, dehydration, or taking medications associated with hypotension. Assess baseline cardiac status, including blood pressure and heart rate, noting rhythm and rate. Teach patient to prevent injury by gradual change in position, and to report any dizziness. Teach patients to avoid dehydration, especially in warm climates. If hypotension noted, assess patient tolerance and need for intervention; discuss management with physician.

V. ALTERATION IN COMFORT related to ASTHENIA, PYREXIA, HEADACHE, INSOMNIA, EDEMA, DIZZINESS, RASH, MYALGIA, MUSCLE CRAMPS, BLURRED VISION

Defining Characteristics: Asthenia (characterized by fatigue, malaise, and weakness) was most common, affecting 65% of patients in clinical trials. Other symptoms included pyrexia (36%), headache (28%), insomnia (27%), arthralgias (26%), edema (26%), dyspnea (22%), dizziness (21%), myalgia (14%), pruritus (11%) and blurred vision (11%).

Nursing Implications: Assess comfort and presence of discomfort, fatigue, peripheral edema, baseline and prior to each treatment. Teach patient that these side effects may occur and to report them. Teach patient local comfort measures as well as energy conservation, and discuss management plan with physician if ineffective.

Drug: cetuximab (Erbitux)

Class: Chimeric (mouse/human) monoclonal antibody targeted against epidermal growth factor receptor (EGFR).

Mechanism of Action: Blocks growth factor (ligand, such as epidermal growth factor and transforming growth factor-alpha) from binding to EGFR, thus preventing dimerization and initiation of cell signaling via receptor tyrosine kinase phosphorylation; thus, the message telling the cell to divide does not occur. In addition to cell growth inhibition, there is induction of apoptosis, and decreased matrix metalloproteinase and vascular endothelial growth factor production. Drug is synergistic with chemotherapy and radiotherapy as it appears to prevent the malignant cell from repairing DNA damage.

Metabolism: Drug is an IgG_1 chimerized antibody, and it is postulated that clearance is via binding of the antibody to EGFR of hepatocytes with internalization of the cetuximab-EGFR complex. Mean elimination half-life is approximately 97 hours (range, 41–213 h). Steady state reached by 3rd weekly infusion. Mean half-life is 114 hours (range 75–188 h). Females have a 25% lower clearance of drug than males, but there was no difference in efficacy. No differences were found related to race, age, and hepatic and renal functional impairment.

Dosage/Range:

- Loading dose of 400 mg/m^2 IV over 2 hours, followed by a weekly maintenance dose of 250 mg/m^2 IV over 1 hour (alone or in combination with irinotecan).
- Premedicate with an H1 antagonist such as diphenhydramine 50 mg IV.

Drug Preparation/Administration: Available in 50 mL vials containing 100 mg of drug, with a concentration of 2 mg/mL. Do not shake or dilute. Solution should be clear and coloreless, and may contain small, white particles of cetuximab that are easily visible.

- Store vials under refrigeration at 2–8°C (36–46°F). Do not freeze. Increased particulate formation may occur at temperatures at or below 0°C. Drug contains no preservatives. Drug prepared in infusion containers are chemically and physically stable for 12 hours at 2–8°C (36–46°F), and for 8 hours at controlled room temperature (20–25°C or 68–77°F). Discard any remaining solution in the infuson container after 8 hours at room temperature, or 12 hours at 2–8°C (36–46°F). Discard any unused portion of the vial.
- Drug must be filtered using a low protein-binding 0.22 μm filter prior to infusion.
- Administer as an IV infusion over 2 hours for a loading dose, and 1 hour for a maintenance dose, using an infusion or syringe pump. Premedicate with an antihistamine before administration, and administer at a maximum of 5 mL/min. Observe patient for 1 hour following infusion.
- Infusion pump: draw up calculated volume of cetuximab from vials using sterile syringe and needle or transfer device, using a new needle for each vial, and inject into sterile, evacuated container or infusion bag.
  - Prime infusion tubing and attach 0.22 μm in-line filter closest to patient.
  - Piggyback cetuximab line into mainline.
  - Maximum infusion rate is 5 mL/min.
  - Flush with 0.9% saline solution at the end of the infusion.
- Syringe pump: draw up calculated volume of cetuximab from vials using sterile syringe and needle, using a new needle for each vial, and place in syringe driver of syringe pump; set rate.
  - Administer through a low protein binding 0.22 μm in-line filter rated for syringe pump, placed closest to patient; piggyback cetuximab line into mainline
  - Connect infusion line, prime line, and start the infusion.
  - Repeat procedure until the calculated volume has been infused, using a new needle and filter for each vial.
  - Maximum infusion rate is 5 mL/min.
  - Flush with 0.9% saline solution at the end of the infusion.
- Dose modification for infusion reactions:

  - Mild to moderate infusion reactions (grade 1–2): reduce infusion rate by 50% for all subsequent infusions.
  - Severe (grade 3–4) stop drug.
- Dose reductions for severe acneform rash:
  - 1st occurrence: delay infusion 1–2 weeks; if improvement, continue at 250 mg/m^2; if no improvement, discontinue cetuximab.
  - 2nd occurrence: delay infusion 1–2 weeks; if improvement, decrease dose to 200 mg/m^2; if no improvement, discontinue cetuximab.
  - 3rd occurrence: delay infusion 1–2 weeks; if improvement, reduce dose to 150 mg/m^2; if no improvement, discontinue cetuximab.
  - 4th occurrence: discontinue cetuximab.
- Irinotecan doses and scheduling when used in combination: 350 mg/m^2 q 3 weeks, 180 mg/m^2 q 2 weeks, or 125 mg/m^2 q week × 4 q 6 weeks with dose modifications as needed.

Drug Interactions:
- Synergy with cytotoxic chemotherapy (e.g., irinotecan, cisplatin) or radiotherapy.

Lab Effects/Interference:
- Unknown.

Special Considerations:
- Indicated for the treatment of EGFR-expressing, metastatic colorectal carcinoma in combination with irinotecan in patients refractory to irinotecan-based chemotherapy; indicated as a single agent in patients who are intolerant to irinotecan-based chemotherapy.
- In clinical trials of patients refractory to irinotecan, cetuximab in combination with irinotecan was shown to have a 23.8% response rate, and in oxaliplatin-irinotecan refractory patients, a 25.8% response rate. Median duration of response was 5.7 months. Response rate to monotherapy was 10.8% overall, with a median duration of 4.2 months (Cunningham et al, 2003).
- EGFR overexpression is associated with more aggressive tumors (poor prognosis, increased risk of metastases, and decreased survival).
- Tumors likely to overexpress EGFR are cancers of the colon and rectum, head and neck, pancreas, lung (NSCLC), breast, and bladder.
- Incidence of severe infusion reactions low (3%) but may be fatal (1/1000). 90% occur during 1st infusion, and are characterized by rapid onset of airway obstruction (stridor, hoarseness, bronchospasm), urticaria, and/or hypotension. Treat with epinephrine, corticosteroids, antihistamines, bronchodilators, oxygen as needed, and keep available. Drug should be discontinued if severe reaction occurs. Mild to moderate reactions require infusion rate reduction and prophylactic diphenhydramine.

- Responses have been shown in irinotecan refractory colorectal cancer when adding cetuximab to irinotecan, cisplatin refractory squamous cell cancer of the head and neck when adding cetuximab to cisplatin, and when added to radiotherapy in the treatment of patients with unresectable squamous cell cancer of the head and neck.
- Early testing in patients with pancreatic, nonsmall cell lung cancer or ovarian cancers is underway.
- Drug is antigenically similar to humanized monoclonal antibodies.
- Very rarely (< 0.5%), interstitial lung disease may occur, which may be complicated with non cardiogenicpulmonary edema and death. Onset is between 4–11th cycle of cetuximab, and is more likely in patients with pre-existing fibrotic lung disease. Hold drug and evaluate patients who develop acute or worsening pulmonary symptoms. Discontinue the drug if interstitial lung disease is found.
- Skin toxicity (acneform rash) is major toxicity; patients should be taught to wear sunscreen and hats, as well as to limit sun exposure. Rash is not acne.
- EGFR overexpression determination should be done by a laboratory with demonstrated proficiency.
- Women of childbearing age should use effective contraception, and for 60 days from the last dose of cetuximab; nursing mothers should not nurse during cetuximab and for 60 days from the last dose of the drug.

Potential Toxicities/Side Effects and the Nursing Process

I. POTENTIAL FOR INJURY related to HYPERSENSITIVITY/ ANAPHYLAXIS and INFUSION REACTION

Defining Characteristics: 19–25% of patients experience an infusion reaction. Rarely it is severe (3% of patients receiving drug in combination with Irinotecan, and 2% In patients receiving monotherapy), characterized by rapid onset of airway obstruction (bronchospams, stridor, hoarseness), urticaria, and/or hypotension. In some cases this may be fatal. Most (90%) occur during the 1st infusion. Mild-to-moderate infusion reactions characterized by chills, fever, dyspnea usually occur during the 1st infusion in 16% of patients receiving combination therapy, and 23% of patients receiving monotherapy. In addition, 73% of patients who received the combination reported asthenia vs 49% who received monotherapy; 33% fever, 9% chills, 7% headache, and 7% mucous membrane disorder (MMD).

Nursing Implications: Ensure patient receives premedication with diphenhydramine as ordered. Assess baseline VS and mental status prior to drug administration, at 15 minutes, and periodically during infusion, as needed. Remain with patient during first 15 minutes of first infusions. Recall signs/symptoms of anaphylaxis, and if these occur, stop drug immediately, notify physician, and assess patient's vital signs. Subjective symptoms are generalized itching, nausea, chest tightness, crampy abdominal pain, difficulty speaking, anxiety, agitation, sense of impending doom, uneasiness, desire to urinate/defecate, dizziness, and chills. Objective signs are flushed appearance; angioedema of face, neck, eyelids, hands, and feet; localized or generalized urticaria; respiratory distress with or without wheezing; hypotension; and cyanosis. Review standing orders or nursing procedures for patient management of anaphylaxis, and be prepared to stop drug immediately, notify physician, monitor VS, and administer ordered medications, which may include epinephrine 1:1000, hydrocortisone sodium succinate, and diphenhydramine. Teach patient to report any unusual symptoms. For mild-to-moderate infusion reactions (grade 1–2), decrease infusion rate permanently by 50%. Drug should be discontinued in patients who experience severe infusion reactions (grade 3/4).

II. POTENTIAL ALTERATION IN BODY IMAGE, SKIN INTEGRITY, COMFORT related to SKIN RASH

Defining Characteristics: Drug inhibits epidermal growth factor receptor, so major toxicity is manifested in the skin. Most patients (88%–90%) develop a mild-to-moderate acne-like rash that is self-limiting. 14% report a grade 3 rash, and in clinical studies 1.6% of patients discontinued treatment due to skin rash. Rash is a sterile, suppurative rash with multiple follicular or pustular lesions that appear during the first 2 weeks of therapy on the face, upper chest and back, but in some cases, extended to the arms. Rash resolves when treatment is stopped, without scar formation. However, in 50% of patients, it takes longer than 28 days to resolve. 7% of patients reported dry skin, which may be associated with fissures and in some cases, inflammation and infection such as blepharitis and cellulitis. Infection can be treated with topical clindamycin, or oral antibiotics. Do not use topical corticosteroid cream. It appears that patients who have significant rash, also have a tumor response.

Nursing Implications: Teach patient that rash most likely will occur due to mechanism of drug action. Assess baseline skin integrity on areas of face, neck, and trunk; assess baseline comfort and satisfaction with body image, and monitor at each treatment. Teach patient to report any distress and assess extent of rash. Drug is held for 1–2 weeks for severe rash, and if it resolves, dose is reduced on and after the 2nd occurrence. If rash does not resolve, drug is stopped. If skin appears to be infected, discuss with physician, the prescription of clindamycin gel (Cleocin T) or oral cephalexin (Keflex) 250 mg PO bid × 3 days, then 250 mg qd × 7 days, for a total of 10 days for skin infection. Rash is not acne, and so usual anti-acne treatment will not be effective.

III. ALTERATION IN NUTRITION, LESS THAN BODY REQUIREMENTS, related to NAUSEA, VOMITING, DIARRHEA, STOMATITIS/ MUCOUS MEMBRANE DISORDER, CONSTIPATION, WEIGHT LOSS

Defining Characteristics: Incidence of mild-to-moderate digestive symptoms include nausea (55% for combination patients, and 29% for monotherapy), diarrhea (72% vs 28%), vomiting (41% vs 25%), stomatitits/mucous membrane disorder (26% vs 11%), weight loss (21% vs 9%), anorexia (36% vs 25%), and constipation (30%).

Nursing Implications: Assess baseline weight and nutritional status. Teach patient that these symptoms may occur, and to report them. Administer antiemetic and other symptom management medications as ordered. Teach patient self-administration of these medications at home. Teach patient dietary modifications to address symptoms such as anorexia (small, frequent high-calorie, high-protein foods, stimulants as permitted by protocol); constipation (high-fiber, high-fluid, high-roughage foods, stool softeners); diarrhea (bananas, rice, applesauce, and toast); nausea (avoid food preparation odors by cooking in zipped plastic bag, or having someone else cook; choose cool, soft, non-spicy, or fatty foods). Assess efficacy of intervention, and revise plan as needed.

IV. POTENTIAL FOR INFECTION AND FATIGUE related to LEUKOPENIA AND ANEMIA

Defining Characteristics: Leukopenia occurs in about 25% of patients (combination vs 1% monotherapy) with 17% grade 3–4 (combination) and anemia in 16% (combination vs 10% monotherapy (4–5% grade 3–4).

Nursing Implications: Assess baseline wbc, hematocrit and hemoglobin, and monitor prior to each treatment, especially if drug is given in combination with irinotecan Teach patient to monitor temperature, and report temperature > 100.5°F. Assess level of fatigue and teach energy baseline and prior to each treatment. Teach patient that fatigue may occur due to anemia, and teach energy conserving strategies such as alternating rest and activity periods.

Drug: denileukin diftitox (ONTAK®)

Class: Fusion protein.

Mechanism of Action: Agent is recombinant DNA-derived cytotoxic protein containing diphtheria toxin fragments, and IL-2. It targets cells with high affinity for IL-2 receptors containing a CD25 component, such as activated T and B lymphocytes, and activated macrophages. The IL-2 portion of the fusion protein binds to the IL-2 receptor on malignant cells, which contain a CD25 component. The diphtheria toxin fragments are brought into the cell through the receptor (receptor-mediated endocytosis) and into the endosomal vesicles. Acidification cleaves the active fragment of diphtheria toxin, which is then actively transported into the cytoplasm. There, it catalyzes a reaction that inhibits protein synthesis and causes cell death within hours.

Metabolism: Distribution phase has half-life of 2–5 minutes, and terminal phase half-life of 70–80 minutes; the development of antibodies to denileukin diftitox significantly increases clearance 2–3 times, with a consequent decrease in mean systemic exposure of about 75%. Metabolized by proteolytic degradation and primarily excreted via the liver and kidneys; excreted material is < 25% of total dose.

Dosage/Range:
- 9 or 18 mcg/kg/day IV daily × 5 days, repeated every 3 weeks × at least 3 cycles.

Drug Preparation:
- Bring ONTAK vial to room temperature (25°C, or 77°F); may thaw in refrigerator at 2–8°C (36–46°F) over less than 24 hours, or at room temperature for 1–2 hours. DO NOT HEAT.
- Mix by gentle swirling. DO NOT SHAKE VIGOROUSLY.
- DO NOT REFREEZE DRUG.
- Inspect solution for clarity and discard if it remains hazy (will be hazy after thawing, but becomes clear when at room temperature).
- Withdraw ordered dose from vial and inject into an empty IV infusion bag; add up to 9 mL of sterile saline without preservative for each 1 mL of ONTAK to the IV bag, for a final concentration of at least 15 mcg/mL.
- Discard any unused portion of the drug.

Drug Administration:
- Give by IV infusion over at least 15 minutes, but less than 80 minutes.
- Slow or stop infusion if infusion reaction occurs, depending upon severity of symptoms.
- DO NOT administer with other drugs, or give through an inline filter.
- Administer prepared IV solution within 6 hours, using a syringe pump or infusion bag.

Drug Interactions:
- Unknown.

Lab Effects/Interference:
- Hypoalbuminemia may occur in up to 83% of patients, with nadir 1–2 weeks after drug administration.

Special Considerations:

- ONTAK is indicated for the treatment of patients with persistent or recurrent cutaneous T-cell lymphoma (CTCL, or mycosis fungoides) whose malignant cells express the CD25 component of the IL-2 receptor.
- Delay administration of drug until serum albumin is ≥ 3.0 g/dL.
- Avoid use during pregnancy unless benefit outweighs risk.
- Nursing mothers should not breast-feed while receiving the drug.
- Adverse reactions tend to be more frequent and/or more severe in the elderly (anorexia, hypotension, anemia, confusion, rash, nausea and/or vomiting).
- The frequency of adverse effects decreases after the second course of therapy.
- CBC, chemistries, including albumin, liver, and renal function studies, should be done baseline and weekly during therapy.

Potential Toxicities/Side Effects and the Nursing Process

I. POTENTIAL FOR INJURY related to HYPERSENSITIVITY OR ANAPHYLAXIS REACTIONS

Defining Characteristics: Acute hypersensitivity reactions occurred in 69% of patients during clinical trials during or within 24 hours of the ONTAK infusion, with 50% occurring during the first day of dosing of each cycle. Reactions were characterized by hypotension (50%), back pain (30%), dyspnea (28%), vasodilation (28%), rash (25%), chest pain/tightness (24%), tachycardia (12%), dysphagia or laryngismus (5%), syncope (3%), allergic reaction (1%), anaphylaxis (1%).

Nursing Implications: Assess baseline VS and mental status prior to drug administration, at 15 minutes, and periodically during infusion. Remain with patient during first 15 minutes of infusion. Recall signs/symptoms of anaphylaxis and, if these occur, stop drug immediately and notify physician. Subjective symptoms are generalized itching, nausea, chest tightness, crampy abdominal pain, difficulty speaking, anxiety, agitation, sense of impending doom, uneasiness, desire to urinate/defecate, dizziness, chills. Objective signs are flushed appearance; angioedema of face, neck, eyelids, hands, feet; localized or generalized urticaria; respiratory distress with or without wheezing, hypotension, cyanosis. Review standing orders or nursing procedure for patient management of anaphylaxis and be prepared to stop drug immediately, notify physician, monitor VS, and administer ordered medications, which may include epinephrine 1:1000, hydrocortisone sodium succinate, and diphenhydramine. Teach patient to report any unusual symptoms.

II. POTENTIAL FOR INJURY related to VASCULAR LEAK SYNDROME

Defining Characteristics: 27% of patients in clinical trial testing developed vascular leak syndrome, characterized by hypotension, edema, and hypoalbuminemia. Onset of symptoms occurs within the first two weeks of infusion and may persist or become more severe after the drug has been stopped. Patients with preexisting cardiac problems are at risk for developing myocardial infarctions. Syndrome is usually self-limiting, but may rarely require management of edema or hypotension. Low serum albumin is a predictor of development of syndrome.

Nursing Implications: Monitor weight, BP, and serum albumin levels baseline and throughout treatment; assess for presence of edema baseline and throughout treatment. Notify physician if edema, hypotension, or serum albumin < 3.0 g/dL. Treatment should be delayed until serum albumin is ≥ 3.0 g/dL.

III. POTENTIAL FOR INFECTION related to LYMPHOPENIA, IMMUNE SUPPRESSION OF MACROPHAGES

Defining Characteristics: Cutaneous T-cell lymphoma increases risk of cutaneous infection, together with drug-induced lymphopenia, and impaired immune function further increases risk. During clinical trials, 48% of patients developed infections (23% severe). Lymphocyte counts < 900 cells/μl occurred in 34% of patients. Counts decreased during days 1–5 (dosing period) with recovery by day 15; subsequent cycles had less lymphopenia and more rapid recovery.

Nursing Implications: Assess baseline WBC, lymphocyte count, and monitor weekly during therapy. Assess skin integrity, potential for infection, and teach patient measures to prevent infection (e.g., keeping skin intact, avoiding sources of infection, good handwashing). Teach patient to report any signs/symptoms of infection (e.g., redness, heat, exudate on skin, T > 100.5, sputum production, dysuria). Assess for signs/symptoms of infection during therapy and at each visit.

IV. ALTERATION IN COMFORT related to FLULIKE SYMPTOMS

Defining Characteristics: 91% of patients developed flulike symptom complex during clinical trials, consisting of fever and chills (81%), asthenia (66%), nausea/vomiting (64%), myalgias (18%), arthralgias (8%). Dehydration occurred in 9% of patients. Symptoms developed within hours to days after having received drug infusion. Symptoms are generally mild to moderate and are responsive to symptom management.

Nursing Implications: Teach patient that flulike symptoms may occur commonly following treatment, and teach symptom management with antipyretics (e.g., acetaminophen) and dietary modification if nausea experienced. Discuss with physician giving patient prescription for antiemetic agent in case nausea is severe or vomiting develops. Discuss use of meperidine, diphenhydramine if patient develops rigors. Teach patient to call nurse or physician if symptoms do not respond, become worse, if unable to take at least 1 qt of fluid orally per day, or new symptoms develop.

V. ALTERATION IN NUTRITION related to DIARRHEA, ANOREXIA, NAUSEA/VOMITING, HYPOALBUMINEMIA

Defining Characteristics: Nausea/vomiting occurs in 64% of patients as part of flulike syndrome, anorexia occurs in 36% of patients, and diarrhea occurs in 29%. Hypoalbuminemia occurs in 83%, weight loss in 14%, and elevated transaminases 61%. Elevation of serum transaminases occurred during first cycle of therapy, and resolved within two weeks. Hypocalcemia (17%) and hypokalemia (6%) have also been reported. Constipation occurred in 9%, dyspepsia 7%, and dysphagia 6%. Rarely, pancreatitis, hyperthyroidism, and hypothyroidism may occur.

Nursing Implications: Assess baseline nutritional status, as well as baseline LFTs and serum albumin, and monitor weekly during therapy. Teach patient to eat high-calorie, high-protein foods. Assess for occurrence of symptoms of nausea, vomiting, diarrhea, anorexia, other problems, and teach patient to report them. Teach patient self-administration of prescribed medications to manage symptoms.

VI. ALTERATION IN COMFORT related to SKIN RASHES, PAIN AT TUMOR SITES

Defining Characteristics: During clinical trials, rash occurred in 34%, pruritus 20%, and sweating 10%. Rashes occurred during/after treatment or were delayed. They were varied, as generalized maculopapular, petechial, vesicular bullous, urticarial, or as eczema.

Nursing Implications: Assess baseline skin integrity and presence of rashes. Assess daily during treatment and weekly thereafter; teach patient to report any skin changes. Assess need for diphenhydramine or other antihistamines for pruritus, and use of topical and/or oral corticosteroids for moderate to severe rashes and discomfort.

VII. POTENTIAL ALTERATION IN CARDIAC OUTPUT related to HYPOTENSION, TACHYCARDIA, THROMBOTIC EVENTS

Defining Characteristics: The following cardiovascular side effects occurred in clinical testing: hypotension (36%), vasodilation (22%), tachycardia (12%), thrombotic events (7%), hypertension (6%), and arrythmia (6%). Two patients with preexisting coronary artery disease developed myocardial infarctions while receiving the drug. Thrombotic events included deep vein thrombosis, pulmonary embolus, arterial thrombosis, and superficial thrombophlebitis.

Nursing Implications: Assess baseline cardiovascular status and presence of risk factor of coronary artery disease. Teach patient to report any chest pain or discomfort, palpitations, pain in calf, heat/redness of calf immediately, or to come to the emergency room if at home. Discuss onset of hypotension, tachycardia with physician, relationship to drug administration, and management strategies. If symptoms severe, stop drug infusion and discuss use of saline hydration to raise BP and decrease HR.

VIII. POTENTIAL FOR FATIGUE AND BLEEDING related to BONE MARROW SUPPRESSION

Defining Characteristics: Anemia occurs in about 18% (6% grades 3 or 4), thrombocytopenia in 8% (2% grades 3 or 4), and leukopenia in 6% (3% grades 3 or 4).

Nursing Implications: Monitor CBC/differential, HCT, and platelet count and assess for signs/symptoms of infection, fatigue, and bleeding baseline prior to treatment, and weekly during treatment. Instruct patient in self-assessment of signs/symptoms of infection, fatigue, bleeding. Transfuse platelet, red cell transfusions per physician's order.

IX. POTENTIAL ALTERATION IN OXYGENATION related to DYSPNEA, COUGH

Defining Characteristics: In clinical trials, 29% of patients reported dyspnea, 26% increased cough, 17% pharyngitis, 13% rhinitis, and 8% "lung disorder."

Nursing Implications: Assess VS, pulmonary exam, and weight prior to each treatment, and at each weekly visit. Teach patient to do daily weights, and to report any SOB, weight gain, increased cough, or other problems. If this occurs, notify physician and discuss obtaining CXR and focused exam. Discuss chest X-ray findings with physician.

X. POTENTIAL SENSORY/PERCEPTUAL ALTERATIONS related to NERVOUSNESS, CONFUSION, INSOMNIA

Defining Characteristics: Nervousness may affect 11%, confusion 8%, and insomnia 9%.

Nursing Implications: Teach patient that these symptoms may occur and to report them. Assess baseline mental status, affect, and sleep pattern prior to each treatment cycle, and weekly during treatment. Discuss need for pharmacologic symptom management if symptoms are severe.

XI. POTENTIAL ALTERATION IN URINE ELIMINATION related to HEMATURIA, ALBUMINURIA, PYURIA

Defining Characteristics: Patients in clinical trials experienced hematuria (10%), albuminuria (10%), and pyuria (10%). 7% had increases in serum creatinine. Rarely, acute renal insufficiency occurs.

Nursing Implications: Assess baseline urinary elimination status, urinalysis, as well as serum renal function studies. Teach patient to report blood in urine, and dysuria, or any problems in voiding. Discuss abnormalities with physician.

Drug: edrecolomab (moAb 17–1A) (investigational)

Class: Monoclonal antibody.

Mechanism of Action: Murine monoclonal antibody that recognizes the human tumor-associated antigen glycoprotein 17–1A or Ep-CAM, that is expressed on epithelial tissues, and in many colon and rectal cancers.

Metabolism: Unknown.

Dosage/Range:
Per protocol in combination with 5-FU/LV.

Drug Preparation/Administration: Per protocol.

Drug Interactions: Unknown.

Lab Effects/Interference: Unknown.

Special Considerations:

- An initial study of 189 patients showed survival benefit of 32% in patients with resected Stage III colon cancer when given in the adjuvant setting (Riethmuller et al, 1994), compared to surgery alone, but these data were not replicated in a later international study of 2761 patients (Punt et al, 2002), which showed that edrecolomab alone is inferior to 5-FU/LV adjuvant chemotherapy and that, when given in combination with 5-FU/LV adjuvant chemotherapy, it did not increase overall survival.

- Drug is well tolerated and did not increase the incidence of neutropenia, diarrhea, or mucositis when combined with 5-FU/LV.

Potential Toxicities/Side Effects and the Nursing Process

I. POTENTIAL FOR INJURY related to HYPERSENSITIVITY/ ANAPHYLAXIS and INFUSION REACTION

Defining Characteristics: 25% of patients experienced a hypersensitivity reaction, causing discontinuation in 4% of patients. Drug is a murine monoclonal antibody, largely made up of mouse antibody. Allergic reactions may be mild characterized by chills, fever, dyspnea, or severe, characterized by rapid onset of airway obstruction (bronchospams, stridor, hoarseness), urticaria, and/or hypotension.

Nursing Implications: Ensure patient receives premedication with diphenhydramine per protocol. Assess baseline VS and mental status prior to drug administration, at 15 minutes, and periodically during infusion, as needed. Remain with patient during first 15 minutes of first infusions. Recall signs/ symptoms of anaphylaxis, and if these occur, stop drug immediately, notify physician, and assess patient's vital signs. Subjective symptoms are generalized itching, nausea, chest tightness, crampy abdominal pain, difficulty speaking, anxiety, agitation, sense of impending doom, uneasiness, desire to urinate/ defecate, dizziness, and chills. Objective signs are flushed appearance; angioedema of face, neck, eyelids, hands, and feet; localized or generalized urticaria; respiratory distress with or without wheezing; hypotension; and cyanosis. Review standing orders or nursing procedures for patient management of anaphylaxis, and be prepared to stop drug immediately, notify physician, monitor VS, and administer ordered medications, which may include epinephrine 1:1000, hydrocortisone sodium succinate, and diphenhydramine. Teach patient to report any unusual symptoms.

Drug: erlotinib (OSI-774, Tarceva™)

Class: Epidermal Growth Factor Receptor (HER1/EGFR) tyrosine kinase inhibitor (quinazoline type).

Mechanism of Action: Mechanism of anti-tumor activity not fully characterized. Inhibits the cytoplasmic protein (tyrosine kinase) domain of the EGFR.

Metabolism: Drug bioavailability is about 60% after oral administration with peak plasma concentration ocurring 4 hours after ingestion. Drug is highly protein-bound (90–95%). It is primarily metabolized by the cytochrome P450 hepatic microsomal enzyme system (CYP3A4). Food can increase drug bioavailability by 100%.

Dosage/Range:

- 150 mg PO q day.

Drug Preparation/Administration:

- Oral, available in 150-, 100-, and 25-mg tablets.
- Dose should be taken on an empty stomach, either 1 hour before meals or 2 hours after meals.

Drug Interactions:

- *Inducers of the CYP3A4* (may increase metabolism of erlotinib and decrease its plasma concentration): rifampin, phenytoin, phenobarbitol, St. John's Wort, carbamazepine, rifapentin, rifabuten. May need to increase dose of erlotinib.
- *Inhibitors of the CYP3A4* (may increase metabolism of erlotinib and increase its plasma concentration): ketoconazole, itraconazole, grapefruit (fruit or juice), clarithromycin, ritonavir, indinavir, atanazavir, nelfinavir, saquinavir, metronidazole, isoniazid, telithromycin, troleandomycin, voriconazole. May need to decrease dose of erlotinib.
- *Warfarin* increases INR and bleeding possible; monitor INR, patient bleeding, and decrease warfarin dose as needed.

Lab Effects/Interference:

- May increase liver function tests (serum transaminases).

Special Considerations:

- Drug is FDA approved for the treatment of patients with locally advanced or metastatic Non-Small Cell lung cancer after failure of at least one prior chemotherapy regimen.
- Infrequently, drug can cause interstitial lung disease (ILD) ($< 1\%$ of patients), which can be serious. This is a class effect, and similar to that of gelfitinib. Drug should be stopped immediately in patients who develop worsening or unexplained pulmonary symptoms, and appropriate diagnostic work-up begun to establish the cause. If ILD is diagnosed, erlotinib should be discontinued.
- Drug can cause conjunctivitis and drying of eyes, ameliorated by artificial tears.
- Patients may require temporary interruption or dose reduction for severe diarrhea that does not resolve with anti-diarrheals, or for severe and intolerable rash; dose modification if refractory or intolerable. Also, consider if patient has severe liver dysfunction.

Potential Toxicities/Side Effects and the Nursing Process

I. ALTERATION IN SKIN INTEGRITY related to RASH

Defining Characteristics: As expected, because EGFR is important in skin function, this is the area of major toxicity. Rash ranges from maculopapular to pustular on the face, neck, chest, back, and arms, affecting up to 75% of patients. Most rashes are mild to moderate (Sandler et al, 2004). Typically, rash begins on days 8–10 of therapy, maximizing in intensity by week 2, and resolving gradually on therapy (often by week 4). Use of skin treatments (corticosteroids, topical clindamycin, or minocycline) have been used with varying results.

Nursing Implications: Assess skin integrity of face, neck, arms, and upper trunk baseline, and regularly during treatment. Teach patient that rash may occur, its usual course, and self-care measures for comfort. Emphasize the need to keep skin with rash clean to prevent infection, and to continue taking erlotinib until told to stop by nurse or physician. Teach patient that skin may become dry, and to use skin emollients or moisturizers. Assess body image intactness, and if rash develops, its threat to body image. Encourage patient to verbalize feelings; provide emotional support, and individualize care plan to patient response.

II. ALTERATION IN ELIMINATION PATTERN related to DIARRHEA

Defining Characteristics: Affects approximately 54% of patients, and is mild to moderate with only 6% of patients experiencing grade 3 diarrhea. Diarrhea usually beginning weeks 3–4. Symptoms may be self-limited or require an anti-diarrheal agent, such as loperamide. Severe diarrhea not responsive to anti-diarrheal medication may require temporary dose-interruption or adjustment if refractory.

Nursing Implications: Assess bowel elimination pattern baseline, and regularly during therapy. Teach patient to report diarrhea; teach patient self-care strategies to manage diarrhea such as dietary modification and self-administration of loperamide; teach patient to minimize potential complications such as dehydration and electrolye depletion. If diarrhea does not resolve or is severe, discuss with physician dose interruption, as well as fluid and electrolyte replacement.

III. SENSORY/PERCEPTUAL ALTERATION, POTENTIAL related to CONJUNCTIVITIS AND EYE DRYNESS

Defining Characteristics: Conjunctivits and eye dryness may occur, and are generally mild to moderate (grades 1–2).

Nursing Implications: Teach patient to report any eye irritation or change in visual acuity. Teach patient to use artificial tears to keep eyes lubricated.

IV. POTENTIONAL ALTERATION IN NUTRITION, LESS THAN BODY REQUIREMENTS related to MUCOSITIS and ANOREXIA

Defining Characteristics: Stomatitis is uncommon, occurring in 17% of patients receiving erlotinib, compared to 3% receiving placebo. Grade 3/4 occurs in <1% of patients. It is usually mild to moderate and is generally self-limited. Anorexia affects about 52% of patients with 8% experiencing grade 3.

Nursing Implications: Assess oral hygiene practices, and status of oral mucosa, gums, and teeth baseline, and regularly throughout therapy. Teach patient to report stomatitis, and to use a systematic cleansing regime as determined by institutional policy.

Drug: gefitinib (Iressa)

Class: Tyrosine kinase inhibitor.

Mechanism of Action: Drug inhibits the intracellular phosphorylation of a number of tyrosine kinases associated with transmembrane cell surface receptors, including the epidermal growth factor receptor (EGFR-TK). This prevents the message for cell division from being sent to the nucleus. Thus cell division, growth, and angiogenesis do not occur.

Metabolism: Absorbed slowly from the gastrointestinal tract following oral administration with peak plasma levels occurring 3–7 hours after dosing. Bioavailability 60%, and unaffected by food. Drug is 90% protein bound (serum albumin). Drug is metabolized via the P450 microenzyme system, primarily the CYP 3A4 subsystem, and excreted in the feces (86%). Elimination half-life 48 hours with steady state plasma level achieved within 10 days.

Dosage/Range:
250 mg po qd. As of 9/15/05, the manufacturer, Astra Zeneca, is limiting availability of the drug to patients who have previously taken the drug and are benefiting, or who have benefited. The drug will be available through the IRESSA access program only. In clinical trials, the drug will be available to patients who are enrolled. If new study data shows an improvement in survival, then the labeling will change.

Drug Preparation: Available as 250 mg tablets in a bottle of 30 tablets.

Drug Administration: Administer with or without food at about the same time each day

- If severe diarrhea or skin reaction, briefly interrupt therapy for up to 14 days, and then resume at same dose.
- If new onset or worsening of pulmonary symptoms (dyspnea, cough, fever), interrupt therapy until pulmonary evaluation can rule out interstitial lung disease. IF interstitial lung disease confirmed, STOP gefitinib and treat pulmonary toxicity.
- If new onset eye pain or other eye symptoms, interrupt therapy and evaluate cause.
- If patient receiving concomitant potent CYP3A4 inducer (e.g., rifampicin or phenytoin), consider increasing dose to 500 mg q d in the absence of severe drug reaction.

Drug Interactions:

- Inducers of CYP3A4 (increase metabolism of gefitinib and decrease its plasma concentrations or AUC by 85%): rifamicin, phenytoin; consider increasing gefitinib dose to 500 mg/da.
- Inhibitors of CYP 3A4 (decrease metabolism of gefitinib and increase its plasma concentration or AUC by 88%): Itraconazole; consider another antifungal or decrease gefitinib if increased toxicity.
- High gastric pH > 5.0 (e.g., ranitidine with sodium bicarbonate: decrease gefitinib AUC by 44%).
- Warfarin: increased INR and bleeding; monitor INR frequently and patient for s/s bleeding and decrease warfarin dose accordingly.

Lab Effects/Interference:

- Asymptomatic elevations in liver function tests (transaminases, bilirubin and alkaline phosphatase).

Special Considerations:

- Indicated as monotherapy for the treatment of patients with locally advanced or metastatic non-small cell lung cancer (NSCLC) after failure of both platinum-based and docetaxel chemotherapies. Given the response rate of 10%, and the fact that there was no survival advantage together with the fact that erlotinib (Tarceva) has since been FDA approved, based on clinical evidence of a survival advantage, gelfitinib is now restricted. Effective 9/15/05, drug is only available to 1) patients who are currently or who have previously taken the drug and are benefiting, or who have benefited and 2) previously enrolled patients or new patients in non-Investigational New Drug (IND) clinical trials approved by an IRB prior to 6/17/05. The drug will be available through the IRESSA access program only.

- Results from two large controlled, randomized clinical trials in first-line treatment of NSCLC showed no benefit from gefitinib added to platinum-based chemotherapy.
- Interstitial lung disease occurs in about 1% of patients. In Japan the incidence was 2%, but in the prospective first-line studies, incidence of interstitial lung disease was equal in treatment and placebo groups. Patients with concurrent idiopathic pulmonary fibrosis whose condition worsens during therapy have an increased mortality compared to those without pulmonary fibrosis.
- Primary side effects are diarrhea, rash, acne, dry skin, nausea, and vomiting.
- No dose reduction necessary for hepatic (related to metastases) or renal dysfunction. No studies have been done in non-cancer-related liver impairment.
- Contraindications: allergy to gefitinib or its components; avoid administration in pregnant women or women who are breast-feeding.
- Drug is associated RARELY with pancreatitits, and allergic reactions including angioedema, urticaria, toxic epidermal necrolysis, and erythema multiforme.
- Patients with specific gene mutations in the EGFR are most likely to respond to the drug (Lynch et al, 2004), and for those patients, ultimately they develop resistance due to a 2nd mutation that develops in this receptor.

Potential Toxicities/Side Effects and the Nursing Process

I. ALTERATION IN OXYGENATION related to INTERSTITIAL LUNG DISEASE (ILD)

Defining Characteristics: Rarely (1%) patients develop interstitial lung disease, with a 33% mortality. In some studies, incidence was similar in treatment and placebo groups. This toxicity has been reported as interstitial pneumonia, pneumonitis, and alveolitis. Onset characterized by dyspnea, sometimes with cough or low-grade fever, and rapidly becoming severe. Incidence increased in patients with prior radiotherapy, prior chemotherapy. Mortality was increased in patients with concurrent pulmonary fibrosis who developed ILD.

Nursing Implications: Assess baseline pulmonary status, and periodically during treatment. Teach patient to report cough, low-grade fever, and shortness of breath (or worsening of pulmonary status). If it develops, discuss with physician pulmonary function tests, and further pulmonary work-up as ordered.

II. ALTERATION IN BOWEL ELIMINATION related to DIARRHEA

Defining Characteristics: Mild to moderate diarrhea occurred in 48% of patients, and in a few patients was severe and associated with dehydration. Drug may be interrupted for up to 14 days if patient develops severe diarrhea, and then restarted when diarrhea resolves.

Nursing Implications: Assess bowel elimination pattern baseline, and regularly during therapy. Teach patient to report diarrhea that does not resolve with anti-diarrheal medication right away. Teach patient self-care strategies to manage diarrhea, including increased oral fluids to 2–3 liters a day, dietary modification and use of anti-diarrheal medications such as loperamide. Discuss with physician dose interruption or reduction for severe diarrhea, as well as fluid and electrolyte replacement and aggressive anti-diarrheal medication.

III. ALTERATION IN SKIN INTEGRITY, POTENTIAL related to RASH, ACNE, DRY SKIN, PRURITUS

Defining Characteristics: As expected, because EGFR is important in skin function, this is the area of major toxicity. Rash occurred in 43% of patients in clinical trials, with acne occurring in 25%, dry skin 13%, pruritis 8% of patients. Rash is manifested as patches of erythema/acneiform (pustular) lesions on the face; with higher doses, it affects the upper torso. Rash resolves quickly after drug discontinuance. Drug may be interrupted for up to 14 days if patient develops severe rash, and then restarted. Ensure that rash is not allergic, and rule out urticaria, toxic epidermal necrolysis, and erythema multiforme that may occur rarely.

Nursing Implications: Assess skin integrity of face, neck, arms, and upper trunk baseline, and regularly during treatment. Teach patient that rash may occur, its usual course, and self-care measures for comfort. Assess body image intactness, and if rash develops, its threat to body image. Encourage patient to verbalize feelings; provide emotional support, and individualize care plan to patient response.

IV. ALTERATION IN NUTRITION, LESS THAN BODY REQUIREMENTS related to NAUSEA, VOMITING, ANOREXIA, WEIGHT LOSS

Defining Characteristics: Nausea affects 13% and vomiting 12% of patients.

Nursing Implications: Assess baseline nutritional status and risk of nausea and vomiting. Teach patient to self-administer antiemetic medications 1 hour prior to taking drug if nausea or vomiting develops. Teach patient to report persistent or continued nausea and/or vomiting. Assess efficacy and discuss change in antiemetic drug with physician if regimen ineffective.

V. ALTERATION IN COMFORT AND ACTIVITY TOLERANCE related to ASTHENIA

Defining Characteristics: Asthenia affects approximately 6% of patients.

Nursing Implications: Assess baseline comfort, energy/activity level, and ability to do self-care. Teach patient that these side effects may occur, and energy conservation strategies to manage them. If patient unable to do ADLs, assess need for home support from outside agency.

VI. SENSORY/PERCEPTUAL ALTERATIONS, POTENTIAL related to VISUAL AND OCULAR CHANGES

Defining Characteristics: Amblyopia occurred in 2% of patients, and conjunctivitis 1%. There are reports of patients with eye pain and corneal erosion/ ulceration, sometimes associated with abnormal eyelash growth. In addition, rarely, corneal membrane sloughing and ocular ischemia/hemorrhage occurred.

Nursing Implications: Teach patient to stop drug and report any eye discomfort or visual changes immediately. Discuss referral of patient to ophthalmologist for evaluation and advice. Discuss drug continuance with physician depending upon cause of problem.

Drug: gemtuzumab ozogamicin for injection (Mylotarg)

Class: Monoclonal antibody conjugated to a cytotoxic antibiotic.

Mechanism of Action: Drug is composed of a recombinant hymanized Ig4 kappa antibody conjugated with a cytotoxic antitumor antibiotic, calicheamicin. The antibody portion of the drug binds to the CD33 antigen found on the cell surface of leukemic blast and immature normal cells in the myeloid cell line but not the pleuripotent stem cell. The CD33 antigen is expressed on more than 80% of patients with acute myeloid leukemia. 98.3% of the amino acids used are of human origin, while the remainder are derived from murine antibody. Once the MoAb binds to the CD33 antibody, the complex is brought inside the cell, calicheamicin is released inside lysosomes within the myeloid cell and then binds to DNA, resulting in DNA double-strand breaks and cell death.

Metabolism: Following first dose, terminal half-lives of total and unconjugated calicheamicin were 45 and 100 hours, while after the second dose 14 days later, the terminal half-life of total calicheamicin was 60 hours, and the area under the concentration-time curve was double that following the first treatment. The cytotoxic drug calicheamicin derivative is hydrolyzed to release it from the monoclonal antibody and forms many metabolites.

Dosage/Range:

9 mg/m^2 given as a 2-hour IV infusion q14 days × 2.

- Premedicate 1 hour before the drug is given with diphenhydramine 50 mg PO and acetaminophen 650–1000 mg PO, with acetaminophen repeated q4h × 2 PRN.

Drug Preparation:
- Protect from direct and indirect sunlight and unshielded fluorescent light during preparation and administration of drug (fluorescent light must be turned off in biological safety cabinet during preparation).
- Allow refrigerated vials to come to room temperature.
- Reconstitute 5 mg vial with 5 mL sterile water for injection, USP, using sterile syringes. Gently swirl the vial to dissolve. Final concentration is 1 mg/mL. While in the amber vial, the reconstituted solution can be refrigerated (2–8°C, 36–36°F) and protected from light for up to 8 hrs.
- Withdraw ordered dose and inject into 100 mL bag of 0.9% Normal Saline Injection, and then place the bag inside an UV-protectant bag. Use the medication immediately.

Drug Administration:
- Premedicate 1 hour before the drug is given with diphenhydramine 50 mg PO and acetaminophen 650–1000 mg PO, with acetaminophen repeated q4h × 2 PRN.
- Administer in light-protected bag IV over 2 hours via separate IV tubing containing a 1.2 micron terminal filter.
- Can be given via peripheral or central IV line.
- DO NOT administer by IVP or bolus.

Drug Interactions:
- Unknown.

Lab Effects/Interference:
- Increased LFTs.
- Hyperglycemia (part of post-infusion syndrome).
- Significant decrease in WBC, Hgb/HCT, platelet count.
- Increased LDH.
- Decreased serum K, Mg.

Special Considerations:
- Drug is indicated for the treatment of patients with CD33 positive acute myeloid leukemia in first relapse who are 60 years or older, and who are not considered candidates for cytotoxic chemotherapy.
- Drug is contraindicated in patients with known hypersensitivity to gemtuzumab ozogamicin or its components (anti-CD33 antibody), calicheamicin derivatives, or inactive ingredients and in pregnant or nursing women.
- Give premedication to prevent post-infusion symptom complex.
- Severe myelosuppression will occur in all patients, and systemic infections must be treated.

- Use cautiously in patients with renal or hepatic dysfunction.
- Women of childbearing age should use effective contraception measures.
- Rarely, patient may develop antibodies to calicheamicin/calicheamicin-linker portion of gemtuzumab ozogamicin (2 patients, after 3 doses of drug, characterized by transient fever, hypotension, dyspnea in 1 patient), but in clinical trials no patient developed antibody responses to the antibody portion of Mylotarg.
- Tumor lysis syndrome may occur commonly in leukemic patients, so patients should be well hydrated, receive allopurinol, and receive alkalinization if at risk (high tumor burden).

Potential Toxicities/Side Effects and the Nursing Process

I. POTENTIAL FOR INJURY related to ACUTE INFUSION-RELATED EVENTS

Defining Characteristics: Patients often experience a post-infusion syndrome characterized by chills (62%), fever (61%), nausea (38%), vomiting (32%), headache (12%), hypotension (11%), hypertension (6%), hypoxia (6%), dyspnea (4%), and hyperglycemia (2%). Syndrome may occur any time within 24 hours after administration, and resolves about 2–4 hours later with supportive therapy of acetaminophen, diphenhydramine, and IV fluids. Patients are less likely to experience this syndrome when receiving the second treatment.

Nursing Implications: Premedicate patient as ordered with acetaminophen and diphenhydramine one hour before drug therapy. Ensure that medications necessary for the management of hypersensitivity/anaphylaxis are readily available (e.g., epinephrine, antihistamines, corticosteroids). Assess baseline VS and monitor frequently during the infusion, and for 4 hours post infusion; keep IV line patent. Monitor VS, and notify physician of abnormalities. Be prepared to provide emergency support as necessary (including IV saline, epinephrine, antihistamines, bronchodilators).

II. POTENTIAL FOR INFECTION, BLEEDING, AND FATIGUE related to BONE MARROW DEPRESSION

Defining Characteristics: Severe (grade 3 or 4) neutropenia occurs in 98% of patients, with recovery of an ANC of 500 cells/micro liter by day 40 (after first dose) in those patients who respond. During treatment phase, 28% developed grades 3 and 4 infections, with 16% experiencing sepsis and 7% pneumonia. 22% of patients developed herpes simplex infection. Thrombocytopenia is common, with 99% of patients developing grades 3 and 4. For those responding to treatment, platelet recovery (25,000/microliter) occurs by day 39 after first day of drug. 23% of patients required platelet transfusions. During treatment phase, bleeding occurred in 15% of patients (grades 3 and 4). These episodes included epistaxis (3%), cerebral hemorrhage (2%), disseminated intravasuclar coagulation (2%), intracranial hemorrhage (2%) and hematuria (1%). Anemia also was common, with 47% of patients developing grades 3 and 4 anemia, and 26% of patients requiring transfusions.

Nursing Implications: Monitor CBC, platelets baseline and regularly during treatment. Assess for signs/symptoms of infection, bleeding, and fatigue baseline, between treatment, and prior to each treatment. Teach patient to self-assess for these, including taking temperature, and instruct to report them immediately. Teach patient measures to minimize infection, bleeding, and fatigue, including avoidance of crowds, and not taking OTC medications containing aspirin. Transfuse red blood cells and platelets as ordered. Teach patient strategies to conserve energy and minimize fatigue.

III. ALTERATION IN NUTRITION, POTENTIAL, related to NAUSEA, MUCOSITIS, VOMITING, HEPATOTOXICITY

Defining Characteristics: Nausea is common, affecting 70% of patients, with 63% developing vomiting. Stomatitis affected 35% of patients, with 4% having grades 3 or 4 toxicity. Transient increases in LFTs occurred, and were usually reversible. In clinical studies, 23% of patients developed grades 3 or 4 hyperbilirubinemia, 9% in levels of ALT, and 17% in levels of AST. In clinical studies, there were deaths reported: one patient died with liver failure as part of multisystem failure related to tumor lysis syndrome, another patient died of persistent jaundice and hepatosplenomegaly five months after treatment, and finally, 4 (of 27) patients died of veno-occlusive disease following stem cell transplantation after Mylotarg administration.

Nursing Implications: Assess baseline nutritional status, integrity of oral mucosa, and liver function studies and regularly after treatment. Administer antiemetic medications prior to chemotherapy to prevent nausea/vomiting, and teach patient self-administration of antiemetics after discharge if drug is given on an outpatient basis. Teach patient to report persistent or continued nausea and/or vomiting. Assess efficacy and discuss change in antiemetic drug with physician if regimen ineffective. Teach patient to assess oral mucosa regularly, use oral hygiene regimen, and report signs/symptoms of stomatitis. If patient develops stomatitis, teach patient self-administration of oral analgesics, antifungals, as ordered and appropriate. Monitor liver function tests, and discuss any abnormalities with physician.

IV. ALTERATION IN BOWEL ELIMINATION related to CONSTIPATION OR DIARRHEA

Defining Characteristics: Diarrhea affects 38% of patients, and constipation 25%.

Nursing Implications: Assess baseline bowel elimination status, and teach patient that alterations may occur. Teach patient self-care measures to manage constipation or diarrhea, and to report persistent or recurrent episodes. Discuss management with physician for refractory constipation or diarrhea. Teach patient dietary modifications such as increased fluid and fiber to prevent constipation, and the BRAT (bananas, rice, applesauce, tea) diet as well as increased hydration to manage diarrhea.

V. ALTERATION IN SKIN INTEGRITY, POTENTIAL, related to RASH, EDEMA, INFECTION

Defining Characteristics: Nonspecific rash affects approximately 22% of patients. 25% of patients had a local reaction, while 16% developed peripheral edema. 22% developed herpes simplex infections.

Nursing Implications: Assess baseline skin integrity, presence of rash or peripheral edema, and history of herpes simplex infections. Teach patient that these side effects may occur and to report them. Discuss with physician prophylactic use of antiviral agent if patient has a history of herpes simplex infections. If patient develops rash, local reaction, or peripheral edema, teach patient local strategies to maintain skin integrity, and use of skin moisturizers to prevent itching or scratching.

Drug: ^{90}Y ibritumomab tiuxetan (Zevalin, IDEC-Y2B8)

Class: Monoclonal antibody chelated to radioisotope ^{90}Y yttrium.

Mechanism of Action: Ibritumomab tiuxetan is a monoclonal antibody that targets the cell surface antigen CD_{20}, which is found on the surface of normal and malignant B-cell lymphocytes. The CD_{20} antigen is also present (expressed) on more than 90% of B-cell non-Hodgkin's lymphoma (NHL) cells but fortunately is not found on normal bone marrow stem cells, pre-B cells, or other normal tissues. The complex is made up of a murine anti-CD_{20} monoclonal antibody conjugate to the linker chelator tiuxetan, which then securely chelates the radioisotope ^{90}Y yttrium. The complex attaches to the CD_{20} receptor, and then the radioisotope delivers high beta energy waves to the malignant cell, causing cell death. The isotope delivers high energy with a short half-life of 64 hours. It appears that if the malignant cells are pretreated with an anti-CD_{20} antibody (e.g., Rituximab), this clears malignant and normal B lymphocytes from the blood, and ^{90}Y ibritumomab tiuxetan is better able to target the lymphoma B-lymphocytes.

Metabolism: ^{90}Y yttrium has a half-life of 64 hours, and effective half-life in the blood of 28 hours, median biological half-life of 47 hours, and median area under the curve (AUC) of 25 hours (Wiseman et al, 1996).

Dosage/Range:
Indium III (gamma emitter) is used to determine biodistribution. 1) Indium III: 5.0 mCi day 1, 2) Rituximab 250 mg/m^2 dl, d7 or 9: 250 mg/m^2; 3) Y-90 dose 0.4 mCi/Kg with maximal total dose of 32.0 mCi, dose reduce to 0.3 mCi/Kg platelet count 100K-149K.

Drug Preparation:
- See package insert.

Drug Administration:
- Day 1: In-111 IV over 10 min using 0.22 micron filter, followed by rituximab IV within 4 hours, initially at 50mg/hr, and gradually increasing the rate in 50 mg/hr increments if no infusion reaction, to a maximum of 400 mg/hr. Premedicate with acetaminophen and antihistamine prior to rituximab.
- Biodistribution imaging 1: 2–24 hr after In-111 injection; image 2: 48–72 hr later; optional image 3; at 90–120 hr.
- If biodistribution acceptable, on day 7–9, rituxan 250 mg/m^2, and within 4 hours, Y-90 Zevalin IV over10 min. Avoid extravasation.

Drug Interactions:
- Increased bone marrow suppression if combined with other myelosuppressive drugs, or drugs interfering with blood clotting.

Lab Effects/Interference:
- Decreased WBC and neutrophil, platelet count, and Hgb/HCT.

Special Considerations:
- FDA indicated for the treatment of patients with relapsed or refractory low-grade, follicular, or transformed B-cell non-Hodgkin's lymphoma, including patients with refractory to rituximab.
- Agent has been shown to clear circulating lymphoma cells with the bcl-2 translocation (bcl-2 [t(14:18)]) (Murray et al, 2000) and predicted response to therapy (80% response rate if these cells were cleared from circulation vs. 20% if the cells were not cleared).
- After treatment, there is rapid reduction in malignant and normal B-cell lymphocytes, with circulating B-cells undetectable for the first 12 weeks, followed by recovery of normal B cells starting in the sixth month after therapy.
- Patient's own circulating antibodies stay within normal range after therapy.
- Rarely, patient may develop an antiantibody response (human antichimeric antibody/human antimouse antibody). Contraindicated in patients with al-

tered biodistribution of Indium-111 Zevalin, patients with ≥ 25% lymphoma marrow involvement or impaired bone marrow reserve.

- 2% incidence of development of secondary malignancy (acute myeloid leukemia, myelodysplastic syndrome). Radiation is a potent carcinogen and mutagen.

Potential Toxicities/Side Effects and the Nursing Process

I. POTENTIAL FOR INJURY related to ANAPHYLAXIS

Defining Characteristics: Rare but potentially life-threatening reaction may occur. Mouse antibodies are used that are foreign and may stimulate anaphylaxis. Rare, fatal anaphylactic reactions have occurred within 24 hours of rituximab dose. Of the reactions, 80% occur during the first rituximab infusion, and within 30–120 minutes of the infusion. Severe infusion reactions include pulmonary infiltrates, acute respiratory distress syndrome, myocardial infarction, ventricular fibrillation, and cardiogenic shock.

Nursing Implications: Assess baseline T, VS. Administer premedications prior to rituximab as ordered, usually acetaminophen and diphenhydramine. Initiate infusion at 50 mg/hr, and increase in 50mg/hr increments q 30 min to a maximum of 400 mg/hr. If patient develops discomfort, slow infusion; stop infusion if reaction is severe. Once symptoms have improved, resume rate at 50% of previous rate. Have emergency equipment and medications nearby, including epinephrine and corticosteroids. Assess patient for signs/symptoms, including generalized flushing andurticaria leading to pallor, cyanosis, bronchospasm, hypotension, unconsciousness. Teach patient to report signs/symptoms, including sense of doom, tickle in throat. If signs/symptoms occur, stop infusion immediately, assess VS, notify physician. Physician may prescribe epinephrine 0.3 mL (1:1000) SQ if hypotensive. Oxygen, antihistamines, corticosteroids may also be used.

II. POTENTIAL FOR INFECTION, BLEEDING, AND FATIGUE related to BONE MARROW SUPPRESSION

Defining Characteristics: Neutropenia common, with 77% incidence, and 25–32% of patients experiencing grade 4 neutropenia, with a median nadir of $900/mm^3$–$1100/mm^3$; Thrombocytopenia incidence 95% with median platelet nadir of $49{,}500/mm^3$; Anemia incidence 61% with median nadir for red blood cells 9.9 g/dL hemoglobin. Nadir occurred around 7–9 weeks after treatment, and duration of cytopenias was 22–35d. Chills and fever were common, affecting 27.5% and 21.6% of patients in one study. There appears to be increased hematologic toxicity in patients with bone marrow involvement by tumor, as expected. Rare fatal cerebral hemorrhage, severe infections.

Nursing Implications: Drug contraindicated in patients with > 25% bone marrow hypocellular bone marrow, or history of failed stem cell collection. Assess baseline CBC, platelet count, and monitor closely during and after therapy at least weekly for the first 12 weeks after treatment. Assess risk for increased hematological toxicity, e.g., whether bone marrow involvement by tumor. Teach patient that blood counts will fall and potential signs/symptoms of infection, bleeding, and fatigue. Teach patient self-care measures including self-assessment for signs/symptoms of infection, bleeding, and anemia; self-care strategies to minimize risk for infection (e.g., avoiding crowds, proximity to people with colds), bleeding (e.g., avoid aspirin-containing OTC medicines), and fatigue (e.g., alternating rest and activity periods), and what/where to report fever, bleeding, signs/symptoms of infection. Most studies show that few patients developed severe infections, and there were few if any deaths from treatment-related infections. Transfuse red blood cells and platelets as ordered.

III. ALTERATION IN COMFORT related to ASTHENIA, NAUSEA, ABDOMINAL PAIN, HEADACHE

Defining Characteristics: Asthenia commonly affects 21.6%, nausea (grades 1 or 2) 21.6%, and abdominal pain and headache 9.8%. Nausea, vomiting, diarrhea, increased cough, dizziness, arthralgia, anxiety may occur.

Nursing Implications: Assess baseline comfort and energy level. Teach patient that these side effects may occur, and strategies to manage them. If the symptom persists or is unresolved, teach patient to report it, and discuss with physician other management strategies.

IV. POTENTIAL FOR INJURY related to RADIATION EXPOSURE

Defining Characteristics: Y-90 Zevalin is a beta-emitter so that patients should protect others from exposure to their body secretions (saliva, stool, blood, urine).

Nursing Implications: Teach patient importance of specific radiation precautions, beginning at the start of treatment, and continuing for 1 week after treatment is completed: use condom during sexual intercourse, refrain from deep kissing; avoid transfer of body fluids; wash hands thoroughly after using the toilet, and continue effective contraception for 12 months following completion of treatment.

Drug: imatinib mesylate (Gleevec, STI 571)

Class: Protein tyrosine kinase inhibitor.

Mechanism of Action: Inhibits sending of message for cell division from abnormal tyrosine kinase encoded by the Philadelphia chromosome (BCR-ABL) in Chronic Myelocytic Leukemia (CML), thus preventing cell proliferation. Drug also inhibits receptor tyrosine kinases for platelet-derived growth factor (PDGF) and stem cell factor (SCF) and thus prevents their respective cell cycle stimulation. Inhibits c-Kit receptor tyrosine kinases as well, which has resulted in marked responses in GIST (gastrointestinal stromal tumors). 15–85% of GISTs have kit mutations; imatinib mesylate selectively inhibits this tyrosine kinase.

Metabolism: Well absorbed after oral administration with 98% bioavailability and Cmax in 2–4 hours after dosing. Elimination half-life of imatinib is 18 hours, and 40 hours for primary active metabolite N-desmethyl derivative. Drug is 95% protein bound. It is metabolized via CYP3A4 hepatic cytochrome P450 enzyme system, with 81% of the dose eliminated in 7 days, primarily via fecal route (68%) and, to a lesser degree, urinary (13%). 25% of drug dose is excreted unchanged in feces and urine.

Dosage/Range:

- 400 mg/da PO (single dose) for patients in chronic phase of CML.
- 600 mg/da PO (single dose) for patients in accelerated phase or blast crisis.
- Treatment continued as long as patient derives benefit from drug.
- If disease progression, failure of hematologic response after 3 months of treatment, or loss of a hematologic remission: increase dose to 600 mg/da (chronic CML), or to 800 mg/da given as 400 mg bid qd (accelerated or blast crisis) if no severe adverse drug reactions occur.
- GIST dosing: 400–600 mg/day.
- Peidatric dosing: 260 mg/m^2/day; if disease progression or no response in 3 months or no cytogenetic response in 6–12 months, or relapse: may increase to 340 mg/m^2/day if no severe drug reaction or treatment complication.

Drug Preparation/Administration:

- Available in hard gelatin 100-mg capsules or scored 100 mg tablets, in bottles of 120.
- Administer dose orally, once daily (unless the total dose is 800 mg, which is given as 400 mg bid), with a meal and a large glass of water.

Drug Interactions:

- CYP3A4 inhibitors (ketoconazole, itraconazole, erythropmycin, clarithromycin) may increase imatinib plasma concentrations; do not coadminister with ketoconazole.

- CYP3A4 substrates (simvastatin): imatinib decreases simvastatin metabolism with simvastatin serum levels increased 2–3.5 times. Use together cautiously, if at all.
- CYP3A4 inducers (dexamethasone, phenytoin, carbamazepine, rifampicin, Phenobarbital, St. John's Wort) may increase metabolism of imatinib so imatinib serum levels are reduced. Use together cautiously, if at all.
- Other CYP3A4 substrates (Cyclosporine, pimozide) increased plasma concentrations if co-administered with imatinib. Do not administer together because drug has a narrow therapeutic window.
- Other CYP3A4 substrates (Triazolo-benzadiazepines, dihydropyridine calcium channel blockers, HMG-CoA reductase inhibitors) may have increased serum levels when given together with imatinib. Use together cautiously, and monitor patient closely.
- Warfarin: Do not give together with imatinib because imatinib inhibits warfarin metabolism by CYP2C9 enzymes. Use low molecular heparin or standard heparin instead.

Lab Effects/Interference:
- Neutropenia, thrombocytopenia.
- Elevated hepatic transaminases (SGOT/AST, SGPT/ALT) and bilirubin.

Special Considerations:
- Imatinib mesylate is indicated for the treatment of patients with CML: 1) initial treatment of newly diagnosed patients with Ph+ chromosome CML, 2) patients in blast crisis, in accelerated phase, or in chronic phase after failure of interferon alpha therapy, 3) patients with metastatic and/or unresectable malignant gastrointestinal stromal tumor (GIST), 4) pediatric patients with chronic phase Ph+ CML recurring after stem cell transplant or resistant to interferon alpha.
- Clinical trials results were remarkable: Chronic phase (n > 500 patients): hematologic complete response (88%), complete cytogenic response (genetic correction) (30%); Accelerated phase (n = 235): hematologic (28%), complete cytogenic response (14%); Blast crisis: hematologic complete response (4%), cytogenic complete response (5%).
- Emerging evidence indicates that resistance can develop with reactivation of the BCR-ABL signal transduction, and, in some patients, an inverted duplicate Philadelphia chromosome with amplification of the BCR-ABL fusion gene occurs (Gorre et al, 2001).
- Drug is teratogeneic. Women should avoid pregnancy or breast-feeding while taking the drug.
- Drug often causes edema that may be serious in some patients. There is increased risk in patients at higher drug doses and in the elderly (> 65 years).
- Drug is associated with neutropenia and thrombocytopenia. Blood counts should be checked weekly for the first month, biweekly for the second

month, and then every 2–3 months as clinically indicated. Patients with accelerated phase CML or blast crisis require closer monitoring.

- Liver function tests (LFTs) should be monitored baseline and monthly or as clinically indicated. Drug should be stopped if bilirubin is increased to 3 times institutional upper limit of normal (IULN), or if liver transaminases is > 5 times IULN and held until these tests have returned to bilirubin < 1.5 times IULN or transaminase levels to < 2.5 times IULN. Drug should then be resumed at a reduced dose (400 mg dose reduced to 300 mg qd, and 600 mg dose reduced to 400 mg qd).
- Use cautiously in patients with liver impairment, and monitor liver function tests closely prior to and throughout treatment.
- Drug modifications for hematologic toxicity: *Chronic phase CML at initial dose of 400 mg/da or GIST at initial dose of 400–600 mg/da:* ANC $< 1000/mm^3$ and/or platelets $< 50,000/mm^3$: stop drug until ANC $\geq 1500/mm^3$ and/or platelets $> 75,000/mm^3$ and then resume at usual dose; if recurrence of ANC $< 1000/mm^3$, and/or platelets $< 50,000/mm^3$, hold until recovered, and reduce dose to 300 mg qd if initial dose 400 mg/da, and 400 mg/da if initial dose was 600 mg/da.
- *Accelerated phase and Blast Crisis:* ANC $< 500/mm^3$ and/or platelets $< 10,000/mm^3$: determine if related to leukemia by bone marrow aspirate/biopsy; if unrelated to leukemia, reduce dose to 400 mg qd; if cytopenia persists 2 weeks, reduce again to 300 mg qd; if cytopenia persists 4 weeks and is still unrelated to leukemia, stop imatinib until ANC $\geq 1000/mm^3$ and platelets $\geq 20/mm^3$, and then resume at 300 mg/da.

Potential Toxicities/Side Effects and the Nursing Process

I. POTENTIAL FOR INFECTION AND BLEEDING related to BONE MARROW DEPRESSION

Defining Characteristics: Neutropenia and thrombocytopenia were common, especially in patients who received higher doses, and in patients with advanced stages of disease (blast crisis and accelerated phase). Median duration of neutropenia was 2–3 weeks, and thrombocytopenia from 3–4 weeks. Dose needs to be held and reduced as noted in *Special Considerations*. Fever affected 14% (chronic phase) to 38% (accelerated phase) of patients. Hemorrhage (CNS and GI) was treated in 13% (chronic phase) to 48% (accelerated phase) of patients.

Nursing Implications: Assess baseline cbc, including wbc and differential and platelet count prior to dosing, as well as at least weekly during first month of treatment, at least every other week for the second month of treatment, and then as clinically indicated and ordered. Discuss dose interruption and reduction as above for neutropenia and thombocytopenia. Teach patient self-assessment of signs/symptoms of infection and bleeding (including epistaxis and development of petechiae), and instruct patient to report them right away. Teach patient self-care measures to minimize risk of infection and bleeding, including avoidance of OTC aspirin-containing medications.

II. ALTERATION IN FLUID AND ELECTROLYTE BALANCE related to FLUID RETENTION, EDEMA, AND HYPOKALEMIA

Defining Characteristics: Fluid retention is common (52% chronic phase and 67% accelerated phase patients), especially in the elderly, and primarily reflects periorbital and lower extremity edema. However, pleural effusions, ascites, rapid weight gain, and pulmonary edema may develop, and in some cases, be life-threatening (pleural effusion, congestive heart failure, renal failure, pericardial effusion, anasarca). Hypokalemia was reported to occur in 2–12% of patients.

Nursing Implications: Assess baseline parameters of weight, presence of edema, pulmonary function, and monitor closely during therapy. Teach patient to monitor weight daily at home, and to report weight gain of 2 pounds in one week, development of edema, or dyspnea. With physician, discuss drug interruption if fluid retention occurs, and the prescription of diuretics.

III. ALTERATION IN NUTRITION, POTENTIAL, LESS THAN BODY REQUIREMENTS, related to NAUSEA, VOMITING, DIARRHEA, HEPATOTOXICITY

Defining Characteristics: Nausea affected 68% of patients with accelerated phase, and 55% with chronic phase; vomiting affected 54% and 28%, respectively. Diarrhea affected 54%, while constipation affected 13%. Dyspepsia affected about 19%.

Nursing Implications: Teach patient to self-administer antiemetics one hour prior to each dose, and to call if nausea/vomiting develop. Discuss with physician more effective antiemetic regime if nausea/vomiting develop. Encourage small, frequent intake of cool, bland foods as tolerated if nausea develops. Refer to dietitian as needed for meal planning.

IV. ALTERATION IN COMFORT related to MUSCLE CRAMPS, MUSCULOSKELETAL PAIN, HEADACHE, FATIGUE, ARTHRALGIA, AND ABDOMINAL PAIN

Defining Characteristics: Muscle cramps are common, affecting 25–46% of patients. Musculoskeletal pain affects 27–37% of patients, headache 24–29% of patients, fatigue 33% of patients, and arthralgias 26% of patients. In clinical studies, abdominal pain affected 20% of patients with chronic phase, and 26% of patients in blast crisis.

Nursing Implications: Teach patient that these events may occur and to report them. Assess baseline comfort, and monitor closely during treatment. Develop plan to assure comfort depending on symptoms reported. Discuss ineffective strategies with physician, and revise plan as needed.

V. ALTERATION IN SKIN INTEGRITY, POTENTIAL, related to RASH

Defining Characteristics: Rash may occur. In clinical studies, 32% of patients with accelerated phase, and 36% of patients in chronic phase CML reported rash. 10% of patients complained of pruritis.

Nursing Implications: Teach patient that rash may occur and to report it. Assess patient skin integrity baseline and regularly during treatment. Teach patient local comfort measures. Discuss rash and management plan with physician, especially if severe.

Drug: lapatinib ditosylate (investigational)

Class: Tyrosine kinase inhibitor.

Mechanism of Action: Drug inhibits tyrosine kinases of both Human Epidermal growth factor Receptor (HER)-1 and HER-2-neu, leading to arrest of cell growth and/or apoptosis in tumor cells that depend upon ErbB1 and ErbB2 cell signaling. Normally, HER-2 dimerizes with other members of the HER family, including HER-1. The message is then sent repeatedly via the tyrosine kinases to the cell nucleus telling the cell to divide. In 20% of patients with breast cancer, HER-2-neu is overexpressed, leading to increased cell proliferation, invasiveness, and conferring a poor prognosis associated with reduced survival. By blockading the tyrosine kinases, the message for repeated cell division is halted.

Dosage/Range:
Per protocol. For example, 1500 mg PO qd.

Drug Preparation/Administration: Oral.

Drug Interactions: Unknown.

Lab Effects/Interference: Unknown.

Special Considerations:

- Drug is being studied in women with metastatic breast cancer who overexpress HER-2-neu, as well as patients with solid tumors, such as NSCLC and colorectal cancers.

Potential Toxicities/Side Effects and the Nursing Process

I. ALTERATION IN COMFORT related to RASH, FATIGUE

Defining Characteristics: Rash is usually mild to moderate. Rash and fatigue are common, with 5% of patients with advanced metastatic breast cancer reporting severe (grade 3) rash and fatigue.

Nursing Implications: Assess patient's baseline comfort, and teach that these symptoms may occur. Assess skin integrity baseline, and during therapy. Teach symptom management strategies to minimize discomfort. Teach patient to notify nurse or physician if fatigue or rash is severe, or does not resolve with local management. Interrupt or delay dose based on protocol.

II. ALTERATION IN NUTRITION, LESS THAN BODY REQUIREMENTS related to DIARRHEA, NAUSEA, VOMITING, ANOREXIA

Defining Characteristics: In patients with metatastic breast cancer studied, diarrhea occurred commonly and was severe (grade 3) in 10% of patients.

Nursing Implications: Assess baseline nutritional status, bowel elimination pattern, and appetite. Inform patient these side effects may occur. Teach self-administration of anti-nausea and anti-diarrheal medications according to protocol, and to notify provider if symptoms persists so dose can be interrupted per protocol. Teach patient dietary modification if nausea and vomiting or diarrhea occur, (e.g., for diarrhea, bananas, rice, applesauce, and toast) and to increase oral fluids to prevent dehydration. Consult dietitian to see patient for dietary counseling for anorexia.

Drug: lenalidomide (Revlimid, CC-5013, investigational)

Class: Immunomodulator with anti-angiogenesis properties.

Mechanism of Action: Drug induces G0/G1 growth arrest and apoptosis, increases expression of genes found on 5q locus including genes involved in cell adhesion. Inhibits COX-2 expression, stimulates T-cell proliferation, as well as the anti-inflammatory cytokines Interleukin-2, Interleukin-10, and Interferon-gamma. Decreases the secretion of proinflammatory cytokines that mediate cell growth and survival (TNF-α, Interleukin-1β, and Interleukin-6); stimulates host natural killer cell immunity (Bartlett et al, 2004).

Metabolism: Unknown.

Dosage/Range:
Per protocol.

Drug Preparation/Administration: Oral, per protocol; for example in multiple myeloma, 25 mg PO qd × 21 days, repeated q 28 days in combination with dexamethasone.

Drug Interactions:
- Bone marrow suppressive agents: additive bone marrow suppression.
- Additive anti-tumor effect when combined with dexamethasone in the treatment of multiple myeloma.

Lab Effects/Interference:

Special Considerations:
- Selectively designed to be more potent (10,000 times) and to have a different adverse event profile than thalidomide; drug is not teratogenic at similar doses, but has been found embryotoxic in animal studies.
- Drug has shown efficacy in treating patients with MDS who are have refractory anemia (5q31–33 chromosomal mutation), so that they achieved transfusion independence.
- Drug does not cause sleepiness, constipation, or peripheral neuropathy like thalidomide.
- Drug may cause tumor lysis syndrome in newly diagnosed multiple myeloma patients with large tumor burdens that lyse quickly when lenalidomide is given.
- Drug is being studied in the treatment of type-1 Complex Regional Pain Syndrome.
- In the treatment of patients with relapsed or refractory multiple myeloma, patients receiving lenalidomide plus dexamethasone had significantly longer TTP (40 to > 60 weeks vs about 20 weeks) and ORR (51.3% vs 22.9%) [Dimopoulous et al, 2004]; and more mature results reported by Fonseca et al (2005) showed a 61% RR compared to 24% with dexamethasone alone, and a 26% CR.
- Drug has hematologic activity in patients with low risk myelodysplastic syndromes who have no response to erythropoietin (List et al, 2005).

Potential Toxicities/Side Effects and the Nursing Process

I. POTENTIAL FOR INFECTION AND BLEEDING related to BONE MARROW SUPPRESSION

Defining Characteristics: Neutropenia occurs in 57% of patients, and thrombocytopenia in 58% of patients studied in multiple myeloma trials.

Nursing Implications: Assess baseline CBC, WBC, differential, and platelet count prior to chemotherapy, as well as signs/symptoms of infection or bleeding. Teach patient the signs/symptoms of infection or bleeding, and to report these immediately, and teach patient self-care measures to minimize risk of infection and bleeding. This includes avoidance of crowds, proximity to people with infections, and OTC aspirin-containing medications. Drug should be used in combination with another agent that does not cause bone marrow suppression, like bortezomib (Velcade) rather than chemotherapy.

II. ALTERATION IN COMFORT related to RASH, FATIGUE, LIGHT-HEADEDNESS AND LEG CRAMPS

Defining Characteristics: Mild rash, light-headedness have been reported, as have fatigue and leg cramps. Pruritis may be limited to the scalp and occur within 1 week of treatment.

Nursing Implications: Assess patient's baseline comfort, and teach patient that these symptoms may occur. Assess skin integrity baseline and during therapy. Teach symptom management strategies to minimize discomfort. Teach patient to notify nurse or physician if fatigue, rash, itching, or leg cramps are severe, or do not resolve with local management.

III. ALTERATION IN NUTRITION, LESS THAN BODY REQUIREMENTS, related to DIARRHEA

Defining Characteristics: In patients with MDS studied, diarrhea occurred in 21% of patients receiving prolonged treatment.

Nursing Implications: Assess baseline bowel elimination pattern, and inform patient diarrhea may occur. Teach self-administration of anti-diarrheals according to protocol, and to notify provider if diarrhea persists for dose interruption. Teach patient dietary modification if diarrhea occurs, (e.g., bananas, rice, applesauce, and toast) and to increase oral fluids to prevent dehydration.

Drug: neovastat (investigational)

Class: Angiogenesis inhibitor made from cartilaginous spine of dogfish shark.

Mechanism of Action: Appears to inhibit Vascular Endothelial Growth Factor (VEGD) signaling, to inhibit matrix metalloproteinases (MMPs), and to induce apoptosis (programmed cell death).

Dosage/Range:
- Per protocol.

Drug Preparation/Administration:
- Available orally in liquid form, taken bid, per protocol.

Drug Interactions:
- Unknown.

Lab Effects/Interference:

- Unknown.

Special Considerations:

- Differs from OTC shark cartilage, which is made primarily from shark fins.
- In a small study of patients with renal cell cancer, patients receiving a higher dose of neovastat survived 16.3 months compared to those receiving a lower dose whose survival was 7.1 months (Bukowski, 2001).
- Well tolerated without reported side effects.
- Clinical trials in patients with lung or ovarian cancer, multiple myeloma, with or without chemotherapy, are ongoing (NCI, others).

Potential Toxicities/Side Effects and Nursing Implications

I. KNOWLEDGE DEFICIT relating to LACK OF KNOWLEDGE, MEDIA MISINFORMATION

Defining Characteristics: Media about shark cartilage has been rife with misinformation, because there is no distinction between the cartilage-derived drug and that sold as an OTC miracle drug. Neovastat is made from shark spine cartilage, and the active substance is found in all animal cartilage. Shark is used because there is a high percentage of cartilage per body weight, and it is abundantly available. OTC shark cartilage is made from shark fins.

Nursing Implications: Assess basic understanding of drug and its mechanism of action, and explain how it differs from OTC shark cartilage. Teach the patient self-administration of the drug. Provide information, and answer questions. Ensure patient makes an informed consent prior to entering the study.

Drug: oblimersen sodium (Gentasense, G3139) (investigational)

Class: Antisense oligonucleotide.

Mechanism of Action: Downregulates Bcl-2 protein, which suppresses apoptosis, thus increasing sensitivity to programmed cell death. Increased levels of Bcl-2 protein are associated with resistance to chemotherapy and radiation, so Bcl-2 is also known as a multidrug-resistance protein. Oblimersen sodium, an antisense oligonucleotide, binds to the first 6 codons of the human Bcl-2 mRNA sequence, causing the degradation of Bcl-2 mRNA, and a reduction in Bcl-2 protein translation. This helps to re-establish apoptosis, or programmed cell death of the cell, and theoretically, sensitivity to chemotherapy or radiotherapy.

Metabolism: Rapidly metabolized in plasma and tissues. Steady state plasma concentratons of oblimersen achieved in 24–48 hours when given as a continuous infusion × 5 (IV)-14 (SQ) days. Plasma concentration directly related to dose. Plasma half-life is 2 hours and is dose independent. Drug excreted essentially unchanged by kidneys into urine.

Dosage/Range:
Per protocol. One study used 7 mg/kg IV continuous infusion daily × 5 days, with chemotherapy given on day 5.

Drug Preparation/Administration: Intravenous or subcutaneous continuous infusion for 5–14 days, given prior to or together with chemotherapy. Half-life of Bcl-2 protein is long. Maximal Bcl-2 protein downregulation reached at 5 days.

Drug Interactions: Synergy with chemotherapy.

Lab Effects/Interference: Unknown.

Special Considerations:
- Being studied in malignant melanoma, 1 chronic lymphocytic leukemia, multiple myeloma, colorectal cancer, small cell lung cancer.
- Toxicity related to Oblimersen sodium: fatigue, thrombocytopenia, pyrexia.
- Patients in study had toxicity from chemotherapy included in treatment as well as infectious complications of venous access devices (VADs).

Potential Toxicities/Side Effects and the Nursing Process

I. POTENTIAL FOR INFECTION AND BLEEDING related to NEUTROPENIA AND THROMBOCYTOPENIA

Defining Characteristics: Risk of neutropenia and thrombocytopenia is increased in combination with bone marrow suppressive chemotherapy.

Nursing Implications: Assess baseline blood counts and platelets. Teach patient to report fever, and signs/symptoms of infection or bleeding right away. Assess medication profile and OTC medications taken. Teach patient to avoid OTC medications containing NSAIDs or aspirin. Teach patient to talk to nurse or physician before beginning any OTC medications.

II. POTENTIAL ALTERATION IN COMFORT related to FATIGUE, PYREXIA

Defining Characteristics: Fatigue and pyrexia appeared to be increased in studies. However, there were also infectious complications of VADs.

Nursing Implications: Teach patient that fatigue and pyrexia may occur and to report pyrexia right away. Teach patient to alternate rest and activity periods, to plan shopping and chores so that it minimizes energy expenditure, and to explore whether family members can help with necessary chores. Teach patient measures to manage pyrexia: acetaminophen, tepid baths, increase oral fluids.

Drug: panitumumab (ABX-EGF) (investigational)

Class: Human monoclonal antibody targeted against epidermal growth factor receptor (EGFR).

Mechanism of Action: Blocks growth factor (ligand, such as epidermal growth factor and transforming growth factor-alpha) from binding to EGFR, thus preventing dimerization and initiation of cell signaling via receptor tyrosine kinase phosphorylation; thus, the message telling the cell to divide does not occur. In addition to cell growth inhibition, there is induction of apoptosis, and decreased matrix metalloproteinase and vascular endothelial growth factor production.

Metabolism: Unknown.

Dosage/Range:
Per protocol; 0.01–5.0 mg/kg IV q wk, 6.0 mg/kg q 2 weeks, and 9.0 mg/kg q 3 weeks are some dosages and frequencies being studied.

Drug Preparation/Administration: Per protocol; administered as IV infusion per protocol. Does not require premedication to prevent hypersensitivity reactions as drug is a human monoclonal antibody.

Drug Interactions: Unknown.

Lab Effects/Interference: Unknown.

Special Considerations:
- Tumors over-expressing epidermal growth factor receptors are colorectal, lung, breast, bladder, pancreas, kidney, head and neck cancers. Principal study is in patients with metasatic colorectal cancer.
- Drug exposure and tolerability similar between weekly, every-other-week, and every-three-week dosing schedules (Weiner LM, 2005).
- Rarely, a patient may develop an infusion reaction. During clinical trials, at least 1 patient developed rigors, dyspnea, wheezing on the day of the 2nd cycle of panitumumab infusion, effectively treated with meperidine, lorazepam, and diphenhydramine. The patient successfully received subsequent treatment with the same premedication (Malik et al, 2005).
- In patients studied, no patient developed HAHA formation (Malik et al, 2005).
- Theoretically, interstitial lung disease, a class effect, may occur; however, this was not seen in clinical trials.

Potential Toxicities/Side Effects and the Nursing Process

I. POTENTIAL ALTERATION IN BODY IMAGE, SKIN INTEGRITY, COMFORT related to SKIN RASH

Defining Characteristics: Drug inhibits epidermal growth factor receptor, so major toxicity is manifested in the skin with 95% of patients experiencing some type of skin toxicity. Most patients (80%, 3% of these grade 3) develop a mild-to-moderate acne-like rash that is self-limiting. 14% report a grade 3 rash, and in clinical studies 1% of patients discontinued treatment due to skin rash. Rash is a sterile, suppurative rash with multiple follicular or pustular lesions that appear during the first 2 weeks of therapy on the face, upper chest and back, but in some cases, extended to the arms. Rash resolves when treatment is stopped, without scar formation. Pruritis affects 34%, dry-skin 26%, acneiform dermatitis 16%, skin desqumation 13%, erythema 11%, paronychia 11%, macular rash 10%, skin fissures 6%, maculopapular rash 7%, popular rash 7%, exfoliative dermatitis 6%. Fissures can become infected; infection can be treated with topical clindamycin, or oral antibiotics. Do not use topical corticosteroid cream. Median time to first skin toxicity was 7 days, and median time to most severe skin toxicity was 12 days in clinical studies.

Nursing Implications: Teach patient that rash most likely will occur due to mechanism of drug action. Assess baseline skin integrity on areas of face, neck, and trunk; assess baseline comfort and satisfaction with body image, and monitor at each treatment. Teach patient to report any distress and assess extent of rash. Consult protocol for drug holiday (e.g., drug may be held for 1–2 weeks for severe rash, and if it resolves, dose reduced on and after the 2nd occurrence. If rash does not resolve, drug may be stopped). If skin appears to be infected, discuss with physician, the prescription of clindamycin gel (Cleocin T) or oral cephalexin (Keflex) 250 mg PO bid × 3 days, then 250 mg qd × 7 days, for a total of 10 days for skin infection. Rash is not acne, and so usual anti-acne treatment will not be effective.

II. ALTERATION IN NUTRITION, LESS THAN BODY REQUIREMENTS, related to NAUSEA, VOMITING, DIARRHEA, STOMATITIS, CONSTIPATION, ANOREXIA, ABDOMINAL PAIN

Defining Characteristics: Incidence of mild-to-moderate digestive symptoms include nausea (39%), diarrhea (36%), abdominal pain (30%), anorexia (27%), vomiting (27%), constipation (25%), stomatitits (18%) in patients on clinical trials.

Nursing Implications: Assess baseline weight and nutritional status. Inform patient that these symptoms may occur, and to report them. Administer antiemetic and other symptom management medications as ordered. Teach patient self-administration of these medications at home. Teach patient dietary modifications to address symptoms such as anorexia (small, frequent high-calorie, high-protein foods, stimulants as permitted by protocol); constipation (high-fiber, high-fluid, high-roughage foods, stool softeners); diarrhea (bananas, rice, applesauce, and toast); nausea (avoid food preparation odors by cooking in zipped plastic bag, or having someone else cook; choose cool, soft, non-spicy, or fatty foods). Teach patient to report any symptoms that do not resolve or improve on the plan. Assess efficacy of intervention, and revise plan as needed.

III. POTENTIAL FOR ALTERATION IN COMFORT related to FATIGUE, DYSPNEA, PERIPHERAL EDEMA, PYREXIA, ARTHRALGIA

Defining Characteristics: In clinical trials, the following symptoms were reported in patients with advanced colorectal cancer: fatigue (51%), cough (18%), dyspnea (14%), peripheral edema (14%), pyrexia (14%), arthralgia (14%), back pain (12%), headache (12%), dizziness (11%), insomnia (11%).

Nursing Implications: Assess patient comfort level, self-care measures baseline and periodically during therapy. Teach patient that these symptoms may arise, either from the drug and/or the treatment. Develop a plan for symptom management, assess efficacy and revise as needed. Assess level of fatigue and teach energy baseline and prior to each treatment. Inform patient that fatigue may occur due to anemia, and teach energy conserving strategies such as alternating restand activity periods.

Drug: pertuzumab (Omnitarg, rhuMab 2C4) (investigational)

Class: First of a new class called Human Epidermal (Growth Factor) Receptor dimerization inhibitors (HDI). Multiple targeted Tyrosine kinase inhibitor, anti-angiogenesis agent.

Mechanism of Action: In order for a growth signal to be sent to the cell nucleus, a growth factor (ligand) attaches to the Human Epidermal Growth Factor Receptor, or HER. The growth factor receptor now needs to dimerize or pair with another growth factor receptor, e.g., HER-2 receptor needs to dimerize or pair with another HER receptor, such as HER-1. Pertuzumab binds to the dimerization domain of HER so the binding of the antibody directly inhibits the ability of HER-2 to dimerize with other HER (EGFR) proteins. This disrupts the activation of downstream effectors so that the growth signal is not sent, notably the AKT pathway (cell survival). Drug is a recombinant, humanized monoclonal antibody.

Metabolism: Unknown.

Dosage/Range:
Per protocol; studies have included doses 0.5–15mg/kg q 3 wk.

Drug Preparation/Administration: Per protocol; IV infusion.

Drug Interactions: Unknown.

Lab Effects/Interference: Unknown.

Special Considerations:

- Drug is being investigated in prostate, NSCLC, metastatc breast, ovarian cancers, but may need to be given with chemotherapy to improve response.
- Drug is targeted against tumors that do not over-express HER-2.
- Side effects varied according to patient population with diarrhea and rash most common in prostate cancer patients studied, and diarrhea, fatigue, nausea, vomiting, and uncommon drop in LVEF in patients with metastatic breast cancer who previously had received anthracyclines (Cortes et al, 2005).

Potential Toxicities/Side Effects and the Nursing Process

I. POTENTIAL ALTERATION IN NUTRITION related to DIARRHEA, NAUSEA, VOMITING

Defining Characteristics: Diarrhea was most common affecting about 50–59% of patients, and ranging in severity from grade 1–3; nausea and vomiting affected patients with metasttic breast cancer, affecting 32% and 23% of women respectively.

Nursing Implications: Assess bowel elimination patterns and nutritional status baseline prior to each treatment. Teach patient to take anti-diarrheal medication per protocol. Administer anti-emetics prior to drug administration per protocol, and teach patient to self-administer anti-emetics as permitted on protocol. Teach patient to report any symptoms that do not resolve or improve with the established plan

II. ACTIVITY INTOLERANCE, POTENTIAL, related to FATIGUE

Defining Characteristics: Fatigue occurs commonly in patients with advanced cancer who were studied.

Nursing Implications: Assess baseline activity and energy level, and teach patient that this symptom may occur. Assess patient's activity patterns, and suggest ways to conserve energy.

Drug: rituximab (Rituxan)

Class: Monoclonal antibody (anti-CD_{20} antibody).

Mechanism of Action: Anti-CD_{20} antibody that is genetically engineered (chimeric monoclonal antibody, or part mouse part human) directed against the CD_{20} antigen found on the surface of normal and malignant B-cell lymphocytes. The CD_{20} antigen is also present (expressed) on more than 90% of B-cell non-Hodgkin's lymphoma (NHL) cells, but fortunately is not found on normal bone marrow stem cells, pre-B cells, or other normal tissues. A section of the rituximab (Fab domain) CD_{20} binds to the CD_{20} antigen on B lymphocytes; another section of the rituximab (Fc domain) calls together other immune effectors, resulting in lysis of the B lymphocyte.

Metabolism: Serum and half-life of drug varies with dose and sequence, and at 375 mg/m^2, the median serum half-life was 76.3 hours after the first infusion, as compared to 205 hours after the fourth infusion. Drug was detected in patient serum up to 3–6 months after completion of treatment.

Dosage/Range:
- 375 mg/m^2 given as IV infusion weekly for × 4 weeks or 8 doses.

Drug Preparation/Administration:
- Do not mix with or dilute with other drugs.
- Store at 2–8°C (36–46°F) and protect vials from direct sunlight.
- Available as 100-mg (10-mL) and 500-mg (50-mL) single-use vials.
- Add ordered dose to 0.9% Sodium Chloride USP or 5% Dextrose, resulting in a final concentration of 1–4 mg/mL; gently invert to mix, and inspect for presence of any particulate matter or discoloration.
- Drug is stable in infusion solution at 2–8°C (36–46°F) for 24 hours, and at room temperature for another 24 hours.
- Must not be given IVB due to risk of hypersensitivity or infusion reactions.
- First infusion: initial infusion rate should be 50 mg/hr; if no hypersensitivity or infusion-related problems occur, increase the infusion rate in 50 mg/hr increments every 30 minutes to a maximum of 400 mg/hr. If infusion or hypersensitivity problems occur, slow or stop the infusion depending on severity. May continue the infusion at half the previous rate once symptoms resolve.
- Second, third, fourth infusions: administer at initial rate of 100 mg/hr, and increase by 100 mg/hr increments every 30 minutes, to a maximum of 400 mg/hr as tolerated.

Drug Interactions:
- None known.

Lab Effects/Interference:

- Decreased lymphocyte count (B cells); decreased IgM and IgG serum levels.

Special Considerations:

- Drug is indicated for the treatment of patients with low-grade or follicular, CD_{20}-positive, B-cell non-Hodgkin's lymphoma who have relapsed or who are refractory to standard therapy, and as initial therapy for patients with bulky disease.
- Severe mucocutaneous reactions may occur, resulting in death. Drug should be stopped if a reaction develops and a skin biopsy performed.
- Contraindicated in patients with known Type 1 hypersensitivity or anaphylactic reactions to murine proteins or product components.
- Infusion reactions common (fever, chills) during the first infusion. Hypotension, bronchospasm, and angioedema may occur. STOP infusion for severe reactions, and manage symptoms with diphenhydramine and acetaminophen, and additional treatment with bronchodilators, epinephrine, or IV saline as indicated. Infusion may be resumed at 50% of the previous rate once symptoms have resolved.
- Emergency medications should be readily available: epinephrine, antihistamines, and corticosteroids.
- STOP infusion if serious cardiac arrhythmias develop; patient should receive cardiac monitoring during and after subsequent infusions of the drug. Patients with a history of arrhythmias and angina should be cardiac monitored during infusion and immediately post-infusion for evidence of recurrence of these problems.
- Monitor CBC, platelet count regularly during therapy.
- Possibility of developing antibodies to the human antimurine (HAMA) and human antichimeric (HACA) exists, and may be as low as 1% incidence; these individuals are at risk for developing allergic/hypersensitivity reactions when treated with rituximab or other MoAbs (murine or chimeric).
- Birth control practices during and for 12 months following therapy should be used by individuals of childbearing potential.
- Women should not breast-feed infants while drug is detectable in the serum.

Potential Toxicities/Side Effects and the Nursing Process

I. POTENTIAL FOR INJURY related to INFUSION-RELATED REACTIONS AND HYPERSENSITIVITY

Defining Characteristics: Infusion-related reactions occurred within 30 minutes to 2 hours of the beginning of the first infusion, and occurred in 80% of patients receiving a first infusion (7% severe), as opposed to 40% of patients (5–10% severe) receiving subsequent infusions. Fever and chills/rigors affect most patients during the initial infusion. Other infusion-related symptoms include: nausea (18%); urticaria (8%); fatigue; headache (14%); pruritus (10%); bronchospasm (8%); dyspnea; sensation of swelling of tongue, throat (13%); hypotension (10%); flushing; and pain at disease site. Infusion-related reactions generally resolve with slowing or interrupting the drug infusion, and/or symptomatic treatment (IV saline, acetaminophen, diphenhydramine). Premedications often reduce the severity and/or occurrence of these reactions. In patients who receive retreatment after having completed at least one course of drug therapy, reactions that occur commonly are: asthenia, throat irritation, flushing, tachycardia, dizziness, respiratory symptoms, pruritus. The incidence of severe hypotension and dyspnea is higher in patients with bulky tumors > 10 cm.

Nursing Implications: Discuss with physician the use of premedications such as acetaminophen and diphenhydramine before drug therapy. Ensure that medications necessary for the management of hypersensitivity/anaphylaxis are readily available (e.g., epinephrine, antihistamines, corticosteroids). Assess baseline VS and monitor frequently during the infusion. Follow infusion rate guide (see Drug Administration section) for first and subsequent infusions. Slow or stop the infusion if severe infusion-related reactions occur. Monitor VS, and notify physician. Be prepared to provide emergency support as necessary (including IV saline, epinephrine, antihistamines, bronchodilators). If/when symptoms resolve, resume the infusion at 50% of the rate of the previous infusion, as directed by the physician.

II. ALTERATION IN ELIMINATION, RENAL, related to TUMOR LYSIS SYNDROME

Defining Characteristics: Patients with high tumor burden receiving rituximab for the first time are at risk for rapid tumor lysis. Tumor lysis syndrome (TLS) occurs as a result of rapid release of intracellular contents into the bloodstream. The risk of TLS appears higher in patients with a high number of circulating lymphocytes, e.g., > 25,000/mm^3.

Nursing Implications: For first infusion, expect patient orders to include: Hydration at 150 mL/hr with or without alkalinization, oral allopurinol, strict monitoring of I/O, daily weight and body balance determination. Monitor baseline and daily BUN, creatinine, K+, phosphorus, uric acid, and calcium. Monitor for renal, cardiac, neuromuscular signs/symptoms hyperkalemia, hyperphosphatemia, hypomagnesemia, hypocalcemia, and elevated uric acid.

III. POTENTIAL FOR INFECTION related to LYMPHOPENIA AND BONE MARROW DEPRESSION

Defining Characteristics: B-cell lymphocytes are reduced in 70–80% of patients, together with a decrease in immunoglobulins in some patients. Bacterial infections that occurred in these patients were not associated with neutropenia, and 9% were severe, involving sepsis due to *Listeria, Staphylococcus*, and polymicrobials; posttreatment infections included rare sepsis, and viral infections (herpes simplex and herpes zoster). Leukopenia occurs in 11% of patients, thrombocytopenia 8%, and neutropenia 7%. Serious bone marrow suppression was uncommon and may occur up to 30 days following treatment. These include severe neutropenia (1.9%), thrombocytopenia (1.3%), and severe anemia (1%). Rarely, transient aplastic anemia or hemolytic anemia may occur. Incidence of neutropenia, thrombocytopenia, anemia, and chest pain was higher, as was the severity, in patients with bulky tumors > 10 cm.

Nursing Implications: Monitor CBC, platelets baseline and regularly during treatment. If the patient develops cytopenia, monitor more frequently. Assess for signs/symptoms of infection, bleeding, fatigue, and chest pain prior to each treatment. Teach patient to self-assess for these, including taking temperature, and instruct to report them immediately. Transfuse red cells and platelets as ordered.

IV. LOSS OF SKIN INTEGRITY, POTENTIAL, related to SEVERE MUCOCUTANEOUS REACTIONS

Defining Characteristics: Severe skin reactions have rarely occurred and, in some cases, ended in death of patient. Skin abnormalities include paraneoplastic pemphigus (uncommon autoimmune disorder, may be related to underlying malignancy), Stevens-Johnson syndrome (may be caused by HSV or other infectious disorder), lichenoid dermatitis, vesiculobullous dermatitis, and toxic epidermal necrolysis. Onset is 1–13 weeks following rituximab exposure.

Nursing Implications: Assess baseline skin and mucous membrane integrity. Teach patient that rarely skin and mucous membrane reactions may occur, and to report any changes right away. Manufacturer recommends stopping rituximab therapy and obtaining skin biopsy to determine cause. Discuss with physician. Teach patient local care strategies depending upon symptoms.

V. ALTERATION IN COMFORT related to ASTHENIA, HEADACHE, NAUSEA, VOMITING, PRURITUS, MYALGIA, AND DIZZINESS

Defining Characteristics: Asthenia occurs in approximately 16% of patients, while headache (14%), nausea (18%), pruritus (10%), vomiting (7%), myalgia (7%), and dizziness (7%) may also occur.

Nursing Implications: Assess baseline comfort prior to each infusion, and tolerance of past infusion. Discuss strategies to manage symptoms. If symptoms are severe, discuss management with physician.

Drug: Sorafenib (BAY 43-9006) (investigational)

Class: Multiple targeted Tyrosine kinase inhibitor, anti-angiogenesis agent.

Mechanism of Action: Drug inhibits a number of tyrosine kinases, including Raf kinase, an enzyme in the RAS pathway (RAS is mutated in about 20–30% of solid tumors), as well as receptor tyrosine kinases VEGFR-2 and PDGFR-β, thus preventing cell proliferation and angiogenesis. First, sorafenib inhibits the signaling cascade in the RAS pathway, blocking uncontrolled cell growth from either excessive stimulation of the RAS pathway, or through mutations of RAS and RAF proteins. In addition, sorafenib inhibits angiogenesis by preventing the message from Vascular Endothelial Growth Factor (VEGF), telling endothelial cells to proliferate and migrate, from reaching the cell nucleus (signal transduction) and angiogenesis is prevented. It also inhibits the message that would be sent to the cell nucleus when the ligand Platelet Derived Growth Factor (PDGF) attaches to it's receptor PDGFR-β; PDGF is necessary for pericytes around the blood vessels to provide external structure during angiogenesis, and when they are not available, angiogenesis is stopped (Onyx, 2005).

Metabolism: Unknown.

Dosage/Range:
Per protocol, varies with other chemotherapy agents administered in combination.

Drug Preparation/Administration: None, oral.

Drug Interactions: Unknown.

Lab Effects/Interference: Unknown.

Special Considerations:
- Drug is being studied in Phase III clinical trials of patients with clear cell metastatic renal cell cancer, as well as patients with malignant melanoma in combination with chemotherapy.
- Drug is well tolerated with principal side effects being hypertension (11% vs 1% placebo), rash (34% vs 13%), hand-foot syndrome (27% vs 5%) and diarrhea (33% vs 10%).
- In patients with malignant melanoma, a specific RAS kinase. BRAF, is mutated in 66% of patients and some patients with colorectal cancer (Onyx Pharmaceuticals, 2005).

Potential Toxicities/Side Effects and the Nursing Process

I. POTENTIAL ALTERATION IN CIRCULATION related to HYPERTENSION

Defining Characteristics: Hypertension occurred in 11% of renal cell cancer patients being studied, compared to 1% receiving placebo.

Nursing Implications: Assess baseline blood pressure, and monitor prior to each treatment cycle. Discuss persistent elevations with physician, and consult protocol.

II. ALTERATION IN SKIN INTEGRITY AND COMFORT related to HAND-FOOT SYNDROME, RASH, POTENTIAL

Defining Characteristics: In renal cell cancer patients being studied, rash occurred in 34% of patients, and hand-foot syndrome in 27% of patients compared to 13% and 5% of patients, respectively, receiving placebo.

Nursing Implications: Assess baseline skin integrity, including soles of feet and palms of hands, and teach patient that these symptoms may occur. Teach patient to self assess all skin areas, and to report rash, as well as redness, swelling, and/or pain anywhere, particularly the soles of feet and palms of hands. Teach patient to avoid activities that increase blood flow in the hands and feet, such as hot showers and baths, and to take tepid showers to reduce likelihood and severity of hand-foot syndrome. Teach patient to avoid constrictive clothing and repetitive movements that can irritate the opposing skin. Teach patient to use skin emollients to prevent skin from drying and cracking.

Drug: sunitinib malate (Sutent, U-11248) (investigational)

Class: Multi-targeted tyrosine kinase inhibitor.

Mechanism of Action: Drug has both anti-tumor and anti-angiogenesis activity. When a growth factor or ligand binds to the receptor on the outside of the cell, it sends a message to the cell nucleus telling the cell to proliferate, make new blood vessels (angiogenesis, by releasing VEGF) and to ignore programmed cell death signals (apoptosis). Protein tyrosine kinases are inside the cell membrane, and then receive the message from outside the cell and send it down through a process called phosphorylation, to the nucleus via multiple signaling pathways, called signal transduction. Sunitinib malate blocks multiple tyrosine kinases, thus preventing the message from getting to the nucleus of the cell via blockage of multiple signaling pathways, and preventing cell division, the formation of new blood vessels, and permitting programmed cell death. The receptor tyrosine kinases blocked are platelet derived growth factor receptor (PDGFR α and β), Vascular endothelial growth factor receptor (VEGFR 1,2,3), c-KIT, and Flt-3 in GastroIntestinal Stomal Tumor (GIST) and VEGF and PDGF pathways in renal cell cancer.

Metabolism: Unknown.

Dosage/Range:
50mg PO qd in 6 week cycles per protocol. Dose reduced for grade 3 and 4 toxicities.

Drug Preparation/Administration: None, oral tablet.

Drug Interactions: Unknown at this time.

Lab Effects/Interference:
- Decreased lymphocyte, neutrophil, red blood cell, and platelet counts; elevated serum lipase and amylase.

Special Considerations:
- Most active in the treatment of Gastrointestinal stromal tumors (GIST) that were refractory to imatinib (Gleevec) and renal cell cancer.
- Hypertension affected 5–14% of patients on clinical trials.

Potential Toxicities/Side Effects and the Nursing Process

I. POTENTIAL FOR INFECTION AND BLEEDING related to NEUTROPENIA AND THROMBOCYTOPENIA

Defining Characteristics: Neutropenia occurred in 39–45% of patients, anemia 25-37% of patients, and thrombocytopenia 18–19% of patients in clinical trials.

Nursing Implications: Assess baseline blood counts and platelets. Teach patient to report fever, and signs/symptoms of infection or bleeding right away. Assess medication profile and OTC medications taken. Teach patient to avoid OTC medications containing NSAIDs or aspirin. Teach patient to talk to nurse or physician before beginning any OTC medications.

II. POTENTIAL ACTIVITY INTOLERANCE related to FATIGUE, DIZZINESS

Defining Characteristics: Fatigue occurred in 22–38% of patients in clinical trials.

Nursing Implications: Teach patient that fatigue may occur and self-care measures. Teach patient to alternate rest and activity periods, to plan shopping and chores to minimize energy expenditure, and to explore whether family members can help with necessary chores.

III. ALTERATION IN NUTRITION, LESS THAN BODY REQUIREMENTS, related to NAUSEA, STOMATITIS, DIARRHEA, ELEVATED AMYLASE AND LIPASE LEVELS

Defining Characteristics: Diarrhea occurred in 16–24% of patients, nausea in 13–19% of patients, and stomatitis in 14–19%, hyperamylasemia in 8-10% (renal cell cancer), and hyperlipasemia in 24–28% (renal cell cancer) of patients in clinical studies.

Nursing Implications: Assess baseline nutritional status, bowel elimination patterns, integrity of oral mucosa, and lipase and amylase function studies regularly during treatment. Teach patient self-administration of anti-diarrheal medications and to report if ineffective. Teach patient self-administration of antiemetics prior to administration of drug. Teach patient to report persistent or continued nausea and/or vomiting. Assess efficacy and discuss change in antiemetic drug with physician if regimen ineffective. Teach patient to assess oral mucosa regularly, use oral hygiene regimen, and report signs/symptoms of stomatitis. If patient develops stomatitis, teach patient self-administration of oral analgesics, antifungals, as ordered and appropriate. Monitor amylase and lipase tests in patients with renal cell cancer, and discuss any abnormalities with physician.

IV. ALTERATION IN SKIN INTEGRITY, POTENTIAL, related to DERMATITIS

Defining Characteristics: In clinical studies, 5–11% of patients complained of dermatologic problems, including skin discoloration and hand-foot syndrome in patients with GIST.

Nursing Implications: Assess patient skin integrity baseline and regularly during treatment. Teach patient local comfort measures. Teach patient to report skin changes and if self-care ineffective, discuss plan with physician, especially if severe.

Drug: suberoylanilide hydroxamic acid (SAHA)

Class: Histone deacetylase (HDAC) inhibitor.

Mechanism of Action: Histone deacetylases work with other regulatory proteins to modulate gene expression (transcriptional activity). By inhibiting selected gene expression of genes involved in cancer, histone deacetylase inhibitors are able to block angiogenesis and cell cycling, and promote apoptosis and differentiation. Drug is cytostatic.

Metabolism: Excellent bioavailability; metabolism unknown.

Dosage/Range:
Per protocol.

Drug Preparation/Administration: Per protocol, administered orally (breast, lung cancers) and intravenously (prostate, breast, colon cancers).

Drug Interactions: Unknown.

Lab Effects/Interference: Unknown.

Special Considerations:

- In Phase I and II clinical trials, SAHA causes accumulation of acetylated histones in peripheral blood mononuclear cells as well as tumor cells, so is being studied in hematologic and solid tumors.
- Synergistic with radiation, tyrosine kinase inhibitors (imatinib), chemotherapy (5-FU), differentiating agents (ATRA).
- As a single agent, demonstrated antitumor activity in cutaneous T-cell lymphoma, diffuse B-cell lymphoma, laryngeal cancer, and mesothelioma.
- Side effects occur after several weeks or months of therapy, and following a drug holiday, drug can be resumed.

Potential Toxicities/Side Effects and the Nursing Process

I. POTENTIAL FOR BLEEDING AND FATIGUE related to BONE MARROW DEPRESSION

Defining Characteristics: In clinical trials, fatigue, anemia and thrombocytopenia were reversible.

Nursing Implications: Monitor CBC, platelet count baseline and periodically during therapy per protocol. Assess for signs and symptoms of bleeding, fatigue, and anemia. Teach patient to self-assess for signs and symptoms of bleeding, anemia, and to call if they occur. Assess patient medication profile, and any OTC medications such as contain aspirin or NSAIDs that would increase risk of bleeding. Teach patient to avoid these drugs, and not to begin any OTC medications without first discussing with nurse or physician. Teach patient to alternate rest and activity periods if feeling fatigued; to organize shopping and chores in a way to minimize energy expenditures.

II. ALTERATION IN NUTRITION, LESS THAN BODY REQUIREMENTS related to DEHYDRATION AND ANOREXIA

Defining Characteristics: In clinical trials, anorexia and dehydration occurred, and were reversible following drug holiday.

Nursing Implications: Assess weight, and baseline nutritional status. Teach patient that anorexia and dehydration can occur, and ways to minimize this effect. Teach patient to identify nutritionally-dense (high calories and protein in the smallest amount) foods and to keep them handy in the refrigerator. Teach patient to eat small, frequent meals and to have a bedtime snack. Teach patient to drink a glass of fluid every hour while awake if patient is at risk for developing dehydration (elderly, forgetful).

Drug: temsirolimus (CCI-779) (investigational)

Class: Protein Kinase Inhibitor.

Mechanism of Action: Drug binds to the immunophilin FKBP and inhibits mTOR (mammalian Target of Rapamycin or FKBP 12) kinase. mTOR is responsible for sensing the nutrients in the cell's environment, and also for organizing actin, trafficking of the membrane, insulin secretion, protein degradation, protein kinase C signaling, and tRNA synthesis. Inhibition of the kinase makes the cell think it is starving and it stops growing (arrests cell growth in G1 phase of the cell cycle). As more is learned about the function of this pathway, it appears that rapamycin and mTOR inhibitors affect only some of mTOR functioning.

Metabolism: Unknown.

Dosage/Range:
Per protocol, but have ranged from 25–250 mg IV weekly; dose reduction for neutropenia, thrombocytopenia, and mucositis.

Drug Preparation/Administration: IV infusion over 30 minutes; premedication with diphenhydraminde 25–50 mg 30 minutes before drug administration. If hypersensitivity occurs, an H2-receptor antagonist is given 30 minutes prior to resuming drug administration.

Drug Interactions: Unknown.

Lab Effects/Interference: Hyperglycemia, hypertriglyceridemia, hypophospatemia; elevated GGT levels; rare neutropenia, thrombocytopenia, anemia.

Special Considerations:
- Drug is well tolerated with most common toxicities: maculopapular rash (76%), mucositis (70%), asthenia (50%) and nausea (43%) when studied in patients with advanced refractory renal cell carcinoma (Atkins et al, 2004); depression is a significant toxicity when the dose of 250 mg IV is used (Chen et al, 2005).
- Drug has shown anti-tumor activity in patients with advanced renal cell and advanced breast cancer. In the treatment of gliobolastoma multiforme, the drug is called a ''smart drug,'' because it targets molecular changes in the malignant cell related to its unfortunate aggressiveness (Galanis et al, 2005).

Potential Toxicities/Side Effects and the Nursing Process

I. POTENTIAL FOR INJURY related to INFUSION-RELATED REACTIONS AND HYPERSENSITIVITY

Defining Characteristics: The incidence of hypersensitivity was uncommon, as most patients received premedicaton with diphenhydramine (Chan et al, 2005).

Nursing Implications: Consult protocol. Discuss with physician the use of premedications such as diphenhydramine before drug therapy. In one study, patients who developed hypersensitivity despite diphenhudramine, the addition of an H2 antagonist 30 minutes prior to resuming the infusion prevented further hypersensitivity. Ensure that medications necessary for the management of hypersensitivity/anaphylaxis are readily available (e.g., epinephrine, antihistamines, corticosteroids). Assess baseline VS and monitor frequently during the infusion, as specified by the infusion. Be prepared to provide emergency support as necessary (including IV saline, epinephrine, antihistamines, bronchodilators). If/when symptoms resolve, resume the infusion at 50% of the rate of the previous infusion, as directed by the physician.

II. POTENTIAL FOR INFECTION AND BLEEDING related to NEUTROPENIA AND THROMBOCYTOPENIA

Defining Characteristics: Although rare, Grade 3 or 4 neutropenia occurred in 7% of patients, thrombocytopenia in 5%, and anemia in 9% of patients in clinical trials comparing doses 75–250 mg weekly.

Nursing Implications: Assess baseline blood counts and platelets. Teach patient to report fever, and signs/symptoms of infection or bleeding right away. Assess medication profile and OTC medications taken. Teach patient to avoid OTC medications containing NSAIDs or aspirin. Teach patient to talk to nurse or physician before beginning any OTC medications.

III. ALTERATION IN SKIN INTEGRITY, POTENTIAL, related to RASH

Defining Characteristics: Maculopapular rash is the most common toxicity, affecting between 51–76%; 33% had acne, 31% had a nail disorder, 19% had dry skin.

Nursing Implications: Assess patient skin integrity, including nails baseline and regularly during treatment. Teach patient self-assessment and local comfort measures. Teach patient to report skin changes and if self-care ineffective, discuss plan with physician, especially if severe.

IV. POTENTIAL ALTERATION IN NUTRITION, LESS THAN BODY REQUIREMENTS, related to MUCOSITIS, NAUSEA, ANOREXIA, DIARRHEA, HYPERGLYCEMIA, HYPERTRIGLYCERIDEMIA

Defining Characteristics: In clinical studies, mucositis affected 70% of patients, nausea 43%, diarrhea 27%, and anorexia 40% of patients; in terms of grade 3 and 4 toxicities, hyperglycemia occurred in 17% of patients, hypophosphatemia 13%, and hypertriglyceridemia in 6% of patients. mTOR is involved in insulin signaling, which possibly explains the hypertriglyceridemia and hypoglycemia.

Nursing Implications: Premedicate with antiemetics per protocol. Encourage small, frequent meals of cool, bland foods, and increase fluid intake. Assess oral mucosa prior to drug administration and instruct patient to report changes. Teach patient oral hygiene measures and self-assessment. Monitor glucose, triglyceride and phosphate serum levels baseline and during therapy per protocol. Notify physician of any abnormalities and discuss implications and management per protocol.

V. ALTERATION IN COMFORT AND ACTIVITY TOLERANCE, POTENTIAL, related to ASTHENIA, SOMNOLENCE AND DEPRESSION

Defining Characteristics: Asthenia affects 50% of patients in clinical studies, depression 17%, but at the higher dose of 250 mg q week, 5% had grade 3 and 4 depression; somnolence 30%, with 6% grade 3 and 4.

Nursing Implications: Assess baseline comfort, mental status, and activity tolerance, and reassess during treatment, asking patient to identify what activities now unable to do, sleep habits, and also feeling state. Discuss alternating rest and activity periods, and also possibility of other family members or friends assisting with energy consuming responsibilities to increase energy reserve. Assess baseline alertness, sleep patterns. Assess other drugs taken, especially those with sedating qualities, and alcohol ingestion. Instruct patient to avoid alcohol and to take drug at bedtime. Assess degree of drowsiness and dizziness for safety of patient. If significant, teach measures to ensure safety.

Drug: thalidomide (investigational)

Class: Inhibitor of TNF-alpha, antiangiogenesis agent.

Mechanism of Action: Drug exerts its immunomodulatory action in an unknown way. Hypothesized that drug may modulate VEGF (vascular epithelial growth factor) by inhibiting neovasculature and thus have an antiangiogenesis effect in malignant tumors.

Metabolism: Well absorbed after oral administration. Mean peak serum level reached at 4–5 hours. Elimination half-life is 4–12 hours, with drug found in the plasma after 24 hours. NOT metabolized using P450 hepatic enzyme system, and has low renal excretion.

Dosage/Range:

- Per protocol.
- Advanced multiple myeloma after relapse (after high-dose chemotherapy): begin dose of 200 mg PO qd, increase dose by 200 mg every 2 weeks up to 800 mg PO qd.

Drug Preparation/Administration:

- Oral, give at bedtime.
- Available for investigational or compassionate use in 50–mg capsules.

Drug Interactions:

- Barbiturates, alcohol, chlorpromazine, reserpine: increased sedation.

Lab Effects/Interference:

- Rare neutropenia.

Special Considerations:

- ABSOLUTE CONTRAINDICATION IS PREGNANCY. Pregnancy tests must be routinely negative prior to beginning therapy in women of childbearing age. Contraception is mandatory in men and women.
- Women taking hormonal contraception as well as any of the following drugs — barbiturates, glucocorticoids, phenytoin, carbamazepine—have decreased efficacy of the hormonal contraception and must use barrier contraception as well.
- Most common side effects are dry skin, occasional tingling of extremities, somnolence, fatigue, constipation, and neutropenia, followed by rash, peripheral neuropathy, lightheadedness, dizziness and edema. Uncommonly, severe rash, DVT, PE, URI and pneumonia, renal insufficiency, severe neutropenia and bradycardia may occur.

Potential Toxicities/Side Effects and the Nursing Process

I. ALTERATION IN SEXUALITY/REPRODUCTION related to POTENTIAL TERATOGENICITY

Defining Characteristics: Drug is teratogenic and a single dose can cause birth defects. Unclear if drug is excreted in semen.

Nursing Implications: Assess reproductive status, sexual activity, and birth control measures used for both men and women. Instruct male patients to use barrier contraception, and women to use both barrier and hormonal contraception. Women of childbearing age must have a negative pregnancy test baseline to begin the drug, and pregnancy test should be repeated every two weeks for two months, then every month. Instruct patient to continue contraception one month after drug is discontinued. Physicians, patients, and pharmacists must participate in drug manufacturer (Celgene, Warren, NJ) STEPS program (System for Thalidomide Education and Prescription Safety).

II. ALTERATION IN SENSORY/PERCEPTUAL PATTERNS related to PERIPHERAL NEUROPATHY

Defining Characteristics: Peripheral neuropathy occurs in about 25% of patients (range, 10–50%). If drug is discontinued at the first sign of neuropathy, symptoms are reversible. Neuropathy is a distal axonal degeneration affecting long and large-diameter motor and sensory axons in hands and feet. Initially, there is numbness of toes/feet, described often as a "tightness around the feet." There may be decreased sensitivity to light touch, pinprick (sensory loss) in hands and feet, muscle cramps, symmetrical sensorimotor neuropathy, painful paresthesias in hands and feet, distal hypoesthesia, proximal weakness in lower limbs, slight postural tremor, leg cramps, absent ankle jerks. If treatment is continued, there is permanent paresthesias of feet and hands, which progresses proximally. Increased risk of occurrence with increased age (> 70 years old) and high total doses > 14 g (40–50 g).

Nursing Implications: Assess baseline neurologic status, especially presence of peripheral neuropathy. Teach patient to stop drug and report immediately dysesthesias, numbness, and/or muscle cramps. Perform assessment for peripheral neuropathy at every visit.

III. ALTERATION IN SENSORY/PERCEPTUAL PATTERNS related to DROWSINESS

Defining Characteristics: Drug has nonbarbiturate sedative qualities, and drowsiness is the most frequent side effect. Tolerance to daytime drowsiness occurs over several weeks of use. Drowsiness and dizziness are more frequent at doses of 20–400 mg/day than at lower doses. HIV-infected patient studies reported drowsiness, dizziness, and mood changes 33–100% of the time.

Nursing Implications: Assess baseline alertness, sleep patterns. Assess other drugs taken, especially those with sedating qualities, and alcohol ingestion. Instruct patient to avoid alcohol and to take drug at bedtime. Assess degree of drowsiness and dizziness and safety of patient. If significant, teach measures to ensure safety. Tell patient that tolerance develops over 2–3 weeks.

IV. ALTERATION IN SKIN INTEGRITY, POTENTIAL, related to RASH

Defining Characteristics: Pruritic, erythematous macular rash may appear over trunk and back 2–13 days after initiation of therapy. Increased incidence in patients with HIV infection with low CD4 counts. Drug rechallenge often results in immediate reaction of rash, tachycardia, and fever. Rash resolves with drug discontinuation.

Nursing Implications: Teach patient to self-assess for rash, and instruct to discontinue drug and report rash to nurse or physician immediately. If necessary, manage symptomatic itching with antihistamines.

V. ALTERATION IN ELIMINATION related to CONSTIPATION

Defining Characteristics: Mild constipation occurs in 3–30% of patients.

Nursing Implications: Instruct patient to prevent constipation by using stool softeners, mild laxatives if needed (e.g., milk of magnesia), and to use bulk (e.g., psyllium). In addition, teach dietary interventions (e.g., increased fiber, fluids of 3 quarts/day), and mild exercise. Instruct patient to report constipation unresponsive to these interventions.

VI. POTENTIAL FOR INFECTION related to NEUTROPENIA

Defining Characteristics: Rare (< 1%) in most patients, but increased incidence of 2–20% in HIV-infected patients. Average onset 6–7 weeks after initiation of treatment (range, 3–12 weeks).

Nursing Implications: Determine baseline WBC and absolute neutrophil count (ANC). Do not initiate therapy if ANC < 750/mm^3. If on treatment, ANC < 750/mm^3, consider drug discontinuance, but drug definitely should be discontinued if ANC < 500/mm^3. Drug may be reinstituted after neutrophil recovery (e.g., G-CSF). WBC and ANC should be monitored closely in HIV-infected patients (e.g., every other week for three months), and then at least every month. If non-HIV-infected patients, monitor baseline and monthly.

Drug: tipifarnib (R115777, Zarnestra)

Class: Farnesyl transferase inhibitor.

Mechanism of Action: Inhibits farnesyl transferase, which activates a cell growth promoting a gene called Ras. Ras acts like a ''light switch,'' that, when turned on, allows growth signals from outside to be passed along to other pathways to reach the cell nucleus, resulting in uncontrolled cell division. It is estimated that 30% of all cancers have a mutated form of the Ras protein, permitting uncontrolled cell growth. Tipifarnib blocks the action of farnesyl transferase, theoretically stopping uncontrolled cell division. As it has effect in tumors that do not have a mutation in the ras gene, it appears to interrupt other signaling pathways involved in cell survival and growth as well.

Metabolism: P450 microenzyme system involved in the drug's metabolism, CYP3A4 and CYP3A5, as well as UDP glucuronosyltransferase isoenzyme UGT1A1. Peak plasm concentration reached after 2 hours.

Dosage/Range:

Per clinical trial protocol.

- acute myelocytic leukemia (aged 65+ with newly diagnosed AML): 300–600 mg PO bid × 3 weeks, 1–3 weeks of recovery.

Drug Preparation/Administration: None, oral

Drug Interactions:

- Unknown.

Lab Effects/Interference:

- Decreased white blood cell, red blood cell, and platelet count.
- Hypokalemia.
- Rare increased LFTs.

Special Considerations:

- Being studied in AML, multiple myeloma, CML, breast cancer, glioma, and myelodysplastic syndrome.
- Phase II trial of newly diagnosed patients aged 65+ with AML presented at ASH 2004: Overall response rate 34%, CR 18%, mean duration of CR 6.4 months (Lancet et al, 2004); appears 3 gene sequence predicts response (Raponi et al, 2004).
- Contraindicated in patients with CHF, unstable angina, cardiac arrythmias, psychiatric problems, allergies to imidazoles, and active infections.

Potential Toxicities/Side Effects and the Nursing Process

I. POTENTIAL FOR BLEEDING AND FATIGUE related to BONE MARROW DEPRESSION

Defining Characteristics: In clinical trials, the following occurred: bone marrow depression 78%, fatigue 54%.

Nursing Implications: Monitor CBC, platelet count baseline and periodically during therapy per protocol. Assess for signs and symptoms of bleeding, fatigue, and anemia. Teach patient to self-assess for signs and symptoms of bleeding, anemia, and to call if they occur. Assess patient medication profile, and any OTC medications such as contain aspirin or NSAIDs that would increase risk of bleeding. Instruct patient to avoid these drugs, and not to begin any OTC medications without first discussing with nurse or physician. Teach patient to alternate rest and activity periods if feeling fatigued and to organize shopping and chores in a way to minimize energy expenditures.

II. ALTERATION IN NUTRITION, LESS THAN BODY REQUIREMENTS related to NAUSEA, DIARRHEA, ANOREXIA, DEHYDRATION, HYPOKALEMIA, AND RARE HEPATOTOXICITY

Defining Characteristics: In clinical trials, nausea occurred in 61% of patients, anorexia 21%, diarrhea 32%, hypokalemia 9%, and hepatotoxicity 5%.

Nursing Implications: Assess weight, bowel elimination status, baseline nutritional status, as well as serum electrolytes and LFTs. Teach patient that nausea, anorexia, and diarrhea can occur; ways to minimize this effect, such as self-administration of anti-nausea and anti-diarrheal medications; and to report symptoms that do not resolve with established plan. Teach patient to identify nutritionally-dense (high calories and protein in the smallest amount) foods and to keep them handy in the refrigerator. Teach patient to eat small, frequent meals and to have a bedtime snack. Teach patient to drink a glass of fluid every hour while awake if patient is at risk for developing dehydration (elderly, forgetful). Monitor electrolytes and LFTs during treatment and discuss abnormalities with the physician.

III. ALTERATION IN SENSORY/PERCEPTUAL PATTERNS related to CENTRAL NEUROTOXICITY, NEUROPATHY, OPTIC NEURITIS

Defining Characteristics: Central neurotoxicity may occur, as well as neuropathy and optic neuritis.

Nursing Implications: Assess baseline neurologic status, especially presence of peripheral neuropathy. Teach patient to stop drug and report immediately dysesthesias, numbness, and/or muscle cramps. Perform assessment for peripheral neuropathy at every visit.

Drug: tositumomab, I^{131} tositumomab (Bexxar™)

Class: Radioimmunotherapeutic agent.

Mechanism of Action: Iodine-I^{131}-labeled anti-B1 murine monoclonal antibody directed against the CD_{20} B-lymphocyte antigen found on the surface of some normal lymphocytes, and lymphocytes in non-Hodgkin's lymphoma (NHL). The agent contains two parts: an IgG_2 murine (mouse) monoclonal antibody directed against the CD_{20} surface antigen, and antibody labeled with iodine-131. The antibody attaches to the CD_{20} surface antigen on the lymphocytes, directly killing the cells by inducing apoptosis, and mediating antibody-dependent cell killing, plus delivering ionizing radiation directly to the cell. Radiation is delivered directly to the tumor cells, as well as some normal cells with CD_{20} antigens.

Metabolism: The median clearance of tositumomab (the monoclonal antibody) is about 68.2 mg/hr but clearance rate increases in patients with a higher tumor burden. Patient specific dosing is based on total body clearance. Radioactive I-131 decays and is excreted in the urine, with 67% of the injected dose excreted after 5 days. At 7 weeks after the therapeutic dose, the median number of circulating CD_{20} positive lymphocytes was zero, and lymphocyte recovery began about 12 weeks after treatment.

Dosage/Range:
Total body dose of 65–75 cGy based on platelet count.

Drug Preparation: See package insert for preparation and radioactivity calibration.

Drug Administration:

- Regimen consists of 4 components administered in 2 steps using the same IV tubing set with in-line 0.22 micron filter throughout the entire dosimetric or therapeutic step. Otherwise, changing the filter can result in loss of drug:
  - **Day-1: At least 24 hours prior to dosimetric dose:** Start saturated solution of potassium iodide (SSKI) 4 drops po tid, Lugol's solution 20 drops po tid, or potassium iodide tablets 130 mg po qd; and continue until 2 weeks after administration of the I-131 tositumomab therapeutic dose. Patient must receive at least 3 doses of SSKI, or 3 doses of Lugol's solution, or 1 dose of potassium iodide 24 hours prior to day 0. Refer to *Workbook for Dosimetry Methodology and Administration* set-up for configuration of tubing using a 3 way stopcock, and shielding.
  - **Day 0: Dosimetric dose**
    - Premedicate patient with acetaminophen 650 mg po and diphenhydramine 50 mg po 30 minutes prior to initial tositumomab.
    - Tositumomab 450 mg in 50 mL 0.9% Sodium Chloride IV infusion over 60 min. Then give Iodine I-131 (containing 5.0 mCi I-131 and 35 mg tositumomab) in 30 mL 0.9% Sodium Chloride IV over 20 min. During either infusion: reduce infusion rate by 50% for mild to moderate infusional reactions; stop if reactions severe. After complete resolution of severe symptoms, resume infusion at 50% slower rate.
    - Post-infusion gamma camera scan is done to determine whole body counts, and then this is repeated over the next week. The whole body counts are used to determine the therapeutic dose.
  - **Day 7–14: Therapeutic dose** (about 1–2 weeks after dosimetric dose):
    - Premedicate patient with acetaminophen 650 mg po and diphenhydramine 50 mg po 30 minutes prior to initial tositumomab.
    - Tositumomab 450 mg in 50 mL 0.9% Sodium Chloride IV over 60 min. Then give calculated I-131 tositumomab IV over 20 min. During

either infusion: reduce infusion rate by 50% for mild to moderate infusional reactions; stop if reactions severe. After complete resolution of severe symptoms, resume infusion at 50% slower rate.
- Dosing: patients with platelet count $\geq$ 150,000/mm^3: dose is activity of I-131 calculated to deliver 75 cGy total body irradiation and 35 mg tositumomab; patients with platelet count 100,000/mm^3 but < 150,000/mm^3: dose is activity of I-131 that will deliver 65 cGy total body irradiation and 35 mg tositumomab.

Drug Interactions:
- Unknown.

Lab Effects/Interference:
- Bone marrow suppressive agents: further depression of red blood cells, white blood cells, and platelets.
- If human anti-murine antibodies (HAMA) develop: interference with accuracy and results of diagnostic tests relying on murine antibody technology may occur.

Special Considerations:
- Indicated for the treatment of patients with CD_{20} positive, follicular, non-Hodgkin's lymphoma, whose disease is refractory to rituximab and has relapsed following chemotherapy.
- In rituximab-resistant patients, 63% responded with a median duration of 25 months.
- Therapeutic regimen should be prescribed by a physician certified or in the process of being certified by Corixa Corporation in dose calculation and administration of BEXXAR.
- Bexxar should be administered only once.
- Contraindicated in patients with known hypersensitivity to murine (mouse) proteins, patients with > 25% lymphoma marrow involvement and/or impaired bone marrow reserve.
- Drug causes fetal harm so avoid use in pregnant women; women who are breast-feeding should discontinue nursing.
- Delayed adverse reactions that can develop are hypothyroidism, HAMA, myelodysplasia/leukemia, and secondary malignancies.
- Oral iodine supplements are given one day prior to dosimetric dose, and continued for 2 weeks after the therapeutic dose (to block the thyroid uptake of I-131).
- Overall summary of responses in 116 patients with low-grade or transformed low-grade NHL showed 78% responses (11.7-month median duration of response), with 46% complete responses (36.5-month median duration of response). 24 patients with no prior chemotherapy had a 100% response, with 71% having a complete response (Vose, 1998).

- The development of human antimouse antibodies (HAMA) was related to extent of prior chemotherapy: in chemonaïve patients, 38% developed HAMA, while only 4% did who received more than one prior chemotherapy regimen.
- Response rate and duration of response were lower in patients aged 65 and older, and duration of severe hematologic toxicity was longer.

Potential Toxicities/Side Effects and the Nursing Process

I. POTENTIAL FOR INJURY related to ANAPHYLAXIS

Defining Characteristics: Rare but potentially life-threatening reaction may occur. Mouse antibodies are used that are foreign and may stimulate anaphylaxis. No grade 4 adverse experiences have been reported. Approximately 8% of patients in clinical trials require slowing of the infusion to manage symptoms.

Nursing Implications: Assess baseline T, VS. If patient develops discomfort, slow infusion per protocol. Have emergency equipment and medications nearby. Assess patient for signs/symptoms, including generalized flushing and urticaria leading to pallor, cyanosis, bronchospasm, hypotension, unconsciousness. Teach patient to report signs/symptoms, including sense of doom, tickle in throat. If signs/symptoms occur, stop infusion immediately, assess VS, notify physician. Physician may prescribe epinephrine 0.3 mL (1:1000) SQ if hypotensive. Oxygen, antihistamines, corticosteroids may also be used.

II. POTENTIAL FOR INFECTION, BLEEDING, AND FATIGUE related to NEUTROPENIA, THROMBOCYTOPENIA, AND ANEMIA

Defining Characteristics: Prolonged Bone marrow suppression is the dose-limiting toxicity. Patients at risk are patients who have been heavily pretreated with minimal bone marrow reserve, who have lower nadir counts with longer times to recovery. The maximum tolerated total body dose is 75 cGy to avoid severe myelosuppression. Nadir counts occur approximately six weeks post-therapy. Median nadirs were ANC 1,000 cells/m^3, platelets 62,000 cells/m^3, and hemoglobin 11.1 gm/dL. Grade 4 toxicity occurred in < 5% of patients: absolute neutropenia < 100 cells/mm^3 (3%), platelet count < 10,000 cells/mm^3 (5%), and Hgb < 6.5% (4%). Supportive use of growth factors and transfusions was 18%, especially in patients heavily pretreated.

Nursing Implications: Assess prior bone marrow suppressive therapy and risk for toxicity. Assess baseline WBC, differential, Hgb/HCT and platelet count, and signs/symptoms of infection, bleeding, or fatigue. Discuss any abnormalities with physician before drug administration. Teach patient signs/symptoms of infection and bleeding, and to report them immediately. Teach patient self-care measures to minimize infection and bleeding, including avoidance of aspirin-containing OTC medication, and oral hygiene regimen. Teach patient signs/symptoms of fatigue, and self-care measures to maximize energy, and to minimize fatigue (e.g., alternate rest and activity periods, organize activities).

III. ALTERATION IN COMFORT related to INFUSION REACTION

Defining Characteristics: Approximately 29% of patients have infusion-related reactions, despite premedication with acetaminophen and diphenhydramine. Symptoms include fever, rigots or chills, sweating, hypotension, dyspnea, bronchospasm and nausea either during or up to 48 hours after the infusion.

Nursing Implications: Assess baseline T, VS, neurological status, and comfort level; monitor q4–6h if patient is in hospital. Assure patient receives premedication and regular dosing of antipyretic (e.g., acetaminophen ± diphenhydramine, nonsteroidal anti-inflammatory drug [NSAID]), and antiemetic as ordered by physician. Teach patient self-care measures, including monitoring T, comfort level, self-administration of prescribed medications prior to dose and regularly postdose, as well as the use of heat or cold for myalgias, anthralgias. Encourage patient to increase oral fluids and alternate rest and activity periods. If patient is in hospital and experiences rigor, discuss with physician IV meperidine (25 mg IV q15 min to maximum 100 mg in 1 hour) and monitor BP for hypotension.

IV. KNOWLEDGE DEFICIT, POTENTIAL, related to RADIATION PRECAUTIONS

Defining Characteristics: The Nuclear Regulatory Commission recommends that patients receiving outpatient I-131 anti-B1 therapy follow measures to prevent radiation contamination of others. Patients may receive outpatient treatment as long as total dose to an individual at 1 meter is < 500 millirem.

Nursing Implications: Teach patient rules of time and distance, and review protocol patient discharge instructions. If in doubt, discuss with radiotherapist or radiation physicist. Patients are advised to sleep alone for at least the first night. Discuss need for longer separation based on dose received. Other teaching is based on dose and should include (1) remain at distances of > 3 feet from other people, except for brief periods as necessary, for at least two days; (2) infants, young children, and pregnant women should not visit the patient; if necessary, visits should be brief, and a distance of at least 9 feet from the patients should be maintained; (3) do not travel by commercial transportation or go on a prolonged automobile trip with others for at least the first two days; (4) have sole use of the bathroom for at least two days; and (5) drink "plenty" of fluids for at least the first two days, e.g., 3+ quarts per day.

Drug: trastuzumab (Humanized anti-*Her*-2 Antibody, rhuMAbHER2, Herceptin)

Mechanism of Action: Recombinant humanized monoclonal antibody targeted against the human epidermal growth factor receptor (*Her*-2). *Her*-2 is overexpressed in a number of cancers, including 25–30% of breast cancers. This monoclonal antibody is believed to act through three different mechanisms: (1) the antagonizing function of the growth-signaling properties of *Her*-2, (2) signaling immune cells to attack and kill malignant cells with this receptor, and (3) synergistic and/or additive effects seen with many chemotherapeutic agents.

Metabolism: Initial studies using a loading dose of 4 mg/kg followed by a weekly maintenance dose of 2 mg/kg, a mean half-life of 5.8 days, with a range of 1–32 days was seen. More recent studies with trastuzumab suggest the half-life may be longer in the 21–28 day range.

Dosage/Range: (in HER-2 positive patients)

- Loading dose: 4 mg/kg IV infusion (never IV push) week 1.
- Maintenance dose: 2 mg/kg IV infusion weekly beginning at week 2 until at least disease progression.

Alternative dosing:

- Loading dose 8 mg/kg IV infusion.
- Maintenance dose: 6 mg/kg IV infusion q 3 weeks.

Drug Preparation:

- Drug is available as a lyophilized sterile powder of 440 mg per vial for parenteral administration. Requires refrigeration at 2–8°C (36–46°F). DO NOT FREEZE.
- Reconstitute with 20 mL of Bacteriostatic Water for Injection, USP, containing 1.1% benzyl alcohol, which is supplied with each vial. DO NOT SHAKE.
- Reconstituted solution contains 22 mg/mL. Further dilute desired dose in 250 mL of 0.9% Sodium Chloride Injection, USP.
- Vial is designed for multiple use, and is stable for 28 days following reconstitution at 2–8°C (36–46°F).

Drug Administration:

- Administered IV infusion; initial loading dose is administered over 90 minutes, and initial maintenance dose (week or dose 2) is administered over 90 minutes. Never give as IV push or bolus.
- Observe patient for 1 hour following completion of initial loading dose, and if well tolerated, observe patient for 30 minutes following completion of initial maintenance dose (week 2). If well tolerated, no further post-infusion observation is needed in subsequent weekly infusions.

- Subsequent maintenance doses are administered over 30 minutes if prior administration was well tolerated without fever, chills.
- Continue to administer over 90 minutes if fever, chills experienced in prior administrations.

Drug Interactions:
- Paclitaxel: 2 fold decrease in trastuzumab clearance in animals and a 1.5 fold increase in trastuzumab serum level in human clinical studies.
- No suggested interactions when combined with cisplatin, doxorubicin, epirubicin plus cyclophosphamide.
- No formal drug interaction studies done.

Lab Effects/Interference:
- None known.

Special Considerations:
- Trastuzumab is indicated in combination with paclitaxel for treatment of patients with metastatic breast cancer whose tumors overexpress the HER2 protein and have not received chemotherapy for their metastatic disease. It may also be given as a single agent in patients who overexpress HER2 protein and who have received one or more chemotherapy regimens for metastatic disease.
- Phase III clinical trials studied co-administration together with doxorubicin/cyclophosphamide and/or paclitaxel, and an increased risk of cardiomyopathy was seen. Left ventricular function should be evaluated prior to and during treatment with trastuzumab therapy.
- FISH appears more accurate in identifying HER2 overexpression.
- Trastuzumab is very well tolerated; given that it is a humanized antibody, no pre-medication is recommended.
- Rarely, trastuzumab may cause hypersensitivity/allergic reactions, so emergency equipment should be available during infusions.
- Trastuzumab at a dose of 6–8 mg/kg q 3 weeks × 1 year in the adjuvant setting was shown to reduce the risk of breast cancer recurrence significantly. Interim analysis of the HERA study (2005) showed that the group receiving trastuzumab for 1–2 yrs after adjuvant chemotherapy in HER-2 positive women had an estimated 2-year survival of 86% compared to 77% for the observation group. $P < 0.01$. Cardiac toxicity was higher in the trastuzumab arm, with CHF occurring 3–4% more commonly in high risk patients in the trastuzumab arm so cardiac function must be monitored (Piccan-Gebart et al, 2005).
- Romond et al (2005) summarized the NSABP B-31 and NCCTG N0931 trials showing that the addition of trastuzumab to paclitaxel (concurrent not sequential) following AC in the adjuvant setting, at 2 years, there was increased disease free and overall survival. Perez (2005) showed that after 4

years on study, 15% of the women treated with trastuzumab plus paclitaxel concurrently had recurrence, compared to 33% of women receiving paclitaxel alone. At this point, there was a 49% improvement in survival (Perez, 2005). While there was increased cardiotoxicity, it was within the 4% acceptable range.

Potential Toxicities/Side Effects and the Nursing Process

I. ALTERATION IN CIRCULATION related to CARDIOMYOPATHY

Defining Characteristics: Trastuzumab administration may result in ventricular dysfunction and congestive heart failure. A significant decrease in left ventricular function was found in patients who received concurrent anthracycline and cyclophosphamide chemotherapy. Incidence in one study with trastuzumab alone was 7%; in combination with paclitaxel it was 11%; paclitaxel alone, 1%; and in combination with doxorubicin (A) and cyclophosphamide (C) it was 28% compared to AC alone (7%). If allowed to progress, failure may be severe, and the following have been reported: severe cardiac failure, death, and mural thrombosis leading to stroke. Rare events described following treatment with trastuzumab were vascular thrombosis, pericardial effusion, heart arrest, hypotension, syncope, hemorrhage, shock, and arrythmia.

Nursing Implications: Assess baseline cardiac function, including apical pulse, BP. Review history, and identify patients at risk who have CHF, hypertension, coronary artery disease, or who are receiving trastuzumab in combination with either paclitaxel or AC. Patients should have baseline ECHO or gated blood pool scan to determine left ventricular ejection fraction, and this should be monitored periodically, especially in patients at risk. Assess for signs and symptoms at each visit: dyspnea, increased cough, paroxysmal nocturnal dyspnea, peripheral edema, S_3 gallop, and decrease in left ventricular function when tested. Teach patient to report cough, weight gain, edema of ankles, difficulty breathing, or need to use more pillows at night. Drug should be discontinued in patients who develop clinically significant congestive heart failure.

II. POTENTIAL FOR INJURY related to HYPERSENSITIVITY

Defining Characteristics: Infusion-related reactions (e.g., fever and/or chills) were reported in about 40% of paients with their first treatment, and > 10% with subsequent infusions. Severe hypersensitivity reactions are rare but have been seen.

Nursing Implications: Assess VS baseline and frequently during infusion, especially during initial loading and maintenance infusions. Observe patient for one hour following completion of loading dose, and 30 minutes after initial maintenance dose if loading dose was well tolerated. If not well tolerated, continue to monitor for 60 minutes until well tolerated. Notify physician if fever, chills develop and assess need for acetaminophen, and slowing of infusion. Although severe allergic reactions are uncommon, have emergency equipment available and nearby, and be prepared to provide emergency support if necessary.

III. ALTERATION IN COMFORT related to PAIN, ASTHENIA, DYSPNEA

Defining Characteristics: Generalized pain may affect 11% of patients, dyspnea 6%, and asthenia 5%. Abdominal pain may specifically affect 3% of patients.

Nursing Implications: Teach patients to report alterations in comfort, especially pain and dyspnea. Distinguish new onset of symptoms versus those experienced prior to treatment due to malignancy. Discuss intensity of symptoms and need for pharmacologic and nonpharmacologic interventions. Monitor response to intervention between weekly treatments, and need for alternative strategies.

Drug: tretinoin (Vesanoid®, ATRA, All-Trans-Retinoic Acid)

Class: Retinoid.

Mechanism of Action: Induces maturation of acute promyelocytic leukemia (APL) cells, thus decreasing proliferation. In patients who achieve a complete response to this therapy, there is an initial maturation of primitive leukemic cells, and then cells in both the bone marrow and peripheral blood are normal, polyclonal blood cells. The exact mechanism is unknown.

Metabolism: This drug is well absorbed orally into the systemic circulation, with peak concentrations in 1–2 hours. Drug is > 95% protein-bound, primarily to albumin. Oxidative metabolism occurs via the cytochrome P450 enzyme system in the liver. Drug is excreted in the urine (63% in 72 hours) and feces (31% in 6 days).

Dosage/Range:
- 45 mg/m^2 per day.

Drug Preparation:
- None: oral.
- Available as 10–mg capsules.
- Protect from light.

Drug Administration:
- Drug is to be used for induction remission only.

- Administer in evenly divided doses until complete remission (CR) is achieved, then for an additional 30 days, or after 90 days of treatment, whichever comes first.

Drug Interactions:

- Drugs that either inhibit or induce the cytochrome P450 hepatic enzyme system potentially will interact with this drug, but there is no data to suggest that these drugs either increase or decrease tretinoin activity.
- Drugs that induce the enzyme system: rifampin, glucocorticoids, phenobarbitol, pentobarbitol; drugs that inhibit the enzyme system: ketoconazole, cimetidine, erythromycin, verapamil, diltiazem, cyclosporin.

Lab Effects/Interference:

- Increased cholesterol and triglyceride levels (60% of patients) and elevated LFTs (50–60% of patients).

Special Considerations:

- Indicated for the induction remission of patients with APL (FAB-M3), characterized by the presence of the t(15:17) translocation and/or presence of the PML/RARα (alpha) gene.
- Absorption is enhanced when taken with food.
- Monitor CBC, platelets, coagulation studies, liver function tests, and triglyceride and cholesterol levels frequently during therapy.

Potential Toxicities/Side Effects and the Nursing Process

I. ALTERATION IN OXYGENATION, POTENTIAL, related to RETINOIC ACID-APL SYNDROME

Defining Characteristics: Syndrome occurs in approximately 25% of patients and varies in severity, but has resulted in death. Syndrome is characterized by fever, dyspnea, weight gain, pulmonary infiltrates on X-ray, and pleural and/or pericardial effusions. May also be accompanied by impaired myocardial contractility, hypotension, ± leukocytosis, and because of progressive hypoxemia and multisystem organ failure, some patients have died. Usually occurs during first month of treatment, but may follow initial drug dose.

Nursing Implications: Assess VS, pulmonary exam, and weight at each visit. Teach patient to do daily weights, and to report any SOB, fever, weight gain. If this occurs, notify physician and discuss obtaining CXR and focused exam. Discuss chest X-ray findings with physician. Be prepared to give high-dose steroids at the first sign of the syndrome, e.g., dexamethasone 10 mg IV q12h × 3 days or until symptom resolution (necessary in 60% of patients). Provide pulmonary and hemodynamic support as necessary. Discuss whether drug should be discontinued based on severity and patient's response to high-dose steroids.

II. ALTERATION IN COMFORT related to VITAMIN A TOXICITY

Defining Characteristics: Almost all patients experience some toxicity, but they do not usually have to discontinue the drug. Toxicity of high-dose vitamin A includes headache (86%) starting the first week of treatment, but fading after that; fever (83%); skin/mucous membrane dryness (77%); bone pain (77%); nausea/vomiting (57%); rash (54%); mucositis (26%); pruritus (20%); increased sweating (20%); visual disturbances (17%); ocular disorders (17%); skin changes (17%); alopecia (14%); changed visual acuity (6%); visual field defects (3%).

Nursing Implications: Teach patient about possible side effects of high-dose vitamin A as above and to report them if they occur. Teach patient symptom management. Assess severity of symptom(s) and discuss with physician symptom management of fever, headache unresponsive to acetaminophen, nausea/vomiting. If headache is severe in a child, have child evaluated for pseudotumor cerebri.

III. POTENTIAL FOR INJURY related to PSEUDOTUMOR CEREBRI

Defining Characteristics: Benign intracranial hypertension has occurred in children treated with retinoids. Early signs and symptoms are papilledema, headache, nausea and vomiting, and visual disturbances.

Nursing Implications: Teach patient/parents to report symptoms. Assess patient for symptomatology on regular basis. If headache is severe, discuss with physician analgesics and therapeutic lumbar puncture.

IV. POTENTIAL DISTURBANCE IN CIRCULATION

Defining Characteristics: The following disturbances may occur: arrythmia (23%), flushing (23%), hypotension (14%), hypertension (11%), phlebitis (11%), cardiac failure (6%); 3% of patients studied developed cardiac arrest, myocardial infarction, enlarged heart, heart murmur, ischemia, stroke, and other serious disturbances.

Nursing Implications: Assess cardiac status baseline and presence of risk factors (e.g., hypertension). Assess VS at each visit and teach patient in a manner not to induce anxiety to report any symptoms such as chest pain, SOB, heart palpitations, or any changes that occur.

V. ALTERATION IN NUTRITION, LESS THAN BODY REQUIREMENTS, related to GI DYSFUNCTION

Defining Characteristics: Some problems are related to APL, and together with drug may emerge, such as GI bleeding/hemorrhage, which may occur in up to 34% of patients. Other GI problems include abdominal pain (31%), diarrhea (23%), constipation (17%), dyspepsia (14%), abdominal distention (11%), hepatosplenomegaly (9%), hepatitis (3%), and ulcer (3%).

Nursing Implications: Assess GI status and presence of GI dysfunction baseline. Teach patient to report any GI disturbances or changes in bowel status. If these occur, assess severity and need for symptom management, or discussion/intervention with physician. Monitor liver function studies frequently during therapy.

VI. SENSORY/PERCEPTUAL ALTERATIONS related to CHANGES IN EAR SENSATION/HEARING

Defining Characteristics: 23% of patients report earache or fullness in ears. Other ear problems that may occur are reversible hearing loss (5%) and irreversible hearing loss (1%).

Nursing Interventions: Teach patient that this may occur and to report it if it occurs. Assess severity and need for intervention.

VII. POTENTIAL FOR INJURY related to CNS, PERIPHERAL NERVOUS SYSTEM CHANGES, AND AFFECT CHANGES

Defining Characteristics: Changes that may occur include dizziness (20%), paresthesias (17%), anxiety (17%), insomnia (14%), depression (14%), confusion (11%), cerebral hemorrhage (9%), agitation (9%), and hallucinations (6%). Rarely, the following may occur: forgetfulness, gait disturbances, convulsions, coma, facial paralysis, tremor, leg weakness, somnolence, slow speech, aphasia, and other CNS changes.

Nursing Implications: Teach patient in a manner that does not cause anxiety to report any changes in affect, sensorium, or functional ability (e.g., to walk, speak). Assess severity of symptom(s) if they arise and potential for injury. If severe, modify patient's environment to minimize risk of injury and discuss medical intervention with physician.

VIII. ALTERED URINARY ELIMINATION, POTENTIAL, related to RENAL CHANGES

Defining Characteristics: Uncommonly, renal insufficiency may occur (11%), dysuria (9%), acute renal failure (3%), urinary frequency (3%), renal tubular necrosis (3%), and enlarged prostate (3%).

Nursing Implications: Assess baseline urinary elimination pattern. Teach patient to report any changes. Monitor BUN/creatinine periodically during therapy and discuss any abnormalities with physician.

Drug: liposomal tretinoin (Atragen®, All-Trans-Retinoic Acid Liposomal, AR-623. LipoATRA, Tretinoin Liposomal) (investigational)

Class: Retinoid.

Mechanism of Action: Induces maturation of acute promyelocytic leukemia (APL) cells, thus decreasing proliferation. In patients who achieve a complete response to this therapy, there is an initial maturation of primitive leukemic cells, and then cells in both the bone marrow and peripheral blood are normal, polyclonal blood cells. The exact mechanism is unknown. Liposomal drug permits IV administration, with less toxicity, as it is believed the liposome overcomes resistance seen with continued oral therapy (possibly due to declining serum levels during oral administration since IV administration of liposome gives higher and more sustained plasma levels of drug (Estey et al, 1999).

Metabolism: IV administration of liposome gives higher and more sustained plasma levels of drug as compared to oral administration. Probably has oxidative metabolism via the cytochrome P450 enzyme system in the liver. Drug is probably excreted in the urine and feces.

Dosage/Range:
- Per research protocol.
- Newly diagnosed acute promyelocytic leukemia (APL) 90 mg/m^2 IV every other day for induction, followed by maintenance with the same dose 3 times a week × 9 months.
- AIDS-related Kaposi's sarcoma: 120 mg/m^2 three times a week × 4 weeks (Bernstein et al, 1998).

Drug Preparation:
- Per research protocol.

Drug Administration:
- IV, per research protocol.

Drug Interactions:
- Drugs that either inhibit or induce the cytochrome P450 hepatic enzyme system potentially will interact with this drug, but there is no data to suggest that these drugs either increase or decrease tretinoin activity.
- Drugs that induce the enzyme system: rifampin, glucocorticoids, phenobarbitol, pentobarbitol; drugs that inhibit the enzyme system: ketoconazole, cimetidine, erythromycin, verapamil, diltiazem, cyclosporin.

Lab Effects/Interference:
- Increased cholesterol and triglyceride levels.
- Elevated LFTs.
- Elevated renal function test.

Special Considerations:

- Has shown effectiveness in the induction remission of patients with APL (FAB-M3) characterized by the presence of the t(15:17) translocation and/or presence of the PML/RARα (alpha) gene. It should be considered in patients relapsing after oral tretinoin, refractory to oral tretinoin and chemotherapy, or unable to take oral tretinoin.
- In one clinical trial, for newly diagnosed patients with APL, time to hematologic complete remission (CR) was a median of 34 days (range, 22–64 days), but at this time only 10% had a molecular CR. However, after an additional three months of therapy, all patients with a hematologic CR achieved a molecular CR (Estey et al, 1999). Complete hematologic remission is defined as $<5\%$ blasts and $<8\%$ promyelocytes in bone marrow (with normal appearing myelocytes), ANC $\geq 1000/mm^3$, and platelet count of $\geq 100,000/mm^3$; molecular remission means the PML-RAR-alpha gene rearrangement has disappeared, as shown by PCR (polymerase chain reaction) at a sensitivity of 10(-4).
- In newly diagnosed APL, high response rates were seen in patients with low white counts, e.g., $<10,000/mm^3$, and were minimal in patients with high white counts (Estey et al, 1999).
- Drug appears to slow progression of lesions in AIDS-related Kaposi's sarcoma.
- Drug is being studied in cancer of the prostate, bladder (superficial), and non-Hodgkin's lymphoma.
- Toxicity profile is less than with oral tretinoin.
- Monitor CBC, platelets, coagulation studies, liver function tests, and triglyceride and cholesterol levels, renal function tests baseline, and frequently during therapy.
- Drug is contraindicated during pregnancy as drug is teratogenic, and women should not breast-feed while taking the drug; drug is contraindicated in patients hypersensitive to tretinoin or any of the liposomal components.
- Drug, as with oral version, can cause retinoic acid-acute promyelocytic leukemia syndrome (RA-APL): fever, dyspnea, joint pain.
- Drug should be used cautiously in patients with renal dysfunction, patients with prior sensitivity to acitretin, etretinate, isotretinoin, or other vitamin A derivatives; and patients with pretherapy leukocytosis, as the risk for developing RA-APL syndrome is increased.

Potential Toxicities/Side Effects and the Nursing Process

I. ALTERATION IN OXYGENATION, POTENTIAL, related to RETINOIC ACID-APL SYNDROME

Defining Characteristics: Syndrome occurs in approximately 25% of patients and varies in severity, but has resulted in death in studies of the oral drug. Syndrome is characterized by fever, dyspnea, weight gain, pulmonary infiltrates on X-ray, and pleural and/or pericardial effusions, and joint pain. May also be accompanied by impaired myocardial contractility, hypotension, ± leukocytosis, and because of progressive hypoxemia and multisystem organ failure, some patients have died in studies using the oral drug. Usually occurs during first month of treatment, but may follow initial drug dose. With liposomal drug, when dose was reduced and it was given with steroids, patients successfully continued/completed liposomal tretinoin treatment.

Nursing Implications: Assess VS, pulmonary exam, and weight at each visit. Teach patient to do daily weights, and to report any SOB, fever, weight gain. If this occurs, notify physician and discuss obtaining CXR and focused exam. Discuss chest X-ray findings with physician. Be prepared to give high-dose steroids at the first sign of the syndrome, e.g., dexamethasone 10 mg IV q12h × 3 days or until symptom resolution (necessary in 60% of patients). Provide pulmonary and hemodynamic support as necessary. Discuss whether drug should be discontinued based on severity and patient's response to high-dose steroids.

II. ALTERATION IN COMFORT related to VITAMIN A TOXICITY

Defining Characteristics: Toxicity is less with liposomal IV drug than when given orally. Almost all patients experience some toxicity, but they do not usually have to discontinue the drug. Toxicity of high-dose vitamin A includes headache starting the first week of treatment (87% incidence in one study), but fading after that; fever; skin/mucous membrane dryness; bone pain; nausea/vomiting; rash; mucositis; pruritus; increased sweating; visual disturbances (ocular disorders); skin changes; alopecia; changed visual acuity; visual field defects.

Nursing Implications: Teach patient about possible side effects of high-dose vitamin A as above and to report them if they occur. Teach patient symptom management. Assess severity of symptom(s) and discuss with physician symptom management of fever, headache unresponsive to acetaminophen, nausea/vomiting. Teach patient to avoid other administration of vitamin A preparations, e.g., beta carotene. If headache is severe in a child, have child evaluated for pseudotumor cerebri.

III. POTENTIAL FOR INJURY related to PSEUDOTUMOR CEREBRI

Defining Characteristics: Benign intracranial hypertension has occurred in children treated with retinoids. Early signs and symptoms are papilledema, headache, nausea and vomiting, and visual disturbances.

Nursing Implications: Teach patient/parents to report symptoms. Assess patient for symptomatology on regular basis. If headache is severe, discuss with physician analgesics and therapeutic lumbar puncture.

IV. POTENTIAL DISTURBANCE IN CIRCULATION

Defining Characteristics: Toxicity is less than in incidence of patients receiving oral tretinoin. The following disturbances may occur: arrythmia, flushing, hypotension, hypertension, phlebitis, cardiac failure; one patient studied developed fatal acute heart failure myocardial infarction occurring day after starting therapy, with death the following day in a patient with a history of coronary artery disease and hypertension, and in whom ACE inhibitor was discontinued day prior to starting liposomal tretinoin. In oral studies, enlarged heart, heart murmur, ischemia, stroke, and other serious disturbances occurred.

Nursing Implications: Assess cardiac status baseline and presence of risk factors (e.g., hypertension). Assess VS at each visit and teach patient, in a manner not to induce anxiety, to report any symptoms such as chest pain, SOB, heart palpitations, or any changes that occur.

V. ALTERATION IN NUTRITION, LESS THAN BODY REQUIREMENTS, related to GI DYSFUNCTION

Defining Characteristics: Toxicity with liposomal tretinoin is less severe or frequent than with oral drug. Some problems are related to APL, and together with drug, may emerge, such as GI bleeding/hemorrhage, abdominal pain, diarrhea, constipation, dyspepsia, abdominal distention, hepatosplenomegaly, hepatitis, and ulcer.

Nursing Implications: Assess GI status and presence of GI dysfunction baseline. Teach patient to report any GI disturbances or changes in bowel status. If these occur, assess severity and need for symptom management, or discuss intervention with physician. Monitor liver function studies frequently during therapy.

VI. SENSORY/PERCEPTUAL ALTERATIONS related to CHANGES IN EAR SENSATION/HEARING

Defining Characteristics: Toxicity with liposomal tretinoin is less severe or frequent than with oral drug. Patients may report earache or fullness in ears, and hearing loss.

Nursing Interventions: Teach patient that this may occur and to report it if it occurs. Assess severity and need for intervention.

VII. POTENTIAL FOR INJURY related to CNS, PERIPHERAL NERVOUS SYSTEM CHANGES, AND AFFECT CHANGES

Defining Characteristics: Toxicity with liposomal tretinoin is less severe or frequent than with oral drug. Changes that may occur include dizziness, paresthesias, anxiety, insomnia, depression, confusion, cerebral hemorrhage, agitation, and hallucinations. Rarely, the following may occur: forgetfulness, gait disturbances, convulsions, coma, facial paralysis, tremor, leg weakness, somnolence, slow speech, aphasia, and other CNS changes.

Nursing Implications: Teach patient in a manner that does not cause anxiety to report any changes in affect, sensorium, or functional ability (e.g., to walk, speak). Assess severity of symptom(s) if they arise and potential for injury. If severe, modify patient's environment to minimize risk of injury and discuss medical intervention with physician.

VIII. ALTERED URINARY ELIMINATION, POTENTIAL, related to RENAL CHANGES

Defining Characteristics: Toxicity with liposomal tretinoin is less severe or frequent than with oral drug. Uncommonly, renal insufficiency may occur, dysuria, acute renal failure, urinary frequency, renal tubular necrosis, and enlarged prostate.

Nursing Implications: Assess baseline urinary elimination pattern. Teach patient to report any changes. Monitor BUN/creatinine periodically during therapy and discuss any abnormalities with physician.

Drug: vatalanib (PTK787/ZK222584)

Class: Angiogenesis inhibitor; protein tyrosine kinase inhibitor.

Mechanism of Action: Drug is a potent inhibitor of all known vascular endothelial growth factor (VEGF) tyrosine kinases (VEGFR-1, 2, 3) that are expressed on endothelial cells; also inhibits c-KIT and platelet-derived growth factor receptor (PDGFR).

Metabolism: Rapidly absorbed in 1–2 hours following oral ingestion; half-life of 4–5 hrs.

Dosage/Range:

Per protocol, eg, 50–1500 mg/day; probably requires multiple dosing per day given half-life of q 4–5 hrs

Drug Preparation: Oral.

Drug Interactions: Unknown

Lab Effects/Interference: Unknown

Special Considerations:

- Drug is being studied in patients with colorectal cancer, and glioblastoma multiforme.
- CONFIRM-1 (Colrectal Oral Novel Therapy for the Inhibition of Angiogenesis and Retarding of Metastases) trial: phase III trial comparing patients with advanced colorectal cancer receiving FOLFOX ± vetalinib. Although there appeared to be a significant difference favoring patients receiving the combination (17% reduction in risk of disease progression) this was not significant when reviewed by central reviewers. Survival data is being accrued. It is questioned that perhaps drug was not given frequently enough (qd instead of bid or more frequent) since the half-life of the drug is only 4–5 hrs.
- CONFIRM 2: Phase III trial comparing patients with metastatic colorectal cancer who have progressed after 1st line irinotecan containing chemotherapy. Overall survival data are expected in mid-2006.
- Grade 3 thrombopenia and Grade 4 neutropenia higher in the patients receiving vatalinib and FOLFOX compared to patients receiving FOLFOX alone.

Potential Toxicities/Side Effects and the Nursing Process

I. ALTERATION IN HEMOSTASIS related to BLEEDING and THROMBOSIS

Defining Characteristics: In the CONFIRM trials, Grade 3 venous thrombosis occurred in 7% of patients compared to 4% in the FOLFOX alone arm, and Grade 4 pulmonary embolism occurred in 6% versus 1% in the FOLFOX only arm.

Nursing Implications: Assess baseline hematologic parameters and monitor during therapy. Teach patient to assess for and report right away signs/symptoms of thrombosis: new swelling, pain, skin warmth and/or change in color (e.g., erythema, mottling) on the legs or thighs; new onset pain in the abdomen; dysnpnea or shortness of breath, rapid heartbeat, chest pain, or pressure that may signal a pulmonary embolism; and any changes in vision, new onset of severe headache, lightheadedness, or dizziness. Assess baseline mental status and neurological signs and monitor during therapy.

II. POTENTIAL ALTERATION IN CIRCULATION related to HYPERTENSION

Defining Characteristics: Grade 3 hypertension occurred in 21% of patients receiving the combination in the CONFIRM trial compared to 6% receiving FOLFOX alone.

Nursing Implications: Assess baseline BP prior to and during treatment, at least for the first treatment, then prior to each drug administration. If the patient has a history of hypertension, monitor BP more closely, although hypertension develops over time rather than during the drug infusion. Blood pressure should continue to be monitored after patient has stopped the drug. Teach patient drug administration, potential side-effects, and self care measures if prescribed antihypertensive medication, such as angiotensin-converting enzyme inhibitors, beta blockers, diuretics, and calcium channel blockers, consult protocol and expect that drug should be permanently discontinued if the patient develops hypertensive crisis (diastolic blood pressure > 120 mm Hg). Drug can be temporarily suspended in patients with severe hypertension until BP can be controlled with medical management per protocol.

III. POTENTIAL FOR ACTIVITY INTOLERANCE related to FATIGUE,

Defining Characteristics: Fatigue occurs commonly in patients with advanced colorectal cancer treated with vatalinib and FOLFOX; dizziness was more common in the patiens receiving the combination, and 7% of patients receiving the combination had grade 3 dizziness compared to 2% receiving FOLFOX alone.

Nursing Implications: Teach patient that fatigue and dizziness may occur and self-care measures. Teach patient to alternate rest and activity periods, to plan shopping and chores to minimize energy expenditure, and to explore whether family members can assist with necessary chores. Teach patient to slowly change position to minimize feeling dizzy, and to hold onto secure objects such as the wall and not a small table, when arising and moving from a sitting to a standing position. Teach patient to report increasing or severe dizziness.

Section 2
Symptom Management

Chapter 6

Pain

Pain in the patient with cancer may result from a variety of stimuli. A careful assessment is critical in order to identify the physical causes and psychosocial factors that modulate pain intensity and perception. Pain can be acute or chronic. Acute pain results from stimuli such as surgical procedures, pathological fractures, and obstruction of a hollow viscus, while chronic pain reflects the more common cancer pain resulting from tissue inflammation caused by tumor, but patients often have both acute and chronic components of pain. Acute pain lasts from minutes to months and ceases when the cause of pain is removed (e.g., pain caused by spinal cord compression is removed when the patient undergoes laminectomy or radiotherapy to relieve the compression). This type of pain is often associated with anxiety, and as well one sees symptoms of sympathetic nervous system arousal (increased heart rate, increased/decreased BP). In contrast, chronic pain lasts from months to years; the cause cannot be removed, and this type of pain is often associated with depression. The long duration of chronic pain dampens sympathetic response, so the patient does not manifest changes in heart rate or BP.

Symptoms often accompanying unrelieved pain are sleeplessness, anorexia (loss of appetite), fatigue, irritability, and fear. Nurses play a critical role in advocating for effective cancer pain management and alleviation of other accompanying symptoms. Fortunately, there are a variety of available analgesic medications, including non-opioid and opioid, adjuvant agents such as antidepressants, as well as nonpharmacologic techniques such as relaxation exercises.

In addition, opioid agents are available in immediate-onset formulations for acute pain, and long-duration agents that allow superior control for chronic pain as long-acting preparations avoid the peaks and valleys of serum levels and relief associated with immediate preparations. While analgesics do not remove the source or stimulus for the pain, they decrease or modulate the impulse so that the pain impulse perceived by the patient is reduced or absent, thus decreasing the distress and discomfort perceived by the patient. *Non-opioid* medications are helpful for mild to moderate pain. Most non-opioid analgesics work peripherally to decrease prostaglandin synthesis (NSAIDs), but some agents may have a central action as well, possibly at the level of the hypothalamus (McEvoy, Litvak, and Welsh, 1992). Pain receptors appear to be sensitized to mechanical and chemical stimulation by prostaglandins, so interruption of prostaglandin synthesis diminishes the painful impulse. For example, bone destruction and pain from metastasis appear to be mediated by prostaglandins, so NSAIDs that inhibit prostaglandin synthesis are first-line analgesics (Foley 2000). In addition, the anti-inflammatory action of NSAIDs contributes to analgesia. Principal side effects of this class are alteration in hemostasis (aspirin inhibits platelet aggregation, while other salicylates may alter hepatic synthesis of blood coagulation factors); alteration in GI mucosal integrity (aspirin and other NSAIDs can erode GI mucosal surface, causing bleeding or ulceration); and altered renal elimination due to inhibition of renal prostaglandins responsible for renal blood flow and function.

Recently, COX-2 inhibitors came upon the health care scene, in relation to the treatment of rheumatoid and osteoarthritis. Their role in the management of cancer-related bony pain is unclear, but the selective inhibition of prostaglandins responsible for inflammation is an achievement that will undoubtedly find a niche. In addition, these agents at slightly higher dosing may have anti-tumor effects as well as they decrease angiogenesis and increase apoptosis ability on the cellular level. NSAIDs achieve their anti-inflammatory effect by inhibiting the enzyme cyclooxygenase (COX), which is necessary for synthesis of prostaglandins and thromboxanes. There are two isoforms of the enzyme, COX-1, which appears to protect the gastric mucosa and is found in most tissues including platelets, and COX-2, which is found in brain and kidney tissue, as well as other body tissues at the site of inflammation. NSAIDs traditionally inhibit both COX-1 and COX-2 isoforms, resulting in a high risk of gastric ulceration and perforation. The risk of gastrointestinal bleeding is significantly less with the selective COX-2 inhibitors but still may occur. In addition, the selective COX-2 inhibitors do not affect bleeding time. The effect of the new COX-2 inhibitors on acute pain remains to be seen. In one study, 50 mg of refecoxib was equally effective as 550 mg of naproxen sodium or 400 mg of ibuprofen. Two other selective COX-2 inhibitors are celecoxib (Celebrex®) and rofecoxib (Vioxx®). Of interest as the applications of these new agents are explored is their possible role in prevention or treatment of colon cancer. An American Cancer Society study (Thun et al, 1991) showed that the regular ingestion of aspirin diminished colon cancer mortality 40% in men and 42% in women over six years. In addition, it appears that prostaglandin E2 may have a role in colon cancer development, and it appears that a COX-2–derived prostanoid promotes survival of colonic adenomas (Lipsky 1999). Currently, research is underway to better define the role of COX-2 inhibitors in the prevention and/or management of colon cancer.

Adjuvant analgesics play a vital role in cancer pain management. These drugs are indicated for purposes other than analgesia but can be combined with primary analgesics to increase analgesia and/or manage symptoms related to pain or the adverse effects of the opioids. There may be wide variations in patient responses. The major classes used as adjuvant drugs are antidepressant (Chapter 9), corticosteroid (Chapter 1), anticonvulsant (Chapter 7), and specialty drugs for bony metastasis (Chapter 10).

The *antidepressants* enhance pain-modulating pathways that are mediated by serotonin and norepinephrine, and, interestingly, clomipramine and amitriptyline have been shown to increase morphine levels (Wilkie, 1995). Not only can these agents help reduce the depression associated with chronic pain, but they can also relieve sleep problems, and often offer significant benefit in the management of neuropathic pain. Most commonly, the tricyclic antidepressants are used, such as amitriptyline and desipramine. The drug selection should be individualized to the patient and the risk for developing side effects. The advent of serotonin-reuptake inhibitors (SSRI) brought great hope to oncology nurses. However, there have been conflicting resports of the efficacy of these SSRIs in managing chronic pain syndromes (Belcheva et al, 1995; Tokunaga et al, 1998). Of the non-tricyclic antidepressants, paroxetine (Paxil) has shown benefit in reducing the painful symptoms of peripheral neuropathy in diabetic patients (Sindrup et al, 1990) and itching in patients with advanced cancer (Zycliz, 1996). In dosing antidepressants, the starting dosage should be low (i.e., 10 mg amitriptyline for the elderly patient, or 25 mg for the young adult) and given at bedtime. The dose should be titrated up slowly to the usually effective range of 50–150 mg. It is important to allow one week between dose titrations to evaluate the benefit of a given dose. Side effects include: sedation, orthostatic hypotension, constipation, dry mouth, dizziness and, less commonly, precipitation of acute angle-closure glaucoma, urinary retention, and arrhythmia.

Corticosteroids are useful in both acute and chronic pain management, such as that associated with metastatic bone pain, neuropathic pain, lymphedema, hepatic capsular distension, and brain metastasis. The dosing is individualized to the etiology of the pain and patient requirements, from low doses to high doses for patients with brain metastasis. It is important to identify patients at risk for peptic ulceration, and then to use corticosteroids cautiously if at all. In addition, patients need to be cautioned not to take concomitant aspirin.

Anticonvulsants may provide analgesia for lancinating, neuropathic pain. Drugs such as gabapentin, carbamazepine, phenytoin, clonazepam, and valproate are often used, and the dosing is the same as that used for seizure prevention.

Specialty drugs for the management of bony metastasis are biphosphonate pamidronate disodium (Aredia) and zolendronate (Zometa), indicated for use in managing pain related to bony metastases. Pamidronate and zolendronate have been shown to inhibit osteoclast activity and reduce pain from bony metastasis. Treatment is given IV every four weeks. Radiopharmaceuticals such as Strontium-89 is taken up in bone mineral preferentially, in sites of metastasis. However, the subsequent development of acute leukemia has limited interest in radiopharmaceutical management of pain.

Opioid analgesics are the cornerstone of management of moderate to severe cancer pain. These drugs, opiate agonists, attach to specific opiate receptors in the limbic system, thalamus, hypothalamus, spinal cord, and organs such as intestines. This leads to altered pain perception at the spinal cord and higher CNS levels. Because of this action, side effects that may occur include suppressed cough reflex; alterations in consciousness and mood (drowsiness, sedation, euphoria, dysphoria, mental clouding); respiratory depression; nausea/vomiting; and constipation. Opiate agonists may cause physical dependence (causing physical signs and symptoms of withdrawal if drug is stopped abruptly after chronic usage) and addiction (psychological dependence). However, addiction is VERY RARE in cancer patients, occurring in less than 0.1% of patients.

Unfortunately, some patients with cancer pain suffer needlessly because health care providers (physicians) underprescribe and (nurses) undermedicate (Marks and Sacher 1973). Chronic cancer pain requires the patient to self-administer opioids "around-the-clock" rather than "as needed (PRN)" to prevent moderate-to-severe pain. Tolerance is the ability to receive larger amounts of a drug without ill effect and to show decreased effect (i.e., pain relief) with continued use of the same drug dose. Tolerance occurs over time, depending on the drug and the route of administration. In addition, tolerance to the respiratory depressant effects of opiates develops over time with chronic usage for prevention of cancer pain. For instance, a patient with severe cancer pain who has been receiving escalating doses over a period of time may require very high doses to finally eliminate or reduce the pain to acceptable levels, as in the case of a patient with head and neck cancer who required 1200 mg/hour of morphine yet was still ambulatory and able to interact with family and friends. According to McCaffery (1982), pain is "whatever the patient says it is, occurring where the patient says it is." Use of quantifiable measurement tools is helpful to identify pain intensity (see Figure 6.1) and pain *relief* in response to intervention. The World Health Organization recommends a two-step approach to cancer pain management, beginning with non-opioids for slight-to-mild pain and adding a opioid as the pain intensity increases. Opioids have different potencies, and when a patient is changed from one opioid to another, it is imperative that equianalgesic dosages be used. Equianalgesic dose tables are based on comparative potencies to morphine (see Table 6.1). Opioids and non-opioids can be combined for additive analgesia. Opioid agonist-antagonists, such as pentazocine (e.g., Talwin), should be used with caution, if at all, since they may cause withdrawal syndrome. NSAIDs and opioid analgesics are available

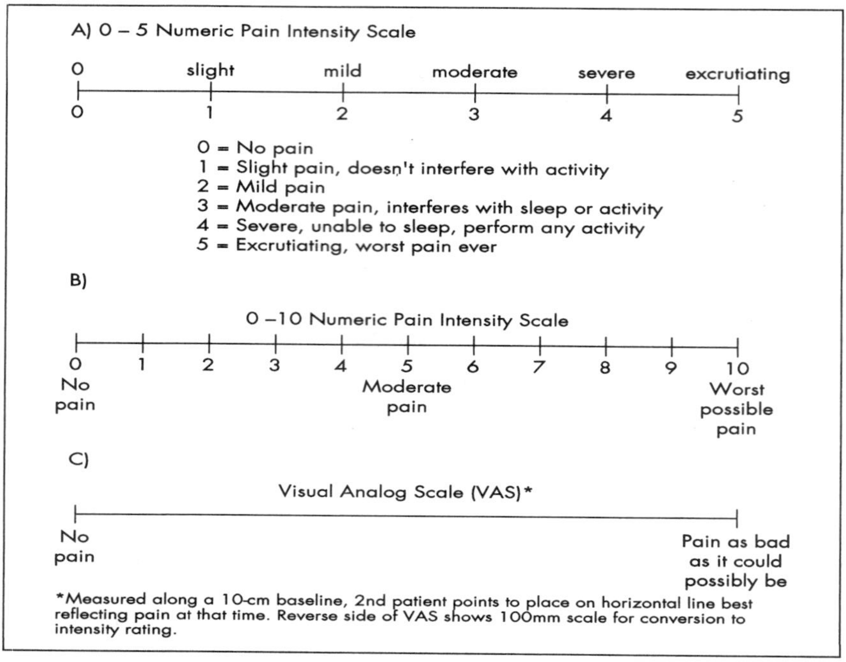

Figure 6.1 Examples of Measurement Tools of Pain Intensity

for oral, parenteral, and rectal administration. The United States Food and Drug Administration (FDA) approved ketorolac in 1996, and it is the only available *parenteral* NSAID. Also, transdermal patch delivery of fentanyl (20 times more potent than morphine) has been available for some time, and an immediate-release oral with mucosal absorption system is available (Actiq). Finally, awareness of the benefits of patient-controlled analgesia (PCA) has made this method of drug delivery for IV analgesics more widely available.

When trying to evaluation an opioid intervention, it is important to again recall that this is the century of genomics. It is now clear that there is considerable genetic polymorphism in the cytochrome P-450 family of enzymes (Bernard & Bruera, 2000), and that this can influence analgesic effect. For example, Payne (1998) states that 15% of Caucasians lack the enzyme CYPD211 that is required to metabolize codeine to morphine, so this group will require higher doses to achieve the same effect. As genotyping becomes more a part of designing a plan of care, it is important to remember this. In addition, as nurses have always done, when one opioid is ineffective, care planning with physician colleagues is to make sure that another opioid from a different class are tried.

Table 6.1 Equianalgesic Dose Table

Drug Opioid Agonist	Approximate Equianalgesic Oral Dose	Approximate Equianalgesic Parenteral Dose	Recommended Starting Dose Adults > 50 kg Body Weight) Oral	Parenteral
Morphine	30 mg q3–4h (around-the-clock dosing) 60 mg q3–4h (single dose or intermittent dosing)	10 mg q3–4h	30 mg q3–4h	10 mg q3–4h
Codeine	130 mg q3–4h	75 mg q3–4h	60 mg q3–4h	60 mg q2h (IM, SQ)
Hydromorphone (Dilaudid)	7.5 mg q3–4h	1.5 mg q3–4h	6 mg q3–4h	1.5 mg q3–4h
Hydrocodone (in Lorcet, Lortab, Vicodin, others)	30 mg q3–4h	Not available	10 mg q3–4h	Not applicable
Levorphanol (Levo-Dromoran)	4 mg q6–8 h	2 mg q6–8 h	4 mg q6–8 h	2 mg q6–8 h
Meperldine (Demerol)	300 mg q2-3h	100 mg q3h	Not recommended	100 mg q3h
Methadone (Dolophine, others)	20 mg q6-8h	10 mg q6-8h	20 mg q6-8h	10 mg q6-8h
Oxycodone (Roxicodone, also in Percocet, Percodan, Tylox, others)	30 mg q3–4h	Not available	10 mg q3–4h	Not applicable
Oxymorphone (Numorphan)	Not available	1 mg q3–4h	Not available	1 mg q3–4h

Source: From AHCPR, Public Health Service, US Department of Health and Human Services. Rockville, MD. AHCPR Publication No. 92-0032.

MANAGEMENT

Numerous practice guidelines are available, and most recently the National Comprehensive Cancer Network (NCCN). Practice emphasize the need for rapid titration of short-acting opioids to manage severe pain, before then determining the optimal analgesic regime to control the patient's pain (Grossman et al, 1999). The recommended guidelines (2002) are available on the Internet at http://www.nccn.org/physician_gls/f_guidelines.html.

New horizons are being explored, and new medications that act directly at the spinal cord level are being studied. Recently, research has identifed alpha-adrenergic receptors for epinephrine at presynaptic and postjunctional sites in the dorsal horn of the spinal cord, located near the opioid receptors. Stimulation of these alpha-2 adrenergic receptors by agonists such as clonidine appears to block the transmission of the pain signal up the spinal cord to the brain, thus blocking pain perception, and this does not compete with opioids at opioid binding sites. One such agent that has been approved is clonidine hydrochloride (Duraclon), which is given along with opioids. Other agents being studied are *N*-methyl-D-aspartate (NMDA) antagonists (such as ketamine and dextromethorphan), which decrease pain due to inflammation and ischemia, and are effective in reducing neuropathic pain. NMDA receptors are found in the brain, spinal cord, and periphery, and are responsible for recognizing neuropathic pain. Unfortunately, side effects such as hallucinations and disassociation may be problematic.

Drugs intended to limit the development of tolerance are ongoing. Mu agonists (e.g., morphine) activate the mu-opioid receptor to inhibit the neuron from passing along incoming pain impulses, thus effecting analgesia. When morphine binds to the mu receptor, it increases the sensitization of the *N*-methyl-D-aspartate receptor, or NMDA receptor, and leads to an overactivation of protein-kinase C. This in turn leads to a desensitization of the mu-opioid receptor so that the effect of morphine is less, and tolerance may develop. By combining morphine with a NMDA antagonist, this stimulates the mu-opioid receptor and at the same time prevents activation of the protein-kinase C, thus preventing desensitization of the mu-opioid receptor, and theoretically increasing analgesia and preventing tolerance.

A second group that is being studied are the calcium channel blockers, which may also offer analgesia. By antagonizing the voltage-sensitive calcium channels in the synaptic membranes of neurons, these *N*-type voltage-sensitive calcium channel (VSCC) antagonists have shown some success in relieving neuropathic pain. Intrathecal administration of selective neuronal channel are being studied and offer promise of relief of chronic intractable pain.

As a nurse negotiating with patients with cancer-related pain around goals, often patients choose a 2–3 on a scale of 0–10 as the goal because they would rather have some pain in exchange for not being too sleepy. One possible intervention that is being studied is the use of modafinil (Provigil) to help treat fatigue and help patients stay awake (NCI, accessed July 2002; Breitbart et al, 1998). This agent could also be useful to help patients try to achieve a goal of pain intensity of 0–1 and not be afraid of becoming too sleepy with a lower quality of life.

References

Algos Pharmaceutical Corporation; *Understanding NMDA-Enhanced Analgesia.* Neptune, NJ: Algos Pharmaceutical Corporation; 1999

Belcheva S, Petkov VD, Konstantinova E, et al. Effects on Nociception of the Calcium and 5-HT Antagonist Dotarizine and Other 5-HT Receptor Agonists and Antagonists. *Acta Physiol Pharmacol Bulg* 1995;21:93–98

Bernard SA, Bruera E. Drug Interactions in Palliative Care. *J Clin Oncol* 2000;18(8): 1780–1799

Breitbart W, Passik S, Payne D. Psychological and Psychiatric Interventions In Pain Control. Doyle D, Hanks GW, MacDonald N, (eds), *Oxford Textbook of Palliative Medicine,* 2nd ed. New York: Oxford University Press;1998;437–454

Eliot L, Geiser R, Loewen G. Steady State Pharmacokinetic Comparison of a New Once-daily, Extended Release Morphine Formulation (Morphelan) and OxyContin Twice Daily. *J Oncol Pharm Pract* 2001;7:1–8

Fan G-H, Zhao J, Wu Y-L, et al. *N*-methyl-D-aspartate Attenuates Opioid Receptor-Mediated G Protein Activation and This Process Involves Protein Kinase C. *Mol Pharmacol* 1998;53:684–690

Ferrell BR, Rivera LM. Cancer Pain Education for Patients. *Semin Oncol Nurs* 1997;13: 42–48

Foley KM. The Treatment of Cancer Pain. *N Engl J Med* 1995;313:84–95

Foley KM. Controlling Cancer Pain. *Hospital Practice* 2000; http://www.hosppract.com/issues/2000/04/foley.htm. Accessed June 26, 2003

Grossman SA, Benedetti C, Payne R, Syrjala K, et al. NCCN Practice Guidelines for Cancer Pain. *Oncology* 1999;13(11A):1–20

Jacox A, Carr DB, Payne R, et al. Management of Cancer Pain. *Clinical Practice Guideline No 9 (AHCPR Pub No 94–0592).* Rockville, MD:Agency for Health Care Policy & Research USDHHS; 1994

Kaiko RF, Wallenstein SL, Rogers AG, et al. Opioids in the Elderly. *Med Clin North Am* 1982;66:1079–1089

Lipsky PE. COX-2 Specific Inhibitors: Basic Science and Clinical Implications. *Am J Med* 1999;106(5B):1–515 (proceeding of a symposium)

Lipsky PE. The Clinical Potential of Cyclooxygenase 2-Specific Inhibitors. *Am J Med* 1999;106(5B):515–575

Marks RM, Sacher EJ. Undertreatment of Medical Inpatients with Opioid Analgesics. *Ann Intern Med* 1973;78:173–181

McCaffery M. Nursing. *Management of the Patient with Pain.* Philadelphia, PA: JB Lippincott Co.; 1982

McEvoy GK, Litvak K, Welsh OH, et al. (eds.) *AHFS Drug Information.* Bethesda, MD: American Society of Health-System Pharmacists; 1992

Merck & Co. Vioxx Package Insert. West Point, NY: Merck & Co; 1992

Miaskowski C. Innovations in Pharmacologic Therapies. *Semin Oncol Nurs* 1997;13: 30–35

National Cancer Institute. Fatigue PDQ: Intervention, Pschostimulants. July 2002; Available at http://www.nci.org. Accessed August 2002

Paice J. Pain, Yarbro CH, Frogge MH, Goodman M, (eds), *Cancer Symptom Management,* 3rd ed. Sudbury, MA: Jones and Bartlett Publishers; 2003

Payne R. Pharmacologic Management of Pain, Section IA3. Berger A, Portenoy RK, Weissman DE, (eds), *Principles and Practice of Supportive Oncology,* Philadelphia, PA: Lippincott-Raven Publishers; 1998

Searle. Celebrex Package Insert. Skokie, IL: Searle Co.; 1999

Syndrup SH, Gram LF, Brosenk EO Jr, et al. The Selective Serotonin Reuptake Inhibitor Paroxetine is Effective in the Treatment of Diabetic Neuropathy Symptoms. *Pain* 1990;42:135–144

Thun MJ, Namboodri MM, Heath CW Jr. Aspirin Use and Reduced Risk of Fatal Colon Cancer. *N Engl J Med* 1991;325:1593–1596

Tokunaga A, Saika M, Senba E. 5-HT2A Receptor Subtype is Involved in the Thermal Hyperalgesic Mechanism of Serotonin in the Periphery. *Pain* 1998;76:349–355

Wilkie D. Neural Mechanisms of Pain: A Foundation for Cancer Pain Assessment and Management. Maguire DB, Yarbro CH, Ferrell BR, (eds), *Cancer Pain Management,* 2nd ed. Sudbury, MA: Jones and Bartlett Publishers;1995;61–87

Zycliz Z, Smits C, Krajnik M. Paroxetine for Pruritis in Advanced Cancer. *J Pain Symptom Management* 1996;16:121–124

NON-OPIOD ANALEGICS

Drug: acetaminophen (Acephen, Actamin, Anacin-3, Apacet, Anesin, Dapa, Datril, Genapap, Genebs, Gentabs, Halenol, Liquiprin, Meda Cap, Panadol, Panex, Suppap, Tempra, Tenol, Ty Caps, Tylenol)

Class: Miscellaneous analgesic/antipyretic.

Mechanism of Action: Appears to inhibit prostaglandin synthesis centrally, thus preventing sensitization of pain receptors to chemical or mechanical stimulation. Mechanism is similar to salicylates but is not uricosuric. May have weak anti-inflammatory effects in nonrheumatoid conditions (e.g., after oral surgery). Reduces fever by direct effect on hypothalamus; heat is lost through vasodilation and increased peripheral blood flow. Analgesic and antipyretic action similar to aspirin.

Metabolism: Rapidly absorbed from GI tract; 25% serum protein-binding. Elimination half-life is 1–3 hours. Metabolized by the liver and excreted in the urine.

Dosage/Range:
325–650 mg every 4–6 hours PRN for pain, discomfort, not to exceed 4 g/24 hours. Some individuals may need increased single doses of 1 g.

Drug Preparation:
- Ensure seals on tamper-resistant package are intact when opening new package.

Drug Administration:
- Oral, rectal, elixir.

Drug Interactions:
- Hepatotoxicity of acetaminophen may be increased by chronic use of high doses of drugs using hepatic microsomal enzyme system: barbiturates, carbamazepine, rifampin, phenytoin, sulfinpyrazone.
- Alcohol: increased risk of hepatic damage with chronic, excessive use.
- Diflunisal: increased acetaminophen serum level; avoid concurrent use.
- Phenothiazines: possible severe hypothermia may occur when used concomitantly.

Lab Effects/Interference:
- None known.

Special Considerations:
- Elixirs contain alcohol (Tylenol, Valadol).
- Contraindicated in patients with known hypersensitivity; use cautiously, if at all, in patients with hepatic or renal dysfunction.
- Chronic ingestion of large doses of acetaminophen may slightly potentiate effects of coumarin and other anticoagulants.

Potential Toxicities/Side Effects and the Nursing Process

I. KNOWLEDGE DEFICIT related to SELF-ADMINISTRATION

Defining Characteristics: Fever curve or excessive fever can be masked by self-dosing with acetaminophen.

Nursing Implications: Instruct patient to report temperature over 38.3°C (101°F) or persistent or recurrent fever. Assess other over-the-counter (OTC) medicines the patient may be taking.

II. POTENTIAL INJURY related to HEPATOTOXICITY

Defining Characteristics: Excessive alcoholic intake and other drugs can increase risk for hepatotoxicity.

Nursing Implications: Assess total acetaminophen dosage/24 hours, taking into account OTC medications. Assess baseline LFTs, especially if the patient has primary hepatoma or liver metastasis. Teach patient to avoid excessive alcohol intake and/or excessive acetaminophen intake.

Drug: aspirin, acetylsalicylic acid (ASA, Aspergum, Bayer Aspirin, Easprin, Ecotrin, Empirin)

Class: Salicylate.

Mechanism of Action: Inhibits prostaglandin synthesis peripherally preventing sensitization of pain receptors by mechanical and chemical stimuli. Also, has anti-inflammatory effect, producing analgesic and antipyretic effects. Central action via hypothalamus unclear.

Metabolism: Rapidly and well absorbed from GI tract, and distributed throughout the body with high concentrations in liver and kidney. Drug is bound to serum proteins, especially albumin. Metabolized by liver and excreted in urine.

Dosage/Range:

- 325–650 mg PO or PR every 4 hours PRN for pain or fever (maximum 3.9 g/day).

Drug Preparation:

- Keep in closed container, away from heat, to prevent drug decomposition.
- Do not use if strong, vinegar-like odor is present. Do not crush enteric-coated aspirin.

Drug Administration:

- Oral or rectal suppositories. Give oral dose with 240 mL water or milk to decrease gastric irritation. Oral solution may be made from effervescent aspirin powders (e.g., Alka-Seltzer); Alka-Seltzer chewable aspirin tablets available.

Drug Interactions:

- Ammonium chloride, ascorbic acid, or methionine (urine acidifiers): Decrease ASA excretion, so increase risk of ASA toxicity.
- Antacids, urinary alkalizers: may increase ASA excretion, so may decrease the ASA effect. Alcohol increases the risk of GI ulceration, bleeding.
- Decreased effect of angiotensin-converting enzyme (ACE) inhibitors. When used together, the effect of anticoagulants may be enhanced (additive hypothrombinemic effect), leading to prolonged bleeding time. DO NOT USE TOGETHER.
- Beta-adrenergic blockers (e.g., propranolol): Possible decrease in antihypertensive effect.
- Corticosteroids: increase in aspirin excretion with decrease in aspirin effect.

- Methotrexate: increase in methotrexate serum levels with increased toxicity. DO NOT USE CONCURRENTLY.
- NSAIDs: decrease in NSAID serum concentration; may have increased incidence of GI side effects. Not recommended to be used together.
- Probenecid, sulfinpyrazone: aspirin (doses ≥ 3 g/day) antagonizes uricosuric drug effect.
- Spirolactone: aspirin may inhibit diuretic effect.
- Sulfonylureas, exogenous insulin: Aspirin may have hypoglycemic effect and may potentiate these drug actions. Monitor for hypoglycemia.
- Valproic acid: aspirin displaces drug and decreases its excretion, resulting in increased serum levels and possible valproic acid toxicity.

Lab Effects/Interference:
- Prolonged bleeding time, leukopenia, thrombocytopenia.

Special Considerations:
- Patients receiving myelosuppressive chemotherapy should be cautioned not to take aspirin due to increased risk of bleeding.
- Patients should be instructed to take drug with food or milk.
- Use cautiously in patients with asthma, rhinitis, or nasal polyps (can cause severe bronchospasm).
- Drug is contraindicated in patients with GI ulcer, GI bleeding, hypersensitivity to aspirin, increased bleeding tendencies.
- Use cautiously in patients with liver damage, hypoprothrombinemia, or with vitamin K deficiency.

Potential Toxicities/Side Effects and the Nursing Process

I. ALTERATION IN NUTRITION, LESS THAN BODY REQUIREMENTS, related to GI TOXICITY

Defining Characteristics: Nausea, dyspepsia (5–25% of patients), heartburn, epigastric discomfort, anorexia, and acute, reversible hepatotoxicity may occur. Risk increases with dose. May potentiate peptic ulcer disease.

Nursing Implications: Teach patient self-administration with 8 oz (240 mL) water or milk. If GI distress develops, discuss use of enteric-coated aspirin (e.g., Ecotrin). If patient receiving high doses of aspirin, monitor LFTs. Drug contraindicated in patients with peptic ulcer disease.

II. POTENTIAL FOR BLEEDING related to INHIBITION OF PLATELET AGGREGATION

Defining Characteristics: Aspirin may cause prolongation of bleeding time, leukopenia, thrombocytopenia, purpura, shortened erythrocyte survival time.

Nursing Implications: Teach patient to avoid aspirin and aspirin-containing drugs if receiving myelosuppressive chemotherapy. Review concurrent medications to identify risk for drug interactions. Monitor Hgb, HCT over time; teach patient signs/symptoms of anemia, and instruct to report them (headache, fatigue, chest pain, irritability). Monitor stool guaiacs.

III. INJURY related to MILD SALICYLISM

Defining Characteristics: Administration of large doses of salicylates may cause salicylism, characterized by dizziness, tinnitus, diminished hearing, nausea, vomiting, diarrhea, mental confusion, CNS depression, headache, sweating, and hyperventilation at serum salicylate concentration 150–300 μg/mL (use in cancer patients usually 100 μg/mL).

Nursing Implications: Teach patient to reduce dose, interrupt dose if signs/symptoms occur. Assess concurrent medications for possible drug interactions.

Drug: celecoxib (Celebrex®)

Class: Nonsteroidal anti-inflammatory drug.

Mechanism of Action: Drug has anti-inflammatory and antipyretic properties effected by inhibition of prostaglandin synthesis via selective inhibition of cyclooxygenase-2 (COX-2) pathway. It does not inhibit the cyclooxygenase-1 (COX-1) isoenzyme.

Metabolism: Following an oral dose, peak serum levels are reached at 3 hours, with a terminal half-life of 11 hours, and with multiple doses, steady-state is reached on or before 5 days. Drug is highly protein-bound (97%) and extensively distributed into tissue. Drug is metabolized in the liver via the cytochrome P450 2C9 system, with little unchanged drug recoverable in the urine or feces. Higher area under the curve (AUC) concentrations are found in the elderly (women > men), in African Americans, and in patients with moderate hepatic dysfunction.

Dosage/Range:
- Adults: 200 mg PO qd, or 100–200 mg PO.
- Patients with moderate hepatic dysfunction or weighing < 50 kg should get lowest dose.

Drug Preparation:
- Oral, available in 100-mg and 200-mg capsules.

Drug Administration:
- Administer orally in morning or evening, without regard to food.

Drug Interactions:

- Celecoxib inhibits cytochrome P450 2D6 system, so when given concurrently with drugs metabolized by this system, may result in increased doses of the second drug; also, celecoxib is metabolized primarily by P450 2C9 system, so if given concomitantly with drugs that inhibit this system, increased serum levels of celecoxib may result (e.g., fluconazole results in 2 × serum levels of celecoxib; use lowest dose possible of celecoxib, if at all).
- Angiotensin converting enzyme (ACE) inhibitors, e.g., lisinopril: may have decreased antihypertensive effect when used together.
- Furosemide, thiazide diuretics: reduced natriuretic effect due to inhibition of renal prostaglandin synthesis; assess diuretic effect and adjust dose as necessary.
- Lithium: use together cautiously, and monitor serum lithium levels if used together.
- Warfarin: monitor INR, PT closely, especially the first few days following initiation of celecoxib therapy or after changing the dose.
- Aspirin: low dose well tolerated, but higher doses may result in GI ulceration or other complications; use only together with low-dose aspirin.
- Methotrexate: no significant interaction.

Lab Effects/Interference:

- Increase in serum chloride, decrease in serum phosphate, and increased BUN; if there is GI bleeding, HCT and Hgb will be reduced. Also, rarely, borderline elevations of liver function tests (e.g., ALT, AST) may occur.

Special Considerations:

- Lowest doses should be used for individuals weighing < 50 kg or those with moderate hepatic impairment. DO NOT ADMINISTER to patients with severe hepatic impairment.
- DO NOT GIVE to pregnant women or nursing mothers unless benefits outweigh risk; DO NOT GIVE to women in last trimester of pregnancy.
- Celecoxib does not affect platelet aggregation or bleeding time. Studies showed significantly fewer GI ulcers in patients receiving celecoxib as compared to naproxen or ibuprofen.
- Indicated for the relief of signs and symptoms of osteoarthritis or rheumatoid arthritis in adults.
- Celecoxib is contraindicated in patients hypersensitive to celecoxib or allergic to sulfonamides, patients with severe hepatic disease, advanced renal disease, or patients who have or have had asthma, urticaria, or allergic-type reactions after taking aspirin or other NSAIDs, as anaphylaxis may occur.
- Use cautiously, if at all, in patients with preexisting asthma, preexisting kidney disease, fluid retention, cardiac failure, hypertension, prior history of ulcer disease or bleeding.

Potential Toxicities/Side Effects and the Nursing Process

I. ALTERATION IN NUTRITION, LESS THAN BODY REQUIREMENTS, related to GI SIDE EFFECTS

Defining Characteristics: Uncommon, but dyspepsia (8.8%), diarrhea (5.6%), abdominal pain (4.1%), nausea (3.4%), and flatulence (2.2%) have occurred. Rarely, the following may occur: diverticulitis, dysphagia, eructation, esophagitis, gastritis, gastroenteritis, gastroesophageal reflux, dry mouth, stomatitis, vomiting, tooth disorder, hemorrhoids, hiatal hernia, melena, vomiting, and tenesmus.

Nursing Implications: Assess history of GI symptoms and history of ulcer disease. Teach patient to take NSAID with meals or milk if possible. Teach patient potential side effects, to report them, and the importance of not taking aspirin. If symptoms are severe, discuss alternative NSAIDs with physician.

II. POTENTIAL FOR BLEEDING related to PEPTIC ULCERATION

Defining Characteristics: Although celecoxib causes fewer GI ulcers ($< 0.1\%$), peptic ulceration and occult GI bleeding can occur and be life-threatening. Increased risk factors: most significant are presence or past history of peptic ulcer, and/or GI bleeding; other risk factors are: smoking, alcoholism, aspirin ingestion, oral corticosteriods, oral anticoagulants, longer duration of NSAID therapy, older age, poor general health status.

Nursing Implications: Assess risk, history of peptic ulcer disease or GI bleeding. Assess baseline Hgb, HCT and presence/absence of occult bleeding by guaiac of stools. Teach patient to report signs and symptoms of abdominal pain, black stools, blood per rectum, epistaxis, menorrhagia. If patient is at risk for bleeding, discuss use of misoprostol to protect GI mucosa with physician. Teach patient to avoid concurrent use of aspirin, other NSAIDs.

III. POTENTIAL SENSORY/PERCEPTUAL ALTERATIONS related to HEADACHE, DIZZINESS

Defining Characteristics: Headache (16%), insomnia (2.3%), dizziness (2%) may occur. Less commonly, migraine, neuralgia, neuropathy, paresthesia, vertigo, deafness, earache, tinnitus, taste perversion may occur.

Nursing Implications: Assess baseline neurologic and mental status. Teach patient to report changes in sensory/perceptual pattern. Teach patient symptom management of headache. If dizziness occurs, teach patient to change position slowly, and other safety measures. Discuss drug continuance with physician for significant symptoms.

IV. ALTERATION IN NUTRITION related to HEPATIC TOXICITY

Defining Characteristics: NSAIDs may cause elevations in LFTs, especially AST and ALK. Very rarely, severe hepatic reactions can occur: jaundice, fatal fulminant hepatitis, liver necrosis, hepatic failure, although this has not been reported with celecoxib.

Nursing Implications: Assess baseline LFTs and monitor periodically during long-term therapy. Teach patient to report the following symptoms immediately and to stop taking drug: nausea, fatigue, lethargy, itching, jaundice, tenderness in the RUQ, and flulike symptoms, so that LFTs can be checked, as well as history and physical exam completed.

V. ALTERATION IN RENAL ELIMINATION related to INHIBITION OF RENAL PROSTAGLANDINS

Defining Characteristics: Long-term use of NSAIDs has rarely resulted in renal papillary necrosis. Rarely, acute renal failure (< 0.1%) may occur in patients with renal insufficiency or in patients with heart failure or liver dysfunction. The following have also been described: albuminuria, cystitis, dysuria, hematuria, urinary frequency, renal calculus, urinary incontinence, and urinary tract infection. Peripheral edema has also been described.

Nursing Implications: Assess baseline renal function. If patient has baseline renal insufficiency, use lowest dose possible initially and assess tolerance. Ensure that patient is well hydrated prior to beginning therapy with celecoxib. Teach patient to report any changes in urinary function, swelling of ankles, or weight gain. Monitor periodic serum BUN, creatinine during chronic therapy.

VI. POTENTIAL FOR INJURY related to ANAPHYLAXIS, ALLERGIC REACTION

Defining Characteristics: Although no patients developed anaphylactioid reactions while receiving celecoxib during clinical testing, there is a risk that this could occur, especially in patients with the "aspirin triad" (asthmatic patients who develop rhinitis with or without nasal polyps or who develop bronchospasm after taking aspirin or NSAIDs). Uncommonly, patients may develop rash, either erythematous or maculopapular (2.2%), dermatitis, photosensitivity reaction, pruritus, or urticaria.

Nursing Implications: Assess baseline allergies, including reaction to aspirin and/or NSAIDs. If patient has asthma and has had a reaction, the patient SHOULD NOT RECEIVE THIS DRUG. Assess baseline skin integrity and presence of lesions. Teach patient to stop drug and report rash immediately. Provide symptomatic relief for rash, pruritus.

Drug: choline magnesium trisalicylate (Trilisate)

Class: Choline and magnesium salicylate combination.

Mechanism of Action: Analgesic effect through peripheral and central pathways, decreasing pain perception. Prostaglandin inhibition probably involved in peripheral mechanism. Antipyretic effect via hypothalamic heat regulation center. Does not interfere with platelet aggregation.

Metabolism: Rapidly absorbed from GI tract. Metabolized by the liver and excreted in the urine.

Dosage/Range:
- Trilisate 750 mg bid or dose-increase to maximum 3200 mg/day.

Drug Preparation:
- Trilisate liquid 5 mL or Trilisate 500-mg tablet contains ASA equivalent of 650 mg.
- Trilisate 750-mg tablet contains 975 mg ASA.
- Trilisate 1000-mg tablet contains 1300 mg ASA.

Drug Administration:
- Oral.

Drug Interactions:
- Antacids, urine alkylinizers: increase salicylate excretion and decrease drug effect. Do not administer with antacids.
- Ammonium chloride, ascorbic acid, methionine (urine acidifiers): decrease salicylate excretion so increase risk of salicylate toxicity.
- Concomitant administration with alcohol, steroids, other NSAIDs may increase GI side effects.
- Corticosteroids: may increase salicylate excretion and decrease Trilisate effect.
- Warfarin: may have increased warfarin levels and increased PT; monitor patient closely, and reduce warfarin dosage as needed.

Lab Effects/Interference:
- Free T4 may be increased with a concurrent decrease in total plasma T4 (does not affect thyroid function).

Special Considerations:
- Drug does not interfere with platelet aggregation.
- Use cautiously in patients with chronic renal failure, gastritis.
- Contraindicated if known hypersensitivity to salicylates.
- Drug contains magnesium, so periodic evaluation of serum magnesium should be performed.

Potential Toxicities/Side Effects and the Nursing Process

I. ALTERATION IN NUTRITION, LESS THAN BODY REQUIREMENTS, related to GI TOXICITY

Defining Characteristics: Fewer GI side-effects than aspirin. Nausea, dyspepsia (5–25% of patients), heartburn, epigastric discomfort, anorexia, and acute reversible hepatotoxicity may occur. Risk increases with dose. May potentiate peptic ulcer disease.

Nursing Implications: Teach patient self-administration with food, or 8 oz (240 mL) water or milk. If patient is receiving antacid, administer antacid two hours after meals and Trilisate before meals. Assess baseline liver and renal function and monitor if patient receiving high doses on ongoing basis. Guaiac stool to assess occult blood, as gastric ulceration may occur.

II. INJURY related to MILD SALICYLISM

Defining Characteristics: Administration of large doses of salicylates may cause salicylism, characterized by dizziness, tinnitus, diminished hearing, nausea, vomiting, diarrhea, mental confusion, CNS depression, headache, sweating, and hyperventilation at serum salicylate concentration 150–300 μg/mL (use in cancer patients usually 100 μg/mL).

Nursing Implications: Teach patient to reduce dose, interrupt dose if signs/symptoms occur. Assess concurrent medications for possible drug interactions.

III. POTENTIAL ALTERATION IN URINARY ELIMINATION related to RENAL PROSTAGLANDIN INHIBITION

Defining Characteristics: Rarely, elevated serum BUN and creatinine may occur.

Nursing Implications: Assess baseline serum BUN, creatinine, and monitor during therapy.

Drug: clonidine hydrochloride (Duraclon)

Class: Antiadrenergic agent.

Mechanism of Action: Acts centrally to stimulate alpha-2-adrenergic receptors in the CNS, thus inhibiting sympathetic vasomotor centers. When given epidurally, the drug is believed to mimic norepinephrine activity at presynaptic and postjunctional alpha-2-adrenoceptors in the dorsal horn of the spinal cord. Is administered together with opioids for severe cancer pain to maximize analgesia. Clonidine HCl shows best efficacy against neuropathic pain.

Metabolism: Drug is highly lipid-soluble and rapidly distributes into extravascular sites and into the CNS; enters the plasma via the epidural veins, leading to hypotensive effect. Drug is metabolized and excreted in the urine (72% of the administered dose in 96 hours, and 40–50% of that is unchanged drug).

Dosage/Range:

To be administered in combination with opioids via epidural route:
- Initial: starting dose is 30 μg/hr.
- May be titrated up to 40 μg/hr or down, based on degree of pain relief and extent of side effects.

Drug Preparation/Administration:
- Preservative-free preparation.
- Given epidurally in combination with opioid via continuous epidural infusion device.

Drug Interactions:
- CNS depressants (e.g., alcohol, barbiturates): potentiation of CNS depression.
- Opioid analgesics: may potentiate hypotension due to clonidine.
- Tricyclic antidepressants: may antagonize hypotensive effect of clonidine.
- Beta-blockers: may exacerbate hypertensive symptoms of clonidine withdrawal.
- Epidural local anesthetics: clonidine may prolong pharmacologic effects of local anesthetic; both motor and sensory blockade.

Lab Effects/Interference:
- None known.

Special Considerations:
- Contraindicated in patients sensitive or allergic to clonidine HCl; epidural administration contraindicated if (1) injection site infection occurs, (2) patient is receiving anticoagulation, (3) patient has bleeding diathesis, (4) administered above the C4 dermatome, (5) patient has severe cardiac disease or is hemodynamically unstable, or (6) used in obstetrical or postoperative analgesia.
- Use cautiously in patients receiving digitalis, calcium channel blockers, and beta-blockers, as there may be additive effects of bradycardia and AV block.
- Severe hypotension may occur during first 2 days of clonidine therapy, especially when drug is infused into the upper thoracic spinal segments—monitor vital signs frequently.
- Do not suddenly withdraw drug, as this may result in nervousness, agitation, headache, tremor, rapid increase in blood pressure; scrupulously maintain drug administration equipment to prevent accidental interruption of drug. Drug dose should be gradually decreased over 2–4 days. If patient is

receiving a beta-blocker, the beta-blocker should be discontinued several days before the gradual discontinuaton of epidural clonidine. Teach patient NOT to discontinue drug on own.

Potential Toxicities/Side Effects and the Nursing Process

I. ALTERED TISSUE PERFUSION related to HYPOTENSION

Defining Characteristics: Hypotension usually occurs within the first four days after beginning epidural clonidine but may also occur throughout treatment. Increased risk in patients receiving infusion into upper-thoracic spinal segments, in women, and in patients who have low body weight. Hypotension may be accentuated by concurrent opiate administration. Clonidine decreases sympathetic CNS outflow, decreasing peripheral resistance, decreasing renal vascular resistance, and decreasing heart rate and BP.

Nursing Implications: Monitor T, BP, HR frequently, especially during first few days of therapy. Notify physician of significant changes. Expect IV fluids to be given to correct hypotension, and if needed, IV ephedrine. Symptomatic bradycardia can be treated with atropine.

II. ALTERED TISSUE PERFUSION related to REBOUND HYPERTENSION

Defining Characteristics: Withdrawal symptoms can occur if drug is interrupted or stopped abruptly; characterized by nervousness, agitation, headache, tremor, rapid increase in BP. Increased risk in patients receiving high drug doses, patients receiving beta-blockers, or patients with a history of hypertension. Rarely, this may result in CVA, hypertensive encephalopathy, or death.

Nursing Implications: Scrupulously manage/maintain catheter and pump to prevent interruption in flow; teach patient catheter and pump care and use; instruct patient never to abruptly discontinue medicine; anticipate physician will discontinue beta-blockers prior to gradual taper of drug over 2–4 days when drug is being discontinued.

III. POTENTIAL FOR INFECTION related to IMPLANTED DEVICE

Defining Characteristics: Implanted epidural catheter may become infected, leading to epidural abcess or meningitis.

Nursing Implications: Scrupulously maintain catheter, using sterile technique; teach patient catheter care and management; monitor for signs/symptoms of infection and teach patient this assessment. If in the hospital, monitor for fever and pain and notify the physician immediately if either is found. Instruct patient to report fever, pain to the physician immediately if at home.

Drug: gabapentin (Neurontin)

Class: Anticonvulsant.

Mechanism of Action: Not clearly understood. Drug is stucturally related to neurotransmitter GABA (gamma-amino-butyric acid), but drug does not bind to GABA receptor sites. It is unclear whether drug has activity at NMDA receptor sites. Drug has been shown to bind to receptor sites in neocortex and hippocampus.

Metabolism: Bioavailability of drug decreases as dose increases, and drug absorption unaffected by food. Drug half-life is 5–7 hours, and drug excreted unchanged in the urine. Plasma clearance may be reduced in elderly and is reduced in renal insufficiency.

Dosage/Range:
- Initial titration: 300 mg on day 1, 300 mg bid on day 2, and 300 mg tid on day 3.
- As needed, dose may be titrated up to 400 mg tid, in increments, to a maximum dose of 600 mg tid (1800 mg total dose per day).
- Dose-reduce in renal insufficiency:

Creatinine Clearance	Drug Dose
30–60 mL/min	300 mg bid
15–30 mL/min	300 mg/day
< 15 mL/min	300 mg every other day

Drug Preparation/Administration:
- Oral, take without regard to food intake.
- Take 1 hour before, or 2 hours after, antacid.
- Take initial dose at bedtime to enhance somnolence and minimize dizziness, fatigue and ataxia.
- Doses should not be separated by > 12 hours (must be tid, e.g., every 8 hours).
- If drug is discontinued or changed to another anticonvulsant, gradually discontinue drug over 1 week.

Drug Interactions:
- Antacids: decrease bioavailability of drug.
- Cimetidine: decreases renal excretion of drug with potential for excess toxicity; monitor patient closely and dose reduce if both drugs must be given concommitantly.

Lab Effects/Interference:
- Urinary protein test using Ames N-Multistix may be falsely positive.
- Drug may cause leukopenia, anemia, thrombocytopenia.

Special Considerations:

- Dose-reduce in patients with renal insufficiency, and consider dose reduction in the elderly.
- Drug helpful in the management of painful peripheral neuropathies.
- Drug may cause dizziness, fatigue, drowsiness, ataxia, so patient should be taught to avoid activities requiring mental acuity, such as driving, until after full effect of drug is known.

Potential Toxicities/Side Effects and the Nursing Process

I. SENSORY/PERCEPTUAL ALTERATIONS related to CNS CHANGES

Defining Characteristics: The most common side effects are somnolence, ataxia, dizziness, and fatigue. Less commonly, nystagmus, tremor, nervousness, dysarthria, amnesia, depression, abnormal thought processes, incoordination, headache, confusion, emotional lability, paresthesia, areflexia, anxiety, hostility, syncope, hypesthesia may occur. Seizures have been reported, as have suicidal tendencies. Other sensory side effects that rarely occur are diplopia, abnormal vision, dry eyes, photophobia, ptosis, and hearing loss.

Nursing Implications: Assess baseline neurological status and document. Instruct patient of general side effects that may occur, and to report them. Assess for suicidal ideation. If significant CNS changes occur, discuss dose reduction or change to an alternative drug with physician. Instruct patient not to drive a car or to do activities that require mental acuity until full effect of drug is known.

II. ALTERATION IN NUTRITION related to GI TOXICITY

Defining Characteristics: Nausea and vomiting may occur. Less commonly, dyspepsia, dry mouth, constipation, increased or decreased appetite, thirst, stomatitis, taste changes, increased salivation, fecal incontinence may occur.

Nursing Implications: Assess patient tolerance of GI side effects. Instruct patient to report side effects. If nausea and vomiting occur, discuss changing to another medication or adding antiemetic agent to regimen if relief of peripheral neuropathy is achieved.

III. ALTERATION IN SKIN INTEGRITY related to RASH

Defining Characteristics: Rash may occur, as may pruritus, acne, alopecia, hirsutism, herpes simplex, dry skin, and increased sweating.

Nursing Implications: Perform baseline skin assessment, and note any areas that are not intact. Teach patient to self-assess for rash, other changes, and to report them. If rash develops, instruct patient to notify provider immediately. If itch occurs, discuss symptomatic management.

IV. ALTERATION IN RESPIRATORY PATTERN related to RHINITIS, COUGH

Defining Characteristics: Rhinitis, pharyngitis, coughing, pneumonia, dyspnea may occur. Rarely, epistaxis and apnea have been reported.

Nursing Implications: Assess baseline respiratory pattern, and instruct patient to report any changes. Discuss any significant changes with physician, and discuss management versus change of drug.

V. ALTERATION IN URINARY ELIMINATION related to URINARY CHANGES

Defining Characteristics: Hematuria, dysuria, frequency, urinary incontinence, cystitis, urinary retention may occur.

Nursing Implications: Assess baseline urinary elimination pattern, and instruct patient of possible side effects and to report them. Discuss symptomatic management, or discuss drug change with physician if changes are significant.

VI. POTENTIAL FOR SEXUAL DYSFUNCTION related to VAGINAL CHANGES AND IMPOTENCE

Defining Characteristics: Vaginal hemorrhage, amenorrhea, dysmenorrhea, menorrhagia, inability to climax, abnormal ejaculation, and impotence have been reported.

Nursing Implications: Assess baseline sexuality, and instruct patient to report any changes. If changes occur, discuss impact and distress caused, and together with physician and patient, discuss drug alternatives.

VII. POTENTIAL ALTERATION IN OXYGENATION related to TACHYCARDIA, HYPOTENSION

Defining Characteristics: Rarely, hypertension, vasodilatation, hypotension, angina pectoris, peripheral vascular disease, palpitation, tachycardia, and appearance of a murmur may occur.

Nursing Implications: Assess baseline cardiovascular status, and instruct patient to notify provider if any changes occur. Instruct patient to report palpitations, fast heart beat, dizziness, or chest pain immediately. If significant changes occur, discuss alternative drug therapy with physician.

Drug: ibuprofen (Advil, Genpril, Haltran, Ibuprin, Midol 200, Nuprin, Rufen)

Class: NSAID.

Mechanism of Action: Peripherally acting analgesic, anti-inflammatory, and antipyretic agent; anti-inflammatory action probably due to prostaglandin inhibition and/or release.

Metabolism: 80% of dose absorbed from GI tract, and absorption rate is slowed by administration with food. Peak serum concentrations with tablet occur in 2 hours; suspension in 1 hour. Highly protein bound (90–99%) and has a plasma half-life of 2–4 hours. Excreted in urine.

Dosage/Range:

200–800 mg every 4–8 hours PRN to maximum of 3200 mg/24 hours.

Drug Preparation:

- Tablets: 200 mg, 300 mg, 400 mg, 600 mg, 800 mg.
- Caplets: 200 mg.
- Oral suspension: 100 mg/5 mL.

Drug Administration:

- Oral.

Drug Interactions:

- Oral anticoagulants, thrombolytic agents: possible increase in PT with increased bleeding; use with caution and monitor patient closely.
- Other NSAIDs: possible increase in GI toxicity; do not administer concomitantly.
- Furosemide, thiazide diuretics: decreased diuretic effect when administered concomitantly.

Lab Effects/Interference:

- Slight decrease in Hgb not exceeding 1 g/dL without signs of bleeding; decrease in Hgb > 1 g/dL may be associated with signs of bleeding.

Special Considerations:

- Contraindicated in patients with known hypersensitivity, asthmatic patients with nasal polyps and other patients who develop bronchospasm or angioedema with aspirin or other NSAIDs, patients with peptic or duodenal ulcer.
- Use cautiously in patients with cardiac or renal dysfunction.

Potential Toxicities/Side Effects and the Nursing Process

I. ALTERATION IN NUTRITION, LESS THAN BODY REQUIREMENTS, related to GI SIDE EFFECTS

Defining Characteristics: Dyspepsia, heartburn, nausea, vomiting, anorexia, diarrhea, constipation, stomatitis, bloating, epigastric and abdominal pain may occur.

Nursing Implications: Assess history of GI symptoms and history of ulcer disease. Teach patient to take NSAID with meals or milk. Teach patient potential side effects, and instruct to report them. If symptoms are severe, discuss alternative NSAIDs with physician.

II. POTENTIAL FOR BLEEDING related to INHIBITION OF PLATELET AGGREGATION

Defining Characteristics: Drug can prolong bleeding time and inhibit platelet aggregation. Peptic ulceration and occult GI bleeding can occur and be life-threatening. Increased risk factors: smoking, alcoholism.

Nursing Implications: Assess risk, history of peptic ulcer disease or GI bleeding. Assess baseline Hgb, HCT, and presence/absence of occult bleeding by guaiac of stools. Instruct patient to report signs/symptoms of abdominal pain, black stools, blood per rectum, epistaxis, menorrhagia. If patient is at risk for bleeding, discuss with physician use of misoprostol to protect GI mucosa. Teach patient to avoid concurrent use of aspirin, other NSAIDs.

III. POTENTIAL SENSORY/PERCEPTUAL ALTERATIONS related to CNS CHANGES

Defining Characteristics: Dizziness, headache, nervousness, fatigue, drowsiness, malaise/light-headedness, anxiety, confusion, mental depression, and emotional lability may occur. Decreased hearing, visual acuity, changes in color vision, conjunctivitis, diplopia, and cataracts have been reported. In addition, though rare, aseptic meningitis has occurred.

Nursing Implications: Assess baseline neurologic and mental status. Instruct patient to report changes in sensory/perceptual pattern, especially VISUAL CHANGES. If visual changes occur, discuss with physician referral to ophthalmologist as soon as possible. Assess for rare occurrence of aseptic meningitis (fever, coma). Discuss drug continuance with physician for significant symptoms.

IV. ALTERATION IN NUTRITION, LESS THAN BODY REQUIREMENTS, related to HEPATIC TOXICITY

Defining Characteristics: Severe and sometimes fatal hepatotoxicity has occurred. Jaundice, hepatitis occur rarely. Borderline increase in LFTs occurs in 15% of patients, while values increase by three times in 1%.

Nursing Implications: Assess baseline LFTs and monitor periodically during long-term therapy. Instruct patient to report jaundice, abdominal pain. Discuss discontinuance of drug with physician for significant toxicity.

V. ALTERATION IN RENAL ELIMINATION related to INHIBITION OF RENAL PROSTAGLANDINS

Defining Characteristics: Acute renal failure may occur rarely within first few days of treatment in patients with preexisting renal dysfunction. Other signs/symptoms of renal dysfunction that may occur rarely are azotemia, cystitis, hematuria, increased serum BUN and creatinine, and decreased creatinine clearance. Peripheral edema has also been described.

Nursing Implications: Assess baseline renal function. Instruct patient to report any changes in urinary function. Monitor periodic serum BUN, creatinine during chronic therapy.

VI. ALTERATION IN SKIN INTEGRITY related to RASH

Defining Characteristics: Rash (urticaria, vesicles, or erythematous macular) may occur, as may Stevens-Johnson syndrome, flushes, alopecia, rectal itching, and acne.

Nursing Implications: Assess baseline skin integrity and presence of lesions. Teach patient to report abnormalities. Provide symptomatic relief for rashes, pruritus.

VII. POTENTIAL FOR FATIGUE AND INFECTION related to BONE MARROW INJURY

Defining Characteristics: Neutropenia, agranulocytosis, aplastic anemia, hemolytic anemia, and THROMBOCYTOPENIA may occur *rarely.*

Nursing Implications: Assess baseline CBC, WBC, differential, and platelet count. Discuss abnormalities with physician. Instruct patient to report severe fatigue, infection, bleeding. Monitor lab values periodically during treatment.

Drug: indomethacin (Indocin, Indocin SR, Indotech)

Class: NSAID, structurally related to sulindac.

Mechanism of Action: Actions similar to other NSAIDs: anti-inflammatory action, probably by inhibition of prostaglandin synthesis, as well as by inhibiting migration of leukocytes to infection site and stabilization of neutrophils so lysosomal enzymes cannot be released; may also interfere with the production of autoantibodies (mediated by prostaglandins). Analgesic and antipyretic effects appear to result from inhibition of prostaglandin synthesis. Probably reduces tumor-associated fever by inhibition of synthesis of prostaglandin (PGE_1) in hypothalamus. However, drug has serious side effects, so should not be used routinely as an antipyretic.

Metabolism: Rapidly and completely absorbed from GI tract. When administered with food or antacid (aluminum and magnesium hydroxide), peak plasma drug concentrations may be slightly decreased or delayed. Drug is 99% bound to plasma proteins. Crosses BBB slightly, and placenta freely. Metabolized by liver, undergoes enterohepatic circulation, and is excreted in urine.

Dosage/Range:
- Capsules: 10 mg, 25 mg, 50 mg, 75 mg, given in 2–4 divided doses.
- Sustained release: 75 mg, given once or bid.
- Oral suspension: 25 mg/5 mL, given in 2–4 divided doses.
- Suppositories: 50 mg, given in 2–4 divided doses.

Drug Preparation:
- Drug is sensitive to light. Store capsules in well-closed containers at temperatures < 40°C (104°F).
- Oral suspension should be stored in tight, light-resistant containers at 30°C (86°F).
- Suppositories should be stored at temperatures < 30°C (86°F).

Drug Administration:
- Give with food or antacid to protect GI mucosa.
- Rectal suppository must remain in rectum for at least 1 hour for maximum absorption.
- Consider reduced dose in patients with renal dysfunction.
- Indocin suspension contains 1% alcohol.

Drug Interactions:
- Indomethacin can displace or be displaced by other protein-bound drugs: oral anticoagulants, hydantoins (e.g., phenytoin), salicylates, sulfonamides, sulfonylureas. Therefore, if taking any of these medications with indomethacin, the patient must be assessed for increased toxicity of each drug.

- Antihypertensive effect of hydralazine, captopril, furosemide, beta-adrenergic blockers, or thiazide diuretics may be decreased.
- NSAIDs: concurrent administration with salicylates does not improve drug effects but increases toxicity (GI, aplastic anemia) so should NOT be given concurrently. Diflunisal may decrease renal excretion of indomethacin and increase risk of GI hemorrhage; AVOID concurrent use.
- Triamterene: may precipitate renal failure. DO NOT USE CONCURRENTLY.
- Digoxin: serum levels may be increased and prolonged, so digoxin levels should be monitored closely.
- Methotrexate, especially HIGH DOSE: increased, prolonged serum methotrexate levels can be fatal; AVOID concurrent use.
- Potassium (K+) supplements, K+ sparing diuretics: indomethacin may increase serum K+ concentrations, especially in the elderly or patients with renal dysfunction. Use with caution and monitor K+ serum levels.
- Lithium: may increase plasma lithium levels; assess patient for lithium toxicity.
- Cyclosporine: possible increased nephrotoxicity; use with caution and monitor renal function.
- Probenecid: increased plasma level and therapeutic effects of indomethacin; decrease indomethacin dose.

Lab Effects/Interference:
- May prolong bleeding time.
- Rarely, hemolytic anemia, leukopenia, thrombocytopenia.

Special Considerations:
- Avoid use or use cautiously in the elderly or in patients with epilepsy, Parkinson's disease, renal dysfunction, mental illness.

Potential Toxicities/Side Effects and the Nursing Process

I. POTENTIAL SENSORY/PERCEPTUAL ALTERATIONS

Defining Characteristics: Dose-related headache occurs in 25–50% of patients (more severe in morning); may be associated with frontal throbbing, vomiting, tinnitus, ataxia, tremor, vertigo, and insomnia. Dizziness, depression, fatigue, and peripheral neuropathy may occur in 3–9% of patients; 1% of patients may have confusion, psychic disturbances, hallucinations, and nightmares. May accentuate epilepsy and Parkinson's disease symptomatology. Blurred vision, corneal and retinal damage, and hearing loss may occur with long-term use.

Nursing Implications: Assess baseline mental and neurologic status. Teach patient to report headache, changes in sensation or perception, and sleep problems. Discuss drug discontinuance with physician if neurologic side effects occur. Patients with visual disturbances or pain, or changes from baseline, should be seen by an ophthalmologist.

II. ALTERATION IN NUTRITION, LESS THAN BODY REQUIREMENTS, related to GI TOXICITY

Defining Characteristics: Nausea, with or without vomiting and indigestion, heartburn, and epigastric pain occur in ~10% of patients. Diarrhea, abdominal pain/distress, and constipation may occur in ~ 3%. Other effects occurring in ~ 1% are anorexia, distension, flatulence, gastroenteritis, rectal bleeding, stomatitis. Severe GI bleeding may occur in 1% of patients, as drug decreases platelet aggregation.

Nursing Implications: Teach patient potential side effects and to self-administer drug with food or antacid. Teach patient to avoid OTC aspirin-containing drugs, alcohol, or steroids, all of which can increase GI toxicity and risk for GI bleeding. Instruct patient to report any signs/symptoms of GI bleeding, abdominal pain immediately, and to stop taking the drug. Guaiac stool for occult blood periodically. If drug must be used, and risk of GI ulceration is high, discuss with physician use of misoprostol to protect the GI mucosa.

III. POTENTIAL FOR INFECTION, FATIGUE, BLEEDING related to BONE MARROW INJURY

Defining Characteristics: Although rare (1%), potential toxicities include hemolytic anemia, bone marrow depression (leukopenia, thrombocytopenia), aplastic anemia, thrombocytopenic purpura. Drug inhibits platelet aggregation but this will reverse to normal within 24 hours of drug discontinuance. May prolong bleeding time, especially in patients with underlying bleeding problems.

Nursing Implications: Assess all medicines the patient is taking and teach patient to avoid OTC aspirin-containing drugs. Teach patient to self-assess and instruct to report signs/symptoms of bleeding, fatigue, and infection.

IV. POTENTIAL FOR ALTERATION IN ELIMINATION PATTERN related to RENAL DYSFUNCTION

Defining Characteristics: Acute interstitial nephritis with hematuria, proteinuria, nephrotic syndrome may occur in 1% of patients. Patients with renal dysfunction may have worsening of renal function. Increased K+ levels may occur in the elderly or in patients with renal dysfunction. Risk increases with long-term therapy.

Nursing Implications: Assess baseline renal status. Discuss alternate drugs if renal dysfunction. Monitor serum K+, sodium (Na+), especially if receiving other drugs that affect serum K+ level (e.g., amphotericin, diuretics), or in the elderly.

V. POTENTIAL FOR ALTERATION IN CARDIAC OUTPUT related to CARDIAC EFFECTS

Defining Characteristics: CHF, tachycardia, chest pain, arrhythmias, palpitations, hypertension, and edema may occur in < 1% of patients.

Nursing Implications: Assess baseline cardiovascular status and monitor periodically while receiving the drug. Assess efficacy of antihypertensive medication due to possible drug interaction.

VI. POTENTIAL FOR INJURY related to DERMATOLOGIC AND SENSITIVITY REACTIONS

Defining Characteristics: Dermatologic effects occur in < 1% of patients and include pruritus, urticaria, rash, exfoliative dermatitis, and Stevens-Johnson syndrome. Allergic reactions occur in < 1%, characterized by asthma in aspirin-sensitive individuals, dyspnea, fever, acute anaphylaxis.

Nursing Implications: Assess baseline dermatologic, pulmonary status, and continue during drug use. Instruct patient to report any adverse reactions immediately.

Drug: ketorolac tromethamine (Toradol)

Class: NSAID.

Mechanism of Action: Inhibits prostaglandin synthesis peripherally to exert analgesic, antiinflammatory, and antipyretic activity.

Metabolism: Drug completely absorbed following PO or IM administration of the drug, with peak serum levels in 44 minutes and 50 minutes, respectively. Drug is extensively bound to serum protein (99%). Terminal half-life is 2.4–9.2 hours. Excreted by the kidney.

Dosage/Range:

- Single dose: IM, 60 mg; IV, 30 mg.
- Multiple dose: IM/IV, 30 mg q6h (maximum daily dose is 120 mg).
- 50% dose reduction for patients aged ≥ 65 years, renally impaired, or weight < 50 kg.
- Oral: for continuation therapy.

- Patients < 65 years old: 20 mg × 1, then 10 mg q4–6h (max 40 mg/24 hours).
- Patients ≥ 65: 10 mg q4–6h (max 40 mg/24 hrs).
- MAXIMUM USE OF KETOROLAC IS 5 DAYS.

Drug Preparation:
- Store at controlled room temperature of 15–30°C (59–86°F) and protect from light.

Drug Administration:
- PO, IM, or IV.

Drug Interactions:
- Other salicylates: displace ketorolac from protein binding. DO NOT USE together or dose-reduce ketorolac.
- Anticoagulants: possible increase in bleeding time; use with caution and monitor closely.
- Furosemide: decreased diuretic response; need to increase diuretic dose.
- Probenecid: causes prolonged, increased serum ketorolac levels; use cautiously, and reduce dose.
- Lithium, methotrexate: theoretically increased serum levels, so should be dose-reduced if given with ketorolac.

Lab Effects/Interference:
- None known.

Special Considerations:
- Drug indicated for the treatment of ACUTE, short-term pain, not chronic pain.
- Concurrent use with other NSAIDs NOT recommended due to risk of additive toxicity.
- Contraindicated in persons with hypersensitivity to ketorolac, or patients with asthma, nasal polyps, angioedema, and bronchospastic reaction to aspirin or other NSAIDs; also in patients with active peptic ulcer disease or GI bleeding, and patients with advanced renal insufficiency.

Equianalgesic Dosing:

Ketorolac	Meperidine		Morphine
IM			
30 or 90 mg	100 mg		12 mg
10 mg	50 mg		6 mg
Ketorolac	**Ibuprofen**	**Aspirin**	**Acetaminophen**
PO			
10 mg	400 mg	650 mg	600 mg

Potential Toxicities/Side Effects and the Nursing Process

I. ALTERATION IN NUTRITION, LESS THAN BODY REQUIREMENTS, related to GI SIDE EFFECTS

Defining Characteristics: Dyspepsia, heartburn, nausea, vomiting, anorexia, diarrhea, constipation, stomatitis, bloating, epigastric and abdominal pain may occur.

Nursing Implications: Assess history of GI symptoms and history of ulcer disease. Teach patient to take NSAID with meals or milk. Teach patient potential side effects and instruct to report them. If symptoms are severe, discuss alternative NSAIDs with physician.

II. POTENTIAL FOR BLEEDING related to INHIBITION OF PLATELET AGGREGATION

Defining Characteristics: Drug can prolong bleeding time and inhibit platelet aggregation. Peptic ulceration and occult GI bleeding can occur and be life-threatening. Increased risk factors: smoking, alcoholism.

Nursing Implications: Assess risk, history of peptic ulcer disease or GI bleeding. Assess baseline Hgb, HCT and presence/absence of occult bleeding by guaiac of stools. Instruct patient to report signs/symptoms of abdominal pain, black stools, blood per rectum, epistaxis, menorrhagia. If patient at risk for bleeding, discuss with physician use of misoprostol to protect GI mucosa. Teach patient to avoid concurrent use of aspirin, other NSAIDs.

III. POTENTIAL SENSORY/PERCEPTUAL ALTERATIONS related to CNS CHANGES

Defining Characteristics: Dizziness, headache, nervousness, fatigue, drowsiness, malaise/light-headedness, anxiety, confusion, mental depression, and emotional lability may occur. Decreased hearing, visual acuity, changes in color vision, conjunctivitis, diplopia, and cataracts have been reported. In addition, though rare, aseptic meningitis has occurred.

Nursing Implications: Assess baseline neurologic and mental status. Instruct patient to report changes in sensory/perceptual pattern, especially VISUAL CHANGES. If visual changes occur, discuss with physician referral to ophthalmologist as soon as possible. Assess for rare occurrence of aseptic meningitis (fever, coma). Discuss drug continuance with physician for significant symptoms.

IV. ALTERATION IN NUTRITION, LESS THAN BODY REQUIREMENTS, related to HEPATIC TOXICITY

Defining Characteristics: Severe and sometimes fatal hepatotoxicity has occurred. Jaundice, hepatitis occur rarely. Borderline increase in LFTs occurs in 15% of patients, while values increase by three times in 1%.

Nursing Implications: Assess baseline LFTs and monitor periodically during long-term therapy. Instruct patient to report jaundice, abdominal pain. Discuss discontinuance of drug with physician for significant toxicity.

V. ALTERATION IN RENAL ELIMINATION related to INHIBITION OF RENAL PROSTAGLANDINS

Defining Characteristics: Acute renal failure may occur rarely within first few days of treatment in patients with preexisting renal dysfunction. Other signs/symptoms of renal dysfunction that may occur rarely are azotemia, cystitis, hematuria, increased serum BUN and creatinine, and decreased creatinine clearance. Peripheral edema has also been described.

Nursing Implications: Assess baseline renal function. Teach patient to report any changes in urinary function. Monitor periodic serum BUN, creatinine during chronic therapy.

VI. ALTERATION IN SKIN INTEGRITY related to RASH

Defining Characteristics: Rash (urticaria, vesicles, or erythematous macular) may occur, as may Stevens-Johnson syndrome, flushes, alopecia, rectal itching, and acne.

Nursing Implications: Assess baseline skin integrity and presence of lesions. Instruct patient to report abnormalities. Provide symptomatic relief for rashes, pruritus.

VII. POTENTIAL FOR FATIGUE AND INFECTION related to BONE MARROW INJURY

Defining Characteristics: Neutropenia, agranulocytosis, aplastic anemia, hemolytic anemia, and thrombocytopenia may occur rarely.

Nursing Implications: Assess baseline CBC, WBC, differential, and platelet count. Discuss abnormalities with physician. Instruct patient to report severe fatigue, infection, bleeding. Monitor lab values periodically during treatment.

Drug: salsalate (Disalcid, Salsalate, Salflex)

Class: Salicylic acid derivative, NSAID.

Mechanism of Action: Hydrolyzed into two molecules of salicylic acid. Has central and peripheral action that decreases pain perception, probably through inhibition of prostaglandin synthesis. Anti-inflammatory action via prostaglandin inhibition.

Metabolism: Absorbed completely from small intestines and widely distributed into body tissues and fluids. Elimination half-life is 1 hour. Metabolized by liver and excreted in urine. Drug DOES NOT accumulate in plasma after multiple doses, unlike salicylates.

Dosage/Range:
- 500 mg q4h or 750 mg q6h, to maximum 3 g/24 hours.

Drug Preparation:
- Not significant.

Drug Administration:
- Oral: Administer with food or 8 oz (240 mL) of water or milk.

Drug Interactions:
- Antacids, urine alkylinizers: increase salicylate excretion and decrease drug effect. Do not administer with antacids.
- Ammonium chloride, ascorbic acid, methionine (urine acidifiers): decrease salicylate excretion, so increase risk of salicylate toxicity.
- Concomitant administration with alcohol, steroids, other NSAIDs may increase GI side effects.
- Corticosteroids may increase salicylate excretion and decrease drug effect.

Lab Effects/Interference:
- Competes with thyroid hormone for protein binding, so plasma T4 may be decreased but thyroid function is unaffected.

Special Considerations:
- Use cautiously if patient has history of GI bleeding, hepatic dysfunction, renal dysfunction, hypoprothrombinemia, vitamin K deficiency, bleeding hypersensitivity.
- Contraindicated if known Salsalate hypersensitivity.

Potential Toxicities/Side Effects and the Nursing Process

I. ALTERATION IN NUTRITION, LESS THAN BODY REQUIREMENTS, related to GI TOXICITY

Defining Characteristics: Fewer GI side effects than aspirin. Nausea, dyspepsia (5–25% of patients), heartburn, epigastric discomfort, anorexia, and acute reversible hepatotoxicity may occur. Risk increases with dose. May potentiate peptic ulcer disease.

Nursing Implications: Teach patient self-administration with food or 8 oz (240 mL) water or milk. If patient is receiving antacid, administer antacid two hours after meal and Salsalate before meal. Assess baseline liver and renal function, and monitor if patient is receiving high doses on ongoing basis.

II. INJURY related to MILD SALICYLISM

Defining Characteristics: Administration of large doses of salicylates may cause salicylism, characterized by dizziness, tinnitus, diminished hearing, nausea, vomiting, diarrhea, mental confusion, CNS depression, headache, sweating, and hyperventilation at serum salicylate concentration 150–300 μg/mL (use in cancer patients usually 100 μg/mL).

Nursing Implications: Teach patient to reduce dose, interrupt dose if signs/symptoms occur. Assess concurrent medications for possible drug interactions.

III. POTENTIAL FOR BLEEDING related to INHIBITION OF PLATELET AGGREGATION, OCCULT BLEEDING, BRUISING

Defining Characteristics: Salsalate may cause prolongation of bleeding time, leukopenia, thrombocytopenia, purpura, shortened erythrocyte survival time.

Nursing Implications: Teach patient to avoid aspirin and Salsalate-containing drugs if receiving myelosuppressive chemotherapy. Review concurrent medications to identify risk for drug interactions. Monitor Hgb, HCT over time; teach patient signs/symptoms of anemia, and instruct to report them (headache, fatigue, chest pain, irritability). Monitor stool guaiacs.

IV. POTENTIAL FOR INJURY related to ALLERGIC REACTION

Defining Characteristics: Rash; hypersensitivity characterized by asthma and anaphylaxis has occurred rarely.

Nursing Implications: Assess for reactions to prior salicylate-containing medications or salsalates. Teach patient to report rash, asthmalike symptoms. If these occur, discuss alternative non-opioid analgesics. Provide systemic support if anaphylaxis occurs.

Drug: ziconotide intrathecal infusion (Prialt)

Class: Selective blocker of neuronal N-type calcium channels in the nerves which normally conduct pain signals from the periphery to the spinal cord.

Mechanism of Action: Synthetic equivalent to a naturally occurring conopeptide found in a marine snail (*Conus magus),* which binds to N-type calcium channels on the primary afferent nerves (A-δ and C) of the dorsal horn of the spinal cord. Voltage sensitive calcium channels (VSCC) permit the cell to regulate the amount of calcium entering and leaving the cell; this directly inflences membrane excitability, among other cellular processes. Ziconotide appears to block these channels so that pain messages from the periphery do not get passed through to the spinal cord and up the spinal cord where pain perception occurs.

Metabolism: Following 1 hour IT administration of 1–10 micrograms of drug, total and peak exposure were variable but dose proportional; as a continuous IT infusion, once a quantifiable serum level of drug is identified, the serum level remains constant at least up to 9 months. Drug is 50% bound to human plasma proteins, and CSF volume of distribution is the same as the total CSF volume of 140 mL. Terminal half-life in the CSF is 4.6 hours, and is cleared from the CSF at approximately the human CSF turnover rate of 0.3–0.4 mL/min. Drug passes across the blood brain barrier into systemic circulation with a serum half-life of 1.3 hrs; Drug is cleaved at multiple sites of the peptide; it is degraded via the ubiquitin-protease system in many organs (kidney, liver, lung) into component amino acids. < 1% of intact ziconotide is recovered in the urine.

Dosage/Range:

- Initial dose no more than 2.4 micrograms (mcg)/day (0.1 mcg/hr) and titrated to patient response.
- Increase dose by up to 2.4 mcg/day (0.1 mcg/hr) at intervals of no more than 2–3 times/week based on patient response, up to recommended MAXIMUM of 19.2 mcg/da (0.8 mcg/hr) by day 21.
- May use dose increases in increments of less than 2.4 mg/da less frequently than 2–3 times a week.
- With each dosage titration ensure that the pump infusion rate is adjusted correctly (either implanted microinfusion device or external microinfusion device and catheter).
- Available in 1, 2, 5 mL vials (100 micrograms/mL) for diluted use; and 20 mL vial (25 micrograms/mL) for undiluted use.
- Diluted ziconotide: use 0.9% Sodium Chloride Injection USP (preservative free) using aseptic procedures to achieve pump manufacturer's recommended concentration.

- Once the appropriate dose has been established, the 100mcg/mL formulation may be used undiluted.
- Store unopened vials at 2°C–8°C (36°F–46°F) but do not freeze; Refrigerate (2°C–8°C) after preparation, protect from light, and use within 24 hours.
- **Initial (naïve) pump priming:** use 2 mL of undiluted 25 mcg/mL formulation to rinse the internal surfaces of the pump; repeat 2× more for a total of 3 rinses.
- **Initial pump fill:** Use undiluted 25 mcg/mL ONLY to fill the naïve pump after priming; begin dosing NO HIGHER than 2.4 mcg/da (0.1mcg/hr). Initial pump fill loses drug through adsorption on internal device surfaces and by dilution in the residual space in the device—this does not occur with subsequent pump filling. Refill the pump reservoir within 14 days of the initial fill to ensure accurate drug administration.
- **Pump Refills:** Fill the pump at least every 40 days if used diluted; if undiluted drug, fill the pump at least every 60 days. Use the Medtronic refill kit to empty the pump contents prior to refill with new drug. If an implanted pump must be surgically replaced while the patient is receiving the drug, the replacement pump should be primed, and the initial drug replaced in 14 days as above.

Drug Preparation:

Zirconotide IT infusion	Initial Fill (expiration)	Refill (expiration)
25 mcg/mL undiluted	14 days	60 days
100 mcg/mL undiluted	N/A	60 days
100 mcg/mL, diluted	N/A	40 days

- Refer to manufacturer's pump manual for specific instructions. When using an external microinfusion device, and filling it the first time, use a concentration of 5 mcg/mL; dilute drug with 0.9% Sodium Chloride USP (preservative free); the flow rate for the external microinfusor usually starts at 0.02 mL/hr to deliver the initial dose rate of 2.4 mcg/day (0.1 mcg/hr).

Drug Administration:

- Continuous IT infusion via Medronic SynchroMed® EL (Medtronic Inc), SynchroMed® II Infusion System (Medtronic Inc), Simms Deltec Cadd Micro® (Ardus Medical, Inc.) External Microinfusion Device and Catheter pumps.
- Most patients continue to receive opioids.
- There is no known antidote for the drug; if overdosage, most patients recover within 24 hours after drug withdrawal; if inadvertent IV or epidural injection of drug, support blood pressure by recumbent positioning, and BP support as needed.

Drug Interactions:

- Additive effect when given with opioid medications as drug does not bind to opiate receptors.
- CNS depressant drugs: increased incidence of CNS adverse events (e.g., dizziness, confusion).

Lab Effects/Interference:

- Increased serum creatine kinase levels (40% of patients) which may be associated with muscle weakness; rare renal failure related to rhabdomyolysis and very high CK elevations.

Special Considerations:

- Severe psychiatric symptoms and neurological impairment may occur during ziconotide IT infusion; patients with a history of psychosis should NOT receive the drug; monitor patients frequently for signs/symptoms of cognitive impairment, hallucinations, or changes in mood or level of consciousness; interrupt or discontinue drug for severe psychiatric or neurological symptoms/signs.
- Drug can be interrupted or discontinued abruptly without risk of withdrawal syndrome.
- Drug is embryotoxic in animals.
- Use cautiously in elderly patients as incidence of confusion is higher; start at lower dose and titrate more slowly.
- Patients should be taught not to engage in hazardous activity, such as operation of heavy machinery.
- Patients should notify provider IMMEDIATELY for any of the following:
  - Change in mental status such as lethargy, confusion, disorientation, decreased alertness.
  - Change in mood or perception, such as hallucinations (e.g., unusual tactile sensations in oral cavity).
  - Symptoms of depression or suicidal ideation.
  - Nausea, vomiting, seizures, fever, headache, and/or stiff neck as these may herald developing meningitis.

Potential Toxicities/Side Effects and the Nursing Process

I. SENSORY/PERCEPTUAL ALTERATIONS related to CNS CHANGES

Defining Characteristics: CNS depression and changes in mental status may occur, including psychiatric symptoms, cognitive impairment and decreased alertness/unresponsiveness. These are characterized by confusion (33%, with a higher incidence in the elderly), memory impairment (22%), speech disorder (14%), aphasia (12%), abnormal thinking (8%), and amnesia (1%). Psychiatric symptoms are more likely to occur in patients with pretreatment psychiatric disorders, and include hallucinations (12%), paranoid ideation (2%), hostility

(2%), delirium (2%), psychosis (1%), and manic reactions (0.4%). Cognitive impairment may be gradual a few weeks after starting therapy. Once dose is interrupted or discontinued, symptoms usually resolve in 2 weeks. Patients may become depressed with suicidal ideation. Other sensory/perceptual alterations include: dizziness (47%), somnolence (22%), abnormal vision (22%), ataxia (16%), abnormal gait (15%), hypertonia (11%), nystagmus (8%), dysesthesia (7%), paresthesia (7%), and vertigo (7%).

Nursing Implications: Assess past medical history for psychiatric and neurological problems. Assess baseline gait, movement, mental, affective, and neurologic status. Assess medication profile to identify other contributions, i.e., CNS depressants, antiepileptics, neuroleptics, sedatives, diuretics. Teach patient and family that these side effects may occur, and instruct patient/family to report any changes. Teach patient/family to notify provider IMMEDIATELY for any of the following:

- Change in mental status such as lethargy, confusion, disorientation, decreased alertness.
- Change in mood or perception, such as hallucinations (e.g., unusual tactile sensations in oral cavity).
- Symptoms of depression or suicidal ideation.

Assess patient safety, and measures to ensure safety. Discuss any significant changes with physician, and need to interrupt/discontinue drug based on severity of symptoms.

OPIOID ANALGESICS

Drug: codeine (as Sulfate or Phosphate); may be combined with acetaminophen (Phenaphen with Codeine, Tylenol with Codeine, Capital and Codeine, Codaphen (Odalan), or with aspirin (Empirin with Codeine, Soma Compound with Codeine, Fiorinal with Codeine)

Class: Opioid analgesic (opioid agonist).

Mechanism of Action: Resembles morphine but has milder action; binds to opiate receptors in CNS (limbic system, thalamus, striatum, hypothalamus, midbrain, spinal cord), altering pain perception at level of spinal cord and higher centers, as well as the emotional response to pain. Also suppresses cough reflex.

Metabolism: Well absorbed after oral or parenteral administration. Metabolized by liver; excreted in urine, and small amount in feces.

Dosage/Range:

- Mild pain: 30 mg q4h (range 15–60 mg), PO, SQ, or IM.

Drug Preparation:
- Store tablets in tight, light-resistant containers at 15–30°C (59–86°F).
- Injection should be protected from light and stored at 15–40°C (59–104°F).
- At home, teach patient to store oral doses in a safe place away from children and pets.

Drug Administration:
- PO, SQ, IM.

Drug Interactions:
- Injection is incompatible with solutions containing aminophylline, ammonium chloride, amobarbital sodium, chlorothiazide sodium, heparin sodium, methicillin sodium, nitrofurantoin, phenobarbital sodium, sodium bicarbonate.
- Alcohol, CNS depressants: additive effects.

Lab Effects/Interference:
- None known.

Special Considerations:
- Parenteral dose is 2/3 oral dose for equianalgesic effect.
- Onset of action after PO or SQ dose is 15–30 minutes, with duration of analgesia 4–6 hours.
- Indicated for relief of mild-to-moderate pain unrelieved by nonopiate analgesia.
- Addition of acetaminophen or aspirin gives additive analgesia.
- Give smallest effective dose to prevent development of tolerance, physical dependency.
- Reduce dose in debilitated patients, or patients receiving other CNS depressants.
- Use with caution in patients with hepatic or renal dysfunction, hypothyroidism, Addison's disease, severe CNS depression, respiratory depression, head injury, elevated intracranial pressure.
- If required, naloxone HCl (Narcan) will reverse opiate toxicity (e.g., respiratory depression). However, it is important that acute withdrawal symptoms be prevented by giving only enough naloxone to reverse respiratory depression and that this be continued for opioid drug half-life.

MANAGEMENT

Potential Toxicities/Side Effects and the Nursing Process

I. SENSORY/PERCEPTUAL ALTERATIONS related to CNS DEPRESSION

Defining Characteristics: Drowsiness, sedation, mood changes, euphoria, dysphoria, dizziness, mental clouding may occur. At high doses, may cause seizures. Miosis (papillary constriction) may occur.

Nursing Implications: Assess baseline neurologic status. Use cautiously, if at all, in patients with head injury, increased intracranial pressure, severe CNS depression, acute alcoholism, or who are elderly or debilitated. Assess other concurrent medications. Use with caution in patients receiving other opioids, tranquilizers, hypnotics, monoamine oxidase (MAO) inhibitors, since increasing CNS depressant effects can occur. Monitor neurologic status closely. Teach patient to avoid driving and operating machinery while taking the medicine, and to AVOID concurrent alcohol.

II. ALTERATION IN OXYGENATION related to RESPIRATORY DEPRESSION

Defining Characteristics: Opiate agonists directly depress respiratory center in brain stem, causing decreased sensitivity and responsiveness to increased pCO2 (CO2 tension in serum). Also may depress deep breathing and reflex to sigh. Tolerance to respiratory depressant effects occurs with chronic use.

Nursing Implications: Assess baseline pulmonary status, and monitor periodically during drug use. Use cautiously in patients with bronchial asthma, chronic obstructive pulmonary disease (COPD), respiratory depression, and monitor closely.

III. ALTERATION IN ELIMINATION related to CONSTIPATION, ILEUS

Defining Characteristics: Opium agonists bind to opiate receptors in bowel, slowing peristalsis, leading to constipation. Untreated constipation may result in bowel perforation.

Nursing Implications: Assess baseline elimination, fluid intake, diet, and exercise patterns. Teach patient about prevention of constipation: goal is to move bowels at least every two days by increasing fluid intake to 3 L/day, following a diet high in fiber (beans, vegetables, fruit), and taking moderate exercise. Assess need for bowel softeners, bulk-forming laxatives, and osmotic cathartics, and discuss prescription with physician. Teach patient self-administration of medications.

IV. ALTERATION IN NUTRITION, LESS THAN BODY REQUIREMENTS, related to GI TOXICITY

Defining Characteristics: Nausea, vomiting, dry mouth may occur. Gastric, biliary, and pancreatic secretions are decreased by opiate agonists; digestion is delayed. Biliary tract muscle tone is increased, and spasm of Oddi's sphincter may occur (morphine > meperidine > codeine).

Nursing Implications: Assess patient tolerance of GI side effects. Teach patient to report side effects. If nausea/vomiting occur, change to another opioid, or premedicate with antiemetic to prevent nausea/vomiting. Assess GI pain, biliary spasm, and consider alternative opioid.

V. ALTERATION IN CARDIAC OUTPUT related to HYPOTENSION, BRADYCARDIA

Defining Characteristics: Orthostatic hypotension, bradycardia due to cholinergic effect, and peripheral vasodilation may occur with rapid IV dosing. There may be histamine-related flushing, pruritus, diaphoresis with chronic drug usage; tolerance develops to this effect.

Nursing Implications: Assess baseline cardiovascular status. Teach patient to change position slowly and to hold onto stable, nearby structure for support as needed. Be careful when giving IV push opioids, and caution patient to remain in supine position for 15–20 minutes after injection. Monitor cardiovascular status after injection.

VI. ALTERATION IN URINE ELIMINATION related to URINARY RETENTION

Defining Characteristics: Increased smooth muscle tone in urinary tract and spasm may occur. Bladder tone is increased, with may cause urgency. Vesical sphincter tone may be increased, leading to difficulty urinating. Increased risk of urinary retention in patients with prostatic hypertrophy or urethral stricture.

Nursing Implications: Assess baseline urinary elimination pattern. Teach patient to increase fluids to 3 L/day, and encourage voiding every 2–3 hours. Instruct patient to report problems with urination.

VII. KNOWLEDGE DEFICIT related to DRUG ADMINISTRATION, POTENTIAL FOR TOLERANCE, AND DEPENDENCY

Defining Characteristics: Psychological dependence (addiction) occurs rarely in patients taking opioid agonists for cancer pain (< 1%). Physical dependence (precipitation of withdrawal symptoms) occurs with chronic use of the drug for the relief of chronic cancer pain. In addition, tolerance, or less analgesic effect over time with the same drug dose, occurs and requires increased dosage of drug.

Nursing Implications: Assess baseline knowledge of opioid analgesics, and attitude about their use for cancer pain management. Teach patient about proper self-administration, possible side effects, and self-care measures. Suggest patient maintain diary of pain intensity, precipitating and alleviating factors, drug dose and time taken, and relief. Teach patient to self-administer opioid agonists for relief of chronic cancer pain around-the-clock, not PRN, to prevent pain. Explain use of prescribed short-acting opioid for rescue or to manage breakthrough pain. Discuss with physician dose increase or change in frequency of administration if tolerance develops. Teach patient that withdrawal symptoms may occur if chronic, around-the-clock dosing is interrupted. Withdrawal (abstinence) symptoms that may be seen are restlessness, lacrimation, rhinorrhea, yawning, perspiration, gooseflesh, restless sleep, mydriasis in first 24 hours. These are followed by twitching and leg spasm; severe aching of the back, abdomen, and legs; cramping in abdomen and legs; hot/cold flashes; insomnia; nausea/vomiting, diarrhea; severe sneezing; and increased heart rate, BP, and temperature (T), which peak at 36–72 hours. Withdrawal syndrome can be prevented by administration of at least 1/4 of previous opioid dose.

VIII. SEXUAL DYSFUNCTION related to IMPOTENCE, ↓ LIBIDO

Defining Characteristics: Opiate agonists may suppress gonadotropin, causing impotence and decreased libido.

Nursing Implications: Assess baseline sexual pattern. Discuss potential toxicity and impact on sexuality. Provide information, emotional support, and referral as needed.

Drug: fentanyl citrate (Oral Transmucosal Fentanyl, Actiq)

Class: Opioid analgesic (opioid agonist).

Mechanism of Action: Fentanyl is a pure opioid agonist that binds to opioid μ-receptors located in the brain, spinal cord, and smooth muscle. The oral transmucosal preparation of the drug is a solid formulation of fentanyl citrate placed on a handle so the drug is sucked. Sucking, the drug dose coats the oral mucosa, through which the drug is rapidly absorbed, reportedly as fast as IV morphine. Onset of analgesia is approximately 5 minutes from onset of administration, with maximum effect in 20–30 minutes.

Metabolism: Initial rapid absorption of about 25% of total dose across buccal mucosa, into systemic circulation, and longer prolonged absorption of swallowed fentanyl (75% of dose) from GI tract. One-third of drug escapes first-pass elimination and enters the systemic circulation for a total of 50% of the total dose that is bioavailable. Following absorption, drug is rapidly distributed to brain, heart, lungs, kidneys, spleen. Plasma binding is 80–85%. The drug is primarily metabolized in the liver, and less than 7% of the dose is excreted in the urine. The terminal elimination half-life is approximately 219 minutes.

Dosage/Range:
Adult:
- Titrate to patient's individual needs: available in six strengths that are color-coded: 200-, 400-, 600-, 800-, 1200-, and 1600-μg fentanyl base.

- Drug CANNOT be used in opioid-naïve patients, and is indicated for the management of chronic pain, especially breakthrough pain in patients who are ALREADY RECEIVING AND WHO ARE TOLERANT to opioid therapy (e.g., taking at least 60 mg of morphine/day, 50 μg/hr of transdermal fentanyl, or an equianalgesic dose of another opioid for a week or longer).
- Patient begins using 200 μg unit for breakthrough pain (BTP) and sucks the medicine for 15 minutes. If the pain is unrelieved, the patient waits an additional 15 minutes then administers a second 200-μg unit. If the pain is unrelieved, the patient waits another 15 minutes and administers a third 200-μg unit. Three units of any dosage is the maximum drug per BTP episode.
- If the patient required two units of 200-μg dosage, then the patient would give 400-μg dose for the next episode of BTP. If using two 200-μg units, the patient would wait 15 minutes between taking units.
- If the patient needed three units of 200-μg dose, the patient would take the 600-μg strength the next dose for BTP.
- The patient should notify the physician if drug is required more than four times per day, so that the long-acting opioid can be increased.

Drug Preparation/Administration:

- Drug is on a handle, sealed in a child-resistant foil pouch that requires scissors to open. The drug dose is color-coded.
- Open foil pack immediately before use. Patient should place drug dose unit in the mouth between cheek and lower gum. Patient should suck, NOT CHEW, the medication over 15 minutes.
- If the patient achieves adequate analgesia or develops excessive side effects, the drug should be removed from the mouth and discarded immediately. The remaining drug is very dangerous if a child or pet ingests it, so maximum precautions must be taken.
- To discard the remaining drug, twist drug off handle using tissue paper, and flush medicine down the toilet. Destroy any medication remaining on the handle by dissolving it under hot water.
- Keep medication away from patient's eyes, skin, or mucous membranes when not sucking the medication, and the patient should wash hands after discarding unused medication portion.
- At home, teach patient to store oral doses in a safe place away from children and pets.

Drug Interactions:

- CNS depressants (e.g., other opioids, alcohol, sedatives, hypnotics, general anesthetics, phenothiazines, tranquilizers, skeletal muscle relaxants, sedating antihistamines) may increase CNS depression (hypoventilation, hypotension, profound sedation, especially in opioid nontolerant patients).

Lab Effects/Interference:

- None known.

Special Considerations:

- CONTRAINDICATED in opioid-nontolerant patients, as life-threatening hypoventilation may occur; in children < 10 kg for management of acute postoperative pain; in patients with hypersensitivity to fentanyl; in patients with head injury and increased intracranial pressure (ICP); and in nursing mothers.
- Administer cautiously to patients with hepatic or renal dysfunction.
- Teach patient drug must be kept out of reach of children as dose can be LETHAL to children.
- Use cautiously in patients with chronic pulmonary disease (degree of hypoventilation), cardiac conduction disease (bradycardia), and the elderly.
- Respiratory depression may be associated with opioids, and patients should be monitored for this. This was not reported in the clinical trials with Actiq.
- Patients should be taught to call nurse or physician if taking four of the same strength units within 60 minutes without relief or if taking drug more than four times per day.
- Once effective dose determined, drug provides rapid relief of BTP.
- Some reported toxicities may be due to advanced malignancy rather than the drug.

Potential Toxicities/Side Effects and the Nursing Process

I. ALTERATION IN OXYGENATION related to HYPOVENTILATION

Defining Characteristics: Dyspnea (10%), increased cough and pharyngitis (3–10%).

Nursing Implications: Assess baseline pulmonary status. Use with caution in patients with COPD, bradycardia, renal or hepatic dysfunction, and in the elderly. Teach patient to report any pulmonary difficulties immediately. Ensure patient knows that if respiratory difficulty develops, the drug must be removed from mouth and discarded immediately; also, to suck and not chew drug. Ensure that patient understands how to handle drug safely to prevent additional absorption of unused drug.

II. SENSORY/PERCEPTUAL ALTERATIONS related to CNS CHANGES

Defining Characteristics: CNS depression and changes in mental status may occur, characterized by somnolence or dizziness (10%); abnormal gait, anxiety, confusion, depression, insomnia, hypesthesia, vasodilation, abnormal vision (3–10% incidence).

Nursing Implications: Assess baseline gait, mental, affective, and neurologic status. Assess medication profile to identify other contributions, i.e., CNS depressants. Instruct patient to report any changes. Assess patient safety, and measures to ensure safety. Discuss any significant changes with physician.

III. ALTERATION IN COMFORT related to HEADACHE, FEVER

Defining Characteristics: Headache, fever, asthenia are reported in ~10% of patients; less commonly, myalgia, pruritus, rash, sweating occur in 3–10% of patients.

Nursing Implications: Assess baseline comfort. Teach patient to report symptoms and manage based on severity. Assess impact on patient's quality of life. If severe, discuss alternative strategies with physician.

IV. ALTERATION IN NUTRITION, LESS THAN BODY REQUIREMENTS, related to NAUSEA/VOMITING

Defining Characteristics: Nausea, vomiting are reported in ~10% of patients; less commonly, anorexia, dehydration, edema, and dyspepsia occur in 3–10% of patients.

Nursing Implications: Assess baseline nutritional status. Teach patient to report nausea, vomiting, anorexia, dyspepsia. Manage symptomatically. Assess severity and impact on quality of life. Discuss severe or unmanaged symptoms with physician.

V. ALTERATION IN ELIMINATION related to CONSTIPATION OR DIARRHEA

Defining Characteristics: Opium agonists bind to opiate receptors in bowel, slowing peristalsis, leading to constipation. Untreated constipation may result in bowel perforation. Opiate receptors in bowel decrease peristalsis. Constipation and diarrhea were each reported in < 10% of patients.

Nursing Implications: Assess baseline elimination, fluid intake, diet, and exercise patterns. Instruct patient regarding prevention of constipation: goal is to move bowels at least every two days by increasing fluids to 3 L/day, following a diet high in fiber (beans, vegetables, fruit), and taking moderate exercise. Assess need for bowel softeners, bulk-forming laxatives, and osmotic cathartics, and discuss prescription with physician. Teach patient self-administration of medications. MUST be started on bowel regimen.

Drug: fentanyl transdermal system (Duragesic)

Class: Opioid analgesic (opioid agonist).

Mechanism of Action: Strong opioid analgesic; 20–30 times more potent than parenteral morphine when given transdermally to opioid-naïve patients. Drug interacts primarily with opioid μ-receptors, found in the brain, spinal cord, and other tissues, causing analgesia and sedation. Duragesic patches provide continuous-released fentanyl from a transdermal reservoir system at a constant amount per unit time. The drug moves from areas of higher concentration (patch) to areas of lower concentration (skin). Initially, the skin under the patch absorbs the fentanyl, and the drug is concentrated in the upper skin layers. The drug gradually enters the systemic circulation, leveling off 2–24 hours later, and remaining fairly constant for the 72-hour application period.

Metabolism: Primarily metabolized by the liver; 75% of IV dose excreted in urine, 9% in feces, and < 10% as unchanged drug. Peak levels occur 24–72 hours after a single application. Half-life is approximately 17 hours (after system removal, serum fentanyl concentrations fall to 50% in approximately 17 hours; range, 13–22 hours).

Dosage/Range:
25 μg/hour is initial dosage for non-opioid-tolerant patients.
Doses for patients currently receiving opioid analgesics who are tolerant can be calculated from the following table:

Duragesic Dose Prescription Based on Daily Morphine Equivalence Dose

Oral 24-hour Morphine (mg/day)	IM 24-hour Morphine (mg/day)	DURAGESIC Dose (μg/hr)
45–134	8–22	25
135–224	23–37	50
225–314	38–52	75
315–404	53–67	100
405–494	68–82	125
495–584	83–97	150
585–674	98–112	175
675–764	113–127	200
765–854	128–142	225
855–944	143–157	250
945–1034	158–172	275
1035–1124	173–187	300

Drug Preparation:
- None.

Drug Administration:

- Apply to nonirritated and nonirradiated skin; clip hair (not shave) as needed. May cleanse with water only and dry completely if necessary. Apply patch immediately after removal from package. Press firmly into place with palm of hand for 10–20 seconds, making sure contact is complete, especially around edges. Patient wears for 72 hours, then changes patch. Some patients may need to reapply new patches every 48 hours. Short-acting opioids must be continued for 24 hours until serum fentanyl level achieved.
- Disposal: at home, patient must fold so adhesive side of system adheres to itself, then flush down toilet. In hospital, used patches must be returned to pharmacy for proper disposal.
- At home, teach patient to store oral doses in a safe place away from children and pets.

Drug Interactions:

- Potentiation of CNS depressant effects, when administered concurrently with other opioids, benzodiazepines, or other CNS depressants.

Lab Effects/Interference:

- None known.

Special Considerations:

- Indications: patients with chronic pain requiring opioid analgesia.
- Contraindicated in patients with known hypersensitivity to fentanyl or adhesives. Use with caution in the following patients: patients with COPD predisposed to hypoventilation; patients with head injuries, brain tumor (very sensitive to effects of CO_2 retention); patients with cardiac disease (may cause bradyarrhythmias); patients with hepatic dysfunction.
- Availability: Dosages: 25 μg/h, 50 μg/h, 75 μg/h, and 100 μg/h. Supplied in one carton containing five individually wrapped patches.

Potential Toxicities/Side Effects and the Nursing Process

I. ALTERATION IN OXYGENATION related to HYPOVENTILATION

Defining Characteristics: Dyspnea, hypoventilation, apnea (3–10% of patients); hemoptysis, pharyngitis, hiccups rare; stertorous breathing, asthma, respiratory dysfunction.

Nursing Implications: Assess baseline pulmonary status. Use with caution in patients with COPD, brain tumors, increased intracranial pressure (ICP), hepatic failure. NEVER exceed 25 μg/h if patient not tolerant to opioids. Must continue to observe patient for 17 hours after dose removed for signs/symptoms of toxicity—same is true if naloxone HCl (Narcan) required to reverse opioid. Theoretically, a temperature of 39°C (102°F) will increase serum fentanyl by 33% due to drug delivery and skin absorption. If patient develops fever, observe for signs/symptoms of overdosage. Elderly patients (> 60–65 years old) may have reduced ability to clear drug, so start at 25 μg/hr unless already tolerant of > 135 mg morphine sulfate/24 hours.

II. SENSORY/PERCEPTUAL ALTERATIONS related to CNS CHANGES

Defining Characteristics: CNS depression and changes in mental status may occur, characterized by somnolence, confusion, depression, asthenia (> 10%), dizziness, nervousness, hallucinations, anxiety, depression, euphoria (3–10%), tremors, abnormal coordination, speech disorder, abnormal thinking, dreams. Rare: aphasia, vertigo, stupor, hypotonia, hypertonia, hostility.

Nursing Implications: Assess baseline mental, neurologic status. Dose of other opioids and benzodiazepines should be 50%. Use cautiously in substance abusers.

III. ALTERATION IN CARDIAC OUTPUT related to ARRYTHMIA, ANGINA

Defining Characteristics: Arrhythmia, chest pain may occur; IV fentanyl has caused bradyarrhythmias.

Nursing Implications: Assess baseline cardiac status, and monitor during drug use. Instruct patient to report palpitations, chest pain.

IV. ALTERATION IN NUTRITION, LESS THAN BODY REQUIREMENTS, related to NAUSEA, VOMITING

Defining Characteristics: Nausea, vomiting, anorexia, dyspepsia, rare abdominal distension.

Nursing Implications: Assess baseline nutritional status. Instruct patient to report nausea, vomiting, anorexia, dyspepsia.

V. ALTERATION IN ELIMINATION related to CONSTIPATION, ILEUS

Defining Characteristics: Opium agonists bind to opiate receptors in bowel, slowing peristalsis, leading to constipation. Untreated constipation may result in bowel perforation. Opiate receptors in bowel decrease peristalsis.

Nursing Implications: Assess baseline elimination, fluid intake, diet, and exercise patterns. Instruct patient regarding prevention of constipation: goal is to move bowels at least every two days, by increasing fluids to 3 L/day, following a diet high in fiber (beans, vegetables, fruit), and taking moderate exercise. Assess need for bowel softeners, bulk-forming laxatives, and osmotic cathartics, and discuss prescription with physician. Teach patient self-administration of medications. MUST be started on bowel regimen.

VI. ALTERATION IN CARDIAC OUTPUT related to HYPOTENSION, BRADYCARDIA

Defining Characteristics: Orthostatic hypotension, bradycardia due to cholinergic effect, and peripheral vasodilation may occur with rapid IV dosing. There may be histamine-related flushing, pruritus, diaphoresis with chronic drug usage; tolerance develops to this effect.

Nursing Implications: Assess baseline cardiovascular status. Teach patient to change position slowly and to hold onto stable, nearby structure for support as needed. Be careful when giving IV push opioids, and caution patient to remain in supine position for 15–20 minutes after injection. Monitor cardiovascular status after injection.

VII. ALTERATION IN URINE ELIMINATION related to URINARY RETENTION

Defining Characteristics: Increased smooth muscle tone in urinary tract and spasm may occur. Bladder tone is increased, which may cause urgency. Vesical sphincter tone may be increased, leading to difficulty urinating. Increased risk of urinary retention in patients with prostatic hypertrophy or urethral stricture. Rare bladder pain, oliguria, urinary frequency.

Nursing Implications: Assess baseline urinary elimination pattern. Teach patient to increase fluids to 3 L/day, and encourage voiding every 2–3 hours. Instruct patient to report problems with urination.

VIII. ALTERATION IN SKIN INTEGRITY/COMFORT related to RASH, PRURITUS

Defining Characteristics: Sweating, pruritus, rash; erythema, papules, itching, edema, exfoliative dermatitis, pustules at application site; headache rare.

Nursing Implications: Teach patient proper drug application and to rotate sites.

Drug: hydromorphone (Dilaudid)

Class: Opioid analgesic (opioid agonist).

Mechanism of Action: Resembles morphine but has milder action; binds to opiate receptors in CNS (limbic system, thalamus, striatum, hypothalamus, midbrain, spinal cord), altering pain perception at level of spinal cord and higher centers as well as the emotional response to pain. Also suppresses cough reflex.

Metabolism: Well absorbed after oral, rectal, and parenteral administration. Onset of action is 15–30 minutes (more rapid than morphine), with a duration of action of 4–5 hours. Metabolized by liver and excreted in urine.

Dosage/Range:
- Use caution in patients who have not received opiates before and have not developed tolerance.
- Moderate pain: oral: 1–6 mg q4–6h; SQ or IM: 2–4 mg q4–6h, 3 mg rectal suppository.
- Severe pain: oral: 4 mg or more q4h; SQ or IM: 4 mg or more, then titrate based on patient response and tolerance.

Drug Preparation:
- Store tablets in tight, light-resistant containers at 15–30°C (59–86°F).
- Injection should be protected from light and stored at 15–40°C (59–104°F).

Drug Administration:
- PO, SQ, IM. Use highly concentrated injectable solution for patients who are tolerant to opiate agonists.
- At home, teach patient to store oral doses in a safe place away from children and pets.

Drug Interactions:
- Alcohol, CNS depressants: Additive effects.

Lab Effects/Interference:
- None known.

Special Considerations:
- Parenteral dose is 1/5 oral dose for equianalgesic effect.
- Indicated for relief of moderate-to-severe pain.
- Additive benefit when combined with acetaminophen or aspirin.
- Give smallest effective dose to prevent development of tolerance, physical dependency.
- Reduce dose in debilitated patients or patients receiving other CNS depressants.
- Use with caution in patients with hepatic or renal dysfunction, hypothyroidism, Addison's disease, severe CNS depression, respiratory depression, head injury, elevated ICP.
- If required, naloxone HCl will reverse opiate toxicity (e.g., respiratory depression). However, it is important that acute withdrawal symptoms be prevented by giving only enough naloxone to reverse respiratory depression and that this be continued for opioid drug half-life.

Potential Toxicities/Side Effects and the Nursing Process

I. SENSORY/PERCEPTUAL ALTERATIONS related to CNS DEPRESSION

Defining Characteristics: Drowsiness, sedation, mood changes, euphoria, dysphoria, dizziness, mental clouding may occur. At high doses, may cause seizures. Miosis (papillary constriction) may occur.

Nursing Implications: Assess baseline neurologic status. Use cautiously, if at all, in patients with head injury, increased ICP, severe CNS depression, acute alcoholism, the elderly, and the debilitated. Assess other concurrent medications. Use with caution in patients receiving other opioids, tranquilizers, hypnotics, MAO inhibitors, since increasing CNS depressant effects can occur. Monitor neurologic status closely. Teach patient to avoid driving and operating machinery while taking the medicine, and to AVOID concurrent alcohol.

II. ALTERATION IN OXYGENATION related to RESPIRATORY DEPRESSION

Defining Characteristics: Opiate agonists directly depress respiratory center in brain stem, causing decreased sensitivity and responsiveness to increased pCO_2. Also may depress deep breathing and reflex to sigh. Tolerance to respiratory depressant effects occurs with chronic use.

Nursing Implications: Assess baseline pulmonary status, and monitor periodically during drug use. Use cautiously in patients with bronchial asthma, COPD, respiratory depression, and monitor closely.

III. ALTERATION IN ELIMINATION related to CONSTIPATION, ILEUS

Defining Characteristics: Opium agonists bind to opiate receptors in bowel, slowing peristalsis, leading to constipation. Untreated constipation may result in bowel perforation.

Nursing Implications: Assess baseline elimination, fluid intake, diet, and exercise patterns. Instruct patient about prevention of constipation: goal is to move bowels at least every two days by increasing fluids to 3 L/day, following a diet high in fiber (beans, vegetables, fruit), and taking moderate exercise. Assess need for bowel softeners, bulk-forming laxatives, and osmotic cathartics, and discuss prescription with physician. Teach patient self-administration of medications.

IV. ALTERATION IN NUTRITION related to GI TOXICITY

Defining Characteristics: Nausea, vomiting, and dry mouth may occur. Gastric, biliary, and pancreatic secretions are decreased by opiate agonists; digestion is delayed. Biliary tract muscle tone is increased, and spasm of Oddi's sphincter may occur (morphine > meperidine > codeine).

Nursing Implications: Assess patient tolerance of GI side effects. Teach patient to report side effects. If nausea/vomiting occur, change to another opioid, or premedicate with antiemetic to prevent nausea/vomiting. Assess GI pain, biliary spasm, and consider alternative opioid.

V. ALTERATION IN CARDIAC OUTPUT related to HYPOTENSION, BRADYCARDIA

Defining Characteristics: Orthostatic hypotension, bradycardia due to cholinergic effect, and peripheral vasodilation may occur with rapid IV dosing. There may be histamine-related flushing, pruritus, diaphoresis with chronic drug usage; tolerance develops to this effect.

Nursing Implications: Assess baseline cardiovascular status. Teach patient to change position slowly and to hold onto stable, nearby structure for support as needed. Be careful when giving IV push opioids, and caution patient to remain in supine position for 15–20 minutes after injection. Monitor cardiovascular status after injection.

VI. ALTERATION IN URINE ELIMINATION related to URINARY RETENTION

Defining Characteristics: Increased smooth muscle tone in urinary tract and spasm may occur. Bladder tone is increased, which may cause urgency. Vesical sphincter tone may be increased, leading to difficulty urinating. Increased risk of urinary retention in patients with prostatic hypertrophy or urethral stricture.

Nursing Implications: Assess baseline urinary elimination pattern. Teach patient to increase fluids to 3 L/day, and encourage voiding every 2–3 hours. Instruct patient to report problems with urination.

VII. KNOWLEDGE DEFICIT related to DRUG ADMINISTRATION, POTENTIAL FOR TOLERANCE, AND DEPENDENCY

Defining Characteristics: Psychological dependence (addiction) occurs rarely in patients taking opioid agonists for cancer pain (< 1%). Physical dependence (precipitation of withdrawal symptoms) occurs with chronic use of the drug for the relief of chronic cancer pain. In addition, tolerance, or less analgesic effect over time with the same drug dose, occurs and requires increased dosage of drug.

Nursing Implications: Assess baseline knowledge of opioid analgesics and attitude about their use for cancer pain management. Teach patient about proper self-administration, possible side effects, and self-care measures. Suggest patient maintain diary of pain intensity, precipitating and alleviating factors, drug dose and time taken, and relief. Teach patient to self-administer opioid agonists for relief of chronic cancer pain around-the-clock, not PRN, to prevent pain. Explain use of prescribed short-acting opioid for rescue or to manage BTP. Discuss with physician dose increase or change in frequency of administration if tolerance develops. Teach patient that withdrawal symptoms may occur if chronic, around-the-clock dosing is interrupted. Withdrawal (abstinence) symptoms that may be seen are restlessness, lacrimation, rhinorrhea, yawning, perspiration, gooseflesh, restless sleep, mydriasis in first 24 hours. These are followed by twitching and leg spasm; severe aching of the back, abdomen, and legs; cramping in abdomen and legs; hot/cold flashes; insomnia; nausea/vomiting, diarrhea; severe sneezing; and increased heart rate, BP, T, which peak at 36–72 hours. Withdrawal syndrome can be prevented by administration of at least 1/4 of previous opioid dose.

VIII. SEXUAL DYSFUNCTION related to IMPOTENCE, ↓ LIBIDO

Defining Characteristics: Opiate agonists may suppress gonadotropin, causing impotence and decreased libido.

Nursing Implications: Assess baseline sexual pattern. Discuss potential toxicity and impact on sexuality. Provide information, emotional support, and referral as needed.

Drug: hydromorphone extended release capsules (Palladone)

Class: Opioid analgesic (opioid agonist, extended release).

Mechanism of Action: Resembles morphine but has milder action; binds to opiate receptors in CNS (limbic system, thalamus, striatum, hypothalamus, midbrain, spinal cord), altering pain perception at level of spinal cord and higher centers as well as the emotional response to pain. Also suppresses cough reflex.

Metabolism: Well absorbed after oral administration, with biphasic absorption: initial, rapid peak with second, braoder peak characterized by therapeutic serum concentration maintained over 24 hours. Two- to three-fold reduction in serum concentration fluctuations compared to immediate release hydromorphone. Terminal half-life of 18 hours, and steady state plasma concentration reached in 2–3 days so dose titration should be every 2–3 days. Metabolized by liver and excreted in urine.

Dosage/Range:

- For use in patients who have received opiates before and who are opioid tolerant; DO NOT USE in patients for whom this is the first opioid product prescribed, or in patients who require opioid analgesia for a short period of time.
- Available in 12, 16, 24, and 32 mg dosage strengths.
- To determine dosage,
  - Use standard equianalgesic dosing table, or conversion table below, to determine equivalent total daily dose of oral hydromorphone in a 24-hour period—these tables provide a ''reasonable starting point'' but have not been verified in well-controlled, multiple-dose trials.
  - Adjust dose as needed based on patient variables.
  - Round off dose to nearest capsule strength.
  - Discontinue all other around-the-clock opioid analgesics when extended release hydromorphone is initiated.
  - Titrate dose based on patient response, recognizing the steady state serum levels require 2–3 days until it is possible to assess full drug effect.
- Dose conversion from other opioids to hydromorphone from manufacturer Purdue Pharma; multiplication factors for converting the daily dose of prior opioids to the daily dose of oral hydromorphone* (mg/day prior opioid X factor = mg/day oral hydromorphone):

Prior Opioid	**ORAL**	**PARENTERAL**
Codeine	0.04	—
Hydrocodone	0.22	–
Hydromorphone	1.00	5.00
Levorphanol	1.88	3.75
Meperidine	0.02	0.10
Methadone	0.38	0.75
Morphine	0.12	0.75
Oxycodone	0.25	–

***To be used only for conversion TO oral hydromorphone. For patients receiving high-dose parenteral opioids, a more conservative conversion is warranted. For example, for high dose parenteral morphine, use 0.38 instead of 0.75 as a multiplication factor, i.e., halve the multiplication factor** (http://www.fda.gov/cder/foi/label/2004/021044lbl.pdf, accessed July 5, 2005.)

Drug Preparation:

- Store capsules at 25°C (77°F), with excursions permitted from 15–30°C (59–86°F). Teach patient to store in a safe place away from children and pets.

Drug Administration:

- Oral; DO NOT crush, open, dissolve or break the capsules–must be swallowed whole as otherwise a potentially lethal rapid release and absorption of hydromorphone will occur.

Drug Interactions:

- Alcohol, CNS depressants: Additive effects.

Lab Effects/Interference:

- None known.

Special Considerations:

- Parenteral dose is 1/5 oral dose for equianalgesic effect.
- Indicated for relief of persistent moderate-to-severe pain in patients requiring continuous, around-the-clock analgesia with a high potency opioid for an extended period of time.
  - Patients MUST be opioid tolerant, and pain must require at least an equivalent opioid dose of 12 mg of hydromorphone a day (24-hour period).
  - For example, the patient must be taking at least 60 mg of oral morphine/day or at least 30 mg of oxycodone/day or at least 8 mg of hydromorphone/day or an equianalgesic dose of another opioid, *for a week or longer.*
- Additive benefit when combined with acetaminophen or aspirin.
- Give smallest effective dose to prevent development of physical dependency. *Adequate dose* is defined as providing effective pain control so the patient requires *2 or less break-through opioid immediate release doses per 24-hour period.*
- Reduce dose in debilitated patients or patients receiving other CNS depressants.
- Use with caution in patients with hepatic or renal dysfunction, hypotension, severe CNS depression, respiratory depression or pulmonary diseases such as Chronic Obstructive Pulmonary Disease, head injury, elevated ICP.
- Contraindicated in patients: requiring opioids on an as needed basis (e.g., PRN); in situations of significant respiratory depression (especially in unmonitored settings); acute or severe bronchial asthma; who have or are suspected of having paralytic ileus; who have known hypersensitivity to hydromorphone or any of the ingredients.

- If required, naloxone HCl will reverse opiate toxicity (e.g., respiratory depression). However, it is important that acute withdrawal symptoms be prevented by giving only enough naloxone to reverse respiratory depression and that this be continued for opioid drug half-life of 18 hours.

Potential Toxicities/Side Effects and the Nursing Process

I. SENSORY/PERCEPTUAL ALTERATIONS related to CNS DEPRESSION

Defining Characteristics: Drowsiness, sedation, mood changes, euphoria, dysphoria, dizziness, mental clouding may occur. At high doses, may cause seizures. Miosis (papillary constriction) may occur.

Nursing Implications: Assess baseline neurologic status. Use cautiously, if at all, in patients with head injury, increased ICP, severe CNS depression, acute alcoholism, the elderly, and the debilitated. Assess other concurrent medications. Use with caution in patients receiving other opioids, tranquilizers, hypnotics, MAO inhibitors, since increasing CNS depressant effects can occur. Monitor neurologic status closely. Teach patient to avoid driving and operating machinery while taking the medicine, and to AVOID concurrent alcohol.

II. ALTERATION IN OXYGENATION related to RESPIRATORY DEPRESSION

Defining Characteristics: Opiate agonists directly depress respiratory center in brain stem, causing decreased sensitivity and responsiveness to increased pCO_2. Also may depress deep breathing and reflex to sigh. Tolerance to respiratory depressant effects occurs with chronic use.

Nursing Implications: Assess baseline pulmonary status, and monitor periodically during drug use. Use cautiously in patients with bronchial asthma, COPD, respiratory depression, and monitor closely.

III. ALTERATION IN ELIMINATION related to CONSTIPATION, ILEUS

Defining Characteristics: Opium agonists bind to opiate receptors in bowel, slowing peristalsis, leading to constipation. Untreated constipation may result in bowel perforation.

Nursing Implications: Assess baseline elimination, fluid intake, diet, and exercise patterns. Instruct patient about prevention of constipation: goal is to move bowels at least every two days by increasing fluids to 3 L/day, following a diet high in fiber (beans, vegetables, fruit), and taking moderate exercise. Assess need for bowel softeners, bulk-forming laxatives, and osmotic cathartics, and discuss prescription with physician. Teach patient self-administration of medications.

IV. ALTERATION IN NUTRITION related to GI TOXICITY

Defining Characteristics: Nausea, vomiting, and dry mouth may occur. Gastric, biliary, and pancreatic secretions are decreased by opiate agonists; digestion is delayed. Biliary tract muscle tone is increased, and spasm of Oddi's sphincter may occur

Nursing Implications: Assess patient tolerance of GI side effects. Teach patient to report side effects. If nausea/vomiting occur, change to another opioid, or premedicate with antiemetic to prevent nausea/vomiting. Assess GI pain, biliary spasm, and consider alternative opioid.

V. ALTERATION IN CARDIAC OUTPUT related to HYPOTENSION, BRADYCARDIA

Defining Characteristics: Orthostatic hypotension, bradycardia due to cholinergic effect, and peripheral vasodilation may occur. There may be histamine-related flushing, pruritus, diaphoresis with chronic drug usage; tolerance develops to this effect.

Nursing Implications: Assess baseline cardiovascular status. Teach patient to change position slowly and to hold onto stable, nearby structure for support as needed. Caution patient to remain in supine position for 15–20 minutes after dose if dizziness occurs. Monitor status closely if patient has other factors contributing to hypotension.

VI. ALTERATION IN URINE ELIMINATION related to URINARY RETENTION

Defining Characteristics: Increased smooth muscle tone in urinary tract and spasm may occur. Bladder tone is increased, which may cause urgency. Vesical sphincter tone may be increased, leading to difficulty urinating. Increased risk of urinary retention in patients with prostatic hypertrophy or urethral stricture.

Nursing Implications: Assess baseline urinary elimination pattern. Teach patient to increase fluids to 3 L/day, and encourage voiding every 2–3 hours. Instruct patient to report problems with urination.

VII. KNOWLEDGE DEFICIT related to DRUG ADMINISTRATION, POTENTIAL FOR TOLERANCE, AND DEPENDENCY

Defining Characteristics: Psychological dependence (addiction) occurs rarely in patients taking opioid agonists for cancer pain ($< 1\%$). Physical dependence (precipitation of withdrawal symptoms) occurs with chronic use of the drug for the relief of chronic cancer pain. In addition, tolerance, or less analgesic effect over time with the same drug dose, occurs and requires increased dosage of drug.

Nursing Implications: Assess baseline knowledge of opioid analgesics and attitude about their use for cancer pain management. Teach patient about proper self-administration, possible side effects, and self-care measures. Suggest patient maintain diary of pain intensity, precipitating and alleviating factors, drug dose and time taken, and relief. Teach patient to self-administer opioid agonists for relief of chronic cancer pain around-the-clock, not PRN, to prevent pain. Explain use of prescribed short-acting opioid for rescue or to manage BTP. Discuss with physician dose increase or change in frequency of administration if tolerance develops. Teach patient that withdrawal symptoms may occur if chronic, around-the-clock dosing is interrupted. Withdrawal (abstinence) symptoms that may be seen are restlessness, lacrimation, rhinorrhea, yawning, perspiration, gooseflesh, restless sleep, mydriasis in first 24 hours. These are followed by twitching and leg spasm; severe aching of the back, abdomen, and legs; cramping in abdomen and legs; hot/cold flashes; insomnia; nausea/vomiting, diarrhea; severe sneezing; and increased heart rate, BP, T, which peak at 36–72 hours. Withdrawal syndrome can be prevented by administration of at least 1/4 of previous opioid dose.

VIII. SEXUAL DYSFUNCTION related to IMPOTENCE, ↓ LIBIDO

Defining Characteristics: Opiate agonists may suppress gonadotropin, causing impotence and decreased libido.

Nursing Implications: Assess baseline sexual pattern. Discuss potential toxicity and impact on sexuality. Provide information, emotional support, and referral as needed.

Drug: levorphanol tartrate opioid (Levo-Dromoran)

Class: Opioid analgesic (opioid agonist).

Mechanism of Action: A synthetic opioid agonist, levorphanol resembles morphine but has milder action; binds to opiate receptors in CNS (limbic system, thalamus, striatum, hypothalamus, midbrain, spinal cord), altering pain perception at level of spinal cord and higher centers, as well as the emotional response to pain. Also suppresses cough reflex.

Metabolism: Well absorbed after oral (peak analgesia 60–90 minutes) or SQ (peak analgesia 20 minutes) administration. Metabolized by liver and excreted in urine.

Dosage/Range:

For moderate to severe pain:

- PO: 2–3 mg PO q6–8h.
- SQ: 2–3 mg SQ q6–8h.

Drug Preparation:

- Store tablets in tight, light-resistant containers at 15–30°C (59–86°F).
- Injectable preparation should be stored at 15–40°C (59–104°F).
- At home, teach patient to store oral doses in a safe place away from children and pets.

Drug Administration:

- PO, SQ, IV.

Drug Interactions:

- Injection incompatible with solutions containing aminophylline, ammonium chloride, amobarbital sodium, chlorothiazide sodium, heparin sodium, methicillin sodium, nitrofurantoin, phenobarbital sodium, sodium bicarbonate.
- Alcohol, CNS depressants: additive effects.

Lab Effects/Interference:

- None known.

Special Considerations:

- Oral dose is twice parenteral dose.
- Produces less nausea, vomiting, constipation than morphine, but more sedation and smooth muscle stimulation.
- Additive benefit when combined with acetaminophen or aspirin.
- Give smallest effective dose to prevent development of tolerance, physical dependency.
- Reduce dose in debilitated patients, or patients receiving other CNS depressants.
- Use with caution in patients with hepatic or renal dysfunction, hypothyroidism, Addison's disease, severe CNS depression, respiratory depression, head injury, elevated ICP.
- If required, naloxone HCl will reverse opiate toxicity (e.g., respiratory depression). However, it is important that acute withdrawal symptoms be prevented by giving only enough naloxone to reverse respiratory depression and that this be continued for opioid drug half-life.

Potential Toxicities/Side Effects and the Nursing Process

I. SENSORY/PERCEPTUAL ALTERATIONS related to CNS DEPRESSION

Defining Characteristics: Drowsiness, sedation, mood changes, euphoria, dysphoria, dizziness, mental clouding may occur. At high doses, may cause seizures. Miosis (papillary constriction) may occur.

Nursing Implications: Assess baseline neurologic status. Use cautiously, if at all, in patients who are elderly, debilitated, have a head injury, increased ICP, severe CNS depression, acute alcoholism. Assess other concurrent medications. Use with caution in patients receiving other opioids, tranquilizers, hypnotics, MAO inhibitors, since increasing CNS depressant effects can occur. Monitor neurologic status closely. Instruct patient to avoid driving and operating machinery while taking the medicine, and to AVOID concurrent alcohol.

II. ALTERATION IN OXYGENATION related to RESPIRATORY DEPRESSION

Defining Characteristics: Opiate agonists directly depress respiratory center in brain stem, causing decreased sensitivity and responsiveness to increased pCO_2. Also may depress deep breathing and reflex to sigh. Tolerance to respiratory depressant effects occurs with chronic use.

Nursing Implications: Assess baseline pulmonary status, and monitor periodically during drug use. Use cautiously in patients with bronchial asthma, COPD, respiratory depression, and monitor closely.

III. ALTERATION IN ELIMINATION related to CONSTIPATION, ILEUS

Defining Characteristics: Opium agonists bind to opiate receptors in bowel, slowing peristalsis, leading to constipation. Untreated constipation may result in bowel perforation.

Nursing Implications: Assess baseline elimination, fluid intake, diet, and exercise patterns. Instruct patient regarding prevention of constipation: goal is to move bowels at least every two days by increasing fluids to 3 L/day, following a diet high in fiber (beans, vegetables, fruit), and taking moderate exercise. Assess need for bowel softeners, bulk-forming laxatives, and osmotic cathartics, and discuss prescription with physician. Teach patient self-administration of medications.

IV. ALTERATION IN NUTRITION, LESS THAN BODY REQUIREMENTS, related to GI TOXICITY

Defining Characteristics: Nausea, vomiting, dry mouth may occur. Gastric, biliary, and pancreatic secretions are decreased by opiate agonists; digestion is delayed. Biliary tract muscle tone is increased, and spasm of Oddi's sphincter may occur (morphine > meperidine > codeine).

Nursing Implications: Assess patient tolerance of GI side effects. Teach patient to report side effects. If nausea/vomiting occur, change to another opioid, or premedicate with antiemetic to prevent nausea/vomiting. Assess GI pain, biliary spasm, and consider alternative opioid.

V. ALTERATION IN CARDIAC OUTPUT related to HYPOTENSION, BRADYCARDIA

Defining Characteristics: Orthostatic hypotension, bradycardia due to cholinergic effect, and peripheral vasodilation may occur with rapid IV dosing. There may be histamine-related flushing, pruritus, and diaphoresis with chronic drug usage; tolerance develops to this effect.

Nursing Implications: Assess baseline cardiovascular status. Teach patient to change position slowly and to hold onto stable, nearby structure for support as needed. Be careful when giving IV push opioids, and caution patient to remain in supine position for 15–20 minutes after injection. Monitor cardiovascular status after injection.

VI. ALTERATION IN URINE ELIMINATION related to URINARY RETENTION

Defining Characteristics: Increased smooth muscle tone in urinary tract and spasm may occur. Bladder tone is increased, which may cause urgency. Vesical sphincter tone may be increased, leading to difficulty urinating. Increased risk of urinary retention in patients with prostatic hypertrophy or urethral stricture.

Nursing Implications: Assess baseline urinary elimination pattern. Teach patient to increase fluids to 3 L/day, and encourage voiding every 2–3 hours. Instruct patient to report problems with urination.

VII. KNOWLEDGE DEFICIT related to DRUG ADMINISTRATION, POTENTIAL FOR TOLERANCE, AND DEPENDENCY

Defining Characteristics: Psychological dependence (addiction) occurs rarely in patients taking opioid agonists for cancer pain (< 1%). Physical dependence (precipitation of withdrawal symptoms) occurs with chronic use of the drug for the relief of chronic cancer pain. In addition, tolerance, or less analgesic effect over time with the same drug dose, occurs and requires increased dosage of drug.

Nursing Implications: Assess baseline knowledge of opioid analgesics, and attitude about their use for cancer pain management. Teach patient about proper self-administration, possible side effects, and self-care measures. Suggest patient maintain diary of pain intensity, precipitating and alleviating factors, drug dose and time taken, and relief. Teach patient to self-administer opioid agonists for relief of chronic cancer pain around-the-clock, not PRN, to prevent pain. Explain use of prescribed short-acting opioid for rescue or to manage BTP. Discuss with physician dose increase or change in frequency of administration if tolerance develops. Teach patient that withdrawal symptoms may occur if chronic, around-the-clock dosing is interrupted. Withdrawal (abstinence) symptoms that may be seen are restlessness, lacrimation, rhinorrhea, yawning, perspiration, gooseflesh, restless sleep, mydriasis in first 24 hours. These are followed by twitching and leg spasm; severe aching of the back, abdomen, and legs; cramping in abdomen and legs; hot/cold flashes; insomnia; nausea/vomiting, diarrhea; severe sneezing; and increased heart rate, BP, and T, which peak at 36–72 hours. Withdrawal syndrome can be prevented by administration of at least 1/4 of previous opioid dose.

VIII. SEXUAL DYSFUNCTION related to IMPOTENCE, ↓ LIBIDO

Defining Characteristics: Opiate agonists may suppress gonadotropin, causing impotence and decreased libido.

Nursing Implications: Assess baseline sexual pattern. Discuss potential toxicity and impact on sexuality. Provide information, emotional support, and referral as needed.

Drug: meperidine hydrochloride (Demerol, Mepergan Fortis)

Class: Opioid analgesic (opioid agonist).

Mechanism of Action: A synthetic opioid agonist, meperidine resembles morphine but has milder action; binds to opiate receptors in CNS (limbic system, thalamus, striatum, hypothalamus, midbrain, spinal cord), altering pain perception at level of spinal cord and higher centers, as well as the emotional response to pain. Also suppresses cough reflex.

Metabolism: After oral administration, metabolized by liver (first pass) with 50–60% reaching systemic circulation; thus oral administration is < 50% as effective as IM dose. After IM dose, 80–85% of drug is absorbed. Peak analgesia is ~ 1 hour after oral administration, 40–60 minutes after SQ, and 30–50 minutes after IM. Duration is 2–4 hours. Drug is 60–80% bound to plasma proteins. Metabolism is by the liver, into metabolites such as normeperidine, and excreted in the urine. Normeperidine has a longer half-life and accumulates in patients with decreased renal function. It is a potent CNS stimulant, producing seizures, agitation, irritability, nervousness, tremors, twitches, and myoclonus.

Dosage/Range:

For moderate to severe pain:

- PO: 50–150 mg q3–4h.
- IM: 50–150 mg q3–4h.
- SQ: 50–150 mg q3–4h.
- IV: 15–35 mg/hr by continuous IV infusion.

Drug Preparation:

- Store tablets in tight, light-resistant containers at 15–30°C (59–86°F).
- Injectable preparation should be stored at 15–40°C (59–104°F).

Drug Administration:

- PO, IM, SQ, IV.
- At home, teach patient to store oral doses in a safe place away from children and pets.

Drug Interactions:

- May increase isoniazid side effects; use concurrently with caution.
- Enhanced toxicity with MAO inhibitors (coma, severe respiratory depression, hypotension), so drug is contraindicated for patients who have received MAO inhibitors in previous 14 days.
- Injection incompatible with solutions containing aminophylline, barbiturates, ephedrine sulfate, heparin sodium, hydrocortisone sodium succinate, methicillin sodium, methylprednisolone sodium succinate, morphine sulfate, tetracycline.
- Alcohol, CNS depressants: additive effects.

Lab Effects/Interference:

- None known.

Special Considerations:

- Drug has many side effects, unfavorable oral to parenteral ratio, so is not recommended in the treatment of cancer-related pain. Drug is NOT used to treat or prevent chronic cancer pain because of short duration of action, bioavailability, and severe risk of neurotoxicity related to metabolite normeperidine.
- Oral meperidine, 50 mg, is equivalent in analgesia (equianalgesic) to acetaminophen 650 mg or aspirin 650 mg.
- Sedative and euphoric effect greater than morphine (equianalgesic dose).
- Oral dose is three times parenteral dose for equianalgesic effect.
- Use with caution in patients with atrial flutter or other supraventricular tachycardias (drug can increase ventricular response rate via vagolytic action).
- Formulation may contain sodium metabisulfite, which may cause anaphylactic or other allergic reactions.
- Additive benefit when combined with acetaminophen or aspirin.

- Give smallest effective dose to prevent development of tolerance, physical dependency.
- Reduce dose in debilitated patients or patients receiving other CNS depressants.
- Use with caution in patients with hepatic or renal dysfunction, hypothyroidism, Addison's disease, severe CNS depression, respiratory depression, head injury, elevated ICP.
- If required, naloxone HCl will reverse opiate toxicity (e.g., respiratory depression). However, it is important that acute withdrawal symptoms be prevented by giving only enough naloxone to reverse respiratory depression and that this be continued for opioid drug half-life.

Potential Toxicities/Side Effects and the Nursing Process

I. SENSORY/PERCEPTUAL ALTERATIONS related to CNS DEPRESSION

Defining Characteristics: Drowsiness, sedation, mood changes, euphoria, dysphoria, dizziness, mental clouding may occur. At high doses, may cause seizures. Miosis (papillary constriction) may occur.

Nursing Implications: Assess baseline neurologic status. Use cautiously, if at all, in the elderly, the debilitated, and patients with head injury, increased ICP, severe CNS depression, acute alcoholism. Assess other concurrent medications. Use with caution in patients receiving other opioids, tranquilizers, hypnotics, MAO inhibitors, since increasing CNS depressant effects can occur. Monitor neurologic status closely. Instruct patient to avoid driving and operating machinery while taking the medicine, and to AVOID concurrent alcohol.

II. ALTERATION IN OXYGENATION related to RESPIRATORY DEPRESSION

Defining Characteristics: Opiate agonists directly depress respiratory center in brain stem, causing decreased sensitivity and responsiveness to increased pCO_2. Also may depress deep breathing and reflex to sigh. Tolerance to respiratory depressant effects occurs with chronic use.

Nursing Implications: Assess baseline pulmonary status, and periodically during drug use. Use cautiously in patients with bronchial asthma, COPD, respiratory depression, and monitor closely.

III. ALTERATION IN ELIMINATION related to CONSTIPATION, ILEUS

Defining Characteristics: Opium agonists bind to opiate receptors in bowel, slowing peristalsis, leading to constipation. Untreated constipation may result in bowel perforation.

Nursing Implications: Assess baseline elimination, fluid intake, diet, and exercise patterns. Instruct patient regarding prevention of constipation: goal is to move bowels at least every two days by increasing fluids to 3 L/day, following a diet high in fiber (beans, vegetables, fruit), and taking moderate exercise. Assess need for bowel softeners, bulk-forming laxatives, and osmotic cathartics, and discuss prescription with physician. Teach patient self-administration of medications.

IV. ALTERATION IN NUTRITION related to GI TOXICITY

Defining Characteristics: Nausea, vomiting, and dry mouth may occur. Gastric, biliary, and pancreatic secretions are decreased by opiate agonists; digestion is delayed. Biliary tract muscle tone is increased, and spasm of Oddi's sphincter may occur (morphine > meperidine > codeine).

Nursing Implications: Assess patient tolerance of GI side effects. Teach patient to report side effects. If nausea/vomiting occur, change to another opioid, or premedicate with antiemetic to prevent nausea/vomiting. Assess GI pain, biliary spasm, and consider alternative opioid.

V. ALTERATION IN CARDIAC OUTPUT related to HYPOTENSION, BRADYCARDIA

Defining Characteristics: Orthostatic hypotension, bradycardia due to cholinergic effect, and peripheral vasodilation may occur with rapid IV dosing. There may be histamine-related flushing, pruritus, diaphoresis with chronic drug usage; tolerance develops to this effect.

Nursing Implications: Assess baseline cardiovascular status. Teach patient to change position slowly and to hold onto stable, nearby structure for support as needed. Be careful when giving IV push opioids, and caution patient to remain in supine position for 15–20 minutes after injection. Monitor cardiovascular status after injection.

VI. ALTERATION IN URINE ELIMINATION related to URINARY RETENTION

Defining Characteristics: Increased smooth muscle tone in urinary tract and spasm may occur. Bladder tone is increased, which may cause urgency. Vesical sphincter tone may be increased, leading to difficulty urinating. Increased risk of urinary retention in patients with prostatic hypertrophy or urethral stricture.

Nursing Implications: Assess baseline urinary elimination pattern. Teach patient to increase fluids to 3 L/day, and encourage voiding every 2–3 hours. Instruct patient to report problems with urination.

VII. KNOWLEDGE DEFICIT related to DRUG ADMINISTRATION, POTENTIAL FOR TOLERANCE, AND DEPENDENCY

Defining Characteristics: Psychological dependence (addiction) occurs rarely in patients taking opioid agonists for cancer pain (< 1%). Physical dependence (precipitation of withdrawal symptoms) occurs with chronic use of the drug for the relief of chronic cancer pain. In addition, tolerance, or less analgesic effect over time with the same drug dose, occurs and requires increased dosage of drug.

Nursing Implications: Assess baseline knowledge of opioid analgesics and attitude about their use for cancer pain management. Teach patient about proper self-administration, possible side effects, and self-care measures. Suggest patient maintain diary of pain intensity, precipitating and alleviating factors, drug dose and time taken, and relief. Teach patient to self-administer opioid agonists for relief of chronic cancer pain around-the-clock, not PRN, to prevent pain. Explain use of prescribed short-acting opioid for rescue or to manage breakthrough pain. Discuss with physician dose increase or change in frequency of administration if tolerance develops. Teach patient that withdrawal symptoms may occur if chronic, around-the-clock dosing is interrupted. Withdrawal (abstinence) symptoms that may be seen are restlessness, lacrimation, rhinorrhea, yawning, perspiration, gooseflesh, restless sleep, mydriasis in first 24 hours. These are followed by twitching and leg spasm; severe aching of the back, abdomen, and legs; cramping in abdomen and legs; hot/cold flashes; insomnia; nausea/vomiting, diarrhea; severe sneezing; and increased heart rate, BP, T, which peak at 36–72 hours. Withdrawal syndrome can be prevented by administration of at least 1/4 of previous opioid dose.

VIII. SEXUAL DYSFUNCTION related to IMPOTENCE, ↓ LIBIDO

Defining Characteristics: Opiate agonists may suppress gonadotropin, causing impotence and decreased libido.

Nursing Implications: Assess baseline sexual pattern. Discuss potential toxicity and impact on sexuality. Provide information, emotional support, and referral as needed.

Drug: methadone (Dolophine, Methadose)

Class: Opioid analgesic (opioid agonist).

Mechanism of Action: A synthetic opioid agonist, methadone resembles morphine but has milder action; binds to opiate receptors in CNS (limbic system, thalamus, striatum, hypothalamus, midbrain, spinal cord), altering pain perception at level of spinal cord and higher centers, as well as the emotional response to pain. Also suppresses cough reflex.

Metabolism: Well absorbed from GI tract; onset and duration of single dose similar to morphine. With chronic administration (physical dependency) half-life is 22–48 hours. Highly tissue-bound; metabolized by liver, excreted by renal filtration, then is reabsorbed (pH dependent).

Dosage/Range:

For moderate to severe pain:

- PO: 5–20 mg q6–8h, or more for severe cancer pain.
- SQ, IM: 2.5–10 mg q3–4h.

Drug Preparation:

- Store tablets in tight, light-resistant containers at 15–30°C (59–86°F).
- Injection should be protected from light and stored at 15–40°C (59–104°F).
- At home, teach patient to store oral doses in a safe place away from children and pets.

Drug Administration:

- PO, IM, SQ.

Drug Interactions:

- Injection incompatible with solutions containing aminophylline, ammonium chloride, amobarbital sodium, chlorothiazide sodium, heparin sodium, methicillin sodium, nitrofurantoin, phenobarbital sodium, sodium bicarbonate.
- Alcohol, CNS depressants: additive effects.

Lab Effects/Interference:

- None known.

Special Considerations:

- Oral dose is twice parenteral dose (equianalgesic effect).
- May produce similar or slightly greater respiratory depression than equivalent doses of morphine.
- Additive benefit when combined with acetaminophen or aspirin.
- Give smallest effective dose to prevent development of tolerance, physical dependency.
- Reduce dose in debilitated patients or patients receiving other CNS depressants.
- Use with caution in patients with hepatic or renal dysfunction, hypothyroidism, Addison's disease, severe CNS depression, respiratory depression, head injury, elevated ICP.
- If required, naloxone HCl will reverse opiate toxicity (e.g., respiratory depression). However, it is important that acute withdrawal symptoms be pre-

vented by giving only enough naloxone to reverse respiratory depression and that this be continued for opioid drug half-life.

Potential Toxicities/Side Effects and the Nursing Process

I. SENSORY/PERCEPTUAL ALTERATIONS related to CNS DEPRESSION

Defining Characteristics: Drowsiness, sedation, mood changes, euphoria, dysphoria, dizziness, mental clouding may occur. At high doses, may cause seizures. Miosis (papillary constriction) may occur.

Nursing Implications: Assess baseline neurologic status. Use cautiously, if at all, in the elderly, the debilitated, and patients with head injury, increased ICP, severe CNS depression, acute alcoholism. Assess other concurrent medications. Use with caution in patients receiving other opioids, tranquilizers, hypnotics, MAO inhibitors, since increasing CNS depressant effects can occur. Monitor neurologic status closely. Instruct patient to avoid driving and operating machinery while taking the medicine, and to AVOID concurrent alcohol.

II. ALTERATION IN OXYGENATION related to RESPIRATORY DEPRESSION

Defining Characteristics: Opiate agonists directly depress respiratory center in brain stem, causing decreased sensitivity and responsiveness to increased pCO2. Also may depress deep breathing and reflex to sigh. Tolerance to respiratory depressant effects occurs with chronic use.

Nursing Implications: Assess baseline pulmonary status, and periodically during drug use. Use cautiously in patients with bronchial asthma, COPD, respiratory depression, and monitor closely.

III. ALTERATION IN ELIMINATION related to CONSTIPATION, ILEUS

Defining Characteristics: Opium agonists bind to opiate receptors in bowel, slowing peristalsis, leading to constipation. Untreated constipation may result in bowel perforation.

Nursing Implications: Assess baseline elimination, fluid intake, diet, and exercise patterns. Instruct patient regarding prevention of constipation: goal is to move bowels at least every two days by increasing fluids to 3 L/day, following a diet high in fiber (beans, vegetables, fruit), and taking moderate exercise. Assess need for bowel softeners, bulk-forming laxatives, and osmotic cathartics, and discuss prescription with physician. Teach patient self-administration of medications.

IV. ALTERATION IN NUTRITION, LESS THAN BODY REQUIREMENTS, related to GI TOXICITY

Defining Characteristics: Nausea, vomiting, and dry mouth may occur. Gastric, biliary, and pancreatic secretions are decreased by opiate agonists; digestion is delayed. Biliary tract muscle tone is increased, and spasm of Oddi's sphincter may occur (morphine > meperidine > codeine).

Nursing Implications: Assess patient tolerance of GI side effects. Instruct patient to report side effects. If nausea/vomiting occur, change to another opioid, or premedicate with antiemetic to prevent nausea/vomiting. Assess GI pain, biliary spasm, and consider alternative opioid.

V. ALTERATION IN CARDIAC OUTPUT related to HYPOTENSION, BRADYCARDIA

Defining Characteristics: Orthostatic hypotension, bradycardia due to cholinergic effect, and peripheral vasodilation may occur with rapid IV dosing. There may be histamine-related flushing, pruritus, diaphoresis with chronic drug usage; tolerance develops to this effect.

Nursing Implications: Assess baseline cardiovascular status. Teach patient to change position slowly and to hold onto stable, nearby structure for support as needed. Be careful when giving IV push opioids, and caution patient to remain in supine position for 15–20 minutes after injection. Monitor cardiovascular status after injection.

VI. ALTERATION IN URINE ELIMINATION related to URINARY RETENTION

Defining Characteristics: Increased smooth muscle tone in urinary tract and spasm may occur. Bladder tone is increased, which may cause urgency. Vesical sphincter tone may be increased leading to difficulty urinating. Increased risk of urinary retention in patients with prostatic hypertrophy or urethral stricture.

Nursing Implications: Assess baseline urinary elimination pattern. Teach patient to increase fluids to 3 L/day, and encourage voiding every 2–3 hours. Instruct patient to report problems with urination.

VII. KNOWLEDGE DEFICIT related to DRUG ADMINISTRATION, POTENTIAL FOR TOLERANCE, AND DEPENDENCY

Defining Characteristics: Psychological dependence (addiction) occurs rarely in patients taking opioid agonists for cancer pain (< 1%). Physical dependence (precipitation of withdrawal symptoms) occurs with chronic use of the drug for the relief of chronic cancer pain. In addition, tolerance, or less analgesic effect over time with the same drug dose, occurs and requires increased dosage of drug.

Nursing Implications: Assess baseline knowledge of opioid analgesics, and attitude about their use for cancer pain management. Teach patient about proper self-administration, possible side effects, and self-care measures. Suggest patient maintain diary of pain intensity, precipitating and alleviating factors, drug dose and time taken, and relief. Teach patient to self-administer opioid agonists for relief of chronic cancer pain around-the-clock, not PRN, to prevent pain. Explain use of prescribed short-acting opioid for rescue or to manage BTP. Discuss with physician dose increase or change in frequency of administration if tolerance develops. Teach patient that withdrawal symptoms may occur if chronic, around the-clock dosing is interrupted. Withdrawal (abstinence) symptoms that may be seen are restlessness, lacrimation, rhinorrhea, yawning, perspiration, gooseflesh, restless sleep, mydriasis in first 24 hours. These are followed by twitching and leg spasm; severe aching of the back, abdomen, and legs; cramping in abdomen and legs; hot/cold flashes; insomnia; nausea/vomiting, diarrhea; severe sneezing; and increased heart rate, BP, T, which peak at 36–72 hours. Withdrawal syndrome can be prevented by administration of at least 1/4 of previous opioid dose.

VIII. SEXUAL DYSFUNCTION related to IMPOTENCE, ↓ LIBIDO

Defining Characteristics: Opiate agonists may suppress gonadotropin, causing impotence and decreased libido.

Nursing Implications: Assess baseline sexual pattern. Discuss potential toxicity and impact on sexuality. Provide information, emotional support, and referral as needed.

Drug: morphine (Astramorph, Avinza, Duramorph, Infumorph, Kadian Morphine Sulfate Sustained Release, MS Contin, MSIR, Morphelan, Oramorph, Roxanol)

Class: Opioid analgesic (opioid agonist).

Mechanism of Action: Binds to opiate receptors in CNS (limbic system, thalamus, striatum, hypothalamus, midbrain, spinal cord). This opioid agonist alters pain perception at level of spinal cord and higher centers, as well as the emotional response to pain. Also suppresses cough reflex.

Metabolism: Variable absorption from GI tract; increased absorption when taken with food. Peak analgesia 60 minutes (oral), 20–60 minutes (rectal), 50–90 minutes (SQ), 30–60 minutes (IM), 20 minutes (IV). Duration is 4–7 hours. Maximum respiratory depression is 30 minutes (IM), 7 minutes (IV), 90 minutes (SQ). Drug is slowly absorbed into systemic circulation after intrathecal (IT) administration. Peak CSF concentrations occur 60–90 minutes after epidural dose. Metabolized by liver and excreted in urine and, to a small degree, feces.

Dosage/Range:

For moderate to severe pain:

- Oral: 10–60 mg PO q3–4h titrated to pain; 10–240 mg sustained release q8–12h, titrated to pain.
- Rectal: 10–60 mg q4h.
- SQ, IM: 4–15 mg q3–4h.
- IV: 1–100 mg/h, and higher, titrated to need in physically dependent patients.
- Intrathecal: dose is 1/10 the epidural dose.
- Epidural: 5 mg q24h.
- At home, teach patient to store oral doses in a safe place away from children and pets.

Drug Preparation:

- Store tablets in tight, light-resistant containers at 15–30°C (59–86°F).
- Injection should be protected from light, and stored at 15–40°C (59–104°F).

Drug Administration:

- Begin morphine therapy using immediate-release oral preparations and increase dose to control pain; once optimal dose identified, convert to sustained-release formulation by dividing 24-hour total morphine dose by 2, giving two (q12h) doses.
- Intrathecal or epidural: use preservative-free morphine only, e.g., Astramorph PF, Duramorph PF, Infumorph; consult individual policies/procedures for administration.

Drug Interactions:

- Injection incompatible with solutions containing aminophylline, ammonium chloride, amobarbital sodium, chlorothiazide sodium, heparin sodium, methicillin sodium, nitrofurantoin, phenobarbital sodium, sodium bicarbonate.
- Alcohol, CNS depressants: additive effects.

Lab Effects/Interference:

- None known.

Special Considerations:

- Oral to parenteral dose is 3–6 to 1 (equianalgesic dose).
- Highly concentrated formulations are available and are for use in continuous infusion pumps.

- Do not crush sustained-release formulations (e.g., MS Contin, Oramorph).
- When epidural or intrathecal route is used, refer to institutional policy/procedure for administration and patient monitoring.
- Additive benefit when combined with acetaminophen or aspirin.
- Give smallest effective dose to prevent development of tolerance, physical dependency.
- Reduce dose in debilitated patients, or patients receiving other CNS depressants.
- Use with caution in patients with hepatic or renal dysfunction, hypothyroidism, Addison's disease, severe CNS depression, respiratory depression, head injury, elevated intracranial pressure.
- If required, naloxone HCl will reverse opiate toxicity (e.g., respiratory depression). However, it is important that acute withdrawal symptoms be prevented by giving only enough naloxone to reverse respiratory depression and that this be continued for opioid drug half-life.
- Kadian as well as Avinza are sustained-release morphine formulated for once-a-day dosing; available in 20-, 50-, and 100-mg tablets (Kadian) and 30-, 60-, 90-, and 120 mg capsules (Avinza).

Potential Toxicities/Side Effects and the Nursing Process

I. SENSORY/PERCEPTUAL ALTERATIONS related to CNS DEPRESSION

Defining Characteristics: Drowsiness, sedation, mood changes, euphoria, dysphoria, dizziness, mental clouding may occur. At high doses, may cause seizures. Miosis (papillary constriction) may occur.

Nursing Implications: Assess baseline neurologic status. Use cautiously, if at all, in the elderly, the debilitated, and patients with head injury, increased intracranial pressure, severe CNS depression, acute alcoholism. Assess other concurrent medications. Use with caution in patients receiving other opioids, tranquilizers, hypnotics, MAO inhibitors, since increasing CNS depressant effects can occur. Monitor neurologic status closely. Instruct patient to avoid driving and operating machinery while taking the medicine, and to AVOID concurrent alcohol.

II. ALTERATION IN OXYGENATION related to RESPIRATORY DEPRESSION

Defining Characteristics: Opiate agonists directly depress respiratory center in brain stem, causing decreased sensitivity and responsiveness to increased pCO2. Also may depress deep breathing and reflex to sigh. Tolerance to respiratory depressant effects occurs with chronic use.

Nursing Implications: Assess baseline pulmonary status, and periodically during drug use. Use cautiously in patients with bronchial asthma, COPD, respiratory depression, and monitor closely.

III. ALTERATION IN ELIMINATION related to CONSTIPATION, ILEUS

Defining Characteristics: Opium agonists bind to opiate receptors in bowel, slowing peristalsis, leading to constipation. Untreated constipation may result in bowel perforation.

Nursing Implications: Assess baseline elimination, fluid intake, diet, and exercise patterns. Instruct patient regarding prevention of constipation: goal is to move bowels at least every two days by increasing fluids to 3 L/day, following a diet high in fiber (beans, vegetables, fruit), and taking moderate exercise. Assess need for bowel softeners, bulk-forming laxatives, and osmotic cathartics, and discuss prescription with physician. Teach patient self-administration of medications.

IV. ALTERATION IN NUTRITION, LESS THAN BODY REQUIREMENTS, related to GI TOXICITY

Defining Characteristics: Nausea, vomiting, and dry mouth may occur. Gastric, biliary, and pancreatic secretions are decreased by opiate agonists; digestion is delayed. Biliary tract muscle tone is increased, and spasm of Oddi's sphincter may occur (morphine > meperidine > codeine).

Nursing Implications: Assess patient tolerance of GI side effects. Teach patient to report side effects. If nausea/vomiting occur, change to another opioid, or premedicate with antiemetic to prevent nausea/vomiting. Assess GI pain, biliary spasm, and consider alternative opioid.

V. ALTERATION IN CARDIAC OUTPUT related to HYPOTENSION, BRADYCARDIA

Defining Characteristics: Orthostatic hypotension, bradycardia due to cholinergic effect, and peripheral vasodilation may occur with rapid IV dosing. There may be histamine-related flushing, pruritus, diaphoresis with chronic drug usage; tolerance develops to this effect.

Nursing Implications: Assess baseline cardiovascular status. Teach patient to change position slowly and to hold onto stable, nearby structure for support as needed. Be careful when giving IV push opioids, and caution patient to remain in supine position for 15–20 minutes after injection. Monitor cardiovascular status after injection.

VI. ALTERATION IN URINE ELIMINATION related to URINARY RETENTION

Defining Characteristics: Increased smooth muscle tone in urinary tract and spasm may occur. Bladder tone is increased, which may cause urgency. Vesical sphincter tone may be increased, leading to difficulty urinating. Increased risk of urinary retention in patients with prostatic hypertrophy or urethral stricture.

Nursing Implications: Assess baseline urinary elimination pattern. Teach patient to increase fluids to 3 L/day, and encourage voiding every 2–3 hours. Instruct patient to report problems with urination.

VII. KNOWLEDGE DEFICIT related to DRUG ADMINISTRATION, POTENTIAL FOR TOLERANCE, AND DEPENDENCY

Defining Characteristics: Psychological dependence (addiction) occurs rarely in patients taking opioid agonists for cancer pain (< 1%). Physical dependence (precipitation of withdrawal symptoms) occurs with chronic use of the drug for the relief of chronic cancer pain. In addition, tolerance, or less analgesic effect over time with the same drug dose, occurs and requires increased dosage of drug.

Nursing Implications: Assess baseline knowledge of opioid analgesics, and attitude about their use for cancer pain management. Teach patient about proper self-administration, possible side effects, and self-care measures. Suggest patient maintain diary of pain intensity, precipitating and alleviating factors, drug dose and time taken, and relief. Teach patient to self-administer opioid agonists for relief of chronic cancer pain around-the-clock, not PRN, to prevent pain. Explain use of prescribed short-acting opioid for rescue or to manage breakthrough pain. Discuss with physician dose increase or change in frequency of administration if tolerance develops. Teach patient that withdrawal symptoms may occur if chronic, around-the-clock dosing is interrupted. Withdrawal (abstinence) symptoms that may be seen are restlessness, lacrimation, rhinorrhea, yawning, perspiration, gooseflesh, restless sleep, mydriasis in first 24 hours. These are followed by twitching and leg spasm; severe aching of the back, abdomen, and legs; cramping in abdomen and legs; hot/cold flashes; insomnia; nausea/vomiting, diarrhea; severe sneezing; and increased heart rate, BP, T, which peak at 36–72 hours. Withdrawal syndrome can be prevented by administration of at least 1/4 of previous opioid dose.

VIII. SEXUAL DYSFUNCTION related to IMPOTENCE, ↓ LIBIDO

Defining Characteristics: Opiate agonists may suppress gonadotropin, causing impotence and decreased libido.

Nursing Implications: Assess baseline sexual pattern. Discuss potential toxicity and impact on sexuality. Provide information, emotional support, and referral as needed.

Drug: oxycodone (Percodan, Endodan, Roxiprin)

Class: Opioid analgesic (opioid agonist).

Mechanism of Action: A synthetic opioid agonist, oxycodone resembles morphine but has milder action; binds to opiate receptors in CNS (limbic system, thalamus, striatum, hypothalamus, midbrain, spinal cord), altering pain perception at level of spinal cord and higher centers, as well as the emotional response to pain. Also suppresses cough reflex.

Metabolism: Onset of analgesia in 10–15 minutes, peaks 30–60 minutes, duration 3–6 hours. Metabolized by liver and kidney; excreted in urine.

Dosage/Range:

For moderate to moderately severe pain:

- 5 mg q6h (Roxicodone).
- 5 mg q6h, combined with acetaminophen: 300 mg (e.g., Oxycet, Percocet, Roxicet caplets), OR 500 mg (e.g., Roxicet caplets, Tylox); OR combined with aspirin: 325 mg (e.g., Percodan, Codoxy, Roxiprin); OR combined with ibuprofen 5 mg/400 mg (e.g., Combunox).
- Oral solution: 5 mg/5 mL (Roxicodone); 20 mg/mL (Roxicodone, Intensol).
- Oxycontin 10-mg, 20-mg, 40-mg (sustained-release) tablets q12h.

Drug Preparation:

- Store tablets in tight, light-resistant containers at 15–30°C (59–86°F) and protect from light.
- At home, teach patient to store oral doses in a safe place away from children and pets.

Drug Administration:

- Oral.

Drug Interactions:

- Alcohol, CNS depressants: additive CNS depressant effects.
- Anticoagulants, chemotherapy: aspirin-oxycodone combination may increase bleeding risk; AVOID concurrent use.

Lab Effects/Interference:

- None known.

Special Considerations:

- Adverse effects are milder than morphine.

- Preparations may contain sodium metabisulfite and may cause allergic reactions, including anaphylaxis and severe asthma-like reactions.
- Additive benefit when combined with acetaminophen or aspirin.
- Give smallest effective dose to prevent development of tolerance, physical dependency.
- Reduce dose in debilitated patients or patients receiving other CNS depressants.
- Use with caution in patients with hepatic or renal dysfunction, hypothyroidism, Addison's disease, severe CNS depression, respiratory depression, head injury, elevated ICP.
- If required, naloxone HCl will reverse opiate toxicity (e.g., respiratory depression). However, it is important that acute withdrawal symptoms be prevented by giving only enough naloxone to reverse respiratory depression and that this be continued for opioid drug half-life.
- Oxycontin is a sustained-release oxycodone preparation that is taken q12h; available in 10-mg, 20-mg, and 40-mg tablets.

Potential Toxicities/Side Effects and the Nursing Process

I. SENSORY/PERCEPTUAL ALTERATIONS related to CNS DEPRESSION

Defining Characteristics: Drowsiness, sedation, mood changes, euphoria, dysphoria, dizziness, mental clouding may occur. At high doses, may cause seizures. Miosis (papillary constriction) may occur.

Nursing Implications: Assess baseline neurologic status. Use cautiously, if at all, in the elderly, the debilitated, and patients with head injury, increased ICP, severe CNS depression, acute alcoholism. Assess other concurrent medications. Use with caution in patients receiving other opioids, tranquilizers, hypnotics, MAO inhibitors, since increasing CNS depressant effects can occur. Monitor neurologic status closely. Instruct patient to avoid driving and operating machinery while taking the medicine, and to AVOID concurrent alcohol.

II. ALTERATION IN OXYGENATION related to RESPIRATORY DEPRESSION

Defining Characteristics: Opiate agonists directly depress respiratory center in brain stem, causing decreased sensitivity and responsiveness to increased pCO_2. Also may depress deep breathing and reflex to sigh. Tolerance to respiratory depressant effects occurs with chronic use.

Nursing Implications: Assess baseline pulmonary status, and periodically during drug use. Use cautiously in patients with bronchial asthma, COPD, respiratory depression, and monitor closely.

III. ALTERATION IN ELIMINATION related to CONSTIPATION, ILEUS

Defining Characteristics: Opium agonists bind to opiate receptors in bowel, slowing peristalsis, leading to constipation. Untreated constipation may result in bowel perforation.

Nursing Implications: Assess baseline elimination, fluid intake, diet, and exercise patterns. Instruct patient regarding prevention of constipation: goal is to move bowels at least every two days by increasing fluids to 3 L/day, following a diet high in fiber (beans, vegetables, fruit), and taking moderate exercise. Assess need for bowel softeners, bulk-forming laxatives, and osmotic cathartics, and discuss preparation with physician. Teach patient self-administration of medications.

IV. ALTERATION IN NUTRITION, LESS THAN BODY REQUIREMENTS, related to GI TOXICITY

Defining Characteristics: Nausea, vomiting, dry mouth may occur. Gastric, biliary, and pancreatic secretions are decreased by opiate agonists; digestion is delayed. Biliary tract muscle tone is increased, and spasm of Oddi's sphincter may occur (morphine > meperidine > codeine).

Nursing Implications: Assess patient tolerance of GI side effects. Teach patient to report side effects. If nausea/vomiting occur, change to another opioid, or premedicate with antiemetic to prevent nausea/vomiting. Assess GI pain, biliary spasm, and consider alternative opioid.

V. ALTERATION IN CARDIAC OUTPUT related to HYPOTENSION, BRADYCARDIA

Defining Characteristics: Orthostatic hypotension, bradycardia due to cholinergic effect, and peripheral vasodilation may occur with rapid IV dosing. There may be histamine-related flushing, pruritus, diaphoresis with chronic drug usage; tolerance develops to this effect.

Nursing Implications: Assess baseline cardiovascular status. Teach patient to change position slowly and to hold onto stable, nearby structure for support as needed. Be careful when giving IV push opioids, and caution patient to remain in supine position for 15–20 minutes after injection. Monitor cardiovascular status after injection.

VI. ALTERATION IN URINE ELIMINATION related to URINARY RETENTION

Defining Characteristics: Increased smooth muscle tone in urinary tract and spasm may occur. Bladder tone is increased, which may cause urgency. Vesical sphincter tone may be increased, leading to difficulty urinating. Increased risk of urinary retention in patients with prostatic hypertrophy or urethral stricture.

Nursing Implications: Assess baseline urinary elimination pattern. Teach patient to increase fluids to 3 L/day, and encourage voiding every 2–3 hours. Instruct patient to report problems with urination.

VII. KNOWLEDGE DEFICIT related to DRUG ADMINISTRATION, POTENTIAL FOR TOLERANCE, AND DEPENDENCY

Defining Characteristics: Psychological dependence (addiction) occurs rarely in patients taking opioid agonists for cancer pain (< 1%). Physical dependence (precipitation of withdrawal symptoms) occurs with chronic use of the drug for the relief of chronic cancer pain. In addition, tolerance, or less analgesic effect over time with the same drug dose, occurs and requires increased dosage of drug.

Nursing Implications: Assess baseline knowledge of opioid analgesics, and attitude about their use for cancer pain management. Teach patient about proper self-administration, possible side effects, and self-care measures. Suggest patient maintain diary of pain intensity, precipitating and alleviating factors, drug dose and time taken, and relief. Teach patient to self-administer opioid agonists for relief of chronic cancer pain around-the-clock, not PRN, to prevent pain. Explain use of prescribed short-acting opioid for rescue or to manage breakthrough pain. Discuss with physician dose increase or change in frequency of administration if tolerance develops. Teach patient that withdrawal symptoms may occur if chronic, around-the-clock dosing is interrupted. Withdrawal (abstinence) symptoms that may be seen are restlessness, lacrimation, rhinorrhea, yawning, perspiration, gooseflesh, restless sleep, mydriasis in first 24 hours. These are followed by twitching and leg spasm; severe aching of the back, abdomen, and legs; cramping in abdomen and legs; hot/cold flashes; insomnia; nausea/vomiting, diarrhea; severe sneezing; and increased heart rate, BP, T, which peak at 36–72 hours. Withdrawal syndrome can be prevented by administration of at least 1/4 of previous opioid dose.

VIII. SEXUAL DYSFUNCTION related to IMPOTENCE, ↓ LIBIDO

Defining Characteristics: Opiate agonists may suppress gonadotropin, causing impotence and decreased libido.

Nursing Implications: Assess baseline sexual pattern. Discuss potential toxicity and impact on sexuality. Provide information, emotional support, and referral as needed.

ADJUVANTS AGENTS

Agent: modafinil (Provigil)

Class: Wakeful promoting agent, symptom management

Mechanism of Action: Promotes wakefulness without generalized CNS stimulation by an unknown mechanism. Drug acts in selected brain areas thought to regulate normal wakefulness in the hypothalamus: increased neuronal activity in tuberomammillary nucleus (wake-promoting center), which then projects into cerebral cortex; decreases activity in the ventrolateral preoptic area (sleep promoting); does not affect suprachiasmatic nucleus (regulated circadian rhythm). Action is different from amphetamines.

Metabolism: Rapidly absorbed from the GI system with peak plasma concentrations in 2–4 hours. Taking with food delays absorption by 1 hour, but does not affect bioavailability. About 60% protein bound (albumin), but at steady state does not displace protein binding of warfarin. Metabolized in the liver, with renal excretion of metabolites. Drug clearance may be reduced in the elderly. Drug is a reversible inhibitor of drug metabolizing enzyme CYP2C19. Elimination half-life 15 hours.

Dosage/Range:
- 200 mg po qd as a single dose in the morning.
- 50% dose reduction in patients with severe liver impairment.
- Consider dose reduction in elderly patients with renal impairment and/or hepatic impairment.

Drug Preparation:
- Oral, available in 100-mg and 200-mg tablets.

Drug Administration:
- Oral, in the morning, with a glass of water.

Drug Interactions:
- Potentially, due to reversible inhibition of CYP2C19 enzyme system
  - —Diazempam, phenytoin, proprandolol: drug may increase serum levels of these drugs; monitor closely for toxicity and dose reduce if needed.
  - —Patients with CYP2C19 deficiency: increased serum levels of tricyclic antidepressants, SSRIs; monitor closely for toxicity and dose reduce if needed.
  - —Patients taking drug chronically may have increased induction of metabolism enzyme CYP3A4, resulting in theoretical decreased serum levels of steroidal contraceptives, cyclosporine, theophylline; monitor closely and dose increase as necessary.
  - —Methylphenidate: delays absorption of modafinil by 1 hour when given together.

—Use in pregnancy or breast-feeding women only if risk outweighs benefit as drug potentially teratogenic.

Lab Effects/Interference:

- Unknown.

Special Considerations:

- Anecdotal success in reducing in non-anemia cancer or HIV-related fatigue (Breitbart).
- Contraindicated in people with a sensitivity to modafinil.
- Contraindicated in patients with history of left ventricular hypertrophy or ischemic EKG changes, chest pain, arrhythmia, or mitral valve prolapse.
- Use with caution in patients who have had a recent MI or unstable angina.
- Use cautiously in patients with a history of psychosis.
- Women using steroidal contraceptives should use alternative or concomitant methods of contraception while taking the drug and for one month following discontinuation of the drug.
- Drug may produce psychoactive and euphoric effects, alterations in mood, perception, thinking, and feelings typical of other CNS stimulants. Drug binds to dopamine reuptake site and causes an increase in extracellular dopamine but no increase in dopamine release. Drug is reinforcing.
- Incidence of insomnia was 3% (placebo 1%).
- Drug is indicated in the treatment of narcolepsy, and does not cause a withdrawal when drug is stopped.

Potential Toxicities/Side Effects (dose and schedule dependent) and the Nursing Process

I. ALTERATION IN COMFORT related to HEADACHE, NAUSEA, DEPRESSION, NERVOUSNESS, RHINITIS

Defining Characteristics: In controlled clinical trials, headache occurred 10% more frequently than placebo, nausea occurred 9% more than placebo, depression 1% more than placebo, rhinitis 11% (placebo 8%), and nervousness 2% more than placebo. The few patients who discontinued the drug did so due to headache (1%), nausea (1%), depression (1%), and nervousness (1%).

Nursing Implications: Teach patient that these effects are rare but may occur. Teach symptom management strategies and if these do not work, to notify provider. If this occurs, discuss drug discontinuance versus more aggressive symptom management if drug is effective in reducing fatigue.

II. ALTERATION IN NUTRITION, POTENTIAL, related to NAUSEA, DRY MOUTH, DIARRHEA, ANOREXIA, THIRST

Defining Characteristics: Although rare, these symptoms may occur: nausea occurs in 13% (placebo 4%), diarrhea 8% (placebo 4%), dry mouth 5% (placebo 1%), anorexia 5% (placebo 1%), and thirst 1%.

Nursing Implications: Perform baseline patient nutritional assessment, history of nausea and vomiting, bowel elimination pattern, oral assessment, and usual appetite. Teach patient these are rare, but to report these side-effects so that they can be evaluated. Teach patient self-care measures, including dietary modification, local comfort measures as well as pharmacologic management as determined by the nurse/physician team. Teach patient to report symptoms that persist and do not respond to the planned therapy.

Chapter 7

Nausea and Vomiting

Nausea and/or vomiting can occur commonly during the course of the cancer experience, related to disease, such as liver metastases, or to treatment, such as with chemotherapy or radiation to the abdomen. In addition, if acute nausea and vomiting were not prevented following cancer chemotherapy, delayed nausea and vomiting often followed. This problem continues. Nausea is often underreported and under-assessed (Wickham, 2003). A replication of the Coates et al (1983) study by de Boer-Dennert et al (1997) showed that patients rated nausea as more distressing than vomiting since much has been done to prevent and control chemotherapy-induced nausea and vomiting (CINV). Complete control of CINV has improved greatly with the advent of serotonin 5-hydroxytryptamine type 3 (5-HT_3) receptor antagonists used in combination with dexamethasone, bringing complete control to about 70% for patients receiving high-dose cisplatin. This new century of genomics has led to the understanding that the effectiveness of many drugs, and in particular, 5-HT_3 receptor antagonists, is influenced by the recipient's genotype. This is because the liver's microenzyme system, Cytochrome P450, and subtypes are determined by an individual's genotype. If the genotype is a ultrarapid metabolizer, the drug is rapidly cleared and eliminated from the body with decreased effect and undertreatment, while slow or poor metabolizers slowly clear the drug from the body with the risk of overtreatment. A study by Kaiser et al (2002) evaluated whether patients who vomited after receiving their first cycle of emetogenic chemotherapy with 5-HT_3 receptor antagonist protection by either ondansetron or tropisetron were either ultrarapid or slow metabolizers of the P450 subsystem CYP 2D6. They found that 30% had nausea and vomiting. The ultrarapid metabolizers had a higher incidence of nausea and vomiting, which was more marked for tropisetron- than ondansetron-receiving patients, and the poor metabolizers had higher serum concentrations and were protected. As we look to the future, not only do we see patients having genotypic evaluation of their tumors for an individualized prescription of anti-cancer treatment, but it will also include individual prescription of antiemetic dose based on genotype.

CHEMOTHERAPY INDUCED NAUSEA AND VOMITING

CINV appears mediated by multiple pathways. Nausea usually precedes vomiting, and is controlled by cerebral and autonomic input, with common accompanying signs and symptoms of tachycardia, pallor, and diaphoresis. Vomiting involves the ejection of stomach contents, and is a critical protection mechanism which helps the body excrete poisons. Most commonly, receptors in the gut enterochromaffin cells are stimulated, and release serotonin. Serotonin binds to 5-HT_3 receptors which stimulate the vagus nerve. This leads to stimulaton of the chemotherapy trigger zone (CTZ) in the area postrema on the floor of the 4th ventricle, leading to activation of the vomiting center (VC) in the medulla, or to stimulation of the vomiting center directly. The 5-HT_3 receptor antagonists, such as dolasetron, granisetron, and ondansetron, block the emetic impulses from reaching the CTZ and VC. In addition, other neuroreceptors in the CTZ can transmit impulses to the VC, such as dopamine, endorphin, and Substance P. Dopamine antagonists include phenothiazines and butyrophenones, and Substance P/Neurokinin1 receptor antagonist antiemetics include aprepitant, which has been newly FDA approved as Emend. Emotional and cognitive factors can influence the occurrence and severity of CINV through a descending pathway from the cerebral cortex to the vomiting center, such as with anticipatory nausea and vomiting. Here a conditioned response is set up based on 3–4 past episodes of severe nausea and/or vomiting. The benzodiazepine lorazepam has been effective in preventing or lessening this effect through the drug's amnesiac qualities.

Dexamethasone has long been known to reduce the incidence of CINV, through a probable anti-inflammatory effect, leading to a closing of spaces in the gut wall that would permit leakage of emetogens into the bloodstream (Wickham, 2003). However, the exact mechanism is unknown.

Delayed nausea and vomiting is difficult to control, but appears to be influenced by slowed gastric emptying. Thus, delayed antiemetic regimes usually include metoclopramide to speed gastric emptying, along with dexamethasone, and a phenothiazine or serotonin antagonist. Recently, it became clear that Substance P and its receptor Neurokinin-1 (NK_1), in the gut and brainstem, were important mediators in delayed CINV. The NK_1 receptors are located near the vomiting center, the "final common pathway" for emesis, so it is expected the NK_1 receptor antagonists will have broader application (Wickham, 2003). Although great strides have been made in the prevention and control of CINV, even with maximal pharmacologic blockade of known pathways, 100% protection is not obtained, so it is clear other pathways await discovery. See Figure 7.1 for a review of pathophysiology of CINV. See Table 7.1 for the emetogenicity of cancer chemotherapy agents, and Table 7.2 for a schematic for antiemetic drugs and doses for CINV.

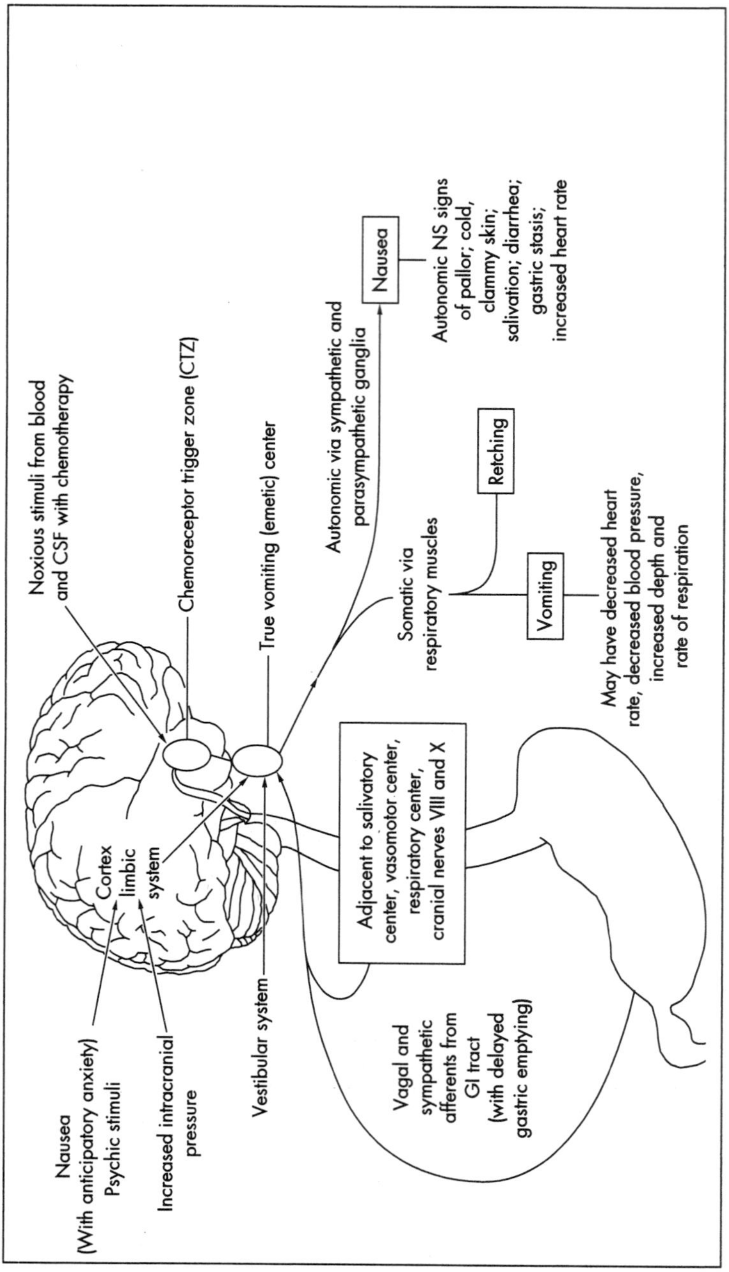

Figure 7.1 The Physiology of Nausea and Vomiting.
Source: Reproduced from Burke MM, Wilkes GM, Ingwersen K et al (1996) *Chemotherapy and the Nursing Process,* Sudbury, MA, Jones and Bartlett Publishers. *Drawing adapted from original by Gail Wilkes.*

Table 7.1 Emetogenic Risk by Antineoplast Agent

High Risk > 90%	Moderate Risk 0–90%	Low Risk 10-30%	Minimal Risk < 10%
Carmustine > 250 mg/m^2	Carmustine < 250 mg/m^2	Aldesleukin (IL=2)	Bleomycin
Cisplatin > 50 mg/m^2	Carboplatin < 250 mg/m^2	Asparaginase	Capecitabine
Cyclophosphamide > 1000 mg/m^2	Cyclophosphamide < 1000 mg/m^2	Docetaxel	Etoposide IV
Dacarbazine > 500 mg/m^2	Cyclophosphamide PO	Doxorubicin < 20 mg/m^2	Fludarabine
Dactinomycin	Cytarabine > 1 g/m^2	Etoposide PO	Methotrexate < 100 mg/m^2
Lomustine > 60 mg/m^2	Doxorubicin	Fluorouracil	Rituximab
Mechlorethamine	Epirubicin	Gemcitabine	Tenoposide IV
Pentostatin	Hexamethylmelamine	Methotrexate > 100mg/m^2	Traztuzumab
Streptozocin	Idarubicin	Mitomycin C	Vinblastine
	Ifosfamide	Mitoxantrone < 12 mg/m^2	Vinorelbine IV
	Irinotecan	Paclitaxel	
	Melphalan	Temozolomide	
	Mitoxantrone > 12 mg/m^2	Thiotepa	
	Procarbazine	Topotecan	
	Oxaliplatin		

Source: From Wickham R (2003) Nausea and Vomiting, Chapter 11. In Yarbro CH, Goodman M, and Frogge MH *Cancer Symptom Mangement*, 3rd ed. Sudbury, MA, Jones and Bartlett Publishers.

MANAGEMENT

CINV can occur *acutely*, during the first 24 hours following chemotherapy administration, *delayed*, occurring after the first 24 hours, or in anticipation (*anticipatory*).

Factors which influence the occurrence and severity of CINV include sex (female has higher risk than male), age (younger have higher risk than older), drug dose and emetogenic potential, combination of drugs versus single agent, history of alcohol intake (increased alcohol intake confers protection), and past experience with nausea and vomiting, such as air sickness, which increase risk.

Delayed nausea and vomiting are influenced by the effectiveness of control/prevention of the acute phase of CINV (Roila, 2000; Koeller et al, 2002), as well as the half-life of the antineoplastic agent. For example, the metabolites of cisplatin continue to be excreted for 3–5 days after drug administration, so protection must be provided for that period of time; and for cyclophosphamide, the half-life is at least 12 hours, so only half the drug is excreted by that time,

Table 7.2 Antiemetic Agents used in CINV

Antiemetic Agent	IV Doses (Acute)	Oral Doses (Acute)	Oral (Delayed)
Serotonin Receptor Antagonists			
• Dolasetron	100 mg or 1.8 mg/kg IV	100 mg (acute)	100 mg qd delayed
• Granisetron	0.01 mg/kg or 1 mg IV	1–2 mg oral (acute)	1 mg bid delayed
• Ondansetron	0.15 mg/kg or 8mg IV	24 mg oral (acute)	8 mg bid delayed
Corticosteroids			
• Dexamethasone	20 mg	20 mg	8 mg bid days 2–4 highly emetogenic 4–8 mg bid days 2–3 moderately emetogenic
Substance P/NK1 Receptor Antagonist			
• Aprepitant		125 mg po day 1 with dexamethasone 12 mg po with serotonin receptor antagonist	80 mg day 2,3 with dexamethasone 8 mg po
Dopamine Receptor Antagonists			
• Metoclopramine			20–40 mg bid-qid
• Prochlorperazine			15–30mg LA spansules bid PRN
Benzodiazepines			
• Lorazepam	0.5–1 mg	1–2 mg	

Source: Modified from Wickham R (2003) Nausea and Vomiting, Chapter 11. In Yarbro CH, Goodman M, and Frogge MH *Cancer Symptom Mangement*, 3rd ed. Sudbury, MA, Jones and Bartlett Publishers.

and full antiemetic protection must continue for at least 24 hours to prevent delayed nausea and vomiting.

Insofar as CINV involves multiple pathways, multiple antiemetics to block these pathways are needed, especially for aggressive antiemesis. Antiemetics must be administered to prevent nausea and vomiting, so the drug(s) should be administered prior to chemotherapy administration in order to block stimulation of the pathways. Oral antiemetics should be administered 30–40 minutes before treatment; rectal (PR) preparations 60 minutes before; intramuscular (IM) injections 20–30 minutes before; and intravenous bolus (IVB) 10–30 minutes prior to chemotherapy (Barton Burke et al, 1997).

In order to better identify treatment approaches for CINV, American Society for Clinical Oncology (ASCO) published "Recommendations for the Use of Antiemetics: Evidence-Based Clinical Practice Guidelines" and stated that "at equivalent doses, serotonin receptor antagonists have equivalent safety and efficacy and can be used intrchangeably based on convenience, availability, and cost" (Gralla et al, 1999). They listed four agents in this class, three of which are commercially available in the United States: dolasetron, granisetron, and ondansetron. In addition, the National Community Network (NCCN) has developed supportive care guidelines for antiemesis, which can be found at http://www.nccn.org/physician_gls/f_guidelines.html. Finally, key members of the Supportive Care in Cancer organization have developed consensus guidelines for the study and prescription of antiemetic care (Koeller et al, 2002).

2003 has seen the advent of a new class of antiemetics for the control of chemotherapy-induced nauseas and vomiting. Aprepitant (Emend) is the first substance P/Neurokinin 1 receptor antagonist indicated for the prevention of acute and delayed nausea and vomiting related to highly emetogenic chemotherapy, in combination with other antiemetic agents. First identified in 1931, and reaching notoriety in 1950 when linked with pain transmission, substance P has continued to be prominent in the symptom management field. Substance P is a member of the tachykinin family of peptides and, together with NK1 receptors, is found in high concentrations in the chemotherapy trigger zone (CTZ, in the medulla oblongata) and the dorsal horn of the spinal cord (posterior column of gray matter), as well as the gut. Substance P is released from peripheral sensory as well as central sensory nerve endings and plays a key role in transmitting noxious sensory information to the brain. Substance P initiates its activity by binding to the Neurokinin 1 (NK_1) receptor, a site distinctly different from the serotonin-mediated $5HT_3$ site (Hesketh, 2001).

In an effort to design a serotonin-antagonist with a long half-life, and activity against delayed chemotherapy-induced nausea and vomiting, palonestron (Aloxi) was created. Recently approved for the prevention of chemotherapy-induced nausea and vomiting, palonestron is the only serotonin-antagonist with an indication for delayed nausea and vomiting.

RADIATION INDUCED NAUSEA AND VOMITING

Radiation therapy to the gastrointestinal tract usually causes nausea and vomiting. Highest risk (90%) is when Total Body Irradiation (TBI) or external beam radiation is administered to the upper or total abdomen or upper hemithorax, with emesis occurring within 10–15 minutes with TBI or hemithorax treatment, and within 1–2 hours when external beam therapy is administered to the upper abdomen (Wickham, 2003). Antiemesis is effective using serotonin-antagonists or phenothiazines.

DISEASE INDUCED NAUSEA AND VOMITING

Site of advanced disease is a strong predictor of the risk for nausea and vomiting. Metastases to the liver is often associated with difficult to control nausea and vomiting. Pressure from ascites or obstruction of a hollow viscus, as with advanced ovarian cancer, can also lead to intractable nausea and vomiting. A factor here, along with advanced pancreatic cancer, may be delayed gastric emptying, or gastric outlet syndrome. Increased intracranial pressure (ICP) from a malignant brain tumor often causes nausea and vomiting. Other conditions related to disease that cause nausea and vomiting include hypercalcemia, hyperglycemia, electrolyte imbalance, and severe constipation. Strategies to relieve nausea and vomiting in these circumstances vary with the cause, and range from aggressive antiemesis to correction of delayed gastric emptying (metoclopramide) or the obstruction (stent if possible, or if not, release of gastric contents via a gastrostomy tube), to correction of electrolyte abnormalities.

In summary then, nausea and/or vomiting can arise from treatment or complications of disease. There are a variety of agents useful for blocking a number of neurotransmitter pathways to prevent or control nausea and vomiting in cancer. Specifically, it is known that chemotherapy stimulates nausea and vomiting via multiple pathways and often, therefore, multiple drugs are necessary for the prevention of nausea and vomiting associated with aggressive chemotherapy. These include a $5HT_3$ receptor (serotonin) antagonist, a corticosteroid (Gralla et al, 1999), and a Substance P/NK 1 receptor antagonist if there is a delayed component anticipated (Koeller et al, 2002).

References

Barnhart ER. *Physicians' Desk Reference.* Oradell, NJ, Medical Economics Data 1998

Barton Burke M, Wilkes G, Berg D, et al. *Cancer Chemotherapy: A Nursing Process Approach,* 2nd ed. Sudbury, MA, Jones and Bartlett Publishers 1997

Barton Burke M, Wilkes G, Ingwersen K. *Chemotherapy Care Plans: Designs for Nursing Care.* Sudbury, MA, Jones and Bartlett Publishers 1997

Coates A, Abraham S, Kaye SB, et al. On the Receivin End–Patient Perception of the Side-Effects of Cancer Chemotherapy. *Eur J Cancer Clin Oncol* 1983;19:203–208

Cotanch PM, Stum S. Progressive Muscle Relaxation as Antiemetic Therapy for Cancer Patients. *Oncol Nurs Forum* 1987;14(1):33–37 de Boer-Dennert M, de Wit R, Schmitz PIM, et al. Patient Perceptions of the Side-effects of Chemotherapy: The Influence of 5HT3 Antagonists. *Br J Cancer* 1997;76: 1055–1061

Gralla RJ, Osoba D, Kris MG, et al. ASCO Special Article: Recommendations for the Use of Antiemetics: Evidence-Based Clinical Practice Guidelines. *J Clin Oncol* 1999;17(9):2971–2994

Hesketh PJ. Potential Role of the NK1 Receptor Antagonists in Chemotherapy-induced Nausea and Vomiting. *Supportive Care in Cancer* 2001;9:350–354

Hesketh PJ, Beck TM, Uhlenhopp M, et al. Adjusting the Dose of Intravenous Ondansetron plus Dexamethasone to the Emetogenic Potential of the Chemotherapy Regimen. *J Clin Oncol* 1995;13(8):2117–2122

Hesketh PJ, Kris MG, Grunberg SM, et al. Proposal for Classifying the Acute Emetogenicity of Cancer Chemotherapy. *J Clin Oncol* 1997;15(1):103–109

Hesketh PJ, Murphy WK, Khojasten A, et al. GR-C507175 (GR38032F): A Novel Compound Effective in the Treatment of Cisplatin-Induced Nausea and Vomiting. *Proc American Society of Clinical Oncologists* 1988;7:280

Hui YF, Ignoffo RJ. Dolasetron: A New 5-Hydroxytryptamine3 Receptor Antagonist. *Cancer Practice* 1997;(Sept/Oct) 5(5):324–327

Kaiser R, Sezer O, Papies A, et al. Patient-tailored Antiemetic Treatment with 5-hydroxytryptamine Type 3 Receptor Antagonists according to Cytochrome P-450 Genotypes. *J Clin Oncol* 2002;20(12):2805–2811

Koeller JM, Aapro MS, Gralla RJ, et al. Antiemetic Guidelines: Creating a More Practical Treatment Approach. *Supportive Care in Cancer* 2002;10:519–522

Nolte MJ, Berkery R, Pizzo B, et al. Assuring the Optimal Use of Serotonin Antagonist Antiemetics: The Process for Development and Implementation of Institutional Antiemetic Guidelines at Memorial Sloan-Kettering Cancer Center. *J Clin Oncol* 1998; 16:771–778

Roila F, Ballatori E, Ruggeri B, et al. Dexamethasone Alone or in Combination with Ondansetron for the Prevention of Delayed Nausea and Vomiting Induced by Chemotherapy. *New Engl J Med* 2000;342(21):1554–1559

Roxane Laboratories. Marinol (Dronabinol) Manufacturer's Information Sheet. Columbus, Ohio: Roxane Laboratories 1986

Rubenstein EB, Gralla RJ, Hainsworth JD, et al. Randomized, Double Blind, Dose-Response Trial across Four Oral Doses of Dolasetron for the Prevention of Acute Emesis after Moderately Emetogenic Chemotherapy. *Cancer* 1997;79(6): 1216–1224

Sylvester RK, Etzell R, Levitt R, et al. Comparison of 16-mg vs 32-mg Ondansetron and Dexamethasone in Patients Receiving Cisplatin. *Proc Am Soc Clin Oncol* 1996; 15:547 (abstract 1781)

Van Belles, Cocquyt V, DeSmet M, et al. Comparison of a Neurokinin-1 Antagonist L-758, 298 to Ondansetron in the Prevention of Cisplatin-induced Emesis. *Proc American Society of Clinical Oncologists* 1998;17:51a (abstract 198)

Wickham R. Nausea and Vomiting, chapter 11. Yarbro CH, Frogge MH, Goodman M, (eds), *Cancer Symptom Management,* 3rd ed. Sudbury, MA: Jones and Bartlett Publishers 2003

Drug: aprepitant (Emend®)

Mechanism of Action: Selective Substance P/Neurokinin 1 (NK_1) receptor antagonist (high affinitiy). Drug has no affinity for $5HT_3$, dopamine, or corticosteroid receptors. Drug crosses the blood brain barrier to saturate brain NK_1 receptors. Drug increases the activity of serotonin receptor antagonists and corticosteroids in preventing acute nausea and vomiting, and inhibits both acute and delayed nausea and vomiting related to cisplatin chemotherapy.

Class: Substance P/Neurokinin 1 Receptor Antagonist.

Dosage/Range:
Day 1, 125 mg po 1 hour before chemotherapy, together with a serotonin (HT3) receptor antagonist and dexamethasone (dose reduced to 12 mg day 1, 8 mg days 2&3); days 2 and 3, 80 mg po each morning.

Drug Preparation/Administration: Oral drug supplied as 1) 80 mg capsules in bottle of 30 capsules or in unit dose packs of 5 capsules, 2) 125 mg tablets in bottle of 30 capsules or in unit dose packs of 5 capsules, and 3) tri-fold pack containing 1–125 mg capsule, and 2–80 mg capsules. Capsules should be stored at room temperature. Day 1, give 125 mg capsule po 1 hour before chemotherapy, and then the 80 mg capsule in the morning on days 2 and 3. Give with or without food.

Drug Interactions:
- Drugs that inhibit the CYP3A4 isoenzyme system can increase the serum level of aprepitant: ketoconazole, itraconazole, nefazodone, troleandomycin, claritromycin, ritonavir, nelfinavir; diltiazem (2-fold increase in aprepitant plasma concentration), so coadminister cautiously and monitor for aprepitant toxicity or dose reduce aprepitant.
- Drugs that strongly induce CYP3A4 isoenzyme system can lower aprepitant serum levels: rifampin, carbamazepine, phenytoin; assess for efficacy of aprepitant and need for drug dose increase.
- Drug is a moderate inhibitor of P450 hepatic isoenzyme system CYP3A4, so the plasma concentrations of the following drugs can theoretically be increased if coadministered:
  - Chemotherapy agents docetaxel, paclitaxel, etoposide, irinotecan, ifosfamide, imatinib, vinorelbine, vinblastine, vincristine.
  - dexamethasone (dose-reduce dexamethasone by 50%).
  - methylprednisolone (dose-reduce 25% if IV, 50% if po).
  - benzodiazepines: midazolam, lorazepam, alprazolam, triazolam.
- Drug is an inducer of CYP2C9, and the plasma concentrations of the following drugs can theoretically be decreased if coadministered:

- Warfarin (34% decrease with 14% decrease in INR; closely monitor INR 7–10 days after 3-day antiemetic regime, and modify warfarin dose as needed.
- Phenytoin, tolbutamide, oral contraceptives.

Lab Effects/Interference: Lab Effects/Interactions: Decreased INR if patient taking warfarin.

Special Considerations:

- Contraindications: do not give concomitantly with pimozide, terfenadine, astemizole, or cisapride; do not give if hypersensitive to aprepitant or any of its components; use cautiously if at all during pregnancy or breast-feeding; no studies have been done in patients with severe liver failure.
- Indications: in combination, with other antiemetic agents, for the prevention of acute and delayed nausea and vomiting associated with initial and repeat courses of highly emetogenic chemotherapy, including high-dose cisplatin.
- Significant drug interactions (see above).
- Drug is well tolerated with few side effects.

Potential Toxicities/Side Effects and the Nursing Process

I. ALTERATION IN NUTRITION, LESS THAN BODY REQUIREMENTS related to CONSTIPATION, DIARRHEA, NAUSEA, ANOREXIA, HICCUPS

Defining Characteristics: Gastrointestinal side effects may occur but are infrequent with the following incidences: constipation (10.3%), diarrhea (10.3%), nausea (12.7%), vomiting (7.5%), hiccups (10.8%), and anorexia (10.1%).

Nursing Implications: Teach patient that these side effects may occur, and to report them if unrelieved by symptom-management measures. Teach patient self-care measures to manage and prevent symptoms.

II. ALTERATION IN COMFORT related to ASTHENIA/FATIGUE, ABDOMINAL PAIN, HEADACHE

Defining Characteristics: Asthenia/fatigue occurred in 17.8% of patients; abdominal pain 4.6%; headache 8.5%.

Nursing Implications: Teach patient that these side effects may occur and measures to minimize their occurrence. Teach energy-conserving measures, management of abdominal pain and headache. Teach patient to report signs and symptoms which worsen or are unrelieved.

Drug: dexamethasone (Decadron)

Class: Glucocorticoid steroid.

Mechanism of Action: May inhibit prostaglandin release by stabilizing lysosomal membranes, thereby interrupting hypothalamic prostaglandin release and subsequent stimulation of nausea and vomiting. Causes demargination of marginated WBCs, with leukocytosis. Decreases inflammation by suppression of migration of polymorphonuclear leukocytes.

Metabolism: Half-life is 3–4 hours; oral dose peaks in 1–2 hours, with duration of two days; IM peaks in 8 hours, with duration of six days.

Dosage/Range:

Adult (as antiemetic):

- Oral: 4 mg q4h × four doses beginning 1–8 hours before chemotherapy.
- IV: 10–20 mg prior to chemotherapy, then q4–6h.

Drug Preparation/Administration:

- Oral: administer with food or milk.
- IV: may be given with H_2-antagonist (e.g., ranitidine) to prevent gastric irritation.

Drug Interactions:

- Indomethacin, aspirin: increased GI irritation and bleeding; avoid concurrent administration.
- Barbiturates, phenytoin, rifampin: decreased dexamethasone effect; increase dose as needed.

Lab Effects/Interference: Lab Effects/Interactions:

- Increased WBC may occur due to demargination.
- Increased serum glucose level.
- May cause decreased K.

Special Considerations:

- Contraindicated in patients with psychosis, hypersensitivity, idiopathic thrombocytopenia, acute glomerulonephritis, amebiasis, fungal infections, and nonasthmatic bronchial disease.
- Indicated in the management of inflammation, allergies, neoplasms, cerebral edema, and in combination antiemetic therapy.
- If patient received dexamethasone chronically, drug must be tapered to prevent withdrawal (i.e., signs/symptoms of adrenal insufficiency, rebound weakness, arthralgia, fever, dizziness, orthostatic hypotension, dyspnea, hypoglycemia).

Potential Toxicities/Side Effects and the Nursing Process

I. ALTERATION IN NUTRITION, LESS THAN BODY REQUIREMENTS, related to GI TOXICITY

Defining Characteristics: Increased appetite, abdominal distension, pancreatitis, GI hemorrhage; diarrhea may occur.

Nursing Implications: Assess baseline nutritional status and monitor throughout therapy. Discuss symptomatic management of diarrhea, abdominal distension, and increased appetite with patient. Assess stool for occult blood and notify physician if positive. Monitor Hgb and HCT values.

II. ALTERATIONS IN SENSORY/PERCEPTUAL PATTERNS related to CHANGES IN MOOD, VASODILATION, CATARACTS

Defining Characteristics: Euphoria, insomnia, depression, flushing, sweating, headache, mood changes, and cataracts may occur.

Nursing Implications: Assess baseline mental status and monitor during therapy. Discuss symptomatic management or drug discontinuance, based on severity, with physician.

III. ALTERATION IN CARDIAC OUTPUT related to CHF

Defining Characteristics: Congestive heart failure (CHF), hypertension, fluid retention, and edema may occur.

Nursing Implications: Assess baseline vital signs (VS), and monitor during therapy. Discuss hypertension with physician, monitor daily weights, and assess for edema.

IV. ALTERATION IN CARBOHYDRATE METABOLISM related to CARBOHYDRATE INTOLERANCE

Defining Characteristics: May cause hyperglycemia, hypokalemia, and carbohydrate intolerance.

Nursing Implications: Assess baseline blood glucose, K, and monitor during therapy. Teach patient signs/symptoms of hyperglycemia (polyuria, polydipsia), especially if receiving drug for extended period.

Drug: diphenhydramine hydrochloride (Benadryl)

Class: Antihistamine.

Mechanism of Action: Inhibits histamine, and has slight, if any, antiemetic activity by blocking the CTZ and decreasing vestibular stimulation. Acts on blood vessels, GI, respiratory systems by competing with histamine for H1-receptor site; decreases allergic response by blocking histamine.

Metabolism: Biologically transformed in the liver; half-life is 2.4–9.3 hours; 80–85% protein-bound; excreted by the kidney. Metabolized in the liver, crosses placenta, and is excreted in breast milk.

Dosage/Range:

Adult:

- Oral: 25–50 mg q4h.
- IM: 25–50 mg q4h.
- IV: 50 mg prior to chemotherapy or 25 mg q4h × 4 doses, beginning prior to antiemetic.

Drug Preparation/Administration:

- Available forms include 25-, 50-mg capsules; elixir 12.5 mg/mL; syrup 12.5 mg/mL; injection available as 10 mg/mL and 50 mg/mL. Administer IM deep in large muscle mass.

Drug Interactions:

- CNS depressants: increased sedation; monitor patient closely.

Lab Effects/Interference: Lab Effects/Interactions:

- None known.

Special Considerations:

- Useful in treatment or prevention of extrapyramidal side effects (EPS) related to antiemetics (dopamine antagonists).
- Contraindicated in patients with prior hypersensitivity to H1-receptor antagonist, acute asthma attack, or lower respiratory tract disease.

Potential Toxicities/Side Effects and the Nursing Process

I. ALTERATIONS IN SENSORY/PERCEPTUAL PATTERNS related to CNS CHANGES

Defining Characteristics: Sedation/drowsiness, dizziness, confusion (especially in the elderly), hyperexcitability, blurred vision/diplopia, tinnitus, dry mouth/nose/throat may all occur.

Nursing Implications: Assess patient's level of consciousness and risk for increased sedation (i.e., elderly, concomitant CNS depressant drugs). Monitor neurologic VS closely if sedated. Instruct patient to avoid alcohol ingestion, operation of equipment, or driving a car while drowsy. Teach strategies to protect safety.

II. ALTERED URINARY ELIMINATION related to URINARY RETENTION, DYSURIA

Defining Characteristics: Urinary retention, dysuria, frequency may occur.

Nursing Implications: Assess baseline urinary elimination pattern. Teach patient potential side effects and instruct to report them. Use drug cautiously in men with prostatic hypertrophy; if side effect occurs, instruct patient not to take drug and discuss with physician.

III. ALTERATION IN COMFORT related to RASH

Defining Characteristics: Rash, urticaria, photosensitivity, hypotension, palpitations may occur.

Nursing Implications: Assess baseline drug allergy history. Instruct patient to report rash, itching, and to avoid sunlight while taking the drug. Assess VS and monitor patient closely for hypotension, especially if patient is elderly or sedated, or taking other sedating drugs.

IV. POTENTIAL FOR INJURY related to BONE MARROW DEPRESSION

Defining Characteristics: Thrombocytopenia, agranulocytosis, hemolytic anemia may occur rarely.

Nursing Implications: Assess baseline CBC, platelet count. Discuss abnormalities with physician.

Drug: dolasetron mesylate (Anzemet)

Class: Serotonin antagonist.

Mechanism of Action: Together with the active metabolite hydrodolasetron, drug is a selective serotonin 5-HT_3 receptor antagonist, blocking transmission of impulses via the vagus nerve peripherally and centrally in the chemotherapy receptor trigger zone (CTZ). Blocks chemotherapy-induced nausea and vomiting produced by the release of serotonin from the enterochromaffin cells of the small intestines, which otherwise would stimulate the 5-HT_3 receptors on the vagus efferents that begin the vomiting reflex.

Metabolism: IV: Parent drug is rapidly eliminated from the plasma and completely metabolized into the major metabolite hydrodolasetron, as is the oral drug. Hydrodolasetron is metabolized by the cytochrome P-450 enzyme system in the liver, with an approximate half-life of 7.3 hours. Oral and orally administered IV solution are bioequivalent, and apparent absolute bioavailability of oral dolasetron is 75%, determined by the active metabolite; 66% of drug is excreted in the urine unchanged, and 33% in the feces. Metabolite is 77% protein-bound.

Dosage/Range:

For the prevention of cancer chemotherapy-induced nausea and vomiting:

Adult:

- IV: 1.8 mg/kg IV, 30 minutes prior to chemotherapy, diluted in 50 mL and infused over a period of up to 15 min, or 100-mg IV fixed dose for most adults given IV over 30 sec.
- Oral: 100 mg given within 1 hour prior to chemotherapy.

Pedi (2–16 years of age):

- IV: the recommended intravenous dosage is 1.8 mg/kg given as a single dose approximately 30 minutes before chemotherapy, up to a maximum of 100 mg. Safety and effectiveness in pediatric patients under 2 years of age have not been established.
- Oral: Anzemet injection mixed in apple or apple-grape juice may be used for oral dosing of pediatric patients. When Anzemet injection is administered orally, the recommended dosage in pediatric patients 2–16 years of age is 1.8 mg/kg, up to a maximum 100-mg dose given within 1 hour before chemotherapy.

For the prevention or treatment of postoperative nausea and/or vomiting:

Adult:

- IV: 12.5 mg given as a single dose 15 minutes before the cessation of anesthesia for prevention, or as soon as nausea or vomiting presents (treatment).
- Oral: 100 mg given within 2 hours before surgery.

Pedi (2–16 years of age):

- IV: 0.35 mg/kg, with a maximum dose of 12.5 mg, given as a single dose 15 minutes prior to the cessation of anesthesia (prevention), or as soon as nausea or vomiting presents (treatment).
- Oral: Anzemet injection mixed in apple or apple-grape juice may be used for oral dosing of pediatric patients. When Anzemet injection is administered orally, the recommended dose is 1.2 mg/kg, up to a maximum 100-mg dose given within 2 hours before surgery.
- Safety and efficacy have not been established for children under 2 years of age.
- Diluted product can be up to 2 hours at room temperature before use. The recommended dose of Anzemet should not be exceeded.

Drug Preparation/Administration:

- Injectable drug available in 100-mg/5-mL single-use vials, and 12.5-mg/0.625 mL single-use vials.
- Tablets available in 50-mg and 100-mg doses, each in a 5-count bottle or blister pack, or in a 10-count unit dose.

- IV dose given IVP over 30 sec or further diluted in 50 mL of 0.9% NS, 5% D_5W, D_5 1/2 NS, D_5LR, LR, or 10% mannitol injection and infused over a period of up to 15 minutes. Diluted drug stable 24 hours at room temperature, or 48 hours refrigerated.
- Oral: administer within 1 hour before chemotherapy, or within 2 hours prior to surgery.

Drug Interactions:

- Anzemet injection has been safely coadministered with other drugs used in chemotherapy and surgery. As with other agents that prolong ECG intervals, caution should be exercised in patients taking other drugs that prolong ECG intervals, particularly QT_c. See Special Considerations section.
- Increased hydrodolasetron serum levels (24%) when given with cimetidine (nonselective inhibitor of cytochrome P-450 enzyme system).
- Decreased hydrodolasetron serum levels (28%) when combined with rifampin (potent inducer of P-450 enzyme system).

Lab Effects/Interference:

- Transient increased liver transaminases (AST, ALT) in < 1% of patients; rare increase in bili, GGT, alk phos.

Special Considerations:

- Administer with caution in patients who have or may develop cardiac conduction defects, especially prolongation of QT interval (e.g., patients with hypokalemia, hypomagnesemia, receiving diuretics, congenital QT syndrome, receiving antiarrhythmic drugs or other drugs causing QT segment prolongation, and with high cumulative doses of anthracycline chemotherapy). Prolongation of PR, QRS, and QT_c intervals was observed in some patients. These changes are mild, transient, asymptomatic, and do not require medical treatment. Of note, other 5-HT_3 antagonists were also associated with similiar electrocardiographic changes.
- Rare anaphylaxis, facial edema, urticaria.
- No dosage modifications necessary in elderly or patients with hepatic or renal impairment.
- IV preparation indicated for highly emetogenic chemotherapy, including high-dose cisplatin; oral dose indicated for prevention of chemotherapy-induced nausea and vomiting due to moderately emetogenic chemotherapy.

MANAGEMENT

Potential Toxicities/Side Effects and Nursing Process

I. ALTERATION IN COMFORT related to HEADACHE

Defining Characteristics: Headache (24%), fever (4%), fatigue (4%), and, rarely, arthralgia, myalgia occur.

Nursing Implications: Assess baseline comfort. Teach patient to report any unusual occurrence. Provide symptomatic management.

II. ALTERATION IN NUTRITION, LESS THAN BODY REQUIREMENTS, related to CONSTIPATION, DYSPEPSIA

Defining Characteristics: Constipation, dyspepsia, anorexia, and, rarely, pancreatitis may occur. In less than 1% of patients, there is an increase in LFTs.

Nursing Implications: Assess baseline weight, nutritional pattern. Instruct patient to report alterations, and manage symptomatically. Discuss alterations in LFTs and/or abdominal pain suggestive of pancreatitis with physician.

III. POTENTIAL ALTERATIONS IN SENSORY/PERCEPTUAL PATTERNS related to VERTIGO, PARESTHESIA

Defining Characteristics: Rarely, flushing, vertigo, paresthesia, agitation, sleep disorder, depersonalization may occur, as may ataxia, twitching, confusion, anxiety, abnormal dreams.

Nursing Implications: Teach patient to report any changes, and assess patient safety. Discuss any significant alterations with physician and consider alternative antiemetics.

Drug: dronabinol (Marinol)

Class: Cannabinoid.

Mechanism of Action: Active ingredient is δ-9-tetrahydrocannabinol (THC). Probably depresses CNS and may disrupt higher cortical input, inhibit prostaglandin synthesis, or bind to opiate receptors in the brain to indirectly block the VC.

Metabolism: Metabolized by the liver.

Dosage/Range:

Adult:

- Oral: 5 mg/m^2–7.5 mg/m^2 1–3 hours prior to chemotherapy, then 2–4 hours postchemotherapy for 4–6 doses per day.

Drug Preparation/Administration:

- If ineffective at above dose and no toxicity, may be increased by 2.5 mg/m^2 to a maximum of 15 mg/m^2/day.

Drug Interactions:

- CNS depressants: increased sedation; avoid concurrent use.

Lab Effects/Interference: Lab Effects/Interactions:

- None known.

Special Considerations:

- More effective than placebo and in some instances may be better than prochlorperazine.
- Indicated in the management of chemotherapy-induced nausea and vomiting refractory to usual antiemetics.
- Can produce physical and psychological dependency.
- May increase appetite.
- May produce dry mouth.

Potential Toxicities/Side Effects and the Nursing Process

I. ALTERATIONS IN SENSORY/PERCEPTUAL PATTERNS related to CNS CHANGES

Defining Characteristics: Mood changes, disorientation, drowsiness, muddled thinking, dizziness, and brief impairment of perception, coordination, and sensory functions may occur. Increased toxicity in elderly (up to 35%).

Nursing Implications: Explain to patient these changes may occur to decrease anxiety, fear. Assess baseline mental status, and monitor during therapy. Assess patient safety and implement measures to ensure this. Avoid use in the elderly.

II. ALTERATION IN CARDIAC OUTPUT related to TACHYCARDIA

Defining Characteristics: Tachycardia, orthostatic hypotension may occur.

Nursing Implications: Assess baseline VS, and monitor during therapy. If hypotension occurs, notify physician and anticipate increasing rate of IV fluids to increase BP.

Drug: droperidol (Inapsine)

Class: Butyrophenone.

Mechanism of Action: Neuroleptic compound that produces a state of quiescence with reduced motor activity, reduced anxiety, and indifference to surroundings. Dopamine antagonist that suppresses CTZ and VC; more potent than phenothiazines. Decreases stimulation of the VC along vestibular pathway.

Metabolism: When given IM/IV, has onset of action in 3–10 minutes, peak 30 minutes, duration 3–6 hours; metabolized in liver, excreted in urine as metabolites; crosses placenta.

Dosage/Range:

Adults:

- IM/IV: 0.5–2.5 mg q4–6h or drip, but reports suggest large loading dose, then intermittent IVB or continuous infusion for 6–10 hours.

Drug Preparation/Administration:

- IM: 2.5 mg/mL.
- IV: 2.5 mg/mL initial reconstitution then further dilute in at least 25 mL 0.9% Sodium Chloride or 5% Dextrose.

Drug Interactions:

- Epinephrine: reversal of vasopressor effects; avoid concurrent use.
- CNS depressants: increased sedation; monitor patient closely.

Lab Effects/Interference:

- None known.

Special Considerations:

- Contraindicated in patients with hypersensitivity or who are pregnant.
- Indicated for premedication prior to surgery; induction and maintenance of general anesthesia; also useful as an antiemetic prior to chemotherapy for some patients.

Potential Toxicities/Side Effects and the Nursing Process

I. ALTERATIONS IN SENSORY/PERCEPTUAL PATTERNS related to SEDATION, RESTLESSNESS

Defining Characteristics: Sedation, restlessness, and EPS may occur, although are less severe than with phenothiazines. Tardive dyskinesia may occur in older patients.

Nursing Implications: Assess baseline level of consciousness and monitor during therapy. Assess for signs/symptoms of EPS (dystonia, tongue protrusion, trismus, opisthotonus), and administer diphenhydramine as ordered.

II. ALTERATION IN OXYGENATION/PERFUSION related to RESPIRATORY DEPRESSION

Defining Characteristics: Can induce respiratory depression when used with narcotic analgesics; rarely, laryngospasm or bronchospasm may occur.

Nursing Implications: Assess baseline pulmonary status and monitor during therapy. Identify risk factors (concomitant narcotics, CNS depressants), notify physician, and hold drug if respiratory depression occurs or is suspected. Be prepared to institute respiratory support if necessary, and to reverse opiate.

III. ALTERATION IN CARDIAC OUTPUT related to TACHYCARDIA

Defining Characteristics: Tachycardia and hypotension may occur.

Nursing Implications: Assess baseline VS, and monitor during therapy. If hypotension occurs, notify physician and anticipate increasing rate of IV fluids to increase BP. Epinephrine should not be used since drug reverses vasopressor effect; rather, metaraminol or norepinephrine should be used.

IV. ALTERATION IN COMFORT related to CHILLS, FACIAL SWEATING

Defining Characteristics: Rarely, chills, facial sweating, and shivering occur.

Nursing Implications: Assess baseline comfort. Teach patient to report any unusual occurrence. Provide symptomatic management.

Drug: granisetron hydrochloride (Kytril)

Class: Serotonin antagonist.

Mechanism of Action: Binds to vagal afferents (serotonin receptors) adjacent to the enterochromaffin cells in the GI mucosa, thus preventing the stimulation of afferent fibers that would otherwise stimulate the VC and CTZ. In addition, granisetron inhibits a positive feedback loop located on the enterochromaffin cells that normally responds to high levels of serotonin released from chemotherapy injury to the gut mucosa by releasing a surge of additional serotonin. Thus, granisetron blocks two pathways of serotonin release to prevent chemotherapy-induced nausea and vomiting.

Metabolism: Rapidly and extensively metabolized by the liver using the P-450 cytochrome enzymes; 12% of unchanged drug is eliminated in the urine at 48 hours. The half-life of IV granisetron in cancer patients is 9 hours.

Dosage/Range:

- IV: 10 μg/kg IV over 5 minutes, beginning within 30 minutes prior to chemotherapy.
- Oral: 1 mg bid (q12h).

Drug Preparation:

- Dilute in 20–50 mL 0.9% Sodium Chloride or 5% Dextrose.

Drug Administration:

- IV infusion over 5 minutes.

- Drug can also be given IV push over 5 minutes.

Drug Interactions:
- None known, but, because the drug is metabolized by the P-450 cytochrome enzymes, drugs that induce or inhibit this may theoretically change the drug serum levels and half-life.

Lab Effects/Interference:
- Rarely, increased AST, ALT.

Special Considerations:
- Useful in the management of high-dose cisplatin, in combination with dexamethasone, either with oral tablets or IV preparation.
- Preliminary study data showed little difference in efficacy between oral dosing of 1 mg bid versus a single dose of 2 mg.
- Both IV and tablet formulation are indicated for the prevention of nausea and vomiting associated with initial and repeat courses of emetogenic chemotherapy, including cisplatin.

Potential Toxicities/Side Effects and the Nursing Process

I. ALTERATION IN COMFORT related to HEADACHE, ASTHENIA, SOMNOLENCE

Defining Characteristics: Side effects are uncommon but may include headache, asthenia, and somnolence.

Nursing Implications: Teach patient that side effects may occur. Headache is usually relieved by OTC analgesics such as acetaminophen.

II. ALTERATION IN ELIMINATION related to CONSTIPATION OR DIARRHEA

Defining Characteristics: A small percentage of patients may experience constipation or diarrhea.

Nursing Implications: Assess baseline elimination pattern. Instruct patient to report alterations. Identify patients at risk, such as those receiving narcotic analgesics for cancer pain, who may develop constipation. Assist patient in modifying bowel regimen.

Drug: haloperidol (Haldol)

Class: Butyrophenone.

Mechanism of Action: Tranquilizer that depresses cerebral cortex, hypothalamus, limbic system (controls activity and aggression); appears to block dopamine receptors in CTZ, giving antiemetic activity.

Metabolism: Metabolized by the liver, excreted in the urine, bile, and crosses placenta. Enters breast milk. Half-life is 21 hours.

Dosage/Range:

Adult:

- Oral: 3–5 mg q2h × 3–4 doses, beginning 30 minutes before chemotherapy.
- IM: 0.5–2 mg (dose-reduce in elderly patients).

Drug Preparation/Administration:

- Available as 0.5-, 1-, 2-, 5-, 10-, 20-mg tablets; injection: 5 mg/mL.

Drug Interactions:

- Epinephrine: reversal of vasopressor effects; avoid concurrent use.
- CNS depressants: increased sedation; monitor patient closely.

Lab Effects/Interference:

- Rarely, increased alk phos, bili, serum transaminases (AST, ALT).
- Rarely, decreased PT (if patient on warfarin).
- Rarely, decreased serum cholesterol.

Special Considerations:

- Indicated for the management of psychotic disorders, short-term treatment of hyperactive children showing excessive motor activity, schizophrenia; may be used in the management of nausea and vomiting.
- Contraindicated in severe toxic CNS depression or comatose states; individuals with hypersensitivity; patients with Parkinson's disease, blood dyscrasias, brain damage, bone marrow depression, and alcohol or barbiturate withdrawal states.
- Shown to be equivalent to THC and superior to phenothiazines when tested as an antiemetic.

Potential Toxicities/Side Effects and the Nursing Process

I. ALTERATIONS IN SENSORY/PERCEPTUAL PATTERNS related to TARDIVE DYSKINESIA

Defining Characteristics: With chronic use, tardive dyskinesia syndrome occurs, characterized by involuntary, dyskinetic movements; sedation, EPS may occur when used as an antiemetic.

Nursing Implications: Assess baseline level of consciousness and monitor during therapy. Assess for signs/symptoms of EPS (dystonia, tongue protrusion, trismus, opisthotonus), and administer diphenhydramine as ordered.

II. ALTERATION IN OXYGENATION related to LARYNGOSPASM

Defining Characteristics: Laryngospasm, respiratory depression occur rarely.

Nursing Implications: Assess baseline pulmonary status and monitor during therapy. Identify risk factors (concomitant narcotics, CNS depressants), notify physician, and hold drug if respiratory depression occurs or is suspected. Be prepared to institute respiratory support if necessary, and to reverse opiate.

III. ALTERATION IN CARDIAC OUTPUT/PERFUSION related to ORTHOSTATIC HYPOTENSION

Defining Characteristics: Orthostatic hypotension may occur and may precipitate angina; also, tachycardia, EKG changes, and rare cardiac arrest may occur.

Nursing Implications: Assess VS baseline, and monitor during therapy. If hypotension occurs, notify physician and anticipate increasing rate of IV fluids to increase BP. Epinephrine should NOT be used since drug reverses vasopressor effect; rather, metaraminol or norepinephrine should be used.

Drug: metoclopramide hydrochloride (Reglan)

Class: Substituted benzamide.

Mechanism of Action: Procainamide derivative without cardiac effects. Acts both centrally and peripherally. Acts peripherally to enhance the action of acetylcholine at muscarinic synapses and in the CNS to antagonize dopamine. Is primarily a dopamine antagonist blocking the CTZ; also stimulates upper GI tract motility, thus increasing gastric emptying, and opposes retrograde peristalsis of retching.

Metabolism: Metabolized by the liver, excreted in the urine, with a half-life of 4 hours.

Dosage/Range:

Adult:

- Oral: 10 mg qid (gastroparesis).
- IV: 2 mg/kg q2h × 3–5 doses OR 3 mg/kg q2h × 2 doses, beginning 30 minutes prior to chemotherapy. Dose-reduce if renal insufficiency.

Drug Preparation/Administration:
- IV: further dilute in 50 mL 0.9% Sodium Chloride or 5% Dextrose and administer over 15 minutes.

Drug Interactions:
- Digoxin: may decrease absorption; monitor digoxin effectiveness and modify dose as needed.
- Aspirin, acetaminophen, tetracycline, ethanol, levodopa, diazepam: may increase absorption; monitor for drug toxicity.
- CNS depressants: increased depressant effects; monitor patient closely.

Lab Effects/Interference:
- None known.

Special Considerations:
- Indicated as an antiemetic to prevent nausea and vomiting from chemotherapy, delayed gastric emptying, gastroesophageal reflux.
- There is an increased incidence of dystonic reactions in men under 35 years old. Consider diphenhydramine q4h or lorazepam and decadron to minimize dystonic reactions.
- Efficacy as an antiemetic: 60% complete protection against high-dose cisplatin, and increased to 66% with the addition of steroids and lorazepam.
- Contraindicated in patients with prior hypersensitivity to this drug, procaine, or procainamide; patients with seizure disorder, pheochromocytoma, GI obstruction.
- Use cautiously in patients with breast cancer, as may increase prolactin levels, and in patients with renal insufficiency.

Potential Toxicities/Side Effects and the Nursing Process

I. ALTERATIONS IN SENSORY/PERCEPTUAL PATTERNS related to SEDATION, EPS

Defining Characteristics: Sedation, akathisia (restlessness), adverse dystonic or extrapyramidal effects may occur; increased risk in patients < 30 years old.

Nursing Implications: Assess baseline neurologic status, and monitor during therapy. Protect patient safety, and keep all necessary patient equipment at the bedside, e.g., commode. Assess for extrapyramidal side effects, and administer diphenhydramine as ordered. In addition, lorazepam administered as part of combination antiemetics helps to decrease akathisia.

II. POTENTIAL FOR ALTERED BOWEL ELIMINATION related to DIARRHEA

Defining Characteristics: Increase in both esophageal sphincter pressure and gastric emptying, leading to diarrhea with high doses. Action antagonized by narcotics.

Nursing Implications: Assess baseline bowel elimination status. Teach patient to report diarrhea, and administer kaolin/pectin as ordered, or other antidiarrheals. Arrange for commode at the bedside if bathroom far from bed. Also, diarrhea may be prevented by administration of dexamethasone as part of antiemetic regimen.

III. ALTERATION IN COMFORT related to DRY/MOUTH, RASH

Defining Characteristics: Dry mouth, rash, urticaria, hypotension may occur.

Nursing Implications: Assess baseline comfort. Teach patient to report rash, urticaria, and treat symptomatically. Monitor VS, and slow infusion rate if hypotensive, as well as replace IV fluids per physician's order.

Drug: ondansetron hydrochloride (Zofran)

Class: Serotonin antagonist.

Mechanism of Action: Selective 5-HT_3 (serotonin) receptor antagonist and may block 5-HT_3 receptors found peripherally on the vagus nerve terminals and centrally in the CTZ, thus preventing chemotherapy-induced vomiting.

Metabolism: Extensively metabolized, with only 5% of parent compound found in urine.

Dosage/Range:

Adults:

- IV: 0.15 mg/kg q4h × 3 doses OR as a single 32-mg dose, beginning 30 minutes prior to chemotherapy.
- Highly emetogenic chemo: 24 mg po 30 minutes before chemotherapy.
- Moderately emetogenic chemotherapy.
- Oral: 8 mg PO bid, beginning 30 minutes before chemotherapy, and continuing for 1–2 days after chemotherapy.

Drug Preparation/Administration:

- IV available as 2 mg/mL or 32 mg/50 mL; mix in 50 mL 5% Dextrose or 0.9% Sodium Chloride and infuse over 15 minutes.
- Note: single-dose ondansetron (> 22 mg) needs to be given over at least 30 minutes to minimize risk of headache/hypotension.

- Tablets available as either regular tablet or ODT (oral disintegrating tablet), which is freeze-dried and dissolves instantly on the tongue, available in 4-mg and 8-mg strengths.
- Available as an oral solution, 4 mg/5 mL.

Drug Interactions:
- None significant.

Lab Effects/Interference:
- Rarely, increased LFTs.

Special Considerations:
- Contraindicated in patients hypersensitive to the drug.
- Does not affect the dopamine system, so does not cause EPS.
- Approved for use to prevent nausea/vomiting related to chemotherapy, radiation therapy to the abdomen or total body, and following surgery (post-operative).

Potential Toxicities/Side Effects and the Nursing Process

I. ALTERATION IN ELIMINATION related to DIARRHEA or CONSTIPATION

Defining Characteristics: Patients may experience diarrhea (22%) or constipation (11%).

Nursing Implications: Assess baseline elimination status. Teach patient to report alterations, and treat symptomatically.

II. ALTERATION IN COMFORT related to HEADACHE

Defining Characteristics: Headache may occur (16%).

Nursing Implications: Assess comfort level. Teach patient to report headache. Administer acetaminophen as ordered.

III. ALTERATION IN NUTRITION, LESS THAN BODY REQUIREMENTS, related to ↑ LFTs

Defining Characteristics: Transient increases in LFTs may occur (5%).

Nursing Implications: Assess LFTs baseline, and monitor during therapy.

Drug: palonosetron (Aloxi)

Class: Serotonin antagonist antiemetic

Mechanism of Action: Selective serotonin antagonist with strong binding affinity to receptor.

Metabolism: Drug is excreted via renal and metabolic pathways

Dosage/Range:

- Single 0.25 mg IV over 30 seconds 30 minutes before the start of chemotherapy
- Give once every 7 days

Drug Preparation/Administration: Draw up in a syringe to administer IVP over 30 seconds; flush line with Normal Saline prior to and after drug administration.

Drug Interactions: None known.

Lab Effects/Interference: Rare prolongation of QTc interval on ECG (> 500 msec, changes > 60 msec from baseline).

Special Considerations:

- Drug is indicated for:
  - Prevention of acute nausea and vomiting associated with initial and repeat courses of moderately and highly emetogenic cancer chemotherapy.
  - Prevention of delayed nausea and vomiting associated with initial and repeat courses of moderately emetogenic cancer chemotherapy.
- Palonosetron has greater potency, higher binding affinity to the 5-HT3 receptor, and has a longer half life (40 hours) than any of the 1st generation serotonin antagonists.
- Drug should be administered with caution to patients with prolonged conduction intervals (QTc), such as patients who have hypokalemia, hypomagnesemia, are taking diuretics, have congenital QT syndrome, taking antiarrhythmic drugs or other drugs leading to QTc prolongation such as arsenic, and cumulative high dose anthracycline therapy.

Potential Toxicities/Side Effects and the Nursing Process

I. ALTERATION IN COMFORT related to HEADACHE

Defining Characteristics: Headache occurs in 9% of patients.

Nursing Implications: Teach patients that this may occur, and to take acetaminophen to relieve headache if it occurs.

II. ALTERATION IN BOWEL ELIMINATION related to CONSTIPATION

Defining Characteristics: Constipation occurs in about 5% of patients

Nursing Implications: Assess baseline bowel elimination status. Teach patients that constipation may occur, and to use usual strategies to prevent constipation. If constipation occurs, teach patient to use bowel softeners, laxatives as needed, and to increase oral fluids, fiber, and exercise to promote peristalsis.

Drug: perphenazine

Class: Phenothiazine.

Mechanism of Action: Antipsychotic agent. Blocks dopamine receptors in CTZ; also decreases vagal stimulation of VC by peripheral afferents.

Metabolism: Metabolized by the liver, excreted in the urine, crosses placenta, enters breast milk.

Dosage/Range:

Adult:

- Oral: 4 mg q4–6h.
- IM/IV: 5 mg IVB q4–6h OR 5 mg IVB then infusion at 1 mg/hour for 10 hours.
- Maximum: 30 mg in 24 hours (inpatient), or 15 mg in 24 hours (outpatient).

Drug Preparation/Administration:

- Further dilute IV drug in 50 mL 0.9% Sodium Chloride, and infuse over 20 minutes.

Drug Interactions:

- Antacids: decreased perphenazine absorption; take 2 hours before or after antacid.
- Antidepressants: increased Parkinsonian symptoms; avoid concomitant use or use cautiously.
- Barbiturates: increased CNS depressant effect; use together cautiously, if at all.

Lab Effects/Interference:

- Rarely, increased LFTs.

Special Considerations:

- Effective in management of nausea and vomiting related to moderately emetogenic drugs.
- Contraindicated in patients hypersensitive to the drug, or who have blood dyscrasias, coma.

- Increased incidence of dystonic reactions in men under 35 years. Consider diphenhydramine or lorazepam and decadron q4h to minimize risk of dystonia.
- Indicated in the treatment of psychotic disorders, schizophrenia, alcoholism, intractable hiccups; and is used to prevent chemotherapy-induced nausea and vomiting.

Potential Toxicities/Side Effects and the Nursing Process

I. ALTERATIONS IN SENSORY PERCEPTUAL PATTERNS related to SEDATION, EPS

Defining Characteristics: Sedation, blurred vision, and EPS reactions may occur, especially dystonia; also, seizure threshold may be lowered.

Nursing Implications: Assess baseline mental status. Instruct patient to report signs/symptoms of EPS, and assess for them during treatment (tongue protrusion, trismus, akathisia or restlessness, tremor, insomnia, dizziness). Administer diphenhydramine as ordered to reverse reaction. Diphenhydramine should be ordered prior to drug to prevent EPS.

II. ALTERATION IN NUTRITION related to CONSTIPATION, ↑ APPETITE, CHOLESTATIC JAUNDICE

Defining Characteristics: Dry mouth, constipation, increased appetite and weight gain, cholestatic jaundice may occur.

Nursing Implications: Assess baseline nutritional patterns, moistness of mucous membranes, and elimination pattern. Assess baseline liver function, and monitor during therapy.

III. ALTERATION IN SKIN INTEGRITY related to RASH

Defining Characteristics: Mild photosensitivity, rash, urticaria, and, rarely, exfoliative dermatitis may occur.

Nursing Implications: Assess baseline skin integrity. Instruct patient to report any changes.

Drug: prochlorperazine (Compazine)

Class: Phenothiazine.

Mechanism of Action: Blocks dopamine receptors in CTZ; also decreases vagal stimulation of VC by peripheral afferents.

Metabolism: Metabolized by liver, excreted in kidney, crosses placenta, excreted in breast milk. Onset of action for oral is 30–40 minutes, duration 3–4 hours; extended-release 30–40 minutes with duration 10–13 hours; PR onset 60 minutes, duration 3–4 hours; and IM onset 10–20 minutes, duration 12 hours.

Dosage/Range:

Adult:

- Oral: 5–25 mg q4–6h; slow-release: 10–75 mg q12h.
- IM/IV: 5–40 mg q3–4h; dilute in 50 mL 5% Dextrose or 0.9% Sodium Chloride and administer IV over 20–30 minutes.
- PR: 25 mg q4–6h.

Drug Preparation/Administration:

- Store in tight, light-resistant containers. Administer IM injection deep into large muscle mass.

Drug Interactions:

- Antacids: decreased prochlorperazine absorption; take 2 hours before or after antacid.
- Antidepressants: increased Parkinsonian symptoms; avoid concomitant use or use cautiously.
- Barbiturates: decreased prochlorperazine effect; may need to increase dose of prochlorperazine.

Lab Effects/Interference:

- Rarely, may cause increased LFTs.

Special Considerations:

- Indicated in the management of chemotherapy-induced nausea and vomiting.
- Increased risk of dystonic reactions in men under 35 years old. Consider diphenyhydramine or lorazepam and decadron q4h to minimize risk of dystonia.
- Dose-reduce in the elderly.
- Use cautiously in combination with CNS depressants.
- Contraindicated in patients with hypersensitivity to phenothiazines or with coma, seizure, encephalopathy.

Potential Toxicities/Side Effects and the Nursing Process

I. ALTERATIONS IN SENSORY PERCEPTUAL PATTERN related to SEDATION, EPS

Defining Characteristics: Sedation, blurred vision, EPS reactions may occur, especially dystonia; also, seizure threshold may be lowered.

Nursing Implications: Assess baseline mental status. Teach patient to report signs/symptoms of EPS and assess for them during treatment (tongue protrusion, trismus, akathisia or restlessness, tremor, insomnia, dizziness). Administer diphenhydramine as ordered to reverse reaction. Diphenhydramine may be ordered prior to drug to prevent EPS.

II. ALTERATION IN NUTRITION related to CONSTIPATION, ↑ APPETITE, CHOLESTATIC JAUNDICE

Defining Characteristics: Dry mouth, constipation, increased appetite and weight gain, cholestatic jaundice may occur.

Nursing Implications: Assess baseline nutritional patterns, moistness of mucous membranes, and elimination pattern. Assess baseline liver function, and monitor during therapy.

III. ALTERATION IN SKIN INTEGRITY related to RASH

Defining Characteristics: Mild photosensitivity, rash, urticaria, and, rarely, exfoliative dermatitis may occur.

Nursing Implications: Assess baseline skin integrity. Teach patient to report any changes.

IV. ALTERATION IN CARDIAC OUTPUT related to ORTHOSTATIC HYPOTENSION

Defining Characteristics: Orthostatic hypotension, tachycardia, and EKG changes may occur.

Nursing Implications: Assess baseline VS prior to and during IV infusions, especially with high doses. Discuss with physician and anticipate increasing IV fluid rate if hypotensive.

Drug: promethazine hydrochloride (Anergan, Phenameth, Phenergan)

Class: Antihistamine; phenothiazine derivative with sedative, antihistamine, and mild antiemetic properties.

Mechanism of Action: Drug is anticholinergic and has CNS depressant effects; specific CNS mechanism is unknown.

Dosage/Range:

Adult:

- Antiemetic: Oral/IM/IV: 12.5–25 mg q4h PRN.

Drug Preparation/Administration:
- Drug must not be given SQ or intraarterially.
- IV: administer a dilute solution < 25 mg/mL, at < 25 mg/min.
- IM: administer deep IM in large muscle mass.

Drug Interactions:
- CNS depressants: increased sedation; avoid concurrent use.
- Epinephrine: may reverse vasopressor effects and further decrease BP; avoid concurrent use.
- Phenothiazines: increased toxicity; avoid concurrent use.

Special Considerations:
- Contraindicated in patients with increased intraocular pressure, prostatic hypertrophy, epilepsy, coma, CNS depression, intestinal obstruction.
- Use cautiously in the elderly and patients with asthma, hypertension, and seizure disorder.

Potential Toxicities/Side Effects and the Nursing Process

I. ALTERATIONS IN SENSORY/PERCEPTUAL PATTERNS related to CONFUSION, RESTLESSNESS

Defining Characteristics: Increased risk in the elderly for confusion, sedation, drowsiness, restlessness, tremors; blurred vision may also occur.

Nursing Implications: Assess baseline level of consciousness, and monitor during therapy. Assess for signs/symptoms of EPS (dystonia, tongue protrusion, trismus, opisthotonus), and administer diphenhydramine as ordered.

II. ALTERATION IN CARDIAC OUTPUT related to HYPOTENSION

Defining Characteristics: Hypotension may occur, especially with high or IV dosing.

Nursing Implications: Assess baseline VS, and monitor during IV administration. Administer drug slowly, and notify physician if hypotension occurs. Anticipate increasing IV fluids.

III. ALTERATION IN NUTRITION, LESS THAN BODY REQUIREMENTS, related to GI SIDE EFFECTS

Defining Characteristics: Dry mouth, nausea, vomiting, and constipation may occur.

Nursing Implications: Assess baseline nutritional status. Instruct patient to report GI side effects. Discuss alternative antiemetic if these occur. Assess elimination status; teach patient importance of diet high in bulk and fiber, increased fluids, and exercise to prevent constipation.

IV. ALTERATION IN URINARY ELIMINATION related to URINARY RETENTION

Defining Characteristics: Urinary retention may occur.

Nursing Implications: Instruct patient to report this symptom; discuss alternative drug with physician for control of emesis.

Drug: scopolamine

Class: Antimuscarinic; used as an antiemetic.

Mechanism of Action: Appears to prevent nausea/vomiting associated with motion sickness by blocking cholinergic impulses, thus preventing stimulation of the VC.

Dosage/Range:

Adult:

- Patch: transdermal patch 1.5 mg q72h.

Drug Preparation/Administration:

- Apply 4 hours prior to time protection is needed.
- Apply to clean and dry hairless area behind ear; remove clear plastic cover, exposing adhesive layer; apply directly to skin behind ear and press firmly; wash hands.

Drug Interactions:

- None significant.

Lab Effects/Interference:

- None known.

Special Considerations:

- Use cautiously in patients with glaucoma, urinary bladder-neck obstruction.
- Wash hands after handling patch to prevent exposure to scopolamine.
- If patch falls off, wash area, then reapply new patch in another location.

Potential Toxicities/Side Effects and the Nursing Process

I. ALTERATION IN MUCOUS MEMBRANE INTEGRITY related to DRY MOUTH

Defining Characteristics: Dry mouth occurs in 67% of patients.

Nursing Implications: Teach patient this may occur. Suggest patient suck ice chips, sugar-free candy, or practice usual oral hygiene regimen more frequently.

II. ALTERATIONS IN SENSORY/PERCEPTUAL PATTERNS related to DROWSINESS, BLURRED VISION

Defining Characteristics: Drowsiness, blurred vision, mydriasis may occur; rarely, disorientation, restlessness, confusion may occur.

Nursing Implications: Assess baseline mental status. Instruct patient to report changes in vision or feeling state. Assess patient safety needs, and provide safe environment.

Drug: thiethylperazine (Torecan)

Class: Phenothiazine derivative; antiemetic.

Mechanism of Action: Blocks stimulation of CTZ and VC.

Metabolism: Metabolized by liver, excreted by kidneys, crosses placenta, and may be excreted in breast milk.

Dosage/Range:

Adult:

- Oral/PR/IM: 10 mg qd-tid.

Drug Preparation/Administration:

- IM: give deep IM into large muscle mass.
- Do not give IV (causes hypotension).

Drug Interactions:

- Barbiturates: may decrease antiemetic effect; increase dose as needed.
- Antacids: may decrease absorption of thiethylperazine; administer 2 hours before or after antacid.
- Epinephrine: may reverse vasopressor effect of epinephrine; avoid concurrent use.

Lab Effects/Interference:

- Rarely, increased LFTs.

Special Considerations:

- Contraindicated in patients with severe CNS depression, coma, prior sensitivity reaction.
- Contraindicated in patients allergic to dye tartazine (FD + C yellow No 5) as it may cause bronchial asthma.
- Torecan injection contains sodium metabisulfite; contraindicated in patients allergic to sulfites.
- Increased risk of dystonic reactions in men under 35 years old. Consider diphenhydramine or lorazepam and decadron every 4 hours to minimize dystonia.

Potential Toxicities/Side Effects and the Nursing Process

I. ALTERATIONS IN SENSORY/PERCEPTUAL PATTERNS related to DROWSINESS, EPS

Defining Characteristics: Drowsiness may occur after IM injection. Rarely, extrapyramidal side effects may occur (i.e., dystonia, torticollis, akathisia, gait disturbances), as may blurred vision and tinnitus.

Nursing Implications: Assess baseline level of consciousness, and monitor during therapy. Assess for signs/symptoms of EPS (dystonia, tongue protrusion, trismus, opisthotonus), and administer diphenhydramine as ordered.

II. ALTERATION IN CARDIAC OUTPUT related to HYPOTENSION

Defining Characteristics: Hypotension may occur after IM dosing; rarely, tachycardia, EKG changes occur.

Nursing Implications: Assess baseline VS, and monitor during IV administration. Administer drug slowly, and notify physician if hypotension occurs. Anticipate increasing IV fluids.

Chapter 8

Anorexia and Cachexia

Anorexia and weight loss may be presenting symptoms of cancer, or symptoms of advanced disease. No other symptoms may cause more powerful distress to a patient than being confronted with weight loss and inability to eat due to anorexia. Consequences of severe anorexia include nutritional depletion and further weight loss, which result in decreased functional status, diminished treatment responses to chemotherapy, and apparent decreased quality of life. Primary cachexia, or wasting syndrome, occurs in at least two-thirds of patients with advanced cancer or human immunodeficiency virus (HIV) disease. The associated extreme weakness and fatigue lead to incapacity, dependency, social isolation, and again, apparent diminished quality of life.

In addition, anorexia and cachexia can be terrifying and frustrating to family members. The patient's spouse may be used to nurturing the patient and preparing meals, and feel rejected and frightened by a loved one's inability to eat. This may symbolize personal failure on the part of the spouse, as well as failure of current treatment to reverse the disease process and a poor prognosis.

Metabolically, cachexia appears to result from chronic, systemic inflammation with the release of acute-phase proteins and orchestration by cytokines such as tumor necrosis factor, IL-1 and IL-6 (Laviano et al, 2002). This leads to the preferential breakdown of skeletal muscle protein and body fat, resulting in the profound wasting syndrome characterized by anorexia, early satiety, weight loss, decreased function, and death (Inui, 2002). Secondary cachexia is simple starvation from decreased food intake or defective nutrient absorption, and results from situations such as nausea, vomiting, and anorexia due to chemotherapy. As expected, patients responding to chemotherapy will show a weight gain.

Pharmacologic agents used to stimulate appetite are varied in mechanism of action, efficacy, and strength of evidence. Corticosteroids have been tried for many years, with usual effect within 1-3 weeks (Ottery et al, 1998; Loprinzi et al, 1999). However, side effects have limited their usefulness, such as insomnia, muscle catabolism, hyperglycemia. Of the studies of pharmacologic agents in the treatment of anorexia and cachexia in cancer, megestrol acetate has shown statistical improvement in nonfluid weight gain (Ottery, 1998). Mantovani et al (1998) suggest that megestrol acetate, in fact, downregulates cytokine production, resulting in increased appetite and anabolism. There appears to be a dose-response effect, and Loprinzi et al (1992) showed optimal weight gain at a dose of 800 mg/day. Patients showed increased appetite, increased food intake, weight gain, and less nausea and vomiting. The incidence of thrombophlebitis was 6%. Loprinzi et al also demonstrated that the weight gain resulting from megestrol acetate is increased fat and lean body mass, not water gain (i.e., edema, ascites).

Thalidomide, an agent originally developed as a nonbarbiturate sedative but which was never marketed as such due to its teratogenicity, has been shown to increase weight gain and lean body mass in HIV-infected individuals with cachexia (Ottery, 1998).

Metoclopramide, at low doses for stimulation of GI motility, has been shown to decrease early satiety and postprandial fullness, and may be helpful for some patients (Kris et al, 1985). Cannabinoid derivatives, such as δ-9-tetrahydrocannabinol (THC) and dronabinol, appear to stimulate appetite and possible weight gain in some patients (Beal et al, 1997; Klausner et al, 1996; Kaplan et al, 1998). Other agents that are being studied are eicosapentaenoic (EPA) acid (fish oil, stabilize acute phase proteins) and melatonin (regulation of circadian rhythm) [Cunningham, 2003].

References

Beal JE, et al. Long-term Efficacy and Safety of Dronabinol for Acquired Immunodeficiency Syndrome-associated Anorexia. *J Pain Symptom Manage.* 1997;14(1):7–14

Brown JK. A Systematic Review of the Evidence on Symptom Management of Cancer-related Anorexia and Cachexia. *Oncol Nurs Forum* 2002;29:517–530

Bruera E, Macmillan K, Kuehn N, et al. A Controlled Trial of Megestrol Acetate on Appetite, Caloric Intake, Nutritional Status, and Other Symptoms in Patients with Advanced Cancer. *Cancer* 1990;66:1279–1282

Chlebowski RT, Bulcavage L, Grosvenor M, et al. Hydrazine Sulfate Influence on Nutritional Status and Survival in NSCLC. *J Clin Oncol* 1990;8:9–15

Cunningham RS. The Anorexia-Cachexia Syndrome, chapter 9. Yarbro CH, Frogge MH, Goodman M, (eds), *Cancer Symptom Management,* 3rd ed. Sudbury, MA: Jones and Bartlett Publishers 2003;137–155

Dreizen S, McCredie KB, Keating MJ, et al. Nutritional Deficiencies in Patients Receiving Cancer Chemotherapy. *Postgrad Med J* 1990;87:163–170

Enck RE. Anorexia and Cachexia: An Update. *Am J Hospice Palliative Care* 1990;7(5): 13–15

Inui A. Cancer Anorexia-Cachexia Syndrome: Current issues in Research and Management. *CACancer J Clin* 2002;52:72–91

Kaplan G, Schambelan M, Gottleib C, et al. Thalidomide Reverses Cachexia in HIV-Wasting Syndrome. *5th International Conf on Retroviruses and Opportunistic Infections, Abstract 476. February 1-5, 1998, Chicago, IL* 1998

Klausner JD, Makonkawkeyoon S, Akarasewi P, et al. The Effect of Thalidomide on the Pathogenesis of Human Immunodeficiency Virus Type 1 and M. tuberculosis Infection. *J Acquir Immune Defic Syndr and Hum Retrovirology* 1996;11:247–257

Kornblith AB, Hollis D, Phillips CA, et al. Effect of Megestrol Acetate upon Quality of Life in Advanced Breast Cancer Patients in a Dose Response Trial. . *Proc American Society of Clinical Oncologists* 1992;11:377

Kris MG, Yeh SDJ, Gralla RJ, et al. Symptomatic Gastroparesis in Cancer Patients: Possible Cause of Anorexia That Can Be Improved with Oral Metoclopramide. *Proc American Society of Clinical Oncologists* 1985;4:267

Laviano A, Russo M, Freda F, et al. Neurochemical Mechanisms for Cancer Cachexia. *Nutrition* 2002;18:100–105

Loprinzi CL, Ellison NM, Schard OJ, et al. Controlled Trial of Megestrol Acetate for the Treatment of Cancer Anorexia and Cachexia. *J Natl Cancer Inst* 1990;82: 1127–1132

Loprinzi CL, Jensen M, Burnham N, et al. Body Composition Changes in Cancer Patients Who GainWeight from Megestrol Acetate. *Proc American Society of Clinical Oncologists* 1992;11:378

Loprinzi CL, Kugler JW, Sloan JA, et al. Randomized Comparison of Megestrol Acetate versus Dexamethasone versus Fluoxymesterone for the Treatment of Cancer Anorexia/Cachexia. *J Clin Oncol* 1999;17:3299–3306

Loprinzi CL, Mailliard J, Schaid D, et al. Dose/Response Evaluation of Megestrol Acetate for the Treatment of Cancer Anorexia/Cachexia: A Mayo Clinic and North Central Cancer Treatment Group Trial. *Proc American Society of Clinical Oncologists* 1992;11:378

Mantovani G, Maccio A, Paola L, et al. Cytokine Activity in Cancer-related Anorexia/ Cachexia: Role of megestrol Acetate and Medroxyprogesterone Acetate. *Semin Oncol* 1998;25 (suppl):45–52

Ottery FD, Walsh D, Strawford A. Pharmacologic Management of Anorexia/Cachexia. *Semin Oncol* 1998;25 (suppl):35–44

Drug: dronabinol (Marinol)

Class: Cannabinoid.

Mechanism of Action: Stimulates appetite in acquired immunodeficiency syndrome (AIDS) patients, leading to trends toward improved body weight and mood.

Metabolism: 90–95% absorption after oral dose, but because of first-pass effect of the liver and high lipid solubility, only about 20% of the dose reaches the systemic circulation. Large area of distribution so that drug continues to be excreted for a long period of time. The appetite stimulation effect may persist for 24 hours from a single dose.

Dosage/Range:
- 2.5 mg bid before lunch and supper, or if patient is intolerant, a single 2.5-mg dose may be taken at bedtime.

Drug Preparation:
- Available in 2.5-, 5-, or 10-mg gel capsules that harden under refrigeration.

Drug Administration:
- Oral.

Drug Interactions:
- Amphetamines, cocaine: additive hypertension, tachycardia.
- Atropine, scopolamine: tachycardia, drowsiness.
- Amitriptyline, tricyclic antidepressants: additive tachycardia, hypertension.
- Barbiturates, CNS depressants, buspirone: drowsiness and additive CNS depression.
- Theophylline: increased metabolism.

Lab Effects/Interference:
- None known.

Special Considerations:
- Drug has antiemetic qualities.

Potential Toxicities/Side Effects and the Nursing Process

I. ALTERATIONS IN SENSORY/PERCEPTUAL PATTERNS related to CNS CHANGES

Defining Characteristics: Drug can cause changes in mood, cognition, memory, and perception. In addition, nervousness, anxiety, confusion, dizziness, depersonalization, euphoria, paranoid reaction, somnolence, and thinking abnormalities can occur. Drug has abuse potential.

Nursing Implications: Assess appropriateness of drug for patient, as this would not be the drug of choice for a substance abuser, either one who is actively using or who has withdrawn and is abstaining because of abuse potential. Teach patient of possible side effects, and self-care strategies to avoid heightened fear or anxiety.

II. POTENTIAL FOR ALTERATION IN OXYGENATION related to SYMPATHOMIMETIC EFFECTS

Defining Characteristics: Tachycardia and conjunctival injection may occur. Drug interactions may cause hypertension.

Nursing Implications: Review patient medication profile to identify any possible drug interactions. Monitor appetite stimulation effects, and weigh these against any sympathomimetic changes.

Drug: megestrol acetate (Megace)

Class: Synthetic progestin.

Mechanism of Action: Alters malignant cell environment in hormonally sensitive tumors, discouraging tumor cell proliferation; appears to stimulate appetite and weight gain in cancer cachexia directly or indirectly through antagonism of TNF. Designated as orphan drug by FDA for management of anorexia, cachexia, or weight loss > 10% of baseline. Approved for AIDS-related cachexia.

Metabolism: Well absorbed from GI tract. Metabolized in liver and excreted by kidneys.

Dosage/Range:
- Optimal dose for management of cachexia is 800 mg/day in a single dose.

Drug Preparation/Administration:
- Store in tight container at temperature < 40°C (104°F).
- Oral administration.

Drug Interactions:
- None.

Lab Effects/Interference:
- Rarely, may increase glucose, lactic dehydrogenase (LDH).

Special Considerations:
- Drug is expensive.
- One-third of patients with metastatic cancer gain weight.
- Weight gain appears to be from increased fat stores rather than water gain (Loprinzi, et al 1992).

Potential Toxicities/Side Effects and the Nursing Process

I. ALTERATIONS IN PERFUSION related to DEEP VEIN THROMBOSIS

Defining Characteristics: Rarely, 6% of patients may experience deep vein thrombosis (DVT) or pulmonary emboli.

Nursing Implications: Assess baseline peripheral vascular status and monitor during therapy. Teach patient to report pain in calf, erythema, shortness of breath, chest pain immediately.

II. ALTERATION IN COMFORT related to CARPAL TUNNEL SYNDROME NIV, TUMOR FLARE

Defining Characteristics: Carpal tunnel syndrome, nausea, vomiting, tumor flare may occur rarely.

Nursing Implications: Instruct patient to report any signs/symptoms. Discuss with patient, physician symptomatic measures.

III. ANXIETY related to ABNORMAL UTERINE BLEEDING

Defining Characteristics: Breakthrough vaginal bleeding, discharge often occur in females, and can cause anxiety.

Nursing Implications: Teach female patient that this is an expected side effect. Encourage patient to verbalize feelings, provide patient with emotional support and information about cause and management.

Drug: thalidomide (Thalomid) (investigational)

Class: Inhibitor of TNF-α; nonbarbiturate sedative.

Mechanism of Action: Selective inhibitor of TNF-α. TNF-α is implicated as a principal mediator in the complex syndrome of HIV or cancer cachexia. TNF-α has been shown to cause effects similar to many of those seen in cancer cachexia: weight loss, anorexia, fever, metabolic abnormalities such as hyperlipidemia, insulin resistance, muscle wasting.

Metabolism: Well absorbed after oral administration. Mean peak serum level reached at 4–5 hours. Elimination half-life is 4–12 hours, with drug found in the plasma after 24 hours. NOT metabolized using P-450 hepatic enzyme system, and has low renal excretion.

Dosage/Range:

Adult:

- 100 mg/day at hs (range 50–200 mg/day).
- If needed, increase by 100 mg/day at intervals of 1–2 weeks.

Drug Preparation/Administration:

- Oral, give at bedtime.
- Available for investigational or compassionate use in 50-mg capsules.

Drug Interactions:

- Barbiturates, alcohol, chlorpromazine, reserpine: increased sedation.

Lab Effects/Interference:

- May slightly increase HIV viral load.
- Rare neutropenia, especially in HIV-infected patients.

Special Considerations:

- Studies in HIV wasting have showed a mean gain of 6.5% in body weight in 3 weeks vs 0.9% in controls (Klausner et al, 1996), and other studies have shown that weight gain is lean body mass (Kaplan et al, 1998).

- ABSOLUTE CONTRAINDICATION IS PREGNANCY. Pregnancy test must be routinely negative prior to beginning therapy in women of child-bearing age. Contraception is mandatory for men and women.
- Women taking hormonal contraception, as well as any of the following—barbiturates, glucocorticoids, phenytoin, carbamazepine—have decreased efficacy of the hormonal contraception and must use barrier contraception as well.
- Drug is being studied in higher doses as an anticancer agent in tumors that are TNF-α dependent (e.g., Kaposi's sarcoma) as well as in other tumors (metastatic breast cancer, prostate cancer); also being studied in graft-versus-host disease.
- Patient must be enrolled in a government-monitored registry, and prescriptions can be written or dispensed by precertified doctors and pharmacists, respectively. Only a 28-day supply will be given, and women must have a negative pregnancy test before next prescription is written.

Potential Toxicities/Side Effects and the Nursing Process

I. ALTERATION IN SEXUALITY/REPRODUCTION related to POTENTIAL TERATOGENICITY

Defining Characteristics: Drug is teratogenic and a single dose can cause birth defects. Unclear if drug is excreted in semen.

Nursing Implications: Assess reproductive status, sexual activity, and birth control measures used for both men and women. Instruct male patients to use barrier contraception, and women to use both barrier and hormonal contraception. Women of childbearing age must have a negative pregnancy test baseline to begin the drug, and pregnancy test should be repeated every two weeks for two months then every month. Instruct patient to continue contraception one month after drug is discontinued. Physicians, patients, and pharmacists must participate in drug manufacturer (Celgene, Warren, NJ) STEPS program (System for Thalidomid Education and Prescription Safety).

II. ALTERATION IN SENSORY/PERCEPTUAL PATTERNS related to PERIPHERAL NEUROPATHY

Defining Characteristics: Peripheral neuropathy occurs in about 25% of patients (range, 10–50%). If drug is discontinued at the first sign of neuropathy, symptoms are reversible. Neuropathy is a distal axonal degeneration affecting long and large-diameter motor and sensory axons in hands and feet. Initially, there is numbness of toes/feet, described often as a "tightness around the feet." There may be decreased sensitivity to light touch, pinprick (sensory loss) in hands and feet, muscle cramps, symmetrical sensorimotor neuropathy, painful paresthesias in hands and feet, distal hypoesthesia, proximal weakness in lower limbs, slight postural tremor, leg cramps, absent ankle jerks. IF treatment is continued, there is permanent paresthesias of feet and hands, which progresses proximally. Increased risk of occurrence with increased age (> 70 years old) and high total doses > 14 g (40–50 g).

Nursing Implications: Assess baseline neurologic status, especially presence of peripheral neuropathy. Teach patient to stop drug and report immediately dysesthesias, numbness, and/or muscle cramps. Perform assessment for peripheral neuropathy at every visit.

III. ALTERATION IN SENSORY/PERCEPTUAL PATTERNS related to DROWSINESS

Defining Characteristics: Drug has nonbarbiturate sedative qualities, and drowsiness is the most frequent side effect. Tolerance to daytime drowsiness occurs over several weeks of use. Drowsiness and dizziness are more frequent at doses of 20–400 mg/day than at lower doses. HIV-infected patient studies reported drowsiness, dizziness, and mood changes 33–100% of the time.

Nursing Implications: Assess baseline alertness, sleep patterns. Assess other drugs taken, especially those with sedating qualities, and alcohol ingestion. Instruct patient to avoid alcohol and to take drug at bedtime. Assess degree of drowsiness and dizziness and safety of patient. If significant, teach measures to ensure safety. Tell patient that tolerance develops over 2–3 weeks.

IV. ALTERATION IN SKIN INTEGRITY, POTENTIAL, related to RASH

Defining Characteristics: Pruritic, erythematous macular rash may appear over trunk and back 2–13 days after initiation of therapy. Increased incidence in patients with HIV infection with low CD4 counts. Drug rechallenge often results in immediate reaction of rash, tachycardia, and fever. Rash resolves with drug discontinuation.

Nursing Implications: Teach patient to self-assess for rash, and instruct to discontinue drug and report rash to nurse or physician immediately. If necessary, manage symptomatic itching with antihistamines.

V. ALTERATION IN ELIMINATION related to CONSTIPATION

Defining Characteristics: Mild constipation occurs in 3–30% of patients.

Nursing Implications: Instruct patient to prevent constipation by using stool softeners, mild laxatives if needed (e.g., milk of magnesia), and to use bulk (e.g., psyllium). In addition, teach dietary interventions (e.g., increased fiber, fluids of 3 qt/day), and mild exercise. Instruct patient to report constipation unresponsive to these interventions.

VI. POTENTIAL FOR INFECTION related to NEUTROPENIA

Defining Characteristics: Rare (< 1%) in most patients, but increased incidence of 2–20% in HIV-infected patients. Average onset 6–7 weeks after initiation of treatment (range, 3–12 weeks).

Nursing Implications: Determine baseline WBC and absolute neutrophil count (ANC). Do not initiate therapy if ANC $< 750/mm^3$. If on treatment, ANC $< 750/ mm^3$, consider drug discontinuance, but definitely drug should be discontinued if ANC $< 500/mm^3$. Drug may be reinstituted after neutrophil recovery (e.g., G-CSF). WBC and ANC should be monitored closely in HIV-infected patients (e.g., every other week for three months), and then at least every month. In non-HIV-infected patients, monitor baseline and monthly.

Chapter 9

Anxiety and Depression

Anxiety and depression in response to uncertainty and hopelessness are frequently associated with the cancer experience. Studies have shown that anxiety increases with the cancer diagnosis and remains elevated to some degree throughout treatment, regardless of modality or setting (Clark, 1990). Nursing efforts are aimed at anxiety-reducing strategies such as helping the patient explore the anxiety and find anxiety-reducing activities (e.g., relaxation exercises, verbalization of feelings). Nurses can also refer patients for specialized support if necessary, and, as appropriate, teach patients and their families about prescribed anxiolytic medications. Depression is an often expected response to the cancer experience, to an actual or perceived loss of health, role, and life. It also may be associated with chronic cancer pain and can clearly adversely affect quality of life. Prominent features may be perceived loss of self-esteem, worthlessness, hopelessness, guilt, and sadness. Symptoms include a change in appetite, sleeplessness, lethargy, and social withdrawal. Nurses use caring and compassion to help patients who are depressed acknowledge and explore their feelings. Through patient teaching and supportive counseling, short-term realistic and achievable goals can often be negotiated by patient and nurse. Now, nurses are helping patients to make the "mountain" more "manageable."

It is generally accepted that depression results from a deficiency in key neurotransmitters, resulting in either an over- or underexpression of neurotransmitters that control the release or breakdown of the neurotransmitters (Barsevick and Much, 2003).

The tricyclic antidepressant (TCA) medications have long been the cornerstone of managing cancer-related depression, partially because of their ability to improve sleeplessness and to enhance analgesia. However, these drugs also have undesirable side effects, such as dry mouth, constipation, and blurred vision. Newer antidepressant medications are now available and have found a firm niche in oncology care. The selective serotonin reuptake inhibitors (SSRIs) are quite effective for many patients and have few side effects, together with a short half-life. More recently, serotonin-norepinephrine reuptake inhibitors (SNRIs) have been developed. An example included in this chapter is venlafaxine, which has shown equal efficacy to fluoxetine (Prozac) without the significant side effects (Silverstone, 1999; Costa SJ, 1998).

Massie and Popkin (1998) suggest principles to guide antidepressant therapy in patients with cancer: start with a lower dose, slowly increase the dose as the therapeutic dose may be lower than that in non-cancer patients, and monitor very carefully for side effects as there may be overlapping toxicity in organ systems (with chemotherapy, the malignancy).

In addition, it is important to do a thorough assessment of herbs used in the management of anxiety and depression, as these may be interact with pharmacologic agents. For example, Mathijssen et al (2002) found that St. John's wort induces the metabolism of SN-38 via the cytochrome P450 CYP3A4 subsystem, lowering serum levels by up 42% with an effect lasting up to 3 weeks. Table 9.1 depicts anti-anxiety and antidepressant agents commonly prescribed.

Table 9.1 Agents Commonly Used in the Management of Anxiety and Depression in Patients with Cancer

Drug	Dose Range (oral)	Half-Life or Onset of Therapeutic Effect	Common Side Effects	Comments
Anti-anxiety				
Alprazolam (Xanax)	0.5–0.6 mg/day (max 2 mg/day)	10–15 hrs half-life	Sedation, confusion, motor incoordination, somnolence	Short half-life
Diazepam (Valium, valrelease)	2–40 mg/day (usual max dose 20 mg/day)	20–70 hrs half-life	Drowsiness, fatigue, lethargy, weakness, rash, vivid dreams, feeling "hung over"	Long half-life, so accumulation of active metabolites; fast absorption
Lorazepam (Ativan)	2–6 mg/day (usual max dose 3 g/day)	10–20 hr half-life	Drowsiness, fatigue, lethargy, weakness, rash, vivid dreams	Short half-life with intermediate absorption
Oxazepam (Serax)	30–120 mg/day (usual max dose 60 mg/day)	5–15 hrs	Drowsiness, fatigue, lethargy, weakness, rash, vivid dreams	Short half life
Antidepressants				
SSRIs				
Paroxetine (Paxil)	10–50 mg	Onset 3–10 days	Nausea, dry mouth, rash, headache, drowsiness, loss of libido, postural hypotension	Caution in elderly, patients with renal or hepatic dysfunction, suicidal ideation

Table 9.1 *(continued)*

Drug	Dose Range (oral)	Half-Life or Onset of Therapeutic Effect	Common Side Effects	Comments
Sertraline (Zoloft)	50–200 mg	Onset 7 days	Same as paroxetine	Same
Fluoxetine (Prozac)	20 mg	Onset 2–4 weeks	Same as paroxetine	Same
TCAs				
Amitriptyline (Elavil)	25–250 mg	Onset 4–6 weeks	Anticholinergic (urinary retention, dry mouth, thirst, blurred vision, sedation) and antihistaminic (sedation); tachycardia, orthostatic hypotension, arrythmia; withdrawal reaction	Caution in patients with suicidal ideation, cardiac/renal or hepatic dysfunction; don't stop drug abruptly; do baseline EKG and assess toxicity
Desipramine (Norpramin)	25–150 mg	4–6 weeks	Same as amitriptyline	Same as amitriptyline; serum level correlates with therapeutic effect
Doxepin (Sinequan)	50–150 mg	4–6 weeks	Same amitriptyline	Same as amitriptyline
Imipramine (Tofranil)	25–150 mg	4–6 weeks	Same amitriptyline	Same as amitriptyline; serum level correlates with therapeutic effect
Nortriptyline (Pamelor)	50–150 mg	4–6 weeks	Same as amitriptyline	Same as amitriptyline; serum level correlates with therapeutic effect
Trazodone (Dyseril)	50–250 mg	1–4 weeks	Same as amitriptyline	Same as amitriptyline

Table 9.1 *(continued)*

Drug	Dose Range (oral)	Half-Life or Onset of Therapeutic Effect	Common Side Effects	Comments
SNRI				
Venlafaxine HCl (Effexor)	75–225 mg/da	1–4 weeks	Emotional lability, vertigo, trismus, nausea	Use cautiously in elderly, patients with cardiac/renal or hepatic dysfunction
Nefazodone HCl (Serzone)	200–600 mg/da	1–4 weeks	Dizziness, drowsiness, dry mouth, headache	Use cautiously in elderly, patients with cardiac/renal or hepatic dysfunction

Modified from: Barsevick AM and Much JK (2003) Depression, chapter 34 in *Cancer Symptom Management,* 3rd ed, Yarbro CH, Frogge MH, Goodman M (eds). Sudbury, MA, Jones and Bartlett Publishers, pp. 668–692; Goebel BH (2003) Anxiety, chapter 33 in *Cancer Symptom Management,* 3rd ed, Yarbro CH, Frogge MH, Goodman M (eds). Sudbury, MA, Jones and Bartlett Publishers, pp. 651–668

MANAGEMENT

References

Barsevick AM, Much JK. Depression, chapter 34. Yarbro CH, Frogge MH, Goodman M, (eds), *Cancer Symptom Management,* 3rd ed. Sudbury, MA: Jones and Bartlett Publishers 2003;668–692

Clark J. Psychosocial Dimensions: The Patient. Groenwald S, Frogge MH, Goodman M, Yarbro CH, (eds), *Cancer Nursing Principles and Practice,* 2nd ed. Sudbury, MA: Jones and Bartlett Publishers 1990

Costa E Silva J. Randomized, Double-blind Comparison of Venlafaxine and Fluoxetine in Outpatients with Major Depression. *J Clin Psychiatry* 1998;59:352–353

Forest Pharmaceuticals. Celexa® package Insert. St. Louis, Forest Pharmaceuticals, Inc 1998

Gerchufsky M. The Art and Science of Prescribing Psychiatric Medications. *ADVANCE for Nurse Practitioners* 1997;4(3):33–36

Goebel BH. Anxiety, chapter 33. Yarbro CH, Frogge MH, Goodman M, (eds), *Cancer Symptom Management,* 3rd ed. Sudbury, MA: Jones and Bartlett Publishers 2003; 651–668

Massie MJ, Popkin MK. Depressive disorders, chapter 10. Holland JC, (eds), *Psycho-Oncology.* New York NY: Oxford University Press 1998;518–540

Mathijssen RH, Verweij J, de Bruijn P, et al. Effects of St. John's Wort on Irinotecan Metabolism. *J Natl Cancer Instit* 2002;94(16):1247–9

Silverstone PH, Ravindran A. Once Daily Venlafaxine Extended Release (XR) Compared with Fluoxetine in Outpatients with Depression and Anxiety. *J Clin Psychiatry* 1999;60:22–24

Drug: alprazolam (Xanax)

Class: Benzodiazepine (anxiolytic).

Mechanism of Action: Binds to benzodiazepine receptors in the CNS (limbic and cortical areas, cerebellum, brain stem, and spinal cord), resulting in the following effects: anxiolytic, ataxia, anticonvulsant, muscle relaxation. Appears to potentiate the effects of γ-aminobutyric acid (GABA).

Metabolism: Well absorbed from GI tract. Widely distributed in body tissues and fluids, including CSF. Crosses placenta and is excreted in breast milk. Highly bound to plasma proteins. Metabolized in liver and excreted in urine. Short elimination time; half-life of 12–15 hours. May produce psychological and physical dependence. Indicated for management of anxiety, the short-term relief of anxiety associated with depression, and panic disorder.

Dosage/Range:

Adult:

- Anxiety: 0.25–0.5 mg PO tid (may gradually increase dose q3–4 days over time to maximum 4 mg/day in divided doses).
- Elderly/debilitated: 0.25 mg PO bid.
- Discontinue drug by decreasing dose by 0.25–0.5 mg q3–7 days.
- Drug should be used for short-term use only (< 4 months).
- Panic: optimal dosage not determined; titrate dose and increase slowly.

Drug Preparation:

- Store in tight, light-resistant containers at 15–30°C (59–86°F).

Drug Administration:

- Orally, in divided doses.
- May take with food if stomach upset occurs.

Drug Interactions:

- CNS depressants (alcohol, anticonvulsants, phenothiazines, opiates): additive CNS depression; avoid concurrent use or use cautiously and monitor carefully.
- Oral contraceptives, isoniazid, ketoconazole, or cimetidine: decrease plasma clearance of alprazolam so may increase effect (e.g., sedation); monitor patient closely.
- Tricyclic antidepressants: increased serum levels of antidepressant possible; use together cautiously.

- Digoxin: may decrease renal excretion of digoxin; monitor for overdosage; may need to decrease digoxin.

Lab Effects/Interference:

- No consistent pattern of interaction between benzodiazepines and laboratory tests.

Special Considerations:

- Wide margin of safety between therapeutic and toxic doses.
- May impair ability to perform activities requiring mental alertness (e.g., driving a car, operating machinery).
- May produce psychological and physical dependence.
- Administer cautiously in patients with liver or renal impairment.
- Use cautiously in patients with chronic pulmonary disease or sleep apnea.
- Contraindicated in patients with depressive neuroses, psychotic reactions (without prominent anxiety), acute alcoholic intoxication (with depressed VS), known hypersensitivity to the drug, or acute angle-closure glaucoma.
- May cause fetal damage so should not be used during pregnancy or if the mother is breast-feeding.
- Withdrawal symptoms (including seizure, delirium) can occur with rapid drug discontinuance in patients taking high or chronic doses.
- If manic episodes or hyperactivity occur soon after drug started, drug should be discontinued.
- Drug should not be used to manage "everyday stress."

Potential Toxicities/Side Effects and the Nursing Process

I. ALTERATIONS IN SENSORY/PERCEPTUAL PATTERNS related to CNS DEPRESSION

Defining Characteristics: CNS depressant effects include drowsiness, fatigue, lethargy, confusion, weakness, headache, which may occur initially and resolve with continued therapy or dose reduction. Vivid dreams, suicidal ideation, and bizarre behavior also may occur. Patient risk factors: elderly, debilitated, liver dysfunction, low serum albumin.

Nursing Implications: Assess baseline neurologic status and risk factors, and monitor during treatment. Instruct patient to report signs/symptoms and discuss drug modification with physician. Evaluate patient satisfaction with drug efficacy. If patient expresses suicidal ideation (more common in panic disorders), refer patient for psychiatric evaluation and drug modification. Instruct patient to avoid alcohol while taking drug. Teach patient prescribed schedule for discontinuing drug when used chronically: assess for signs/symptoms of withdrawal (increased anxiety, rebound insomnia; may also include agitation, dysphoria, nausea/vomiting, irritability, muscle cramps, hallucinations, seizures).

II. ALTERATION IN NUTRITION, LESS THAN BODY REQUIREMENTS, related to GI SIDE EFFECTS

Defining Characteristics: Nausea, vomiting, weight increase or decrease, dry mouth, constipation may occur; also, elevated serum LFTs.

Nursing Implications: Assess baseline nutrition and elimination patterns and LFTs, and monitor during therapy. Discuss abnormalities and drug modification with physician. Teach patient to self-administer prescribed antiemetics as appropriate.

III. POTENTIAL FOR INJURY related to DECREASE IN MENTAL ALERTNESS, PHYSICAL COORDINATION

Defining Characteristics: Drug may cause drowsiness, dizziness, and impair physical coordination, mental alertness.

Nursing Implications: Assess other medications that may increase risk (e.g., opiates, phenothiazenes) and response to drug. Instruct patient to avoid potentially hazardous activities, including driving a car, operating machinery.

IV. ALTERATIONS IN CARDIAC OUTPUT related to RHYTHM DISTURBANCES, VASODILATION

Defining Characteristics: Drug may cause bradycardia, tachycardia, hyper- or hypotension, palpitations, edema.

Nursing Implications: Assess baseline VS, and monitor during therapy. Discuss abnormalities with physician. Instruct patient to report dizziness on standing or other changes.

V. ALTERATIONS IN SKIN INTEGRITY related to RASH

Defining Characteristics: Urticaria, pruritus, rash (morbilliform, urticarial, or maculopapular) may occur.

Nursing Implications: Assess baseline skin integrity, and instruct patient to report changes. Teach symptomatic skin management, and discuss drug discontinuance with physician if severe.

Drug: amitriptyline hydrochloride (Elavil)

Class: Tricyclic antidepressant.

Mechanism of Action: Blocks reuptake of neurotransmitters at neuronal membrane, thus increasing available serotonin, norepinephrine in CNS, and potentiating their effects. Appears to have analgesic effect separate from antidepressant action. May increase bioavailability of morphine. Indicated in the treatment of depressive (affective) mood disorders. Also used as an adjuvant analgesic in cancer pain management.

Metabolism: Well absorbed from GI tract. Distributed to lungs, heart, brain, liver; highly bound to plasma, proteins. Plasma half-life of 10–50 hours. Metabolized in liver, excreted in urine and, to a lesser degree, in bile and feces.

Dosage/Range:

Adult:

- Oral: 25–100 mg PO hs divided or single dose; may increase to 200–300 mg/day (300 mg maximum).
- Cancer pain: 25 mg/day hs; may increase by 25 mg of 1–2 days to 75–150 mg, when desired relief level is reached; may start at 10 mg in elderly.
- Elderly: 30 mg/day in divided doses.
- Intramuscular (IM): 20–30 mg qid or as single dose at bedtime.

Drug Preparation/Administration:

- Oral: store in well-closed containers at 15–30°C (59–86°F); store Elavil 10-mg capsules away from light. Administer as a single bedtime dose.
- IM: administer IM in large muscle mass; change to oral as soon as possible.

Drug Interactions:

- Monamine oxidase inhibitors (MAOIs): increased excitation, hyperpyrexia, seizures; use together cautiously (especially if high dose is used).
- CNS depressants (alcohol, sedatives, hypnotics): increase CNS depression; use together cautiously.
- Sympathomimetic (epinephrine, amphetamines): increased hypertension; AVOID concurrent use.
- Cimetidine methylphenidate: increased amitriptyline levels, increased toxicity; use cautiously and monitor for increased toxicity.
- Warfarin: may increase PT; monitor closely and decrease dose of warfarin as needed.

Lab Effects/Interference:

- None known; bone marrow depression uncommon.

Special Considerations:

- Antidepressant effect may take two weeks or longer.
- Adjuvant analgesic useful in cancer pain management.
- May also decrease depression associated with chronic cancer pain and promote improved sleep.
- Contraindicated in patients with myocardial infarction, seizure disorder, or benign prostatic hypertrophy.
- Use cautiously in patients with urine retention, narrow-angle glaucoma, hyperthyroidism, hepatic dysfunction, or suicidal ideation.

- Drug should be gradually discontinued rather than abruptly withdrawn to prevent anxiety, malaise, dizziness, nausea/vomiting.
- May be helpful in treating hiccups.
- Increased anticholinergic side effects in elderly.

Potential Toxicities/Side Effects and the Nursing Process

I. ALTERATIONS IN SENSORY/PERCEPTUAL PATTERNS related to DROWSINESS, FATIGUE, EPS

Defining Characteristics: Drowsiness, dizziness, weakness, lethargy, and fatigue are common; confusion, disorientation, hallucinations may occur in the elderly. Extrapyramidal symptoms may occur (fine tremor, rigidity, dystonia, dysarthria, dysphagia), as may peripheral neuropathy and blurred vision.

Nursing Implications: Assess baseline gait, neurologic and mental status, and monitor during therapy. Instruct patient to report signs/symptoms; discuss benefit/risk ratio with physician. Assess for signs/symptoms of suicidal ideation; if they occur, refer for psychiatric evaluation. Inform patient that drowsiness, dizziness will resolve after 1–2 weeks; instruct to avoid hazardous activities while drowsy (e.g., driving a car, operating machinery).

II. ALTERATION IN CARDIAC OUTPUT related to POSTURAL HYPOTENSION, TACHYCARDIA

Defining Characteristics: Postural hypotension, EKG changes, tachycardia, hypertension may occur.

Nursing Implications: Assess baseline orthostatic BP, heart rate, and monitor during therapy. Instruct patient to report abnormalities, including postural dizziness, palpitations. Drug should be stopped several days before surgery to prevent hypertensive crisis, especially if high dose.

III. ALTERATION IN NUTRITION, LESS THAN BODY REQUIREMENTS, related to GI SIDE EFFECTS

Defining Characteristics: Dry mouth, anorexia, nausea, vomiting, diarrhea, abdominal cramping may occur; also, elevated LFTs.

Nursing Implications: Assess baseline nutrition and elimination patterns and LFTs, and monitor during therapy. Discuss abnormalities with physician, and discuss drug modification. Teach patient to self-administer prescribed antiemetics as appropriate. LFTs should be repeated, and if still elevated, the drug should be discontinued. Teach patient to take full dose at bedtime. Suggest patient use sugar-free hard candy, frequent ice chips, or artificial saliva for dry mouth.

IV. ALTERATION IN URINARY ELIMINATION related to URINARY RETENTION

Defining Characteristics: Urinary retention may occur. Increased risk if patient has history of urinary retention.

Nursing Implications: Assess baseline urinary elimination pattern and risk. Assess for urinary retention, and instruct patient to report signs/symptoms. Discuss alternative drug with physician if this occurs.

V. ALTERATIONS IN SKIN INTEGRITY related to ALLERGY

Defining Characteristics: Urticaria, erythema, rash, and photosensitivity may occur.

Nursing Implications: Assess baseline drug allergy history and skin integrity. Instruct patient to report skin changes. If angioedema of face, tongue develops, discuss drug discontinuance with physician. Instruct patient to avoid sunlight or to use sunblock protection.

Drug: bupropion hydrochloride (Wellbutrin)

Class: Aminoketone antidepressant.

Mechanism of Action: Unknown. Does block reuptake of serotonin, norepinephrine, and dopamine weakly; does not inhibit MAO; has CNS stimulant effects.

Metabolism: Peak plasma level 2 hours after oral administration, and it appears that only a small percentage of the dose reaches the systemic circulation. Half-life about 14 hours (8–24 hours average). Four major metabolites, with significantly longer elimination half-lives. Primarily excreted in the urine (87%) and to a lesser extent in the feces (10%).

Dosage/Range:

Adult:

- Initial dose: 100 mg bid for at least 3 days.
- Based on response, may increase to usual dose of 100 mg tid (300 mg total dose/day).
- If after 4 weeks of treatment there is no clinical response, may increase to a maximum of 450 mg/day (150 mg tid).

Drug Preparation/Administration:

- Available in 75-mg and 100-mg tablets.
- Protect tablets from light and moisture.
- Ensure at least 4 hours between doses (optimally, give in morning and evening).

Drug Interactions:
- Because of extensive drug metabolism by liver, when given with other drugs that have hepatic metabolism may have decreased effect of that drug (e.g., carbamazepine, cimetidine, phenobarbital, phenytoin).
- MAOIs may increase drug toxicity.
- Use cautiously in patients receiving L-dopa, starting with small initial dose, and slowly increasing dose.
- Use cautiously in patients receiving other seizure-threshold-lowering drugs, starting with small initial dose, and slowly and gradually increasing dose.
- Bupropion, (Zyban; smoking cessation aid): DO NOT USE TOGETHER, as will increase risk of seizures.

Lab Effects/Interference:
- Rarely, anemia and pancytopenia.

Special Considerations:
- Contraindicated in patients with seizure disorder, present/past history of bulimia, or anorexia nervosa.
- Contraindicated in patients receiving MAOI; if MAOI is discontinued, wait at least 14 days before starting bupropion HCl.
- Risk of seizures for patients receiving drug at a dose of 450 mg is 0.4% and appears related to dose and predisposing factors, such as prior seizure, head trauma, CNS tumor, and concomitant medications that lower seizure threshold (e.g., antipsychotics, other antidepressants, abrupt cessation of a benzodiazepine medication, use or abrupt cessation of alcohol).
- Avoid alcohol when taking drug.
- Can precipitate manic episodes in patients with bipolar manic depression or can activate latent psychoses.
- Use cautiously, if at all, in individuals who are underweight, as drug may cause weight loss of at least 2.25 kg (5 lb) (28% of patients), and most patients do not gain weight (only 9% of patients gain weight).
- Drug contains same ingredient found in burpropion, which is used in smoking cessation. DO NOT USE TOGETHER.
- Use cautiously in patients with a recent history of myocardial infarction or unstable heart disease.

Potential Toxicities/Side Effects and the Nursing Process

I. ALTERATIONS IN SENSORY/PERCEPTUAL PATTERNS related to RESTLESSNESS, AGITATION, INSOMNIA

Defining Characteristics: Many patients experience increased restlessness, agitation, anxiety, and insomnia, especially after initiation of therapy. This may be severe enough to require treatment with sedative/hypnotic or drug discontinuation. Restlessness, agitation, hostility, decreased concentration, ataxia, incoordination, confusion, paranoia, anxiety, manic episodes in bipolar manic depressives, migraine, insomnia, euphoria, and psychoses may occur. Akathesia, dyskinesia, dystonia, muscle spasms, bradykinesia, and sensory disturbances may occur.

Nursing Implications: Assess baseline gait, neurologic and mental status, and monitor during therapy. Teach patient to report signs/symptoms; discuss benefit/risk ratio with physician. Assess for signs/symptoms of suicidal ideation; if they occur, refer for psychiatric evaluation. Inform patient that drowsiness, dizziness will resolve after 1–2 weeks; instruct to avoid hazardous activities while drowsy (e.g., driving a car, operating machinery). Instruct patient to avoid alcohol ingestion, as this may precipitate seizures.

II. ALTERATION IN CARDIAC OUTPUT related to CHANGES IN BP, HR

Defining Characteristics: Dizziness, tachycardia, hypertension or hypotension, palpitations, edema, syncope, and cardiac arrhythmias may occur.

Nursing Implications: Assess baseline orthostatic BP, heart rate, presence of peripheral edema, and monitor during therapy. Patient should have a baseline EKG. Instruct patient to report abnormalities including postural dizziness, palpitations. Discuss any significant changes with physician, and discuss interventions. If the patient has had a recent myocardial infarction, expect that dose of drug may be reduced.

III. ALTERATION IN NUTRITION, LESS THAN BODY REQUIREMENTS, related to GI SIDE EFFECTS

Defining Characteristics: Dry mouth, anorexia, nausea, vomiting, diarrhea, constipation, weight loss of up to 2.25 kg (5 lb), dyspepsia, weight gain and increased appetite, increased salivation, taste changes, stomatitis may occur rarely.

Nursing Implications: Assess baseline nutrition and elimination patterns, weight, and monitor during therapy. Discuss abnormalities with physician, and discuss drug modification. Teach patient to self-administer prescribed antiemetics as appropriate. Suggest patient use sugar-free hard candy, frequent ice chips, or artificial saliva for dry mouth.

IV. ALTERATION IN URINARY ELIMINATION related to URINARY RETENTION

Defining Characteristics: Urinary retention, frequency, and nocturia may occur. Increased risk in patients with history of urinary retention.

Nursing Implications: Assess baseline urinary elimination pattern and risk. Assess for urinary retention, and instruct patient to report signs/symptoms. Discuss alternative drug with physician if this occurs.

V. ALTERATIONS IN SKIN INTEGRITY related to ALLERGY

Defining Characteristics: Urticaria, erythema, rash, pruritus may occur.

Nursing Implications: Assess baseline drug allergy history and skin integrity. Instruct patient to report skin changes. If angioedema of face or tongue develops, tell patient to stop drug and discuss drug discontinuance with physician.

VI. POTENTIAL SEXUAL DYSFUNCTION related to IMPOTENCE, IRREGULAR MENSES

Defining Characteristics: Impotence in men and irregular menses in women may occur.

Nursing Considerations: Assess baseline sexual functioning. Inform patient that alterations may occur, and instruct to report them. If severe, discuss dysfunction with physician, and whether another antidepressant would provide equal benefit with less dysfunction.

Drug: buspirone hydrochloride (BuSpar)

Class: Antianxiety agent.

Mechanism of Action: Unclear; drug is considered a midbrain modulator and affects many neurotransmitters (serotonin, dopamine, and cholinergic and noradrenergic systems).

Metabolism: Rapid and complete GI absorption. Food may delay absorption but does not affect total serum drug level. Distributed to body tissues and fluids, especially brain. Metabolized in liver and excreted in urine.

Dosage/Range:
Adult:
- Oral: 10–15 mg in 2–3 divided doses.
- May be increased in 5-mg increments every 2–4 days to achieve goal (maximum 60 mg/day).
- Maintenance: usual is 5–10 mg tid.

Drug Preparation/Administration:
- Store tablets in tight, light-resistant containers at < 30°C (86°F).
- Administer with food.

Drug Interactions:
- MAOIs: increased BP; AVOID CONCURRENT USE.
- Haloperidol: increased haloperidol serum levels; AVOID CONCURRENT USE or reduce haloperidol dose.
- Alcohol: may increase fatigue, drowsiness, dizziness; AVOID CONCURRENT USE.
- Other CNS depressants (analgesics, sedatives): may increase fatigue, drowsiness, dizziness; AVOID CONCURRENT USE.

Lab Effects/Interference:
- None known.

Special Considerations:
- Selective anxiolytic; causes little sedation or psychomotor dysfunction.
- Anxiolytic effect comparable to oral diazepam.
- Onset slower, so patients should be told to expect full anxiolytic effect in 3–4 weeks.
- Use with caution if renal insufficiency; dose-reduce in anuric patients.

Potential Toxicities/Side Effects and the Nursing Process

I. ALTERATIONS IN SENSORY/PERCEPTUAL PATTERNS related to DIZZINESS, DROWSINESS

Defining Characteristics: Far less sedation than with other anxiolytics. May cause dizziness, drowsiness, headache in 10% of patients; fatigue, nightmares, weakness, paresthesia occur less frequently.

Nursing Implications: Assess baseline neurologic status, and monitor during therapy. Instruct patient to report signs/symptoms, and discuss drug modification with physician. Instruct patient to avoid alcohol while taking drug.

II. ALTERATION IN NUTRITION, LESS THAN BODY REQUIREMENTS, related to GI SIDE EFFECTS

Defining Characteristics: Nausea occurs in 8% of patients; less common is dry mouth, vomiting, diarrhea, or constipation.

Nursing Implications: Assess baseline nutrition and elimination patterns, and monitor during therapy. Instruct patient to report signs/symptoms.

Drug: citalopram hydrobromide (Celexa®)

Class: Antidepressant.

Mechanism of Action: Selective serotonin reuptake inhibitor (SSRI) with unique structure unlike other antidepressants (racemic bicyclic phthalane derivative).

Drug inhibits the reuptake of neurotransmitter serotonin in the CNS, thus potentiating serotonin activity in the CNS and relieving depressive symptoms.

Metabolism: Steady-state plasma level reached in one week. Bioavailability is 80% following single daily dose, unaffected by food intake, and peak plasma level is reached in 4 hours. Metabolism is primarily hepatic, with a terminal half-life of 25 hours. Renal excretion accounts for 20% of drug excretion. In the elderly, drug is more slowly cleared, with increases in area under the curve (AUC) by 23% and half-life by 30%. Patients with hepatic dysfunction have reduced drug clearance (37%), with half-life of drug extended to 8 hours.

Dosage/Range:

- Adult: 20 mg qd, increased 40 mg qd after at least 1 week.
- Patients with hepatic dysfunction or elderly: 20 mg qd.
- If changing to or from monamine oxidase inhibitor therapy, wait at least 14 days between drugs.

Drug Preparation:

- Oral: available in 20-mg (pink) and 40-mg (white) oval, scored tablets.

Drug Administration:

- Administer orally in morning or evening, without regard to food.

Drug Interactions:

- Monamine oxidase inhibitors: potential for serious, sometimes fatal interactions (hyperthermia, rigidity, myoclonus, autonomic instability, mental status changes, including coma). DO NOT USE TOGETHER, and if changing to/from citaloprom HBr, drugs MUST be separated by at least 14 days.
- Alcohol: possible potentiation of depression of cognitive and motor function; DO NOT USE TOGETHER.
- Cimetidine: increases AUC of citaloprom HBr by 43%. Use together with caution, if at all; assess for toxicity and reduce dose as needed if must use together.
- Lithium: use together cautiously, and monitor serum lithium levels if used together.
- Warfarin: monitor INR, PT closely.
- Carbamazepine, ketoconazole, itraconazole, fluconazole, erythromycin: possible increase in clearance of citaloprom HBr, monitor drug effectiveness and increase dose as needed.

- Metoprolol: may increase metoprolol levels; monitor BP and HR.
- Tricyclic antidepressants, e.g., imipramine: possible increases in plasma tricyclic antidepressant level; use together cautiously, if at all.

Lab Effects/Interference:
- Infrequently, increased liver function tests, alk phos, and abnormal glucose tolerance test.
- Rarely, bilirubinemia, hypokalemia, and hypoglycemia.

Special Considerations:
- At high doses in animals, drug is teratogenic, and, in some tests, mutagenic and carcinogenic (> 20 times the human maximum dose). DO NOT give to pregnant women or nursing mothers.
- Most responses occur within 1–4 weeks of therapy, but if no benefit has yet occurred, patients should be taught to continue taking medicine as prescribed.
- Use cautiously in patients with a seizure disorder, and monitor closely during therapy.

Potential Toxicities/Side Effects and the Nursing Process

I. ALTERATION IN NUTRITION related to GI SIDE EFFECTS

Defining Characteristics: Nausea (21%) and dry mouth (20%) are common. Less common are diarrhea (8%), dyspepsia (5%), vomiting (4%), and abdominal pain (3%). Infrequent are gastritis, stomatitis, eructation, dysphagia, teeth grinding, change in weight, and gingivitis. The following were rare: colitis, cholecystitis, gastroesophageal reflux, diverticulitis, and hiccups.

Nursing Implications: Assess baseline nutrition and elimination patterns, and monitor during therapy. Discuss abnormalities with physician, and discuss drug modification. Teach patient to self-administer prescribed antiemetics as appropriate. Suggest patient use sugar-free hard candy, frequent ice chips, or artificial saliva for dry mouth.

II. ALTERATION IN CARDIAC OUTPUT, POTENTIAL, related to CHANGES IN BLOOD PRESSURE

Defining Characteristics: Tachycardia, postural hypotension, and hypotension are common. The following are infrequent: hypertension, bradycardia, peripheral edema, angina, arrythmias, flushing, and cardiac failure. Rarely, transient ischemic attacks, phlebitis, changes in cardiac conduction (atrial fibrillation, bundle branch block), and cardiac arrest.

Nursing Implications: Assess baseline orthostatic BP, heart rate, and monitor during therapy. Teach patient to report abnormalities, including postural dizziness, palpitations. Discuss significant changes with physician. If patient has orthostatic hypotension, teach patient to change position slowly and to hold on to support.

III. SENSORY/PERCEPTUAL ALTERATIONS related to CHANGES IN MENTAL STATUS

Defining Characteristics: The following may occur: somnolence (18%), insomnia (15%), agitation (3%), impaired concentration, amnesia, apathy, confusion, taste perversion, abnormal ocular accommodation, and possibly worsening depression and suicide attempt. Infrequently, increased libido, aggressive reaction, depersonalization, hallucination, euphoria, paranoia, emotional lability, and panic reaction may occur.

Nursing Implications: Assess baseline gait, neurologic, affective, and mental status, and monitor during therapy. Teach patient to report signs and symptoms; discuss benefit/risk ratio with physician. Assess for signs and symptoms of suicidal ideation; if they occur, refer for psychiatric evaluation. Teach patient that drowsiness may occur, and teach to avoid hazardous activities while drowsy (e.g., driving a car, operating machinery).

IV. POTENTIAL FOR INJURY related to DRUG OVERDOSE

Defining Characteristics: Although rare, drug overdoses have resulted in fatalities (total drug 3920 mg and 2800 mg in two cases resulting from this drug only) while other total doses of 6000 mg have not resulted in death. Symptoms resulting from overdose include: dizziness, sweating, nausea, vomiting, tremor, somnolence, sinus tachycardia, amnesia, confusion, coma, convulsions, hyperventilation, cyanosis, rhabdomyolysis, and EKG changes (QT interval prolongation, nodal rhythm, and ventricular arrythmias).

Nursing Implications: Teach patient self-administration schedule and to keep drug in tightly closed container out of reach of children and pets. Teach patient not to double doses if a dose is missed. Give prescriptions in smallest number of pills possible (e.g., one month's worth at a time). In the event of an overdosage, teach patient to come to nearest emergency department where focus is on maintaining a patent airway and oxygenation, gastric evacuation by lavage and use of activated charcoal, and close monitoring of cardiac and overall status. Because of large area of drug distribution, dialysis is unlikely to be beneficial.

V. ALTERATIONS IN SKIN INTEGRITY related to RASH, SKIN CHANGES

Defining Characteristics: Rash and pruritus may occur. Less commonly, photosensitivity, urticaria, eczema, acne, dermatitis, alopecia, and dry skin may occur. Rarely, angioedema, epidermal necrolysis, erythema multiforme have been reported.

Nursing Implications: Assess baseline skin integrity. Teach patient to report skin changes. If angioedema of face, tongue develops, discuss drug discontinuance with physician. Assess impact of changes on patient and discuss strategies to minimize distress and preserve skin integrity and comfort.

VI. SEXUAL DYSFUNCTION, POTENTIAL, related to ↓ LIBIDO, IMPOTENCE, ANORGASMIA

Defining Characteristics: While difficult to separate from sexual dysfunction related to depression, the following have been reported in men: decreased ejaculation disorder (6.1%), libido (3.8%), and impotence (2.8%), and in women: decreased libido (1.3%) and anorgasmia (1.1%). Dysmenorrhea and amenorrhea may occur in female patients.

Nursing Implications: Assess baseline sexual functioning. Teach patient that alterations may occur and to report them. If severe, discuss dysfunction with physician and whether an antidepressant other than a SSRI would provide equal benefit with less dysfunction.

VII. ALTERATION IN URINE ELIMINATION related to CHANGES IN PATTERNS

Defining Characteristics: Polyuria is common. Less commonly, the following may occur: urinary frequency, incontinence, retention, and dysuria. Rarely, hematuria, liguria, pyelonephritis, renal calculus, and renal pain have been reported.

Nursing Implications: Assess baseline urinary elimination pattern and risk for alterations. Assess for changes in urinary elimination and teach patient to report signs and symptoms. Discuss alternative drug with physician if severe or bothersome symptoms occur.

Drug: clonazepam (Klonopin)

Class: Benzodiazepine.

Mechanism of Action: Appears to enhance the activity of γ-aminobutyric acid (GABA), which inhibits neurotransmitter activity in the CNS. Drug is able to suppress absence seizures (petit mal) and decrease the frequency, amplitude, and duration of minor motor seizures. Unclear mechanism in relieving panic episodes.

Metabolism: Completely absorbed after oral administration, with peak plasma levels of 1–2 hours. Drug half-life is 18–60 hours (typically 30–40 hours), and therapeutic serum level is 20–80 ng/mL; 80% protein-bound, metabolized by the liver via the P-450 cytochrome enzyme system, and inactive metabolites are excreted in the urine.

Dosage/Range:

Adult (panic attacks):

- Initial: 0.25 mg bid.
- May increase as needed to target dose of 1 mg/day after at least 3 days on the previous dose. Some individuals may require doses of up to 4 mg/day in divided doses, and dose is titrated up to that dose in increments of 0.125–0.25 mg bid every 3 days until panic disorder is controlled or as limited by side effects.
- Withdrawal of treatment must be gradual, with a decrease of 0.125 mg bid every 3 days until drug is completely withdrawn.

Adult (seizure disorders):

- Initial dose: 1.5 mg/day in 3 divided doses.
- Dosage may be increased in increments of 0.5–1 mg every 3 days until seizures are controlled or as limited by side effects.
- Maximum recommended daily dose is 20 mg/day.

Drug Preparation/Administration:

- Oral.
- Available in 0.5-, 1-, and 2-mg tablets.
- Discontinuance of drug when used for panic attacks: gradually discontinue, by 0.125 mg bid every 3 days, until drug is completely withdrawn.

Drug Interactions:

- CNS depressants (narcotics, barbiturates, hypnotics, anxiolytics, phenothiazines): potentiation of CNS depressive effects; use together cautiously, if at all, and monitor patient closely.
- Alcohol: potentiates CNS depressant effects; DO NOT use together.
- Phenobarbital: increases hepatic metabolism of clonazepam so that decreased serum levels lead to decreased clonazepam effect; assess patient for drug efficacy and need for increased drug dose.
- Phenytoin: increased hepatic metabolism of clonazepam so that decreased serum levels lead to decreased clonazepam effect; assess patient for drug efficacy and need for increased drug dose.
- Valproic acid: increased risk of absence seizure activity.

Lab Effects/Interference:

- Rarely, anemia, leukopenia, thrombocytopenia, eosinophilia.
- Transient elevation of liver function studies (serum transaminases and alk phos).

Special Considerations:

- Contraindicated during pregnancy, for breast-feeding mothers, and patients with severe liver dysfunction or acute narrow-angle glaucoma.

- May cause psychological and physical dependency.

I. ALTERATIONS IN SENSORY/PERCEPTUAL PATTERNS related to CNS DEPRESSION

Defining Characteristics: CNS depressant effects include drowsiness (37%), and, less commonly, dizziness (8%); abnormal coordination (6%); ataxia (5%); dysarthria (2%); depression (7%); memory disturbance (4%); nervousness (3%); decreased intellectual ability (2%); emotional lability; confusion; paresthesia; feeling of drunkenness; paresis; tremor; head fullness; hyperactivity, or hypoactivity. Rarely, suicidal ideation.

Nursing Implications: Assess baseline gait, neurologic status, affects, and monitor during treatment. Instruct patient to report signs/symptoms, and discuss drug modification with physician. Evaluate patient satisfaction with drug efficacy. Instruct patient to avoid alcohol while taking drug. Instruct patient prescribed schedule for discontinuing drug when used chronically: assess for signs/symptoms of withdrawal. Assess patient risk for suicide, and if at risk, refer to psychiatry for supportive counseling.

II. ALTERATION IN NUTRITION, LESS THAN BODY REQUIREMENTS, related to GI SIDE EFFECTS

Defining Characteristics: Constipation (1%), decreased appetite (1%), and less commonly, abdominal pain, flatulence, increased salivation, dyspepsia, decreased appetite; also elevated serum transaminases and alk phos.

Nursing Implications: Assess baseline nutrition and elimination patterns and serum transaminases, alk phos, and monitor during therapy. Assess degree of discomfort and interference with nutrition. Discuss significant abnormalities with physician and discuss drug modification.

III. INJURY related to DECREASE IN MENTAL ALERTNESS, PHYSICAL COORDINATION

Defining Characteristics: Drug may cause drowsiness, dizziness, and impair physical coordination, mental alertness.

Nursing Implications: Assess other medications that may increase risk (e.g., opiates, phenothiazenes) and response to drug. Instruct patient to avoid potentially hazardous activities, including driving a car, operating machinery. Instruct patient to avoid alcohol.

IV. ALTERATIONS IN CARDIAC OUTPUT related to POSTURAL HYPOTENSION

Defining Characteristics: Drug may cause postural hypotension, palpitations, chest pain, edema.

Nursing Implications: Assess baseline VS, and monitor during therapy. Discuss abnormalities with physician. Instruct patient to report dizziness on standing or other changes, and to change position slowly and hold on to support if this occurs.

V. ALTERATIONS IN SKIN INTEGRITY related to SKIN DISORDERS

Defining Characteristics: Acne flare, xeroderma, contact dermatitis, pruritus, skin disorders may occur.

Nursing Implications: Assess baseline skin integrity, and instruct patient to report changes. Teach symptomatic skin management, and discuss drug discontinuance with physician if severe.

VI. SEXUAL DYSFUNCTION related to CHANGES IN LIBIDO, MENSTRUAL IRREGULARITIES

Defining Characteristics: Loss or increase in libido, menstrual irregularities in women; decreased ejaculation in men.

Nursing Implications: Assess baseline sexual functioning. Inform patient that alterations may occur, and instruct to report them. If severe, discuss dysfunction with physician, and whether another antidepressant would provide equal benefit with less dysfunction.

VII. ALTERATION IN ELIMINATION, URINARY, related to DYSURIA, BLADDER DYSFUNCTION

Defining Characteristics: Dysuria, polyuria, cystitis, urinary incontinence, bladder dysfunction, urinary retention, urine discoloration, and urinary bleeding may occur uncommonly.

Nursing Implications: Assess baseline urinary elimination pattern. Instruct patient to report any changes. Discuss impact on patient, and severity, and discuss significant problems with physician.

Drug: desipramine hydrochloride (Norpramin, Pertofrane)

Class: Tricyclic antidepressant.

Mechanism of Action: Blocks reuptake of neurotransmitters at neuronal membrane, thus increasing available serotonin, norepinephrine in CNS, and potentiating their effects. Appears to have analgesic effect separate from antidepressant action. May increase bioavailability of morphine. Indicated in the treatment of depressive (affective) mood disorders. Also used as an adjuvant analgesic in cancer pain management.

Metabolism: Well absorbed from GI tract. Highly protein-bound. Plasma half-life of 7–60 hours. Metabolized in liver, and primarily excreted in urine.

Dosage/Range:

Adult:

- Oral: 75–150 mg hs, or in divided doses.
- May be gradually increased to 300 mg/day if needed.
- Elderly: 25–50 mg/day, maximum 150 mg/day.

Drug Preparation/Administration:

- Store in tight containers at < 40°C (104°F).
- Administer as a single bedtime dose.

Drug Interactions:

- MAOIs: increased excitation, hyperpyrexia, seizures; use together cautiously (especially if high dose used).
- Sympathomimetic (epinephrine, amphetamines): increased hypertension; AVOID concurrent use.
- Cimetidine methylphenidate: increased amitriptyline levels, increased toxicity; use cautiously and monitor for increased toxicity.
- Warfarin: may increase PT; monitor closely and decrease dose of warfarin as needed.
- Barbiturates: may decrease desipramine serum level; monitor for decreased antidepressant effect; may need increased dose.
- Alcohol: may antagonize antidepressant effects; AVOID CONCURRENT USE.

Lab Effects/Interference:

- Rarely, altered liver function studies.
- Rarely, increased or decreased serum glucose levels.
- Rarely, increased pancreatic enzymes.
- Rarely, bone marrow depression with agranulocytosis, eosinophilia, purpura, thrombocytopenia.

Special Considerations:

- Antidepressant effect may take two weeks or longer.

- Adjuvant analgesic useful in cancer pain management.
- May also decrease depression associated with chronic cancer pain and promote improved sleep.
- Contraindicated in patients with myocardial infarction, seizure disorder, or benign prostatic hypertrophy.
- Use cautiously in patients with urine retention, narrow-angle glaucoma, hyperthyroidism, hepatic dysfunction, or suicidal ideation.
- Drug should be gradually discontinued rather than abruptly withdrawn to prevent anxiety, malaise, dizziness, nausea/vomiting.
- May be helpful in treating hiccups.
- Increased anticholinergic side effects in elderly.

Potential Toxicities/Side Effects and the Nursing Process

I. ALTERATIONS IN SENSORY/PERCEPTUAL PATTERNS related to DROWSINESS, EPS

Defining Characteristics: Drowsiness, dizziness, weakness, lethargy, fatigue are common; confusion, disorientation, hallucinations may occur in the elderly. Extrapyramidal symptoms may occur (fine tremor, rigidity, dystonia, dysarthria, dysphagia), as may peripheral neuropathy and blurred vision. Less sedation than amitriptyline.

Nursing Implications: Assess baseline gait, neurologic and mental status, and monitor during therapy. Instruct patient to report signs/symptoms; discuss benefit/risk ratio with physician. Assess for signs/symptoms of suicidal ideation; if they occur, refer for psychiatric evaluation. Inform patient that drowsiness, dizziness will resolve after 1–2 weeks; instruct to avoid hazardous activities while drowsy (e.g., driving a car, operating machinery).

II. ALTERATION IN CARDIAC OUTPUT related to POSTURAL HYPOTENSION, TACHYCARDIA

Defining Characteristics: Postural hypotension, EKG changes, tachycardia, hypertension may occur. Less severe than with other tricyclics.

Nursing Implications: Assess baseline orthostatic BP, heart rate, and monitor during therapy. Instruct patient to report abnormalities, including postural dizziness, palpitations. Drug should be stopped several days before surgery to prevent hypertensive crisis, especially if high dose is used.

III. ALTERATION IN NUTRITION, LESS THAN BODY REQUIREMENTS, related to GI SIDE EFFECTS

Defining Characteristics: Dry mouth, anorexia, nausea, vomiting, diarrhea, abdominal cramping may occur; also, elevated LFTs.

Nursing Implications: Assess baseline nutrition and elimination patterns and LFTs, and monitor during therapy. Discuss abnormalities with physician, and discuss drug modification. Teach patient to self-administer prescribed antiemetics as appropriate. LFTs should be repeated, and if still elevated, the drug should be discontinued. Instruct patient to take full dose at bedtime. Suggest patient use sugar-free hard candy, frequent ice chips, or artificial saliva for dry mouth.

IV. ALTERATION IN URINARY ELIMINATION related to URINARY RETENTION

Defining Characteristics: Urinary retention may occur. Increased risk in patients with history of urinary retention.

Nursing Implications: Assess baseline urinary elimination pattern and risk. Assess for urinary retention, and instruct patient to report signs/symptoms. Discuss alternative drug with physician if this occurs.

V. ALTERATIONS IN SKIN INTEGRITY related to ALLERGY

Defining Characteristics: Urticaria, erythema, rash, and photosensitivity may occur.

Nursing Implications: Assess baseline drug allergy history and skin integrity. Instruct patient to report skin changes. If angioedema of face or tongue develops, discuss drug discontinuance with physician. Instruct patient to avoid sunlight or to use sunblock protection.

Drug: diazepam (Valium)

Class: Benzodiazepine (anxiolytic).

Mechanism of Action: Binds to benzodiazepine receptors in the CNS (limbic and cortical areas, cerebellum, brain stem, and spinal cord), resulting in the following effects: anxiolytic, ataxia, anticonvulsant, muscle relaxation. Appears to potentiate the effects of GABA.

Metabolism: Well absorbed from GI tract. Widely distributed in body tissues and fluids, including CSF. Crosses placenta and is excreted in breast milk. Highly bound to plasma proteins. Metabolized in liver and excreted in urine. Half-life of 20–80 hours. May produce psychological and physical dependence. Indicated for management of anxiety, the relief of reflex spasm or spasticity, and as an anticonvulsant for termination of status epilepticus.

Dosage/Range:
Adult:

- Oral: 2–10 mg tid-qid or 15–30 mg/day extended-release preparation.
- Intravenous (IV) (tension): 5–10 mg IV, maximum 30 mg/8 h.
- IV (seizures): 5–10 mg IV, maximum 30 mg; may repeat in 2–4 hours if needed.
- IV (status epilepticus): 5–20 mg slow IV push (IVP) (2–5 mg/min), q5–10 min, maximum 60 mg.
- IV (elderly, debilitated): 2–5 mg slow IVP.

Drug Preparation/Administration:
- Oral: protect tablets from light and store at 15–30°C (59–86°F).
- IV: do not administer with other drugs; drug may absorb to sides of plastic syringe or to plastic IV bag and tubing if added to IV infusion bag; consult hospital pharmacist for IV infusion protocol; administer IVP slowly 2–5 mg/min; have emergency equipment available.

Drug Interactions:
- CNS depressants (alcohol, anticonvulsants, phenothiazines, opiates): additive CNS depression; avoid concurrent use or use cautiously and monitor carefully.
- Oral contraceptives, isoniazid, ketoconazole, or cimetidine: decrease plasma clearance of diazepam so may increase effect (e.g., sedation); monitor patient closely.
- Tricyclic antidepressants: increased serum levels of antidepressant possible; use together cautiously.
- Digoxin: may decrease renal excretion of digoxin; monitor for overdosage; may need to decrease digoxin.
- Levodopa: may decrease levodopa effect; monitor patient response; may have to increase levodopa dose.

Lab Effects/Interference:
- Rarely, altered liver function studies.
- Rarely, neutropenia.

Special Considerations:
- Wide margin of safety between therapeutic and toxic doses.
- May impair ability to perform activities requiring mental alertness (e.g., driving a car, operating machinery).
- May produce psychological and physical dependence.
- Administer cautiously in patients with liver or renal impairment.
- Use cautiously in patients with chronic pulmonary disease or sleep apnea.
- Contraindicated in patients with depressive neuroses, psychotic reactions (without prominent anxiety), acute alcoholic intoxication (with depressed VS), known hypersensitivity to the drug, or acute angle-closure glaucoma.
- May cause fetal damage, so should not be used during pregnancy or if the mother is breast-feeding.

- Withdrawal symptoms (including seizure, delirium) can occur with rapid drug discontinuance in patients taking high or chronic doses.

Potential Toxicities/Side Effects and the Nursing Process

I. ALTERATIONS IN SENSORY/PERCEPTUAL PATTERNS relating to CNS DEPRESSION

Defining Characteristics: CNS depressant effects include drowsiness, fatigue, lethargy, confusion, weakness, headache, which may occur initially and resolve with continued therapy or dose reduction. Vivid dreams, visual disturbances, slurred speech, "hangover," and bizarre behavior may also occur. Patient risk factors: elderly, debilitated, liver dysfunction, low serum albumin.

Nursing Implications: Assess baseline neurologic status and risk factors, and monitor during treatment. Instruct patient to report signs/symptoms and discuss drug modification with physician. Evaluate patient satisfaction with drug efficacy. Instruct patient to avoid alcohol while taking drug. Teach patient prescribed schedule for discontinuing drug when used chronically: assess for signs/symptoms of withdrawal (increased anxiety, rebound insomnia; may also include agitation, dysphoria, nausea/vomiting, irritability, muscle cramps, hallucinations, seizures).

II. ALTERATION IN NUTRITION, LESS THAN BODY REQUIREMENTS, related to GI SIDE EFFECTS

Defining Characteristics: Nausea, vomiting, abdominal discomfort may occur; also, elevated LFTs.

Nursing Implications: Assess baseline nutrition and elimination patterns and LFTs, and monitor during therapy. Discuss abnormalities with physician and discuss drug modification. Teach patient to self-administer prescribed antiemetics as appropriate.

III. INJURY related to DECREASE IN MENTAL ALERTNESS, PHYSICAL COORDINATION

Defining Characteristics: Drug may cause drowsiness, dizziness, and impair physical coordination, mental alertness.

Nursing Implications: Assess other medications that may increase risk (e.g., opiates, phenothiazines) and response to drug. Instruct patient to avoid potentially hazardous activities, including driving a car, operating machinery.

IV. ALTERATIONS IN PERFUSION related to CARDIOPULMONARY COMPROMISE

Defining Characteristics: Drug may cause transient hypotension, bradycardia, cardiovascular collapse, respiratory depression.

Nursing Implications: Assess baseline VS; have resuscitation equipment nearby. Monitor q5–15 min and before IV dose of drug. Discuss abnormalities with physician.

V. ALTERATIONS IN SKIN INTEGRITY related to RASH

Defining Characteristics: Urticaria, rash may occur; also phlebitis, pain at injection site.

Nursing Implications: Assess baseline skin integrity, and instruct patient to report changes. Teach symptomatic skin management, and discuss drug discontinuance with physician if severe. Assess IV site for evidence of pain, phlebitis, and change site; apply heat as needed.

Drug: doxepin hydrochloride (Sinequan)

Class: Antidepressant of the dibenzoxepine tricyclic class.

Mechanism of Action: Appears to exert adrenergic effect at the synapses, preventing deactivation of norepinephrine by reuptake into the nerve terminals.

Metabolism: Metabolized in the liver by the P-450 enzyme system, into active metabolite. Effective serum level of doxepin and metabolite is 100–200 ng/mL. Takes 2–8 days to reach steady-state.

Dosage/Range:

Adult:

- Initial dose of 75 mg/day is recommended; in elderly, dose should start at 25–50 mg/day.
- Dose may be titrated up or down based on response. Usual dose is 75 mg/day to 150 mg/day.
- Patients with mild symptoms may require only 25 mg/day to 50 mg/day.
- Patients with severe symptoms may require gradual titration up to 300 mg/day.

Drug Preparation/Administration:

- Oral, taken in a single dose (maximum 150-mg dose) or in divided doses. Single dose given at bedtime enhances sleep.
- Available in 10-, 25-, 50-, 75-, 100-, and 150-mg capsules.
- If changing a patient from MAOI to doxepin HCl, wait at least 14 days before the careful initiation of doxepin.

Drug Interactions:
- Alcohol: do not use concomitantly, as increases drug toxicity.
- MAOI: severe reaction, including death may occur; DO NOT USE TOGETHER.
- Cimetidine: increased serum levels of drug and anticholinergic side effects (severe dry mouth, urinary retention, blurred vision); avoid concurrent use.
- Tolazamide: may cause severe hypoglycemia; monitor patient's serum glucose carefully.

Lab Effects/Interference:
- Rarely, eosinophilia, bone marrow depression (e.g., agranulocytosis, leukopenia, thrombocytopenia, purpura).
- Increased or decreased blood glucose levels.

Special Considerations:
- Contraindicated in patients with glaucoma or urinary retention.
- Antianxiety effect appears before the antidepressant effect, which takes 2–3 weeks.
- Most sedating of antidepressants, so useful in enhancing sleep, and single dose (up to 150 mg) should be taken at bedtime.
- Recommended for the treatment of depression accompanied by anxiety and insomnia, depression associated with organic illness or alcohol, psychotic depressive disorders with associated anxiety.

Potential Toxicities/Side Effects and the Nursing Process

I. ALTERATIONS IN SENSORY/PERCEPTUAL related to DROWSINESS, EPS

Defining Characteristics: Drowsiness, which may disappear as therapy continues. Rarely, dizziness, confusion, disorientation, hallucinations, numbness, paresthesia, ataxia, extrapyramidal symptoms, seizures, blurred vision, tardive dyskinesia, tremor may occur.

Nursing Implications: Assess baseline gait, neurologic, affective and mental status, and monitor during therapy. Instruct patient to report signs/symptoms; discuss benefit/risk ratio with physician and measures to reduce extrapyramidal side effects if they occur. Assess for signs/symptoms of suicidal ideation; if they occur, refer for psychiatric evaluation. Inform patient that drowsiness will decrease after 1–2 weeks, and instruct to avoid hazardous activities while drowsy (e.g., driving a car, operating machinery). Instruct patient to avoid alcohol while taking drug.

II. ALTERATION IN CARDIAC OUTPUT related to BLOOD PRESSURE CHANGES

Defining Characteristics: Hypotension or hypertension, tachycardia may occur.

Nursing Implications: Assess baseline orthostatic BP, heart rate, and monitor during therapy. Instruct patient to report abnormalities, including postural dizziness, palpitations.

III. ALTERATION IN NUTRITION, LESS THAN BODY REQUIREMENTS, related to GI SIDE EFFECTS

Defining Characteristics: Dry mouth, anorexia, nausea, vomiting, diarrhea, indigestion, taste changes, aphthous stomatitis may occur rarely.

Nursing Implications: Assess baseline nutrition and elimination patterns. Discuss abnormalities with physician, and discuss drug modification. Teach patient to self-administer prescribed antiemetics as appropriate. Instruct patient to take full dose at bedtime (if 150 mg or less). Suggest patient use sugar-free hard candy, frequent ice chips, or artificial saliva for dry mouth.

IV. ALTERATION IN URINARY ELIMINATION related to URINARY RETENTION

Defining Characteristics: Urinary retention may occur. Increased risk in patients with history of urinary retention.

Nursing Implications: Assess baseline urinary elimination pattern and risk. Assess for urinary retention, and instruct patient to report signs/symptoms. Discuss alternative drug with physician if this occurs.

V. ALTERATIONS IN SKIN INTEGRITY related to ALLERGY

Defining Characteristics: Urticaria, erythema, rash, and photosensitivity may occur.

Nursing Implications: Assess baseline drug allergy history and skin integrity. Instruct patient to report skin changes. If severe changes occur, discuss drug discontinuance with physician. Instruct patient to avoid sunlight or to use sunblock protection.

VI. SEXUAL DYSFUNCTION related to CHANGES IN LIBIDO

Defining Characteristics: Increased or decreased libido, testicular swelling, gynecomastia in males; enlargement of breasts and galactorrhea in women.

Nursing Implications: Assess baseline sexual functioning. Inform patient that alterations may occur, and instruct to report them. If severe, discuss dysfunction with physician and whether another antidepressant would provide equal benefit with less dysfunction.

Drug: fluoxetine hydrochloride (Prozac)

Class: Antidepressant.

Mechanism of Action: Inhibits CNS neuronal uptake of serotonin.

Metabolism: Well absorbed after oral administration, and peak serum levels occur in 6–8 hours. Peak plasma concentrations are 15–55 ng/mL. Time to steady-state in serum level is 2–4 weeks; 94.5% protein-bound. Drug is extensively metabolized in the liver to norfluoxetine and other metabolites using P-450 enzyme pathway; inactive metabolites are excreted in the urine. Elimination half-life is 1–3 days when administered acutely, and 4–6 days with chronic administration.

Dosage/Range:

Adult (for depression):

- 20 mg/day initially.
- After several weeks of therapy, if no response, may increase dose gradually to a maximum dose of 80 mg/day.
- Patients with hepatic dysfunction, elderly, or patients with concurrent diseases: start at lower dose or give less frequently.
- Weekly 90 mg tablets: begin 7 days after last 20-mg daily dose.

Drug Preparation/Administration:

- Give orally with or without food in the morning; with higher doses, e.g., 80 mg/day, may give two doses, one in the morning and one at noon.
- Available in pulvules of 10 mg and 20 mg; liquid/oral solution available as 20 mg/5 mL; weekly 90-mg tablets.
- Allow at least 14 days between stopping an MAOI and beginning fluoxetine; when stopping fluoxetine to begin an MAOI, wait at least five weeks before beginning the MAOI.

Drug Interactions:

- Alcohol: DO NOT USE CONCOMITANTLY, as increases impaired judgment, thinking, and motor skills.
- Tricyclic antidepressants (TCA): decreased metabolism and increased serum levels of TCA; monitor for increased toxicity and dose-reduce TCA as necessary when drug is given concomitantly with fluoxetine.
- MAOIs: when drug is given concomitantly or within a short time period, severe, potentially life-threatening interactions may occur, including symptoms resembling neuroleptic malignant syndrome. DO NOT GIVE

TOGETHER, AND END SEPARATELY, as stated in Administration section.
- Buspirone: reduced effects of buspirone; assess need to increase dose.
- Carbamazepine: increased serum levels of carbamazepine, with potential increased toxicity; monitor closely and dose-reduce as necessary.
- Cyproheptadine: decreased fluoxetine serum levels, so that effect was reduced or reversed; avoid concomitant administration if possible.
- Dextromethorphan: increased risk of hallucinations.
- Diazepam: increased diazepam half-life with increased circulating serum levels, leading to increased toxicity (e.g., excessive sedation or impaired psychomotor skills); dose-reduce diazepam or avoid concurrent administration.
- Digoxin: displaces fluoxetine from plasma protein binding, leading to increased fluoxetine serum levels and effect; monitor for toxicity and dosereduce as necessary.
- Lithium: increased lithium serum levels leading to possible increased neurotoxicity; monitor patient closely, and reduce lithium dose as needed.
- Phenytoin: increased phenytoin serum levels; monitor effect and serum levels, and modify dose accordingly.
- Thioridazine: DO NOT administer together. Discontinue fluoxetine at least 5 weeks before starting thioridazine.
- Tryptophan: increased risk of CNS toxicity (e.g., headache, sweating, dizziness, agitation, aggressiveness) and peripheral toxicity (e.g., nausea, vomiting); use together cautiously if at all; avoid if possible.
- Warfarin: displaces fluoxetine from plasma protein binding sites, leading to increased fluoxetine serum levels, and effect; monitor for toxicity and dosereduce as necessary.

Lab Effects/Interference:
- None known.

Special Considerations:
- Weekly dosing is for patients whose depression is stable on daily dosing. Diarrhea and cognitive changes are more common with weekly dosing.
- May take up to four weeks of therapy before benefit is seen.
- Possibility of suicide attempt may exist in depression and persist until depression managed by drug; monitor high-risk patients closely and give smallest prescription of tablets possible to ensure frequent follow-up and reduce the risk of overdosage.
- Has slight-to-no anticholinergic, sedative, or orthostatic hypotensive side effects.
- Avoid use in women who are pregnant or breast-feeding.
- Drug is also indicated for treatment of obsessive-compulsive disorder and bulimia disorder.

Potential Toxicities/Side Effects and the Nursing Process

I. ALTERATIONS IN SKIN INTEGRITY related to RASH

Defining Characteristics: Urticaria, rash may occur (7%). In initial trials, in one-third of patients developing rash, rash was associated with fever, leukocytosis, arthralgias, edema, carpal tunnel syndrome, respiratory distress, lymphadenopathy, proteinuria, and/or mildly elevated liver transaminase levels that required drug discontinuation, which largely resolved symptoms.

Nursing Implications: Assess baseline skin integrity, and instruct patient to report rash immediately. Discuss drug discontinuance with physician if severe or associated with other symptoms as above. Teach symptomatic skin management.

II. ALTERATIONS IN SENSORY/PERCEPTUAL PATTERNS related to CNS EFFECTS

Defining Characteristics: CNS effects include headache and, less commonly, activation of mania or hypomania, insomnia, anxiety, decreased ability to concentrate, tremor, sensory disturbances, abnormal dreams, nervousness, dizziness, fatigue, sedation, lightheadedness, blurred vision. Rarely, seizures may occur. Patients at risk for suicide may commit suicide during initial period of treatment.

Nursing Implications: Assess baseline neurologic status and risk factors, and monitor during treatment. Instruct patient to report signs/symptoms, and discuss drug modification with physician. Evaluate patient satisfaction with drug efficacy. Instruct patient to avoid alcohol while taking drug. Assess suicide risk, and if at high risk, monitor closely, provide supportive counseling, and prescribe only small numbers of pills to prevent overdosage. May take up to four weeks for therapeutic effect to be seen.

III. ALTERATION IN NUTRITION, LESS THAN BODY REQUIREMENTS, related to GI SIDE EFFECTS

Defining Characteristics: Nausea and, less commonly, vomiting, diarrhea, constipation, dry mouth, dyspepsia, anorexia, abdominal discomfort, flatulence, taste changes, gastroenteritis, and increased hunger may occur. Significant weight loss can occur in underweight, depressed patients.

Nursing Implications: Assess baseline nutrition and elimination patterns. Discuss abnormalities with physician and discuss drug modification. Teach patient to self-administer prescribed antiemetics as appropriate. If patient is losing weight, instruct patient to report this immediately, and discuss benefit of continuation of drug with physician.

IV. INJURY related to DECREASE IN MENTAL ALERTNESS, PHYSICAL COORDINATION

Defining Characteristics: Drug may cause drowsiness, dizziness, and impair physical coordination, mental alertness.

Nursing Implications: Assess other medications that may increase risk (e.g., opiates, phenothiazines) and response to drug. Instruct patient to avoid potentially hazardous activities, including driving a car, operating machinery.

V. SEXUAL DYSFUNCTION, POTENTIAL, related to IMPOTENCE

Defining Characteristics: Sexual dysfunction, impotence, anorgasmia may occur.

Nursing Implications: Assess baseline sexual functioning. Inform patient that alterations may occur, and instruct to report them. If severe, discuss dysfunction with physician, and whether another antidepressant would provide equal benefit with less dysfunction.

VI. ALTERATION IN OXYGENATION, POTENTIAL, related to ALTERED BREATHING PATTERNS

Defining Characteristics: Bronchitis, upper respiratory infections, pharyngitis, cough, dyspnea, rhinitis, nasal congestion, and sinusitis may occur infrequently.

Nursing Implications: Assess baseline respiratory status, and instruct patient to report any changes. Discuss serious changes with physician, and interventions necessary.

VII. ALTERATION IN COMFORT, POTENTIAL, related to PAIN

Defining Characteristics: Pain in muscles, joints, or back may occur; flulike symptoms are infrequent, as are asthenia, chest pain, and limb pain.

Nursing Implications: Assess baseline comfort level; instruct patient to report any changes. Discuss symptom management strategies, unless severe, and then discuss benefit of changing to another antidepressant medicine.

Drug: imipramine pamoate (Tofranil-PM)

Class: Tricyclic antidepressant.

Mechanism of Action: Blocks reuptake of neurotransmitters at neuronal membrane, thus increasing available serotonin, norepinephrine in CNS, and potentiating their effects. Appears to have analgesic effect separate from antidepressant action. May increase bioavailability of morphine. Indicated in the treatment of depressive (affective) mood disorders. Also used as an adjuvant analgesic in cancer pain management.

Metabolism: Completely absorbed from GI tract; highly protein bound. Plasma half-life is 8–16 hours. Metabolized in liver; excreted in urine and, to lesser degree, in bile and feces.

Dosage/Range:

Adult:

- Oral: 75–100 mg/day (may increase on patient response, to maximum 300 mg; reduce dose in elderly, 30–40 mg/day, to maximum 100 mg).
- IM: used only when oral route cannot be used.

Drug Preparation/Administration:

- Oral: store in well-closed containers at 15–30°C (59–86°F). Administer as a single bedtime dose.
- IM: administer IM in large muscle mass; change to oral as soon as possible.

Drug Interactions:

- MAOIs: increased excitation, hyperpyrexia, seizures; use together cautiously (especially if high dose is used).
- CNS depressants (alcohol, sedatives, hypnotics): increase CNS depression; use together cautiously.
- Sympathomimetic (epinephrine, amphetamines): increased hypertension; AVOID concurrent use.
- Cimetidine methylphenidate: increased imipramine levels, increased toxicity; use cautiously and monitor for increased toxicity.
- Warfarin: may increase PT; monitor closely and decrease dose of warfarin as needed.
- Barbiturates: may decrease imipramine level; monitor patient response; may need to increase dose.

Lab Effects/Interference:

- Increased metanephrine (Pisano test).
- Decreased urinary 5-HIAA.

Special Considerations:

- Antidepressant effect may take two weeks or longer.
- Adjuvant analgesic useful in cancer pain management.
- May also decrease depression associated with chronic cancer pain and promote improved sleep.
- Contraindicated in patients with myocardial infarction, seizure disorder, or benign prostatic hypertrophy.
- Use cautiously in patients with urine retention, narrow-angle glaucoma, hyperthyroidism, hepatic dysfunction, or suicidal ideation.

- Drug should be gradually discontinued rather than abruptly withdrawn to prevent anxiety, malaise, dizziness, nausea/vomiting.
- May be helpful in treating hiccups.
- Increased anticholinergic side effects in elderly.
- Some preparations may contain sodium bisulfite, which can cause allergic reactions, including anaphylaxis, in hypersensitive individuals. Check ingredients. Assess allergy history.

Potential Toxicities/Side Effects and the Nursing Process

I. ALTERATIONS IN SENSORY/PERCEPTUAL PATTERNS related to DROWSINESS, CNS EFFECT

Defining Characteristics: Drowsiness, dizziness, weakness, lethargy, fatigue are common; confusion, disorientation, hallucinations may occur in the elderly. Extrapyramidal symptoms may occur (fine tremor, rigidity, dystonia, dysarthria, dysphagia), as may peripheral neuropathy and blurred vision.

Nursing Implications: Assess baseline gait, neurologic and mental status, and monitor during therapy. Instruct patient to report signs/symptoms; discuss benefit/risk ratio with physician. Assess for signs/symptoms of suicidal ideation; if they occur, refer for psychiatric evaluation. Inform patient that drowsiness, dizziness will resolve after 1–2 weeks; instruct to avoid hazardous activities while drowsy (e.g., driving a car, operating machinery).

II. ALTERATION IN CARDIAC OUTPUT related to POSTURAL HYPOTENSION, TACHYCARDIA

Defining Characteristics: Postural hypotension, EKG changes, tachycardia, hypertension may occur.

Nursing Implications: Assess baseline orthostatic BP, heart rate, and monitor during therapy. Instruct patient to report abnormalities, including postural dizziness, palpitations. Drug should be stopped several days before surgery to prevent hypertensive crisis (especially if high dose is used).

III. ALTERATION IN NUTRITION related to GI SIDE EFFECTS

Defining Characteristics: Dry mouth, anorexia, nausea, vomiting, diarrhea, and abdominal cramping may occur; also, elevated LFTs.

Nursing Implications: Assess baseline nutrition and elimination patterns and LFTs, and monitor during therapy. Discuss abnormalities with physician, and discuss drug modification. Teach patient to self-administer prescribed antiemetics as appropriate. LFTs should be repeated, and if still elevated, the drug should be discontinued. Instruct patient to take full dose at bedtime. Suggest patient use sugar-free hard candy, frequent ice chips, or artificial saliva for dry mouth.

IV. ALTERATION IN URINARY ELIMINATION related to URINARY RETENTION

Defining Characteristics: Urinary retention may occur. Increased risk in patients with history of urinary retention.

Nursing Implications: Assess baseline urinary elimination pattern and risk. Assess for urinary retention, and instruct patient to report signs/symptoms. Discuss alternative drug with physician if this occurs.

V. ALTERATIONS IN SKIN INTEGRITY related to ALLERGY

Defining Characteristics: Urticaria, erythema, rash, photosensitivity may occur.

Nursing Implications: Assess baseline drug allergy history and skin integrity. Instruct patient to report skin changes. If angioedema of face, tongue develops, discuss drug discontinuance with physician. Instruct patient to avoid sunlight or to use sunblock protection.

Drug: lorazepam (Ativan)

Class: Benzodiazepine (anxiolytic).

Mechanism of Action: Binds to benzodiazepine receptors in the CNS (limbic and cortical areas, cerebellum, brain stem, and spinal cord), resulting in the following effects: anxiolytic, ataxia, anticonvulsant, muscle relaxation. Appears to potentiate the effects of GABA.

Metabolism: Well absorbed from GI tract. Widely distributed in body tissues and fluids, including CSF. Crosses placenta and is excreted in breast milk. Highly bound to plasma proteins. Metabolized in liver and excreted in urine. Short half-life of 10–20 hours. May produce psychological and physical dependence. Indicated for management of anxiety and short-term relief of anxiety associated with depression.

Dosage/Range:
Adult:
- Oral: 1–6 mg/day in divided doses (maximum 10 mg/day).
- IM: 0.044 mg/kg or 2 mg, whichever is smaller (initial dose).
- IV: 0.044 mg/kg (up to 2 mg) given 15–20 minutes prior to surgery; 1.4 mg/m^2 given 30 minutes prior to chemotherapy; or 0.05 mg/kg (maximum 4 mg) if perioperative amnesia is desired.

- Use maximum dose (2 mg) in patients > 50 years old.

Drug Preparation/Administration:

- Oral: may administer with food to decrease stomach upset; has been given sublingually for more rapid onset (investigational).
- IM and IV: store drug in refrigerator until use.
- IM: administer undiluted, deep IM in large muscle mass (e.g., gluteus maximus).
- IV: dilute in equal volume of 0.9% Sodium Chloride or 5% Dextrose for IVP administration (administer slowly; not > than 2 mg/min) OR dilute in 50 mL 0.9% Sodium Chloride or 5% Dextrose immediately prior to administering IVB over 15 minutes.

Drug Interactions:

- CNS depressants (alcohol, anticonvulsants, phenothiazines, opiates): additive CNS depression; avoid concurrent use or use cautiously and monitor carefully.
- Oral contraceptives, isoniazid, ketoconazole: decrease plasma clearance of lorazepam so may increase effect (e.g., sedation); monitor patient closely.
- Tricyclic antidepressants: increased serum levels of antidepressant possible; use together cautiously.
- Digoxin: may decrease renal excretion of digoxin; monitor for overdosage; may need to decrease digoxin.

Lab Effects/Interference:

- Rarely, leukopenia, elevated LDH.
- Less frequently, elevated liver function studies.

Special Considerations:

- Wide margin of safety between therapeutic and toxic doses.
- May impair ability to perform activities requiring mental alertness (e.g., driving a car, operating machinery).
- May produce psychological and physical dependence.
- Administer cautiously in patients with liver or renal impairment.
- Use cautiously in patients with chronic pulmonary disease or sleep apnea.
- Contraindicated in patients with depressive neuroses, psychotic reactions (without prominent anxiety), acute alcoholic intoxication (with depressed VS), known hypersensitivity to the drug, or acute angle-closure glaucoma.
- May cause fetal damage, so should not be used during pregnancy or if the mother is breast-feeding.
- Withdrawal symptoms (including seizure, delirium) can occur with rapid drug discontinuance in patients taking high or chronic doses.
- If manic episodes or hyperactivity occur soon after drug started, drug should be discontinued.
- Drug should not be used to manage "everyday stress."

- Causes anterograde amnesia.

Potential Toxicities/Side Effects and the Nursing Process

I. ALTERATIONS IN SENSORY/PERCEPTUAL PATTERNS related to CNS DEPRESSION

Defining Characteristics: CNS depressant effects include drowsiness, fatigue, lethargy, confusion, weakness, headache, which may occur initially and resolve with continued therapy or dose reduction. Vivid dreams, suicidal ideation, and bizarre behavior may also occur. Patient risk factors: elderly, debilitated, liver dysfunction, low serum albumin.

Nursing Implications: Assess baseline neurologic status and risk factors, and monitor during treatment. Instruct patient to report signs/symptoms and discuss drug modification with physician. Evaluate patient satisfaction with drug efficacy. If patient expresses suicidal ideation (more common in panic disorders), refer patient for psychiatric evaluation and drug modification. Instruct patient to avoid alcohol while taking drug. Teach patient prescribed schedule for discontinuing drug when used chronically; assess for signs/symptoms of withdrawal (increased anxiety, rebound insomnia; may also include agitation, dysphoria, nausea/vomiting, irritability, muscle cramps, hallucinations, seizures).

II. ALTERATION IN NUTRITION, LESS THAN BODY REQUIREMENTS, related to GI SIDE EFFECTS

Defining Characteristics: Nausea, vomiting, weight increase or decrease, dry mouth, constipation may occur; also elevated serum LFTs.

Nursing Implications: Assess baseline nutrition and elimination patterns and LFTs, and monitor during therapy. Discuss abnormalities with physician and discuss drug modification. Teach patient to self-administer prescribed antiemetics as appropriate.

III. INJURY related to DECREASE IN MENTAL ALERTNESS, PHYSICAL COORDINATION

Defining Characteristics: Drug may cause drowsiness, dizziness, and impair physical coordination, mental alertness. Sedation, amnesia may last hours, impaired thinking and coordination 24–48 hours, and longer in the elderly.

Nursing Implications: Assess other medications that may increase risk (e.g., opiates, phenothiazenes) and response to drug. Instruct patient to avoid potentially hazardous activities, including driving a car, operating machinery. For 8 hours following IV injection, assess level of consciousness and instruct patient to call nurse for assistance in ambulating if needed. Instruct patient to avoid alcohol for 24–48 hours after drug injection.

IV. ALTERATIONS IN CARDIAC OUTPUT related to CHANGES IN BP, HR

Defining Characteristics: Drug may cause bradycardia, tachycardia, hypertension or hypotension, palpitations, edema.

Nursing Implications: Assess baseline VS, and monitor during therapy. Discuss abnormalities with physician. Instruct patient to report dizziness upon standing or other changes.

V. ALTERATIONS IN SKIN INTEGRITY related to RASH

Defining Characteristics: Urticaria, pruritus, rash (morbilliform, urticarial, or maculopapular) may occur.

Nursing Implications: Assess baseline skin integrity, and instruct patient to report changes. Teach symptomatic skin management, and discuss drug discontinuance with physician if severe.

Drug: mirtazapine (Remeron)

Class: Antidepressant.

Mechanism of Action: Centrally active presynaptic a2-antagonist, which increases central noradrenergic and serotonergic neurotransmission (via 5-HT1 receptors). Drug also blocks 5-HT2 and 5-HT3 receptors that contribute to antidepressant action. Thus, drug increases brain levels of both serotonin and norepinephrine. Antagonizes histamine H1 causing some sedation but has limited anticholinergic or cardiovascular effects.

Metabolism: Active ingredient mirtazapine is rapidly absorbed from the GI tract with > 50% bioavailability. Peak plasma level is reached in about 2 hours, with approximately 85% of drug protein bound. Mean elimination half-life is 20–40 hours with rare variation (up to 65 hours vs shorter in young men). Steady state reached in 3–4 days. Drug extensively metabolized (demethylation, oxidation, conjugation) and eliminated via urine and feces in a few days. Renal or hepatic insufficiency can delay drug clearance.

Dosage/Range:

Adults:

- 15 mg po qd to start, increasing in 2–4 weeks to a maximum of 45 mg qd if no response.
- If no response at maximal dose in 2–4 weeks, stop drug.

- Monitor elderly patients during dose titration. Use lowest dose, and monitor patients with renal or hepatic insufficiency closely due to reduced drug clearance.
- Response should be seen in 2–4 weeks of treatment at optimal dose.
- Once a response is obtained, drug is usually continued until the patient is symptom free for 4–6 months, and then the drug is gradually discontinued.

Drug Preparation/Administration:

- Tablets available in 15-, 30-, and 45-mg strengths, as well as in SolTab Orally Disintegrating Tablets (ODT), which dissolve on the tongue within 30 seconds.
- Administer tablets in a single daily dose at bedtime or in 2 divided doses (morning and evening).
- Administer SolTab ODT with or without water, to be chewed or allowed to disintegrate on the tongue.
- Store drug in the dark at 2–30 degrees C.

Drug Interactions:

- Alcohol: AVOID concurrent use as potentiation of CNS depressant effects.
- Monamine Oxidase Inhibitors (MAOI): AVOID concurrent use; DO NOT start mirtazapine until at least 2 weeks after the cessation of MAOI, and do not start a MAOI until at least 2 weeks after cessation of mirtazapine.
- Benzodiazepines: Potentiate CNS depressant effects of drug. Use together cautiously, if at all.

Lab Effects/Interference:

- Transient increase in hepatic ransaminases (SGOT/AST and SGPT/ALT).

Special Considerations:

- Rarely, granulocytopenia or agranulocytosis may occur, usually after 4–6 weeks of treatment.
- Possibility of suicide attempt may exist in depression and persist until depression is managed by drug. Monitor high-risk patients closely and give smallest prescription of tablets to ensure frequent follow-up and reduce the risk of overdosage.
- Avoid use in women who are pregnant or breast-feeding.
- Discontinue the drug if jaundice develops.
- Abrupt termination of drug after long-term therapy can result in nausea, headache, and malaise.
- Patients requiring close monitoring for toxicity: include those with epilepsy or organic brain syndrome; hepatic or renal insufficiency; heart disease, including conduction disturbances, and angina pectoris, or history of myocardial infarction; hypotension; prostatic hypertrophy or other voiding (micturition) disturbances; acute narrow angle glaucoma; and diabetes mellitus.

Potential Toxicities/Side Effects and the Nursing Process

I. ALTERATION IN NUTRITION, MORE THAN BODY REQUIREMENTS, related to INCREASED APPETITE, WEIGHT GAIN, EDEMA

Defining Characteristics: Increased appetite and weight gain are common. Peripheral edema may occur, resulting in increased weight. Drug may be chosen for its appetite stimulation in patients with advanced cancer who are depressed and losing weight.

Nursing Implications: Assess baseline nutrition pattern and weight, and monitor during therapy. Assess baseline fluid status and presence of edema, and monitor during therapy. Teach patient that these side effects may occur and to report them, especially edema. If patient develops significant edema, assess cardiopulmonary status (heart rate, orthostatic blood pressure, respiratory rate at rest and with activity, oxygen saturation). Discuss significant edema with physician.

II. ALTERATIONS IN SENSORY/PERCEPTUAL PATTERNS related to CNS EFFECTS

Defining Characteristics: CNS effects include drowsiness and sedation, especially during the first few weeks of treatment. Rarely, seizure, tremor, or myoclonus may occur. Worsening of psychotic symptoms may occur in patients with schizophrenia or other psychotic disturbances, and paranoid thoughts may become intensified. Mania may become activated in patients with manic depressive psychosis. Patients at risk for suicide may attempt/commit suicide during initial period of treatment.

Nursing Implications: Assess baseline neurologic status and risk factors, and monitor during treatment. Instruct patient to report signs/symptoms, and discuss drug modification with physician. Evaluate patient satisfaction with drug efficacy. Teach patient to avoid alcohol while taking drug, and to avoid benzodiazepines unless physician feels benefits outweigh risks. Assess suicide risk, and if at high risk, monitor closely, provide supportive counseling, and prescribe only a small number of pills to prevent overdosage. May take up to 4 weeks for therapeutic effect to be seen.

III. POTENTIAL FOR INJURY related to DECREASE IN MENTAL ALERTNESS, PHYSICAL COORDINATION, ORTHOSTATIC HYPOTENSION

Defining Characteristics: Drug may cause drowsiness, decreased mental alertness, and orthostatic hypotension.

Nursing Implications: Assess other medications patient is taking that may increase the risk (e.g., opiates, phenothiazines) and response to drug. Instruct patient to avoid potentially hazardous activities, such as driving a car or other vehicle, and operating machinery. Assess baseline orthostatic blood pressure and heart rate, and monitor during therapy. Teach patient that orthostatic hypotension may occur, and to report symptoms such as dizziness when changing position. Teach patient self-care measures to minimize risk of injury, such as changing position slowly over the course of 5 minutes, going from lying to sitting, and then from sitting to standing positions, holding on to walls or fixed railings when walking, and removing scatter rugs from walkways.

IV. POTENTIAL FOR INFECTION, BLEEDING, AND FATIGUE related to RARE BONE MARROW DEPRESSION

Defining Characteristics: Rare granulocytopenia or agranulocytosis may occur, usually after 4–6 weeks of treatment. If it occurs, it is usually reversible following drug discontinuance.

Nursing Implications: Teach patient that this rare side effect may occur. Instruct patient to stop the drug and to report signs and symptoms of infection, such as fever, sore throat, productive cough, or dysuria right away. If the patient develops any signs and symptoms of infection, the drug should be stopped and a complete blood count with differential checked. Assess baseline cbc/differential, and periodically during therapy, especially at 4–6 weeks after drug initiated.

V. POTENTIAL ALTERATION IN SKIN INTEGRITY related to EXANTHEMA

Defining Characteristics: Rarely, skin rash resembling chicken pox, measles, or rubella may develop.

Nursing Implications: Assess baseline skin integrity, and instruct patient to report rash immediately. Discuss drug cessation or discontinuance with physician. Teach patient symptomatic skin management.

Drug: nefazodone HCl (Serzone)

Class: Antidepressant, synthetically derived phenylpiperazine.

Mechanism of Action: Appears to inhibit neuronal uptake of serotonin and norepinephrine. Drug occupies central serotonin (5-HT2) receptors and acts as an antagonist. In addition, it antagonizes α-adrenergic receptors, that may explain the associated postural hypotension.

Metabolism: Rapidly and completely absorbed after oral administration, but extensively metabolized by the liver using the P-450 cytochrome enzyme system. Food delays absorption and decreases bioavailability by 20%. Peak plasma concentrations occur at 1 hour, and half-life of the drug is 2–4 hours. Drug is extensively protein-bound (> 99%). Time to steady-state is 4–5 days. Only 1% of drug is excreted unchanged in the urine.

Dosage/Range:

Adult:

- Initial: 200 mg/day, administered in two divided doses.
- If no or slight response, increase dose by 100–200 mg/day in two divided doses after at least one week at the previous dose; usual dose requirements are 300–600 mg/day in two divided doses.
- Elderly (especially women) or debilitated patients: begin at 50% of dose or 100 mg/day in two divided doses, and titrate up to therapeutic dose very slowly and gradually.

Drug Preparation/Administration:

- Oral, total dose given in two divided, bid doses on an empty stomach.
- Available in 100-, 150-, 200-, and 250-mg tablets.
- If changing from an MAOI to nefazodone HCl, allow at least 14 days after discontinuance of the MAOI before starting nefazodone; if changing from nefazodone to an MAOI, allow at least 7 days after stopping nefazodone before starting the MAOI.

Drug Interactions:

- Terfenadine, astemizole, cisapride: are metabolized by the P-450 hepatic enzyme system; nefazodone can inhibit their metabolism, resulting in QT elongation and potential cardiac arrest; DO NOT GIVE CONCOMITANTLY WITH NEFAZODONE.
- MAOIs: may cause symptoms resembling neuroleptic malignant syndrome, including death. DO NOT USE CONCURRENTLY. See administration guidelines above when changing from/to MAOIs.
- Alprazolam: increased serum levels of alprazolam; monitor effect and toxicity, and determine need for dose reduction.
- Digoxin: increased plasma levels of digoxin; assess effect and toxicity, and need for dose reduction of digoxin.
- Propranolol: decreased plasma levels of propranolol; assess effect and need for increased dosage.
- Triazolam: increased plasma levels of triazolam; assess effect, toxicity, and need for dosage reduction.

Lab Effects/Interference:

- Rarely, increased AST, ALT, LDH.
- Rarely, decreased HCT, anemia, leukopenia.

- Rarely, hypercholesterolemia, hypoglycemia.

Special Considerations:

- Contraindications: coadministration with terfenadine, astemizole, cisapride, or MAOIs.
- Drug produces slight anticholinergic effects, moderate sedation, and slight orthostatic hypotension.
- May take several weeks until therapeutic effect is known.
- Use with caution in patients recovering from myocardial infarction, who have unstable heart disease and are taking digoxin, and patients with a history of mania.
- Monitor patients at risk for suicide carefully, as attempts may be made during initial period before significant antidepressant effects of the drug are seen.
- Avoid use during pregnancy or in nursing mothers.

Potential Toxicities/Side Effects and the Nursing Process

I. ALTERATIONS IN SENSORY/PERCEPTUAL PATTERNS related to DROWSINESS, DIZZINESS

Defining Characteristics: Dizziness (17% incidence), drowsiness (25%), insomnia (17%), lightheadedness (10%), activation of mania or hypomania, agitation, blurred vision (9%), confusion (7%), decreased concentration (3%), memory impairment (4%), paresthesia (4%), ataxia (2%), incoordination (2%), psychomotor retardation (2%), tremor (1%), hypertonia (1%), vertigo, twitching, hallucinations, abnormal dreams (3%), and paranoia may occur. Neuroleptic malignant syndrome is rare (e.g., hyperthermia, seizures).

Nursing Implications: Assess baseline gait, neurologic and mental status, and monitor during therapy. Instruct patient to report signs/symptoms; depending upon severity and dysfunction, discuss benefit/risk ratio with physician. Assess for signs/symptoms of suicidal ideation; if they occur, refer for psychiatric evaluation. Inform patient that drowsiness, dizziness will resolve after 1–2 weeks; instruct to avoid hazardous activities while drowsy (e.g., driving a car, operating machinery).

II. ALTERATION IN CARDIAC OUTPUT related to POSTURAL HYPOTENSION, TACHYCARDIA

Defining Characteristics: Infrequent postural hypotension (4% incidence), hypotension (2%), tachycardia, hypertension, syncope, ventricular ectopic beats, angina pectoris, and CVA may occur rarely.

Nursing Implications: Assess baseline orthostatic BP, heart rate, and monitor during therapy. Instruct patient to report abnormalities, including postural dizziness, palpitations. If patient has orthostatic hypotension, teach patient to change position slowly and to hold on to supportive structure. If symptoms are significant, discuss changing to another antidepressant with physician.

III. ALTERATION IN NUTRITION, LESS THAN BODY REQUIREMENTS, related to GI SIDE EFFECTS

Defining Characteristics: Dry mouth (25% incidence), nausea (22%), vomiting (rare), diarrhea (5%), constipation (14%), dyspepsia (9%), and rarely eructation, gastritis, stomatitis, peptic ulceration, rectal hemorrhage have been reported.

Nursing Implications: Assess baseline nutrition and elimination patterns and LFTs, and monitor during therapy. Discuss abnormalities with physician, and discuss drug modification. Teach patient to self-administer prescribed antiemetics, and other symptom management interventions as ordered. Suggest patient use sugar-free hard candy, frequent ice chips, or artificial saliva for dry mouth.

IV. ALTERATION IN URINARY ELIMINATION related to URINARY FREQUENCY

Defining Characteristics: Infrequently, (2% incidence) urinary frequency, urinary retention, and urinary tract infections may occur.

Nursing Implications: Assess baseline urinary elimination pattern and risk. Assess for urinary frequency, retention, and infection, and instruct patient to report signs/symptoms. Discuss alternative drug with physician if this occurs.

V. ALTERATION IN COMFORT related to HEADACHE

Defining Characteristics: Headache (36% incidence), asthenia (11%), arthralgia (1%) may occur.

Nursing Implications: Assess baseline comfort. Instruct patient to report unrelieved symptoms, and consider symptom-management strategies. Discuss severe discomfort that is unrelieved with physician and consider alternative antidepressant therapy.

Drug: nortriptyline hydrochloride (Aventyl, Pamelor)

Class: Tricyclic antidepressant.

Mechanism of Action: Blocks reuptake of neurotransmitters at neuronal membrane, thus increasing available serotonin, norepinephrine in CNS, and potentiating their effects. May increase bioavailability of morphine. Indicated in the treatment of depressive (affective) mood disorders. Also used as an adjuvant analgesic in cancer pain management.

Metabolism: Distributed to lungs, heart, brain, liver; highly bound to plasma, proteins. Plasma half-life is 16–90 hours. Metabolized in liver, excreted in urine, and, to a lesser degree, in bile and feces.

Dosage/Range:

Adult:

- Oral: 75–100 mg/day (maximum 100 mg or serum levels should be monitored; therapeutic dose: 50–150 mg/mL).
- Elderly: 30–50 mg/day.

Drug Preparation/Administration:

- Store oral solution in tight, light-resistant containers; store tablets in tight containers; keep at temperature of 15–30°C (59–86°F).
- Administer in single bedtime dose.

Drug Interactions:

- MAOIs: increased excitation, hyperpyrexia, seizures; use together cautiously (especially if high dose is used).
- CNS depressants (alcohol, sedatives, hypnotics): increase CNS depression; use together cautiously.
- Sympathomimetic (epinephrine, amphetamines): increased hypertension; AVOID concurrent use.
- Cimetidine methylphenidate: increased nortriptyline levels, increased toxicity; use cautiously and monitor for increased toxicity.
- Warfarin: may increase PT; monitor closely and decrease dose of warfarin as needed.
- Barbiturates: may decrease nortriptyline levels; monitor patient response; may need to increase dose.

Lab Effects/Interference:

- Rarely, bone marrow depression (agranulocytosis, eosinophilia, purpura, thrombocytopenia).
- Rarely, increased or decreased serum glucose levels.

Special Considerations:

- Antidepressant effect may take two weeks or longer.
- Adjuvant analgesic useful in cancer pain management.
- May also decrease depression associated with chronic cancer pain and promote improved sleep.
- Contraindicated in patients with myocardial infarction, seizure disorder, or benign prostatic hypertrophy.
- Use cautiously in patients with urine retention, narrow-angle glaucoma, hyperthyroidism, hepatic dysfunction, or suicidal ideation.

- Drug should be gradually discontinued rather than abruptly withdrawn to prevent anxiety, malaise, dizziness, nausea/vomiting.
- May be helpful in treating hiccups.
- Increased anticholinergic side effects in elderly.
- Some preparations may contain sodium bisulfite, which can cause allergic reactions, including anaphylaxis, in hypersensitive individuals. Check ingredients and assess allergy history.

Potential Toxicities/Side Effects and the Nursing Process

I. ALTERATIONS IN SENSORY/PERCEPTUAL PATTERNS related to DROWSINESS, DIZZINESS

Defining Characteristics: Drowsiness, dizziness, weakness, lethargy, fatigue are common; confusion, disorientation, hallucinations may occur in the elderly. Extrapyramidal symptoms may occur (fine tremor, rigidity, dystonia, dysarthria, dysphagia), as may peripheral neuropathy and blurred vision.

Nursing Implications: Assess baseline gait, neurologic and mental status, and monitor during therapy. Instruct patient to report signs/symptoms; discuss benefit/risk ratio with physician. Assess for signs/symptoms of suicidal ideation; if they occur, refer for psychiatric evaluation. Inform patient that drowsiness, dizziness will resolve after 1–2 weeks; instruct to avoid hazardous activities while drowsy (e.g., driving a car, operating machinery).

II. ALTERATION IN CARDIAC OUTPUT related to POSTURAL HYPOTENSION, TACHYCARDIA

Defining Characteristics: Low incidence of postural hypotension; EKG changes, tachycardia, and hypertension may occur.

Nursing Implications: Assess baseline orthostatic BP, heart rate, and monitor during therapy. Instruct patient to report abnormalities, including postural dizziness, palpitations. Drug should be stopped several days before surgery to prevent hypertensive crisis (especially if high dose is used).

III. ALTERATION IN NUTRITION, LESS THAN BODY REQUIREMENTS, related to GI SIDE EFFECTS

Defining Characteristics: Dry mouth, anorexia, nausea, vomiting, diarrhea, abdominal cramping may occur; also, elevated LFTs.

Nursing Implications: Assess baseline nutrition and elimination patterns and LFTs, and monitor during therapy. Discuss abnormalities with physician, and discuss drug modification. Teach patient to self-administer prescribed antiemetics as appropriate. LFTs should be repeated, and if still elevated, the drug should be discontinued. Instruct patient to take full dose at bedtime. Suggest patient use sugar-free hard candy, frequent ice chips, or artificial saliva for dry mouth.

IV. ALTERATION IN URINARY ELIMINATION related to URINARY FREQUENCY

Defining Characteristics: Urinary retention may occur. Increased risk if history of urinary retention.

Nursing Implications: Assess baseline urinary elimination pattern and risk. Assess for urinary retention, and instruct patient to report signs/symptoms. Discuss alternative drug with physician if this occurs.

V. ALTERATIONS IN SKIN INTEGRITY related to ALLERGY

Defining Characteristics: Urticaria, erythema, rash, photosensitivity may occur.

Nursing Implications: Assess baseline drug allergy history and skin integrity. Instruct patient to report skin changes. If angioedema of face, tongue develops, discuss drug discontinuance with physician. Instruct patient to avoid sunlight or to use sunblock protection.

Drug: oxazepam (Serax)

Class: Benzodiazepine (anxiolytic).

Mechanism of Action: Binds to benzodiazepine receptors in the CNS (limbic and cortical areas, cerebellum, brain stem, and spinal cord), resulting in the following effects: anxiolytic, ataxia, anticonvulsant, muscle relaxation. Appears to potentiate the effects of GABA.

Metabolism: Well absorbed from GI tract. Widely distributed in body tissues and fluids, including CSF. Crosses placenta and is excreted in breast milk. Highly bound to plasma proteins. Metabolized in liver and excreted in urine. Short half-life of 5–20 hours. May produce psychological and physical dependence. Indicated for management of anxiety, the short-term relief of anxiety associated with depression, and alcohol withdrawal.

Dosage/Range:

Adult:

- Oral: 10–30 mg tid–qid.
- Elderly: 10 mg tid OR 15 mg tid–qid.

Drug Preparation/Administration:

- Store tablets in tight container at < 40°C (104°F).

Drug Interactions:
- CNS depressants (alcohol, anticonvulsants, phenothiazines, opiates): additive CNS depression; avoid concurrent use or use cautiously and monitor carefully.
- Oral contraceptives, isoniazid, ketoconazole, or cimetidine: decrease plasma clearance of oxazepam, so may increase effect (e.g., sedation); monitor patient closely.
- Tricyclic antidepressants: increased serum levels of antidepressant possible; use together cautiously.
- Digoxin: may decrease renal excretion of digoxin; monitor for overdosage; may need to decrease digoxin.

Lab Effects/Interference:
- Rarely, leukopenia.
- Rarely, altered liver function studies.

Special Considerations:
- Wide margin of safety between therapeutic and toxic doses.
- May impair ability to perform activities requiring mental alertness (e.g., driving a car, operating machinery).
- May produce psychological and physical dependence.
- Administer cautiously in patients with liver or renal impairment.
- Use cautiously in patients with chronic pulmonary disease or sleep apnea.
- Contraindicated in patients with depressive neuroses, psychotic reactions (without prominent anxiety), acute alcoholic intoxication (with depressed VS), known hypersensitivity to the drug, or acute angle-closure glaucoma.
- May cause fetal damage, so should not be used during pregnancy or if the mother is breast-feeding.
- Withdrawal symptoms (including seizure, delirium) can occur with rapid drug discontinuance in patients taking high or chronic doses.
- If manic episodes or hyperactivity occur soon after drug started, drug should be discontinued.
- Drug should not be used to manage "everyday stress."
- Serax 15-mg tablet contains dye tartrazine, which may cause allergic reactions in sensitive individuals, especially if sensitive to aspirin.

Potential Toxicities/Side Effects and the Nursing Process

I. ALTERATIONS IN SENSORY/PERCEPTUAL PATTERNS related to CNS DEPRESSION

Defining Characteristics: CNS depressant effects include drowsiness, fatigue, lethargy, weakness. Cumulative effects are less, as there is a short plasma half-life. Risk factors: elderly, debilitated, liver dysfunction, low serum albumin.

Nursing Implications: Assess baseline neurologic status and risk factors, and monitor during treatment. Instruct patient to report signs/symptoms. Instruct patient to avoid alcohol while taking drug. Teach patient prescribed schedule for discontinuing drug when drug is used chronically.

II. ALTERATION IN NUTRITION, LESS THAN BODY REQUIREMENTS, related to GI SIDE EFFECTS

Defining Characteristics: Nausea, vomiting, weight increase or decrease, dry mouth, constipation may occur; also, elevated LFTs.

Nursing Implications: Assess baseline nutrition and elimination patterns and LFTs, and monitor during therapy. Discuss abnormalities with physician and discuss drug modification. Teach patient to self-administer prescribed antiemetics as appropriate.

III. INJURY related to DECREASE IN MENTAL ALERTNESS, PHYSICAL COORDINATION

Defining Characteristics: Drug may cause drowsiness, dizziness, and impair physical coordination, mental alertness.

Nursing Implications: Assess other medications that may increase risk (e.g., opiates, phenothiazenes) and response to drug. Instruct patient to avoid potentially hazardous activities, including driving a car, operating machinery.

IV. ALTERATIONS IN CARDIAC OUTPUT related to TRANSIENT HYPOTENSION

Defining Characteristics: Transient hypotension may occur.

Nursing Implications: Assess baseline VS, and monitor during therapy. Discuss abnormalities with physician. Instruct patient to report dizziness on standing or other changes.

V. ALTERATIONS IN SKIN INTEGRITY related to RASH

Defining Characteristics: Urticaria, pruritus, rash (morbilliform, urticarial, or maculopapular) may occur.

Nursing Implications: Assess baseline skin integrity, and instruct patient to report changes. Teach symptomatic skin management, and discuss drug discontinuance with physician if severe.

Drug: paroxetine hydrochloride (Paxil)

Class: Antidepressant with mechanism of action different from selective serotonin reuptake inhibitors, tricyclic, or tetracyclic antidepressants.

Mechanism of Action: Appears to potentiate serotonergic activity of the CNS by potent and selective inhibition of serotonin reuptake by the neurons.

Metabolism: Completely absorbed after oral administration and metabolized to some degree by the P-450 hepatic enzyme system. Distributed throughout the body, including the CNS, and is extensively protein-bound (95%). Increased serum levels occur in patients with hepatic or renal dysfunction (twofold), and in elderly patients. Time to peak plasma levels 5.2 hours, and time to reach steady-state is 10–24 days. Largely excreted in the urine (64%) over a 10-day period, and approximately 36% is excreted in the feces.

Dosage/Range:

Adult (depression):

- Initial: 20 mg/day PO in the morning. Initial response may be delayed; if no response, may increase dose in 10 mg/day increments after an interval of at least one week, to a maximum of 50 mg/day.
- Patients who are elderly, or who have severe hepatic or renal dysfunction: initial dose of 10 mg/day, with increased dose adjustments made after at least one week, in 10 mg/day increments up to a maximum of 40 mg/day.

Drug Preparation/Administration:

- Oral, available in 10-, 20-, 30-, and 40-mg tablets.
- Administer as a single daily dose, usually in the morning.
- Allow at least 14 days when changing from an MAOI to paroxetine, or when changing from paroxetine to an MAOI.

Drug Interactions:

- Tryptophan: when administered concomitantly, headache, nausea, sweating and dizziness may occur; avoid concomitant administration.
- MAOIs: reactions including death have occurred (hyperthermia, rigidity, myoclonus, autonomic instability, mental status changes including delirium/coma); allow at least 14 days between changing to or from paroxetine to an MAOI.
- Warfarin: increased bleeding despite a normal PT; give together cautiously if at all.
- Sumatriptan: may cause hyperreflexia, weakness; incoordination may occur; monitor patient closely.
- Drugs inhibiting the P-450 cytochrome hepatic metabolic pathway (e.g., cimetidine): paroxetine serum levels may be increased by up to 50%; assess response and toxicity carefully and need to decrease paroxetine dosage.

- Drugs inducing the P-450 cytochrome hepatic metabolic pathway (e.g., phenobarbital, phenytoin): paroxetine serum levels may be reduced by up to 25–50%; assess response and need to increase paroxetine dosage.
- Drugs metabolized by the P-450 cytochrome hepatic metabolic pathway (other antidepressant medications, phenothiazines, type 1C antiarrhythmics): paroxetine may inhibit the metabolism of these drugs, resulting in increased toxicity.
- Tricyclic antidepressants should be given together with caution, and the dose of the tricyclic antidepressant may need to be reduced.
- Drugs that are highly bound to plasma proteins: paroxetine may displace the other drug from serum proteins, thus increasing the serum level of the other drug, resulting in toxicity. Give together cautiously and monitor/reduce drug as needed.
- Alcohol: avoid concurrent administration.
- Lithium, digoxin: use together cautiously; digoxin levels may be reduced.
- Procyclidine: increased anticholinergic effects possible; decrease dose of procyclidine if necessary to coadminister.
- Theophylline: may elevate serum theophylline levels; monitor and adjust dose accordingly.

Lab Effects/Interference:
- None known.

Special Considerations:
- Drug excreted in breast milk; drug should be administered cautiously, if at all, in breast-feeding mothers.
- Drug is teratogenic, so women of childbearing age should use contraception if sexually active.
- Drug indicated for the treatment of depression, panic disorder, obsessive/compulsive disorder.

Potential Toxicities/Side Effects and the Nursing Process

I. ALTERATIONS IN SENSORY/PERCEPTUAL PATTERNS related to DIZZINESS, SOMNOLENCE

Defining Characteristics: Somnolence, dizziness, insomnia, tremor, nervousness, and asthenia occur in more than 5% of patients. Less common are headache, agitation, seizures, anxiety, activation of mania or hypomania, paresthesia, confusion, impaired concentration, emotional lability, depression.

Nursing Implications: Assess baseline neurologic status, affective state, and risk factors, and monitor during treatment. Instruct patient to avoid alcohol while taking drug. Assess effect on elderly and/or patients with hepatic or renal dysfunction. Inform patient that daytime drowsiness may occur, and instruct to use caution if driving or operating heavy machinery. Assess for symptoms at each visit, and instruct patient to report changes. If symptoms occur, discuss strategies to ensure patient safety and comfort.

II. ALTERATION IN NUTRITION, LESS THAN BODY REQUIREMENTS, related to GI SIDE EFFECTS

Defining Characteristics: Nausea and decreased appetite may occur.

Nursing Implications: Assess baseline nutrition status, and instruct patient to report any nausea or loss of appetite. Discuss measures to reduce nausea and/or stimulate appetite.

III. ALTERATION IN COMFORT related to SWEATING

Defining Characteristics: Sweating may occur.

Nursing Implications: Inform patient that this may occur, and assess impact on patient and need for intervention.

IV. SEXUAL DYSFUNCTION, POTENTIAL, related to EJACULATORY DISTURBANCES

Defining Characteristics: Incidence of ejaculatory disturbances is 13%; other disorders may occur (10%), including erectile difficulties, delayed ejaculation/ orgasm, impotence, and other sexual dysfunction.

Nursing Implications: Assess baseline sexual functioning. Inform patient that alterations may occur, and instruct to report them. If severe, discuss dysfunction with physician, and whether another antidepressant would provide equal benefit with less dysfunction.

Drug: sertraline hydrochloride (Zoloft)

Class: Antidepressant.

Mechanism of Action: Inhibits CNS neuronal uptake of serotonin.

Metabolism: Undergoes extensive first-pass metabolism by the liver and is excreted in the urine (45% by 9 days) and the feces (40–45%). Time to peak plasma levels is 4.5–8.4 hours, and peak plasma levels are 20–55 ng/mL. Food reduces time to reach peak serum levels. Highly protein bound (98%). Time to steady-state plasma levels is 7 days, but is increased to 2–3 weeks in the elderly.

Dosage/Range:

Adult:

- Initial: 50 mg/day.

- If no response after a period of 1–2 weeks, may titrate gradually up to a maximum dose of 200 mg/day.

Drug Preparation/Administration:
- Oral, once daily in morning or evening.
- Available in 25-, 50-, and 100-mg tablets.
- When changing from an MAOI to sertraline HCl, wait at least 14 days after stopping the MAOI before initiating sertraline; when changing from sertraline HCl to an MAOI, wait at least 14 days after stopping sertraline before beginning the MAOI.

Drug Interactions:
- MAOIs: severe reactions, similar to neuroleptic malignant syndrome, including death may occur; DO NOT ADMINISTER CONCURRENTLY; see Administration section.
- Alcohol: DO NOT give concurrently.
- Benzodiazepines: decreased metabolism of benzodiazepine drugs, which are metabolized by the P-450 enzyme system in the liver, resulting in increased serum levels and toxicity; monitor for toxicity and adjust dose accordingly.
- Tolbutamide: decreased clearance with increased serum levels; monitor blood sugar levels closely.
- Warfarin: increased PT and delayed normalization of same; monitor PT values closely.
- CNS active drugs: monitor effects closely and modify drug doses accordingly (e.g., lithium).

Lab Effects/Interference:
- Increased AST or ALT, total cholesterol, triglycerides.
- Decreased serum uric acid.

Potential Toxicities/Side Effects and the Nursing Process

I. ALTERATIONS IN SENSORY/PERCEPTUAL PATTERNS related to HEADACHE, INSOMNIA

Defining Characteristics: Commonly, headache, insomnia. Less commonly, drowsiness, dizziness, agitation, nervousness, anxiety, tremor, fatigue, impaired concentration, paresthesia, yawning, hypoesthesia, twitching, confusion, abnormal coordination (ataxia), abnormal gait, hyperesthesia, hyperkinesia, abnormal dreams, amnesia, apathy, hallucinations. Suicidal ideation or attempt is uncommon, but patients at risk may attempt suicide during initial treatment before therapeutic effects of drug are felt.

Nursing Implications: Assess baseline gait, neurologic, affective, and mental status, and monitor during therapy. Instruct patient to report signs/symptoms;

discuss benefit/risk ratio with physician. Assess for signs/symptoms of suicidal ideation; if they occur, refer for psychiatric evaluation. Inform patient that drowsiness may occur, and instruct to avoid hazardous activities while drowsy (e.g., driving a car, operating machinery).

II. ALTERATION IN CARDIAC OUTPUT, POTENTIAL, related to CHANGES IN BP

Defining Characteristics: Rarely, palpitations, edema, hypertension or hypotension, peripheral ischemia, postural hypotension, tachycardia, and syncope may occur.

Nursing Implications: Assess baseline orthostatic BP, heart rate, and monitor during therapy. Instruct patient to report abnormalities, including postural dizziness, palpitations. Discuss significant changes with physician. If patient has orthostatic hypotension, teach patient to change position slowly and to hold on to support.

III. ALTERATION IN NUTRITION, LESS THAN BODY REQUIREMENTS, related to GI SIDE EFFECTS

Defining Characteristics: Nausea and diarrhea are common. Less common are dry mouth, constipation, dyspepsia, increased or decreased appetite, vomiting, increased salivation, abdominal pain, gastroenteritis, dysphagia, eructation, taste changes; also, elevated LFTs.

Nursing Implications: Assess baseline nutrition and elimination patterns and LFTs, and monitor during therapy. Discuss abnormalities with physician, and discuss drug modification. Teach patient to self-administer prescribed antiemetics as appropriate. Suggest patient use sugar-free hard candy, frequent ice chips, or artificial saliva for dry mouth.

IV. ALTERATION IN URINARY ELIMINATION related to URINARY FREQUENCY

Defining Characteristics: Urinary frequency, dysuria, urinary incontinence, nocturia, polyuria may occur.

Nursing Implications: Assess baseline urinary elimination pattern and risk. Assess for changes in urinary elimination, and instruct patient to report signs/symptoms. Discuss alternative drug with physician if this occurs.

V. ALTERATIONS IN SKIN INTEGRITY related to RASH

Defining Characteristics: Maculopapular rash, acne, facial edema, pruritus, excessive sweating, alopecia, and dry skin may occur rarely.

Nursing Implications: Assess baseline skin integrity. Instruct patient to report skin changes. If angioedema of face, tongue develops, discuss drug discontinuance with physician. Assess impact of changes on patient and discuss strategies to minimize distress.

VI. SEXUAL DYSFUNCTION, POTENTIAL, related to MENSTRUAL IRREGULARITY, ↓ LIBIDO

Defining Characteristics: Menstrual disorders, dysmenorrhea, intermenstrual bleeding, sexual dysfunction, decreased libido may occur.

Nursing Implications: Assess baseline sexual functioning. Inform patient that alterations may occur, and instruct to report them. If severe, discuss dysfunction with physician, and whether another antidepressant would provide equal benefit with less dysfunction.

Drug: trazodone hydrochloride (Desyrel, Trialodine)

Class: Antidepressant.

Mechanism of Action: Appears to selectively inhibit the uptake of serotonin by brain synaptosomes and potentiates the behavioral changes induced by the serotonin precursor, 5-hydroxytryptophan.

Metabolism: Well absorbed after oral administration, with peak plasma levels occuring at 1 hour when taken on an empty stomach and at 2 hours when taken with food. Metabolized by the liver and excreted in the urine and feces. Time to steady-state is 3–7 days. Elimination half-life initially is 3–6 hours, followed by slower phase with a half-life of 5–9 hours.

Dosage/Range:

Adult:

- Initial dose of 150 mg in divided doses.
- Increase dose by 50 mg/day q3–4 days (maximum outpatient dosage is 300 mg/day, and inpatient is 600 mg/day in divided doses).

Maintenance:

- Lowest possible dose; once therapeutic effect reached, may be able to gradually reduce dose.

Elderly:

- 75 mg/day in divided doses; increase dose as needed and tolerated, every 3–4 days.

Drug Preparation/Administration:

- Oral administration, shortly after a meal or light snack, in divided doses.
- If drowsiness, may take majority of dose at bedtime.

Drug Interactions:

- Alcohol, CNS depressants: increased CNS depression; DO NOT GIVE TOGETHER.
- Antihypertensives: additive hypotension; evaluate and modify dose of antihypertensive as needed.
- Barbiturates: increased CNS depression; avoid concomitant use.
- Clonidine: reduced effect of clonidine; assess need for increased clonidine dosage.
- Digoxin: trazodone may increase serum digoxin levels; assess effects, and need to decrease digoxin dosage.
- MAOIs: initiate combined therapy cautiously and monitor patient for toxicity.
- Phenytoin: serum phenytoin levels may be increased; monitor levels and therapeutic effect and need for reduced phenytoin dosage.

Lab Effects/Interference:

- Occasional decreased WBC and neutrophil count.

Special Considerations:

- 75% of patients will respond within 2 weeks of therapy, and the remainder within 2–4 weeks.
- Drug causes moderate sedative effects and orthostatic hypotension, with slight anticholinergic effects.
- Contraindicated in patients during recovery from myocardial infarction, or patients receiving electroshock therapy.
- Elderly may be more vulnerable to sedative and hypotensive effects of drug.

Potential Toxicities/Side Effects and the Nursing Process

I. SEXUAL DYSFUNCTION related to PRIAPISM

Defining Characteristics: Priapism (prolonged or inappropriate penile erection) may occur, and has required surgical intervention in some cases, and in others there was permanent dysfunction.

Nursing Implications: Teach male patients that this may occur. If it does, patient should immediately discontinue the drug and call physician. Make certain the patient understands the instructions and knows how to contact the physician. If priapism has persisted for 24 hours or more, a urologist should be consulted.

II. ALTERATIONS IN SENSORY/PERCEPTUAL PATTERNS related to CNS DEPRESSION

Defining Characteristics: CNS depressant effects include drowsiness, fatigue, nightmares, confusion, anger, excitement, decreased ability to concentrate, disorientation, insomnia, nervousness, impaired memory, dizziness, lightheadedness; rarely, hallucinations, impaired speech, hypomania, incoordination, tremors, paresthesias may occur.

Nursing Implications: Assess baseline gait, neurologic status, affective state, and risk factors, and monitor during treatment. Instruct patient to report worsening depression, and assess for any suicidal ideation. Instruct patient to avoid alcohol while taking drug. Assess effect on elderly and/or debilitated patients (cognition, motor function, other sensitivities). Assess effect of drug side effects on patient, and weigh against benefit. Inform patient that daytime drowsiness may occur, and instruct to use caution if driving or operating heavy machinery. If sleep problems, have patient take majority of dose at bedtime to enhance sleep.

III. ALTERATION IN NUTRITION, LESS THAN BODY REQUIREMENTS, related to GI SIDE EFFECTS

Defining Characteristics: Diarrhea, nausea, vomiting, flatulence may occur rarely.

Nursing Implications: Assess baseline nutrition status, and instruct the patient to report any nausea or vomiting. If required, discuss with physician antiemetic to manage symptoms. If severe, discuss alternative antidepressant medications.

IV. INJURY related to DECREASE IN MENTAL ALERTNESS, PHYSICAL COORDINATION

Defining Characteristics: Drug may cause drowsiness, dizziness, blurred vision, and impair physical coordination, mental alertness.

Nursing Implications: Assess baseline mental alertness, and teach patient to assess tolerance of medication before driving a car or operating heavy machinery. Assess medication profile to identify other medications that may increase risk (e.g., opiates, phenothiazenes) and response to drug.

V. ALTERATION IN OXYGENATION, POTENTIAL, related to CHANGES IN BP, SYNCOPE

Defining Characteristics: Rarely, hypotension or hypertension, syncope, palpitations, tachycardia, shortness of breath, and chest pain may occur.

Nursing Implications: Assess baseline cardiovascular status, and vital signs, and monitor during therapy at each visit. Instruct patient to report any palpitations, chest pain, or any changes in condition. Discuss significant symptoms with the physician. If patient is hypotensive and receiving antihypertensive medication, discuss with physician discontinuing or dose-reducing the antihypertensive medication. Prior to elective surgery, because interaction with anesthesia is unknown, temporarily discontinue drug.

Drug: venlafaxine hydrochloride (Effexor)

Class: Serotonin-norepinephrine reuptake inhibitor (SNRI) antidepressant.

Mechanism of Action: Appears to potentiate neurotransmitter activity by inhibiting neuronal serotonin and norepinephrine reuptake.

Metabolism: Well absorbed after oral administration, and eliminated via the kidneys; time to reach steady-state is 3–4 days. Drug and metabolite half-lives are 5 ± 2 and 11 ± 2 hours. Increased drug serum levels in patients with renal or hepatic dysfunction.

Dosage/Range:

Adult (indicated for the treatment of depression and generalized anxiety disorder):

- Initial (extended-release capsule): 75 mg once a day, at the same time each day; if indicated, can start dose at 37.5 mg once daily for 4–7 days, increasing to 75-mg capsule strength; if no response after adequate trial at 75 mg per day, may increase dose in 75-mg increments after at least a 4-day trial at the previous dose, up to a maximum of 225 mg per day in a single dose.
- Initial (immediate-release tablets): 75 mg/day in two or three divided doses.
- If little or no response, dose may be increased in dose increments of up to 75 mg/day after at least 4 days at the previous dose, to 150 mg/day, and up to a maximum of 225 mg/day for moderately depressed patients. Severely depressed patients may need up to 350–375 mg/day in three divided doses.
- Patients with hepatic dysfunction: daily dose should be reduced at least 50%.
- Patients with renal impairment: Mild to moderate dysfunction: reduce daily dose by 25%; patients receiving hemodialysis: 50% dose reduction; dose is given after dialysis.

Drug Preparation/Administration:

- XL capsule available in 37.5-mg, 75-mg, and 150-mg strengths.
- Immediate-release tablets available as 25-, 37.5-, 50-, 75-, and 100-mg tablets.
- Drug should be administered orally with food in a single dose in morning or at night (same time every day) for extended-release capsule, or in two to three divided doses for tablets.
- When changing from an MAOI to venlafaxine HCl, wait at least 14 days after MAOI is stopped; when stopping venlafaxine HCl and beginning an MAOI, wait at least 7 days.

- When discontinuing drug after > 1 week of therapy, taper dose. If more than 6 weeks of therapy, taper over 2 weeks.

Drug Interactions:
- MAOIs: tremor, myoclonus, diaphoresis, nausea, vomiting, flushing, dizziness, hyperthermia resembling neuroleptic malignant syndrome, and may be fatal. DO NOT USE TOGETHER. See Administration section.
- Cimetidine: may increase venlafaxine HCl serum levels that are significant in patients with existing hypertension, hepatic dysfunction, or who are elderly; use with caution in these patients and monitor closely.
- Haloperidol: may increase haloperidol serum levels; monitor patient when drugs are administered concomitantly.

Lab Effects/Interference: Lab Effects/Interactions:
- Infrequent increased alk phos, creatinine, transaminases AST, ALT.
- Infrequent hyperglycemia with glycosuria, hyperlipemia, bilirubinemia, hyperuricemia, hypercholesterolemia, hypoglycemia, hypokalemia, hyperkalemia, hyperphosphatemia, hyponatremia, hypophosphatemia, hypoproteinemia, uremia, albuminuria.

Special Considerations:
- Avoid drug use during pregnancy and in nursing mothers.
- Dose-reduce in patients with hepatic or renal dysfunction.
- Use caution in patients with mania.
- Use for more than 4–6 weeks has not been evaluated.
- Contraindicated in patients receiving MAOIs.
- Studies have shown equal efficacy to fluoxetine (Costa, 1998; Silverstone and Ravindran, 1999).
- Serious adverse reactions have occurred in patients changing from MAOIs to venlafaxine HCl or from venlafaxine to an MAOI. It is imperative to wait 14 days changing from MAOIs to venlafaxine HCl or 7 days after stopping venlafaxine before starting an MAOI.

Potential Toxicities/Side Effects and the Nursing Process

I. ALTERATION IN OXYGENATION, POTENTIAL, related to CHANGES IN BP

Defining Characteristics: Rarely, hypertension, vasodilation, tachycardia, postural hypotension, angina, extrasystoles, syncope, thrombophlebitis, peripheral edema occur. Migraine headaches are frequent.

Nursing Implications: Assess baseline weight, presence of peripheral edema, cardiac status and vital signs, and monitor during therapy at each visit. Instruct patient to report any edema, palpitations, chest pain, or any changes in condition. Discuss any symptoms with the physician depending on severity.

II. ALTERATIONS IN SENSORY/PERCEPTUAL PATTERNS related to EMOTIONAL LABILITY, VERTIGO

Defining Characteristics: Emotional lability, trismus, vertigo occur frequently; infrequently, apathy, ataxia, circumoral paresthesia, CNS stimulation, euphoria, hallucinations, hostility, blurred vision, abnormal accommodation, photophobia, tinnitus, taste perversion, manic reaction, psychosis, sleep disturbance, abnormal dreams, and stupor may occur.

Nursing Implications: Assess baseline neurologic status, affective state, and risk factors, and monitor during treatment. Instruct patient to avoid alcohol while taking drug. Assess effect on elderly and/or patients with hepatic or renal dysfunction. Assess for symptoms at each visit, and instruct patient to report changes. If symptoms occur, discuss strategies to ensure patient safety and comfort.

III. ALTERATION IN NUTRITION, LESS THAN BODY REQUIREMENTS, related to GI SIDE EFFECTS

Defining Characteristics: Nausea (37% of patients), anorexia (11%), constipation (15%) may occur. Less commonly, dry mouth, diarrhea, dyspepsia, flatulence, dysphagia, melena, gastroenteritis, and eructation may occur.

Nursing Implications: Assess baseline nutrition and gastrointestinal functional status, and instruct the patient to report any GI disturbances or changes. Discuss measures to reduce nausea and/or stimulate appetite.

IV. SEXUAL DYSFUNCTION, POTENTIAL, related to EJACULATORY DISTURBANCES

Defining Characteristics: Incidence of ejaculatory disturbances is 12%, and other disorders may occur (1–6%), including erectile difficulties, delayed ejaculation/orgasm, impotence, and other sexual dysfunction. Rarely, women with uterine fibroids may develop enlargement, uterine hemorrhage, or vaginal hemorrhage; in addition, women may develop vaginitis and metrorrhagia and, rarely, amenorrhea.

Nursing Implications: Assess baseline sexual functioning. Inform patient that alterations may occur, and instruct to report them. If severe, discuss dysfunction with physician, and whether another antidepressant would provide equal benefit with less dysfunction.

V. ALTERATION IN COMFORT related to PAIN

Defining Characteristics: Malaise, neck pain, hangover-like effect, arthritis, bone pain may occur infrequently.

Nursing Implications: Assess baseline comfort level. Instruct patient to report any changes in comfort, and discuss strategies to reduce discomfort.

VI. ALTERATION IN OXYGENATION, POTENTIAL, related to altered BREATHING PATTERNS

Defining Characteristics: Bronchitis, dyspnea may occur frequently; infrequently, asthma, chest congestion, hyperventilation, laryngitis may occur.

Nursing Implications: Assess baseline respiratory status, and instruct patient to report any changes. Discuss serious changes with physician, and interventions necessary.

VII. ALTERATION IN SKIN INTEGRITY, POTENTIAL, related to RASH

Defining Characteristics: Infrequently, acne, alopecia, brittle nails, contact dermatitis, dry skin, maculopapular rash, urticaria, and herpes simplex and zoster may occur.

Nursing Implications: Assess baseline skin integrity, and instruct patient to report any changes. Discuss serious changes with the physician, and need for changing to another antidepressant depending on severity.

VIII. POTENTIAL FOR INJURY related to EFFECTS ON BLOOD CELL ELEMENTS

Defining Characteristics: Frequently, ecchymosis may occur; less commonly, anemia, leucocytosis, leukopenia, lymphadenopathy, lymphocytosis, thrombocytopenia, thrombocythemia may occur.

Nursing Implications: Assess baseline CBC and presence of bruising on skin. Instruct patient to report any bleeding, bruising, infection, or any changes in condition. Check CBC as indicated and discuss any changes with physician.

IX. ALTERATION IN URINARY ELIMINATION related to DYSURIA

Defining Characteristics: Frequently, dysuria, hematuria, metorrhagia, impaired urination, or vaginitis may occur. Infrequently, albuminuria, kidney calculus, cystitis, nocturia, bladder pain, kidney pain, polyuria, prostatitis, pyelonephritis, pyuria, incontinence, urinary urgency may occur.

Nursing Implications: Assess baseline urinary status. Instruct patient to report any changes, and discuss interventions with physician.

Drug: zolpidem tartrate (Ambien)

Class: Benzodiazepinelike hypnotic.

Mechanism of Action: Despite a chemical structure unlike the benzodiazepines, it selectively binds to one of the GABA complexes that the benzodiazepines nonselectively bind to, producing deep sleep (stages 3 and 4) without muscle relaxant or anticonvulsant properties.

Metabolism: Well absorbed from GI tract, with 70% of drug reaching the systemic circulation. Absorption and distribution affected by food intake. Widely distributed in body tissues and fluids, including CSF. Crosses placenta and is excreted in breast milk. Highly bound to plasma proteins. Metabolized in liver and excreted in urine, bile, and feces. Onset of action in 7–27 minutes, with a peak of 0.5–2.3 hours, and duration of 6–8 hours. Elimination half-life is 1.7–2.5 hours.

Dosage/Range:

Adult (for insomnia):

- Oral: 10–20 mg PO at hs.
- Elderly or debilitated individuals: 5 mg PO.

Drug Preparation/Administration:

- Store tablets in tight container at < 40°C (104°F).
- Administer on an empty stomach immediately before bedtime.

Drug Interactions:

- CNS depressants (e.g., alcohol, phenothiazines): additive CNS depression; avoid concurrent use or use cautiously and monitor carefully.

Lab Effects/Interference:

- None.

Special Considerations:

- Indicated for the short-term treatment of insomnia, generally 7–10 days of use.
- Contraindications: nursing mothers.
- Administer cautiously in patients with liver or renal dysfunction, pregnancy, pulmonary compromise, or who are depressed.
- May cause increased depression in patients who are already depressed.

Potential Toxicities/Side Effects and the Nursing Process

I. ALTERATIONS IN SENSORY/PERCEPTUAL PATTERNS related to CNS DEPRESSION

Defining Characteristics: CNS depressant effects include drowsiness, fatigue, lethargy, drugged feeling, depression, anxiety, irritability.

Nursing Implications: Assess baseline neurologic status, affective state, and risk factors, and monitor during treatment. Instruct patient to report worsening depression, and assess for any suicidal ideation. Instruct patient to avoid alcohol while taking drug. Assess effect on elderly and/or debilitated patients (cognition, motor function, other sensitivities). Assess effect of drug side effects on patient, and weigh against benefit. Inform patient that daytime drowsiness may occur, and instruct to use caution if driving or operating heavy machinery.

II. ALTERATION IN NUTRITION, LESS THAN BODY REQUIREMENTS, related to GI SIDE EFFECTS

Defining Characteristics: Nausea, vomiting, dyspepsia may occur.

Nursing Implications: Assess baseline nutrition status, and instruct the patient to report any nausea or vomiting.

III. INJURY related to DECREASE IN MENTAL ALERTNESS, PHYSICAL COORDINATION

Defining Characteristics: Drug may cause drowsiness, dizziness, diplopia, and impair physical coordination, mental alertness. At doses > 10 mg, patients may experience anterograde amnesia or memory impairment.

Nursing Implications: Assess other medications that may increase risk (e.g., opiates, phenothiazenes) and response to drug. Instruct patient to avoid potentially hazardous activities, including driving a car, operating machinery.

Section 3
Complications

Chapter 10

Hypercalcemia

Hypercalcemia is a metabolic complication of malignant disease and is evidenced by a serum calcium of > 10.5 mg/dL. Potentially fatal, hypercalcemia occurs in 10–20% of patients with cancer, principally in patients with breast cancer, multiple myeloma, squamous cell cancers of head and neck and esophagus, prostate cancer, and adult T-cell lymphoma. Hypercalcemia is compounded by problems of advanced disease, such as immobility and dehydration.

In reviewing normal calcium homeostasis, calcium is found primarily in bone. As such, 99% of the body's calcium is in the form of insoluble crystals, giving the human skeleton strength and durability. The remaining 1% is distributed between the body's intracellular and extracellular fluids: 45% is ionized in the serum, 45% is bound by protein, and 10% is found in insoluble complexes.

The ionized fraction of calcium is necessary for excitation of nerves, voluntary skeletal muscle, cardiac muscle, and involuntary muscles in the gut. If the body has too much ionized calcium, there is decreased excitability of these tissues. For instance, symptoms of early hypercalcemia (calcium of 10–12 mg/dL) are fatigue, lethargy, constipation, anorexia, nausea and vomiting, and polyuria. Later symptoms, when the calcium is > 12 mg/dL, are altered mental status, coma, decreased deep tendon reflexes, increased cardiac contractility, and oliguric renal failure. In contrast, if there is too little ionized calcium in the body, there is increased excitability of nerves and muscle. The body attempts to regain more calcium to raise the level of ionized calcium by "raiding" the bone matrix.

Because 45% of the calcium outside of bone is bound to albumin, it is important to correct the value of ionized calcium in the serum if the albumin is low (normally bound calcium is now free in the serum, and the serum level may be actually higher than the laboratory value). The formula to determine ionized serum calcium, corrected for low serum albumin is:

$$\text{Corrected serum calcium} = \text{measured total serum calcium (mg/dL)} + [4.0 - \text{serum albumin (g/dL)}] \times 0.8$$

For example, a patient has a serum calcium of 10.0 mg/dL but has a serum albumin of 2.2 (normal is 3.5–5.5 g/dL). The corrected serum calcium is 10.0 mg/dL + (4.0 − 2.2 = 1.8 g/dL) × 0.8 = 10.0 + 1.44 = 11.44. Thus, a serum calcium level that appears normal may be abnormal (high) in the presence of a low serum albumin level.

The human skeleton undergoes constant remodeling, where there is an exquisite balance between bone formation and bone resorption (breakdown). Bone formation is mediated by osteoblasts and bone resorption by osteoclasts. Calcium balance is maintained by a number of factors. First, parathyroid hormone (PTH) released by the parathyroid gland increases serum calcium levels by stimulating bone resorption, increasing renal absorption of calcium, and stimulating the production of $1,25(OH)_2D_3$, which increases the intestinal absorption of calcium. In contrast, calcitonin balances these effects by reducing serum calcium: it inhibits bone resorption (breakdown) and decreases renal absorption of calcium. Normally, intestinal absorption of calcium is balanced by an approximately equal loss of calcium through urinary excretion. In most individuals before midlife, bone formation balances bone resorption.

There are many potential causes of hypercalcemia of malignancy. These include:

- Secretion of parathyroid-related protein by tumor.
- Secretion of other bone-resorbing substances by tumor (i.e., cytokines, transforming growth factor [TGF-α], IL-1, tumor necrosis factor [TNF]).
- Conversion of 25-hydroxyvitamin D_3 to 1,25-dihydroxyvitamin D_3 by tumor.
- Local effects of osteolytic bony metastasis.

Therapeutic efforts to lower serum calcium in hypercalcemia of malignancy are based on rehydration to restore glomerular filtration and excretion of calcium (normally up to 600 mg/day), and drugs that promote calcium excretion or inhibit osteoclastic bone resorption. General management principles are based on palliation of symptoms, since usually the patient has advanced malignancy. Diet restriction of calcium is not necessary, as calcium absorbed from the gut is often less than normal and patients are malnourished. Patients with T-cell lymphoma, who have increased 1,25-dihydroxyvitamin D_3, are an exception to this rule. These patients have high levels of 1,25-dihydroxyvitamin D_3 and should avoid intake of dairy products. It is important for patients to bear weight if possible, since immobility increases osteoclastic activity and decreases osteoblastic activity. Since calcium is a potent diuretic, patients are often dehydrated with the loss of sodium and water. Further, as the serum calcium increases, the distal renal tubules become less able to retain sodium, and there is further sodium loss from the kidneys. Patients are usually rehydrated with 3–4 liters per day of 0.9% Sodium Chloride over 48 hours to restore fluid volume. Loop diuretics are administered, such as furosemide (Lasix), which increase calcium excretion. Thiazide diuretics are avoided, since they increase tubular reabsorption of calcium. This usually provides symptomatic improvement, but it is important to monitor the patient closely for possible fluid overload on the one hand, or intravascular dehydration with electrolyte imbalance on the other.

There are a number of drugs that inhibit osteoclastic bone activity. Oral phosphates inhibit bone resorption and stimulate bone formation, as well as precipitate calcium. However, the side effect of diarrhea limits the usefulness of the drug. Glucocorticoids have an unpredictable effect, and their value is limited by side effects of high drug doses. However, they are often used in steroid-responsive malignancies such as multiple myeloma and lymphoma. Calcitonin inhibits bone resorption and promotes urinary calcium excretion with a rapid, but brief, response (2–3 days). Plicamycin (Mithramycin) inhibits osteoclastic bone resorption by killing the osteoclasts. It is potent, lowering calcium in 24–72 hours, but rebound hypercalcemia often occurs within one week. The high toxicity of the drug prevents wide usage. The biphosphonates have potent hypocalcemic activity, binding tightly to the calcified bone matrix. Some of the drugs inhibit lymphokine- and prostaglandin-mediated bone resorption, and the drugs vary in their inhibition of bone mineralization. Etidronate (Didronel) inhibits osteoclastic resorption, but with long-term use the drug inhibits bone mineralization, causing osteomalacia and pathologic fractures. Pamidronate (Aredia) and zolendronic acid (Zometa) inhibit bone resorption at low doses without decreasing mineralization, and normalizing serum calcium in 80–90% of patients within 48–96 hours (Fitton and McTavish, 1991). Zolendronic acid has been found superior to pamidronate (Major et al, 2001). Pamidronate and zolendronic acid are effective in reducing pain from bony metastases, and decrease the incidence of bone metastasis in patients with multiple myeloma or breast cancer. Zolendronic acid was shown to reduce skeletal events in patients with prostate cancer (Berenson et al, 1996).

Once symptomatic hypercalcemia is resolved, the malignant disease is treated if appropriate to prevent recurrence (e.g., with chemotherapy or radiotherapy to lytic bone lesions). Nursing implications revolve around management of the patient receiving aggressive hydration and hypocalcemic medications. Patient education is prominent, as patients and their families are taught about the disease, as well as self-assessment of signs and symptoms of hypercalcemia, fluid balance, activity, and oral care.

References

Bajorunas OR. Clinical Manifestations of Cancer-Related Hypercalcemia. *Semin Oncol* 1990;17:16–25

Berenson JR, Lichtenstein A, Porter L, et al. Efficacy of Pamidronate in Reducing Skeletal Events in Patients with Advanced Multiple Myeloma. *N Engl J Med* 1996; 334:488–493

Berenson JR, Rosen LS, Howell A. Zoledronic Acid Reduces Skeletal-related Events in Patients with Osteolytic Metastases. A Double-blind, Randomized Dose-response Study. *Cancer* 2001;91:144–154

Bilezikian JP. Management of Acute Hypercalcemia. *N Engl J Med* 1992;326(18): 1196–1203

Fitton A, McTavish D. Pamidronate: A Review of its Pharmacological Properties and Therapeutic Efficacy in Resorptive Bone Disease. *Drugs* 1991;41(2):289–318

Major P, Lortholary A, Hon J. Zoledronic Acid is Superior to Pamidronate in the Treatment of Hypercalcemia of Malignancy: A Pooled Analysis of Two Randomized, Controlled Clinical Trials. *J Clin Oncol* 2001;19:558–567

Novartis. Zometa Package Insert. East Hanover, NJ: Novartis; 2003

Solimandro DA, Bressler LR, Kintzel PE, Geraci MC. *Drug Information Handbook for Oncology*. Cleveland, OH: Lexi-Comp Inc.; 2000

Drug: calcitonin-salmon (Calcimar, Miacalcin)

Class: Thyroid hormone.

Mechanism of Action: Inhibits bone absorption (breakdown) by inhibiting bone osteoclasts and blocking osteolysis. Decreases high serum calcium concentrations in hypercalcemia of malignancy, beginning 2 hours after dose and lasting 6–8 hours. Promotes renal excretion of calcium, phosphate; also, acts on GI tract to decrease volume, acidity of gastric fluid, and enzyme content in pancreatic fluid.

Metabolism: Rapidly converted to smaller fragments by kidneys; excreted in urine.

Dosage/Range:

Adult (hypercalcemia):

- Subcutaneous (SQ) or intramuscular (IM): 4 IU/kg q12h × 2 days; if no effect, increase dose to 8 IU/kg q12h × 2 days, then to 8 IU q6h (maximum).

Drug Preparation/Administration:

- Refrigerate for 2–6 hours (36–43°F, 2–6°C).
- Reconstitute according to manufacturer's recommendations.
- If allergy suspected, perform skin test first: withdraw 0.05 mL of the 200 IU/mL solution in tuberculin syringe, then fill syringe with 1 mL 0.9% Sodium Chloride. After mixing, discard 0.9 mL; inject 0.1 mL intradermally on forearm and inspect for urticaria, wheal at 15 minutes.

Drug Interactions:

- None.

Lab Effects/Interference:

- Decreased alk phos.
- Decreased 24-hour urinary excretion of hydroxyproline.
- Casts in urine (indicate kidney damage).
- Decreased Ca++.

Special Considerations:

- Calcitonin-salmon consists of a foreign protein, so allergic reactions may occur. Perform skin test first if sensitivity is suspected. Do not use drug if wheal forms.
- It is unknown whether drug crosses placenta or is excreted in breast milk; use cautiously in pregnancy or breast-feeding.
- Patient should receive adequate saline hydration to keep urinary output at ~2 L/day throughout treatment.
- 80% of patients have reduction in calcium in 24 hours.
- Antibodies to drug may develop with long-term use.
- Rapid onset of action and mild side effects.
- Short duration of response.

Potential Toxicities/Side Effects and the Nursing Process

I. INJURY related to HYPERSENSITIVITY

Defining Characteristics: Rare hypersensitivity may occur.

Nursing Implications: Perform skin testing as ordered when sensitivity suspected; if positive, suggest use of human calcitonin or other hypocalcemic agent. Assess for signs/symptoms of hypersensitivity (generalized itching, agitation, dizziness, nausea, sense of impending doom, urticaria, angioedema, respiratory distress, hypotension). If this develops, stop drug immediately, notify physician, maintain IV access, and be prepared to administer epinephrine, hydrocortisone, diphenhydramine.

II. ALTERATION IN NUTRITION, LESS THAN BODY REQUIREMENTS, related to GI SIDE EFFECTS

Defining Characteristics: Transient nausea/vomiting is mild and tolerance develops; anorexia, diarrhea, epigastric discomfort, and abdominal pain may occur as well.

Nursing Implications: Assess baseline nutrition and elimination patterns. Since nausea/vomiting may occur within 30 minutes after injection, administer at bedtime to decrease distress.

III. ALTERATION IN COMFORT related to DRUG EFFECTS

Defining Characteristics: Flushing of face, hands, feet may occur soon after injection, as well as tingling of palms and soles. Rarely, rash (maculopapular), erythema, urticaria, headache, chills have developed. Inflammation may occur at IM or SQ injection site.

Nursing Implications: Assess comfort level. Administer drug at bedtime if possible. If symptoms are uncomfortable, consider symptomatic relief measures (e.g., heat, cold). Reassure patient that flushing lasts ~1 hour and is transient. Assess rash if severe; discuss with physician drug discontinuance.

IV. ALTERATIONS IN ELECTROLYTES related to HYPOCALCEMIA, HYPERCALCEMIA

Defining Characteristics: Rarely, if drug is very effective, hypocalcemia may occur; conversely, if drug is ineffective, hypercalcemia may occur.

Nursing Implications: Monitor serum Ca+ closely. Assess for signs/symptoms of hypocalcemia (muscle twitching, spasm tetany, seizures) and hypercalcemia (bone pain, nausea, vomiting, polyuria, polydipsia, constipation, bradycardia, lethargy, muscle weakness, psychosis). Notify physician, recheck serum calcium immediately, and institute corrective measures as ordered.

Drug: cinacalcet HCl (Sensipar)

Class: Hypocalcemic agent

Mechanism of Action: The calcium-sensing receptor on the surface of the chief cell of the parathyroid gland regulates PTH secretion. PTH is responsible for telling the bones to break down bone (osteoclastic) and release calcium into the blood when it is needed. Cinacalcet HCl directly decreases PTH levels by increasing the sensitivity of calcium-sensing receptors to activation by extracellular calcium. As PTH levels decrease, the level of calcium in the blood decreases.

Metabolism: Oral drug is well absorbed, and maximum plasma levels are achieved in 2–6 hours. Drug AUC levels are increased 82% when ingested with a high fat meal. Drug is metabolized by CYP3A4, CYP2D6, and CYP1A2 enzymes of the P450 microenzyme system. Drug is excreted in the urine (80%) primarily, and to a lesser degree in the feces (15%). Drug is poorly excreted in patients with moderate-to-severe hepatic impairment, with a half-life prolonged 33% and 70% respectively. Drug is highly protein bound so hemodialysis does not treat over dosage.

Dosage/Range:
30 mg PO bid, titrated every 2–4 weeks through sequential doses of 30 mg PO bid, then 60 mg PO bid, then 90 mg PO bid, and 90 mg tid or quid as necessary to normalize serum calcium levels.
- Monitor patients with moderate or severe hepatic impairment closely.
- Do not administer if serum calcium is < 8.4 mg/dL.
- Monitor calcium levels frequently during dose titration.

Drug Preparation/Administration:
- Drug available in 30, 60, and 90 mg tablets.
- Administer with food or shortly after a meal.

Drug Interactions:
- Drug is a potent inhibitor of CYP2D6: Dosage adjustment may be needed for flecainide, vinblastine, thioridazine, tricyclic antidepressants.
- Ketoconazole: increased AUC by 2.3 times of cinacalcet HCl.
- Amitriptyline: increased amitriptyline and nortriptyline by 20% in CYP2D6 extensive metabolizers.
- Warfarin: no effect.

Lab Effects/Interference:
- Hypocalcemia
- Hyperphosphatemia

Special Considerations:
- Drug is indicated for treatment of hypercalcemia in patients with parathyroid carcinoma.
- Patients should be monitored for signs and symptoms of hypocalcemia.
- Drug should not be used by pregnant or breast-feeding mothers, unless benefit outweighs risk.

Potential Toxicities/Side Effects and the Nursing Process

I. POTENTIAL FOR INJURY related to HYPOCALCEMIA

Defining Characteristics: Drug lowers serum calcium. Signs and symptoms of hypocalcemia are paresthesia, myalgias, cramping, tetany, and seizures.

Nursing Implications: Assess baseline serum calcium, phosphate, magnesium levels, as well as PTH level. Develop a plan for titration with the patient, and frequency of laboratory monitoring. Teach patient symptoms of hypocalcemia, and to report them right away if they occur. Serum calcium should be assessed within 1 week after initiation or dose adjustment. Once dose has been established, serum calcium should be assessed q month. If serum calcium > 7.5 mg/dL but < 8.4 mg/dL, or if symptoms of hypocalcemia occur, discuss with physician the addition of calcium-containing phosphate binders and/or vitamin D sterols to raise the serum calcium. If the serum calcium falls to < 7.5 mg/dL or if symptoms of hypocalcemia persist, stop drug until serum calcium level reaches 8.0 mg/dL and/or symptoms resolve. Resume dose per physician, at next lowest dose of drug.

II. ALTERATION IN NUTRITION, LESS THAN BODY REQUIREMENTS, related to GI SIDE EFFECTS

Defining Characteristics: Nausea (31%), vomiting (27%) are most common adverse effects, but diarrhea may also occur (21%).

Nursing Implications: Assess baseline nutritional and elimination status, and monitor during treatment. Ensure adequate hydration and urinary output of 2 L/day. Teach patient to administer oral antiemetics prior to taking drug, and as needed between drug doses. Assess food preferences, and suggest small, frequent feedings. Teach patient to report symptoms that worsen or do not resolve with supportive care.

III. ALTERATION IN COMFORT related to MYALGIA AND DIZZINESS

Defining Characteristics: Myalgia affects about 15% of patients and dizziness 10% of patients.

Nursing Implications: Assess baseline hydration, comfort status, and teach patient that these side effects may occur. Teach patient to change position slowly if dizziness occurs, and to notify nurse or physician if dizziness worsens or does not resolve. Teach patient symptom management strategies such as local application of heat for myalgias, and to notify provider if myalgias worsen.

Drug: etidronate disodium (Didronel)

Class: Biphosphonate; hypocalcemic agent.

Mechanism of Action: Inhibits osteoclastic bone resorption (bone breakdown), thereby decreasing calcium release, and serum calcium levels. Indicated in the management of hypercalcemia of malignancy.

Metabolism: Oral absorption is variable and decreased by food. Following IV injection, drug is distributed into bone, then excreted unchanged in the urine.

Dosage/Range:

Adult (hypercalcemia of malignancy):

- IV (induction): 7.5* mg/kg/day × 3 days (may increase to 7 days; if hypercalcemia recurs, wait at least 7 days before treatment using same induction regimen).
- Oral (maintenance): 20 mg/kg/day beginning on day after last IV dose, for up to 90 days if effective.

Drug Preparation/Administration:

- Oral: give as single oral dose (may be advised if GI distress); give at least 2 hours before or after a meal.
- IV: dilute drug in at least 250 mL 0.9% Sodium Chloride and infuse over at least 2 hours.

Drug Interactions:

- Nephrotoxic drugs: additive nephrotoxicity; AVOID concurrent use.

Lab Effects/Interference:

- Decreased P, decreased Mg.
- Abnormal renal function tests.
- Decreased Ca.

Special Considerations:

- Saline hydration should be maintained during treatment to keep urinary output at 2 L/day.
- Use with caution.
- It is unknown whether drug crosses placenta or is excreted in breast milk; use with caution, if at all, in pregnant or breast-feeding women.
- 60–70% response rate when given with hydration and diuresis, and one-half of this when based on corrected calcium value.

Potential Toxicities/Side Effects and the Nursing Process

I. ALTERATIONS IN NUTRITION, LESS THAN BODY REQUIREMENTS, related to GI SIDE EFFECTS

Defining Characteristics: Diarrhea, nausea, vomiting, abdominal discomfort, and guaiac-positive stools may occur rarely.

Nursing Implications: Assess baseline nutritional and elimination status and monitor during treatment. Instruct patient to report nausea and vomiting, and consider dividing dose (if oral) or slowing infusion rate >2 hours. Guaiac stools and notify physician if positive.

*Dose reduction necessary in patients with renal insufficiency.

II. ALTERATION IN URINE ELIMINATION related to NEPHROTOXICITY

Defining Characteristics: Drug is nephrotoxic and may cause rises in serum BUN and creatinine. Increased risk when concurrent nephrotoxic drugs administered.

Nursing Implications: Assess baseline hydration status and total body fluid balance to ensure adequate urinary output (> 2 L/day). Assess baseline serum BUN and creatinine, and monitor throughout treatment. Dose reduction necessitated by renal insufficiency.

III. ALTERATIONS IN ELECTROLYTES related to HYPOCALCEMIA, HYPERCALCEMIA

Defining Characteristics: Rarely, if drug is very effective, hypocalcemia may occur; conversely, if drug is ineffective, hypercalcemia may occur. Increased sodium phosphate levels may occur during oral therapy but are less frequent with IV dosing (serum phosphate levels are inversely proportional to serum calcium).

Nursing Implications: Monitor serum calcium closely. Assess for signs/symptoms of hypocalcemia (muscle twitching, spasm tetany, seizures) and hypercalcemia (bone pain, nausea, vomiting, polyuria, polydipsia, constipation, bradycardia, lethargy, muscle weakness, psychosis). Notify physician, recheck serum calcium immediately, and institute corrective measures as ordered.

Drug: furosemide (Lasix)

Class: Loop diuretic.

Mechanism of Action: Inhibits renal reabsorption of sodium and chloride in proximal loop of Henle. Useful in management of edema, hypertension related to CHF or renal disease, and with 0.9% Sodium Chloride IV hydration/diuresis to increase renal excretion of calcium in patients with hypercalcemia of malignancy.

Metabolism: Variable GI absorption of oral drug. Diuretic effect of oral dose occurs within 30–60 minutes, lasting 6–8 hours; with IV dose, occurs within 5 minutes, maximal 20–60 minutes, and lasts 2 hours. Highly protein-bound. Slight hepatic metabolism and is excreted in urine.

Dosage/Range:

- Edema: 20–80 mg PO in morning; if no response, dose-increase in 20–40 mg increments q6–8h.

- Hypertension: 10–20 mg PO bid, increasing to 40 mg bid based on BP response.
- Hypercalcemia: 80–100 mg IV q1–2h.

Drug Preparation/Administration:
- Oral: store in tight, light-resistant containers.
- IV: slow IVP over 1–2 minutes (use multidose vial or draw up drug from ampule through filtered needles).

Drug Interactions:
- Ascorbic acid, tetracycline, epinephrine form a precipitate; DO NOT give together with IV.
- Diuretics: enhanced diuretic effect; dose-reduce furosemide.
- Digoxin: toxicity enhanced by furosemide-induced hypokalemia; keep potassium level 4.5–5.0 mEq/dL.
- Drugs causing potassium loss (corticosteroids, amphotericin B): enhanced hypokalemia; monitor potassium level closely.
- Antidiabetic agents: decreases effect of insulin or oral hypoglycemics; monitor blood glucose and adjust antidiabetic drug as needed.
- Indocin: may decrease diuretic effect; monitor patient response and increase furosemide dose as needed.
- Aminoglycosides: increased ototoxicity; use cautiously.
- High doses of salicylates: increase salicylate toxicity at lower doses; monitor carefully and decrease salicylate dose.

Lab Effects/Interference:
- Decreased potassium, decreased chloride, decreased sodium, increased uric acid.
- Rarely, anemia, thrombocytopenia, neutropenia, leukopenia.

Special Considerations:
- Contraindicated in anuric patients and patients hypersensitive to the drug.
- May produce profound diuresis and electrolyte depletion.
- Should not be used by pregnant women, and breast-feeding should be interrupted during drug therapy.
- Use with caution in patients with liver cirrhosis.

Potential Toxicities/Side Effects and the Nursing Process

I. ALTERATIONS IN FLUID AND ELECTROLYTE BALANCE related to HYDRATION/DIURESIS

Defining Characteristics: Aggressive hydration with 0.9% Sodium Chloride and IV furosemide is used to promote calcium excretion. Hypokalemia, hypochloremia, hyperuricemia, hypomagnesemia may occur.

Nursing Implications: Assess baseline electrolyte (K+, Mg++, Cl−, Ca++), renal BUN, creatinine, and fluid balance, and monitor during therapy. Strictly monitor intake/output (I/O), assess daily weights, and maintain total body fluid balance (I = O). Administer prescribed replacement electrolytes. Assess for signs/symptoms of hypokalemia. Assess orthostatic BP, heart rate, and monitor during therapy.

II. ALTERATION IN SENSORY/PERCEPTUAL PATTERNS related to OTOTOXICITY, CNS EFFECTS

Defining Characteristics: Tinnitus and reversible or permanent hearing impairment may occur, often related to high doses of drug given IVP (high serum drug concentrations). Headache, vertigo, paresthesias can occur.

Nursing Implications: Assess baseline hearing (ability to hear spoken voice) and neurologic status. Teach patient to report tinnitus, decreased hearing, and any other symptoms. Discuss administration of high doses as IV infusion (4 mg/min).

III. ALTERATIONS IN SKIN INTEGRITY related to RASH, SENSITIVITY

Defining Characteristics: Purpura, photosensitivity, rash, urticaria, pruritus, exfoliative dermatitis, erythema multiforme may occur. Anaphylaxis has occurred in patients allergic to sulfonamides.

Nursing Implications: Assess drug allergies, especially to furosemide and sulfonamides. Assess baseline skin integrity, and instruct patient to report changes. Discuss drug discontinuance if severe reaction occurs.

COMPLICATIONS

Drug: gallium nitrate (Ganite)

Class: Hypocalcemic agent.

Mechanism of Action: Inhibits calcium release from bone by inhibiting bone resorption and turnover. Indicated for the treatment of hypercalcemia of malignancy refractory to hydration.

Metabolism: Excreted by kidneys.

Dosage/Range:
Adult:
- IV: Severe hypercalcemia: 200 mg/m² as continuous 24-hour infusion × 5 days (or when serum calcium normalizes if before 5 days). Moderate hypercalcemia: 100 mg/m² as continuous 24-hour infusion × 5 days (or less if patient achieves normal serum calcium).

Drug Preparation/Administration:
- Dilute daily dose in 1 L 0.9% Sodium Chloride or 5% Dextrose injection and infuse over 24 hours (42 mL/hour) via infusion pump.

Drug Interactions:
- Nephrotoxic drugs (amphotericin B, aminoglycosides, cisplatin): additive nephrotoxicity; avoid concurrent use.

Lab Effects/Interference:
- Increased BUN, creatinine.
- Decreased calcium; transient decrease in phosphorus, decrease bicarbonate.
- Rarely, anemia, leukopenia.

Special Considerations:
- Contraindicated in patients with severe renal dysfunction (serum creatinine > 2.5 mg/dL).
- Unknown if drug crosses placenta or is excreted in breast milk; use cautiously in pregnancy, and suggest mother interrupt breast-feeding while taking drug.
- 92% patient response (reduction in serum calcium corrected for albumin), lasting for 7.5 days.
- Saline hydration to maintain urinary output of 2 L/day should be maintained during treatment.

Potential Toxicities/Side Effects and the Nursing Process

I. ALTERATION IN URINE ELIMINATION related to NEPHROTOXICITY

Defining Characteristics: Increased serum BUN, creatinine in 13% of patients. Decreased risk if concurrent administration of other nephrotoxic drugs.

Nursing Implications: Assess baseline hydration status and total body fluid balance to ensure adequate urinary output (> 2 L/day). Assess baseline serum BUN and creatinine, and monitor throughout treatment. Dose reduction necessitated by renal insufficiency. Drug should NOT be given if serum creatinine > 2.5 mg/dL.

II. ALTERATIONS IN ELECTROLYTES related to HYPOCALCEMIA, HYPERCALCEMIA

Defining Characteristics: Rarely, if drug is very effective, hypocalcemia may occur; conversely, if drug is ineffective, hypercalcemia may occur. Transient hypophosphatemia occurs in up to 79% of hypercalcemic patients after treatment with drug. Also, decreased serum bicarbonate occurs in 40–50% of patients.

Nursing Implications: Monitor serum calcium closely. Assess for signs/symptoms of hypocalcemia (muscle twitching, spasm tetany, seizures) and hypercalcemia (bone pain, nausea, vomiting, polyuria, polydipsia, constipation, bradycardia, lethargy, muscle weakness, psychosis). Notify physician, recheck serum calcium immediately, and institute corrective measures as ordered. Monitor serum phosphate levels, and administer replacement oral phosphates as ordered.

III. ALTERATIONS IN NUTRITION, LESS THAN BODY REQUIREMENTS, related to GI SIDE EFFECTS

Defining Characteristics: Diarrhea, nausea, vomiting, constipation may occur.

Nursing Implications: Assess baseline nutritional and elimination status, and monitor during treatment. Instruct patient to report nausea and vomiting. Administer ordered antiemetics. Ensure adequate hydration with urinary output >2 L/day.

Drug: pamidronate disodium (Aredia)

Class: Biphosphonate; hypocalcemic agent.

Mechanism of Action: Probably inhibits osteoclast activity in bone (bone breakdown) and may also block dissolution of minerals (hydroxyapatite) in bone, thus preventing calcium release from bone. Does not inhibit bone formation or bone mineralization. Indicated for the treatment of hypercalcemia of malignancy, in conjunction with adequate hydration.

Metabolism: Excreted by kidneys.

Dosage/Range:

Adult (hypercalcemia of malignancy):

- IV(moderate hypercalcemia, 12–13.5 mg/dL corrected): 60–90 mg as continuous infusion over 24 hours.
- IV (severe hypercalcemia >13.5 mg/dL): 90 mg as continuous infusion over 24 hours.

Osteolytic bone metastases of breast cancer:

- 90 mg in 250 mL of IV fluid via 2-hour infusion q3–4 weeks.

Osteolytic lesions of multiple myeloma:

- 90 mg in 500 mL IV fluid via 4-hour infusion every month.

Drug Preparation/Administration:

- Reconstitute by adding 10 mL sterile water for injection to 30-mg vial. Further dilute in 1 L 0.9% Sodium Chloride or 5% Dextrose injection as per manufacturer's directions.
- Infuse over 2–24 hours via infusion pump or rate controller.

Drug Interactions:

- None.

Lab Effects/Interference:

- Decreased calcium.
- Decreased K+, decreased Mg, decreased P (phosphate).

Special Considerations:

- Saline hydration to maintain urinary output of 2 L/day should be maintained during treatment.
- Clinical studies show 64% of patients have corrected serum calcium levels by 24 hours after beginning therapy, and after 7 days 100% of the 90-mg group had normal corrected levels. For some (33–53%), normal or partially corrected calciums in 60-mg and 90-mg groups persisted × 14 days.
- Has been shown to reduce bony metastasis in patients with multiple myeloma and to reduce pain.
- Patients with preexisting anemia, leukopenia, or thrombocytopenia should be monitored closely for 2 weeks after pamidronate disodium treatment.

Potential Toxicities/Side Effects and the Nursing Process

I. ALTERATIONS IN NUTRITION, LESS THAN BODY REQUIREMENTS, related to GI SIDE EFFECTS

Defining Characteristics: Nausea, vomiting, abdominal discomfort, constipation, and anorexia may occur rarely.

Nursing Implications: Assess baseline nutritional and elimination status and monitor during treatment. Ensure adequate hydration and urinary output of 2 L/day. Administer ordered antiemetics. Administer oral phosphates as cathartics if ordered. Assess food differences and offer small, frequent feedings.

II. ALTERATION IN ELECTROLYTES related to HYPOCALCEMIA, HYPERCALCEMIA

Defining Characteristics: Rarely, if drug is very effective, hypocalcemia may occur; conversely, if drug is ineffective, hypercalcemia may occur. Hypokalemia, hypomagnesemia, hypophosphatemia may occur.

Nursing Implications: Monitor serum calcium closely. Assess for signs/symptoms of hypocalcemia (muscle twitching, spasm tetany, seizures) and hypercalcemia (bone pain, nausea, vomiting, polyuria, polydipsia, constipation, bradycardia, lethargy, muscle weakness, psychosis). Notify physician, recheck serum calcium immediately, and institute corrective measures as ordered. Monitor serum potassium, magnesium, phosphate levels and notify physician of abnormalities.

III. ALTERATIONS IN COMFORT related to LOCAL VEIN IRRITATION

Defining Characteristics: Transient fever (1°C or 3°F elevation) may occur 24–48 hours after drug administration (27% of patients), local reactions (pain, irritation, phlebitis) are common with 90-mg dose.

Nursing Implications: Assess baseline temperature, and monitor during and after infusion. Administer antipyretics as ordered. Assess IV site and restart new IV as needed for 90-mg dose in large vein where drug can be rapidly diluted. Apply warm packs as needed to site.

IV. ALTERATIONS IN FLUID BALANCE related to AGGRESSIVE HYDRATION

Defining Characteristics: Patients receive aggressive saline hydration to ensure urinary output of 2 L/day. Hypertension may occur. Patients with history of heart disease or renal insufficiency are at risk for fluid overload.

Nursing Implications: Assess baseline hydration status, total body fluid balance; monitor q4h. Discuss with physician need for diuretics once hydrated to keep body fluid balance equal (I = O). Monitor vital signs q4h during hydration, and notify physician of changes.

Drug: zoledronic acid (Zometa)

Class: Third-generation bisphosphonate.

Mechanism of Action: Inhibits bone resorption. Inhibits tumor related osteoclast activity in bone (bone breakdown) and may also block dissolution of minerals (hydroxyapatite) in bone, thus preventing calcium release from bone. Does not inhibit bone formation or bone mineralization. Drug is very rapidly taken up in the bone, but very slowly released. Drug appears to inhibit endothelial cell proliferation and to inhibit the beta fibroblast growth factor (βFGF)-mediated angiogenesis.

Metabolism: Drug is primarily eliminated intact via the kidney. Long terminal half life in plasma of 167 hours. Rapid injection results in 30% increase in serum drug concentration and renal damage.

Dosage/Range:
4 mg (maximum dose)

Drug Preparation/Administration:
- Drug is available in 4-mg vials. Reconstitute drug by adding 5 mL sterile water for injection, USP.
- Further dilute in 100 ml 5% dextrose injection, USP or 0.9% Sodium Chloride Injection, USP.
- Administer IV over *at least* 15 minutes.
- Assure that patient has been adequately rehydrated prior to drug administration, and the BUN and creatinine are WNL.
- Patients who require retreatment and who have had altered renal status after receiving the drug (manufacturer's recommendations):
- Normal serum creatinine prior to receiving drug, but have an increase of 0.5 mg/dL within 2 weeks of their next dose: hold drug until serum creatinine is at least within 10% of their baseline value.
- Abnormal serum creatinine prior to receiving drug: but have an increase of 1.0 mg/dL within 2 weeks of next dose, drug should be held until serum creatinine is at least within 10% of their baseline value.

Drug Interactions:
- Incompatible with calcium-containing fluids, such as Lactated Ringer's.
- Use cautiously together with aminoglycoside antibiotics, as there may be an additive effect resulting in hypocalcemia for prolonged periods.
- Use cautiously together with loop diuretics as the risk of hypocalcemia may be increased.

Lab Effects/Interference:
- Hypocalcemia.
- Hypophosphatemia.
- Hypomagnesemia.
- Increased BUN and serum creatinine.

Special Considerations:
- Indicated for the treatment of hypercalcemia of malignancy. Indicated for the treatment of patients with multiple myeloma and patients with documented bone metastases from solid tumors, in conjunction with standard antineoplastic therapy. Indicated for patients with prostate cancer who have progressed after treatment with at least one hormonal therapy.
- Serum creatinine must be monitored prior to each treatment, and abnormal values discussed with physician, as risk must be weighed against benefit.
- As compared to pamidronate in the management of hypercalcemia of malignancy, Zometa had a 45.3% response rate by day 4, and an 82.6% response rate by day 7, as compared to a 33.3% response rate and a 63.6% response rate, respectively, when pamidronate was given. Time to relapse was 30 days with Zometa, and 17 days with pamidronate (package insert for Zometa, Novartis, 2001).

- Use drug cautiously in patients who have aspirin-sensitive asthma, as well as in elder patients.
- Use drug in pregnant or nursing women only if benefit outweighs risk.

Potential Toxicities/Skin Effects and the Nursing Process

I. ALTERATION IN COMFORT, related to FEVER, NAUSEA AND VOMITING, INSOMNIA, AND FLU-LIKE SYMPTOMS

Defining Characteristics: Fever occurred in 44% of patients during clinical trials. Flu-like symptoms of chills, bone pain, and/or arthralgias and myalgias may occur less commonly. Nausea occurred in 29% of patients, and vomiting 14%. Insomnia affects 15%.

Nursing Implications: Assess baseline comfort and temperature. Teach patient that these side effects may occur and to report them. Administer or teach patient self-administration of acetaminophen or over-the-counter NSAIDs as appropriate to manage fever, arthralgias myalgias, if they occur. Teach patient to report if symptoms do not resolve. Administer antiemetics as ordered to minimize nausea and vomiting.

II. ALTERATION IN BOWEL ELIMINATION PATTERN related to CONSTIPATION, DIARRHEA, ABDOMINAL PAIN, AND ANOREXIA

Defining Characteristics: Diarrhea affected 17% of patients in clinical trials, while 27% developed constipation. 16% of patients developed abdominal pain, and 9% anorexia.

Nursing Implications: Assess baseline bowel elimination status, and teach patient to report alterations. Teach patient to use diet modifications depending upon changes, and over-the-counter antidiarrheals or laxatives as necessary. Teach patient to report persistent diarrhea or constipation (lasting more than 24 hours), presence of blood, abdominal cramping, or pain.

III. ALTERATION IN ACTIVITY TOLERANCE related to ANEMIA, FATIGUE

Defining Characteristics: Anemia occurred in 22% of patients during clinical trials.

Nursing Implications: Assess baseline hemoglobin and hematocrit. Teach patient to report fatigue, and discuss strategies to conserve energy, such as alternating rest and activity. Discuss with physician transfusion if symptoms are severe.

IV. ALTERATION IN FLUID AND ELECTROLYTE BALANCE related to CHANGES IN RENAL EXCRETION

Defining Characteristics: Drug will cause renal dysfunction with rise in serum creatinine if drug is given rapidly or in less than 15 minutes. Hypophosphatemia occurred in 13% of patients during clinical trials, hypokalemia in 12%, and hypomagnesemia in 10%.

Nursing Implications: Assess baseline renal function and electrolytes prior to initial therapy, post therapy, and prior to any additional therapy as needed. Hold drug if renal abnormalities do not correct, as indicated in administration section.

Chapter 11
Infection

Patients with cancer are susceptible to infection because chemotherapy, radiation therapy, or the malignancy itself results in immunosuppression. Risk for infection results from damage to the bone marrow stem cells that form blood cell elements. Leukocytes, or white blood cells (WBCs), are composed of five different cell types; they are further divided into cells that contain granules in their cytoplasm (granulocytes) and those that do not. Granulocytes include the neutrophils, basophils, and eosinophils. Neutrophils fight infection against invading micro-organisms by migrating to the site of infection. See Figure 11.1 for maturation of the formed blood cell elements. The absolute neutrophil count [ANC], the number of neutrophils in the body, determines the risk for infection. This calculation is shown in Table 11.1.

The risk of infection increases as the number of neutrophils decreases, as shown in Table 11.2. The longer the duration of neutropenia, the greater the risk for infection. Infection and fever in a neutropenic patient represent a medical emergency, and, if untreated, can result in sepsis and death within 48 hours. Initial therapy with third-generation cephalosporins containing a β-lactam ring (i.e., ceftazidime) or combination therapy with broadspectrum antibiotics should be instituted immediately. Fortunately, the use of colony stimulating factor (CSFs), such as granulocyte-colony stimulating factor (G-CSF) and granulocyte-macrophage colony stimulating factor (GM-CSF), has helped to reduce the incidence of febrile neutropenia.

Gram-negative bacilli are responsible for a high incidence of life-threatening infections (*Escherichia coli*, *Klebsiella* spp., *Proteus* spp., and *Pseudomonas aeruginosa*). However, gram-positive organisms such as *Staphylococcus epidermidis* and streptococci have become more prominent, probably due to a decrease in gram-negative sepsis resulting from prompt empiric antimicrobial therapy against gram-negative organisms, as well as the wide use of central venous access lines that become infected by gram-positive organisms.

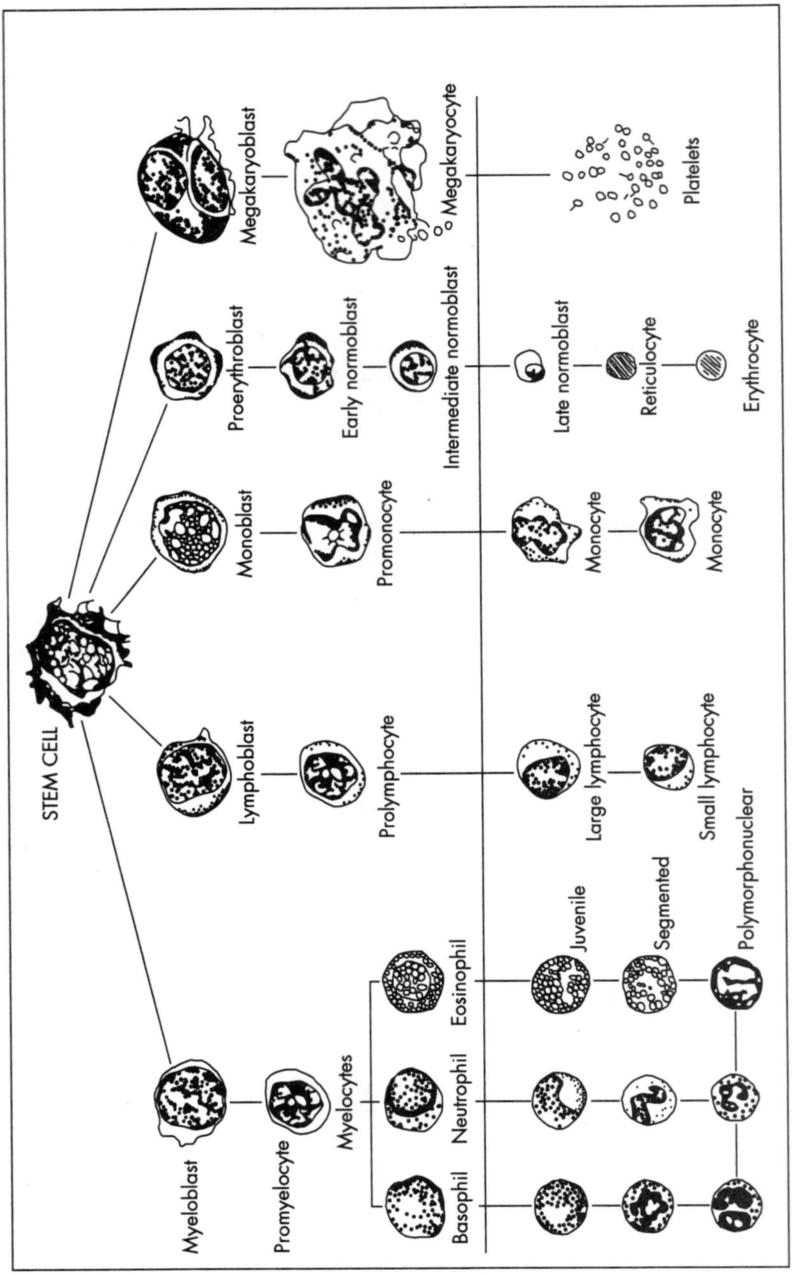

Figure 11.1 The development of formed blood cell elements

Table 11.1 Calculation of Absolute Neutrophil Count (ANC)

Patient Example	Normal Values
1. Lab results: total white blood count (WBC) = 4000/mm^3	5000–10,000/mm^3
neutrophils = 40	50–70%
lymphocytes = 50	20–40%
monocytes = 6	2–6%
eosinophils = 1	0.5–1%
bands = 2	
2. Total WBC × % (neutrophils + bands)	2500–7000/mm^3
4000 × % (40 + 2) =	
4000 × 42/100 =	
4000 × 0.42 = 1680/mm^3	
3. Assessment: low but no significant risk	

Table 11.2 Relative Risk of Infection

Risk	Number/Neutrophils
No significant risk	> 1500–2000/mm^3
Minimal risk	1000–1500/mm^3
Moderate risk	500–1000/mm^3
Severe risk	< 500/mm^3

Disease-related immunosuppression is related to defects in the cell-mediated immunity (thymus-dependent lymphocytes), such as with certain lymphomas. This leads to an increased risk for bacterial infections (*Mycobacterium, Nocardia asteroides, Legionella, Salmonella*), as well as infections caused by fungi (*Cryptococcus, Histoplasma, Candida, Aspergillus*), parasites (*Pneumocystis carinii* pneumonia, *Toxoplasma gondii*), and viruses (varicella zoster, cytomegalovirus). Other malignancies may have defects in the humoral immune system (B lymphocytes), as in multiple myeloma and chronic lymphocytic leukemia (CLL). Patients with these malignancies are at risk for infection from bacteria (*Streptococcus pneumoniae, Haemophilus influenzae, Neisseria meningitidis, Klebsiella pneumoniae, Staphylococcus aureus*) and certain enteroviruses.

Another antibiotic-related concern is the emergence of antibiotic resistance, such as vancomycin-resistant enterococci (VRE) and methacillin-resistant *Staphylococcus aureus* (MRSA). Since 1989, US hospitals report a rapid increase in the incidence of infection and colonization with vancomycin-resistant enterococci (VRE). This increase poses important problems, including (a) the lack of available antimicrobial therapy for VRE infections, since most VRE infections are also resistant to drugs previously used to treat these infections (e.g., aminoglycosides and ampicillin), and (b) the possibility that the vancomycin-resistant genes present in VRE can be transferred to other gram-positive microorganisms (e.g., *Staphylococcus aureus*).

The increased risk for VRE infection and colonization is associated with previous vancomycin and/or multiantimicrobial therapy, severe underlying disease or immunosuppression, and intraabdominal surgery. Because enterococci are found in the normal gastrointestinal and female genital tracts, most enterococcal infections are attributed to endogenous sources within the patient. Whenever possible, empiric antimicrobial therapy should be modified based on culture and sensitivity results so that the most specific therapy is administered.

The Food and Drug Administration (FDA) has approved tigecycline, the first of a new class of agents called glycylcyclines. The drug is indicated for the treatment of complicated intra-abdominal infections and complicated skin and skin structure infections in adults. Approval of this first-in-class agent is opportune as the need for new antimicrobial options is increasing.

Antimicrobial medications are intended to kill or to inhibit the growth of the organism without harming the patient. Antimicrobial agents may be bacteriostatic (inhibit growth of organisms) or bactericidal (kill microorganisms). Drug activity varies, so that at low concentrations a drug may be bacteriostatic, but bactericidal at higher concentrations. Usually antimicrobial drugs target some difference between the microorganism and the host. Overall, antibiotics are prescribed based on patient factors—the condition of the renal and hepatic systems, as well as drug allergies, the spectrum of antibiotic activity, and the site of infection.

This section focuses on antimicrobial medications used to treat infections in patients with cancer: antibacterial, antiviral, and antifungal. These drugs target specific cellular mechanisms of the infectious agent. For example, sulfonamide antibiotics inhibit para-aminobenzoic acid, an essential requirement for nucleic acid synthesis in many bacteria but not in humans. Penicillins and the cephalosporins contain a β-lactam ring that disrupts the synthesis of peptidoglycan. Peptidoglycan gives shape and strength to the bacterial cell wall. Table 11.3 provides an overview of one of the oldest (penicillins/cephalosporins) as well as the newest groups of antibacterials (streptogramins/oxazolidinones).

Table 11.3 Comparison of Antibiotic Categories

Antibacterial Category	Examples	Mechanism of Action, Including Differences Among or Between Categories or Unique Characteristics
Penicillins		Penicillins are derived from the fungus *Penicillium* and contain a β-lactam ring.
Natural penicillins	• penicillin V • penicillin G	The first group comprises natural penicillins, which are active against many aerobic Gram-positive cocci (*S. aureus, Streptococcus*), Gram-negative aerobic cocci (*N. meningitidis,* some *H. influenzae*), and some spirochetes. However, they are resistant to *Pseudomonas,* most *Enterobacter,* and to bacteria that produce the enzyme penicillinase, which inactivates the penicillin molecule.
Penicillinase-resistant penicillins	• cloxacillin • dicloxacillin • nafcillin • oxacillin	The second group contains the penicillinase-resistant penicillins. These are semisynthetic drugs that can withstand the action of the enzyme penicillinase and continue to exert their antibiotic action. They are primarily used to treat *S. aureus* and *S. epidermidis* strains that secrete penicillinase; they also have some activity against Gram-negative bacteria and spirochetes.
Aminopenicillins	• amoxicillin • ampicillin • bacampicillin	The third group includes the aminopenicillins; this group has heightened activity against Gram-negative bacteria as compared to the first two groups. These drugs are resistant to penicillinase-producing bacteria.
Extended-spectrum penicillins	• carbenicillin • mezlocillin • piperacillin • ticarcillin	The fourth group is composed of the extended-spectrum penicillins; drugs in this group have enhanced activity against gram-negative bacilli, both aerobic and nonaerobic.

(continued)

Table 11.3 *(continued)*

Antibacterial Category	Examples	Mechanism of Action, Including Differences Among or Between Categories or Unique Characteristics
Cephalosporins		The cephalosporins are derived from cephalosporin C (produced by a fungus) and have broad bactericidal activity. They contain a β-lactam ring and may also be referred to as β-lactam antibiotics. Bacterial resistance can develop, and a major mechanism is the development by the bacteria of an enzyme, β-lactamase, which inactivates the cephalosporin antibiotic by destroying the β-lactam ring.
First generation	• cefadroxil • cefalothin • cefazolin • cephalexin • cephapirin • cephradine	First-generation cephalosporins are active against Gram-positive cocci (*Staphylococcus* and *Streptococcus*) and have only limited activity against Gram-negative bacteria (e.g., *E. coli*); they have no activity against enterococci.
Second generation	• cefaclor • cefamandole • cefmetazole • cefonicid • ceforanide • cefotetan • cefoxitin • cefprozil • cefuroxime • cefuroxime • axetil	Second-generation cephalosporins are active against the same organisms as the first-generation drugs but are slightly more active against Gram-negative bacteria. In addition, they are active against *H. influenzae*

(continued).

Table 11.3 *(continued)*

Antibacterial Category	Examples	Mechanism of Action, Including Differences Among or Between Categories or Unique Characteristics
Third generation	• cefdinir • cefixime • cefoperazone • cefotaxime • cefpodoxime • ceftazidime • ceftibuten • ceftizoxime • ceftriaxone • loracarbef	Third-generation cephalosporins are less active against gram-positive organisms but have broader activity against Gram-negative organisms than either first- or second-generation drugs.
Fourth generation	• cefepime	Fourth-generation cephalosporins are projected to have many attributes including: • Extended spectrum of activity for Gram-negative and Gram-positive organisms (different from third-generation cephalosporins) • Minimal β-lactamase activity due to rapid periplasmic penetration and high penicillin-binding protein (PBP) access • Spectrum of activity to include Gram-negative organisms with multiple drug resistance patterns (*Enterobacter* and *Klebsiella*)

(continued)

Table 11.3 *(continued)*

Antibacterial Category	Examples	Mechanism of Action, Including Differences Among or Between Categories or Unique Characteristics
Streptogramins	• quinupristin/ dalfopristin	This new class of antibiotics, the streptogramin group, is a separate family of antimicrobials. Synercid is an intravenous combination of two semisynthetic, water-soluble derivatives of naturally occurring pristinamycin. The two distinct compounds are quinupristin and dalfopristin, derived from pristinamycin I and pristinamycin II. These two compounds work synergistically to kill susceptible bacteria through a two-pronged attack on protein synthesis in bacterial cells. Each component of the drug binds irreversibly to different sites on the bacterial cell's ribosomal subunit to form a stable quinupristin-ribosome-dalfopristin complex, which disables the cell's ability to make cellular protein. Without the ability to manufacture new proteins, the bacterial cell dies.
Oxazolidinones	• linezolid	Inhibits initiation of protein synthesis by binding to a site on bacterial 23S ribosomal RNA of the 50S subunit. This mechanism of inhibiting protein synthesis is not shared by other antibacterials. Cross-resistance is unlikely.
Macrolides	• azithromycin • clarithromycin • erythromycin	Binds to 50S ribosomal subunit resulting in inhibition of protein synthesis. In some cases the drug metabolite is twice as active as the parent compound.
Lipopeptides	• daptomycin	Derived from the fermentation of *Streptomyces roseosporus*. The mechanism of action is not fully understood. Binds to bacterial membranes and causes a rapid depolarization of membrane potential. This loss of membrane potential leads to inhibition of protein, DNA, and RNA synthesis resulting in bacterial cell death.
Ketolide	telithromycin	Similar to that of macrolides and is related to the 50S-ribosomal subunit binding with inhibition of bacterial protein synthesis. Telithromycin appears to have greater affinity for the ribosomal binding site than macrolides. It concentrates in phagocytes where it exhibits activity against intracellular respiratory pathogens.

Within the past few years, the FDA approved daptomycin and telithromycin. These new antibiotics have largely been developed by making minor modifications to an existing class of drugs. Daptomycin is the first drug in a new structural class, the cyclic lipopeptides. Its mode of action is to rapidly kill gram-positive bacteria by disrupting multiple aspects of bacterial membrane function. Telithromycin, a first-in-class antibiotic group called the ketolides, is structurally related to the macrolide antibiotics and specifically designed to offer optimal spectrum activity for the first-line treatment of upper and lower respiratory tract infections. The latest antibiotic group, the glycylcyclines, is structurally similar to the tetracyclines and tigecycline is the first agent in this class to be FDA-approved for the treatment of MRSA.

Another class of antimicrobial agents, the echinocandins or glucan synthesis inhibitors, has recently been added to the options available for treating opportunistic fungal infections. Caspofungin, the first-in-class, inhibits the synthesis of a key component of the fungal cell wall. Caspofungin demonstrates fungicidal activity against *Candida* species; it is indicated for the treatment of invasive *Aspergillus* in patients who are refractory to, or intolerant of, other therapies. Ideal candidates for this drug are patients with amphotericin B–induced nephrotoxicity. Caspofungin appears to be well tolerated.

The latest FDA-approved anti-fungal agent is micafungin. This drug inhibits the synthesis of 1,3-β-D-glucan, an essential component of fungal cell walls, which is not present in mammalian cells. It is indicated for the treatment of patients with esophageal candidiasis and as prophylaxis of *Candida* infections in patients undergoing hematopoietic stem cell transplantation.

COMPLICATIONS

References

American Thoracic Society. Guidelines for the management of adults with hospital-acquired, ventilatory-associated and health care-associated pneumonia. *Am J of Respiratory Critical Care* 2005;171:388–416171:388–416

Ampicillin sodium/sulbactam sodium. Available at http://hcunviweb05/mdxcgi/quiklocn.exe?CTL=E:/Mdx/mdxcgi/MEGAT.SYS&SET=1C573 June 2005

Antman KD, Griffin JD, Elias A, et al. Effect of Recombinant Human Granulocyte-Macrophage Colony Stimulating Factor on Chemotherapy-Induced Myelosuppression. *N Engl J Med* 1998;319(19):593–598

Aumercier M, Bouhallab S, Capmau M, et al. RP 59500: A Proposed Mechanism for Its Bactericidal Activity. *J Antimicrob Chemother* 1992;30 (Suppl A):9–14

Bodey G, Buckley M, Sathe YS, et al. Quantitative Relationship between Circulating Leukocytes and Infections in Patients with Acute Leukemia. *Ann Intern Med* 1966; 64(2):328–340

Brandt B. A Nursing Protocol for the Client with Neutropenia. *Oncol Nurs Forum* 1984;11(2):24–28

Carlson AC. Infection Prophylaxis in the Patient with Cancer. *Oncol Nurs Forum* 1985; 12(3):60

Cubicin. Product Information. Cubist Pharmaceutical Inc. September 2003

Cunningham R. Infection Prophylaxis for the Patient with Cancer. *Oncol Nurs Forum* 1990;17(1) (Suppl 1):16–19

Declomycin. Product Information. Lederle Pharmaceutical Division, American Cynamid Co. Pearl River, NY: 2003

Declomycin, Available at http://www.rxmed.com/b.main/b2.pharmaceutical/b2.1monographs/CPS-%20Monographs. Accessed June 2004

Drugs.com. Drug Information Online. Daptomycin. Available at http://www.drugs.com/MTM/daptomycin.html. Accessed June 2004

Gemifloxacin mesylate [package insert]. http://hcunviweb05/mdxcgi/quiklocn.exe?CTL=E:/Mdx/mdxcgi/MEGAT.SYS&SET=1C573. June 2005

Goh K.P., Management of hyponatremia. *AM Fam Physician* 2004;69(10):2387–2394

Hughes WT, Armstrong D, Bodey GP, et al. Guidelines for the Use of Antimicrobial Agents in Neutropenic Patients with Unexplained Fever. *J Infect Dis* 1989;161: 381–396

Ketek. Product Information.Aventis Pharmaceutical Inc. March 2004

Kucers A, Bennett N. *The Use of Antibiotics: A Comprehensive Review with Clinical Analysis,* 4th ed. Philadelphia, PA: JB Lippincott Co.; 1987

Medline. Drug Information: Daptomycin. Available at http://www.nlm.nih.gov/medline. Accessed June 2004

Meropenem [package insert]. http://hcunviweb05/mdxcgi/quiklocn.exe?CTL=E:/Mdx/mdxcgi/MEGAT.SYS&SET=1C573. June 2005

Mycamine [Package Insert]. Osaka Japan: Fujisawa Pharmaceutical Company LTD; 2005

Morstyn G, Campbell L, Souza LM, et al. Effect of Granulocyte Colony Stimulating Factor on Neutropenia Induced by CytotoxicChemotherapy. *Lancet* 1988;1:667–671

Pizzo PA, Hathorn MD, Hiemenz J, et al. A Randomized TrialComparing Ceftazidime Alone with Combination Antibiotic Therapy in Cancer Patients with Fever and Neutropenia. *N Engl J Med* 1986;315:552–558

Recommendations for Preventing the Spread of Vancomycin Resistance (Sept 22, 1994). *Recommendations of the Hospital Infection Control Practices Advisory Committee (HICPAC) MMWR (Morbidity and Mortality Weekly Report)* 44 (RR-12):1–712

Rifaximin [package insert]. http://hcunviweb05/mdxcgi/quiklocn.exe?CTL=E:/Mdx/mdxcgi/MEGAT.SYS&SET=1C573. June 2005

Rostad ME. Current Strategies for Managing Myelosuppression in Patients with Cancer. *Oncol Nurs Forum* 1991;18(2):7–15

Telithromycin. Thompson Center Watch. Clinical Trials Listing Service. Drugs approved by the FDA. Available at http://www.mcromedex.com/products/updates/drugdex_updates/de/tilithromycinfull.html. Accessed June 2004

Telithromycin. Available at http://www.centerwatch.com/patient/drugs/dru853.html. Accessed June 2004

Tygacil [package insert]. Philadelphia, PA: Wyeth Pharmaceuticals, Inc.; 2005.

United States Pharmacopoeia Drug Information for Health Care Professionals. Rockville, MD: 18th ed.
The United States Pharmacopoeia Convention, Inc.; 1998
VHA Pharmacy Benefits Management Strategic Healthcare Group and Medical Advisor Panel. Daptomycin.
Warner-Lambert Co. Omnicef Package Insert. Morris Plains, NJ: Parke-Davis; 1998
Wujik D. Infection. Groenwald SL, Frogge MH, Goodman M, Yarbro CH, (eds), *Cancer Symptom Management.* Sudbury, MA: Jones and Bartlett; 1996;289–308

ANTIBIOTICS

Drug: amikacin sulfate (Amikin)

Class: Aminoglycoside antibacterial antibiotic.

Mechanism of Action: Synthetic antibiotic derived from kanamycin; bactericidal, most probably by inhibition of protein synthesis. Active against aerobic microorganisms: many sensitive gram-negative organisms (including *Acinetobacter, Citrobacter, Enterobacter, E. coli, Klebsiella, Proteus, Pseudomonas, Salmonella, Serratia*, and *Shigella*), and some sensitive gram-positive organisms (*S. aureus* and *S. epidermidis*). Over time, bacterial resistance may develop, either naturally or acquired.

Metabolism: Well absorbed following parenteral administration, but variability in absorption after IM injection (peak serum level 0.5–2 hours, duration 8–12 hours). Widely distributed into body fluids. Minimally protein-bound. Readily crosses placenta and into breast milk. Drug excreted unchanged in the urine.

Dosage/Range:
- 15 mg/kg/day given in 8-hour or 12-hour doses IV or IM.
- Desired peak serum concentration is 15–30 μg/mL, and trough serum concentration is 5–10 μg/mL. DOSE-REDUCE IF RENAL IMPAIRMENT.

Drug Preparation:
- Store injectable at < 40°C (104°F).
- Potency not affected by pale yellow color that may develop.
- Stable for 24 hours at concentrations of 0.25 and 5 mg/mL in 0.9% Sodium Chloride, 5% Dextrose.

Drug Administration:
- IV: in 100–200 mL IV fluid (e.g., 0.9% Sodium Chloride or 5% Dextrose injection), infused over 30–60 minutes.

Drug Interactions:

- Increased risk of toxicity with other ototoxic drugs: acyclovir, other aminoglycosides, amphotericin B, bacitracin, cephalosporins, colistin, cisplatin, ethacrynic acid, furosemide, vancomycin.
- Potentiation of neuromuscular blockade when given concurrently with general anesthetics (succinylcholine, tubocurarine) — use cautiously; observe for signs/symptoms of respiratory depression.
- Synergism with extended-spectrum penicillins, but must be administered separately.

Lab Effects/Interference:

- Serum ALT, serum alk phos, serum AST, serum bili, and serum LDH values all may be increased.
- BUN and serum creatinine values may be increased.
- Serum Ca+, serum Mg+, serum K+, and serum Na+ concentrations may be decreased.

Special Considerations:

- Used as first-line treatment in short-term treatment of serious gram-negative infections (e.g., septicemia, respiratory tract infections).
- Use against gram-positive organisms only as second-line treatment.
- Use in pregnancy only if infection is life-threatening and no safer drug exists; drug crosses placenta and may cause fetal toxicity.

Potential Toxicities/Side Effects and the Nursing Process

I. ALTERATIONS IN SENSORY/PERCEPTUAL PATTERNS related to OTOTOXICITY

Defining Characteristics: Damage to eighth cranial nerve (auditory) may result in dizziness, nystagmus, vertigo, ataxia (vestibular damage) and less commonly, tinnitus, roaring sound in ears, and impaired hearing (auditory damage). Hearing loss usually begins with high-frequency loss, followed by clinical hearing loss, then permanent hearing loss if damage continues. Increased risk in elderly or renally impaired patients.

Nursing Implications: Assess baseline hearing (ability to hear spoken voice) and continue during therapy. Teach patient potential side effects, and instruct patient to report any hearing/perceptual problems (e.g., tinnitus, vertigo, decreased hearing). Discuss drug discontinuance and audiogram with physician to confirm hearing dysfunction if symptoms arise. Assess for increased risk if given concurrently with other ototoxic medications (e.g., cisplatin, furosemide).

II. ALTERATION IN URINARY ELIMINATION related to NEPHROTOXICITY

Defining Characteristics: Renal damage characterized by tubular necrosis with increased serum BUN, creatinine; decreased urine creatinine clearance and specific gravity; proteinuria and casts in urine. Azotemia usually not associated with oliguria. Rarely, electrolyte wasting with hypomagnesemia, hypocalcemia, and hypokalemia may occur. Renal dysfunction usually reversible after drug discontinuance. Increased risk in elderly and in patients with preexisting renal dysfunction. Risk is low in well-hydrated patients with normal renal function when normal doses given.

Nursing Implications: Assess baseline renal function and electrolytes, and monitor periodically during therapy. Discuss any abnormalities with physician, as drug should be dose-reduced or discontinued if renal dysfunction develops. Assess baseline total body fluid balance, weight, and monitor periodically during antibiotic therapy. Monitor hydration status to keep patient well hydrated. Assess drug peak and trough levels as ordered so that drug dosage is correctly titrated. Increased risk of toxicity if peak serum concentration > 30–35 μg/mL. Draw blood for peak drug concentration 30 minutes after end of 30-minute infusion or at the end of a 60-minute infusion; draw trough immediately before next dose.

III. ALTERATIONS IN SENSORY/PERCEPTUAL PATTERNS related to CNS EFFECTS, NEUROMUSCULAR BLOCKADE

Defining Characteristics: Headache, tremor, lethargy may occur. Peripheral neuropathy or encephalopathy (numbness, skin tingling, muscle twitching) may occur rarely. Neuromuscular blockade is dose related, self-limiting, and uncommon: risk is greater with topical application or when drug is administered to patient with neuromuscular disease (myasthenia gravis) or hypocalcemia.

Nursing Implications: Assess baseline neurologic status. Assess coexisting risk factors, neuroblockade medications. Teach patient about side effects, and instruct to report headache, tremor, lethargy. Observe for respiratory depression. If signs/symptoms arise, discuss drug discontinuance with physician.

IV. POTENTIAL FOR INJURY related to HYPERSENSITIVITY

Defining Characteristics: Rash, urticaria, pruritus, fever, and eosinophilia have occurred rarely. CROSS-SENSITIVITY between AMINOGLYCOSIDES exists!

Nursing Implications: Assess for drug allergies to any aminoglycoside—amikacin, gentamycin, kanamycin, neomycin, netilmicin, streptomycin, tobramycin—prior to drug administration. Instruct patient to report any allergic reactions. Assess for signs/symptoms of allergic reaction after drug dose.

V. ALTERATION IN NUTRITION, LESS THAN BODY REQUIREMENTS, related to GI SIDE EFFECTS

Defining Characteristics: Nausea, vomiting, anorexia have occurred rarely. Also, transient hepatomegaly with elevated LFTs—AST, ALT, LDH, alk phos—has occurred.

Nursing Implications: Assess baseline nutritional status, preexisting nausea/vomiting, anorexia. Assess baseline LFTs and monitor periodically during treatment. Instruct patient to report side effects. Provide symptomatic interventions if side effects occur; discuss with physician use of alternative drug(s).

VI. POTENTIAL FOR FATIGUE, INFECTION, AND BLEEDING related to BONE MARROW INJURY

Defining Characteristics: Anemia, leukopenia, granulocytopenia, and thrombocytopenia may occur. Also, patients receiving antibiotics are at risk for overgrowth of nonsusceptible microorganisms, such as fungi (superinfection). Rare.

Nursing Implications: Assess baseline CBC, differential, and monitor periodically during treatment. Instruct patient to report signs/symptoms of fatigue, infection, or bleeding immediately. Assess for signs/symptoms of superinfection. Discuss any adverse effects with physician.

Drug: amoxicillin (Amoxil, Polymox, Trimox, Wymox; amoxicillin plus potassium clavulanate is Augmentin)

Class: Penicillin (aminopenicillin antibiotic); β-lactam.

Mechanism of Action: Semisynthetic antibiotic prepared from fungus *Penicillium.* Contains β-lactam ring and is bactericidal by inhibiting cell wall synthesis. Aminopenicillins have increased activity against gram-negative bacilli (*H. influenzae, E. coli*), as well as some activity against gram-positive bacilli (*Streptococci* and *Staphylococci*). Used for treatment of infections of upper and lower respiratory tract, genitourinary (GU) tract, and skin by sensitive organisms.

Metabolism: Well absorbed from GI tract; rate of absorption slowed by food but total amount of drug absorbed remains unchanged. Widely distributed in body tissues and fluids. Crosses placenta and is found in breast milk. Excreted in urine and bile.

Dosage/Range:

Adult:

- 125–500 mg PO q8h 48–72 hours after infection eradicated; for uncomplicated urinary tract infection, may use single dose of 3 gm PO.
- Drug dose should be reduced if severe renal failure occurs.
- Augmentin dose: mild to moderate infection: 500 mg PO 2 × /day; severe infection: 875 mg PO 2 × /day

Drug Preparation/Administration:

- Store capsules in tight container at 15–30°C (59–86°F).
- Administer on empty stomach.

Drug Interactions:

- Aminoglycosides: synergism.
- Aminoglycosides (e.g., gentamicin): incompatible when mixed together; administer at separate sites at different times. Also, penicillinase-resistant penicillins can inactivate aminoglycoside serum samples from patients receiving both drugs.
- Rifampin: possible antagonism, only at high doses of penicillin.
- Probenecid: increased serum level of penicillin; may be co-administered to exert this effect.
- Allopurinol: increased incidence of rash; avoid concurrent administration if possible.
- Clavulanic acid (β-lactamase inhibitor): synergistic bactericidal effect. Amoxicillin plus potassium clavulanate = Augmentin.

Lab Effects/Interference:

Major clinical significance:

- Urine glucose: high urinary concentrations of a penicillin may produce false-positive or falsely elevated test results with copper-reduction tests (Benedict's, Clinitest, or Fehling's); glucose enzymatic tests (Clinistix or Testape) are not affected.

Clinical significance:

- Coombs' tests: false-positive result may occur during therapy with any penicillin.
- ALT, alk phos, AST, serum bili, and serum LDH values may be increased.
- Estradiol, total conjugated estriol, estriol-glucuronide, or conjugated estrone concentrations may be transiently decreased in pregnant women following administration of amoxicillin.
- WBC: leukopenia or neutropenia is associated with the use of all penicillins; the effect is more likely to occur with prolonged and severe hepatic function impairment.

Special Considerations:

- Contraindicated in patients with prior hypersensitivity to penicillins. Use with caution in patients sensitive to other β-lactams (e.g., cephalosporins) since partial cross-allergenicity exists.
- Obtain ordered specimen and send for culture and sensitivity prior to first antibiotic dose.
- Consider alternative antibiotic therapy if eosinophilia, drug fever or rash, arthralgia, hematuria, or unexplained rise in BUN and serum creatinine occur.
- Monitor electrolytes and renal, hepatic, and hematologic laboratory parameters during extended treatment periods.
- Use with caution in pregnancy or with nursing women.
- Amoxicillin rash may occur that is distinct from drug-allergic rash; increased risk if concurrent use of allopurinol.
- Less diarrhea as a GI side effect than ampicillin.
- May cause false-positive with Clinitest glucose testing.

Potential Toxicities/Side Effects and the Nursing Process

I. POTENTIAL FOR INJURY related to HYPERSENSITIVITY REACTION

Defining Characteristics: Urticaria, pruritus, rash (maculopapular or erythematous), fever and chills, eosinophilia, myalgia, edema, erythema, angioedema, Stevens-Johnson syndrome, and exfoliative skin reactions occur in 5% of patients. Increased risk in individuals allergic to cephalosporin antibiotics. A nonimmunologic rash may occur 3–14 days after drug started, characterized as a generalized erythematous/maculopapular rash, and worse over pressure areas of elbows and knees. Rash usually subsides in 6–14 days, even if drug is continued. If drug is stopped, resolves in 1–7 days.

Nursing Implications: Assess allergy to cephalosporin antibiotics and penicillin: if patient states "yes," determine actual response, e.g., "swollen lips = angioedema." If angioedema, patient SHOULD NOT receive drug. Discuss other patient responses with physician to determine whether drug should be given. Assess baseline skin condition, including integrity and allergy history to drugs. Instruct patient to report rash, itching, other skin changes. Teach patient skin care and symptomatic measures as appropriate. If skin rash develops, discuss drug discontinuance with physician. If rash progresses, drug should be discontinued, as fatal Stevens-Johnson syndrome may develop. Be prepared to treat severe acute hypersensitivity reactions with airway management, oxygen, epinephrine, corticosteroids, antihistamines as ordered.

II. ALTERATION IN NUTRITION, LESS THAN BODY REQUIREMENTS, related to GI SIDE EFFECTS

Defining Characteristics: Nausea, vomiting, diarrhea, anorexia may occur; rarely, pseudomembranous colitis caused by *Clostridium difficile* resistant to the antibiotic occurs. Rarely, transient increases in LFTs—AST, ALT, alk phos, bili—may occur.

Nursing Implications: Assess baseline nutritional status. Instruct patient to report GI disturbances. Administer and instruct patient to self-administer antiemetics as needed and as ordered. Teach patient importance of nutritious diet, and suggest small, frequent, high-calorie, high-protein meals as appropriate. Assess baseline LFTs and monitor periodically during treatment. Discuss abnormalities and drug interruption with physician.

III. FUNGAL SUPERINFECTION related to OVERGROWTH of ENDOGENOUS MICROORGANISMS

Defining Characteristics: Vaginal candidiasis, vaginitis may occur as endogenous bacteria are eliminated, and normal fungal population expands.

Nursing Implications: Teach female patient to report vaginal itching or discharge. Discuss appropriate antifungal treatment with physician. Teach perineal hygiene and symptomatic management.

IV. ALTERATIONS IN PROTECTIVE MECHANISMS (RARE) related to TRANSIENT LEUKOPENIA

Defining Characteristics: Rarely, transient leukopenia, lymphocytosis, anemia, eosinophilia may occur. Prolonged PT, prolonged activated partial thromboplastin time (APTT), and hypoprothrombinemia have occurred rarely, especially in elderly or debilitated patients, or in individuals with vitamin K deficiency.

Nursing Implications: Assess baseline laboratory parameters, and monitor periodically during treatment. Assess patient for response to antibiotics. Discuss abnormalities with physician.

V. KNOWLEDGE DEFICIT related to SELF-ADMINISTRATION OF MEDICATION

Defining Characteristics: Increased compliance when patient is instructed in self-care activities.

Nursing Implications: Assess knowledge regarding infection and planned treatment. Teach drug action, potential side effects, and when and how to take drug (take medication as directed, 1 hour before or 2 hours after food). Instruct patient to report any possible drug side effects that occur.

Drug: ampicillin sodium/sulbactam sodium (UNASYN)

Class: Penicillin (aminopenicillin antibiotic).

Mechanism of Action: Semisynthetic antibiotic prepared from fungus *Penicillium.* Contains β-lactam ring and is bactericidal by inhibiting cell wall synthesis. Aminopenicillins have increased activity against gram-negative bacilli *(H. influenzae, E. coli),* as well as some activity against gram-positive bacilli *(Streptococci* and *Staphylococci).* Although sulbactam alone possesses little useful antibacterial activity, whole organism studies have shown that sulbactam restores ampicillin activity against beta-lactamase producing strains of bacteria. Used for treatment of infections of the skin, intra-abdominal infections, and gynecologic infections by sensitive organisms. In combination with sulbactam there is irreversible inhibition of beta lactamases, thus making ampicillin effective against beta lactamase bacteria that would otherwise be resistant to it.

Metabolism: Metabolism: Well absorbed from GI tract, but rate and amount of drug absorbed is decreased with food. Widely distributed in body tissues and fluids. Crosses placenta and is found in breast milk. Excreted in urine and bile.

Dosage/Range:

Adult:

- Dose modification necessary if renal impairment occurs. See manufacturer's package insert.
- UNASYN: 1.5–3 grams ampicillin and 0.5–1 gram sulbactam IV/IM every 6 hours (dose not to exceed 4 g sulbactam a day).

Drug Preparation/Administration:

- IV dilute with Normal Saline only, give over 10–30 minutes.
- IM: reconstitute per manufacturer's directions and use within 1 hour after reconstitution.

Drug Interactions:

- Aminoglycosides: synergism.
- Aminoglycosides (e.g., gentamicin): incompatible when mixed together; administer at separate sites at different times. Also, penicillinase-resistant penicillins can inactivate aminoglycoside serum samples from patients receiving both drugs.
- Rifampin: possible antagonism, only at high doses of ampicillin.
- Probenecid: decreases renal tubular secretion of ampicillin and sulbactam.
- Oral contraceptives: may decrease efficacy of contraceptive and increase incidence of breakthrough bleeding. Suggest additional use of barrier contraception.

- Sulbactam: broadens antibacterial coverage of ampicillin against resistant beta lactamase-producing microorganisms.
- Concurrent administration of allopurinal and ampicillin increases the incidence of rashes.

Lab Effects/Interference:

- Urine glucose: high urinary concentrations of a penicillin may produce false-positive or falsely elevated test results with copper-reduction tests (Benedict's Clinitest, or Fehling's); glucose enzymatic tests (Clinistix or Testape) are not affected
- Estradiol, total conjugated estriol, estriol-glucuronide or conjugated estrone concentrations may be transiently decreased in pregnant women following administration of ampicillin.
- Increased AST (SGOT), ALT (SGPT), alkaline phosphatase, and LDH.
- Decreased serum albumin and total protein.
- WBC: leukopenia or neutropenia is associated with the use of all penicillins; the effect is more likely to occur with prolonged and severe hepatic function impairment.
- BUN and serum creatinine: increased concentrations have been associated with ampicillin.

Special Considerations:

- Contraindicated in patients with prior hypersensitivity to penicillins. Use with caution in patients sensitive to other β-lactams (e.g., cephalosporins) since partial cross-allergenicity exists.
- Obtain ordered specimen and send for culture and sensitivity prior to first antibiotic dose.
- Consider alternative antibiotic therapy if eosinophilia, drug fever or rash, arthralgia, hematuria, or unexplained rise in BUN and serum creatinine occur.
- Monitor electrolytes and renal, hepatic, and hematologic laboratory parameters during extended treatment periods.
- Use with caution in pregnancy or with nursing women.
- Renal dysfunction: Unasyn dose must be reduced.

Potential Toxicities/Side Effects and the Nursing Process

I. POTENTIAL FOR INJURY related to HYPERSENSITIVITY REACTION and LOCAL REACTIONS (pain at injection site & thrombophlebitis)

Defining Characteristics: Urticaria, pruritus, rash (maculopapular or erythematous), fever and chills, eosinophilia, myalgia, edema, erythema, angioedema, Stevens-Johnson syndrome, and exfoliative skin reactions occur in 5% of patients. Increased risk in individuals allergic to cephalosporin antibiotics.

Nursing Implications: Assess allergy to cephalosporin antibiotics and penicillin: if patient states "yes," determine actual response, e.g., "swollen lips = angioedema." If angioedema, patient SHOULD NOT receive drug. Discuss other patient responses with physician to determine whether drug should be given. Assess baseline skin condition, including integrity and allergy history to drugs. Instruct patient to report rash, itching, other skin changes. Teach patient skin care and symptomatic measures as appropriate. If skin rash develops, discuss drug discontinuance with physician. If rash progresses, drug should be discontinued, as fatal Stevens-Johnson syndrome may develop. Be prepared to treat severe acute hypersensitivity reactions with airway management, oxygen, epinephrine, corticosteroids, antihistamines as ordered.

II. ALTERATION IN NUTRITION, LESS THAN BODY REQUIREMENTS, related to GI SIDE EFFECTS

Defining Characteristics: Nausea, vomiting, diarrhea may occur; rarely, pseudomembranous colitis caused by *C. difficile* resistant to the antibiotic occurs. Rarely, transient increases in LFTs—AST, ALT, alk phos, bili—may occur.

Nursing Implications: Assess baseline nutritional status. Instruct patient to report GI disturbances. Administer and teach patient to self-administer antiemetics as needed and as ordered. Teach patient importance of nutritious diet, and suggest small, frequent, high-calorie, high-protein meals as appropriate. Assess baseline LFTs, and monitor periodically during treatment. Discuss abnormalities and drug interruption with physician.

III. FUNGAL SUPERINFECTION related to REDISTRIBUTION OF ENDOGENOUS MICROORGANISMS

Defining Characteristics: Vaginal candidiasis, vaginitis may occur as endogenous bacteria are eliminated, and normal fungal population expands.

Nursing Implications: Instruct female patient to report vaginal itching or discharge. Discuss appropriate antifungal treatment with physician. Teach perineal hygiene and symptomatic management.

IV. KNOWLEDGE DEFICIT related to SELF-ADMINISTRATION OF MEDICATION

Defining Characteristics: Increased compliance when patient is instructed in self-care activities.

Nursing Implications: Assess knowledge regarding infection and planned treatment. Teach about drug action, potential side effects, and when and how to take drug. (Take medication as directed, 1 hour before or 2 hours after food.) Instruct patient to report any possible drug side effects.

Drug: azithromycin (Zithromax)

Class: Antibacterial (macrolide).

Mechanism of Action: Azithromycin binds to the 50S ribosomal subunit of the 70S ribosome of susceptible organisms, thereby inhibiting RNA-dependent protein synthesis. Bactericidal for *S. pyogenes, S. pneumoniae,* and *H. influenzae.* It is bacteriostatic for staphylococci and most aerobic gram-negative species.

Metabolism: Rapidly and widely distributed throughout the body; concentrates intracellulary, resulting in tissue concentrations 10 to 100 times those in plasma and serum. Rapidly absorbed with decreased absorption when given with food. Concentrates intracellularly, resulting in tissue concentration 10 to 100 times those in plasma or serum. Azithromycin is highly concentrated in phagocytes and fibroblasts. Over 50% of the dose is eliminated through biliary excretion as unchanged drug; approximately 4.5% of the dose is excreted unchanged in the urine within 72 hours.

Dosage/Range:
- Oral: loading dose of 500 mg as a single dose on day 1, then 250 mg once a day on days 2–5.
- No adjustment in dose is required in patients with mild renal function impairment. No data available for patients with more severe renal function impairment.
- IV: if indicated, 500 mg may be given daily × 1–2 days, then followed by oral therapy 250 mg to complete course.

Drug Preparation:
- Reconstitute 500-mg vial with 4.8 mL sterile water for concentration of 100 mg/mL.
- Further dilute with 250 or 500 mL of compatible IV solution.

Drug Administration:
- Oral: give at least 1 hour before and 2 hours after meals.
  Give at least 1 hour before and 2 hours after aluminum- and magnesium-containing antacids.
- IV: infuse 500 mg/500 mL over 3 hours and 500 mg/250 mL over 1 hour.

Drug Interactions:
- Concurrent use with antacids has decreased the peak serum concentration by approximately 24%.

Lab Effects/Interference:
- Serum SGPT, serum SGOT values may be increased.
- Creatinine clearance ≥ 40 mL per minute is desired.

Special Considerations:

- Do not use when there is a known hypersensitivity to erythromycins or other macrolides.
- Use with caution in patients with severe, impaired hepatic function.

Potential Toxicities/Side Effects and the Nursing Process

I. POTENTIAL FOR INJURY related to HYPERSENSITIVITY

Defining Characteristics: Rarely, serious allergic reactions such as anaphylaxis and angioedema have been known to occur. Fever, joint pain, skin rash, urticaria, pruritus, difficulty breathing, swelling of face, mouth, neck, hands, and feet have occurred rarely.

Nursing Implications: Assess for drug allergies to erythromycin or macrolide antibiotic prior to drug administration. Teach patient to report any allergic reactions. Assess for signs/symptoms of allergic reaction after drug dose.

II. ALTERATION IN NUTRITION related to GI SIDE EFFECTS

Defining Characteristics: Abdominal pain, diarrhea, nausea, and vomiting have occurred rarely.

Nursing Implications: Assess baseline nutritional status, preexisting nausea/vomiting, anorexia. Assess baseline LFTs and monitor periodically during treatment. Teach patient to report side effects. Provide symptomatic interventions if side effects occur; discuss with physician use of alternative drug(s).

III. ALTERATION IN URINARY ELIMINATION related to ACUTE INTERSTITIAL NEPHRITIS

Defining Characteristics: Risk is low, but patient may manifest symptoms of acute interstitial nephritis—fever, joint pain, skin rash.

Nursing Implications: Assess baseline renal function and electrolytes, and monitor periodically during therapy. Monitor hydration status to keep patient well hydrated.

IV. SENSORY/PERCEPTUAL ALTERATIONS related to CNS EFFECTS OF DIZZINESS AND HEADACHE

Defining Characteristics: Dizziness and headache may occur.

Nursing Implications: Assess baseline neurological status. Teach patient about side effects and to report dizziness or headache. If signs/symptoms arise, discuss drug discontinuance with physician.

Drug: aztreonam (Azactam)

Class: Antibacterial (systemic).

Mechanism of Action: Bactericidal by inhibition of cell wall synthesis, which results in cell wall disintegration, lysis, and cell death. Narrow-spectrum of activity against aerobic, gram-negative microorganisms (*Enterobacteriaceae* and *P. aeruginosa*). Used to treat gram-negative infections of urinary and lower respiratory tract, septicemia, and gynecologic and intraabdominal infections.

Metabolism: Poorly absorbed from GI tract. Widely distributed in body tissue and fluids, including CSF and peritoneal fluid. Crosses placenta and is excreted in breast milk. Partially metabolized, and excreted primarily in urine.

Dosage/Range:
- Given IV or IM (IV preferred for doses > 1 g, and for serious infections).
- Adults: 500 mg–2 g IV/IM q6–12h (maximum 8 g/day).
- Dose modification needed for renal dysfunction (creatinine clearance < 30 mL/min); may need to modify dosage in hepatic impairment.

Drug Preparation/Administration:
- IV: reconstitute by adding 10 mL sterile water for injection or compatible IV fluid. Further dilute by adding to a volume of IV fluid (50 mL for each gram of drug) so final concentration is < 20 mg/mL. Administer over 20–60 minutes. Flush line with plain IV fluid before and after drug infusion to prevent incompatibilities.
- IM: reconstitute drug with 3 mL for each gram of drug using sterile or bacteriostatic water for injection, or 0.9% Sodium Chloride. Do not mix with local anesthetics. Administer deep IM in large muscle mass (e.g., gluteus maximus).

Drug Interactions:
- Probenecid: increased serum concentrations of antibiotic; monitor and decrease dose if needed.
- Aminoglycosides, penicillins: may have synergistic antibacterial effect against some organisms.
- Nephrotoxic drugs (aminoglycosides, colistin, vancomycin): may increase risk of renal dysfunction; avoid if possible.
- Magnesium, calcium: incompatible in IV fluid.
- Oral anticoagulants, ASPIRIN: may increase risk of bleeding.
- Alcohol: disulfiramlike reaction (flushing, throbbing headache, dyspnea, nausea, vomiting, diaphoresis, chest pain, palpitation, hyperventilation, tachycardia, hypertension, syncope, weakness, blurred vision) when alcohol is ingested within 48–72 hours of aztreonam; does not occur if alcohol is ingested prior to first antibiotic dose. If no alcohol prior to first dose, avoid alcohol for 72 hours after last dose.

Lab Effects/Interference:

- Coombs' (antiglobulin) tests may become positive during therapy.
- Serum ALT, serum alk phos, serum AST, and serum LDH values may be transiently increased during therapy.
- Serum creatinine concentrations may be transiently increased during therapy.
- PTT and PT may be prolonged during therapy.

Special Considerations:

- Obtain and send specimen for culture and sensitivity prior to first drug dose.
- May cause false-positive Clinitest glucose result.
- Use with caution in patients with renal or hepatic dysfunction.
- Drug crosses placenta and is excreted in breast milk. Use with caution if patient is pregnant; weigh potential risks and benefits carefully if lactating; suggest interruption of breast-feeding during antibiotic therapy.
- Use cautiously if prior immediate hypersensitivity reaction to penicillins or cephalosporins; little risk of cross-allergenicity, but monitor patient closely.
- Comparable antiinfective effectiveness to aminoglycosides against gram-negative organisms without ototoxicity or nephrotoxicity.

Potential Toxicities/Side Effects and the Nursing Process

I. ALTERATIONS IN SKIN INTEGRITY related to ALLERGY HYPERSENSITIVITY REACTION

Defining Characteristics: 1–2% incidence of rash that is mild, transient, pruritic, and/or erythematous. Less than 1% of patients develop purpura, erythema multiforme, urticaria, or exfoliative dermatitis. Less than 1% incidence occurs of immediate hypersensitivity reaction characterized by angioedema, bronchospasm, severe shock. Little cross-allergenicity with penicillins, cephalosporins (less than 1%).

Nursing Implications: Assess baseline skin integrity and presence of drug allergies; if anaphylactic reaction to penicillins or cephalosporins, monitor patient closely during drug infusions. Instruct patient to report immediately signs/symptoms of rash, pruritus, shortness of breath, and adverse sensation. Teach patient skin care and symptomatic measures as appropriate. If skin rash develops, discuss drug discontinuance with physician. If rash progresses, especially in HIV-infected patients, drug should be discontinued, as fatal Stevens-Johnson syndrome may develop. Be prepared to treat severe acute hypersensitivity reactions with airway management, oxygen, epinephrine, corticosteroids, antihistamines as ordered.

II. ALTERATION IN NUTRITION, LESS THAN BODY REQUIREMENTS, related to GI SIDE EFFECTS

Defining Characteristics: Nausea, vomiting, diarrhea, anorexia may occur; rarely, pseudomembranous colitis caused by *C. difficile* resistant to the antibiotic occurs. Rarely, transient increases in LFTs—AST, ALT, alk phos—may occur. May develop taste alteration and halitosis.

Nursing Implications: Assess baseline nutritional status. Instruct patient to report GI disturbances. Administer and teach patient to self-administer antiemetics as needed and as ordered. Teach patient importance of nutritious diet, and suggest small, frequent, high-calorie, high-protein meals as appropriate. Assess baseline LFTs, and monitor periodically during treatment. Discuss abnormalities and drug interruption with physician. Encourage oral hygiene after meals and at bedtime.

III. FUNGAL SUPERINFECTION related to REDISTRIBUTION OF ENDOGENOUS MICROORGANISMS

Defining Characteristics: Vaginal candidiasis, vaginitis may occur as endogenous bacteria are eliminated, and normal fungal population expands.

Nursing Implications: Instruct female patient to report vaginal itching or discharge. Discuss appropriate antifungal treatment with physician. Teach perineal hygiene and symptomatic management.

IV. ALTERATIONS IN PROTECTIVE MECHANISMS (RARE) related to PANCYTOPENIA

Defining Characteristics: Pancytopenia, neutropenia, thrombocytopenia, anemia, leukocytosis, thrombocytosis may occur rarely. Eosinophilia occurs in 11% of patients. May have slight prolongation of bleeding time with high doses (e.g., 2-gm IV q6h).

Nursing Implications: Assess baseline laboratory parameters, and monitor periodically during treatment. Assess patient for response to antibiotics. Discuss abnormalities with physician. Assess for signs/symptoms of bleeding. If taking anticoagulants, assess for increased PT, signs/symptoms of bleeding.

V. ALTERATIONS IN SENSORY/PERCEPTUAL PATTERNS related to DIZZINESS, SOMNOLENCE

Defining Characteristics: Dizziness, headache, somnolence, seizures occur rarely.

Nursing Implications: Assess baseline neurologic function and comfort, and monitor during treatment. Instruct patient to report any changes. Discuss any abnormalities with physician.

VI. ALTERATIONS IN COMFORT related to LOCAL INJECTION IRRITATION

Defining Characteristics: 2–3% incidence of phlebitis and thrombophlebitis when administering IV; 3% incidence of pain and swelling at injection site when given IM.

Nursing Implications: Rotate IM injection sites, and administer drug deep IM in large muscle mass (e.g., gluteus maximus). Use IM injection when IV administration is not possible. Change IV sites q48h, and assess for signs/symptoms of phlebitis prior to each administration. Administer drug slowly. Apply warm packs to increase comfort.

VII. ALTERATIONS IN CARDIAC OUTPUT related to CARDIOVASCULAR CHANGES

Defining Characteristics: Rare, ~1% incidence of hypotension, transient EKG changes (e.g., premature ventricular contractions), bradycardia, flushing, and chest pain.

Nursing Implications: Assess baseline heart rate and BP; monitor during therapy, at least with initial dose.

Drug: carbenicillin indanyl sodium (Geocillin, Geopen)

Class: Extended-spectrum penicillin antibacterial.

Mechanism of Action: Semisynthetic penicillin prepared from fungus *Penicillium*. Contains β-lactam ring and is bactericidal by inhibiting cell wall synthesis. Active against gram-positive and gram-negative organisms, but most active against *Pseudomonas* and *Proteus,* except those that have developed resistance to carbenicillin.

Metabolism: After oral administration, rapidly converted to carbenicillin by hydrolysis. Widely distributed in body tissues and fluids. Crosses placenta and is excreted in breast milk. Excreted via urine and bile.

Dosage/Range:

Adult:

- 1 tablet (382 mg).

Urinary tract infections:

- *Escherichia coli Proteus* species *Enterobacter:* 1–2 tabs QID (QID = 4 times a day).
- *Pseudomonas, Enterococcus:* 2 tabs QID.
- *Prostatitis* due to *Escherichia coli, Proteus mirabilis, Enterobacter, Enterococcus:* 2 tabs QID.

Drug Preparation/Administration:
- Oral, none.

Drug Interactions:
- Probenecid: increased serum level of penicillin; may be coadministered to exert this effect.

Lab Effects/Interference:
Major clinical significance:
- Urine glucose: high urinary concentrations of a penicillin may produce falsepositive or falsely elevated test results with copper sulfate tests (Benedict's, Clinitest, or Fehling's); glucose enzymatic tests (Clinistix or Testape) are not affected.
- PTT and PT: an increase has been associated with intravenous carbenicillin.

Clinical significance:
- Coombs' (direct antiglobulin) tests: false-positive result may occur during therapy with any penicillin.
- ALT, alk phos, AST, and serum LDH values may be decreased.
- WBC: leukopenia or neutropenia is associated with the use of all penicillins; the effect is more likely to occur with prolonged therapy and severe hepatic function impairment.

Special Considerations:
- Contraindicated in patients with prior hypersensitivity to penicillins. Use with caution in patients sensitive to other β-lactams (e.g., cephalosporins) since partial cross-allergenicity exists.
- Obtain ordered specimen and send for culture and sensitivity prior to first antibiotic dose.
- Consider alternative antibiotic therapy if eosinophilia, drug fever or rash, arthralgia, hematuria, or unexplained rise in BUN and serum creatinine occur.
- Use with caution in pregnancy or with nursing women.

Potential Toxicities/Side Effects and the Nursing Process

I. POTENTIAL FOR INJURY related to HYPERSENSITIVITY REACTION

Defining Characteristics: Urticaria, pruritus, rash (maculopapular or erythematous), fever and chills, eosinophilia, myalgia, edema, erythema, angioedema, Stevens-Johnson syndrome, and exfoliative skin reactions occur in 5% of patients. Increased risk in individuals allergic to cephalosporin antibiotics.

Nursing Implications: Assess allergy to cephalosporin antibiotics and penicillin: if patient states "yes," determine actual response, e.g., "swollen lips = angioedema." If angioedema, patient SHOULD NOT receive drug. Discuss other patient responses with physician to determine whether drug should be given.

Assess baseline skin condition, including integrity and allergy history to drugs. Instruct patient to report rash, itching, other skin changes. Teach patient skin care and symptomatic measures as appropriate. If skin rash develops, discuss drug discontinuance with physician. If rash progresses, drug should be discontinued, as fatal Stevens-Johnson syndrome may develop.

II. ALTERATION IN NUTRITION, LESS THAN BODY REQUIREMENTS, related to GI SIDE EFFECTS

Defining Characteristics: Nausea, vomiting, diarrhea may occur; rarely, "furry" tongue, abdominal cramps, transient increases in LFTs—AST, ALT, alk phos, bili—may occur.

Nursing Implications: Assess baseline nutritional status. Instruct patient to report GI disturbances. Administer and teach patient to self-administer antiemetics as needed and as ordered. Teach patient importance of nutritious diet, and suggest small, frequent, high-calorie, high-protein meals as appropriate. Assess baseline LFTs and monitor periodically during treatment. Discuss abnormalities and drug interruption with physician.

III. FUNGAL SUPERINFECTION related to REDISTRIBUTION OF ENDOGENOUS MICROORGANISMS

Defining Characteristics: Vaginal candidiasis, vaginitis may occur as endogenous bacteria are eliminated, and normal fungal population expands.

Nursing Implications: Instruct female patient to report vaginal itching or discharge. Discuss appropriate antifungal treatment with physician. Teach perineal hygiene and symptomatic management.

IV. ALTERATIONS IN PROTECTIVE MECHANISMS (RARE) related to LEUKOPENIA

Defining Characteristics: Rarely, transient leukopenia, lymphocytosis, anemia, eosinophilia may occur. Prolonged PT, prolonged APTT, and hypoprothrombinemia have occurred rarely, especially in elderly or debilitated patients, or in individuals with vitamin K deficiency.

Nursing Implications: Assess baseline laboratory parameters, and monitor periodically during treatment. Assess patient for response to antibiotics. Discuss abnormalities with physician. Assess for signs/symptoms of bleeding.

Drug: cefaclor (Ceclor)

Class: Second-generation cephalosporin antibiotic.

Mechanism of Action: Semisynthetic derivative of cephalosporin C (produced by fungus); contains β-lactam ring and is related to penicillins and cephamycins (e.g., cefoxitin). Bactericidal through inhibition of cell wall synthesis, with resulting cell wall instability and cell lysis. Active against organisms causing lower respiratory tract infections (*H. influenzae, Klebsiella, Proteus, S. aureus, Streptococcus pneumoniae*); urinary tract infections (*Enterobacter, E. coli*); skin and soft tissue infections (*S. aureus, E. coli*); septicemia; and biliary infections. (Active against *H. influenzae, S. pneumoniae, Streptococcus pyogenes, E. coli, Proteus mirabilis, Klebsiella,* and staphylococci.)

Metabolism: Well absorbed from GI tract; delayed GI absorption if taken with food, but total amount of drug absorption is the same. Widely distributed in body tissues, fluids except CSF; readily crosses placenta and is excreted in breast milk. Unchanged drug rapidly excreted by the kidneys.

Dosage/Range:
- Oral: 250–500 mg q8h (maximum total 4 gm/day).

Drug Preparation/Administration:
- Store in tight container at 15–30°C (59–86°F).

Drug Interactions:
- Probenecid: increased serum concentrations of cefaclor, but does not usually require dose reduction of antibiotic.

Lab Effects/Interference:

Major clinical significance:
- Coombs' (antiglobulin) tests: a positive reaction frequently appears in patients who receive large doses of cephalosporins; hemolysis rarely occurs, but it has been reported; test may be positive in neonates whose mothers received cephalosporins before delivery.
- Urine glucose: cefaclor may produce false-positive or falsely elevated test results with copper sulfate tests (Benedicts, Clinitest, or Fehling's); glucose enzymatic tests (Clonistix or Testape) are not affected.
- PT: may be prolonged; cephalosporins may inhibit vitamin K synthesis by suppressing gut flora.

Clinical significance:
- Serum ALT, serum alk phos, serum AST, serum bili, or serum LDH values may be increased.
- BUN and serum creatinine concentrations may be increased.

- CBC or platelet count: transient leukopenia, neutropenia, agranulocytosis, thrombocytopenia, eosinophilia, lymphocytosis, and thrombocytosis have been seen on rare occasions.

Special Considerations:
- Use cautiously if renal impairment is present.
- Contraindicated if hypersensitive to other cephalosporins, or if has had angioedema response to penicillin.
- Urine glucose testing with Clinitest may result in false-positive.

Potential Toxicities/Side Effects and the Nursing Process

I. POTENTIAL FOR INJURY related to HYPERSENSITIVITY REACTION

Defining Characteristics: Urticaria, pruritus, rash (maculopapular or erythematous), fever and chills, eosinophilia, myalgia, edema, erythema, angioedema, Stevens-Johnson syndrome, and exfoliative skin reactions occur in 5% of patients. Increased risk in individuals allergic to penicillin.

Nursing Implications: Assess allergy to cephalosporin antibiotics and penicillin: if patient states "yes," determine actual response, e.g., "swollen lips = angioedema." If angioedema, patient SHOULD NOT receive drug. Discuss other patient responses with physician to determine whether drug should be given. Assess baseline skin condition, including integrity and allergy history to drugs. Instruct patient to report rash, itching, and other skin changes. Teach patient skin care and symptomatic measures as appropriate. If skin rash develops, discuss drug discontinuance with physician. If rash progresses, drug should be discontinued, as fatal Stevens-Johnson syndrome may develop. Be prepared to treat severe acute hypersensitivity reactions with airway management, oxygen, epinephrine, corticosteroids, antihistamines as ordered.

II. ALTERATION IN NUTRITION, LESS THAN BODY REQUIREMENTS, related to GI SIDE EFFECTS

Defining Characteristics: Nausea, vomiting, diarrhea, and anorexia may occur; rarely, pseudomembranous colitis caused by *C. difficile* resistant to the antibiotic occurs. May cause transient increases in LFTs.

Nursing Implications: Assess baseline nutritional status. Instruct patient to report GI disturbances. Administer and teach patient to self-administer antiemetics as needed and as ordered. Teach patient importance of nutritious diet, and suggest small, frequent, high-calorie, high-protein meals as appropriate. Assess baseline LFTs and monitor periodically during treatment. Discuss abnormalities and drug interruption with physician.

III. FUNGAL SUPERINFECTION related to REDISTRIBUTION OF ENDOGENOUS MICROORGANISMS

Defining Characteristics: Vaginal candidiasis, vaginitis may occur as endogenous bacteria are eliminated, and normal fungal population expands.

Nursing Implications: Instruct female patient to report vaginal itching or discharge. Discuss appropriate antifungal treatment with physician. Teach perineal hygiene and symptomatic management.

IV. ALTERATIONS IN PROTECTIVE MECHANISMS (RARE) related to CHANGES IN BLOOD CELL ELEMENTS, CLOTTING FACTOR

Defining Characteristics: Rarely, transient leukopenia, lymphocytosis, anemia, eosinophilia may occur. Prolonged PT, prolonged APTT, and hypoprothrombinemia have occurred rarely, especially in elderly or debilitated patients, or in individuals with vitamin K deficiency.

Nursing Implications: Assess baseline laboratory parameters, and monitor periodically during treatment. Assess patient for response to antibiotics. Discuss abnormalities with physician.

V. ALTERATIONS IN SENSORY/PERCEPTUAL PATTERNS related to DIZZINESS, SOMNOLENCE

Defining Characteristics: Dizziness, headache, somnolence occur rarely.

Nursing Implications: Assess baseline neurologic function and comfort, and monitor during treatment. Instruct patient to report any changes. Discuss any abnormalities with physician.

VI. KNOWLEDGE DEFICIT related to SELF-ADMINISTRATION OF MEDICATION

Defining Characteristics: Increased compliance when patient is instructed in self-care activities.

Nursing Implications: Assess knowledge regarding infection and planned treatment. Teach about drug action, potential side effects, and when and how to take drug. Instruct patient to report any possible side effects that occur.

Drug: cefadroxil (Duracef)

Class: First-generation cephalosporin antibacterial.

Mechanism of Action: Semisynthetic derivative of cephalosporin C, contains beta-lactam ring, and is related to penicillins and cephamycins. Bactericidal through inhibition of cell wall synthesis by binding to one or more of the penicillin-binding proteins (PBPs) that in turn inhibit the final transpeptidation step of peptidoglycan synthesis in bacterial cell walls, thus inhibiting cell wall biosynthesis. Bacteria eventually lyse due to ongoing activity of cell wall autolytic enzymes (autolysins and murein hydrolases) while cell wall assembly is arrested.

Metabolism: Well absorbed from GI tract; delayed GI absorption if taken with food, but total amount of drug absorption is the same. Widely distributed in body tissues, fluids except cerebrospinal fluid; readily crosses placenta and is excreted in breast milk. Unchanged drug rapidly excreted by the kidneys.

Dosage/Range:
- Adults: 1–2 g/day every 12 hours.
- Dose reduce if creatinine clearance is reduced per manufacturer's recommendations.

Drug Preparation/Administration:
- Store suspension in refrigerator, discard after 14 days.
- Oral administration.

Drug Interactions:
- Furosemide and aminoglycosides increase nephrotic potential and increase toxicity.
- Probenecid may decrease cephalosporin elimination and increase effect.

Lab Effects/Interference:
- Serum SGPT, serum Alk Phos, serum SGOT, serum bilirubin, or serum LDH—values may be increased
- BUN and serum creatinine—concentrations may be increased

Special Considerations:
- Use with caution in patients with renal dysfunction—dose reduction required if severe impairment exists.
- Contraindicated in patients hypersensitive to other cephalosporin antibiotics
- Use cautiously if sensitive to penicillin; contraindicated if angioedema reaction to penicillin.
- Obtain ordered specimen and send for culture and sensitivity prior to first drug dose.

Potential Toxicities/Side Effects and the Nursing Process

I. POTENTIAL FOR INJURY related to HYPERSENSITIVITY REACTION

Defining Characteristics: Urticaria, pruritis, rash (maculopapular or erythematous), fever and chills, eosinophilia, myalgia, edema, erythema, angioedema. Increased risk in individuals allergic to penicillin.

Nursing Implications: Assess allergy to cephalosporin antibiotics and penicillin: if patient states "yes," determine actual response, e.g., "swollen lips = angioedema." If angioedema, patient SHOULD NOT receive drug. Discuss other patient responses with physician to determine whether drug should be given. Assess baseline skin condition, including integrity and allergy history to drugs. Teach patient to report rash, itching, other skin changes. Teach patient skin care and symptomatic measures as appropriate. If skin rash develops, discuss drug discontinuance with physician.

II. ALTERATION IN NUTRITION, LESS THAN BODY REQUIREMENTS related to GI SIDE EFFECTS

Defining Characteristics: Nausea and vomiting and diarrhea and anorexia may occur. Rarely, transient increases in LFTs—AST (SGOT), ALT (SGPT), ALKPHOS, BR—may occur.

Nursing Implications: Assess baseline nutritional status. Teach patient to report GI disturbances. Administer and teach patient to self-administer medication as needed and as ordered. Teach patient importance of nutritious diet, and suggest small, frequent, high-calorie, high-protein meals as appropriate. Assess baseline LFTs and monitor periodically during treatment. Discuss abnormalities and drug interruption with physician.

III. FUNGAL SUPERINFECTION related to REDISTRIBUTION OF ENDOGENOUS MICROORGANISMS

Defining Characteristics: Vaginal moniliasis, vaginitis may occur as endogenous bacteria are eliminated and normal fungal population expands.

Nursing Implications: Teach female patient to report vaginal itching or discharge. Discuss appropriate antifungal treatment with physician. Teach perineal hygiene and symptomatic management.

Drug: cefamandole nafate (Mandol)

Class: Second-generation cephalosporin antibacterial.

Mechanism of Action: Semisynthetic derivative of cephalosporin C (produced by fungus); contains β-lactam ring and is related to penicillins and cephamycins (e.g., cefoxitin). Bactericidal through inhibition of cell wall synthesis, with resulting cell wall instability and cell lysis. Active against organisms causing lower respiratory tract infections (*H. influenzae, Klebsiella, Proteus, S. aureus, S. pneumoniae*); urinary tract infections (*Enterobacter, E. coli*); skin and soft tissue infections (*S. aureus, E. coli*); septicemia; and biliary infections.

Metabolism: Not absorbed from GI tract, so must be given IV or IM. Rapidly hydrolyzed to active metabolite. Widely distributed to body tissues and fluids except CSF; 65–75% bound to serum proteins. Readily crosses placenta and is excreted in breast milk. Rapidly excreted by kidneys in urine.

Dosage/Range:

Adult:

- 500 mg–1 g q4–8h; severe infections: 1–2 g q4–6h.
- Dose modification if renal impairment, based on creatinine clearance: refer to manufacturer's package insert.

Drug Preparation/Administration:

- Store powder for injection at T < 40°C (104°F). Reconstituted solution stable for 24 hours at room temperature, or 96 hours refrigerated.
- IV or deep IM injection. IV: reconstitute with 10 mL sterile water for injection, 5% Dextrose or 0.9% Sodium Chloride injection, then further dilute in 100-mL piggyback set and infuse over 30 minutes. IM: reconstitute 1-g vial with 3 mL sterile or bacteriostatic water for injection, 0.9% Sodium Chloride. Administer deep IM into large muscle mass (e.g., gluteus maximus).

Drug Interactions:

- Probenecid: increased serum concentrations of antibiotic; monitor and decrease dose if needed.
- Aminoglycosides, penicillins: may have synergistic antibacterial effect against some organisms.
- Nephrotoxic drugs (aminoglycosides, colistin, vancomycin): may increase risk of renal dysfunction; avoid if possible.
- Magnesium, calcium: incompatible in IV fluid.
- Oral anticoagulants, ASPIRIN: may increase risk of bleeding.
- Alcohol: disulfiramlike reaction (flushing, throbbing headache, dyspnea, nausea, vomiting, diaphoresis, chest pain, palpitations, hyperventilation, tachycardia, hypertension, syncope, weakness, blurred vision) when alcohol ingested within 48–72 hours of cefamandole; does not occur if alcohol ingested prior to first antibiotic dose. If no alcohol prior to first dose, avoid alcohol for 72 hours after last dose.

Lab Effects/Interference:

Major clinical significance:

- Coombs' (antiglobulin) tests: a positive reaction frequently appears in patients who receive large doses of cephalosporins; hemolysis rarely occurs, but it has been reported; test may be positive in neonates whose mothers received cephalosporins before delivery.
- Urine glucose: cefamandole may produce false-positive or falsely elevated test results with copper sulfate tests (Benedicts, Clinitest, or Fehling's); glucose enzymatic tests (Clonistix or Testape) are not affected.

- PT: may be prolonged; cephalosporins may inhibit vitamin K synthesis by suppressing gut flora; also, cephalosporins with the NMTT side chain (cefamandole) have been associated with an increased incidence of hypoprothrombinemia; patients who are critically ill, malnourished, or have liver function impairment may be at the highest risk of bleeding.

Clinical significance:

- Urine protein may produce false-positive tests for proteinuria with acid and denaturization-precipation tests.
- Serum ALT, serum alk phos, serum AST, serum bili, or serum LDH values may be increased.
- BUN and serum creatinine concentrations may be increased.
- CBC or platelet count: transient leukopenia, neutropenia, agranulocytosis, thrombocytopenia, eosinophilia, lymphocytosis, and thrombocytosis have been seen on rare occasions.

Special Considerations:

- Use cautiously if renal impairment is present.
- Contraindicated if hypersensitive to other cephalosporins, or if has had angioedema response to penicillin.
- Urine glucose testing with Clinitest may result in false-positive.

Special Considerations:

- Use with caution in patients with renal dysfunction—dose reduction required if severe impairment exists.
- Use cautiously if history of colitis exists.
- Contraindicated in patients hypersensitive to other cephalosporin antibiotics.
- Use cautiously if sensitive to penicillin; contraindicated if angioedema reaction to penicillin.
- Obtain ordered specimen and send for culture and sensitivity prior to first drug dose.
- May cause false-positive direct Coombs' test.
- May cause false-positive Clinitest glucose result.

Potential Toxicities/Side Effects and the Nursing Process

I. POTENTIAL FOR INJURY related to HYPERSENSITIVITY REACTION

Defining Characteristics: Urticaria, pruritus, rash (maculopapular or erythematous), fever and chills, eosinophilia, myalgia, edema, erythema, angioedema, Stevens-Johnson syndrome, and exfoliative skin reactions occur in 5% of patients. Increased risk in individuals allergic to penicillin.

Nursing Implications: Assess allergy to cephalosporin antibiotics and penicillin: if patient states "yes," determine actual response, e.g., "swollen lips = angioedema." If angioedema, patient SHOULD NOT receive drug. Discuss other patient responses with physician to determine whether drug should be given. Assess baseline skin condition, including integrity and allergy history to drugs. Instruct patient to report rash, itching, other skin changes. Teach patient skin care and symptomatic measures as appropriate. If skin rash develops, discuss drug discontinuance with physician. If rash progresses, drug should be discontinued, as fatal Stevens-Johnson syndrome may develop. Be prepared to treat severe acute hypersensitivity reactions with airway management, oxygen, epinephrine, corticosteroids, antihistamines as ordered.

II. ALTERATION IN NUTRITION, LESS THAN BODY REQUIREMENTS, related to GI SIDE EFFECTS

Defining Characteristics: Nausea, vomiting, diarrhea, anorexia may occur; rarely, pseudomembranous colitis caused by *C. difficile* resistant to the antibiotic occurs. Rarely, transient increases in LFTs—AST, ALT, alk phos, bili—may occur.

Nursing Implications: Assess baseline nutritional status. Instruct patient to report GI disturbances. Administer and teach patient to self-administer antiemetics as needed and as ordered. Teach patient importance of nutritious diet, and suggest small, frequent, high-calorie, high-protein meals as appropriate. Assess baseline LFTs, and monitor periodically during treatment. Discuss abnormalities and drug interruption with physician.

III. FUNGAL SUPERINFECTION related to REDISTRIBUTION OF ENDOGENOUS MICROORGANISMS

Defining Characteristics: Vaginal candidiasis, vaginitis may occur as endogenous bacteria are eliminated and normal fungal population expands.

Nursing Implications: Teach female patient to report vaginal itching or discharge. Discuss appropriate antifungal treatment with physician. Teach perineal hygiene and symptomatic management.

IV. ALTERATIONS IN PROTECTIVE MECHANISMS (RARE) related to TRANSIENT LEUKOPENIA

Defining Characteristics: Rarely, transient leukopenia, lymphocytosis, anemia, eosinophilia may occur. Prolonged PT, prolonged APTT, and hypoprothrombinemia have occurred rarely, especially in elderly or debilitated patients, or in individuals with vitamin K deficiency.

Nursing Implications: Assess baseline laboratory parameters, and monitor periodically during treatment. Assess patient for response to antibiotics. Discuss abnormalities with physician. Assess for signs/symptoms of bleeding. If they occur, especially in elderly or debilitated patients, discuss vitamin K administration with physician. Instruct patient to avoid aspirin. If taking oral anticoagulants, assess for increased PT, signs/symptoms of bleeding.

V. ALTERATIONS IN SENSORY/PERCEPTUAL PATTERNS related to DIZZINESS, HEADACHE, SOMNOLENCE

Defining Characteristics: Dizziness, headache, somnolence occur rarely.

Nursing Implications: Assess baseline neurologic function and comfort, and monitor during treatment. Instruct patient to report any changes. Discuss any abnormalities with physician.

VI. ALTERATIONS IN COMFORT related to LOCAL INJECTION IRRITATION

Defining Characteristics: Pain, induration, sterile abscesses may form in IM injection sites; phlebitis may develop in IV sites.

Nursing Implications: Rotate IM injection sites, and administer drug deep IM in large muscle mass (e.g., gluteus maximus). Use IM injection when IV administration is not possible. Change IV sites q48h, and assess for signs/symptoms of phlebitis prior to each administration. Administer drug slowly. Apply warm packs to increase comfort.

Drug: cefazolin sodium (Ancef)

Class: First-generation cephalosporin antibacterial.

Mechanism of Action: Semisynthetic derivative of cephalosporin C (produced by fungus); contains β-lactam ring and is related to penicillins and cephamycins (e.g., cefoxitin). Bactericidal through inhibition of cell wall synthesis, with resulting cell wall instability and cell lysis. Active against many gram-positive aerobic cocci (*S. aureus,* groups A and B streptococci); some susceptible gramnegative organisms (*E. coli, H. influenzae, Klebsiella, Proteus*); and gramnegative organisms causing intraabdominal and biliary infections.

Metabolism: Not absorbed from GI tract so must be given IV or IM. Widely distributed to body tissues and fluids, including bile; 74–86% bound to serum proteins. Excreted unchanged in urine. Crosses placenta and is excreted in breast milk.

Dosage/Range:
- IV is same as IM.
- Adults: 250 mg–1.5 g q6–8h (maximum 12 g/day in life-threatening infections).

- May give loading dose of 500 mg.
- Dose-reduce if serum creatinine = 1.5 mg/dL according to manufacturer's package insert.

Drug Preparation/Administration:
- Store powder at < 40°C (104°F) and protect from light. Is available as frozen solution that should be stored at T < −20°C (−4°F).
- Reconstitute powder with sterile water for injection, bacteriostatic water for injection, or 0.9% Sodium Chloride; solution stable for 24 hours at room temperature or 96 hours at 5°C (41°F).
- Further dilute in 50–100 mL 0.9% Sodium Chloride or 5% Dextrose for IV administration.
- For IM administration, reconstitute with 2–2.5 mL sterile or bacteriostatic water for injection or 0.9% Sodium Chloride injection. Administer deep IM in large muscle mass (e.g., gluteus maximus).

Drug Interactions:
- Probenecid: increased serum concentrations of antibiotic; monitor and decrease dose if needed.
- Aminoglycosides, penicillins: may have synergistic antibacterial effect against some organisms.
- Nephrotoxic drugs (aminoglycosides, colistin, vancomycin): may increase risk of renal dysfunction; avoid if possible.

Lab Effects/Interference:
Major clinical significance:
- Coombs' (antiglobulin) tests: a positive reaction frequently appears in patients who receive large doses of cephalosporins; hemolysis rarely occurs, but it has been reported; test may be positive in neonates whose mothers received cephalosporins before delivery.
- Urine glucose: cefazolin may produce false-positive or falsely elevated test results with copper sulfate tests (Benedicts, Clinitest, or Fehling's); glucose enzymatic tests (Clonistix or Testape) are not affected.
- PT may be prolonged; cephalosporins may inhibit vitamin K synthesis by suppressing gut flora.

Clinical significance:
- Serum ALT, serum alk phos, serum AST, serum bili, or serum LDH values may be increased.
- BUN and serum creatinine concentrations may be increased.
- CBC or platelet count: transient leukopenia, neutropenia, agranulocytosis, thrombocytopenia, eosinophilia, lymphocytosis, and thrombocytosis have been seen on rare occasions.

Special Considerations:

- Used in treatment of serious infections of respiratory tract, urinary tract, skin and soft tissues, and biliary tree.
- Use with caution in patients with renal dysfunction—dose reduction required if severe impairment exists.
- Use cautiously if history of colitis exists.
- Contraindicated in patients hypersensitive to other cephalosporin antibiotics.
- Use cautiously if sensitive to penicillin; contraindicated if angioedema reaction to penicillin.
- Obtain ordered specimen and send for culture and sensitivity prior to first drug dose.
- May cause false-positive direct Coombs' test.
- May cause false-positive Clinitest glucose result.

Potential Toxicities/Side Effects and the Nursing Process

I. POTENTIAL FOR INJURY related to HYPERSENSITIVITY REACTION

Defining Characteristics: Urticaria, pruritus, rash (maculopapular or erythematous), fever and chills, eosinophilia, myalgia, edema, erythema, angioedema, Stevens-Johnson syndrome, and exfoliative skin reactions occur in 5% of patients. Increased risk in individuals allergic to penicillin.

Nursing Implications: Assess allergy to cephalosporin antibiotics and penicillin: if patient states "yes," determine actual response, e.g., "swollen lips = angioedema." If angioedema, patient SHOULD NOT receive drug. Discuss other patient responses with physician to determine whether drug should be given. Assess baseline skin condition, including integrity and allergy history to drugs. Instruct patient to report rash, itching, other skin changes. Teach patient skin care and symptomatic measures as appropriate. If skin rash develops, discuss drug discontinuance with physician. If rash progresses, drug should be discontinued, as fatal Stevens-Johnson syndrome may develop. Be prepared to treat severe acute hypersensitivity reactions with airway management, oxygen, epinephrine, corticosteroids, antihistamines as ordered.

II. ALTERATION IN NUTRITION, LESS THAN BODY REQUIREMENTS, related to GI SIDE EFFECTS

Defining Characteristics: Nausea, vomiting, diarrhea, anorexia may occur; rarely, pseudomembranous colitis caused by *C. difficile* resistant to the antibiotic occurs. Rarely, transient increases in LFTs—AST, ALT, alk phos, bili—may occur.

Nursing Implications: Assess baseline nutritional status. Instruct patient to report GI disturbances. Administer and teach patient to self-administer antiemetics as needed and as ordered. Teach patient importance of nutritious diet, and suggest small, frequent, high-calorie, high-protein meals as appropriate. Assess baseline LFTs, and monitor periodically during treatment. Discuss abnormalities and drug interruption with physician.

III. FUNGAL SUPERINFECTION related to REDISTRIBUTION OF ENDOGENOUS MICROORGANISMS

Defining Characteristics: Vaginal candidiasis, vaginitis may occur as endogenous bacteria are eliminated and normal fungal population expands.

Nursing Implications: Teach female patient to report vaginal itching or discharge. Discuss appropriate antifungal treatment with physician. Teach perineal hygiene and symptomatic management.

IV. ALTERATIONS IN PROTECTIVE MECHANISMS (RARE) related to CHANGES IN FORMED BLOOD CELL ELEMENTS

Defining Characteristics: Rarely, transient leukopenia, lymphocytosis, anemia, eosinophilia may occur. Prolonged PT, prolonged APTT, and hypoprothrombinemia have occurred rarely, especially in elderly or debilitated patients, or in individuals with vitamin K deficiency.

Nursing Implications: Assess baseline laboratory parameters, and monitor periodically during treatment. Assess patient for response to antibiotics. Discuss abnormalities with physician. Assess for signs/symptoms of bleeding. If they occur, especially in elderly or debilitated patients, discuss vitamin K administration with physician. Instruct patient to avoid aspirin. If taking oral anticoagulants, assess for increased PT, signs/symptoms of bleeding.

V. ALTERATIONS IN SENSORY/PERCEPTUAL PATTERNS related to DIZZINESS, SOMNOLENCE

Defining Characteristics: Dizziness, headache, somnolence occur rarely.

Nursing Implications: Assess baseline neurologic function and comfort, and monitor during treatment. Teach patient to report any changes. Discuss any abnormalities with physician.

VI. ALTERATIONS IN COMFORT related to LOCAL INJECTION IRRITATION

Defining Characteristics: Pain, induration, sterile abscesses may form in IM injection sites; phlebitis may develop in IV sites.

Nursing Implications: Rotate IM injection sites, and administer drug deep IM in large muscle mass (e.g., gluteus maximus). Use IM injection when IV administration is not possible. Change IV sites q48h, and assess for signs/symptoms of phlebitis prior to each administration. Administer drug slowly. Apply warm packs to increase comfort.

Drug: cefdinir (Omnicef)

Class: Cephalosporin broad-spectrum antibiotic.

Mechanism of Action: Inhibits cell wall synthesis, thus destroying microorganisms. Stable in presence of some β-lactamase enzymes, so active against many microorganisms that are resistant to the penicillins and other cephalosporin antibiotics.

Metabolism: Well absorbed from the GI tract following oral dosing, with maximal plasma concentration in 2–4 hrs. Drug largely unmetabolized and eliminated by the kidneys. Mean plasma half-life is 1.7 hours. Dose must be adjusted in patients with severe renal dysfunction or who receive hemodialysis.

Dosage/Range:

Adults with:

- Community-acquired pneumonia: 300 mg PO q12h × 10 days.
- Acute exacerbation of chronic bronchitis: 300 mg PO q12h or 600 mg PO q24h × 10 days.
- Acute maxillary sinusitis: 300 mg PO q12h or 600 mg PO q24h × 10 days.
- Pharyngitis/tonsilitis: 300 mg PO q12h × 5–10 days or 600 mg PO q24h × 10 days.
- Uncomplicated skin/skin structures: 300 mg PO q12h × 10 days.
- Patients with renal insufficiency (creatinine clearance < 30 mL/min) is 300 mg PO q24h.
- Patients on hemodialysis: 300 mg PO every other day with 300 mg given at the end of each dialysis.

Drug Preparation:

- Oral, available as 300-mg tablets or oral suspension that, when reconstituted as directed, results in 125 mg/5 mL in 60- or 100-mL bottles.

Drug Administration:

- Take orally without regard to meals or food intake.

Drug Interactions:

- Antacids containing magnesium or aluminum decrease absorption of cefdinir; take cefdinir at least 2 hours before or after the antacid.

- Iron or iron supplements decrease absorption by up to 80%; separate drugs by at least 2 hours.
- Probenecid inhibits the renal excretion of cefdinir, increasing peak plasma levels by 54% and prolonging half-life by 50%; decrease cefdinir dose if must use together.

Lab Effects/Interference:

- False-positive reaction for ketones in testing using nitroprusside.
- False-positive test for glucose in the urine using Clinitest, Benedict's solution, or Fehling's solution (suggest using Clinistix or Testape).
- False-positive Coombs' test (rare).
- Increased gamma glutamyltransferase (1%); rarely other liver function tests.

Special Considerations:

Indicated for the treatment of adults with mild-tomoderate infections:

- Community-acquired pneumonia caused by *Haemophilus influenzae* (including β-lactamase–producing strains), penicillin-susceptible strains of *Streptococcus pneumoniae, Moraxella catarrhalis* (including β-lactamase–producing strains).
- Acute exacerbation of chronic bronchitis cased by *Haemophilus influenzae,* (including β-lactamase–producing strains), penicillin-susceptible strains of *Streptococcus pneumoniae, Moraxella catarrhalis* (including β-lactamase–producing strains).
- Acute maxillary sinusitis caused by *Haemophilus influenzae* (including β-lactamase–producing strains), penicillin-susceptible strains of *Streptococcus pneumoniae, Moraxella catarrhalis* (including β-lactamase–producing strains).
- Pharyngitis/tonsillitis caused by *Streptococcus pyogenes.*
- Uncomplicated skin and skin structure infections caused by *Staphylococcus aureus* (including β-lactamase–producing strains) and *Streptococcus pyogenes.*
- Contraindicated in patients with an allergy to the cephalosporin class of antibiotics as well as penicillin (cross-sensitivity in 10% of patients).
- Use cautiously, if at all, in patients with a history of colitis.
- Use in pregnancy only when benefits outweigh risks.
- If patient has severe renal dysfunction as evidenced by creatinine clearance < 30 mL/min, the dose should be reduced to 300 mg q day.
- Diabetic patients should know that the oral suspension has 2.86 g of sucrose per teaspoon.

Potential Toxicities/Side Effects and the Nursing Process

I. ALTERATION IN NUTRITION related to GI SIDE EFFECTS

Defining Characteristics: Diarrhea occurs in approximately 16% of patients, and nausea in 3%. Less common are abdominal discomfort (1%), vomiting < 1%, anorexia (< 1%). The following rarely occur: dyspepsia, flatulence, constipation, abnormal stools (red-colored in patients taking iron). As with all antibiotics, psuedomembranous colitis may occur, ranging in severity from mild to life-threatening. Treatment with antibiotics changes the intestinal microflora, so *Clostridiaum difficile* bacteria may overgrow. Once diagnosis is made, mild diarrhea may stop with cessation of drug; if moderate to severe, it will require, in addition, hydration, electrolyte replacement, nutritional support, and antibacterial coverage against *C. difficile.*

Nursing Implications: Assess baseline nutritional and elimination status. Teach patient to report GI disturbances. Teach patient to report diarrhea immediately, consider whether this is pseudomembranous colitis, and send stool specimen for *C. difficile;* if positive, discuss drug discontinuance with physician. Administer and teach patient to self-administer antiemetics, antidiarrheals as needed and as ordered. Teach patient importance of nutritious diet, and suggest small, frequent, high-calorie, high-protein meals as appropriate. Assess baseline LFTs and monitor periodically during treatment. Discuss abnormalities and drug interruption with physician.

II. SENSORY/PERCEPTUAL ALTERATIONS related to CNS EFFECTS

Defining Characteristics: Headaches occur in 2% of patients, and less common (< 1%) are dizziness, asthenia, insomnia, somnolence.

Nursing Implications: Assess baseline neurological function and comfort, and monitor during treatment. Teach patient to report any changes. Teach patient how to manage symptoms. If unrelieved or persistent, discuss any abnormalities with physician.

III. ALTERATION IN SKIN INTEGRITY related to ALLERGY/HYPERSENSITIVITY

Defining Characteristics: Uncommonly (< 1%) rash and pruritus may occur; other manifestations include eosinophilia, urticaria, flushing, fever, chills, photosensitivity, angioedema. Rarely, Stevens-Johnson reaction, toxic epidermal necrolysis, and exfoliative dermatitis have occurred. Anaphylactic reactions have occurred rarely.

Nursing Implications: Assess baseline skin condition, including integrity and drug allergy history. Teach patient to report rash, itching, other skin changes. Teach patient skin care and symptomatic measures as appropriate. If skin rash develops, discuss drug discontinuance with physician. If rash progresses, drug should be discontinued, as fatal Stevens-Johnson syndrome may develop. Be prepared to treat severe acute hypersensitivity reactions with airway management, oxygen, epinephrine, corticosteroids, antihistamines as ordered.

IV. FUNGAL SUPERINFECTION related to REDISTRIBUTION OF ENDOGENOUS MICROORGANISMS

Defining Characteristics: Vaginal moniliasis, vaginitis may occur as endogenous bacteria are eliminated and normal fungal population expands.

Nursing Implications: Teach female patient to report vaginal itching or discharge. Discuss appropriate antifungal treatment with physician. Teach perineal hygiene and symptomatic management.

Drug: cefditoren pivoxil (Spectracef)

Class: Cephalosporin antibacterial

Mechanism of Action: Semisynthetic derivative of cephalosporin C, contains beta-lactam ring, and is related to penicillins and cephamycins. Bactericidal through inhibition of cell wall synthesis, with resulting cell wall instability and cell lysis.

Metabolism: Well absorbed from GI tract.

Dosage/Range:
- Oral (adult 12 years and older): 200–400 mg q 12 hours
- Dose modification if renal impairment, based on creatinine clearance—refer to manufacturer's recommendations.
- Dose modification if hepatic impairment, based on LFTs—refer to manufacturer's recommendations.

Drug Preparation/Administration:
- Take with food.

Drug Interactions:
- Probenecid: increased serum concentrations of antibiotic; monitor and decrease dose if needed.
- Histamine H_2 antagonists: Famotidine decreases oral absorption; concomitant use should be avoided.
- Nephrotoxic drugs: may increase risk of renal dysfunction; avoid if possible.
- Magnesium- and aluminum-containing antacids decrease oral absorption; concomitant use should be avoided.

Lab Effects/Interference:
- Serum ALT (SGPT), serum Alk Phos, serum AST (SGOT), and serum bilirubin—values may be increased.
- BUN and serum creatinine—concentrations may be increased.

Special Considerations:
- Use cautiously if renal impairment is present.
- Contraindicated if hypersensitive to other cephalosporins, or if has had angioedema response to penicillin.

Potential Toxicities/Side Effects and the Nursing Process

I. POTENTIAL FOR INJURY related to HYPERSENSITIVITY REACTION

Defining Characteristics: Urticaria, pruritis, rash (maculopapular or erythematous), fever and chills, eosinophilia, myalgia, edema, erythema, angioedema. Increased risk in individuals allergic to penicillin.

Nursing Implications: Assess allergy to cephalosporin antibiotics and penicillin: if patient states "yes," determine actual response, e.g., "swollen lips = angioedema." If angioedema, patient SHOULD NOT receive drug. Discuss other patient responses with physician to determine whether drug should be given. Assess baseline skin condition, including integrity and allergy history to drugs. Teach patient to report rash, itching, other skin changes. Teach patient skin care and symptomatic measures as appropriate. If skin rash develops, discuss drug discontinuance with physician.

II. ALTERATION IN NUTRITION, LESS THAN BODY REQUIREMENTS, related to GI SIDE EFFECTS

Defining Characteristics: Nausea, vomiting, diarrhea, and anorexia may occur.

Nursing Implications: Assess baseline nutritional status. Teach patient to report GI disturbances. Administer and teach patient to self-administer antiemetics as needed and as ordered. Teach patient importance of nutritious diet, and suggest small, frequent, high-calorie, high-protein meals as appropriate. Discuss abnormalities and drug interruption with physician.

III. FUNGAL SUPERINFECTION related to REDISTRIBUTION OF ENDOGENOUS MICROORGANISMS

Defining Characteristics: Vaginal moniliasis, vaginitis may occur as endogenous bacteria are eliminated and normal fungal population expands.

Nursing Implications: Teach female patient to report vaginal itching or discharge. Discuss appropriate antifungal treatment with physician. Teach perineal hygiene and symptomatic management.

Drug: cefepime (Maxipime)

Class: Fourth-generation cephalosporin antibacterial.

Mechanism of Action: Exerts bactericidal action by inhibiting cell wall synthesis. Highly resistant to hydrolysis by β-lactamases, and exhibits rapid penetration into gram-negative bacterial cells. Active against gram-negative and grampositive organisms. Spectrum of activity includes gram-negative organisms with multiple drug resistance patterns (*Enterobacter* and *Klebsiella.*) Drug is used for treatment of infections in lower respiratory tract, skin, abdomen, and urinary tract.

Metabolism: Given intramuscularly and parenterally. Widely distributed into body tissues and fluids. Serum protein binding is less than 19% and is independent of its concentration in the serum. Excreted in urine. The average elimination half-life is approximately 2 hours.

Dosage/Range:

Adult:

- IV and IM are similar.
- Mild–mod UTI: 0.5–1 g IV or IM q12h × 7–10 days.
- Severe UTI, Klebsiella pneumonia: 2 g IV q12h × 10 days.
- Mod–severe pneumonia: 1–2 g IV q12h × 10 days.
- Febrile neutropenia: 2 g IV q8h × 7 days or neutrophil recovery.

Drug Preparation/Administration:

- IV or IM: add diluent recommended by manufacturer into vial.

Drug Interactions:

- Solutions of cefepime should not be added to solutions of metronidazole, vancomycin hydrochloride, gentamicin sulfate, tobramycin sulfate, or netilmicin sulfate and aminophylline because of potential side effects. If necessary, administer each drug separately.

Lab Effects/Interference:

Major clinical significance:

- Coombs' (antiglobulin) tests: a positive reaction has appeared in clinical trials without evidence of hemolysis.
- PT or PTT: may be prolonged; cephalosporins may inhibit vitamin K synthesis by suppressing gut flora.

Clinical significance:

- Serum SGPT, serum alk phos, serum SGOT, serum bilirubin, or serum LDH: values may be increased.
- BUN and serum creatinine: concentrations may be increased.
- CBC or platelet count: transient leukopenia, neutropenia, agranulocytosis, thrombocytopenia, eosinophilia, lymphocytosis, and thrombocytosis have been seen on rare occasions.

Special Considerations:
- Contraindicated in patients hypersensitive to other cephalosporin antibiotics.
- Use cautiously if sensitive to penicillin; contraindicated if angioedema reaction to penicillin.
- Obtain specimen and send for culture and sensitivity prior to first drug dose.
- May cause false-positive Clinitest glucose result.

Potential Toxicities/Side Effects and the Nursing Process

I. POTENTIAL FOR INJURY related to HYPERSENSITIVITY REACTION

Defining Characteristics: Urticaria, pruritus, rash (maculopapular or erythematous), fever and chills, eosinophilia, myalgia, edema, erythema, angioedema, Stevens-Johnson syndrome, and exfoliative skin reactions occur in 5% of patients. Increased risk in individuals allergic to penicillin.

Nursing Implications: Assess allergy to cephalosporin antibiotics and penicillin: if patient states "yes," determine actual response, e.g., "swollen lips = angioedema." If angioedema, patient SHOULD NOT receive drug. Discuss other patient responses with physician to determine whether drug should be given. Assess baseline skin condition, including integrity and allergy history to drugs. Teach patient to report rash, itching, other skin changes. Teach patient skin care and symptomatic measures as appropriate. If skin rash develops, discuss drug discontinuance with physician. If rash progresses, drug should be discontinued, as fatal Stevens-Johnson syndrome may develop. Be prepared to treat severe acute hypersensitivity reactions with airway management, oxygen, epinephrine, corticosteroids, antihistamines as ordered.

II. ALTERATION IN NUTRITION, LESS THAN BODY REQUIREMENTS, related to GI SIDE EFFECTS

Defining Characteristics: Nausea, vomiting, diarrhea, constipation, abdominal pain, and dyspepsia may occur; rarely, pseudomembranous colitis caused by *C. difficile* resistant to the antibiotic occurs. Rarely, transient increases in LFTs—AST (SGOT), ALT (SGPT), alk phos, BR—may occur.

Nursing Implications: Assess baseline nutritional status. Teach patient to report GI disturbances. Administer and teach patient to self-administer antiemetics, antidiarrheals as needed and as ordered. Teach patient importance of nutritious diet, and suggest small, frequent, high-calorie, high-protein meals as appropriate. Assess baseline LFTs and monitor periodically during treatment. Discuss abnormalities and drug interruption with physician.

III. FUNGAL SUPERINFECTION related to REDISTRIBUTION OF ENDOGENOUS MICROORGANISMS

Defining Characteristics: Vaginal moniliasis, vaginitis may occur as endogenous bacteria are eliminated and normal fungal population expands.

Nursing Implications: Teach female patient to report vaginal itching or discharge. Discuss appropriate antifungal treatment with physician. Teach perineal hygiene and symptomatic management.

IV. ALTERATIONS IN PROTECTIVE MECHANISMS (RARE) related to CHANGES IN FORMED BLOOD CELL ELEMENTS

Defining Characteristics: Rarely, transient leukopenia, lymphocytosis, anemia, eosinophilia may occur. Prolonged PT, prolonged APTT, and hypoprothrombinemia have occurred rarely, especially in elderly or debilitated patients, or in individuals with vitamin K deficiency.

Nursing Implications: Assess baseline laboratory parameters and monitor periodically during treatment. Assess patient for response to antibiotics. Discuss abnormalities with physician. Assess for signs and symptoms of bleeding. If they occur, especially in elderly or debilitated patients, discuss vitamin K administration with physician. Teach patient to avoid aspirin. If taking oral anticoagulants, assess for increased PT, signs and symptoms of bleeding.

V. SENSORY/PERCEPTUAL ALTERATIONS related to DIZZINESS, SOMNOLENCE

Defining Characteristics: Dizziness, headache, somnolence occur rarely.

Nursing Implications: Assess baseline neurological function and comfort, and monitor during treatment. Teach patient to report any changes. Discuss any abnormalities with physician.

Drug: cefixime (Suprax)

Class: Third-generation cephalosporin antibacterial.

Mechanism of Action: Semisynthetic derivative of cephalosporin C (produced by fungus); contains β-lactam ring and is related to penicillins and cephamycins (e.g., cefoxitin). Bactericidal through inhibition of cell wall synthesis, with resulting cell wall instability and cell lysis. Active against sensitive gramnegative bacteria (e.g., urinary tract infections caused by *E. coli, Proteus, H. influenzae*), as well as *S. pneumoniae* and *H. influenzae* related to acute bronchitis and acute exacerbations of chronic bronchitis.

Metabolism: 30–50% absorbed from GI tract; rate of absorption slowed by food but does not affect total dose absorbed; 65–70% protein-bound. Eliminated unchanged in urine, and to a lesser degree in bile and feces.

Dosage/Range:

- Adult: 400 mg/day PO (single, or two divided doses q12h).
- Duration: 5–10 days for uncomplicated urinary tract infection or upper respiratory infection; 10–14 days for lower respiratory tract infections.
- Dose-reduce if creatinine clearance < 60 mL/min per manufacturer's package insert.

Drug Preparation/Administration:

- Store tablets in tight container at 15–30°C (59–86°F).
- Oral administration.

Drug Interactions:

- Probenecid: increased serum concentrations of antibiotic; monitor and decrease dose if needed.

Lab Effects/Interference:

Major clinical significance:

- Coombs' (antiglobulin) tests: a positive reaction frequently appears in patients who receive large doses of cephalosporins; hemolysis rarely occurs, but it has been reported; test may be positive in neonates whose mothers received cephalosporins before delivery.
- PT: may be prolonged; cephalosporins may inhibit vitamin K synthesis by suppressing gut flora.

Clinical significance:

- Serum ALT, serum alk phos, serum AST, serum bili, or serum LDH values may be increased.
- BUN and serum creatinine concentrations may be increased.
- CBC or platelet count: transient leukopenia, neutropenia, agranulocytosis, thrombocytopenia, eosinophilia, lymphocytosis, and thrombocytosis have been seen on rare occasions.

Special Considerations:

- Use with caution in patients with renal dysfunction; dose reduction required if severe impairment exists.
- Use cautiously if history of colitis exists.
- Contraindicated in patients hypersensitive to other cephalosporin antibiotics.

- Use cautiously if sensitive to penicillin; contraindicated if angioedema reaction to penicillin.
- Obtain ordered specimen and send for culture and sensitivity prior to first drug dose.
- May cause false-positive direct Coombs' test.
- May cause false-positive Clinitest glucose result.

Potential Toxicities/Side Effects and the Nursing Process

I. POTENTIAL FOR INJURY related to HYPERSENSITIVITY REACTION

Defining Characteristics: Urticaria, pruritus, rash (maculopapular or erythematous), fever and chills, eosinophilia, myalgia, edema, erythema, angioedema, Stevens-Johnson syndrome, and exfoliative skin reactions occur in 5% of patients. Increased risk in individuals allergic to penicillin.

Nursing Implications: Assess allergy to cephalosporin antibiotics and penicillin: if patient states "yes," determine actual response, e.g., "swollen lips = angioedema." If angioedema, patient SHOULD NOT receive drug. Discuss other patient responses with physician to determine whether drug should be given. Assess baseline skin condition, including integrity and allergy history to drugs. Instruct patient to report rash, itching, other skin changes. Teach patient skin care and symptomatic measures as appropriate. If skin rash develops, discuss drug discontinuance with physician. If rash progresses, drug should be discontinued, as fatal Stevens-Johnson syndrome may develop. Be prepared to treat severe acute hypersensitivity reactions with airway management, oxygen, epinephrine, corticosteroids, antihistamines as ordered.

II. ALTERATION IN NUTRITION, LESS THAN BODY REQUIREMENTS, related to GI SIDE EFFECTS

Defining Characteristics: Nausea, vomiting, diarrhea, anorexia may occur; rarely, pseudomembranous colitis caused by *C. difficile* resistant to the antibiotic occurs. Rarely, transient increases in LFTs—AST, ALT, alk phos, bili—may occur.

Nursing Implications: Assess baseline nutritional status. Instruct patient to report GI disturbances. Administer and teach patient to self-administer antiemetics as needed and as ordered. Teach patient importance of nutritious diet, and suggest small, frequent, high-calorie, high-protein meals as appropriate. Assess baseline LFTs and monitor periodically during treatment. Discuss abnormalities and drug interruption with physician.

III. FUNGAL SUPERINFECTION related to REDISTRIBUTION OF ENDOGENOUS MICROORGANISMS

Defining Characteristics: Vaginal candidiasis, vaginitis may occur as endogenous bacteria are eliminated, and normal fungal population expands.

Nursing Implications: Teach female patient to report vaginal itching or discharge. Discuss appropriate antifungal treatment with physician. Teach perineal hygiene and symptomatic management.

IV. ALTERATIONS IN PROTECTIVE MECHANISMS (RARE) related to TRANSIENT LEUKOPENIA

Defining Characteristics: Rarely, transient leukopenia, lymphocytosis, anemia, eosinophilia may occur. Prolonged PT, prolonged APTT, and hypoprothrombinemia have occurred rarely, especially in elderly or debilitated patients, or in individuals with vitamin K deficiency.

Nursing Implications: Assess baseline laboratory parameters, and monitor periodically during treatment. Assess patient for response to antibiotics. Discuss abnormalities with physician. Assess for signs/symptoms of bleeding. If they occur, especially in elderly or debilitated patients, discuss vitamin K administration with physician. Instruct patient to avoid aspirin. If taking oral anticoagulants, assess for increased PT, signs/symptoms of bleeding.

V. ALTERATIONS IN SENSORY/PERCEPTUAL PATTERNS related to DIZZINESS, SOMNOLENCE

Defining Characteristics: Dizziness, headache, somnolence occur rarely.

Nursing Implications: Assess baseline neurologic function and comfort, and monitor during treatment. Instruct patient to report any changes. Discuss any abnormalities with physician.

Drug: cefoperazone sodium (Cefobid)

Class: Third-generation cephalosporin antibacterial.

Mechanism of Action: Semisynthetic derivative of cephalosporin C, contains beta-lactam ring, and is related to penicillins and cephamycins. Bactericidal through inhibition of cell wall synthesis, with resulting cell wall instability and cell lysis.

Metabolism: Not absorbed from GI tract so must be given IV or IM. Widely distributed in body fluids, including bile and cerebrospinal fluid at high doses, and body tissues. Metabolized by liver and excreted by kidneys into urine.

Dosage/Range:
- IV route when possible, but IV and IM doses are the same.
- Adults: 2–12 gm q 6–12 hours IM/IV; MAX 16 gm/day.
- Pediatrics: 100–150 mg/kg/day q 8–12 hours IV; MAX 6 gm/day.

Drug Preparation/Administration:
- Store vial containing powder at < 30°C (86°F).
- IV: Reconstitute with sterile water for injection, and further dilute in 50–100 mL of 0.9% Sodium Chloride or 5% Dextrose injection and infuse over 15–30 minutes at maximum concentration of 50 mg/ml.
- IM: Reconstitute by adding sterile or bacteriostatic water for injection. Depending on dose, divide dose and give in separate IM sites; may need to administer large doses to avoid discomfort. Administer IM injections deeply into large muscle (e.g., gluteus maximus).

Drug Interactions:
- Probenecid: increased serum concentrations of antibiotic; monitor and decrease dose if needed.
- Aminoglycosides, penicillins: may have synergistic antibacterial effect against some organisms.
- Nephrotoxic drugs (aminoglycosides, colistin, vancomycin): may increase risk of renal dysfunction; avoid if possible.
- Heparin and warfarin-cephalosporins may inhibit vitamin K synthesis by suppressing gut flora.
- Typhoid vaccine.

Lab Effects/Interference:
- PT: may be prolonged; cephalosporins may inhibit vitamin K synthesis by suppressing gut flora.
- Serum SGPT, serum Alk Phos, serum SGOT, serum bilirubin, or serum LDH: values may be increased.
- BUN and serum creatinine: concentrations may be increased.

Special Considerations:
- Use with caution in patients with renal dysfunction; dose reduction required if severe impairment exists.
- Contraindicated in patients hypersensitive to other cephalosporin antibiotics.
- Use cautiously if sensitive to penicillin; contraindicated if angioedema reaction to penicillin.
- Obtain ordered specimen and send for culture and sensitivity prior to first drug dose.

Potential Toxicities/Side Effects and the Nursing Process

I. POTENTIAL FOR INJURY related to HYPERSENSITIVITY REACTION

Defining Characteristics: Urticaria, pruritis, rash (maculopapular or erythematous), fever and chills, eosinophilia, myalgia, edema, erythema, and angioedema. Increased risk in individuals allergic to penicillin.

Nursing Implications: Assess allergy to cephalosporin antibiotics and penicillin: if patient states "yes," determine actual response, e.g., "swollen lips = angioedema." If angioedema, patient SHOULD NOT receive drug. Discuss other patient responses with physician to determine whether drug should be given. Assess baseline skin condition, including integrity and allergy history to drugs. Teach patient to report rash, itching, or other skin changes. Teach patient skin care and symptomatic measures as appropriate. If skin rash develops, discuss drug discontinuance with physician.

II. ALTERATION IN NUTRITION, LESS THAN BODY REQUIREMENTS, related to GI SIDE EFFECTS

Defining Characteristics: Diarrhea or anorexia may occur.

Nursing Implications: Assess baseline nutritional status. Teach patient to report GI disturbances. Administer and teach patient to self-administer antidiarrheal agent as needed and as ordered.

III. FUNGAL SUPERINFECTION related to REDISTRIBUTION OF ENDOGENOUS MICROORGANISMS

Defining Characteristics: Vaginal moniliasis, vaginitis may occur as endogenous bacteria are eliminated and normal fungal population expands.

Nursing Implications: Teach female patient to report vaginal itching or discharge. Discuss appropriate antifungal treatment with physician. Teach perineal hygiene and symptomatic management.

IV. ALTERATIONS IN PROTECTIVE MECHANISMS (RARE)

Defining Characteristics: Prolonged PT, prolonged APTT, and hypoprothrombinemia have occurred rarely, especially in elderly or debilitated patients, or in individuals with vitamin K deficiency.

Nursing Implications: Assess baseline laboratory parameters, and monitor periodically during treatment. Assess patient for response to antibiotics. Discuss abnormalities with physician. Assess for signs/symptoms of bleeding. If they occur, especially in elderly or debilitated patients, discuss vitamin K administration with physician. Teach patient to avoid aspirin. If taking oral anticoagulants, assess for increased PT, signs/symptoms of bleeding.

V. ALTERATIONS IN COMFORT related to LOCAL INJECTION IRRITATION

Defining Characteristics: Pain, induration, and sterile abscesses may form in IM injection sites; phlebitis may develop in IV sites.

Nursing Implications: Rotate IM injection sites, and administer drug deep IM in large muscle mass (e.g., gluteus maximus). Use IM injection when IV administration is not possible. Change IV sites q 48 hours, and assess for signs/symptoms of phlebitis prior to each administration. Administer drug slowly. Apply warm packs to increase comfort.

Drug: cefotaxime sodium (Claforan)

Class: Third-generation cephalosporin antibacterial.

Mechanism of Action: Semisynthetic derivative of cephalosporin C (produced by fungus); contains β-lactam ring and is related to penicillins and cephamycins (e.g., cefoxitin). Bactericidal through inhibition of cell wall synthesis, with resulting cell wall instability and cell lysis. Active against gramnegative cocci (*Enterobacter,* some strains of *Pseudomonas, E. coli, Klebsiella, Serratia*), as well as gram-positive *S. aureus* and *Staphylococcus epidermidis*, and *S. pneumoniae.* Used to treat serious lower respiratory tract, urinary tract, gynecologic, CNS, blood, and skin infections caused by sensitive bacteria.

Metabolism: Not absorbed from GI tract, so must be given IV or IM. Widely distributed in body fluids, including bile and CSF at high doses, and body tissues. Crosses placenta and is excreted in breast milk. Metabolized by liver and excreted by kidneys into urine.

Dosage/Range:

- IV route when possible, but IV and IM doses are the same.
- Adults: 1–2 g q6–8h (severe, 2 g q4h) × 48–72 hours after infection eradicated.

Drug Preparation/Administration:

- Store vial containing powder at < 30°C (86°F).
- Frozen injection should be stored at < −20°C (−4°F).
- IV: reconstitute with 10 mL sterile water for injection, and further dilute in 50–100 mL of 0.9% Sodium Chloride or 5% Dextrose injection and infuse over 20–30 minutes.
- IM: reconstitute by adding 2–5 mL sterile or bacteriostatic water for injection. Depending on dose, divide dose and give in separate IM sites; may need to administer large doses (2 g) IV to avoid discomfort. Administer IM injections deeply into large muscle (e.g., gluteus maximus).

Drug Interactions:

- Probenecid: increased serum concentrations of antibiotic; monitor and decrease dose if needed.
- Aminoglycosides, penicillins: may have synergistic antibacterial effect against some organisms.
- Nephrotoxic drugs (aminoglycosides, colistin, vancomycin): may increase risk of renal dysfunction; avoid if possible.

Lab Effects/Interference:

Major clinical significance:

- Coombs' (antiglobulin) tests: a positive reaction frequently appears in patients who receive large doses of cephalosporins; hemolysis rarely occurs, but it has been reported, test may be positive in neonates whose mothers received cephalosporins before delivery.
- PT: may be prolonged; cephalosporins may inhibit vitamin K synthesis by suppressing gut flora.

Clinical significance:

- Serum ALT, serum alk phos, serum AST, serum bili, or serum LDH values may be increased.
- BUN and serum creatinine concentrations may be increased.
- CBC or platelet count: transient leukopenia, neutropenia, agranulocytosis, thrombocytopenia, eosinophilia, lymphocytosis, and thrombocytosis have been seen on rare occasions.

Special Considerations:

- Use with caution in patients with renal dysfunction; dose reduction required if severe impairment exists.
- Use cautiously if history of colitis exists.
- Contraindicated in patients hypersensitive to other cephalosporin antibiotics.
- Use cautiously if sensitive to penicillin; contraindicated if angioedema reaction to penicillin.
- Obtain ordered specimen and send for culture and sensitivity prior to first drug dose.
- May cause false-positive direct Coombs' test.

Potential Toxicities/Side Effects and the Nursing Process

I. POTENTIAL FOR INJURY related to HYPERSENSITIVITY REACTION

Defining Characteristics: Urticaria, pruritus, rash (maculopapular or erythematous), fever and chills, eosinophilia, myalgia, edema, erythema, angioedema, Stevens-Johnson syndrome, and exfoliative skin reactions occur in 5% of patients. Increased risk in individuals allergic to penicillin.

Nursing Implications: Assess allergy to cephalosporin antibiotics and penicillin: if patient states "yes," determine actual response, e.g., "swollen lips = angioedema." If angioedema, patient SHOULD NOT receive drug. Discuss other patient responses with physician to determine whether drug should be given. Assess baseline skin condition, including integrity and allergy history to drugs. Instruct patient to report rash, itching, other skin changes. Teach patient skin care and symptomatic measures as appropriate. If skin rash develops, discuss drug discontinuance with physician. If rash progresses, drug should be discontinued, as fatal Stevens-Johnson syndrome may develop. Be prepared to treat severe acute hypersensitivity reactions with airway management, oxygen, epinephrine, corticosteroids, antihistamines as ordered.

II. ALTERATION IN NUTRITION, LESS THAN BODY REQUIREMENTS, related to GI SIDE EFFECTS

Defining Characteristics: Nausea, vomiting, diarrhea, anorexia may occur; rarely, pseudomembranous colitis caused by *C. difficile* resistant to the antibiotic occurs. Rarely, transient increases in LFTs—AST, ALT, alk phos, bili—may occur.

Nursing Implications: Assess baseline nutritional status. Instruct patient to report GI disturbances. Administer and teach patient to self-administer antiemetics as needed and as ordered. Teach patient importance of nutritious diet, and suggest small, frequent, high-calorie, high-protein meals as appropriate. Assess baseline LFTs, and monitor periodically during treatment. Discuss abnormalities and drug interruption with physician.

III. FUNGAL SUPERINFECTION related to REDISTRIBUTION OF ENDOGENOUS MICROORGANISMS

Defining Characteristics: Vaginal candidiasis, vaginitis may occur as endogenous bacteria are eliminated and normal fungal population expands.

Nursing Implications: Instruct female patient to report vaginal itching or discharge. Discuss appropriate antifungal treatment with physician. Teach perineal hygiene and symptomatic management.

IV. ALTERATIONS IN PROTECTIVE MECHANISMS (RARE) related to TRANSIENT LEUKOPENIA

Defining Characteristics: Rarely, transient leukopenia, lymphocytosis, anemia, eosinophilia may occur. Prolonged PT, prolonged APTT, and hypoprothrombinemia have occurred rarely, especially in elderly or debilitated patients, or in individuals with vitamin K deficiency.

Nursing Implications: Assess baseline laboratory parameters, and monitor periodically during treatment. Assess patient for response to antibiotics. Discuss abnormalities with physician. Assess for signs/symptoms of bleeding. If they occur, especially in elderly or debilitated patients, discuss vitamin K administration with physician. Instruct patient to avoid aspirin. If taking oral anticoagulants, assess for increased PT, signs/symptoms of bleeding.

V. ALTERATIONS IN SENSORY/PERCEPTUAL PATTERNS related to DIZZINESS, SOMNOLENCE

Defining Characteristics: Dizziness, headache, somnolence occur rarely.

Nursing Implications: Assess baseline neurologic function and comfort, and monitor during treatment. Instruct patient to report any changes. Discuss any abnormalities with physician.

VI. ALTERATIONS IN COMFORT related to LOCAL INJECTION IRRITATION

Defining Characteristics: Pain, induration, and sterile abscesses may form in IM injection sites; phlebitis may develop in IV sites.

Nursing Implications: Rotate IM injection sites, and administer drug deep IM in large muscle mass (e.g., gluteus maximus). Use IM injection when IV administration is not possible. Change IV sites q48h, and assess for signs/symptoms of phlebitis prior to each administration. Administer drug slowly. Apply warm packs to increase comfort.

Drug: cefotetan (Cefotan)

Class: Second-generation cephalosporin antibiotic.

Mechanism of Action: Semisynthetic derivative of cephalosporin C; contains beta-lactam ring, and is related to penicillins and cephamycins. Bactericidal through inhibition of cell wall synthesis by binding to one or more of the penicillin-binding proteins (PSPs) that in turn inhibit the final transpeptidation step of peptidoglycan synthesis in bacterial cell walls, thus inhibiting cell wall biosynthesis. Bacteria eventually lyse due to ongoing activity of cell wall autolytic enzymes (autolysins and murein hydrolases) while cell wall assembly is arrested.

Metabolism: Widely distributed in body tissues, fluids except cerebrospinal fluid; readily crosses placenta and is excreted in breast milk. Unchanged drug rapidly excreted by the kidneys.

Dosage/Range:
- Oral (adult): 1–6 g/day in divided doses every 12 hours, usual dose: 1–2 g every 12 hours for 5–10 days; 1–2 g may be given every 24 hours for urinary tract infection.
- Oral (child): 20–40 mg/kg/dose q 12 hours.

Drug Preparation/Administration:
- Refrigerate suspension.

Drug Interactions:
- Probenecid: increased serum concentrations of cefotetan but does not usually require dose reduction of antibiotic.
- Aminoglycosides and furosemide can increase nephrotoxicity.
- Disulfiram-like reaction has been reported when taken within 72 hours of ethanol consumption.

Lab Effects/Interference:
- Serum ALT (SGPT), serum Alk Phos, serum AST (SGOT), and serum bilirubin—values may be increased.
- BUN and serum creatinine—concentrations may be increased.

Special Considerations:
- Use cautiously if renal impairment is present.
- Contraindicated if hypersensitive to other cephalosporins, or if has had angioedema response to penicillin.

Potential Toxicities/Side Effects and the Nursing Process

I. POTENTIAL FOR INJURY related to HYPERSENSITIVITY REACTION

Defining Characteristics: Urticaria, pruritis, rash (maculopapular or erythematous), fever and chills, eosinophilia, myalgia, edema, erythema, angioedema. Increased risk in individuals allergic to penicillin.

Nursing Implications: Assess allergy to cephalosporin antibiotics and penicillin: if patient states "yes," determine actual response, e.g., "swollen lips = angioedema." If angioedema, patient SHOULD NOT receive drug. Discuss other patient responses with physician to determine whether drug should be given. Assess baseline skin condition, including integrity and allergy history to drugs. Teach patient to report rash, itching, and other skin changes. Teach patient skin care and symptomatic measures as appropriate. If skin rash develops, discuss drug discontinuance with physician.

II. ALTERATION IN NUTRITION, LESS THAN BODY REQUIREMENTS related to GI SIDE EFFECTS

Defining Characteristics: Nausea, vomiting, diarrhea, and anorexia may occur. May cause transient increases in LFTs.

Nursing Implications: Assess baseline nutritional status. Teach patient to report GI disturbances. Administer and teach patient to self-administer antiemetics as needed and as ordered. Teach patient importance of nutritious diet, and suggest small, frequent, high-calorie, high-protein meals as appropriate. Assess baseline LFTs and monitor periodically during treatment. Discuss abnormalities and drug interruption with physician.

III. FUNGAL SUPERINFECTION related to REDISTRIBUTION OF ENDOGENOUS MICROORGANISMS

Defining Characteristics: Vaginal moniliasis, vaginitis may occur as endogenous bacteria are eliminated, and normal fungal population expands.

Nursing Implications: Teach female patient to report vaginal itching or discharge. Discuss appropriate antifungal treatment with physician. Teach perineal hygiene and symptomatic management.

IV. KNOWLEDGE DEFICIT related to SELF-ADMINISTRATION OF MEDICATION

Defining Characteristics: Increased compliance when patient is instructed in self-care activities.

Nursing Implications: Assess knowledge re: infection and planned treatment. Teach about drug action, potential side effects, and when and how to take drug. Teach patient to report any possible side effects that occur.

Drug: cefoxitin sodium (Mefoxin)

Class: Considered second-generation cephalosporin based on activity spectrum; technically, a cephamycin antibacterial.

Mechanism of Action: β-lactam antibiotic that inhibits bacterial cell wall synthesis, leading to cell lysis. Active against sensitive gram-negative bacteria causing lower respiratory infections (*H. influenzae, E. coli, Klebsiella*); GU infections (*E. coli, Klebsiella, Proteus*); septicemia; pelvic infections (*E. coli, Neisseria gonorrheae*); or skin infections (*E. coli, Klebsiella*). Also, some grampositive infections, including lower respiratory tract infections (*S. aureus, S. pneumoniae,* streptococci).

Metabolism: Not absorbed from GI tract, so must be administered IV or IM.

Dosage/Range:
- IV route preferred; IV and IM dosages the same.
- Adult: 1–2 g q6–8h (maximum 12 g/day in divided doses).

- Dose-reduce for renal compromise (based on manufacturer's package insert).

Drug Preparation/Administration:
- Store sterile powder at < 30°C (86°F); frozen injection should be stored at < −20°C (−4°F).
- IV: reconstitute drug by adding 10 mL sterile water for injection. Further dilute in 50–100 mL 0.9% Sodium Chloride or 5% Dextrose injection and infuse over 30–60 minutes.
- IM: reconstitute drug by adding 2 mL sterile water for injection or 0.5% or 1% lidocaine HCl injection without epinephrine to 1 g of cefoxitin. Administer IM deeply into large muscle mass (e.g., gluteus maximus). Using proper technique, ensure that injection is not into blood vessel. (Make certain patient is NOT ALLERGIC to lidocaine.)

Drug Interactions:
- Probenecid: increased serum concentrations of antibiotic; monitor and decrease dose if needed.
- Aminoglycosides, penicillins: may have synergistic antibacterial effect against some organisms.
- Nephrotoxic drugs (aminoglycosides, colistin, vancomycin): may increase risk of renal dysfunction; avoid if possible.
- Magnesium, calcium: incompatible in IV fluid.
- Oral anticoagulants, ASPIRIN: may increase risk of bleeding.
- Alcohol: disulfiramlike reaction (flushing, throbbing headache, dyspnea, nausea, vomiting, diaphoresis, chest pain, palpitation, hyperventilation, tachycardia, hypertension, syncope, weakness, blurred vision) when alcohol ingested within 48–72 hours of cefoxitin; does not occur if alcohol ingested prior to first antibiotic dose. If no alcohol prior to first dose, avoid alcohol for 72 hours after last dose.

Lab Effects/Interference:

Major clinical significance:
- Coombs' (antiglobulin) tests: a positive reaction frequently appears in patients who receive large doses of cephalosporins; hemolysis rarely occurs, but it has been reported; test may be positive in neonates whose mothers received cephalosporins before delivery.
- Urine glucose: some cephalosporins (cefoxitin) may produce false-positive or falsely elevated test results with copper sulfate tests (Benedict's, Fehling's, or Clinitest); glucose enzymatic tests (Clinistix and Testape) are not affected.
- PT: may be prolonged; cephalosporins may inhibit vitamin K synthesis by suppressing gut flora.

Clinical significance:

- Serum and urine creatinine may falsely elevate test values when the Jaffe reaction is used; serum samples should not be obtained within 2 hours of administration.
- Serum ALT, serum alk phos, serum AST, serum bili, or serum LDH values may be increased.
- BUN and serum creatinine concentrations may be increased.
- CBC or platelet count: transient leukopenia, neutropenia, agranulocytosis, thrombocytopenia, eosinophilia, lymphocytosis, and thrombocytosis have been seen on rare occasions.

Special Considerations:

- Use with caution in patients with renal dysfunction; dose reduction required if severe impairment exists.
- Use cautiously if history of colitis exists.
- Contraindicated in patients hypersensitive to other cephalosporin antibiotics.
- Use cautiously if sensitive to penicillin; contraindicated if angioedema reaction to penicillin.
- Obtain ordered specimen and send for culture and sensitivity prior to first drug dose.
- May cause false-positive direct Coombs' test.
- May cause false-positive Clinitest glucose result.

Potential Toxicities/Side Effects and the Nursing Process

I. POTENTIAL FOR INJURY related to HYPERSENSITIVITY REACTION

Defining Characteristics: Urticaria, pruritus, rash (maculopapular or erythematous), fever and chills, eosinophilia, myalgia, edema, erythema, angioedema, Stevens-Johnson syndrome, and exfoliative skin reactions occur in 5% of patients. Increased risk in individuals allergic to penicillin.

Nursing Implications: Assess allergy to cephalosporin antibiotics and penicillin: if patient states "yes," determine actual response, e.g., "swollen lips = angioedema." If angioedema, patient SHOULD NOT receive drug. Discuss other patient responses with physician to determine whether drug should be given. Assess baseline skin condition, including integrity and allergy history to drugs. Instruct patient to report rash, itching, and other skin changes. Teach patient skin care and symptomatic measures as appropriate. If skin rash develops, discuss drug discontinuance with physician. If rash progresses, drug should be discontinued, as fatal Stevens-Johnson syndrome may develop. Be prepared to treat severe acute hypersensitivity reactions with airway management, oxygen, epinephrine, corticosteroids, antihistamines as ordered.

II. ALTERATION IN NUTRITION, LESS THAN BODY REQUIREMENTS, related to GI SIDE EFFECTS

Defining Characteristic: Nausea, vomiting, diarrhea, anorexia may occur; rarely, pseudomembranous colitis caused by *C. difficile* resistant to the antibiotic occurs. Rarely, transient increases in LFTs—AST, ALT, alk phos, bili—may occur.

Nursing Implications: Assess baseline nutritional status. Instruct patient to report GI disturbances. Administer and teach patient to self-administer antiemetics as needed and as ordered. Teach patient importance of nutritious diet, and suggest small, frequent, high-calorie, high-protein meals as appropriate. Assess baseline LFTs and monitor periodically during treatment. Discuss abnormalities and drug interruption with physician.

III. FUNGAL SUPERINFECTION related to REDISTRIBUTION OF ENDOGENOUS MICROORGANISMS

Defining Characteristics: Vaginal candidiasis, vaginitis may occur as endogenous bacteria are eliminated and normal fungal population expands.

Nursing Implications: Instruct female patient to report vaginal itching or discharge. Discuss appropriate antifungal treatment with physician. Teach perineal hygiene and symptomatic management.

IV. ALTERATIONS IN PROTECTIVE MECHANISMS (RARE) related to TRANSIENT LEUKOPENIA

Defining Characteristics: Rarely, transient leukopenia, lymphocytosis, anemia, eosinophilia may occur. Prolonged PT, prolonged APTT, and hypoprothrombinemia have occurred rarely, especially in elderly or debilitated patients, or in individuals with vitamin K deficiency.

Nursing Implications: Assess baseline laboratory parameters, and monitor periodically during treatment. Assess patient for response to antibiotics. Discuss abnormalities with physician. Assess for signs/symptoms of bleeding. If they occur, especially in elderly or debilitated patients, discuss vitamin K administration with physician. Instruct patient to avoid aspirin. If taking oral anticoagulants, assess for increased PT, signs/symptoms of bleeding.

V. ALTERATIONS IN SENSORY/PERCEPTUAL PATTERNS related to DIZZINESS, SOMNOLENCE

Defining Characteristics: Dizziness, headache, somnolence occur rarely.

Nursing Implications: Assess baseline neurologic function and comfort, and monitor during treatment. Instruct patient to report any changes. Discuss any abnormalities with physician.

VI. ALTERATIONS IN COMFORT related to LOCAL INJECTION IRRITATION

Defining Characteristics: Pain, induration, sterile abscesses may form in IM injection sites; phlebitis may develop in IV sites.

Nursing Implications: Rotate IM injection sites, and administer drug deep IM in large muscle mass (e.g., gluteus maximus). Use IM injection when IV administration is not possible. Change IV sites q48h, and assess for signs/symptoms of phlebitis prior to each administration. Administer drug slowly. Apply warm packs to increase comfort.

Drug: cefpodoxime proxetil (Vantin)

Class: Cephalosporin antibacterial.

Mechanism of Action: Semisynthetic derivative of cephalosporin C, contains beta-lactam ring, and is related to penicillins and cephamycins. Bactericidal through inhibition of cell wall synthesis, with resulting cell wall instability and cell lysis.

Metabolism: Well absorbed from GI tract.

Dosage/Range:
- Oral (adult 13 years and older): 100–400 mg q 12 hours.
- Oral (gonorrhea indication): 200-mg single dose.
- Oral (child 6 months–12 years): 10 mg/kg/daily (divided QD-BID), (MAX 400 mg/day).
- Dose modification if renal impairment, based on creatinine clearance: refer to manufacturer's recommendations.

Drug Preparation/Administration:
- Take with food.

Drug Interactions:
- Probenecid: increased serum concentrations of antibiotic; monitor and decrease dose if needed.
- Aminoglycosides, penicillins: may have synergistic antibacterial effect against some organisms.
- Nephrotoxic drugs: may increase risk of renal dysfunction; avoid if possible.
- Magnesium and aluminum.

Lab Effects/Interference:
- Serum ALT (SGPT), serum Alk Phos, serum AST (SGOT), and serum bilirubin: values may be increased.
- BUN and serum creatinine: concentrations may be increased.

Special Considerations:

- Use cautiously if renal impairment is present.
- Contraindicated if hypersensitive to other cephalosporins, or if has had angioedema response to penicillin.

Potential Toxicities/Side Effects and the Nursing Process

I. POTENTIAL FOR INJURY related to HYPERSENSITIVITY REACTION

Defining Characteristics: Urticaria, pruritis, rash (maculopapular or erythematous), fever and chills, eosinophilia, myalgia, edema, erythema, angioedema. Increased risk in individuals allergic to penicillin.

Nursing Implications: Assess allergy to cephalosporin antibiotics and penicillin: if patient states "yes," determine actual response, e.g., "swollen lips = angioedema." If angioedema, patient SHOULD NOT receive drug. Discuss other patient responses with physician to determine whether drug should be given. Assess baseline skin condition, including integrity and allergy history to drugs. Teach patient to report rash, itching, other skin changes. Teach patient skin care and symptomatic measures as appropriate. If skin rash develops, discuss drug discontinuance with physician.

II. ALTERATION IN NUTRITION, LESS THAN BODY REQUIREMENTS, related to GI SIDE EFFECTS

Defining Characteristics: Nausea, vomiting, diarrhea, and anorexia may occur.

Nursing Implications: Assess baseline nutritional status. Teach patient to report GI disturbances. Administer and teach patient to self-administer antiemetics as needed and as ordered. Teach patient importance of nutritious diet, and suggest small, frequent, high-calorie, high-protein meals as appropriate. Discuss abnormalities and drug interruption with physician.

III. FUNGAL SUPERINFECTION related to REDISTRIBUTION OF ENDOGENOUS MICROORGANISMS

Defining Characteristics: Vaginal moniliasis, vaginitis may occur as endogenous bacteria are eliminated and normal fungal population expands.

Nursing Implications: Teach female patient to report vaginal itching or discharge. Discuss appropriate antifungal treatment with physician. Teach perineal hygiene and symptomatic management.

Drug: cefprozil (Cefzil)

Class: Second-generation cephalosporin antibiotic.

Mechanism of Action: Semisynthetic derivative of cephalosporin C; contains beta-lactam ring, and is related to penicillins and cephamycins. Bactericidal through inhibition of cell wall synthesis, with resulting cell wall instability and cell lysis.

Metabolism: Well absorbed from GI tract; delayed GI absorption if taken with food, but total amount of drug absorption is the same. Widely distributed in body tissues and fluids, except cerebrospinal fluid; readily crosses placenta and is excreted in breast milk. Unchanged drug rapidly excreted by the kidneys.

Dosage/Range:
- Oral (adult 13 years and older): 250–500 mg q 12–24 hours.
- Oral (child 7 months–12 years): 7.5–15 mg/kg q 12 hours (MAX 1 gm/day).

Drug Preparation/Administration:
- Refrigerate suspension.
- Discard after 14 days.

Drug Interactions:
- Probenecid: increased serum concentrations of cefprozil but does not usually require dose reduction of antibiotic.
- Aminoglycosides, penicillins: may have synergistic antibacterial effect against some organisms.
- Typhoid vaccine.

Lab Effects/Interference:
- Serum ALT (SGPT), serum Alk Phos, serum AST (SGOT), and serum bilirubin: values may be increased.
- BUN and serum creatinine: concentrations may be increased.

Special Considerations:
- Use cautiously if renal impairment is present.
- Contraindicated if hypersensitive to other cephalosporins, or if has had angioedema response to penicillin.

Potential Toxicities/Side Effects and the Nursing Process

I. POTENTIAL FOR INJURY related to HYPERSENSITIVITY REACTION

Defining Characteristics: Urticaria, pruritis, rash (maculopapular or erythematous), fever and chills, eosinophilia, myalgia, edema, erythema, angioedema. Increased risk in individuals allergic to penicillin.

Nursing Implications: Assess allergy to cephalosporin antibiotics and penicillin: if patient states "yes," determine actual response, e.g., "swollen lips = angioedema." If angioedema, patient SHOULD NOT receive drug. Discuss other patient responses with physician to determine whether drug should be given. Assess baseline skin condition, including integrity and allergy history to drugs. Teach patient to report rash, itching, and other skin changes. Teach patient skin care and symptomatic measures as appropriate. If skin rash develops, discuss drug discontinuance with physician.

II. ALTERATION IN NUTRITION, LESS THAN BODY REQUIREMENTS, related to GI SIDE EFFECTS

Defining Characteristics: Nausea, vomiting, diarrhea, and anorexia may occur. May cause transient increases in LFTs.

Nursing Implications: Assess baseline nutritional status. Teach patient to report GI disturbances. Administer and teach patient to self-administer antiemetics as needed and as ordered. Teach patient importance of nutritious diet, and suggest small, frequent, high-calorie, high-protein meals as appropriate. Assess baseline LFTs and monitor periodically during treatment. Discuss abnormalities and drug interruption with physician.

III. FUNGAL SUPERINFECTION related to REDISTRIBUTION OF ENDOGENOUS MICROORGANISMS

Defining Characteristics: Vaginal moniliasis, vaginitis may occur as endogenous bacteria are eliminated and normal fungal population expands.

Nursing Implications: Teach female patient to report vaginal itching or discharge. Discuss appropriate antifungal treatment with physician. Teach perineal hygiene and symptomatic management.

IV. KNOWLEDGE DEFICIT related to SELF-ADMINISTRATION OF MEDICATION

Defining Characteristics: Increased compliance when patient is instructed in self-care activities.

Nursing Implications: Assess knowledge regarding infection and planned treatment. Teach about drug action, potential side effects, and when and how to take drug. Teach patient to report any possible side effects that occur.

Drug: ceftazidime (Fortaz, Tazicef, Tazidime)

Class: Third-generation cephalosporin antibacterial.

Mechanism of Action: Semisynthetic derivative of cephalosporin C (produced by fungus); contains β-lactam ring and is related to penicillins and cephamycins (e.g., cefoxitin). Bactericidal through inhibition of cell wall synthesis, with resulting cell wall instability and cell lysis. Active against sensitive microorganisms causing lower respiratory tract, urinary tract, skin, bone and joint, gynecologic, intraabdominal infections. These include primarily gram-negative bacteria (*Enterobacter, E. coli, Klebsiella, Proteus, Serratia,* and *Pseudomonas*) and, to a lesser degree, some gram-positive bacteria (*S. aureus, S. epidermidis,* streptococci).

Metabolism: Not absorbed from GI tract so must be administered parenterally. Small degree of protein binding (5–24%). Widely distributed in body fluids (including CSF and bile) and body tissues. Crosses placenta and is excreted unchanged in urine.

Dosage/Range:

- IV and IM doses are the same.
- Adult: maximum 6 g/d.
- Uncomplicated pneumonia, skin/structure infections: 0.5–1 g IV q8h.
- Bone, joint infection: 2 g q12h.
- Severe GYN, abdominal infections or febrile neutropenia: 2 g IV q8h.
- Lung infection by pseudomonas in patients with cystic fibrosis: 30–50 mg/kg q8h.
- Dose should be reduced in renal insufficiency according to manufacturer's package insert.

Drug Preparation/Administration:

- Store sterile powder vials at 15–30°C (59–86°F) and protect from light; frozen injection containers should be stored at < −20°C (−4°F).
- IV: reconstitute according to manufacturer's package insert, as some preparations contain sodium carbonate. Further dilute in 100 mL of 0.9% Sodium Chloride or 5% Dextrose and infuse over 30–60 minutes.
- IM: reconstitute according to manufacturer's package insert, which may suggest the addition of 0.5–1% lidocaine HCl to decrease discomfort. Make certain patient is NOT ALLERGIC to lidocaine. Administer deep IM in large muscle mass (e.g., gluteus maximus).

Drug Interactions:

- Probenecid: increased serum concentrations of antibiotic; monitor and decrease dose if needed.
- Aminoglycosides, penicillins: may have synergistic antibacterial effect against some organisms.
- Nephrotoxic drugs (aminoglycosides, colistin, vancomycin): may increase risk of renal dysfunction; avoid if possible.
- Sodium bicarbonate: incompatible; DO NOT administer concurrently through same IV site.

Lab Effects/Interference:
Major clinical significance:
- Coombs' (antiglobulin) tests: a positive reaction frequently appears in patients who receive large doses of cephalosporins; hemolysis rarely occurs, but it has been reported; test may be positive in neonates whose mothers received cephalosporins before delivery.
- PT: may be prolonged; cephalosporins may inhibit vitamin K synthesis by suppressing gut flora.

Clinical significance:
- Serum ALT, serum alk phos, serum AST, serum bili, or serum LDH values may be increased.
- BUN and serum creatinine concentrations may be increased.
- CBC or platelet count: transient leukopenia, neutropenia, agranulocytosis, thrombocytopenia, eosinophilia, lymphocytosis, and thrombocytosis have been seen on rare occasions.

Special Considerations:
- Empiric use in management of febrile neutropenic patient appears to be as effective as combination antibiotic regimens; vancomycin may need to be added to ceftazidime to better cover gram-positive bacteria (e.g., *S. epidermidis*).
- Has excellent coverage against *P. aeruginosa.*
- Use with caution in patients with renal dysfunction; dose reduction required if severe impairment exists.
- Use cautiously if history of colitis exists.
- Contraindicated in patients hypersensitive to other cephalosporin antibiotics.
- Use cautiously if sensitive to penicillin; contraindicated if angioedema reaction to penicillin.
- Obtain specimen and send for culture and sensitivity prior to first drug dose.
- May cause false-positive direct Coombs' test.
- May cause false-positive Clinitest glucose result.

Potential Toxicities/Side Effects and the Nursing Process

I. POTENTIAL FOR INJURY related to HYPERSENSITIVITY REACTION

Defining Characteristics: Urticaria, pruritus, rash (maculopapular or erythematous), fever and chills, eosinophilia, myalgia, edema, erythema, angioedema, Stevens-Johnson syndrome, and exfoliative skin reactions occur in 5% of patients. Increased risk in individuals allergic to penicillin.

Nursing Implications: Assess allergy to cephalosporin antibiotics and penicillin: if patient states "yes," determine actual response, e.g., "swollen lips = angioedema." If angioedema, patient SHOULD NOT receive drug. Discuss other patient responses with physician to determine whether drug should be given. Assess baseline skin condition, including integrity and allergy history to drugs. Instruct patient to report rash, itching, other skin changes. Teach patient skin care and symptomatic measures as appropriate. If skin rash develops, discuss drug discontinuance with physician. If rash progresses, drug should be discontinued, as fatal Stevens-Johnson syndrome may develop. Be prepared to treat severe acute hypersensitivity reactions with airway management, oxygen, epinephrine, corticosteroids, antihistamines as ordered.

II. ALTERATION IN NUTRITION, LESS THAN BODY REQUIREMENTS, related to GI SIDE EFFECTS

Defining Characteristics: Nausea, vomiting, diarrhea, anorexia may occur; rarely, pseudomembranous colitis caused by *C. difficile* resistant to the antibiotic occurs. Rarely, transient increases in LFTs—AST, ALT, alk phos, bili—may occur.

Nursing Implications: Assess baseline nutritional status. Instruct patient to report GI disturbances. Administer and teach patient to self-administer antiemetics as needed and as ordered. Teach patient importance of nutritious diet, and suggest small, frequent, high-calorie, high-protein meals as appropriate. Assess baseline LFTs, and monitor periodically during treatment. Discuss abnormalities and drug interruption with physician.

III. FUNGAL SUPERINFECTION related to REDISTRIBUTION OF ENDOGENOUS MICROORGANISMS

Defining Characteristics: Vaginal candidiasis, vaginitis may occur as endogenous bacteria are eliminated, and normal fungal population expands.

Nursing Implications: Instruct female patient to report vaginal itching or discharge. Discuss appropriate antifungal treatment with physician. Teach perineal hygiene and symptomatic management.

IV. ALTERATIONS IN PROTECTIVE MECHANISMS (RARE) related to TRANSIENT LEUKOPENIA

Defining Characteristics: Rarely, transient leukopenia, lymphocytosis, anemia, eosinophilia may occur. Prolonged PT, prolonged APTT, and hypoprothrombinemia have occurred rarely, especially in elderly or debilitated patients, or in individuals with vitamin K deficiency.

Nursing Implications: Assess baseline laboratory parameters, and monitor periodically during treatment. Assess patient for response to antibiotics. Discuss abnormalities with physician.

V. ALTERATIONS IN SENSORY/PERCEPTUAL PATTERNS related to DIZZINESS, SOMNOLENCE

Defining Characteristics: Dizziness, headache, somnolence occur rarely.

Nursing Implications: Assess baseline neurologic function and comfort, and monitor during treatment. Instruct patient to report any changes. Discuss any abnormalities with physician.

VI. ALTERATIONS IN COMFORT related to LOCAL INJECTION IRRITATION

Defining Characteristics: Pain, induration, sterile abscesses may form in IM injection sites; phlebitis may develop in IV sites.

Nursing Implications: Rotate IM injection sites, and administer drug deep IM in large muscle mass (e.g., gluteus maximus). Use IM injection when IV administration is not possible. Change IV sites q48h, and assess for signs/symptoms of phlebitis prior to each administration. Administer drug slowly. Apply warm packs to increase comfort.

Drug: ceftibuten (Cedax)

Class: Third-generation cephalosporin antibacterial.

Mechanism of Action: Semisynthetic derivative of cephalosporin C, contains beta-lactam ring, and is related to penicillins and cephamycins. Bactericidal through inhibition of cell wall synthesis, with resulting cell wall instability and cell lysis.

Metabolism: Well absorbed from GI tract; delayed GI absorption if taken with food, but total amount of drug absorption is the same. Widely distributed in body tissues and fluids, except cerebrospinal fluid; readily crosses placenta and is excreted in breast milk. Unchanged drug rapidly excreted by the kidneys.

Dosage/Range:
- Adults: 400 mg orally QD × 10 days.
- Dose reduce if creatinine clearance is reduced per manufacturer's recommendations.

Drug Preparation/Administration:
- Store suspension in refrigerator; discard after 14 days.
- Oral administration.

Drug Interactions:
- Aminoglycosides, penicillins: may have synergistic antibacterial effect against some organisms.

- Typhoid vaccine.

Lab Effects/Interference:

- Serum SGPT, serum Alk Phos, serum SGOT, serum bilirubin, or serum LDH: values may be increased.
- BUN and serum creatinine: concentrations may be increased.

Special Considerations:

- Use with caution in patients with renal dysfunction; dose reduction required if severe impairment exists.
- Contraindicated in patients hypersensitive to other cephalosporin antibiotics.
- Use cautiously if sensitive to penicillin; contraindicated if angioedema reaction to penicillin.
- Obtain ordered specimen and send for culture and sensitivity prior to first drug dose.

Potential Toxicities/Side Effects and the Nursing Process

I. POTENTIAL FOR INJURY related to HYPERSENSITIVITY REACTION

Defining Characteristics: Urticaria, pruritis, rash (maculopapular or erythematous), fever and chills, eosinophilia, myalgia, edema, erythema, angioedema. Increased risk in individuals allergic to penicillin.

Nursing Implications: Assess allergy to cephalosporin antibiotics and penicillin: if patient states "yes," determine actual response, e.g., "swollen lips = angioedema." If angioedema, patient SHOULD NOT receive drug. Discuss other patient responses with physician to determine whether drug should be given. Assess baseline skin condition, including integrity and allergy history to drugs. Teach patient to report rash, itching, other skin changes. Teach patient skin care and symptomatic measures as appropriate. If skin rash develops, discuss drug discontinuance with physician.

II. ALTERATION IN NUTRITION, LESS THAN BODY REQUIREMENTS, related to GI SIDE EFFECTS

Defining Characteristics: Nausea, vomiting, diarrhea, and anorexia may occur. Rarely, transient increases in LFTs—AST (SGOT), ALT (SGPT), ALK-PHOS, BR—may occur.

Nursing Implications: Assess baseline nutritional status. Teach patient to report GI disturbances. Administer and teach patient to self-administer medication as needed and as ordered. Teach patient importance of nutritious diet, and suggest small, frequent, high-calorie, high-protein meals as appropriate. Assess baseline LFTs and monitor periodically during treatment. Discuss abnormalities and drug interruption with physician.

III. FUNGAL SUPERINFECTION related to REDISTRIBUTION OF ENDOGENOUS MICROORGANISMS

Defining Characteristics: Vaginal moniliasis, vaginitis may occur as endogenous bacteria are eliminated and normal fungal population expands.

Nursing Implications: Teach female patient to report vaginal itching or discharge. Discuss appropriate antifungal treatment with physician. Teach perineal hygiene and symptomatic management.

Drug: ceftriaxone sodium (Rocephin)

Class: Third-generation cephalosporin antibacterial.

Mechanism of Action: Semisynthetic derivative of cephalosporin C (produced by fungus); contains β-lactam ring and is related to penicillins and cephamycins (e.g., cefoxitin). Bactericidal through inhibition of cell wall synthesis, with resulting cell wall instability and cell lysis. Active primarily against gram-negative cocci (*H. influenzae, Enterobacter, E. coli, Klebsiella, Proteus, Pseudomonas*) and, to a lesser degree, gram-positive cocci (*S. aureus* and streptococci). Drug is used for treatment of infections in lower respiratory tract, skin, bone and joint, abdomen, urinary tract, and pelvis (gonorrhea), as well as for treatment of meningitis and sepsis.

Metabolism: Not absorbed from GI tract and must be given parenterally. Widely distributed into body tissues and fluids, including bile and CSF. Crosses placenta and excreted in breast milk. Protein binding depends on drug concentration, and varies from 58–96%. Excreted in urine and feces to a lesser extent. Has long half-life.

Dosage/Range:

- IV and IM doses same.
- 1–2 g/day, or in equally divided doses q12h.
- CNS infections may require maximum recommended of 4 g/day in divided doses.

Drug Preparation/Administration:

- Store vial of sterile drug powder at ≤ 25°C (77°F) and protect from light. Frozen injection containers should be stored at ≤ −20°C (−4°F).
- IV: Add diluent recommended by manufacturer into vial, then further dilute in 100 mL 0.9% Sodium Chloride or 5% Dextrose. Infuse over 30–60 minutes.
- IM: Add 0.9–7.2 mL of sterile or bacteriostatic water for injection, or 1% lidocaine HCl without epinephrine to appropriate vial, resulting in 250

mg/mL. Administer deep IM into large muscle mass (e.g., gluteus maximus). Make certain patient is NOT ALLERGIC to lidocaine.

Drug Interactions:

- Probenecid: increased serum concentrations of antibiotic; monitor and decrease dose if needed.
- Aminoglycosides, penicillins: may have synergistic antibacterial effect against some organisms.
- Nephrotoxic drugs (aminoglycosides, colistin, vancomycin): may increase risk of renal dysfunction; avoid if possible.

Lab Effects/Interference:

Major clinical significance:

- Coombs' (antiglobulin) tests: a positive reaction frequently appears in patients who receive large doses of cephalosporins; hemolysis rarely occurs, but it has been reported; test may be positive in neonates whose mothers received cephalosporins before delivery.
- PT: may be prolonged; cephalosporins may inhibit vitamin K synthesis by suppressing gut flora.

Clinical significance:

- Serum ALT, serum alk phos, serum AST, serum bili, or serum LDH values may be increased.
- BUN and serum creatinine concentrations may be increased.
- CBC or platelet count: transient leukopenia, neutropenia, agranulocytosis, thrombocytopenia, eosinophilia, lymphocytosis, and thrombocytosis have been seen on rare occasions.

Special Considerations:

- Use cautiously if history of colitis exists.
- Contraindicated in patients hypersensitive to other cephalosporin antibiotics.
- Use cautiously if sensitive to penicillin; contraindicated if angioedema reaction to penicillin.
- Obtain specimen and send for culture and sensitivity prior to first drug dose.
- May cause false-positive direct Coombs' test.
- May cause false-positive Clinitest glucose result.

Potential Toxicities/Side Effects and the Nursing Process

I. POTENTIAL FOR INJURY related to HYPERSENSITIVITY REACTION

Defining Characteristics: Urticaria, pruritus, rash (maculopapular or erythematous), fever and chills, eosinophilia, myalgia, edema, erythema, angioedema, Stevens-Johnson syndrome, and exfoliative skin reactions occur in 5% of patients. Increased risk in individuals allergic to penicillin.

Nursing Implications: Assess allergy to cephalosporin antibiotics and penicillin: if patient states "yes," determine actual response, e.g., "swollen lips = angioedema." If angioedema, patient SHOULD NOT receive drug. Discuss other patient responses with physician to determine whether drug should be given. Assess baseline skin condition, including integrity and allergy history to drugs. Instruct patient to report rash, itching, other skin changes. Teach patient skin care and symptomatic measures as appropriate. If skin rash develops, discuss drug discontinuance with physician. If rash progresses, drug should be discontinued, as fatal Stevens-Johnson syndrome may develop. Be prepared to treat severe acute hypersensitivity reactions with airway management, oxygen, epinephrine, corticosteroids, antihistamines as ordered.

II. ALTERATION IN NUTRITION, LESS THAN BODY REQUIREMENTS, related to GI SIDE EFFECTS

Defining Characteristics: Nausea, vomiting, diarrhea, anorexia may occur; rarely, pseudomembranous colitis caused by *C. difficile* resistant to the antibiotic occurs. Rarely, transient increases in LFTs—AST, ALT, alk phos, bili—may occur.

Nursing Implications: Assess baseline nutritional status. Instruct patient to report GI disturbances. Administer and teach patient to self-administer antiemetics, antidiarrheals as needed and as ordered. Teach patient importance of nutritious diet, and suggest small, frequent, high-calorie, high-protein meals as appropriate. Assess baseline LFTs and monitor periodically during treatment. Discuss abnormalities and drug interruption with physician.

III. FUNGAL SUPERINFECTION related to REDISTRIBUTION OF ENDOGENOUS MICROORGANISMS

Defining Characteristics: Vaginal candidiasis, vaginitis may occur as endogenous bacteria are eliminated and normal fungal population expands.

Nursing Implications: Instruct female patient to report vaginal itching or discharge. Discuss appropriate antifungal treatment with physician. Teach perineal hygiene and symptomatic management.

IV. ALTERATIONS IN PROTECTIVE MECHANISMS (RARE) related to TRANSIENT LEUKOPENIA

Defining Characteristics: Rarely, transient leukopenia, lymphocytosis, anemia, eosinophilia may occur. Prolonged PT, prolonged APTT, and hypoprothrombinemia have occurred rarely, especially in elderly or debilitated patients, or in individuals with vitamin K deficiency.

Nursing Implications: Assess baseline laboratory parameters, and monitor periodically during treatment. Assess patient for response to antibiotics. Discuss abnormalities with physician. Assess for signs/symptoms of bleeding. If they occur, especially in elderly or debilitated patients, discuss vitamin K administration with physician. Instruct patient to avoid aspirin. If taking oral anticoagulants, assess for increased PT, signs/symptoms of bleeding.

V. ALTERATIONS IN SENSORY/PERCEPTUAL PATTERNS related to DIZZINESS, SOMNOLENCE

Defining Characteristics: Dizziness, headache, somnolence occur rarely.

Nursing Implications: Assess baseline neurologic function and comfort, and monitor during treatment. Instruct patient to report any changes. Discuss any abnormalities with physician.

VI. ALTERATIONS IN COMFORT related to LOCAL INJECTION IRRITATION

Defining Characteristics: Pain, induration, and sterile abscesses may form in IM injection sites; phlebitis may develop in IV sites.

Nursing Implications: Rotate IM injection sites, and administer drug deep IM in large muscle mass (e.g., gluteus maximus). Use IM injection when IV administration is not possible. Change IV sites q48h, and assess for signs/symptoms of phlebitis prior to each administration. Administer drug slowly. Apply warm packs to increase comfort.

Drug: cefuroxime (Ceftin; Kefurox; Zinacef)

Class: Second-generation cephalosporin antibiotic.

Mechanism of Action: Semisynthetic derivative of cephalosporin C; contains beta-lactam ring, and is related to penicillins and cephamycins. Bactericidal through inhibition of cell wall synthesis by binding to one or more of the penicillin-binding proteins (PSPs) that in turn inhibit the final transpeptidation step of peptidoglycan synthesis in bacterial cell walls, thus inhibiting cell wall biosynthesis. Bacteria eventually lyse due to ongoing activity of cell wall autolytic enzymes (autolysins and murein hydrolases) while cell wall assembly is arrested.

Metabolism: Widely distributed in body tissues, fluids; crosses blood-brain barrier, therapeutic concentrations achieved in cerebrospinal fluid even when meninges are not inflamed; readily crosses placenta and is excreted in breast milk. Unchanged drug rapidly excreted by the kidneys.

Dosage/Range:
- Oral (adult): 250–500 mg twice daily for 10 days.
- IM & IV (adult): 750 mg to 1.5 g/dose every 8 hours or 100–150 mg/kg/day in divided doses every 6–8 hours; maximum dose—6 g/24 hours.

Drug Preparation/Administration:
- Refrigerate suspension; solution stable for 48 hours.
- IV infusion in NS or D5W solution stable for 7 days when refrigerated.

Drug Interactions:
- Probenecid: increased serum concentrations of cefotetan, but does not usually require dose reduction of antibiotic.
- Aminoglycosides: can increase nephrotoxicity.

Lab Effects/Interference:
- Serum ALT (SGPT), serum Alk Phos, serum AST (SGOT), and serum bilirubin—values may be increased.
- BUN and serum creatinine—concentrations may be increased.

Special Considerations:
- Use cautiously if renal impairment is present.
- Contraindicated if hypersensitive to other cephalosporins, or if has had angioedema response to penicillin.

Potential Toxicities/Side Effects and the Nursing Process

I. POTENTIAL FOR INJURY related to HYPERSENSITIVITY REACTION

Defining Characteristics: Urticaria, pruritis, rash (maculopapular or erythematous), fever and chills, eosinophilia, myalgia, edema, erythema, angioedema. Increased risk in individuals allergic to penicillin.

Nursing Implications: Assess allergy to cephalosporin antibiotics and penicillin: if patient states "yes," determine actual response, e.g., "swollen lips = angioedema." If angioedema, patient SHOULD NOT receive drug. Discuss other patient responses with physician to determine whether drug should be given. Assess baseline skin condition, including integrity and allergy history to drugs. Teach patient to report rash, itching, and other skin changes. Teach patient skin care and symptomatic measures as appropriate. If skin rash develops, discuss drug discontinuance with physician.

II. ALTERATION IN NUTRITION, LESS THAN BODY REQUIREMENTS, related to GI SIDE EFFECTS

Defining Characteristics: Nausea, vomiting, diarrhea, and anorexia may occur. May cause transient increases in LFTs.

Nursing Implications: Assess baseline nutritional status. Teach patient to report GI disturbances. Administer and teach patient to self-administer antiemetics as needed and as ordered. Teach patient importance of nutritious diet, and suggest small, frequent, high-calorie, high-protein meals as appropriate. Assess baseline LFTs and monitor periodically during treatment. Discuss abnormalities and drug interruption with physician.

III. FUNGAL SUPERINFECTION related to REDISTRIBUTION OF ENDOGENOUS MICROORGANISMS

Defining Characteristics: Vaginal moniliasis, vaginitis may occur as endogenous bacteria are eliminated and normal fungal population expands.

Nursing Implications: Teach female patient to report vaginal itching or discharge. Discuss appropriate antifungal treatment with physician. Teach perineal hygiene and symptomatic management.

IV. KNOWLEDGE DEFICIT related to SELF-ADMINISTRATION OF MEDICATION

Defining Characteristics: Increased compliance when patient is instructed in self-care activities.

Nursing Implications: Assess knowledge re: infection and planned treatment. Teach about drug action, potential side effects, and when and how to take drug. Teach patient to report any possible side effects that occur.

Drug: cephalexin (Biocef; Keflex; Keftab)

Class: First-generation cephalosporin antibacterial.

Mechanism of Action: Semisynthetic derivative of cephalosporin C, contains beta-lactam ring, and is related to penicillins and cephamycins. Bactericidal through inhibition of cell wall synthesis by binding to one or more of the penicillin-binding proteins (PBPs) that in turn inhibits the final transpeptidation step of peptidoglycan synthesis in bacterial cell walls, thus inhibiting cell wall biosynthesis. Bacteria eventually lyse due to ongoing activity of cell wall autolytic enzymes (autolysins and murein hydrolases) while cell wall assembly is arrested.

Metabolism: Well absorbed from GI tract; delayed GI absorption if taken with food, but total amount of drug absorption is the same. Widely distributed in body tissues, fluids except cerebrospinal fluid; readily crosses placenta and is excreted in breast milk. Unchanged drug rapidly excreted by the kidneys.

Dosage/Range:
- Adults: 250–1000 mg every 6 hours, maximum—4 g/day.
- Dose reduce if creatinine clearance is reduced per manufacturer's recommendations.

Drug Preparation/Administration:
- Store suspension in refrigerator, discard after 14 days.
- Oral administration.

Drug Interactions:
- Aminoglycosides increase nephrotic potential and increase toxicity.
- Probenecid may decrease cephalosporin elimination and increase effect.

Lab Effects/Interference:
- Serum SGPT, serum Alk Phos, serum SGOT, serum bilirubin, or serum LDH—values may be increased.
- BUN and serum creatinine—concentrations may be increased.

Special Considerations:
- Use with caution in patients with renal dysfunction—dose reduction required if severe impairment exists.
- Contraindicated in patients hypersensitive to other cephalosporin antibiotics.
- Use cautiously if sensitive to penicillin; contraindicated if angioedema reaction to penicillin.
- Obtain ordered specimen and send for culture and sensitivity prior to first drug dose.

Potential Toxicities/Side Effects and the Nursing Process

I. POTENTIAL FOR INJURY related to HYPERSENSITIVITY REACTION

Defining Characteristics: Urticaria, pruritis, rash (maculopapular or erythematous), fever and chills, eosinophilia, myalgia, edema, erythema, angioedema. Increased risk in individuals allergic to penicillin.

Nursing Implications: Assess allergy to cephalosporin antibiotics and penicillin: if patient states "yes," determine actual response, e.g., "swollen lips = angioedema." If angioedema, patient SHOULD NOT receive drug. Discuss other patient responses with physician to determine whether drug should be given. Assess baseline skin condition, including integrity and allergy history to drugs. Teach patient to report rash, itching, other skin changes. Teach patient skin care and symptomatic measures as appropriate. If skin rash develops, discuss drug discontinuance with physician.

II. ALTERATION IN NUTRITION, LESS THAN BODY REQUIREMENTS, related to GI SIDE EFFECTS

Defining Characteristics: Nausea and vomiting and diarrhea and anorexia may occur. Rarely, transient increases in LFTs—AST (SGOT), ALT (SGPT), ALKPHOS, BR—may occur.

Nursing Implications: Assess baseline nutritional status. Teach patient to report GI disturbances. Administer and teach patient to self-administer medication as needed and as ordered. Teach patient importance of nutritious diet, and suggest small, frequent, high-calorie, high-protein meals as appropriate. Assess baseline LFTs and monitor periodically during treatment. Discuss abnormalities and drug interruption with physician.

III. FUNGAL SUPERINFECTION related to REDISTRIBUTION OF ENDOGENOUS MICROORGANISMS

Defining Characteristics: Vaginal moniliasis, vaginitis may occur as endogenous bacteria are eliminated and normal fungal population expands.

Nursing Implications: Teach female patient to report vaginal itching or discharge. Discuss appropriate antifungal treatment with physician. Teach perineal hygiene and symptomatic management.

Drug: cephapirin (Cefadyl; Cephapirin Sodium)

Class: First-generation cephalosporin antibacterial.

Mechanism of Action: Semisynthetic derivative of cephalosporin C, contains beta-lactam ring, and is related to penicillins and cephamycins. Bactericidal through inhibition of cell wall synthesis by binding to one or more of the penicillin-binding proteins (PBPs) that in turn inhibit the final transpeptidation step of peptidoglycan synthesis in bacterial cell walls, thus inhibiting cell wall biosynthesis. Bacteria eventually lyse due to ongoing activity of cell wall autolytic enzymes (autolysins and murein hydrolases) while cell wall assembly is arrested.

Metabolism: Well absorbed from GI tract; delayed GI absorption if taken with food, but total amount of drug absorption is the same. Widely distributed in body tissues, fluids except cerebrospinal fluid; readily crosses placenta and is excreted in breast milk. Unchanged drug rapidly excreted by the kidneys.

Dosage/Range:
- Adults: 500–1000 mg every 6 hours, maximum—4 g/day
- Dose reduce if creatinine clearance is reduced per manufacturer's recommendations.

Drug Preparation/Administration:
- Reconstituted solution is stable for 10 days when refrigerated.
- IV infusion in NS or D5W solution stable for 10 days when refrigerated.

Drug Interactions:
- Aminoglycosides increase nephrotic potential and increase toxicity.
- Probenecid may decrease cephalosporin elimination and increase effect.

Lab Effects/Interference:
- Serum SGPT, serum Alk Phos, serum SGOT, serum bilirubin, or serum LDH—values may be increased.
- BUN and serum creatinine—concentrations may be increased.

Special Considerations:
- Use with caution in patients with renal dysfunction—dose reduction required if severe impairment exists.
- Contraindicated in patients hypersensitive to other cephalosporin antibiotics.
- Use cautiously if sensitive to penicillin; contraindicated if angioedema reaction to penicillin.
- Obtain ordered specimen and send for culture and sensitivity prior to first drug dose.

Potential Toxicities/Side Effects and the Nursing Process

I. POTENTIAL FOR INJURY related to HYPERSENSITIVITY REACTION

Defining Characteristics: Urticaria, pruritis, rash (maculopapular or erythematous), fever and chills, eosinophilia, myalgia, edema, erythema, angioedema. Increased risk in individuals allergic to penicillin.

Nursing Implications: Assess allergy to cephalosporin antibiotics and penicillin: if patient states "yes," determine actual response, e.g., "swollen lips = angioedema." If angioedema, patient SHOULD NOT receive drug. Discuss other patient responses with physician to determine whether drug should be given. Assess baseline skin condition, including integrity and allergy history to drugs. Teach patient to report rash, itching, other skin changes. Teach patient skin care and symptomatic measures as appropriate. If skin rash develops, discuss drug discontinuance with physician.

II. ALTERATION IN NUTRITION, LESS THAN BODY REQUIREMENTS, related to GI SIDE EFFECTS

Defining Characteristics: Nausea and vomiting and diarrhea and anorexia may occur. Rarely, transient increases in LFTs—AST (SGOT), ALT (SGPT), ALKPHOS, BR—may occur.

Nursing Implications: Assess baseline nutritional status. Teach patient to report GI disturbances. Administer and teach patient to self-administer medication as needed and as ordered. Teach patient importance of nutritious diet, and suggest small, frequent, high-calorie, high-protein meals as appropriate. Assess baseline LFTs and monitor periodically during treatment. Discuss abnormalities and drug interruption with physician.

III. FUNGAL SUPERINFECTION related to REDISTRIBUTION OF ENDOGENOUS MICROORGANISMS

Defining Characteristics: Vaginal moniliasis, vaginitis may occur as endogenous bacteria are eliminated and normal fungal population expands.

Nursing Implications: Teach female patient to report vaginal itching or discharge. Discuss appropriate antifungal treatment with physician. Teach perineal hygiene and symptomatic management.

Drug: cephradine (Anspor, Velosef)

Class: First-generation cephalosporin antibacterial.

Mechanism of Action: Semisynthetic derivative of cephalosporin C (produced by fungus); contains β-lactam ring and is related to penicillins and cephamycins (e.g., cefoxitin). Bactericidal through inhibition of cell wall synthesis, with resulting cell wall instability and cell lysis. Active against many gram-positive aerobic cocci (streptococci, staphylococci) and has limited gram-negative activity (*Klebsiella, H. influenzae, E. coli, Proteus*). Used in treatment of infections of respiratory tract, GU tract, skin, bone and joint, and in meningitis, sepsis.

Metabolism: Poorly absorbed from GI tract so must be given parenterally. Widely distributed throughout body tissues and fluids, including CSF; 65–79% protein-bound. Crosses placenta and is excreted in breast milk. Metabolized in liver and kidneys and is excreted in the urine.

Dosage/Range:
- Adult: 500 mg–1 g IM or IV q4–6h; and in life-threatening infections, 2 g q4h.
- Dose reduction in renal insufficiency according to manufacturer's package insert.

Drug Preparation/Administration:
- Store vial of powder for injection at < 40°C (< 104°F), and frozen injection containers at ≤ −20° (−4°F).

- IV: Reconstitute with at least 10 mL sterile water for injection according to manufacturer's package insert. Further dilute in 100 mL 0.9% Sodium Chloride or 5% Dextrose injection and administer over 30–60 minutes.
- IM: Reconstitute each gram of drug with 4 mL sterile water for injection. Administer deep IM in large muscle mass (e.g., gluteus maximus).

Drug Interactions:

- Probenecid: increased serum concentrations of antibiotic; monitor and decrease dose if needed.
- Aminoglycosides, penicillins: may have synergistic antibacterial effect against some organisms.
- Nephrotoxic drugs (aminoglycosides, colistin, vancomycin): may increase risk of renal dysfunction; avoid if possible.

Lab Effects/Interference:

Major clinical significance:

- Coombs' (antiglobulin) tests: a positive reaction frequently appears in patients who receive large doses of cephalosporins; hemolysis rarely occurs, but it has been reported; test may be positive in neonates whose mothers received cephalosporins before delivery.
- Urine glucose: some cephalosporins (cephradine) may produce a false-positive or falsely elevated test results with copper sulfate tests (Benedict's, Fehling's, or Clinitest); glucose enzymatic tests (Clinistix and Testape) are not affected.
- PT: may be prolonged; cephalosporins may inhibit vitamin K synthesis by suppressing gut flora.

Clinical significance:

- Serum ALT, serum alk phos, serum AST, serum bili, or serum LDH values may be increased.
- BUN and serum creatinine concentrations may be increased.
- CBC or platelet count: transient leukopenia, neutropenia, agranulocytosis, thrombocytopenia, eosinophilia, lymphocytosis, and thrombocytosis have been seen on rare occasions.

Special Considerations:

- Use with caution in patients with renal dysfunction; dose reduction required if severe impairment exists.
- Use cautiously if history of colitis exists.
- Contraindicated in patients hypersensitive to other cephalosporin antibiotics.
- Use cautiously if sensitive to penicillin; contraindicated if angioedema reaction to penicillin.
- Obtain specimen and send for culture and sensitivity prior to first drug dose.
- May cause false-positive direct Coombs' test.

- May cause false-positive Clinitest glucose result.

Potential Toxicities/Side Effects and the Nursing Process

I. POTENTIAL FOR INJURY related to HYPERSENSITIVITY REACTION

Defining Characteristics: Urticaria, pruritus, rash (maculopapular or erythematous), fever and chills, eosinophilia, myalgia, edema, erythema, angioedema, Stevens-Johnson syndrome, and exfoliative skin reactions occur in 5% of patients. Increased risk in individuals allergic to penicillin.

Nursing Implications: Assess allergy to cephalosporin antibiotics and penicillin: if patient states "yes," determine actual response, e.g., "swollen lips = angioedema." If angioedema, patient SHOULD NOT receive drug. Discuss other patient responses with physician to determine whether drug should be given. Assess baseline skin condition, including integrity and allergy history to drugs. Instruct patient to report rash, itching, other skin changes. Teach patient skin care and symptomatic measures as appropriate. If skin rash develops, discuss drug discontinuance with physician. If rash progresses, drug should be discontinued, as fatal Stevens-Johnson syndrome may develop. Be prepared to treat severe acute hypersensitivity reactions with airway management, oxygen, epinephrine, corticosteroids, antihistamines as ordered.

II. ALTERATION IN NUTRITION, LESS THAN BODY REQUIREMENTS, related to GI SIDE EFFECTS

Defining Characteristics: Nausea, vomiting, diarrhea, anorexia may occur; rarely, pseudomembranous colitis caused by *C. difficile* resistant to the antibiotic occurs. Rarely, transient increases in LFTs—AST, ALT, alk phos, bili—may occur.

Nursing Implications: Assess baseline nutritional status. Instruct patient to report GI disturbances. Administer and teach patient to self-administer antiemetics as needed and as ordered. Teach patient importance of nutritious diet, and suggest small, frequent, high-calorie, high-protein meals as appropriate. Assess baseline LFTs and monitor periodically during treatment. Discuss abnormalities and drug interruption with physician.

III. FUNGAL SUPERINFECTION related to REDISTRIBUTION OF ENDOGENOUS MICROORGANISMS

Defining Characteristics: Vaginal candidiasis, vaginitis may occur as endogenous bacteria are eliminated and normal fungal population expands.

Nursing Implications: Instruct female patient to report vaginal itching or discharge. Discuss appropriate antifungal treatment with physician. Teach perineal hygiene and symptomatic management.

IV. ALTERATIONS IN PROTECTIVE MECHANISMS (RARE) related to TRANSIENT LEUKOPENIA

Defining Characteristics: Rarely, transient leukopenia, lymphocytosis, anemia, eosinophilia may occur. Prolonged PT, prolonged APTT, and hypoprothrombinemia have occurred rarely, especially in elderly or debilitated patients, or in individuals with vitamin K deficiency.

Nursing Implications: Assess baseline laboratory parameters, and monitor periodically during treatment. Assess patient for response to antibiotics. Discuss abnormalities with physician.

V. ALTERATIONS IN SENSORY/PERCEPTUAL PATTERNS related to DIZZINESS, SOMNOLENCE

Defining Characteristics: Dizziness, headache, somnolence occur rarely.

Nursing Implications: Assess baseline neurologic function and comfort, and monitor during treatment. Instruct patient to report any changes. Discuss any abnormalities with physician.

VI. ALTERATIONS IN COMFORT related to LOCAL INJECTION IRRITATION

Defining Characteristics: Pain, induration, sterile abscesses may form in IM injection sites; phlebitis may develop in IV sites.

Nursing Implications: Rotate IM injection sites, and administer drug deep IM in large muscle mass (e.g., gluteus maximus). Use IM injection when IV administration is not possible. Change IV sites q48h, and assess for signs/symptoms of phlebitis prior to each administration. Administer drug slowly. Apply warm packs to increase comfort.

VII. KNOWLEDGE DEFICIT related to SELF-ADMINISTRATION OF MEDICATION

Defining Characteristics: Increased compliance when patient is instructed in self-care activities.

Nursing Implications: Assess knowledge about infection and planned treatment. Teach about drug action, potential side effects, and when and how to take drug. Teach patient to report any side effects that occur.

Drug: ciprofloxacin (Cipro)

Class: Fluoroquinolone.

Mechanism of Action: Antiinfective; appears to inhibit DNA replication in susceptible bacteria. Has a broad spectrum, and is active against most gramnegative bacteria (e.g., *Enterobacter, Pseudomonas*), some gram-positive organisms (e.g., methicillin-resistant staphylococci), and some mycobacteria.

Metabolism: Well absorbed from GI tract; rate decreased by food but not extent of absorption. Widely distributed in body tissues and fluids with highest concentrations in organs, such as liver, kidneys, and lungs. Partially metabolized in liver; excreted in urine and feces. Crosses placenta and is excreted in breast milk.

Dosage/Range:
- 250–750 mg q12h × 1–2 weeks.
- IV: 200–400 mg q12h × 1–2 weeks (IV used if patient unable to take oral formulation).
- Dose modification necessary if renal impairment exists.

Drug Preparation/Administration:
- Oral: Take drug with 1 large glass of fluid, preferably 2 hours after meal/food. Encourage oral fluids of 2–3 qt(liters)/day.
- IV: Further dilute drug in 0.9% Sodium Chloride or 5% Dextrose in water to final concentration of < 2 mg/mL. Administer over 60 minutes.

Drug Interactions:
- Antacids (containing magnesium, aluminum, or calcium): decrease oral ciprofloxacin serum level; do not administer concurrently. If must administer antacids, administer at least 2 hours apart.
- Other antiinfectives: potential synergism with clindamycin, aminoglycosides, β-lactam antibiotics against certain organisms.
- Probenecid: 50% increase in ciprofloxacin serum levels; decrease ciprofloxacin dose if given concurrently.
- Theophylline: increases theophylline serum level; avoid if possible since fatal reactions have occurred. Otherwise, monitor theophylline level very closely and decrease theophylline dose as needed.
- Caffeine: delays caffeine clearance from body. Instruct patient to limit coffee, tea, soft drinks, especially if CNS side effects.

Lab Effects/Interference:
- Serum ALT, serum alk phos, serum AST, and serum LDH values may be increased.

Special Considerations:

- Used in the treatment of infections of urinary and lower respiratory tract, skin, bone and joint, and GI tract, as well as gonorrhea.
- Contraindicated in pregnancy and in women who are breast-feeding.
- Obtain ordered specimen for culture and sensitivity prior to first drug dose.
- Use cautiously in patients with seizure disorders.
- Use cautiously in patients receiving concurrent theophylline, as cardiopulmonary arrest has occurred.

Potential Toxicities/Side Effects and the Nursing Process

I. ALTERATION IN NUTRITION, LESS THAN BODY REQUIREMENTS, related to GI SIDE EFFECTS

Defining Characteristics: 2–10% incidence of nausea, vomiting, abdominal discomfort, diarrhea, anorexia.

Nursing Implications: Assess baseline nutritional and elimination status. Instruct patient to report GI disturbances. Administer and teach patient to selfadminister antiemetics, antidiarrheals as needed and as ordered. Teach patient importance of nutritious diet, and suggest small, frequent, high-calorie, high-protein meals as appropriate. Assess baseline LFTs and monitor periodically during treatment. Discuss abnormalities and drug interruption with physician. Assess whether taking other hepatotoxic drugs. (See Special Considerations section.)

II. ALTERATIONS IN SENSORY/PERCEPTUAL PATTERNS related to CNS EFFECTS

Defining Characteristics: 1–2% incidence of headache, restlessness. Dizziness, hallucinations, and seizures may also occur. Exacerbated by caffeine, as ciprofloxacin delays caffeine excretion.

Nursing Implications: Assess baseline neurologic function and comfort, and monitor during treatment. Instruct patient to report any changes. Discuss any abnormalities with physician. Teach patient to limit or restrict all caffeinecontaining fluids, medications, e.g., tea, coffee, soft drinks containing caffeine.

III. ALTERATION IN SKIN INTEGRITY related to ALLERGY/HYPERSENSITIVITY

Defining Characteristics: 1–4% incidence of rash; other manifestations include eosinophilia, urticaria, flushing, fever, chills, photosensitivity, angioedema. Fatal hypersensitivity reactions have occurred rarely. Direct exposure to sunlight can cause sunburn (moderate to severe phototoxicity).

Nursing Implications: Assess baseline skin condition, including integrity and drug allergy history. Instruct patient to report rash, itching, other skin changes. Teach patient skin care and symptomatic measures as appropriate. If skin rash develops, discuss drug discontinuance with physician. If rash progresses, especially in HIV-infected patients, drug should be discontinued as fatal Stevens-Johnson syndrome may develop. Be prepared to treat severe acute hypersensitivity reactions with airway management, oxygen, epinephrine, corticosteroids, antihistamines as ordered. Instruct patient to avoid excessive sun exposure and to use skin protection factor (SPF) 15 or higher.

IV. ALTERATION IN URINARY ELIMINATION related to RENAL TOXICITY

Defining Characteristics: Increased BUN and creatinine, crystal and stone formation in urine, interstitial nephritis, and renal failure may occur.

Nursing Implications: Assess baseline renal function; expect that drug dose will be decreased in presence of renal dysfunction. Instruct patient to take drug with at least 8 oz (240 mL) of water, and to increase oral fluids to 2–3 qt/day.

V. ALTERATION IN COMFORT related to IV ADMINISTRATION

Defining Characteristics: Drug may cause pain, inflammation, and rare thrombophlebitis at IV site.

Nursing Implications: Change IV site q48h. Assess for phlebitis, discomfort, and IV patency prior to each administration. Administer drug slowly over 60–90 minutes in large volume of 5% Dextrose (see Drug Preparation/Administration). Apply heat to promote comfort.

VI. FUNGAL SUPERINFECTION related to REDISTRIBUTION OF ENDOGENOUS MICROORGANISMS

Defining Characteristics: Vaginal candidiasis, vaginitis may occur as endogenous bacteria are eliminated and normal fungal population expands.

Nursing Implications: Instruct female patient to report vaginal itching or discharge. Discuss appropriate antifungal treatment with physician. Teach perineal hygiene and symptomatic management.

Drug: clarithromycin (Biaxin; Biaxin XL)

Class: Antibacterial (macrolide).

Mechanism of Action: Clarithromycin exerts its antibacterial action by binding to 50S ribosomal subunit resulting in inhibition of protein synthesis. The

14-OH metabolite of clarithromycin is twice as active as the parent compound against certain organisms.

Metabolism: Rapidly and widely distributed throughout the body. Highly stable in presence of gastric acid (unlike erythromycin); food delays but does not affect extent of absorption. Widely distributed in body tissues but does not cross blood brain barrier into CSF. Metabolized by liver and excreted by kidneys into urine.

Dosage/Range:

- Adults: Usual dosage 250–500 mg every 12 hours or 1000 mg (two 500 mg extended release tablets) once daily for 7–14 days.
- Children ≥ 6 months: 15 mg/kg/day divided every 12 hours for 10 days.

Drug Preparation/Administration:

- Store tablets and granules for oral suspension at controlled room temperature.
- Reconstituted oral suspension should not be refrigerated because it might gel.
- Microencapsulated particles of clarithromycin in suspension are stable for 14 days when stored at room temperature.

Drug Interactions:

- Alfentanil (and possible other narcotic analgesics): Serum levels may be increased by clarithromycin—monitor for increased effect.
- Astemizole: Concomitant use is contraindicated—may lead to QT prolongation or torsade de pointes.
- Benzodiazepines (those metabolized CYP3A4, including alprazolam and triazolam): Serum levels may be increased by clarithromycin—somnolence and confusion have been reported.
- Bromocriptine: Serum levels may be increased by clarithromycin—monitor for increased effect.
- Buspirone: Serum levels may be increased by clarithromycin—monitor.
- Calcium channel blockers (felodipine, verapamil, and potentially others metabolized by CYP3A4): Serum levels may be increased by clarithromycin—monitor.
- Carbamazepine: Serum levels may be increased by clarithromycin—monitor.
- Cisapride: Serum levels may be increased by clarithromycin—monitor.
- Cilostazol: Serum levels may be increased by clarithromycin—monitor.
- Clozapine: Serum levels may be increased by clarithromycin—monitor.
- Cyclosporine: Serum levels may be increased by clarithromycin—monitor serum levels.
- Delavirdine: Serum levels may be increased by clarithromycin.

- Digoxin: Serum levels may be increased by clarithromycin; digoxin toxicity and potentially fatal arrhythmias have been reported; monitor digoxin levels.
- Dispyramide: Serum levels may be increased by clarithromycin—monitor.
- Ergot alkaloids: Concurrent use may lead to acute ergot toxicity (severe peripheral vasospasm and dysesthesia).
- Fluconazole: Increases clarithromycin levels and AUC by ~25%.
- Indinavir: Serum levels may be increased by clarithromycin—monitor.
- Loratadine: Serum levels may be increased by clarithromycin—monitor.
- Neuromuscular-blocking agents: May be potentate by clarithromycin (case reports)
- Oral contraceptives: Serum levels may be increased by clarithromycin—monitor.
- Phenytoin: Serum levels may be increased by clarithromycin; other evidence suggests phenytoin levels may be decreased in some patients—monitor.
- Pimozide: Serum levels may be increased, leading to malignant arrhythmias; concomitant use is contraindicated.
- Quinolone antibiotics (sparfloxacin, gatifloxacin, or moxifloxacin): Concomitant use may increase the risk of malignant arrhythmias—avoid concomitant use.
- Rifabutin: Serum levels may be increased by clarithromycin—monitor.
- Ritonavir: Concurrent use results in a 77% increase in clarithromycin levels (100% increase in metabolite levels); may be given together without dosage adjustment in patients with normal renal function; dosage of clarithromycin must be decreased in renal impairment.
- Sildenafil: Serum levels may be increased by clarithromycin—monitor.
- Tacrolimus: Serum levels may be increased by clarithromycin—monitor serum concentrations.
- Terfenadine: Serum levels may be increased by clarithromycin; may lead to QT prolongation, ventricular tachycardia, ventricular fibrillation or torsade de pointes; concomitant use is contraindicated.
- Theophylline: Serum levels may be increased by clarithromycin (by as much as 20%)—monitor.
- Valproic acid (and derivatives): Serum levels may be increased by clarithromycin—monitor.
- Warfarin: Effects may be potentiated—monitor INR closely and adjust warfarin dose as needed or choose another antibiotic.
- Zidovudine: Peak levels (but not AUC) of zidovudine may be increased—other studies suggest levels may be decreased.
- St. John's Wort: May decrease clarithromycin levels.
- CYP3A3/4 enzyme substrate—CYP1A2 and 3A3/4 enzyme inhibitor.

Lab Effects/Interference:
- PT/INR—may be prolonged.
- Serum SGPT, serum Alk Phos, serum SGOT, serum bilirubin, or serum LDH—values may be increased.
- BUN and serum creatinine—concentrations may be increased.

Special Considerations:
- Use with caution in patients with renal dysfunction—dose reduction required if severe impairment exists.
- Do not use when there is known hypersensitivity to erythromycins or other macrolides.
- Obtain ordered specimen and send for culture and sensitivity prior to first drug dose.

Potential Toxicities/Side Effects and the Nursing Process

I. POTENTIAL FOR INJURY related to HYPERSENSITIVITY REACTION

Defining Characteristics: Urticaria, pruritis, rash (maculopapular or erythematous), fever and chills, eosinophilia, myalgia, edema, erythema, angioedema.

Nursing Implications: Assess allergy to erythromycin: if patient states "yes," determine actual response, e.g., "swollen lips = angioedema." If angioedema, patient SHOULD NOT receive drug. Discuss other patient responses with physician to determine whether drug should be given. Assess baseline skin condition, including integrity and allergy history to drugs. Teach patient to report rash, itching, other skin changes. Teach patient skin care and symptomatic measures as appropriate. If skin rash develops, discuss drug discontinuance with physician.

II. ALTERATION IN NUTRITION, LESS THAN BODY REQUIREMENTS, related to GI SIDE EFFECTS

Defining Characteristics: Abdominal pain, diarrhea, nausea, and vomiting may occur.

Nursing Implications: Assess baseline nutritional status, preexisting nausea/vomiting, anorexia. Assess baseline LFTs and monitor periodically during treatment. Teach patient to report GI disturbances. Administer and teach patient to self-administer symptomatic interventions if side effects occur; discuss with physician use of alternative drug(s).

III. FUNGAL SUPERINFECTION related to REDISTRIBUTION OF ENDOGENOUS MICROORGANISMS

Defining Characteristics: Vaginal moniliasis, vaginitis may occur as endogenous bacteria are eliminated and normal fungal population expands.

Nursing Implications: Teach female patient to report vaginal itching or discharge. Discuss appropriate antifungal treatment with physician. Teach perineal hygiene and symptomatic management.

IV. ALTERATIONS IN PROTECTIVE MECHANISMS (RARE)

Defining Characteristics: Prolonged PT, prolonged INR, and hypoprothrombinemia have occurred rarely, especially in elderly or debilitated patients, or in individuals with vitamin K deficiency.

Nursing Implications: Assess baseline laboratory parameters, and monitor periodically during treatment. Assess patient for response to antibiotics. Discuss abnormalities with physician. Assess for signs/symptoms of bleeding. If they occur, especially in elderly or debilitated patients, discuss vitamin K administration with physician. Teach patient to avoid aspirin. If taking oral anticoagulants, assess for increased PT, signs/symptoms of bleeding.

Drug: clindamycin phosphate (Cleocin)

Class: Antibacterial (systemic); antiprotozoal.

Mechanism of Action: Bacteriostatic or bactericidal depending on drug concentration or when used against highly susceptible organisms; binds to bacterial ribosomes and prevent peptide bond formation, thus inhibiting protein synthesis. Active against gram-positive cocci (e.g., staphylococci, streptococci) and some anaerobic gram-positive and gram-negative bacilli (e.g., clostridia, mycobacteria).

Metabolism: Well absorbed (90% of dose) from GI tract. Food may delay absorption but does not affect amount absorbed. Widely distributed in body tissues and fluids, including bile. Crosses placenta and is excreted in breast milk. Excreted in urine, bile, and feces.

Dosage/Range:

Adult:

- Oral: 150–450 mg PO q6h; IM/IV: 300 mg q6–12h (maximum 2.7 g/day).

Drug Preparation/Administration:

- Oral: Administer with 8 oz (240 mL) of water to prevent esophageal irritation.
- IM: Single dose should not exceed 600 mg.

- Further dilute in 0.9% Sodium Chloride or 5% Dextrose in water to final concentration < 12 mg/mL, and infuse over 20 minutes (600-mg dose) or 30–40 minutes (1.2-g dose). Maximum 1.2 gm in single 1-hour period. May be given as continuous infusion.

Drug Interactions:
- Neuromuscular blocking agents (tubocurarine, ether, pancuronium): may increase neuromuscular blockade; use concurrently with caution.
- Erythromycin: decreases bactericidal activity of clindamycin.
- Kaolin: decreases GI absorption of clindamycin. Avoid concurrent administration, or administer at least 2 hours apart.

Lab Effects/Interference:
- Serum ALT, serum alk phos, and serum AST concentrations may be increased.

Special Considerations:
- Contraindicated in patients with hypersensitivity to clindamycin or lincomycin; contraindicated in patients with history of colitis.
- Can cause severe, sometimes fatal colitis. Stop drug if diarrhea develops, or if necessary, continue only under close monitoring and endoscopy.
- Used in the treatment of serious infections of respiratory tract, skin/soft tissues, female pelvic/genital tract. May be used investigationally with other drugs in treatment of *Mycobacterium avium* complex (MAC); also may be used to treat *P. carinii* pneumonia, cryptosporidiosis, and toxoplasmosis in AIDS patients.
- Also used for prophylaxis of bacterial endocarditis in penicillin-allergic, erythromycin-intolerant patients.
- DO NOT GIVE rapid IVB: cardiopulmonary arrest has occurred.
- Avoid use in pregnant or breast-feeding women.

Potential Toxicities/Side Effects and the Nursing Process

I. ALTERATION IN NUTRITION, LESS THAN BODY REQUIREMENTS, related to GI SIDE EFFECTS

Defining Characteristics: Nausea, vomiting, diarrhea, abdominal pain, and tenesmus may occur. Flatulence, bloating, anorexia, and esophagitis may occur as well. Fatal pseudomembranous colitis has occurred, characterized by severe diarrhea, abdominal cramping, and melena. Usually begins 2–9 days after drug is initiated.

Nursing Implications: Assess elimination and nutrition pattern, baseline and during therapy. Instruct patient to report diarrhea and/or abdominal pain immediately. Discuss drug discontinuance with physician if diarrhea occurs. Guaiac stool for occult blood, and notify physician if positive. If severe diarrhea develops, discuss management plan including endoscopy, fluid and electrolyte replacement. Do not administer antiperistaltic agents such as opiates and diphenoxylate with atropine (Lomotil), since it may worsen condition. Assess for nausea/vomiting, and administer prescribed antiemetic medications. Encourage small, frequent feedings as tolerated. Instruct patient to take oral dose with a full glass of water.

II. ALTERATION IN SKIN INTEGRITY related to HYPERSENSITIVITY

Defining Characteristics: Maculopapular rash, urticaria may occur. Rarely, erythema multiforme may occur. Increased risk of allergic reaction in asthma patients. Anaphylaxis may rarely occur.

Nursing Implications: Assess baseline allergy history. Assess baseline skin integrity. Instruct patient to report rash, pruritus. Teach patient symptomatic management of rash, pruritus. Assess for hypersensitivity reaction: if it occurs, monitor vital signs (VS), discontinue drug, notify physician, and institute supportive measures.

III. ALTERATION IN COMFORT related to LOCAL ADMINISTRATION EFFECTS

Defining Characteristics: IM administration may cause pain, induration, sterile abscesses, and transient increase in creatine phosphokinase (CPK) due to muscle injury. IV administration may cause erythema, pain, swelling, and thrombophlebitis.

Nursing Implications: Administer maximum 600-mg dose IM deeply in large muscle mass (e.g., gluteus maximus). Rotate sites. Assess IV site prior to each dose for phlebitis or swelling, and change site at least q48h. Administer dose slowly: 300–600 mg in 50 mL over 20–30 minutes, and 900–1200-mg dose in 100 mL IV over 40–60 minutes. Apply heat to painful IV sites as ordered.

IV. ALTERATION IN HEPATIC FUNCTION related to TRANSIENT INCREASE LFTs

Defining Characteristics: Transient increases in serum bili, AST, alk phos have occurred.

Nursing Implications: Assess baseline LFTs, and monitor during therapy.

V. FUNGAL SUPERINFECTION related to REDISTRIBUTION OF ENDOGENOUS MICROORGANISMS

Defining Characteristics: Vaginal candidiasis, vaginitis may occur as endogenous bacteria are eliminated, and normal fungal population expands.

Nursing Implications: Instruct female patient to report vaginal itching or discharge. Discuss appropriate antifungal treatment with physician. Teach perineal hygiene and symptomatic management.

Drug: co-trimoxazole; trimethoprim and sulfamethoxazole (Bactrim, Bactrim DS, Cotrim, Septra)

Class: Sulfonamide antibacterial (systemic); antiprotozoal.

Mechanism of Action: Bactericidal by preventing folic acid synthesis so microorganism cannot undergo cell division (sequential inhibition of folic acid synthesis, first by sulfamethoxazole, then by trimethoprim). Active against gram-positive bacteria (streptococci, *S. aureus, Nocardia*), gram-negative bacteria (*Enterobacter, E. coli, Proteus, Klebsiella, Shigella*), and protozoa (*P. carinii*).

Metabolism: Rapidly absorbed from GI tract. Widely distributed into body tissues and fluids; crosses the placenta and is excreted in breast milk. Highly protein-bound. Metabolized by the liver and excreted in the urine.

Dosage/Range:

Adult:

- Oral: Trimethoprim 160 mg and sulfamethoxazole 800 mg (double-strength tablet DS) q12h × 7–14 days (depending on infection).
- Oral: *P. carinii* pneumonia prophylaxis: 1 DS tablet twice daily 2 days per week (typically consecutive) or 1 DS tablet every other day.
- IV: 10–20 mg/kg in two to four divided doses q6–8h (usually 21 days for *P. carinii* pneumonia in AIDS patients).
- Dose modification if renal impairment exists.

Drug Preparation:

- Oral tablets should be stored in tight, light-resistant containers; vials of powder for injection and suspension should be stored at 15–30°C (59–86°F).

Drug Administration:

- Oral: Administer with full (8 oz or 240 mL) glass of water.
- IV: Add each 5 mL of drug to 125 mL of 5% Dextrose in water ONLY. Stable for 6 hours. If patient is fluid restricted, can mix each 5 mL in 75 mL of 5% Dextrose immediately prior to administration and give within 2 hours. DO NOT REFRIGERATE. Administer over 60–90 minutes.

Drug Interactions:

- Warfarin: increases PT. Monitor PT closely and decrease dose of warfarin as needed.

- Sulfonylureas: increases hypoglycemic effect. Monitor blood glucose closely and reduce sulfonylurea dose as needed.
- Phenytoin: increases and prolongs serum levels. Monitor serum phenytoin level closely and reduce dose as needed.
- Thiazide diuretics (in elderly): increases toxicity (thrombocytopenia with purpura). AVOID CONCURRENT USE.
- Cyclosporine: decreases cyclosporine effect; increases risk of nephrotoxicity. AVOID CONCURRENT USE when possible.
- Methotrexate: increases methotrexate level and potential toxicity (e.g., bone marrow depression). Monitor levels or decrease methotrexate dose as needed.
- Oral contraceptives: decreases contraceptive effect. Monitor for breakthrough bleeding and counsel patient to use barrier contraceptive in addition during antibiotic therapy.
- Ammonium chloride or ascorbic acid: causes antibiotic drug precipitation in kidneys. AVOID CONCURRENT USE.

Lab Effects/Interference:

- Jaffe alkaline picrate reaction overestimation of creatinine by 10%.

Special Considerations:

- Drug is teratogenic, so should not be used in pregnant women if avoidable.
- Drug is excreted in breast milk and can cause kernicterus in infants. Alternative drug should be used or mother should interrupt breast-feeding during drug use.
- Contraindicated if patient has porphyria.
- Contraindicated in patients with hypersensitivity to sulfites, sulfonamides, or to trimethoprim.
- Contraindicated if severe renal failure (creatinine clearance < 15 mL/minute).
- Use with caution at reduced dosage in patients with glucose-6-phosphate dehydrogenase deficiency (G6PD); hemolysis may occur. Also, use with caution in patients with impaired renal or hepatic function, severe allergy, bronchial asthma, and blood dyscrasias.
- Use cautiously in patients with known hypersensitivity to sulfonamide-derivative drugs such as thiazides, acetazolamide, tolbutamide.
- Increased incidence of adverse side effects in AIDS patients, especially allergic, hematologic reactions. Monitor closely for toxicity.
- Drug is first line treatment for *P. carinii* pneumonia; it is at least as effective as pentamidine, with a cure rate of 70–80%.
- Send specimen for culture and sensitivity prior to initial drug dose, as appropriate.

Potential Toxicities/Side Effects and the Nursing Process

I. ALTERATION IN SKIN INTEGRITY related to HYPERSENSITIVITY REACTION

Defining Characteristics: Skin reactions ranging from mild maculopapular rash with urticaria, pruritus to erythema multiforme, exfoliative dermatitis, and Stevens-Johnson syndrome. Risk for rash is increased in AIDS patients; usually occurs 7–14 days after beginning drug. Other allergic manifestations include fever, chills, photosensitivity, angioedema, and anaphylaxis.

Nursing Implications: Assess for prior hypersensitivity to drug. Assess for signs/symptoms of drug allergy. Instruct patient to report rash, allergic reaction immediately. Discuss any drug continuance with physician if rash appears. Teach patient symptomatic management of discomfort and skin irritation. Be prepared to treat severe acute hypersensitivity reactions with airway management, oxygen, epinephrine, corticosteroids, antihistamines as ordered.

II. POTENTIAL FOR INFECTION, BLEEDING, AND FATIGUE related to HEMATOLOGIC TOXICITY

Defining Characteristics: Leukopenia, neutropenia, and thrombocytopenia are common in AIDS patients. Agranulocytosis, aplastic and megaloblastic anemia, thrombocytopenia, hemolytic anemia, neutropenia, hypoprothrombinemia, and eosinophilia may occur less commonly. Increased risk exists in folate-deficient patients: elderly, alcoholic, malnourished; also, patients receiving folate antimetabolites, e.g., phenytoin, methotrexate, or thiazide diuretics; or in patients with renal dysfunction.

Nursing Implications: Assess baseline risk, CBC, and monitor CBC periodically during treatment. Assess for and teach patient to monitor signs/symptoms of infection, bleeding, fatigue, and to report these. If side effects occur, discuss with physician use of folinic acid (leucovorin).

III. ALTERATIONS IN NUTRITION, LESS THAN BODY REQUIREMENTS, related to GI TOXICITY

Defining Characteristics: Nausea, vomiting, and anorexia are most common; pseudomembranous colitis, glossitis, stomatitis, abdominal pain, diarrhea may occur.

Nursing Implications: Assess GI function. Teach patient to assess for and instruct to report GI side effects, and to administer prescribed antiemetics or antidiarrheals as needed. Assess oral mucosa, and if stomatitis develops, discuss with physician use of leucovorin (folinic acid). Teach patient oral hygiene. Take drug with 8 oz (240 mL) water to prevent esophageal ulcerations. Discuss food preferences, use of spices, and suggest small, frequent meals if anorexia develops.

IV. SENSORY/PERCEPTUAL DYSFUNCTION related to FATIGUE, WEAKNESS

Defining Characteristics: Headache, vertigo, insomnia, fatigue, weakness, mental depression, seizures, and hallucinations may occur.

Nursing Implications: Assess baseline neurologic function and comfort, and monitor during treatment. Instruct patient to report any changes. Discuss any abnormalities with physician.

V. ALTERATION IN URINARY ELIMINATION related to RENAL TOXICITY

Defining Characteristics: Increased BUN and creatinine, crystal and stone formation in urine, interstitial nephritis, and renal failure may occur.

Nursing Implications: Assess baseline renal function; expect that drug dose will be decreased in presence of renal dysfunction. Instruct patient to take drug with at least 8 oz water and to increase oral fluids to 2–3 qt (liters)/day.

VI. ALTERATION IN COMFORT related to IV ADMINISTRATION

Defining Characteristics: Drug may cause pain, inflammation, and rare thrombophlebitis at IV site.

Nursing Implications: Change IV site q48h. Assess for phlebitis, discomfort, and IV patency prior to each administration. Administer drug slowly over 60–90 minutes in large volume of 5% Dextrose (see Drug Administration). Apply heat to promote comfort.

VII. FUNGAL SUPERINFECTION related to REDISTRIBUTION OF ENDOGENOUS MICROORGANISMS

Defining Characteristics: Vaginal candidiasis, vaginitis may occur as endogenous bacteria are eliminated and normal fungal population expands.

Nursing Implications: Instruct female patient to report vaginal itching or discharge. Discuss appropriate antifungal treatment with physician. Teach perineal hygiene and symptomatic management.

Drug: daptomycin (Cubicin)

Class: Cyclic lipopeptide antibiotic

Mechanism of Action: This antibiotic is the first in a new structural class. It is derived from the fermentation of *Streptomyces roseosporus*. The mechanism of action is not fully understood. Daptomycin binds to bacterial membranes and causes a rapid depolarization of membrane potential. This loss of membrane potential leads to inhibition of protein, DNA, and RNA synthesis resulting in bacterial cell death. It acts against Gram-positive bacteria, and retains in vitro potency against isolates resistant to methicillin, vancomycin, and linezolid.

Metabolism: Excreted by the kidney. Renal excretion is primary route of elimination.

Dosage/Range:
Adult: 4 mg/kg by IV infusion q d for 7–14 days
Drug dose should be reduced or adjusted in patients with severe renal insufficiency.

Drug Preparation/Administration:
- 0.9% sodium chloride injection
- Administer over 30 minutes

Drug Interactions:
- Tobramycin: interaction between daptomycin and tobramycin is unknown. Caution is warranted when daptomycin is co-administered with tobramycin.
- Warfarin: anticoagulant activity in patients receiving daptomycin and warfarin should be monitored for the first several days.

Lab Effects/Interference:
- There are no reported drug-laboratory test interactions.

Special Considerations:
- Contraindicated in patients with known hypersensitivity to daptomycin.
- Obtain ordered specimen and send for culture and sensitivity prior to first antibiotic dose.
- Consider alternative antibiotic therapy if anemia, drug rash or fever, arthralgia, or unexplained rise in BUN and serum creatinine occur.

Potential Toxicities/Side Effects and the Nursing Process

I. ALTERATION IN NUTRITION, LESS THAN BODY REQUIREMENTS, related to GI SIDE EFFECTS

Defining Characteristics: Constipation, nausea, diarrhea, vomiting, dyspepsia

Nursing Implications: Assess baseline nutritional status, preexisiting nausea/vomiting, anorexia. Assess baseline bowel pattern. Administer symptomatic interventions if side effects occur; discuss with physician use of alternative drug(s).

II. POTENTIAL FOR INJURY related to HYPERSENSITIVITY REACTION

Defining Characteristics: Rash, urticaria, pruritis, and fever can occur in individuals with hypersensitivity to daptomycin.

Nursing Implications: Assess for drug allergies prior to drug administration. Instruct patient to report any allergic reactions. Assess for signs/symptoms of allergic reaction after drug dose.

III. SENSORY/PERCEPTUAL ALTERATIONS related to CNS EFFECTS OF DIZZINESS AND HEADACHE

Defining Characteristics: Dizziness, headache and insomnia may occur.

Nursing Implications: Assess baseline neurological status. Teach patient about side effects and to report dizziness or headache. If signs/symptoms arise, discuss drug discontinuance with physican.

Drug: demeclocycline hydrochloride (Declomycin)

Class: Antibacterial (systemic); tetracycline; antiprotozoal

Mechanism of Action: Bacteriostatic but may be bactericidal at high concentrations. Binds to bacterial ribosomes and prevents protein synthesis. Active against broad range of Gram-negative and Gram-positive organisms. Demeclocycline hydrochloride may also be used in special cases of fluid retention (SIADH). A syndrome of polyuria, polydipesia, and weakness has been shown to be nephrogenic, dose-dependent, and reversible on discontinuation of therapy.

Metabolism: Absorbed from the GI tract. Widely distributed into body tissues and fluids. Crosses placenta and is excreted in breast milk. Concentrated in the liver, excreted into the bile. The rate of demeclocycline hydrochloride clearance is less than half that of tetracycline.

Dosage/Range:
Adult: Oral: 150 mg q 6 hours or 300 mg q 12 hours
- Duration of therapy depends on indication
- As treatment for hyponatremia: 600–1200 mg daily.
- Drug dose should be reduced or adjusted in patients with hepatic or renal insufficiency.

Drug Preparation/Administration:

- Oral: Take 1 hour before meals or 2 hours after meals. Dose reduce in patients with renal and liver impairment.

Drug Interactions:

- Oral anticoagulants: increase PT. Monitor patient closely and decrease anticoagulant dose as needed.
- Concurrent use of tetracyclines with oral contraceptives may render oral contraceptives less effective. Advise patient to use barrier contraceptive as well during a course of tetracycline therapy.
- Methoxyflurane: fatal renal toxicity has been reported with concurrent use.
- Iron preparations: decreases oral absorption. Administer iron preparations 3 hours after or 2 hours before any tetracycline.
- Antacids & antidiarrheals: may decrease absorption of tetracyclines. Avoid concurrent use.

Lab Effects/Interference:

- There are no reported drug-laboratory test interactions.
- SGPT, alk phos, Amylase, SGOT, and bilirubin: serum concentrations may be increased.

Special Considerations:

- Avoid use in pregnant or lactating women.
- Contraindicated in patients with known hypersensitivity to tetracyclines.
- Obtain ordered specimen and send for culture and sensitivity prior to first antibiotic dose.

Potential Toxicities/Side Effects and the Nursing Process

I. ALTERATION IN NUTRITION related to GI SIDE EFFECTS

Defining Characteristics: Anorexia, nausea, vomiting, diarrhea, glossitis, dysphagia, enterocolitis, pancreatitis.

Nursing Implications: Assess baseline nutritional status. Assess for and teach patient to report any symptoms. Administer and teach patient self-administration of prescribed antiemetic or antidiarrheal medication as appropriate. Administer and teach to self-administer oral dose with at least 8 oz of water at least 1 hour before or 2 hours after a meal or sleep.

II. ALTERATION IN SKIN INTEGRITY related to RASH, PHOTOSENSITIVITY

Defining Characteristics: Maculopapular and erythematous rash may occur. Photosensitivity risk (exaggerated sunburn) persists 1–2 days after completion of drug therapy.

Nursing Implications: Teach patient about potential side effects, to avoid sunlight during drug therapy, and to report rash, and other abnormalities. Teach symptomatic skin care as appropriate.

III. INJURY related to HYPERSENSITIVITY

Defining Characteristics: Urticaria, angioneurotic edema, anaphylaxis may occur; also fever, arthralgias, eosinophilia, and pericarditis.

Nursing Implications: Assess drug allergy history. Assess baseline allergy history. Assess baseline skin integrity. Teach patient to report rash, pruritis, Teach patient symptomatic management of rash, pruritis. Assess for hypersensitivity reacton: if it occurs, monitor VS, discontinues drug, notify physician, and institute supportive measures.

IV. FUNGAL SUPERINFECTION related to REDISTRIBUTION OF ENDOGENOUS MICROORGANISMS

Defining Characteristics: Vaginal moniliasis, vaginitis may occur as endogenous bacteria are eliminated and normal fungal population expands.

Nursing Implications: Teach female patient to report vaginal itching or discharge. Discuss appropriate antifungal treatment with physician. Teach perineal hygiene and symptom management.

Drug: dicloxacillin sodium (Dycill, Dynapen, Pathocil)

Class: Penicillin antibacterial.

Mechanism of Action: Semisynthetic antibiotic prepared from fungus *Penicillium.* Contains β-lactam ring and is bactericidal by inhibiting cell wall synthesis. Penicillinase-resistant and active against penicillin-resistant staphylococci, which produce the enzyme penicillinase. Used to treat upper and lower respiratory tract and skin infections.

Metabolism: Well absorbed from GI tract, but food decreases rate and extent of absorption. Widely distributed through body tissues and fluids; crosses placenta and is excreted in breast milk; 95–99% bound to serum proteins. Excreted in urine and bile.

Dosage/Range:

- Adult: 125 mg–500 mg PO q6h × 14 days (but depends on severity of infection).

Drug Preparation:

- Store in tight containers at < 40°C (104°F).

Drug Administration:

- Oral: administer at least 1 hour before or 2 hours after meals.

Drug Interactions:

- Aminoglycosides: synergism.
- Rifampin: possible antagonism, only at high doses of penicillin.
- Probenecid: increased serum level of penicillin; may be coadministered to exert this effect.

Lab Effects/Interference:

Major clinical significance:

- Urine glucose: high urinary concentrations of a penicillin may produce false-positive or falsely elevated test results with copper sulfate tests (Benedict's, Clinitest, or Fehling's); glucose enzymatic tests (Clinistix or Tes-tape) are not affected

Clinical significance:

- Coombs' (direct antiglobulin) test: false-positive result may occur during therapy with any penicillin.
- ALT, alk phos, AST, serum LDH values may be increased.
- WBC: leukopenia or neutropenia is associated with the use of all penicillins; the effect is more likely to occur with prolonged therapy and severe hepatic function impairment.

Special Considerations:

- Contraindicated in patients with prior hypersensitivity to penicillins. Use with caution in patients sensitive to other β-lactams (e.g., cephalosporins) since partial cross-allergenicity exists.
- Obtain ordered specimen and send for culture and sensitivity prior to first antibiotic dose.
- Consider alternative antibiotic therapy if eosinophilia, drug fever or rash, arthralgia, hematuria, or unexplained rise in BUN and serum creatinine occur.
- Monitor electrolytes and renal, hepatic, and hematologic laboratory parameters during extended treatment periods.
- Use with caution in pregnancy or with nursing women.

Potential Toxicities/Side Effects and the Nursing Process

I. POTENTIAL FOR INJURY related to HYPERSENSITIVITY REACTION

Defining Characteristics: Urticaria, pruritus, rash (maculopapular or erythematous), fever and chills, eosinophilia, myalgia, edema, erythema, angioedema, Stevens-Johnson syndrome, and exfoliative skin reactions occur in 5% of patients. Increased risk exists in individuals allergic to cephalosporin antibiotics.

Nursing Implications: Assess allergy to cephalosporin antibiotics and penicillin: if patient states "yes," determine actual response, e.g., "swollen lips = angioedema." If angioedema, patient SHOULD NOT receive drug. Discuss other patient responses with physician to determine whether drug should be given. Assess baseline skin condition, including integrity and allergy history to drugs. Instruct patient to report rash, itching, and other skin changes. Teach patient skin care and symptomatic measures as appropriate. If skin rash develops, discuss drug discontinuance with physician. If rash progresses, drug should be discontinued as fatal Stevens-Johnson syndrome may develop. Be prepared to treat severe acute hypersensitivity reactions with airway management, oxygen, epinephrine, corticosteroids, antihistamines as ordered.

II. ALTERATION IN NUTRITION, LESS THAN BODY REQUIREMENTS, related to GI SIDE EFFECTS

Defining Characteristics: Nausea, vomiting, diarrhea may occur; rarely, pseudomembranous colitis caused by *C. difficile* resistant to the antibiotic occurs. Rarely, transient increases in LFTs—AST, ALT, alk phos, bili—may occur.

Nursing Implications: Assess baseline nutritional status. Instruct patient to report GI disturbances. Administer and teach patient to self-administer antiemetics as needed and as ordered. Teach patient importance of nutritious diet, and suggest small, frequent, high-calorie, high-protein meals as appropriate. Assess baseline LFTs, and monitor periodically during treatment. Discuss abnormalities and drug interruption with physician.

III. FUNGAL SUPERINFECTION related to REDISTRIBUTION OF ENDOGENOUS MICROORGANISMS

Defining Characteristics: Vaginal candidiasis, vaginitis may occur as endogenous bacteria are eliminated and normal fungal population expands.

Nursing Implications: Instruct female patient to report vaginal itching or discharge. Discuss appropriate antifungal treatment with physician. Teach perineal hygiene and symptomatic management.

IV. ALTERATIONS IN PROTECTIVE MECHANISMS (RARE) related to TRANSIENT LEUKOPENIA

Defining Characteristics: Rarely, transient leukopenia, lymphocytosis, anemia, eosinophilia may occur. Prolonged PT, prolonged APTT, and hypoprothrombinemia have occurred rarely, especially in elderly or debilitated patients, or in individuals with vitamin K deficiency.

Nursing Implications: Assess baseline laboratory parameters, and monitor periodically during treatment. Assess patient for response to antibiotics. Discuss abnormalities with physician.

V. KNOWLEDGE DEFICIT related to SELF-ADMINISTRATION OF MEDICATION

Defining Characteristics: Increased compliance when patient is instructed in self-care activities.

Nursing Implications: Assess knowledge about infection and planned treatment. Teach about drug action, potential side effects, and when and how to take drug (take medication as directed, 1 hour before or 2 hours after food). Instruct patient to report any possible drug side effects that occur.

Drug: doxycycline hyclate (Vibramycin, Doryx, MonoDox)

Class: Antibacterial (systemic); antiprotozoal.

Mechanism of Action: Bacteriostatic but may be bactericidal at high concentrations. Binds to bacterial ribosomes and prevents protein synthesis. Active against broad range of gram-positive and gram-negative bacteria, Chlamydia, and Mycoplasma.

Metabolism: Absorbed (60%–80%) from GI tract. Widely distributed into body tissues and fluids. Crosses placenta and is excreted in breast milk. Excreted unchanged in urine.

Dosage/Range:

Adult:

- Oral: 100 mg q12 hours for the first day, then 100–200 mg once daily, or 50–100 mg q12 hours. Duration of therapy depends on indication.
- IV: 200 mg QD or 100 mg q12 hours for the first day, then 100–200 mg QD or 50–100 mg q12 hours. Duration of therapy depends on indication.

Drug Preparation/Administration:

- Oral: may be taken with food, water, milk, or carbonated beverages.
- IV: add 10 mL sterile water for injection to 100-mg vial or 20 mL to each 200-mg vial. Further dilute in 100 to 1000 mL or in 200 to 2000 ml, respectively, of lactated Ringer's injection or 5% dextrose and lactated Ringer's injection. Infuse over 1 to 4 hours.
- CONCENTRATIONS LESS THAN 100 MCG PER ML OR GREATER THAN 1 MG PER ML ARE NOT RECOMMENDED.
- AVOID RAPID ADMINISTRATION.

- Solution stable for 6 hours, so use after mixing. Avoid exposure to heat or sunlight. Convert to oral preparation as soon as possible as there is risk of thrombophlebitis.
- DO NOT ADMINISTER INTRAMUSCULARLY OR SUBCUTANEOUSLY.

Drug Interactions:
- Hepatotoxic drugs: may increase hepatotoxicity if given concurrently. Assess baseline and periodically during treatment.
- Iron preparations: decrease oral and possibly IV absorption. Administer iron preparations 3 hours after or 2 hours before any tetracycline.
- Oral anticoagulants: increase PT. Monitor patient closely and decrease anticoagulant dose as needed.
- Antidiarrheals (containing kaolin, pectate, or bismuth): may decrease absorption of tetracyclines. Avoid concurrent use.
- Oral contraceptives: decreased effectiveness of contraceptive and increased incidence of breakthrough bleeding. Advise patient to use barrier contraceptive as well during a course of tetracycline therapy.
- Lithium: may decrease lithium levels. Monitor serum levels and increase dose as needed.

Lab Effects/Interference:
- Urine catecholamine determinations: may produce false elevations of urinary catecholamines because of interfering fluorescence in the Hingerty method.
- SGPT, alk phos, Amylase, SGOT, and bilirubin: serum concentrations may be increased.

Special Considerations:
- Use cautiously in patients with myasthenia gravis: may increase muscle weakness.
- Avoid use in pregnant or lactating women.
- Obtain ordered specimen for culture and sensitivity prior to first dose.
- IV preparation contains ascorbic acid and may cause false-positive result using Clinitest, or false-negative result when using Clinistix and Testape.
- Drug has affinity for ischemic, necrotic tissue, and may localize in tumors.

Potential Toxicities/Side Effects and the Nursing Process

I. ALTERATION IN NUTRITION related to GI SIDE EFFECTS

Defining Characteristics: Nausea, vomiting, diarrhea, anorexia, abdominal discomfort, epigastric burning and distress, glossitis, black hairy tongue may occur.

Nursing Implications: Assess baseline nutritional status. Assess for and teach patient to report any symptoms. Administer and teach patient self-administration of prescribed antiemetic or antidiarrheal medication as appropriate. Administer and teach patient to self-administer oral dose with at least 8 oz of water taken at least 1 hour before lying down for sleep.

II. ALTERATION IN SKIN INTEGRITY related to RASH, PHOTOSENSITIVITY

Defining Characteristics: Maculopapular and erythematous rashes may occur. Rarely, exfoliative dermatitis, onycholyis, and nail discoloration. Photosensitivity risk (exaggerated sunburn) persists 1–2 days after completion of drug therapy.

Nursing Implications: Each patient about potential side effects, to avoid sunlight during drug therapy, and to report rash, other abnormalities. Teach symptomatic skin care as appropriate.

III. INJURY related to HYPERSENSITIVITY

Defining Characteristics: Urticaria, angioneurotic edema, anaphylaxis may occur; also, fever, rash, arthralgias, eosinophilia, and pericarditis.

Nursing Implications: Assess drug allergy history. Assess baseline allergy history. Assess baseline skin integrity. Teach patient to report rash, pruritus. Teach patient symptomatic management of rash, pruritus. Assess for hypersensitivity reaction: if it occurs, monitor VS, discontinue drug, notify physician, and institute supportive measures.

IV. FUNGAL SUPERINFECTION related to REDISTRIBUTION OF ENDOGENOUS MICROORGANISMS

Defining Characteristics: Vaginal moniliasis, vaginitis may occur as endogenous bacteria are eliminated, and normal fungal population expands.

Nursing Implications: Teach female patient to report vaginal itching or discharge. Discuss appropriate antifungal treatment with physician. Teach perineal hygiene and symptomatic management.

V. ALTERATION IN HEPATIC FUNCTION

Defining Characteristics: Associated with high IV doses (> 2 gm/day): hepatotoxicity and cholestasis may occur.

Nursing Implications: Assess baseline LFTs and monitor during therapy.

VI. INFECTION AND BLEEDING related to NEUTROPENIA, THROMBOCYTOPENIA

Defining Characteristics: Neutropenia, leukocytosis, leukopenia, atypical lymphocytes, thrombocytopenia, thrombocytopenic purpura, hemolytic anemia occur rarely with long-term therapy.

Nursing Implications: Assess baseline WBC, hematocrit, and platelets, and monitor periodically during long-term therapy.

VII. ALTERATION IN COMFORT related to LOCAL ADMINISTRATION EFFECTS

Defining Characteristics: IM administration may cause pain, induration due to muscle injury. IV administration may cause erythema, pain, swelling, and thrombophlebitis.

Nursing Implications: Rotate sites. Apply ice as ordered to painful buttock. Assess IV site prior to each dose for phlebitis or swelling and change site at least q 48 hours. Apply heat to painful IV sites as ordered.

VIII. SENSORY/PERCEPTUAL ALTERATION

Defining Characteristics: Light-headedness, dizziness, headache may occur.

Nursing Implications: Assess baseline neurological status. Teach patient to report any changes and discuss them with physician.

Drug: ertapenem sodium (Invanz)

Class: antibiotic, carbapenem.

Mechanism of Action: The bactericidal activity results from the inhibition of cell wall synthesis. Penetrates the cell wall of most gram-positive and gram-negative bacteria to reach penicillin-binding protein (PBP) targets.

Metabolism: Widely distributed in body tissues and fluids, excreted in urine.

Dosage/Range:

Adult:

- Acute Pelvic Infection: 1 gram IV/IM once a day for 3–10 days
- Community Acquired Pneumonia: 1 gram IV/IM once a day for 10–14 days
- Intrabdominal infection: 1 gram IV/IM once a day for 5–14 days
- Skin/Skin Structure Infections: 1 gram IV/IM once a day for 7–14 days
- Urinary Tract Infections: 1 gram IV/IM once a day for 10–14 days
- Adjust dose in patients with renal impairment and on hemodialysis

Drug Preparation/Administration:

- IV infusion for up to 14 days.
- IV infusion for up to 14 days.
- IM injection for up to 7 days.
- DO NOT DILUTE WITH Diluents containing dextrose.

Drug Interactions:

- Probenecid competes with ertapenem for active tubular secretion; increasing AUC by 25% and reducing the plasma and renal clearances by 20% and 35% respectively.

Lab Effects/Interference:

- Ertapenem posses the characteristic low toxicity of the beta-lactam group of antibiotics.
- Periodically assess organ system function: renal, hepatic & hematopoietic.

Potential Toxicities/Side Effects and the Nursing Process

I. POTENTIAL FOR INJURY related to HYPERSENSITIVITY REACTION and LOCAL REACTIONS (pain at injection site)

Defining Characteristics: Urticaria, pruritus, rash (maculopapular or erythematous), fever and chills, eosinophilia, myalgia, edema, erythema, angioedema.

Nursing Implications: Assess allergy to cephalosporin antibiotics and penicillin; if patient states ''yes,'' determine actual response, e.g., ''swollen lips = angioedema.'' If angioedema, patient SHOULD NOT receive drug. Discuss other patient responses with physician to determine whether drug should be given. Assess baseline skin condition, including integrity and allergy history to drugs. Instruct patient to report rash, itching, and other skin changes. Teach patient skin care and symptomatic measures as appropriate. If skin rash develops, discuss drug discontinuance with physician. Be prepared to treat severe acute hypersensitivity reactions with airway management, oxygen, epinephrine, corticosteroids, antihistamines as ordered.

II. ALTERATION IN NUTRITION, LESS THAN BODY REQUIREMENTS, related to GI SIDE EFFECTS

Defining Characteristics: Nausea, vomiting, diarrhea may occur; rarely, pseudomembranous colitis caused by antibiotic resistance occurs.

Nursing Implications: Assess baseline nutritional status. Instruct patient to report GI disturbances. Administer and teach patient to self-administer antiemetics as needed and as ordered. Teach patient importance of nutritious diet, and suggest small, frequent, high-calorie, high-protein meals as appropriate. Assess baseline LFTs, and monitor periodically during treatment. Discuss abnormalities and drug interruption with physician.

III. FUNGAL SUPERINFECTION related to REDISTRIBUTION OF ENDOGENOUS MICROORGANISMS

Defining Characteristics: Vaginal candidiasis, vaginitis may occur as endogenous bacteria are eliminated, and normal fungal population expands.

Nursing Implications: Instruct female patient to report vaginal itching or discharge. Discuss appropriate antifungal treatment with physician. Teach perineal hygiene and symptomatic management.

Drug: erythromycin (ERYC, E-Mycin, Illotycin, Erythrocin)

Class: Antibacterial (macrolide).

Mechanism of Action: Erythromycin is a broad spectrum antibiotic with activity against gram-positive and gram-negative bacteria, and other infectious agents, including *Chlamydia trachomatis,* mycoplasmas (*Mycoplasma pneumoniae* and *Ureaplasma urealyticum*), and spirochetes (*Treponema pallidum* and *Borrelia* species). Erythromycin has good activity against *S. pyogenes, Streptococcus pneumoniae (group A beta-hemolytic streptococci)*, and *Straphylococcus aureus*.

Erythromycin is a bacteriostatic macrolide antibiotic. It may be bactericidal in high concentrations or when used against highly susceptible organisms. It is thought to penetrate the bacterial cell membrane and to reversibly bind to the 50 S ribosomal subunit. It does not directly inhibit peptide formation rather, it inhibits the translocation of peptides from the acceptor site on the ribosome to the donor site, inhibiting subsequent protein synthesis. Effective against actively dividing organisms.

Metabolism: 90% of the drug is metabolized by the liver; may accumulate in patients with severe hepatic disease. Primarily excreted into the bile. Between 2 to 5% is excreted unchanged by the kidneys following oral administration; 12 to 15% excreted unchanged following IV administration. Erythromycins cross the placental barrier in pregnancy; can be found in breast milk.

Dosage/Range:
- Oral: 250 mg once q6h for 10 days; or 500 mg q6h for 10 days; or 333 mg q8h
- IV: 500 mg q6h; up to 1000 mg q6h (Legionnaires' Disease).

Drug Preparation:
- Further dilute in 0.9% Sodium Chloride to a concentration of 1–5 mg/mL (500 mg/100 mL, 1000 mg/250 mL).
- Reconstitute 500 mg or 1 g vials with 10 or 20 mL, respectively, of sterile water for injection only (no preservatives).

Drug Administration:

- Must not be given IV push.
- Intermittent IV infusion over 1 hour is appropriate.

Drug Interactions:

- Use of alcohol concurrently with IV erythromycin increases peak blood alcohol concentrations by 40%; this is thought to be related to rapid gastric emptying, less exposure to alcohol dehydrogenase in the gastric mucosa, and slower small intestine transit time.
- Concurrent use of astemizole or terfenadine with erythromycins is contraindicated and may increase risk of cardiotoxicity, such as *torsades de points*, ventricular tachycardia, and death.
- Erythromycins may inhibit carbamazepine and valproic acid metabolism, resulting in increased anticonvulsant plasma concentration and toxicity.
- Concurrent use of chloramphenicol, lincomycins, and erythromycins is not recommended due to their antagonizing effects. It is best to avoid concurrent use of bactericidal and bacteriostatic drugs until culture and sensitivity results are determined.
- Erythromycin can increased cyclosporin plasma concentrations and may increase the risk of nephrotoxicity.
- Erythromycins inhibit the metabolism of ergotamine and increase the vasospasm associated with ergotamines.
- Simultaneous administration of erythromycin and lovastatin should be used with caution since concurrent use may increase the risk of rhabdomyolysis.
- Concurrent use of midazolam and triazolam with erythromycins can increase the pharmacological effect of these drugs.
- Erythromycins may cause prolonged prothrombin time and increased risk of hemorrhage, especially in the elderly.
- Use of erythromycins and xanthines (i.e., Aminophylline, caffeine, Oxtriphylline, and Theophylline) may lead to increased serum levels of xanthines and toxicity.

Lab Effects/Interference:

- Serum SGPT, serum SGOT serum bilirubin, and alkaline phosphatase—values may be increased by all erythromycins.
- Urinary catecholamines may produce false positive results when patient is on erythromycin.

Special Considerations:

- Do not use when there is a known hypersensitivity to erythromycins.
- Use with caution in patients with impaired hepatic function.
- Patients with a history of hearing loss, may be at risk of further hearing loss especially if hepatic or renal function is present or if on high dose erythromycins, or if patient is elderly.

Potential Toxicities/Side Effects and the Nursing Process

I. ALTERATION IN NUTRITION related to GI SIDE EFFECTS

Defining Characteristics: Nausea, vomiting, anorexia have occurred frequently. Also, transient increase LFTs—AST (SGOT), ALT (SGPT), LDH, ALK-PHOS, BR—has occurred. Hepatotoxicity (fever, nausea, skin rash, stomach pain, severe and unusual tiredness or weakness, yellow eyes or skin, and vomiting) has occurred less frequently. Pancreatitis (severe abdominal pain, nausea and vomiting) has occurred but is rare.

Nursing Implications: Assess baseline nutritional status, preexisting nausea/vomiting, anorexia. Assess baseline LFTs and monitor periodically during treatment. Teach patient to report side effects. Provide symptomatic interventions if side effects occur; discuss with physician use of alternative drug(s).

II. POTENTIAL FOR INJURY related to HYPERSENSITIVITY REACTION

Defining Characteristics: Urticaria, pruritus, rash (maculopapular or erythematous), fever and chills, eosinophilia, myalgia, edema, erythema, angioedema.

Nursing Implications: Assess for drug allergies to erythromycin or macrolide antibiotic prior to drug administration. Teach patient to report any allergic reactions. Assess for signs/symptoms of allergic reaction after drug dose. Assess baseline skin integrity and presence of drug allergies; monitor patient closely during drug infusions. Teach patient to report immediately signs/symptoms of rash, pruritus, shortness of breath, any adverse sensation. Teach patient skin care and symptomatic measures as appropriate. If skin rash develops, discuss drug discontinuance with physician. If rash progresses, especially in human immunodeficiency virus (HIV)-infected patients, drug should be discontinued as fatal Stevens-Johnson syndrome may develop. Be prepared to treat severe acute hypersensitivity reactions with airway management, oxygen, epinephrine, corticosteroids, antihistamines as ordered.

III. ALTERATIONS IN COMFORT related to LOCAL INJECTION IRRITATION

Defining Characteristics: Incidence of phlebitis, thrombophlebitis, and pain when administering IV.

Nursing Implications: Change IV sites q 48 hours, and assess for signs/symptoms of phlebitis prior to each administration. Administer drug slowly. Apply warm packs to increase comfort.

IV. ALTERATIONS IN CARDIAC OUTPUT related to CARDIOVASCULAR CHANGES

Defining Characteristics: Rare incidence of cardiac arrhythmias, electrocardiogram (EKG) changes (e.g., QT prolongation), torsades de points (irregular or slow heart rate: recurrent fainting, sudden death).

Nursing Implications: Assess baseline heart rate and blood pressure (BP); monitor during therapy, at least with initial dose.

V. SENSORY/PERCEPTUAL ALTERATIONS related to OTOTOXICITY

Defining Characteristics: Damage to eighth cranial nerve (auditory) may result in dizziness, nystagmus, vertigo, ataxia (vestibular damage), and more commonly tinnitus, roaring sound in ears, and impaired hearing (auditory damage). Hearing loss usually begins with high-frequency loss, followed by clinical hearing loss, then permanent hearing loss if damage continues. Increased risk in elderly, renally, hepatically impaired patients.

Nursing Implications: Assess baseline hearing (ability to hear spoken voice) and continue to assess during therapy. Teach patient potential side effects, and instruct patient to report any hearing/perceptual problems (e.g., tinnitus, vertigo, decreased hearing). Discuss drug discontinuance and audiogram with physician to confirm hearing dysfunction if symptoms arise. Assess for increased risk if given concurrently with other ototoxic medications (e.g., cisplatin, furosemide).

VI. FUNGAL SUPERINFECTION related to REDISTRIBUTION OF ENDOGENOUS MICROORGANISMS

Defining Characteristics: Vaginal candidiasis (sore mouth or tongue; white patches in mouth and/or tongue); vaginitis (vaginal candidiasis); vaginal itching and discharge may occur as endogenous bacteria are eliminated and normal fungal population expands.

Nursing Implications: Teach female patient to report vaginal itching or discharge. Discuss appropriate antifungal treatment with physician. Teach perineal hygiene and symptomatic management.

Drug: gatifloxacin (Tequin)

Class: Quinolone.

Mechanism of Action: Gatifloxacin is a broad-spectrum anti-infective, active against a wide range of aerobic gram-positive and gram-negative organisms. Acts intracellularly by inhibiting DNA gyrase (bacterial topoisomerase IV).

Metabolism: Widely distributed to most body fluids and tissues with highest concentrations in organs such as kidneys, gallbladder, lungs, liver, gynecological tissue, prostatic tissue, phagocytic cells, urine, sputum, and bile. Well absorbed from GI tract. Metabolized in liver; excreted in urine and feces. Crosses placenta and is excreted in breast milk.

Dosage/Range:
- 400 mg PO or IV QD.

Drug Preparation/Administration:
- Oral: Take drug with large glass of water; preferably 2 hours after meal/food. Encourage oral fluids of 2–3 qt (liters)/day.
- IV: Further dilute drug in 0.9% Sodium Chloride or 5% Dextrose in water to final concentration of 2 mg/mL.

Drug Interactions:
- Antacids (containing magnesium, aluminum, or calcium) and iron decrease absorption of serum level of gatifloxacin; do not administer concurrently. If must administer antacids or iron, administer at least 4 hours apart. The administration of antacids containing aluminum, magnesium, calcium, sucralfate, zinc, or iron may substantially reduce the absorption of gatofloxacin; do not administer concurrently.
- Serum digoxin concentrations should be monitored; gatifloxacin may raise serum levels in some patients.
- Probenecid: decreases the renal tubular secretion of gatifloxacin resulting in a prolonged elimination half-life and increased risk of toxicity.
- Gatifloxacin may have the potential to prolong the Q-T interval of the EKG in some patients. Gatifloxacin should not be used in patients with prolonged Q-T interval; patients with uncorrected hypokalemia; and patients taking quinidine, procanamide, amiodrone, and sotalol (antiarrhythmic agents).
- Increased intracranial pressure and psychosis have been reported along with CNS stimulation.
- Hypersensitivity reactions have been reported.

Lab Effects/Interference:
- Serum SGPT, serum Alk Phos, serum SGOT, and serum LDH: values may be increased.

Special Considerations:
- Used in treatment of infections of urinary and lower respiratory tracts, skin, bone and joint, and GI tract, as well as gonorrhea.
- Contraindicated in pregnancy or in women who are breast-feeding.
- Obtain ordered specimen for culture and sensitivity prior to first drug dose.
- Use cautiously in patients with seizure disorders.
- Used in the treatment of infections or most bacterial infections.

Potential Toxicities/Side Effects and the Nursing Process

I. ALTERATION IN NUTRITION related to GI SIDE EFFECTS

Defining Characteristics: Incidence of nausea, vomiting, abdominal discomfort, diarrhea, anorexia.

Nursing Implications: Assess baseline nutritional and elimination status. Teach patient to report GI disturbances. Administer and teach patient to self-administer antiemetics and antidiarrheals as needed and as ordered. Teach patient importance of nutritious diet, and suggest small, frequent, high-calorie, high-protein meals as appropriate. Assess baseline LFTs and monitor periodically during treatment. Discuss abnormalities and drug interruption with physician. Assess taking other hepatotoxic drugs (see Special Considerations).

II. SENSORY/PERCEPTUAL ALTERATIONS related to CNS EFFECTS

Defining Characteristics: Incidence of headache, restlessness. Dizziness, hallucinations, and seizures may also occur. Exacerbated by caffeine as quinolones delay caffeine excretion.

Nursing Implications: Assess baseline neurological function and comfort, and monitor during treatment. Teach patient to report any changes. Discuss any abnormalities with physician. Teach patient to limit or restrict all medications and caffeine-containing fluids (e.g., tea, coffee, caffeinated soft drinks).

III. ALTERATION IN SKIN INTEGRITY related to ALLERGY/HYPERSENSITIVITY

Defining Characteristics: Incidence of rash; other manifestations include eosinophilia, urticaria, flushing, fever, chills, photosensitivity, angioedema. Fatal hypersensitivity reactions have occurred rarely. Direct exposure to sunlight can cause sunburn (moderate to severe phototoxicity).

Nursing Implications: Assess baseline skin condition, including integrity and drug allergy history. Teach patient to report rash, itching, other skin changes. Teach patient skin care and symptomatic measures as appropriate. If skin rash develops, discuss drug discontinuance with physician. Be prepared to treat severe acute hypersensitivity reactions with airway management, oxygen, epinephrine, corticosteroids, antihistamines as ordered. Teach patient to avoid excessive sun exposure and to use skin protection factor (SPF) 15 or higher. If rash progresses, especially in HIV-infected patients, drug should be discontinued as fatal Stevens-Johnson syndrome may develop.

IV. FUNGAL SUPERINFECTION related to REDISTRIBUTION OF ENDOGENOUS MICROORGANISMS

Defining Characteristics: Vaginal moniliasis, vaginitis may occur as endogenous bacteria are eliminated and normal fungal population expands.

Nursing Implications: Teach female patient to report vaginal itching or discharge. Discuss appropriate antifungal treatment with physician. Teach perineal hygiene and symptomatic management.

V. ALTERATION IN URINARY ELIMINATION related to RENAL TOXICITY

Defining Characteristics: Increased BUN and creatinine, crystal and stone formation in urine, interstitial nephritis, and renal failure may occur.

Nursing Implications: Assess baseline renal function; expect that drug dose will be decreased in presence of renal dysfunction. Teach patient to take drug with at least 8 oz of water, and to increase oral fluids to 2–3 qt/day.

VI. ALTERATION IN COMFORT related to IV ADMINISTRATION

Defining Characteristics: Drug may cause pain, inflammation, and rare thrombophlebitis at IV site.

Nursing Implications: Change IV site q 48 hours. Assess for phlebitis, discomfort, and IV patency prior to each administration. Administer drug slowly over 60–90 minutes in large volume of 5% Dextrose (see Drug Preparation/Administration). Apply heat to promote comfort.

Drug: gemifloxacin mesylate (Factive)

Class: Quinolone.

Mechanism of Action: Gemifloxacin is a broad-spectrum anti-infective, active against a wide range of aerobic gram-positive and gram-negative organisms. Acts inhibiting DNA synthesis through the inhibition of DNA gyrase and topoisomerase IV, which are essential for bacterial growth.

Metabolism: Widely distributed to most body fluids and tissues after oral administration. Gemifloxacin penetrates well into lung tissues and fluids. Well absorbed from GI tract. Metabolized to a limited extent in the liver; excreted in urine and feces. The safety in pregnant women has not been established. The drug is excreted in breast milk in animal studies.

Dosage/Range:
- 320 mg orally once a day for 5–7 days.

Drug Preparation/Administration:
- Oral: Take drug with or without food. Take with large glass of water; encourage oral fluids of 2–3 qt (liters)/day.

Drug Interactions:
- Antacids (containing magnesium, aluminum, or calcium) and iron decrease absorption of serum level of gemifloxacin; do not administer concurrently. If must administer antacids or iron, administer at least 3 hours before or 2 hours after. The administration of antacids containing aluminum, magnesium, calcium, sucralfate, zinc, or iron may substantially reduce the absorption of gemifloxacin; do not administer concurrently.
- Probenecid: decreases the renal tubular secretion of gemifloxacin resulting in a prolonged elimination half-life and increased risk of toxicity.
- Gemifloxacin may have the potential to prolong the Q-T interval of the EKG in some patients. Gemifloxacin should not be used in patients with prolonged Q-T interval; patients with uncorrected hypokalemia or hypomagnesemia; and patients taking quinidine, procanamide, amiodrone, and sotalol (Class 1A antiarrhythmic agents).
- Increased intracranial pressure and psychosis have been reported along with CNS stimulation.
- Hypersensitivity reactions have been reported.
- Fluroquinolones have been shown to cause arthropathy and osteochondrosis in animal studies. Discontinue if patient experiences pain, inflammation, or rupture of a tendon. Elderly patients, athletes, and patients taking corticosteroids are more prone to tendonitis.
- Pseudomembranous colitis has been reported and may range from mild to life-threatening.

Lab Effects/Interference:
- Serum SGPT, serum Alk Phos, serum SGOT, and serum LDH: values may be increased.

Special Considerations:
- Used in treatment of infections of lower respiratory tracts.
- Contraindicated in pregnancy or in women who are breast-feeding.
- Obtain ordered specimen for culture and sensitivity prior to first drug dose.
- Use cautiously in patients with seizure disorders.
- Used in the treatment of infections or most bacterial infections.

Potential Toxicities/Side Effects and the Nursing Process

I. ALTERATION IN NUTRITION related to GI SIDE EFFECTS

Defining Characteristics: Incidence of nausea, vomiting, abdominal discomfort, diarrhea, anorexia.

Nursing Implications: Assess baseline nutritional and elimination status. Teach patient to report GI disturbances. Administer and teach patient to self-administer antiemetics and antidiarrheals as needed and as ordered. Teach patient importance of nutritious diet, and suggest small, frequent, high-calorie, high-protein meals as appropriate. Assess baseline LFTs and monitor periodically during treatment. Discuss abnormalities and drug interruption with physician. Assess taking other hepatotoxic drugs.

II. SENSORY/PERCEPTUAL ALTERATIONS related to CNS EFFECTS

Defining Characteristics: Incidence of headache, restlessness. Dizziness, hallucinations, and seizures may also occur. Exacerbated by caffeine as quinolones delay caffeine excretion.

Nursing Implications: Assess baseline neurological function and comfort, and monitor during treatment. Teach patient to report any changes. Discuss any abnormalities with physician. Teach patient to limit or restrict all medications and caffeine-containing fluids (e.g., tea, coffee, caffeinated soft drinks).

III. ALTERATION IN SKIN INTEGRITY related to ALLERGY/ HYPERSENSITIVITY

Defining Characteristics: Incidence of rash; other manifestations include eosinophilia, urticaria, flushing, fever, chills, photosensitivity, angioedema. Fatal hypersensitivity reactions have occurred rarely. Direct exposure to sunlight can cause sunburn (moderate to severe phototoxicity).

Nursing Implications: Assess baseline skin condition, including integrity and drug allergy history. Teach patient to report rash, itching, and other skin changes. Teach patient skin care and symptomatic measures as appropriate. If skin rash develops, discuss drug discontinuance with physician. Be prepared to treat severe acute hypersensitivity reactions with airway management, oxygen, epinephrine, corticosteroids, antihistamines as ordered. Teach patient to avoid excessive sun exposure and to use skin protection factor (SPF) 15 or higher. If rash progresses, especially in HIV-infected patients, drug should be discontinued as fatal Stevens-Johnson syndrome may develop.

IV. FUNGAL SUPERINFECTION related to REDISTRIBUTION OF ENDOGENOUS MICROORGANISMS

Defining Characteristics: Vaginal moniliasis, vaginitis may occur as endogenous bacteria are eliminated and normal fungal population expands.

Nursing Implications: Teach female patient to report vaginal itching or discharge. Discuss appropriate antifungal treatment with physician. Teach perineal hygiene and symptomatic management.

V. ALTERATION IN URINARY ELIMINATION related to RENAL TOXICITY

Defining Characteristics: Increased BUN and creatinine, crystal and stone formation in urine, interstitial nephritis, and renal failure may occur.

Nursing Implications: Assess baseline renal function; expect that drug dose will be decreased in presence of renal dysfunction. Teach patient to take drug with at least 8 oz of water, and to increase oral fluids to 2–3 qt/day.

Drug: gentamicin sulfate (Garamycin, Gentamicin)

Class: Aminoglycoside antibacterial.

Mechanism of Action: Derived from *Micromonospora*; bactericidal, most probably by inhibition of protein synthesis. Active against aerobic microorganisms: many sensitive gram-negative organisms (including *Acinetobacter, Brucella, Citrobacter, Enterobacter, E. coli, Klebsiella, Proteus, Pseudomonas, Salmonella, Serratia,* and *Shigella*) and some sensitive gram-positive organisms (*S. aureus* and *S. epidermidis*). Over time, bacterial resistance may develop, either naturally or acquired.

Metabolism: Well absorbed following IV administration, but variability in absorption after IM injection (peak serum level 0.5–2 hours, duration 8–12 hours). Widely distributed into body fluids. Minimally protein-bound. Readily crosses placenta and into breast milk. Drug excreted unchanged in the urine.

Dosage/Range:
- IM, IV: Loading dose, 2 mg/Kg, then 3–6 mg/Kg/day in one daily dose, 2 equal doses in split 8-hour dosing.
- IT: 4–8 mg (preservative-free).
- Desired peak serum concentration 4–10 μg/mL, and trough serum concentration is 1–2 μg/mL.
- DOSE REDUCTION IF RENAL DYSFUNCTION.

Drug Preparation:
- Store injectable at < 40°C (104°F). Stable for 24 hours at room temperature in 0.9% Sodium Chloride or 5% Dextrose.

Drug Administration:
- Do not mix with other drugs.
- IV: Mix in 50–200 mL 0.9% Sodium Chloride or 5% Dextrose injection and infuse over 30 minutes to 2 hours. Can also be given IM.

Drug Administration:

- Increased risk of toxicity with other ototoxic drugs: acyclovir, other aminoglycosides, amphotericin B, bacitracin, cephalosporins, colistin, cisplatin, ethacrynic acid, furosemide, vancomycin.
- Potentiation of neuromuscular blockade when given concurrently with general anesthetics (succinylcholine, tubocurarine); use cautiously, observe for signs/symptoms of respiratory depression.
- Synergism with extended-spectrum penicillins, but must be administered separately.

Lab Effects/Interference:

- Serum ALT, serum alk phos, serum AST, serum bili, and serum LDH values may be increased.
- BUN and serum creatinine concentrations may be increased.
- Serum Ca++, serum Mg++, serum K+, and serum Na+ concentrations may be decreased.

Special Considerations:

- Used as first-line treatment in short-term treatment of serious gram-negative infections (e.g., septicemia, respiratory tract infections).
- Use against gram-positive organisms only as second-line treatment.
- Use in pregnancy only if infection is life-threatening and no safer drug exists; drug crosses placenta and may cause fetal toxicity.

Potential Toxicities/Side Effects and the Nursing Process

I. ALTERATIONS IN SENSORY/PERCEPTUAL PATTERNS related to OTOTOXICITY

Defining Characteristics: Damage to eighth cranial nerve (auditory) may result in dizziness, nystagmus, vertigo, ataxia (vestibular damage), and more commonly tinnitus, roaring sound in ears, and impaired hearing (auditory damage). Hearing loss usually begins with high-frequency loss, followed by clinical hearing loss, then permanent hearing loss if damage continues. Increased risk in elderly or renally impaired patients.

Nursing Implications: Assess baseline hearing (ability to hear spoken voice) and continue to access during therapy. Teach patient potential side effects and instruct patient to report any hearing/perceptual problems (e.g., tinnitus, vertigo, decreased hearing). Discuss drug discontinuance and audiogram with physician to confirm hearing dysfunction if symptoms arise. Assess for increased risk if given concurrently with other ototoxic medications (e.g., cisplatin, furosemide).

II. ALTERATION IN URINARY ELIMINATION related to NEPHROTOXICITY

Defining Characteristics: Renal damage characterized by tubular necrosis with increased serum BUN, creatinine; decreased urine creatinine clearance and specific gravity; proteinuria and casts in urine. Azotemia usually not associated with oliguria. Rarely, electrolyte wasting with hypomagnesemia, hypocalcemia, and hypokalemia may occur. Renal dysfunction is usually reversible after drug discontinuance. Increased risk exists in elderly and if preexisting renal dysfunction. Risk low in well-hydrated patients with normal renal function when normal doses given.

Nursing Implications: Assess baseline renal function and electrolytes, and monitor periodically during therapy. Discuss any abnormalities with physician, as drug should be dose-reduced or discontinued if renal dysfunction develops. Assess baseline total body fluid balance, weight, and monitor periodically during antibiotic therapy. Monitor hydration status to keep patient well hydrated. Assess drug peak and trough levels as ordered so that drug dosage is correctly titrated. Increased risk of toxicity if peak serum concentration > 10–12 μg/mL. Draw blood for peak drug concentration 30 minutes after end of 30-minute infusion or at the end of a 60-minute infusion; draw trough immediately before next dose.

III. ALTERATIONS IN SENSORY/PERCEPTUAL PATTERNS related to CNS EFFECTS, NEUROMUSCULAR BLOCKADE

Defining Characteristics: Headache, tremor, lethargy may occur. Peripheral neuropathy or encephalopathy (numbness, skin tingling, muscle twitching) may occur rarely. Neuromuscular blockade is dose-related, self-limiting, and uncommon; risk is greater with topical application or when drug is administered to patient with neuromuscular disease (myasthenia gravis) or hypocalcemia.

Nursing Implications: Assess baseline neurologic status. Assess coexisting risk factors, neuromuscular blockade medications. Teach patient about side effects and to report headache, tremor, lethargy. Observe for respiratory depression. If signs/symptoms arise, discuss drug discontinuance with physician.

IV. POTENTIAL FOR INJURY related to HYPERSENSITIVITY

Defining Characteristics: Rash, urticaria, pruritus, fever, eosinophilia have occurred rarely. CROSS-SENSITIVITY between AMINOGLYCOSIDES exists!

Nursing Implications: Assess for drug allergies to any aminoglycoside—amikacin, gentamicin, kanamycin, neomycin, netilmicin, streptomycin, tobramycin—prior to drug administration. Instruct patient to report any allergic reactions. Assess for signs/symptoms of allergic reaction after drug dose.

V. ALTERATION IN NUTRITION, LESS THAN BODY REQUIREMENTS, related to GI SIDE EFFECTS

Defining Characteristics: Nausea, vomiting, anorexia have occurred rarely. Also, transient hepatomegaly with increased LFTs—AST, ALT, LDH, alk phos, bili—has occurred.

Nursing Implications: Assess baseline nutritional status, preexisting nausea/vomiting, anorexia. Assess baseline LFTs and monitor periodically during treatment. Instruct patient to report side effects. Provide symptomatic interventions if side effects occur; discuss with physician use of alternative drug(s).

VI. POTENTIAL FOR FATIGUE, INFECTION, AND BLEEDING related to BONE MARROW INJURY

Defining Characteristics: Anemia, leukopenia, granulocytopenia, and thrombocytopenia may occur. Also, patients receiving antibiotics are at risk for overgrowth of nonsusceptible microorganisms, such as fungi (superinfection). Rare.

Nursing Implications: Assess baseline CBC, differential, and monitor periodically during treatment. Instruct patient to report signs/symptoms of fatigue, infection, or bleeding immediately. Assess for signs/symptoms of superinfection. Discuss any adverse effects with physician.

Drug: imipenem/cilastatin sodium (Primaxin)

Class: Antibacterial. Imipenem is a β-lactam antibiotic, carbapenem type; cilastatin inhibits an enzyme in the kidneys that breaks down imipenem, increasing drug potency and protecting kidneys.

Mechanism of Action: Semisynthetic derivative of cephalosporin C (produced by fungus); contains β-lactam ring and is related to penicillins and cephamycins (e.g., cefoxitin). Bactericidal through inhibition of cell wall synthesis, with resulting cell wall instability and cell lysis. Active against most anaerobic and aerobic gram-positive and gram-negative organisms. These include *Staphylococcus, Streptococcus, E. coli, P. aeruginosa, Proteus, Klebsiella, Enterobacter.* Some activity against *Mycobacterium.* Resists hydrolysis by β-lactamase enzymes produced by microorganisms, so resistance to these organisms is much less than other β-lactam antibiotics (e.g., cephalosporins, penicillins). Used in treatment of serious infections of lower respiratory tract, urinary tract, abdomen, female pelvis, skin, bone, and joint, as well as polymicrobial infections and infections resistant to other antibiotics.

Metabolism: Not well absorbed from GI tract, so must be given IV. Incompletely absorbed after IM injection. Widely distributed in body tissues and fluids, including bile; does not result in significant CSF drug levels. Crosses placenta and is excreted in breast milk. Cilastatin decreases renal metabolism of imipenem; both drugs are excreted in urine, and to a lesser degree in feces.

Dosage/Range:

Adult:

- IV: 250 mg–1 g q6–8h (maximum 50 mg/kg or 4 g/day, whichever is less).
- IM (if unable to give IV): 500–750 mg q12h (maximum 1.5 g/day). Reduce dose if renal insufficiency, according to manufacturer's package insert.

Drug Preparation/Administration:

- Store vial of sterile powder at < 30°C (86°F).
- IV: Reconstitute according to manufacturer's package insert and further dilute in 100 mL 0.9% Sodium Chloride or 5% Dextrose injection. Infuse over 60 minutes for each gram of drug administered. Slow infusion if nausea/vomiting develop.
- IM: Reconstitute drug with lidocaine HCl 1% injection (without epinephrine) as directed by package insert. Administer deep IM in large muscle mass (e.g., gluteus maximus). Assess allergy to lidocaine. IM preparation SHOULD NOT BE USED FOR IV ADMINISTRATION.

Drug Interactions:

- Probenecid: increases serum concentrations of imipenem. DO NOT USE CONCURRENTLY.
- Aminoglycosides: may have synergistic antimicrobial effect.
- β-lactam antibiotics (cephalosporins, extended-spectrum penicillins): Antagonism. Imipenem stimulates production of β-lactamase enzymes by the bacteria that inactivate the cephalosporins and penicillins. DO NOT USE CONCURRENTLY.
- Ganciclovir: may decrease seizure threshold. Do not use concurrently unless critical for life-saving treatment.
- Co-trimoxazole: possible synergy against *Nocardia asteroides*.
- Chloramphenicol: possible antagonism. Consider chloramphenicol administration 2+ hours after imipenem (requires clinical study).

Lab Effects/Interference:

- Serum ALT, serum alk phos, and serum AST values may be transiently increased.

Clinical significance:

- Coombs' (direct antiglobulin) tests: may occur during therapy.
- Serum LDH values may be transiently increased.

- Serum bili, BUN concentrations, and serum creatinine concentrations may be transiently increased.
- HCT and Hgb concentrations may be decreased.

Special Considerations:

- Contraindicated in patients hypersensitive to imipenem or cilastatin. Use cautiously in patients sensitive to penicillin or other β-lactams, as partial cross-allergenicity exists.
- Do not give IM preparation reconstituted with 1% lidocaine if hypersensitive to lidocaine.
- Drug may cause false-positive glucose determination when using Clinitest.
- Ensure specimen sent for culture and sensitivity prior to first antibiotic dose.
- Drug has significantly broad antibacterial properties.
- Drug dosage needs to be reduced if severe renal insufficiency.
- Slow IV infusion if nausea/vomiting develops.

Potential Toxicities/Side Effects and the Nursing Process

I. POTENTIAL FOR INJURY related to HYPERSENSITIVITY REACTION

Defining Characteristics: Urticaria, pruritus, rash (maculopapular or erythematous), fever and chills, eosinophilia, myalgia, edema, erythema, angioedema, Stevens-Johnson syndrome, and exfoliative skin reactions occur in 5% of patients. Increased risk in individuals allergic to penicillin.

Nursing Implications: Assess allergy to cephalosporin antibiotics and penicillin: if patient states "yes," determine actual response, e.g., "swollen lips = angioedema." If angioedema, discuss with physician RISK versus benefit prior to drug administration, as there is partial cross-allergenicity. Discuss other patient responses with physician to determine whether drug should be given. Assess baseline skin condition, including integrity and allergy history to drugs. Instruct patient to report rash, itching, other skin changes. Teach patient skin care and symptomatic measures as appropriate. If skin rash develops, discuss drug discontinuance with physician. If rash progresses, drug should be discontinued, as fatal Stevens-Johnson syndrome may develop. Be prepared to treat severe acute hypersensitivity reactions with airway management, oxygen, epinephrine, corticosteroids, antihistamines as ordered.

II. ALTERATION IN NUTRITION, LESS THAN BODY REQUIREMENTS, related to GI SIDE EFFECTS

Defining Characteristics: Nausea, vomiting occurs more frequently than diarrhea, anorexia; rarely, pseudomembranous colitis caused by *C. difficile* resistant to the antibiotic occurs. Rarely, transient increases in LFTs—AST, ALT, alk phos, bili—may occur.

Nursing Implications: Assess baseline nutritional status. Instruct patient to report GI disturbances. Administer and teach patient to self-administer antiemetics as needed and as ordered. Teach patient importance of nutritious diet and suggest small, frequent, high-calorie, high-protein meals as appropriate. Assess baseline LFTs and monitor periodically during treatment. Discuss abnormalities and drug interruption with physician.

III. FUNGAL SUPERINFECTION related to REDISTRIBUTION OF ENDOGENOUS MICROORGANISMS

Defining Characteristics: Vaginal candidiasis, vaginitis may occur as endogenous bacteria are eliminated and normal fungal population expands.

Nursing Implications: Instruct female patient to report vaginal itching or discharge. Discuss appropriate antifungal treatment with physician. Teach perineal hygiene and symptomatic management.

IV. ALTERATIONS IN PROTECTIVE MECHANISMS (RARE) related to TRANSIENT LEUKOPENIA

Defining Characteristics: Rarely, transient leukopenia, lymphocytosis, anemia, eosinophilia may occur. Prolonged PT, prolonged APTT, and hypoprothrombinemia have occurred rarely, especially in elderly or debilitated patients, or in individuals with vitamin K deficiency.

Nursing Implications: Assess baseline laboratory parameters, and monitor periodically during treatment. Assess patient for response to antibiotics. Discuss abnormalities with physician.

V. ALTERATIONS IN SENSORY/PERCEPTUAL PATTERNS related to DIZZINESS, SOMNOLENCE

Defining Characteristics: Dizziness, headache, somnolence, seizures occur rarely. Most seizures have occurred in patients with preexisting CNS problems, those who had received higher-than-recommended IV doses, the elderly, and patients with impaired renal function.

Nursing Implications: Assess baseline neurologic function and comfort, and monitor during treatment. Instruct patient to report any changes. Discuss any abnormalities with physician. Institute seizure precautions. If seizures occur, discuss with physician anticonvulsant therapy or discontinuance of antibiotic.

VI. ALTERATIONS IN COMFORT related to LOCAL INJECTION IRRITATION

Defining Characteristics: Pain, induration, sterile abscesses may form in IM injection sites; phlebitis may develop in IV sites.

Nursing Implications: Rotate IM injection sites, and administer drug deep IM in large muscle mass (e.g., gluteus maximus). Use IM injection when IV administration is not possible. Change IV sites q48h, and assess for signs/symptoms of phlebitis prior to each administration. Administer drug slowly. Apply warm packs to increase comfort.

Drug: kanamycin sulfate (Kantrex)

Class: Aminoglycoside antibacterial.

Mechanism of Action: Synthetic antibiotic derived from *Streptomyces;* bactericidal, most probably by inhibition of protein synthesis. Active against aerobic microorganisms: many sensitive gram-negative organisms (including *Acinetobacter, Citrobacter, Enterobacter, E. coli, Klebsiella, Proteus, Salmonella, Serratia, and Shigella)* and some sensitive gram-positive organisms (*S. aureus* and *S. epidermidis).* Over time, bacterial resistance may develop, either naturally or acquired.

Metabolism: Well absorbed following parenteral administration, but variable absorption after IM injection (peak serum level 0.5–2 hours, duration 8–12 hours). Widely distributed into body fluids. Minimally protein-bound. Readily crosses placenta and into breast milk. Drug excreted unchanged in the urine.

Dosage/Range:
- IM, IV: 15 mg/kg/day in equally divided doses at 8- or 12-hour intervals.
- Desired peak serum concentration 15–30 μg/mL, and trough serum concentration is 5–10 μg/mL.
- DOSE REDUCTION IF RENAL IMPAIRMENT.

Drug Preparation:
- Store capsules in tight containers at temperature < 40°C (104°F).
- Injection should be stored at < 40°C (104°F), preferably 15–30°C (59–86°F).
- Mix 500 mg in 100–200 mL of IV infusion solution. Stable for 24 hours at room temperature in 0.9% Sodium Chloride or 5% Dextrose. DO NOT MIX WITH OTHER MEDICATIONS.

Drug Administration:
- Deep IM: upper outer quadrant of buttock.
- IV: Infuse over 30–60 minutes.
- Orally (pre-op bowel sterilization): 1 g PO qh × four doses, then q4h × four doses.
- Wound irrigation: 2–2.5 mg/mL in 0.9% Sodium Chloride irrigant.

Drug Interactions:

- Increased risk of toxicity with other ototoxic drugs: acyclovir, other aminoglycosides, amphotericin B, bacitracin, cephalosporins, colistin, cisplatin, ethacrynic acid, furosemide, vancomycin.
- Potentiation of neuromuscular blockade when given concurrently with general anesthetics (succinylcholine, tubocurarine); use cautiously, observe for signs/symptoms of respiratory depression.
- Synergism with extended-spectrum penicillins, but must be administered separately.

Lab Effects/Interference:

- Serum ALT, serum alk phos, serum AST, serum bili, and serum LDH values may be increased.
- BUN and serum creatinine concentrations may be increased.
- Serum Ca++, serum Mg++, serum K+, and serum Na+ concentrations may be decreased.

Special Considerations:

- Used as first-line treatment in short-term treatment of serious gram-negative infections (e.g., septicemia, respiratory tract infections).
- Use against gram-positive organisms only as second-line treatment.
- Use in pregnancy only if infection is life-threatening and no safer drug exists; drug crosses placenta and may cause fetal toxicity.

Potential Toxicities/Side Effects and the Nursing Process

I. ALTERATIONS IN SENSORY/PERCEPTUAL PATTERNS related to OTOTOXICITY

Defining Characteristics: Damage to eighth cranial nerve (auditory) may result in dizziness, nystagmus, vertigo, ataxia (vestibular damage), and less commonly tinnitus, roaring sound in ears, and impaired hearing (auditory damage). Hearing loss usually begins with high-frequency loss, followed by clinical hearing loss, then permanent hearing loss if damage continues. Increased risk in elderly or renally impaired patients.

Nursing Implications: Assess baseline hearing (ability to hear spoken voice) and continue during therapy. Teach patient potential side effects, and instruct patient to report any hearing/perceptual problems (e.g., tinnitus, vertigo, decreased hearing). Discuss drug discontinuance and audiogram with physician to confirm hearing dysfunction if symptoms arise. Assess for increased risk if given concurrently with other ototoxic medications (e.g., cisplatin, furosemide).

II. ALTERATION IN URINARY ELIMINATION related to NEPHROTOXICITY

Defining Characteristics: Renal damage characterized by tubular necrosis with increased serum BUN, creatinine; decreased urine creatinine clearance and specific gravity; proteinuria and casts in urine. Azotemia usually not associated with oliguria. Rarely, electrolyte wasting with hypomagnesemia, hypocalcemia, and hypokalemia may occur. Renal dysfunction usually reversible after drug discontinuance. Increased risk exists in elderly and if there is preexisting renal dysfunction. Risk is low in well-hydrated patients with normal renal function when normal doses given.

Nursing Implications: Assess baseline renal function and electrolytes, and monitor periodically during therapy. Discuss any abnormalities with physician, as drug should be dose-reduced or discontinued if renal dysfunction develops. Assess baseline total body fluid balance, weight, and monitor periodically during antibiotic therapy. Monitor hydration status to keep patient well hydrated. Assess drug peak and trough levels as ordered so that drug dosage is correctly titrated. Increased risk of toxicity if peak serum concentration > 30–35 μg/mL. Draw blood for peak drug concentration 30 minutes after end of 30-minute infusion or at the end of a 60-minute infusion; draw trough immediately before next dose.

III. ALTERATIONS IN SENSORY/PERCEPTUAL PATTERNS related to CNS EFFECTS, NEUROMUSCULAR BLOCKADE

Defining Characteristics: Headache, tremor, lethargy may occur. Peripheral neuropathy or encephalopathy (numbness, skin tingling, muscle twitching) may occur rarely. Neuromuscular blockade is dose-related, self-limiting, and uncommon; risk is greater with topical application or when drug is administered to patient with neuromuscular disease (myasthenia gravis) or hypocalcemia.

Nursing Implications: Assess baseline neurologic status. Assess coexisting risk factors, neuromuscular blockade medications. Teach patient about side effects, and instruct to report headache, tremor, lethargy. Observe for respiratory depression. If signs/symptoms arise, discuss drug discontinuance with physician.

IV. POTENTIAL FOR INJURY related to HYPERSENSITIVITY

Defining Characteristics: Rash, urticaria, pruritus, fever, eosinophilia have occurred rarely. CROSS-SENSITIVITY between AMINOGLYCOSIDES exists!

Nursing Implications: Assess for drug allergies to any aminoglycoside—amikacin, gentamicin, kanamycin, neomycin, netilmicin, streptomycin, tobramycin—prior to drug administration. Instruct patient to report any allergic reactions. Assess for signs/symptoms of allergic reaction after drug dose.

V. ALTERATION IN NUTRITION, LESS THAN BODY REQUIREMENTS, related to GI SIDE EFFECTS

Defining Characteristics: Nausea, vomiting, anorexia have occurred rarely. Also, transient hepatomegaly with increased LFTs—AST, ALT, alk phos—has occurred.

Nursing Implications: Assess baseline nutritional status, preexisting nausea/vomiting, anorexia. Assess baseline LFTs and monitor periodically during treatment. Instruct patient to report side effects. Provide symptomatic interventions if side effects occur; discuss with physician use of alternative drug(s).

VI. POTENTIAL FOR FATIGUE, INFECTION, AND BLEEDING related to BONE MARROW INJURY

Defining Characteristics: Anemia, leukopenia, granulocytopenia, and thrombocytopenia may occur. Also, patients receiving antibiotics are at risk for overgrowth of nonsusceptible microorganisms, such as fungi (superinfection). Rare.

Nursing Implications: Assess baseline CBC, differential, and monitor periodically during treatment. Instruct patient to report signs/symptoms of fatigue, infection, or bleeding immediately. Assess for signs/symptoms of superinfection. Discuss any adverse effects with physician.

Drug: levofloxacin (Levaquin)

Class: Fluoroquinolone antibiotic.

Mechanism of Action: Drug is a synthetic, broad-spectrum antibacterial agent. Inhibits DNA gyrase (bacterial topoisomerase II), which is necessary for DNA replication, transcription, and repair. Has activity against a wide range of gramnegative and gram-positive bacteria, as well as against some bacteria resistant to β-lactam antibiotics.

Metabolism: Drug is well absorbed from the GI tract without regard to food, with 99% bioavailability; peak serum levels occur in 1–2 hours. Steady-state is reached in 48 hours. Drug is not extensively metabolized, with 87% of drug excreted largely unchanged in the urine at 48 hours. Terminal half-life is 6–8 hours.

Dosage/Range:

- 500 mg qd × 7 days (acute bacterial exacerbation of chronic bronchitis), × 7–14 days (community-acquired pneumonia), × 7–10 days (uncomplicated skin and skin structure infection), × 10–14 days (acute maxillary sinusitis), × 10 days (uncomplicated UTI, acute pyelonephritis).

Drug Preparation:

- Oral, available in 250-mg and 500-mg tablets.
- IV: Administer over 60 min to prevent hypotension; IV available in premixed 250-mg or 500-mg bags, or 20-mL vial containing 500 mg that is further diluted in 5% Dextrose, 0.9% Sodium Chloride.

Drug Administration:

- Administer without regard to food.
- Dose-reduce if renal compromise (see Special Considerations section).
- Administer oral doses at least 2 hours before or 2 hours after antacids containing magnesium or aluminum, as well as sucralfate, metal cations such as iron, and multivitamins containing zinc.

Drug Interactions:

- Antacids containing magnesium or aluminum, sucralfate, iron, multivitamins containing zinc: may decrease serum levels of levofloxacin; take any of these agents at least 2 hours before or 2 hours after levofloxacin.
- Theophylline: possible increase in theophylline serum levels; monitor levels and change dose accordingly.
- Warfarin: theoretically could enhance effects of oral anticoagulants; monitor INR closely and modify dose accordingly.
- NSAIDs: possible increase in the risk of CNS stimulation and seizures; assess patient risk for seizures, and use cautiously if at all in patients at risk.
- Antidiabetic agents: changes in glucose (hyper- or hypoglycemia); monitor blood sugar closely, and modify dose accordingly.

Lab Effects/Interference:

- Decreased glucose, decreased lymphocytes.

Special Considerations:

- Indicated for the treatment of acute maxillary sinusitis due to *Streptococcus pneumoniae, Haemophilus influenzae, Moraxella catarrhalis;* acute bacterial exacerbation of chronic bronchitis due to *Staphylococcus aureus, Streptococcus pneumoniae, Haemophilus influenzae, Haemophilus parainfluenzae,* or *Moraxella catarrhalis;* community-acquired pneumonia due to *Staphylococcus aureus, Streptococcus pneumoniae, Haemophilus influenzae, Haemophilus parainfluenzae, Klebsiella pneumoniae, Moraxella catarrhalis, Chlamydia pneumoniae, Legionella pneumonophila,* or *Mycoplasma pneumoniae.*

- Active against the above as well as aerobic gram-positive *Enterococcus faecalis* and *Streptococcus pyogenes* and aerobic gram-negative microorganisms *Enterobacter cloacae, Escherichia coli, Proteus mirabilis,* and *Pseudomonas aeruginosa.*
- Dose modifications for renal dysfuncion:

Acute Bacterial Exacerbation of:	**Chronic Bronchitis, Community-Acquired**	**Pneumonia, Acute Maxillary Sinusitis, Uncomplicated Skin Infections**
Renal status	Initial dose	Subsequent dose
Cr cl 20–49 mL/min	500 mg	250 mg q24h
Cr cl 10–19 mL/min	500 mg	250 mg q48h
Hemodialysis	500 mg	250 mg q48h
CAPD	500 mg q48h	250 mg q48h
Uncomplicated UTI/Acute Pyelonephritis		
Cr cl 10–19 mL/min	250 mg	250 mg q48h

- Use drug cautiously, if at all, in the following patients: (1) known or suspected CNS or seizure disorder (e.g., severe cerebral arteriosclerosis or epilepsy); (2) possess factors lowering seizure threshold (e.g., renal dysfunction, other drug therapy); (3) pregnant or nursing mothers; (4) children < 18 years old.
- Obtain ordered specimen for culture and sensitivity prior to first drug dose.

Potential Toxicities/Side Effects and the Nursing Process

I. ALTERATION IN NUTRITION related to GI SIDE EFFECTS

Defining Characteristics: 0.1–3.0% incidence of nausea, vomiting, abdominal discomfort, diarrhea, anorexia. As with all antibiotics, pseudomembranous colitis may occur, ranging in severity from mild to life-threatening. Treatment with antibiotics changes the intestinal microflora, so *C. difficile* bacteria may overgrow. Once diagnosis is made, mild diarrhea may stop with cessation of drug; if moderate to severe, it will require hydration, electrolyte replacement, nutritional support, and antibacterial coverage against *C. difficile.*

Nursing Implications: Assess baseline nutritional and elimination status. Teach patient to report GI disturbances. Teach patient to report diarrhea immediately, and consider whether this is pseudomembranous colitis and send stool specimen for *C. difficile;* if positive, discuss drug discontinuance with physician. Administer and teach patient to self-administer antiemetics, antidiarrheals as needed and as ordered. Teach patient importance of nutritious diet, and suggest small, frequent, high-calorie, high-protein meals as appropriate. Assess baseline LFTs and monitor periodically during treatment. Discuss abnormalities and drug interruption with physician.

II. SENSORY/PERCEPTUAL ALTERATIONS related to CNS EFFECTS

Defining Characteristics: 1–2% incidence of insomnia, dizziness, taste perversion, headache, nervousness, anxiety, tremors, and seizures may also occur.

Nursing Implications: Assess baseline neurological function and comfort, and monitor during treatment. Teach patient to report any changes. Discuss any abnormalities with physician. Teach patient to avoid caffeine-containing fluids, medications, e.g., tea, coffee, soft drinks.

III. ALTERATION IN SKIN INTEGRITY related to ALLERGY/HYPERSENSITIVITY

Defining Characteristics: 1–4% incidence of rash; other manifestations include eosinophilia, urticaria, flushing, fever, chills, photosensitivity, angioedema. Fatal hypersensitivity reactions have occurred rarely. Direct exposure to sunlight can cause sunburn (moderate-to-severe phototoxicity).

Nursing Implications: Assess baseline skin condition, including integrity and drug allergy history. Teach patient to report rash, itching, other skin changes. Teach patient skin care and symtomatic measures as appropriate. If skin rash develops, discuss drug discontinuance with physician. If rash progresses, especially in HIV-infected patients, drug should be discontinued, as fatal Stevens-Johnson syndrome may develop. Be prepared to treat severe acute hypersensitivity reactions with airway management, oxygen, epinephrine, corticosteroids, antihistamines as ordered. Teach patient to avoid excessive sun exposure and to use skin protection factor (SPF) 15 or higher.

IV. FUNGAL SUPERINFECTION related to REDISTRIBUTION OF ENDOGENOUS MICROORGANISMS

Defining Characteristics: Vaginal moniliasis, vaginitis may occur as endogenous bacteris are eliminated and normal fungal population expands.

Nursing Implications: Teach female patient to report vaginal itching or discharge. Discuss appropriate antifungal treatment with physician. Teach perineal hygiene and symptomatic management.

Drug: linezolid (Zyvox)

Class: Oxazolidinone class of antibiotic.

Mechanism of Action: Linezolid inhibits initiation of protein synthesis by preventing the formation of the fmet-tRNA:mRNA:30S subunit ternary complex. Oxazolidinones bind to the 50S subunit in a region shared with the peptidyl transferase inhibitor chloramphenicol. Oxazolidinones are not peptidyl transferase inhibitors, and it is not known which specific ribosome reaction is inhibited by 50S subunit binding. Linezolid has a specific mechanism of action against bacteria resistant to other antibiotics, including methicillin-resistant *Staphylococcus aureus* (MRSA), multi-resistant strains of *Streptococcus pneumoniae,* and vancomycin-resistant (VRE) *enterococcus faecium.*

Metabolism: Primarily metabolized by oxidation of the morpholine ring, resulting in two inactive carboxylic acid metabolites. Only about 30% of a dose is excreted unchanged in the urine.

Dosage/Range:
- Oral: 400–600 mg q12h for 10 to 14 days; up to 28 days for VRE.
- IV: 600 mg q12h for 10–14 days; up to 28 days for VRE.

Drug Preparation:
- Available in single-use, ready-to-use infusion bags.

Drug Administration:
- IV infusion over 30–120 minutes.

Drug Administration:
- Linezolid has the potential to interact with adrenergic (phenylpropanolamine, pseudoephedrine) and serotonergic agents since it is a reversible, nonselective monoamine oxidase inhibitor.
- Large quantities of foods or beverages with high tyramine content should be avoided.

Lab Effects/Interference:
- Thrombocytopenia has been seen when this drug is administered long-term (up to 28 days).

Special Considerations:
- IV and PO doses are the same.

Potential Toxicities/Side Effects and the Nursing Process

I. ALTERATION IN NUTRITION related to GI SIDE EFFECTS

Defining Characteristics: Nausea, vomiting, anorexia have occurred frequently.

Nursing Implications: Assess baseline nutritional status, preexisting nausea/vomiting, anorexia. Teach patient to report side effects. Provide symptomatic interventions if side effects occur; discuss with physician use of alternative drug(s).

II. POTENTIAL FOR INJURY related to HYPERSENSITIVITY REACTION

Defining Characteristics: Urticaria, pruritus, rash (maculopapular or erythematous), fever and chills, eosinophilia, myalgia, edema, erythema, angioedema.

Nursing Implications: Assess for drug allergies to erythromycin or macrolide antibiotic prior to drug administration. Teach patient to report any allergic reactions. Assess for signs/symptoms of allergic reaction after drug dose. Assess baseline skin integrity and presence of drug allergies; monitor patient closely during drug infusions. Teach patient to report immediately signs/symptoms of rash, pruritus, shortness of breath, any adverse sensation. Teach patient skin care and symptomatic measures as appropriate. If skin rash develops, discuss drug discontinuance with physician. If rash progresses, especially in human immunodeficiency virus (HIV)-infected patients, drug should be discontinued, as fatal Stevens-Johnson syndrome may develop. Be prepared to treat severe acute hypersensitivity reactions with airway management, oxygen, epinephrine, corticosteroids, antihistamines as ordered.

III. ALTERATION IN COMFORT related to HEADACHE

Defining Characteristics: Headache has occurred in some patients.

Nursing Implications: Assess baseline hearing (ability to hear spoken voice) and continue to assess during therapy. Teach patient potential side effects, and instruct patient to report any hearing/perceptual problems (e.g., tinnitus, vertigo, decreased hearing). Discuss drug discontinuance and audiogram with physician to confirm hearing dysfunction if symptoms arise. Assess for increased risk if given concurrently with other ototoxic medications (e.g., cisplatin, furosemide).

IV. FUNGAL SUPERINFECTION related to REDISTRIBUTION OF ENDOGENOUS MICROORGANISMS

Defining Characteristics: Vaginal or oral candidiasis (sore mouth or tongue; white patches in mouth and/or tongue); vaginitis (vaginal candidiasis); vaginal itching and discharge may occur as endogenous bacteria are eliminated and normal fungal population expands.

Nursing Implications: Teach female patient to report vaginal itching or discharge. Discuss appropriate antifungal treatment with physician. Teach perineal hygiene and symptomatic management.

Drug: meropenem (Merrem)

Class: antibiotic, carbapenem.

Mechanism of Action: The bactericidal activity results from the inhibition of cell wall synthesis. Penetrates the cell wall of most gram-positive and gram-negative bacteria to reach penicillin-binding protein (PBP) targets.

Metabolism: Widely distributed in body tissues and fluids, excreted in urine.

Dosage/Range:

Adult:

- Intrabdominal infection: 1 gram IV every 8 hours.
- Meningitis: bacterial 2 grams IV every 8 hours.

Drug Preparation/Administration:

- IV bolus, dilute with 5–20 ml. Sterile Water for Injection and give over 3–5 minutes,
- IV infusion dilute with D5W or normal saline, infuse over 15–30 minutes, maximum concentration 50 mg/ml

Drug Interactions:

- Probenecid competes with meropenem for active tubular secretion and thus inhibits the renal excretion of meropenem.
- Meropenem may reduce serum levels of valproic acid to subtherapeutic levels.

Lab Effects/Interference:

- Meropenem posses the characteristic low toxicity of the beta-lactam group of antibiotics.
- Periodically assess organ system function; renal, hepatic & hematopoietic.

Potential Toxicities/Side Effects and the Nursing Process

I. POTENTIAL FOR INJURY related to HYPERSENSITIVITY REACTION and LOCAL REACTIONS (pain at injection site)

Defining Characteristics: Urticaria, pruritus, rash (maculopapular or erythematous), fever and chills, eosinophilia, myalgia, edema, erythema, angioedema.

Nursing Implications: Assess allergy to cephalosporin antibiotics and penicillin: if patient states ''yes,'' determine actual response, e.g., ''swollen lips = angioedema.'' If angioedema, patient SHOULD NOT receive drug. Discuss other patient responses with physician to determine whether drug should be given. Assess baseline skin condition, including integrity and allergy history to drugs. Instruct patient to report rash, itching, and other skin changes. Teach patient skin care and symptomatic measures as appropriate. If skin rash develops, discuss drug discontinuance with physician. Be prepared to treat severe acute hypersensitivity reactions with airway management, oxygen, epinephrine, corticosteroids, antihistamines as ordered.

II. ALTERATION IN NUTRITION, LESS THAN BODY REQUIREMENTS, related to GI SIDE EFFECTS

Defining Characteristics: Nausea, vomiting, diarrhea may occur; rarely, pseudomembranous colitis caused by antibiotic resistance occurs.

Nursing Implications: Assess baseline nutritional status. Instruct patient to report GI disturbances. Administer and teach patient to self-administer antiemetics as needed and as ordered. Teach patient importance of nutritious diet, and suggest small, frequent, high-calorie, high-protein meals as appropriate. Assess baseline LFTs, and monitor periodically during treatment. Discuss abnormalities and drug interruption with physician.

III. FUNGAL SUPERINFECTION related to REDISTRIBUTION OF ENDOGENOUS MICROORGANISMS

Defining Characteristics: Vaginal candidiasis, vaginitis may occur as endogenous bacteria are eliminated, and normal fungal population expands.

Nursing Implications: Instruct female patient to report vaginal itching or discharge. Discuss appropriate antifungal treatment with physician. Teach perineal hygiene and symptomatic management.

Drug: metronidazole hydrochloride (Flagyl)

Class: Antibacterial (systemic); antiprotozoal.

Mechanism of Action: Disrupts DNA, inhibits nucleic acid synthesis in susceptible organisms. Active against anaerobic gram-negative (*Bacteroides*) and gram-positive bacilli (*Clostridium*), and protozoa (*Trichomonas, Giardia*).

Metabolism: Well absorbed after oral administration; rate affected by food, but not amount absorbed. Oral and IV serum levels are similar. Widely distributed in body tissues and fluids, including CSF, placenta, breast milk. Excreted in urine (60–80%) and feces.

Dosage/Range:

Adult:

- Oral: 250–750 mg PO tid × 7–10 days or single dose of 2 g PO (trichomoniasis).
- Pseudomembranous colitis: 250 mg PO qid × 7–14 days or 500 mg PO tid × 7–14 days.

- IV: Loading dose of 15 mg/kg IV over 1 hour (1 g); then maintenance dose of 7.5 mg/kg IV (500 mg) q8h (maximum 4 g/day).

Drug Preparation/Administration:
- Oral: Store in light-resistant container at < 30°C (86°F).
- IV: Protect from light and freezing. Reconstitute according to manufacturer's package insert. Further dilute with 0.9% Sodium Chloride or 5% Dextrose to concentration of ≤ 8 mg/mL. Do not use aluminum needles. Administer over 30–60 minutes. May be given as continuous or intermittent infusion.

Drug Interactions:
- Coumarin anticoagulants: increase anticoagulant effect. Avoid concurrent use if possible; otherwise, monitor PT closely and decrease anticoagulant drug dose as needed.
- Alcohol: inhibits alcohol metabolism, causing a disulfiram-like reaction (flushing, headache, nausea, vomiting, abdominal cramps, diaphoresis). Avoid alcohol and alcohol-containing medications for 48 hours after last metronidazole dose.
- Disulfiram: causes acute psychoses and confusion. Avoid concurrent use and separate use by 2 weeks.
- Phenobarbital/phenytoin: decrease metronidazole activity. Monitor effectiveness and increase metronidazole dose as needed.
- Cimetidine: increases metronidazole levels with potential for increased toxicity. Avoid concurrent administration.

Lab Effects/Interference:
- Serum ALT, serum AST, and LDH: metronidazole has a high absorbance at the wavelength at which NADH is determined; therefore, elevated liver enzyme concentrations may appear to be suppressed by metronidazole when measured by continuous-flow methods based on endpoint decrease.

Special Considerations:
- Carcinogenic in rodents, so drug is used only when necessary.
- Contraindicated in first trimester of pregnancy and administered only as salvage therapy in second and third trimesters when other agents have failed; lactating mothers should interrupt breast-feeding during treatment with drug.
- Use with caution in patients with a history of blood dyscrasias, CNS disorders/dysfunction, hepatic dysfunction, or alcoholism.
- May interfere with laboratory determinations of LFTs (AST, ALT, LDH).

Potential Toxicities/Side Effects and the Nursing Process

I. ALTERATION IN NUTRITION, LESS THAN BODY REQUIREMENTS, related to GI SIDE EFFECTS

Defining Characteristics: Nausea (with/without headache), anorexia, dry mouth, metallic taste in mouth have occurred; less frequently, vomiting, diarrhea, epigastric distress, or constipation. Rare pseudomembranous colitis.

Nursing Implications: Assess baseline nutritional and elimination status. Instruct patient to report GI disturbances. Administer and teach patient to self-administer antiemetics, antidiarrheals as needed and as ordered. Teach patient importance of nutritious diet, and suggest small, frequent, high-calorie, high-protein meals as appropriate. Assess baseline LFTs and monitor periodically during treatment. Discuss abnormalities and drug interruption with physician. Assess whether taking other hepatotoxic drugs (see Special Considerations section). Instruct patient to avoid alcohol and alcohol-containing medications for 48 hours after last drug dose.

II. ALTERATIONS IN SENSORY/PERCEPTUAL PATTERNS related to PERIPHERAL NEUROPATHY

Defining Characteristics: Peripheral neuropathy (numbness, tingling, paresthesia) is reversible with drug discontinuance. Headache, dizziness, ataxia, confusion, mood changes have also occurred.

Nursing Implications: Assess baseline neurologic function and comfort, and monitor during treatment. Instruct patient to report any changes. Discuss abnormalities and drug discontinuance with physician.

III. ALTERATIONS IN SKIN INTEGRITY related to SENSITIVITY REACTIONS

Defining Characteristics: Urticaria, erythematous rash, pruritus, flushing, transient joint pain may occur.

Nursing Implications: Assess drug allergy history. Assess baseline skin integrity. Instruct patient to report rash, pruritus. Teach patient symptomatic management of rash, pruritus.

IV. ALTERATIONS IN URINARY ELIMINATION related to DYSURIA

Defining Characteristics: Urethral burning, dysuria, cystitis, polyuria, incontinence, sensation of pelvic pressure may occur with oral dose. Urine may be dark or reddish-brown.

Nursing Implications: Assess baseline elimination status. Instruct patient to report side effects, and to increase oral fluids to 2–3 qt (liters)/day. Reassure patient urine color change is related to drug and will disappear when drug therapy is completed.

V. ALTERATIONS IN SEXUALITY related to DECREASED LIBIDO, DYSPAREUNIA

Defining Characteristics: Decreased libido, dyspareunia, dryness of vagina and vulva may occur.

Nursing Implications: Assess pattern of sexuality. Inform patient and partner that these effects, if they occur, are temporary. Suggest frequent perineal hygiene as needed to relieve dryness and use of lubricants during intercourse.

VI. FUNGAL SUPERINFECTION related to REDISTRIBUTION OF ENDOGENOUS MICROORGANISMS

Defining Characteristics: Vaginal candidiasis, vaginitis may occur as endogenous bacteria are eliminated and normal fungal population expands.

Nursing Implications: Instruct female patient to report vaginal itching or discharge. Discuss appropriate antifungal treatment with physician. Teach perineal hygiene and symptomatic management.

VII. ALTERATIONS IN COMFORT related to PHLEBITIS

Defining Characteristics: Phlebitis and thrombophlebitis may occur with IV administration.

Nursing Implications: Assess IV site prior to each dose for phlebitis, erythema, swelling, and change site at least q48h. Apply heat to painful IV site as ordered.

Drug: mezlocillin sodium (Mezlin)

Class: Antibacterial (extended spectrum penicillin).

Mechanism of Action: Semisynthetic antibiotic prepared from fungus *Penicillium.* Contains β-lactam ring and is bactericidal by inhibiting cell wall synthesis. Active against most gram-positive (except penicillinase-producing strains) and most gram-negative bacilli. Used in the treatment of serious gram-negative infections, especially *P. aeruginosa*–related infections of lower respiratory tract, urinary tract, and skin.

Metabolism: Poorly absorbed from GI tract, so must be given parenterally. Widely distributed in body tissues and fluids. Crosses placenta and is excreted in breast milk. Excreted via urine and bile.

Dosage/Range:

Adult:

- IV: 200–300 mg/kg/day in four to six divided doses (usual dose 3 g q4–6h).
- Dose modification if severe renal insufficiency; refer to manufacturer's package insert.

Drug Preparation/Administration:

- IV: Reconstitute each gram with at least 10 mL sterile water for injection. Further dilute in 50–100 mL 0.9% Sodium Chloride or 5% Dextrose injection. Administer over 30 minutes.
- IM: Reconstitute each gram with 3–4 mL sterile water for injection or 0.5–1% lidocaine HCl (without epinephrine). Maximum dose is 2 g. Divide dose into two injections, as needed, and administer deep IM in large muscle mass. Administer slowly. Make certain patient is NOT ALLERGIC to lidocaine.

Drug Interactions:

- Aminoglycosides: synergism.
- Aminoglycosides (e.g., gentamicin): incompatible when mixed together; administer at separate sites at different times. Also, penicillinase-resistant penicillins can inactivate aminoglycoside serum samples from patients receiving both drugs.
- Clavulanic acid (inhibits β-lactamase): increases antibacterial action.
- Probenecid: increased serum level of mezlocillin; may be coadministered to exert this effect.

Lab Effects/Interference:

Major clinical significance:

- Urine glucose: high urinary concentrations of a penicillin may produce false-positive or falsely elevated test results with copper sulfate tests (Benedict's, Clinitest, or Fehling's); glucose enzymatic tests (Clinistix or Tes-tape) are not affected.

Clinical significance:

- Coombs' (direct antiglobulin) test: false-positive result may occur during therapy with any penicillin.
- Urine protein: high urinary concentrations of mezlocillin may produce false-positive protein reactions (pseudoproteinuria) with the sulfosalicylic acid and boiling test, the acetic acid test, the biuret reaction, and the nitric acid test; bromophenol blue reagent test strips (Multistix) are reportedly unaffected.
- ALT, alk phos, AST, serum LDH values may be increased.
- Serum bili: an increase has been associated with mezlocillin.
- BUN and serum creatinine: an increase has been associated with mezlocillin.

- Serum K+: hypokalemia may occur following the administration of parenteral mezlocillin, which may act as a non-reabsorbable anion in the distal renal tubules; this may cause an increase in pH and result in increased urinary K+ loss. The risk of hypokalemia increases with the use of larger doses.
- Serum Na+: hypernatremia may occur following administration of large doses of parenteral mezlocillin because of the high Na+ content of these medications.
- WBC: leukopenia or neutropenia is associated with the use of all penicillins; the effect is more likely to occur with prolonged therapy and severe hepatic function impairment.

Special Considerations:

- Contraindicated in patients with prior hypersensitivity to penicillins. Use with caution in patients sensitive to other β-lactams (e.g., cephalosporins) since partial cross-allergenicity exists.
- Obtain ordered specimen, and send for culture and sensitivity test prior to first antibiotic dose.
- Consider alternative antibiotic therapy if eosinophilia, drug fever or rash, arthralgia, hematuria, or unexplained rise in BUN and serum creatinine occur.
- Monitor electrolytes and renal, hepatic, and hematologic laboratory parameters during extended treatment periods.
- Use with caution in pregnancy or with nursing women.
- Na content is 1.85 mEq/g of drug.

Potential Toxicities/Side Effects and the Nursing Process

I. POTENTIAL FOR INJURY related to HYPERSENSITIVITY REACTION

Defining Characteristics: Urticaria, pruritus, rash (maculopapular or erythematous), fever and chills, eosinophilia, myalgia, edema, erythema, angioedema, Stevens-Johnson syndrome, and exfoliative skin reactions occur in 5% of patients. Increased risk in individuals allergic to cephalosporin antibiotics.

Nursing Implications: Assess allergy to cephalosporin antibiotics and penicillin: if patient states "yes," determine actual response, e.g., "swollen lips = angioedema." If angioedema, patient SHOULD NOT receive drug. Discuss other patient responses with physician to determine whether drug should be given. Assess baseline skin condition, including integrity and allergy history to drugs. Instruct patient to report rash, itching, and other skin changes. Teach patient skin care and symptomatic measures as appropriate. If skin rash develops, discuss drug discontinuance with physician. If rash progresses, drug should be discontinued, as fatal Stevens-Johnson syndrome may develop. Be prepared to treat severe acute hypersensitivity reactions with airway management, oxygen, epinephrine, corticosteroids, antihistamines as ordered.

II. ALTERATION IN NUTRITION, LESS THAN BODY REQUIREMENTS, related to GI SIDE EFFECTS

Defining Characteristics: Nausea, vomiting, diarrhea may occur; rarely, pseudomembranous colitis caused by *C. difficile* resistant to the antibiotic occurs. Rarely, transient increases in LFTs—AST, ALT, alk phos, bili—may occur.

Nursing Implications: Assess baseline nutritional status. Instruct patient to report GI disturbances. Administer and teach patient to self-administer antiemetics as needed and as ordered. Teach patient importance of nutritious diet, and suggest small, frequent, high-calorie, high-protein meals as appropriate. Assess baseline LFTs, and monitor periodically during treatment. Discuss abnormalities and drug interruption with physician.

III. FUNGAL SUPERINFECTION related to REDISTRIBUTION OF ENDOGENOUS MICROORGANISMS

Defining Characteristics: Vaginal candidiasis, vaginitis may occur as endogenous bacteria are eliminated and normal fungal population expands.

Nursing Implications: Instruct female patient to report vaginal itching or discharge. Discuss appropriate antifungal treatment with physician. Teach perineal hygiene and symptomatic management.

IV. ALTERATIONS IN PROTECTIVE MECHANISMS (RARE) related to TRANSIENT LEUKOPENIA

Defining Characteristics: Rarely, transient leukopenia, lymphocytosis, anemia, eosinophilia may occur. Prolonged PT, prolonged APTT, and hypoprothrombinemia have occurred rarely, especially in elderly or debilitated patients, or in individuals with vitamin K deficiency.

Nursing Implications: Assess baseline laboratory parameters, and monitor periodically during treatment. Assess patient for response to antibiotics. Discuss abnormalities with physician. Assess for signs/symptoms of bleeding.

V. ALTERATIONS IN SENSORY/PERCEPTUAL PATTERNS related to DIZZINESS, SOMNOLENCE

Defining Characteristics: Dizziness, headache, somnolence occur rarely. Neuromuscular irritability and seizures may occur with high drug serum levels.

Nursing Implications: Assess baseline neurologic function and comfort, and monitor during treatment. Instruct patient to report any changes. Discuss any abnormalities with physician. Institute seizure precautions.

VI. ALTERATIONS IN COMFORT related to LOCAL INJECTION IRRITATION

Defining Characteristics: Vein irritation (pain, erythema), phlebitis, and thrombophlebitis may occur at IV administration site.

Nursing Implications: Change IV sites q48h, and assess for signs/symptoms of phlebitis prior to each administration. Administer drug slowly. Apply warm packs to increase comfort. Discuss central line with patient and physician to facilitate administration.

VII. ALTERATION IN FLUID AND ELECTROLYTE BALANCE related to HYPOKALEMIA AND INCREASED SODIUM INTAKE

Defining Characteristics: Prolonged therapy may cause hypokalemia; also, drug is prepared as sodium salt. Frequent IV infusions increase fluid intake.

Nursing Implications: Assess baseline electrolytes, fluid balance, weight, and monitor throughout therapy. Monitor renal function studies, especially if patient has preexisting renal dysfunction.

Drug: minocycline hydrochloride (Minocin, Vectrin, Dynacin)

Class: Antibacterial (systemic); antiprotozoal.

Mechanism of Action: Bacteriostatic, but may be bactericidal at high concentrations. Binds to bacterial ribosomes and prevents protein synthesis. Active against broad range of gram-positive and gram-negative bacteria, Chlamydia, and Mycoplasma.

Metabolism: Absorbed (60%–80%) from GI tract. Widely distributed into body tissues and fluids. Crosses placenta and is excreted in breast milk. Excreted unchanged in urine.

Dosage/Range:

Adult:

- Oral: 200 mg initially, then 100 mg q12h for 5–15 days; or 100–200 mg initially, then 50 mg q6h for 5–15 days.
- IV: 200 mg initially, then 100 mg q12h for 5–15 days (depends on indication).
- Dose modification necessary if renal dysfunction exists.

Drug Preparation/Administration:

- Oral: may be taken with food, water, or milk.
- IV: add 5–10 mL sterile water for injection to 100-mg vial. Further dilute in 500 to 1000 mL of 0.9% Sodium Chloride injection, Dextrose injection, Dextrose and Sodium Chloride injections, Ringer's injection, or lactated

Ringer's injection. Do not use other calcium-containing solutions, since precipitate may form.

- AVOID RAPID ADMINISTRATION.
- Solution stable for 24 hours at room temperature. Avoid exposure to heat or sunlight. Convert to oral preparation as soon as possible, as there is risk of thrombophlebitis.
- DO NOT ADMINISTER INTRAMUSCULARLY or SUBCUTANEOUSLY.

Drug Interactions:

- Hepatotoxic drugs: may increase hepatotoxicity if given concurrently. Assess baseline and periodically during treatment.
- Iron preparations: decrease oral and possibly IV absorption. Administer iron preparations 3 hours after or 2 hours before any tetracycline.
- Oral anticoagulants: increase PT. Monitor patient closely and decrease anticoagulant dose as needed.
- Antidiarrheals (containing kaolin, pectate, or bismuth): may decrease absorption of tetracyclines. Avoid concurrent use.
- Oral contraceptives: decreased effectiveness of contraceptive and increased incidence of breakthrough bleeding. Advise patient to use barrier contraceptive as well during a course of tetracycline therapy.
- Lithium: may decrease lithium levels. Monitor serum levels and increase dose as needed.

Lab Effects/Interference:

- Urine catecholamine determinations: may produce false elevations of urinary catecholamines because of interfering fluorescence in the Hingerty method.
- SGPT, alk phos, amylase, SGOT, and bilirubin: serum concentrations may be increased.

Special Considerations:

- May cause dizziness, lightheadedness, or unsteadiness (CNS toxicity).
- Pigmentation of skin and mucous membranes may occur.
- Use cautiously in patients with myasthenia gravis: may increase muscle weakness.
- Avoid use in pregnant or lactating women.
- Obtain ordered specimen for culture and sensitivity prior to first dose.
- IV preparation contains ascorbic acid and may cause false-positive result using Clinitest, or false-negative when using Clinistix and Testape.
- Drug has affinity for ischemic, necrotic tissue, and may localize in tumors.

Potential Toxicities/Side Effects and the Nursing Process

I. ALTERATION IN NUTRITION related to GI SIDE EFFECTS

Defining Characteristics: Nausea, vomiting, diarrhea, anorexia, abdominal discomfort, epigastric burning and distress, glossitis, black hairy tongue may occur.

Nursing Implications: Assess baseline nutritional status. Assess for and teach patient to report any symptoms. Administer and teach patient self-administration of prescribed antiemetic or antidiarrheal medication as appropriate. Administer and teach patient to self-administer oral dose with at least 8 oz of water taken at least 1 hour before lying down for sleep.

II. ALTERATION IN SKIN INTEGRITY related to RASH, PHOTOSENSITIVITY

Defining Characteristics: Maculopapular and erythematous rashes may occur. Rarely, exfoliative dermatitis, onycholysis, and nail discoloration. Photosensitivity risk (exaggerated sunburn) persists 1–2 days after completion of drug therapy.

Nursing Implications: Teach patient about potential side effects, to avoid sunlight during drug therapy, and to report rash, other abnormalities. Teach symptomatic skin care as appropriate.

III. INJURY related to HYPERSENSITIVITY

Defining Characteristics: Urticaria, angioneurotic edema, anaphylaxis may occur; also, fever, rash, arthralgias, eosinophilia, and pericarditis.

Nursing Implications: Assess drug allergy history. Assess baseline allergy history. Assess baseline skin integrity. Teach patient to report rash, pruritus. Teach patent symptomatic management of rash, pruritus. Assess for hypersensitivity reaction; if it occurs, monitor VS, discontinue drug, notify physician, and institute supportive measures.

IV. FUNGAL SUPERINFECTION related to REDISTRIBUTION OF ENDOGENOUS MICROORGANISMS

Defining Characteristics: Vaginal moniliasis, vaginitis may occur as endogenous bacteria are eliminated and normal fungal population expands.

Nursing Implications: Teach female patient to report vaginal itching or discharge. Discuss appropriate antifungal treatment with physician. Teach perineal hygiene and symptomatic management.

V. ALTERATION IN HEPATIC FUNCTION

Defining Characteristics: Associated with high IV doses (> 2 g/day): hepatotoxicity and cholestasis may occur.

Nursing Implications: Assess baseline LFTs and monitor during therapy.

VI. INFECTION AND BLEEDING related to NEUTROPENIA, THROMBOCYTOPENIA

Defining Characteristics: Neutropenia, leukocytosis, leukopenia, atypical lymphocytes, thrombocytopenia, thrombocytopenic purpura, hemolytic anemia occur rarely with long-term therapy.

Nursing Implications: Assess baseline WBC, HCT, and platelets, and monitor periodically during long-term therapy.

VII. ALTERATION IN COMFORT related to LOCAL ADMINISTRATION EFFECTS

Defining Characteristics: IM administration may cause pain, induration due to muscle injury. IV administration may cause erythema, pain, swelling, and thrombophlebitis.

Nursing Implications: Rotate sites. Apply ice as ordered to painful buttock. Assess IV site prior to each dose for phlebitis or swelling, and change site at least q48h. Apply heat to painful IV sites as ordered.

VIII. SENSORY/PERCEPTUAL ALTERATION

Defining Characteristics: Light-headedness, dizziness, headache may occur.

Nursing Implications: Assess baseline neurological status. Teach patient to report any changes and discuss them with physician.

Drug: moxifloxacin (ABC Pack; Avelox)

Class: Antibiotic; Quinolone.

Mechanism of Action: Moxifloxacin is a broad-spectrum anti-infective, active against a wide range of aerobic gram-positive and gram-negative organisms. Acts intracellularly by inhibiting DNA gyrase and bacterial topoisomerase IV. DNA gyrase is required for DNA replication and transcription, DNA repair, recombination, and transposition; inhibition is bactericidal.

Metabolism: Widely distributed to most body fluids and tissues with highest concentrations in organs, such as kidneys, gallbladder, lungs, liver, gynecological tissue, prostatic tissue, phagocytic cells, urine, sputum, and bile. Well absorbed from GI tract. Metabolized in liver; excreted in urine and feces. Crosses placenta and is excreted in breast milk.

Dosage/Range:
- 400 mg PO or IV QD.

Drug Preparation/Administration:
- Oral: Take drug with large glass of water, preferably 2 hours after meal/food. Encourage oral fluids of 2–3 qt (liters)/day.
- IV: Further dilute drug in 0.9% Sodium Chloride or 5% Dextrose in water to final concentration of 2 mg/mL. Administer over 60 minutes, do not infuse by rapid or bolus intravenous infusion.
- Do not refrigerate.

Drug Interactions:
- Antacids (containing magnesium, aluminum, or calcium) and iron decrease absorption of serum level of moxifloxacin; do not administer concurrently. If must administer antacids or iron, administer at least 4 hours apart. The administration of antacids containing aluminum, magnesium, calcium, sucralfate, zinc, or iron may substantially reduce the absorption of moxifloxacin; do not administer concurrently.
- Serum digoxin concentrations should be monitored; moxifloxacin may raise serum levels in some patients.
- Probenecid: decreases the renal tubular secretion of moxifloxacin, resulting in a prolonged elimination half-life and increased risk of toxicity.
- Moxifloxacin may have the potential to prolong the Q-T interval of the EKG in some patients. Moxifloxacin should not be used in patients with prolonged Q-T interval; patients with uncorrected hypokalemia; and patients on quinidine, procanamide, amiodrone, and sotalol (antiarrhythmic agents).
- Increased intracranial pressure and psychosis has been reported along with CNS stimulation.
- Hypersensitivity reactions have been reported.

Lab Effects/Interference:
- Serum SGPT, serum Alk Phos, serum SGOT, and serum LDH—values may be increased.

Special Considerations:
- Used in the treatment of respiratory tract infections (acute bacterial exacerbation of chronic bronchitis, acute bacterial sinusitis, and commonly acquired pneumonia).
- Used in the treatment of uncomplicated infections of the skin and skin structures.
- Contraindicated in pregnancy or women who are breast-feeding.
- Obtain ordered specimen for culture and sensitivity prior to first drug dose.

- Use cautiously in patients with seizure disorders.

Potential Toxicities/Side Effects and the Nursing Process

I. ALTERATION IN NUTRITION related to GI SIDE EFFECTS

Defining Characteristics: Incidence of nausea, vomiting, abdominal discomfort, diarrhea, anorexia.

Nursing Implications: Assess baseline nutritional and elimination status. Teach patient to report GI disturbances. Administer and teach patient to self-administer antiemetics, antidiarrheals as needed and as ordered. Teach patient importance of nutritious diet, and suggest small, frequent, high-calorie, high-protein meals as appropriate. Assess baseline LFTs and monitor periodically during treatment. Discuss abnormalities and drug interruption with physician.

II. SENSORY/PERCEPTUAL ALTERATIONS related to CNS EFFECTS

Defining Characteristics: Incidence of headache, restlessness. Dizziness, hallucinations, and seizures may also occur. Exacerbated by caffeine as quinolones delay caffeine excretion.

Nursing Implications: Assess baseline neurological function and comfort, and monitor during treatment. Teach patient to report any changes. Discuss any abnormalities with physician. Teach patient to limit or restrict all caffeine-containing fluids, medications, e.g., tea, coffee, soft drinks.

III. ALTERATION IN SKIN INTEGRITY related to ALLERGY/HYPERSENSITIVITY

Defining Characteristics: Incidence of rash; other manifestations include eosinophilia, urticaria, flushing, fever, chills, photosensitivity, angioedema. Fatal hypersensitivity reactions have occurred rarely. Direct exposure to sunlight can cause sunburn (moderate to severe phototoxicity).

Nursing Implications: Assess baseline skin condition, including integrity and drug allergy history. Teach patient to report rash, itching, and other skin changes. Teach patient skin care and symptomatic measures as appropriate. If skin rash develops, discuss drug discontinuance with physician. Be prepared to treat severe acute hypersensitivity reactions with airway management, oxygen, epinephrine, corticosteroids, antihistamines as ordered. Teach patient to avoid excessive sun exposure and to use skin protection factor (SPF) 15 or higher. If rash progresses, especially in HIV-infected patients, drug should be discontinued as fatal Stevens-Johnson syndrome may develop.

IV. FUNGAL SUPERINFECTION related to REDISTRIBUTION OF ENDOGENOUS MICROORGANISMS

Defining Characteristics: Vaginal moniliasis, vaginitis may occur as endogenous bacteria are eliminated and normal fungal population expands.

Nursing Implications: Teach female patient to report vaginal itching or discharge. Discuss appropriate antifungal treatment with physician. Teach perineal hygiene and symptomatic management.

V. ALTERATION IN URINARY ELIMINATION related to RENAL TOXICITY

Defining Characteristics: Increased BUN and creatinine, crystal and stone formation in urine, interstitial nephritis, and renal failure may occur.

Nursing Implications: Assess baseline renal function; expect that drug dose will be decreased in presence of renal dysfunction. Teach patient to take drug with at least 8 oz of water, and to increase oral fluids to 2–3 qt/day.

VI. ALTERATION IN COMFORT related to IV ADMINISTRATION

Defining Characteristics: Drug may cause pain, inflammation, and rare thrombophlebitis at IV site.

Nursing Implications: Change IV site q 48 hours. Assess for phlebitis, discomfort, and IV patency prior to each administration. Administer drug slowly over 60–90 minutes in large volume of 5% Dextrose (see Drug Preparation/Administration). Apply heat to promote comfort.

Drug: nafcillin sodium (Unipen)

Class: Antibacterial (systemic).

Mechanism of Action: Semisynthetic antibiotic. Contains β-lactam ring and is bactericidal by inhibiting cell wall synthesis. Penicillinase-resistant penicillin; active against penicillin-resistant staphylococci that produce the enzyme penicillinase.

Metabolism: Incompletely absorbed from GI tract; rapidly absorbed when given IM or IV. Widely distributed in body tissues and fluid, including bile. Crosses placenta and is excreted in breast milk; 70–90% bound to serum proteins. Metabolized in liver, excreted in bile, and to a lesser degree in the urine.

Dosage/Range:

Adult:

- Oral: 500 mg–1 g PO q6h.

- IM/IV: 500 mg–2 g q4h.

Drug Preparation/Administration:
- Oral: Reconstitute per manufacturer's recommendation or by capsules or tablets. Administer 1 hour before meals or 2 hours after meals.
- IM: Reconstitute with sterile or bacteriostatic water for injection, and give deep IM in large muscle (e.g., gluteus maximus).
- IV: Reconstitute with sterile water for injection or 0.9% Sodium Chloride for injection according to manufacturer's package insert. Further dilute in 100 mL IV solution and infuse over 40–60 minutes.

Drug Interactions:
- Aminoglycosides: synergism.
- Aminoglycosides (e.g., gentamicin): incompatible when mixed together; administer at separate sites at different times. Also, penicillinase-resistant penicillins can inactivate aminoglycoside serum samples from patients receiving both drugs.
- Rifampin: possible antagonism, only at high doses of penicillin.
- Probenecid: increased serum level of nafcillin; may be coadministered to exert this effect.

Lab Effects/Interference:
Major clinical significance:
- Urine glucose: high urinary concentrations of a penicillin may produce false-positive or falsely elevated test results with copper sulfate tests (Benedict's, Clinitest, or Fehling's); glucose enzymatic tests (Clinistix or Testape) are not affected.

Clinical significance:
- Coombs' (direct antiglobulin) test: false-positive result may occur during therapy with any penicillin.
- ALT, alk phos, AST, serum LDH: values may be increased.
- WBC: leukopenia or neutropenia is associated with the use of all penicillins; the effect is more likely to occur with prolonged therapy and severe hepatic function impairment.

Special Considerations:
- Contraindicated in patients with prior hypersensitivity to penicillins. Use with caution in patients sensitive to other β-lactams (e.g., cephalosporins) since partial cross-allergenicity exists.
- Obtain ordered specimen and send for culture and sensitivity prior to first antibiotic dose.
- Consider alternative antibiotic therapy if eosinophilia, drug fever or rash, arthralgia, hematuria, or unexplained rise in BUN and serum creatinine occur.

- Monitor electrolytes and renal, hepatic, and hematologic laboratory parameters during extended treatment periods.
- Use with caution in pregnancy or with nursing women.

Potential Toxicities/Side Effects and the Nursing Process

I. POTENTIAL FOR INJURY related to HYPERSENSITIVITY REACTION

Defining Characteristics: Urticaria, pruritus, rash (maculopapular or erythematous), fever and chills, eosinophilia, myalgia, edema, erythema, angioedema, Stevens-Johnson syndrome, and exfoliative skin reactions occur in 5% of patients. Increased risk in individuals allergic to cephalosporin antibiotics.

Nursing Implications: Assess allergy to cephalosporin antibiotics and penicillin: if patient states "yes," determine actual response, e.g., "swollen lips = angioedema." If angioedema, patient SHOULD NOT receive drug. Discuss other patient responses with physician to determine whether drug should be given. Assess baseline skin condition, including integrity and allergy history to drugs. Instruct patient to report rash, itching, other skin changes. Teach patient skin care and symptomatic measures as appropriate. If skin rash develops, discuss drug discontinuance with physician. If rash progresses, drug should be discontinued, as fatal Stevens-Johnson syndrome may develop. Be prepared to treat severe acute hypersensitivity reactions with airway management, oxygen, epinephrine, corticosteroids, antihistamines as ordered.

II. ALTERATION IN NUTRITION, LESS THAN BODY REQUIREMENTS, related to GI SIDE EFFECTS

Defining Characteristics: Nausea, vomiting, diarrhea may occur; rarely, pseudomembranous colitis caused by *C. difficile* resistant to the antibiotic occurs. Rarely, transient increases in LFTs—AST, ALT, alk phos, bili—may occur.

Nursing Implications: Assess baseline nutritional status. Instruct patient to report GI disturbances. Administer and teach patient to self-administer antiemetics, antidiarrheals as needed and as ordered. Teach patient importance of nutritious diet, and suggest small, frequent, high-calorie, high-protein meals as appropriate. Assess baseline LFTs and monitor periodically during treatment. Discuss abnormalities and drug interruption with physician.

III. FUNGAL SUPERINFECTION related to REDISTRIBUTION OF ENDOGENOUS MICROORGANISMS

Defining Characteristics: Vaginal candidiasis, vaginitis may occur as endogenous bacteria are eliminated and normal fungal population expands.

Nursing Implications: Instruct female patient to report vaginal itching or discharge. Discuss appropriate antifungal treatment with physician. Teach perineal hygiene and symptomatic management.

IV. ALTERATIONS IN PROTECTIVE MECHANISMS (RARE) related to TRANSIENT LEUKOPENIA

Defining Characteristics: Rarely, transient leukopenia, lymphocytosis, anemia, eosinophilia may occur. Prolonged PT, prolonged APTT, and hypoprothrombinemia have occurred rarely, especially in elderly or debilitated patients, or in individuals with vitamin K deficiency.

Nursing Implications: Assess baseline laboratory parameters, and monitor periodically during treatment. Assess patient for response to antibiotics. Discuss abnormalities with physician.

V. ALTERATIONS IN COMFORT related to PHLEBITIS

Defining Characteristics: Phlebitis and thrombophlebitis may occur with IV administration. Increased risk in elderly.

Nursing Implications: Assess IV site prior to each dose for phlebitis, erythema, swelling, and change site at least q48h. Apply heat to painful IV site as ordered.

Drug: oxacillin sodium (Bactocill, Prostaphlin)

Class: Antibacterial (systemic).

Mechanism of Action: Semisynthetic antibiotic. Contains β-lactam ring and is bactericidal by inhibiting cell wall synthesis. Penicillinase-resistant penicillin and active against penicillin-resistant staphylococci, which produce the enzyme penicillinase.

Metabolism: Incompletely absorbed from GI tract; rapidly absorbed when given IM or IV. Widely distributed in body tissues and fluid, including bile. Crosses placenta and is excreted in breast milk; 89–94% bound to serum proteins. Metabolized in liver, excreted in urine.

Dosage/Range:

Adult:

- Oral: 500 mg–1 g PO q6h.
- IM/IV: 500 mg–2 g q4h.

Drug Preparation/Administration:

- Oral: Reconstitute per manufacturer's package insert or by capsules or tablets. Administer 1 hour before meals or 2 hours after meals.

- IM: Reconstitute with sterile or bacteriostatic water for injection, and give deep IM in large muscle (e.g., gluteus maximus).
- IV: Reconstitute with sterile water for injection or 0.9% Sodium Chloride for injection according to manufacturer's package insert. Further dilute in 100 mL IV solution and infuse over 40–60 minutes.

Drug Interactions:

- Aminoglycosides: synergism.
- Aminoglycosides (e.g., gentamicin): incompatible when mixed together; administer at separate sites at different times. Also, penicillinase-resistant penicillins can inactivate aminoglycoside serum samples from patients receiving both drugs.
- Rifampin: possible antagonism, only at high doses of oxacillin.
- Probenecid: increased serum level of oxacillin; may be coadministered to exert this effect.

Lab Effects/Interference:

Major clinical significance:

- Urine glucose: high urinary concentrations of a penicillin may produce false-positive or falsely elevated test results with copper sulfate tests (Benedict's, Clinitest, or Fehling's); glucose enzymatic tests (Clinistix or Testape) are not affected.

Clinical significance:

- Coombs' (direct antiglobulin) test: false-positive result may occur during therapy with any penicillin.
- ALT, alk phos, AST, serum LDH values may be increased.
- WBC: leukopenia or neutropenia is associated with the use of all penicillins; the effect is more likely to occur with prolonged therapy and severe hepatic function impairment.

Special Considerations:

- Contraindicated in patients with prior hypersensitivity to penicillins. Use with caution in patients sensitive to other β-lactams (e.g., cephalosporins) since partial cross-allergenicity.
- Obtain ordered specimen and send for culture and sensitivity prior to first antibiotic dose.
- Consider alternative antibiotic therapy if eosinophilia, drug fever or rash, arthralgia, hematuria, or unexplained rise in BUN and serum creatinine occur.
- Monitor electrolytes and renal, hepatic, and hematologic laboratory parameters during extended treatment periods.
- Use with caution in pregnant or nursing women.

Potential Toxicities/Side Effects and the Nursing Process

I. POTENTIAL FOR INJURY related to HYPERSENSITIVITY REACTION

Defining Characteristics: Urticaria, pruritus, rash (maculopapular or erythematous), fever and chills, eosinophilia, myalgia, edema, erythema, angioedema, Stevens-Johnson syndrome, and exfoliative skin reactions occur in 5% of patients. Increased risk in individuals allergic to cephalosporin antibiotics.

Nursing Implications: Assess allergy to cephalosporin antibiotics and penicillin: if patient states "yes," determine actual response, e.g., "swollen lips = angioedema." If angioedema, patient SHOULD NOT receive drug. Discuss other patient responses with physician to determine whether drug should be given. Assess baseline skin condition, including integrity and allergy history to drugs. Instruct patient to report rash, itching, and other skin changes. Teach patient skin care and symptomatic measures as appropriate. If skin rash develops, discuss drug discontinuance with physician. If rash progresses, drug should be discontinued, as fatal Stevens-Johnson syndrome may develop. Be prepared to treat severe acute hypersensitivity reactions with airway management, oxygen, epinephrine, corticosteroids, antihistamines as ordered.

II. ALTERATION IN NUTRITION, LESS THAN BODY REQUIREMENTS, related to INCREASED LFTs

Defining Characteristics: Oral lesions may occur, as may hepatitis (rare) and increased LFTs.

Nursing Implications: Assess baseline oral mucosa, and LFTs—AST, ALT, alk phos, bili. Teach patient to practice oral hygiene after meals and at bedtime, and instruct to report any oral lesions. Monitor LFTs periodically during treatment, and discuss abnormalities with physician.

III. FUNGAL SUPERINFECTION related to REDISTRIBUTION OF ENDOGENOUS MICROORGANISMS

Defining Characteristics: Vaginal candidiasis, vaginitis may occur as endogenous bacteria are eliminated and normal fungal population expands.

Nursing Implications: Instruct female patient to report vaginal itching or discharge. Discuss appropriate antifungal treatment with physician. Teach perineal hygiene and symptomatic management.

IV. ALTERATIONS IN PROTECTIVE MECHANISMS (RARE) related to TRANSIENT LEUKOPENIA

Defining Characteristics: Rarely, transient leukopenia, lymphocytosis, anemia, eosinophilia may occur. Prolonged PT, prolonged APTT, and hypoprothrombinemia have occurred rarely, especially in elderly or debilitated patients, or in individuals with vitamin K deficiency.

Nursing Implications: Assess baseline laboratory parameters, and monitor periodically during treatment. Assess patient for response to antibiotics. Discuss abnormalities with physician.

V. ALTERATIONS IN COMFORT related to PHLEBITIS

Defining Characteristics: Phlebitis and thrombophlebitis may occur with IV administration. Increased risk in elderly.

Nursing Implications: Assess IV site prior to each dose for phlebitis, erythema, swelling, and change site at least q48h. Apply heat to painful IV site as ordered.

VI. ALTERATIONS IN URINARY ELIMINATION related to RENAL DAMAGE

Defining Characteristics: Interstitial nephritis, transient proteinuria, hematuria may occur.

Nursing Implications: Assess baseline liver, renal function tests (e.g., serum BUN, creatinine, and urinalysis), and monitor during therapy.

VII. ALTERATIONS IN SENSORY/PERCEPTUAL PATTERNS related to NEUROPATHY

Defining Characteristics: Neuropathy, seizures, neuromuscular irritability may occur rarely.

Nursing Implications: Assess baseline neurologic function and comfort, and monitor during treatment. Instruct patient to report any changes. Discuss any abnormalities with physician.

Drug: penicillin G (PenG Potassium, PenG Sodium, Intravenous; PenVK, Oral Preparation)

Class: Natural penicillin.

Mechanism of Action: Produced by fermentation of *Penicillium chrysogenum.* Active against many gram-positive bacteria (streptococci, staphylococci) but resistant to *S. aureus* and *S. epidermidis* strains that produce penicillinases. Also active against some gram-negative bacteria (*Neisseria, H. influenzae*), and spirochetes.

Metabolism: Decreased oral absorption, but IM or IV absorption is quite rapid and complete. Widely distributed in body tissues and fluids; 45–68% bound to proteins. Eliminated in urine and bile.

Dosage/Range:
- Oral: 250–500 mg qid.
- IV: 200,000–4 million U q4h.
- Dose modification may be necessary in patients with renal impairment.

Drug Preparation/Administration:
- Oral: Administer at least 1 hour before or 2 hours after meals.
- IM: Reconstitute drug as directed. Administration of greater than 100,000 U is likely to result in some discomfort. Give IM deep in large muscle mass.
- IV: Reconstitute drug as directed. Further dilute in 0.9% Sodium Chloride or 5% Dextrose in water, and administer over 1–2 hours.

Drug Interactions:
- Aminoglycosides: synergism.
- Aminoglycosides (e.g., gentamicin): incompatible when mixed together; administer at separate sites at different times. Also, penicillinase-resistant penicillins can inactivate aminoglycoside serum samples from patients receiving both drugs.
- Rifampin: possible antagonism, only at high doses of penicillin.
- Probenecid: increased serum level of penicillin; may be coadministered to exert this effect.

Lab Effects/Interference:

Major clinical significance:
- Urine glucose: high urinary concentrations of a penicillin may produce false-positive or falsely elevated test results with copper sulfate tests (Benedict's, Clinitest, or Fehling's); glucose enzymatic tests (Clinistix or Testape) are not affected.

Clinical significance:
- Coombs' (direct antiglobulin) test: false-positive result may occur during therapy with any penicillin.
- ALT, alk phos, AST, serum LDH values may be increased.
- Serum K+: hyperkalemia may occur following administration of parenteral penicillin G potassium because of the high potassium content.
- Serum Na+: hypernatremia may occur following administration of large doses of parenteral penicillin G sodium because of the high sodium content.
- WBC: leukopenia or neutropenia is associated with the use of all penicillins; the effect is more likely to occur with prolonged therapy and severe hepatic function impairment.

Special Considerations:

- Contraindicated in patients with prior hypersensitivity to penicillins. Use with caution in patients sensitive to other β-lactams (e.g., cephalosporins) since partial cross-allergenicity exists.
- Obtain ordered specimen and send for culture and sensitivity test prior to first antibiotic dose.
- Consider alternative antibiotic therapy if eosinophilia, drug fever or rash, arthralgia, hematuria, or unexplained rise in BUN and serum creatinine occur.
- Monitor electrolytes and renal, hepatic, and hematologic laboratory parameters during extended treatment periods.
- Hyperkalemia may occur with high dose therapy: monitor serum K+.
- Use with caution in pregnant or nursing women.
- Penicillin G benzathine should never be given IV (suspension); give IM only.

Potential Toxicities/Side Effects and the Nursing Process

I. POTENTIAL FOR INJURY related to HYPERSENSITIVITY REACTION

Defining Characteristics: Urticaria, pruritus, rash (maculopapular or erythematous), fever and chills, eosinophilia, myalgia, edema, erythema, angioedema, Stevens-Johnson syndrome, and exfoliative skin reactions occur in 5% of patients. Increased risk exists in individuals allergic to cephalosporin antibiotics.

Nursing Implications: Assess allergy to cephalosporin antibiotics and penicillin: if patient states "yes," determine actual response, e.g., "swollen lips = angioedema." If angioedema, patient SHOULD NOT receive drug. Discuss other patient responses with physician to determine whether drug should be given. Assess baseline skin condition, including integrity and allergy history to drugs. Instruct patient to report rash, itching, and other skin changes. Teach patient skin care and symptomatic measures as appropriate. If skin rash develops, discuss drug discontinuance with physician. If rash progresses, drug should be discontinued, as fatal Stevens-Johnson syndrome may develop. Be prepared to treat severe acute hypersensitivity reactions with airway management, oxygen, epinephrine, corticosteroids, antihistamines as ordered.

II. ALTERATION IN NUTRITION, LESS THAN BODY REQUIREMENTS, related to GI SIDE EFFECTS

Defining Characteristics: Rarely, nausea, vomiting, diarrhea, and pseudomembranous colitis caused by *C. difficile* resistant to the antibiotic may occur. Rarely, transient increases in LFTs—AST, ALT, alk phos, bili—may occur.

Nursing Implications: Assess baseline nutritional status. Instruct patient to report GI disturbances. Administer and teach patient to self-administer antiemetics as needed and as ordered. Teach patient importance of nutritious diet, and suggest small, frequent, high-calorie, high-protein meals as appropriate. Assess baseline LFTs and monitor periodically during treatment. Discuss abnormalities and drug interruption with physician.

III. FUNGAL SUPERINFECTION related to REDISTRIBUTION OF ENDOGENOUS MICROORGANISMS

Defining Characteristics: Vaginal candidiasis, vaginitis may occur as endogenous bacteria are eliminated and normal fungal population expands.

Nursing Implications: Instruct female patient to report vaginal itching or discharge. Discuss appropriate antifungal treatment with physician. Teach perineal hygiene and symptomatic management.

IV. ALTERATIONS IN PROTECTIVE MECHANISMS (RARE) related to RARE LEUKOPENIA

Defining Characteristics: Rarely, hemolytic anemia, leukopenia, thrombocytopenia may occur.

Nursing Implications: Assess baseline laboratory parameters, and monitor periodically during treatment. Assess patient for response to antibiotics. Discuss abnormalities with physician.

V. ALTERATIONS IN SENSORY/PERCEPTUAL PATTERNS related to NEUROPATHY

Defining Characteristics: Neuropathy, seizures may occur with high doses.

Nursing Implications: Assess baseline neurologic function and comfort, and monitor during treatment. Instruct patient to report any changes. Discuss any abnormalities with physician.

VI. ALTERATIONS IN COMFORT related to LOCAL INJECTION IRRITATION

Defining Characteristics: Pain, induration may form in IM injection sites; phlebitis may develop in IV sites.

Nursing Implications: Rotate IM injection sites, and administer drug deep IM in large muscle mass (e.g., gluteus maximus). Use IM injection when IV administration is not possible. Change IV sites q48h, and assess for signs/symptoms of phlebitis prior to each administration. Administer drug slowly. Apply warm packs to increase comfort.

Drug: piperacillin sodium (Pipracil); combined with tazobactam sodium (Zosyn)

Class: Antibacterial (systemic) (extended-spectrum penicillin).

Mechanism of Action: Semisynthetic antibiotic prepared from fungus *Penicillium.* Contains β-lactam ring and is bactericidal by inhibiting cell wall synthesis. Active against most gram-positive (except penicillinase-producing strains) and most gram-negative bacilli. Used in the treatment of serious gram-negative infections, especially *P. aeruginosa*–related infections of lower respiratory tract, urinary tract, and skin. When combined with tazobactam sodium, which inhibits β-lactamases, piperacillin sodium is effective against resistant bacteria.

Metabolism: Poorly absorbed from GI tract, so must be given parenterally. Widely distributed in body tissues and fluids. Crosses placenta and is excreted in breast milk. Excreted via urine and bile.

Dosage/Range:
- IV route preferred.

Adult:

piperacillin sodium:
- IV: 3–4 g q4–6h (maximum 24 g, but higher doses may be used in severe infection); IM: maximum 2 g/per dose.

Zosyn:
- 3 g piperacillin and 0.375 g tazobactam (3.375 g)–4 g piperacillin and 0.50 g tazobactam (4.50 g) q6h IV × 7–10 days.
- Moderate-to-severe pneumonia caused by piperacillin-resistant s. aureus that produces β-lactamase: 3.375 g IV q6h plus aminoglycoside × 7–10 days.
- Dose modification necessary if severe renal insufficiency exists.

Drug Preparation/Administration:
- IV: Reconstitute each gram of drug with at least 5 mL of sterile or bacteriostatic water. Further dilute in 50–100 mL 0.9% Sodium Chloride or 5% Dextrose injection and infuse over 30 minutes.
- IM: Reconstitute with 2 mL of sterile or bacteriostatic water, or 0.5–1.0% lidocaine HCl (without epinephrine), with final concentration 1 g/2.5 mL. Administer as deep IM injection in large muscle mass (e.g., gluteus maximus). Make certain patient is NOT ALLERGIC to lidocaine.

Drug Interactions:
- Aminoglycosides: synergism.
- Aminoglycosides (e.g., gentamicin): incompatible when mixed together; administer at separate sites at different times. Also, penicillinase-resistant penicillins can inactivate aminoglycoside serum samples from patients receiving both drugs.

- Clavulanic acid (inhibits β-lactamase): increases antibacterial action.
- Probenecid: increased serum level of piperacillin; may be coadministered to exert this effect.
- Tazobactam: inhibits β-lactamase, thus broadening drug's antimicrobial effectiveness.

Lab Effects/Interference:

Major clinical significance:

- Urine glucose: high urinary concentrations of a penicillin may produce false-positive or falsely elevated test results with copper sulfate tests (Benedict's, Clinitest, or Fehling's); glucose enzymatic tests (Clinistix or Tes-tape) are not affected.
- PTT and PT: an increase has been associated with intravenous piperacillin.

Clinical significance:

- Coombs' (direct antiglobulin) test: false-positive result may occur during therapy with any penicillin.
- Urine protein: high urinary concentrations of piperacillin may produce false-positive protein reactions (pseudoproteinuria) with the sulfosalicyclic acid and boiling test; bromophenol blue reagent test strips (Multistix) are reportedly unaffected.
- ALT, alk phos, AST, serum LDH values may be increased.
- Serum bili: an increase has been associated with piperacillin.
- BUN and serum creatinine: increased concentrations have been associated with piperacillin.
- Serum K+: hypokalemia may occur following administration of parenteral piperacillin, which may act as a non-reabsorbable anion in the distal tubals; this may cause an increase in pH and result in increased urinary potassium loss: the risk of hypokalemia increases with use of larger doses.
- WBC: leukopenia or neutropenia is associated with the use of all penicillins; the effect is more likely to occur with prolonged therapy and severe hepatic function impairment.

Special Considerations:

- Contraindicated in patients with prior hypersensitivity to penicillins. Use with caution in patients sensitive to other β-lactams (e.g., cephalosporins), since partial cross-allergenicity exists.
- Obtain ordered specimen, and send for culture and sensitivity test prior to first antibiotic dose.
- Consider alternative antibiotic therapy if eosinophilia, drug fever or rash, arthralgia, hematuria, or unexplained rise in BUN and serum creatinine occur.
- Monitor electrolytes and renal, hepatic, and hematologic laboratory parameters during extended treatment periods.
- Use with caution in pregnant or nursing women.

- Low Na content: 1.98 mEq/g of drug.
- Increased activity against *P. aeruginosa*.

Potential Toxicities/Side Effects and the Nursing Process

I. POTENTIAL FOR INJURY related to HYPERSENSITIVITY REACTION

Defining Characteristics: Urticaria, pruritus, rash (maculopapular or erythematous), fever and chills, eosinophilia, myalgia, edema, erythema, angioedema, Stevens-Johnson syndrome, and exfoliative skin reactions occur in 5% of patients. Increased risk exists in individuals allergic to cephalosporin antibiotics.

Nursing Implications: Assess allergy to cephalosporin antibiotics and penicillin: if patient states "yes," determine actual response, e.g., "swollen lips = angioedema." If angioedema, patient SHOULD NOT receive drug. Discuss other patient responses with physician to determine whether drug should be given. Assess baseline skin condition, including integrity and allergy history to drugs. Instruct patient to report rash, itching, other skin changes. Teach patient skin care and symptomatic measures as appropriate. If skin rash develops, discuss drug discontinuance with physician. If rash progresses, drug should be discontinued, as fatal Stevens-Johnson syndrome may develop. Be prepared to treat severe acute hypersensitivity reactions with airway management, oxygen, epinephrine, corticosteroids, antihistamines as ordered.

II. ALTERATION IN NUTRITION, LESS THAN BODY REQUIREMENTS, related to GI SIDE EFFECTS

Defining Characteristics: Nausea, vomiting, diarrhea may occur; rarely, pseudomembranous colitis caused by *C. difficile* resistant to the antibiotic occurs. Rarely, transient increases in LFTs—AST, ALT, alk phos, bili—may occur.

Nursing Implications: Assess baseline nutritional status. Instruct patient to report GI disturbances. Administer and teach patient to self-administer antiemetics as needed and as ordered. Teach patient importance of nutritious diet, and suggest small, frequent, high-calorie, high-protein meals as appropriate. Assess baseline LFTs and monitor periodically during treatment. Discuss abnormalities and drug interruption with physician.

III. FUNGAL SUPERINFECTION related to REDISTRIBUTION OF ENDOGENOUS MICROORGANISMS

Defining Characteristics: Vaginal candidiasis, vaginitis may occur as endogenous bacteria are eliminated and normal fungal population expands.

Nursing Implications: Instruct female patient to report vaginal itching or discharge. Discuss appropriate antifungal treatment with physician. Teach perineal hygiene and symptomatic management.

IV. ALTERATIONS IN PROTECTIVE MECHANISMS (RARE) related to HEMATOLOGIC ABNORMALITIES

Defining Characteristics: Rarely, transient leukopenia, lymphocytosis, anemia, eosinophilia may occur. Prolonged PT, prolonged APTT, and hypoprothrombinemia have occurred rarely, especially in elderly or debilitated patients, or in individuals with vitamin K deficiency.

Nursing Implications: Assess baseline laboratory parameters, and monitor periodically during treatment. Assess patient for response to antibiotics. Discuss abnormalities with physician. Assess for signs/symptoms of bleeding.

V. ALTERATIONS IN SENSORY/PERCEPTUAL PATTERNS related to DIZZINESS, SOMNOLENCE

Defining Characteristics: Dizziness, headache, somnolence occur rarely. Neuromuscular irritability and seizures may occur with high drug serum levels.

Nursing Implications: Assess baseline neurologic function and comfort, and monitor during treatment. Instruct patient to report any changes. Discuss any abnormalities with physician. Institute seizure precautions.

VI. ALTERATIONS IN COMFORT related to LOCAL INJECTION IRRITATION

Defining Characteristics: Vein irritation (pain, erythema), phlebitis, and thrombophlebitis may occur at IV administration site.

Nursing Implications: Change IV sites q48h, and assess for signs/symptoms of phlebitis prior to each administration. Administer drug slowly. Apply warm packs to increase comfort. Discuss central line with patient and physician to facilitate administration.

VII. ALTERATION IN FLUID AND ELECTROLYTE BALANCE related to HYPOKALEMIA AND INCREASED SODIUM INTAKE

Defining Characteristics: Prolonged therapy may cause hypokalemia; also, drug is prepared as sodium salt. Frequent IV infusions increase fluid intake.

Nursing Implications: Assess baseline electrolytes, fluid balance, weight, and monitor throughout therapy. Monitor renal function studies, especially if patient has preexisting renal dysfunction.

Drug: quinupristin and dalfopristin (Synercid)

Class: Macrolide-lincoasmide-streptogram (MLS) class of antibiotic.

Mechanism of Action: Synercid inhibits bacterial protein synthesis by each component irreversibly binding to different sites on the 50S bacterial ribosome subunit to form stable quinupristin-ribosome-dalfopristin tertiary complex. Quinupristin inhibits peptide chain formation and results in early termination, while dalfopristin directly interferes with peptidyl transferase and inhibits peptide chain elongation. Active against gram-positive aerobic microorganisms, e.g., *Entercoccus faecium,* including vancomycin- and teicoplanin-resistant organisms and vancomycin-resistant, but teicoplanin-susceptible organisms; staphylococci; streptococci; some anaerobes and respiratory pathogens.

Metabolism: Quinupristin and dalfopristin are rapidly converted in the liver to several active metabolites. Quinupristin is broken down into two active metabolites: one glutathione-conjugated metabolite and one cysteine-conjugated metabolite. Dalfopristin has one active metabolite formed by drug hydrolysis. Elimination half-life is approximately 0.9 and 0.75 hours for quinupristin and dalfopristin, respectively. Protein binding for quinupristin ranges from 55–78%, and from 11–26% for dalfopristin. Excreted in feces (75–77%) and urine (15% of quinupristin and 19% dalfopristin).

Dosage/Range:

- Recommended dose is 7.5 mg/kg of actual body weight in D5W over 60 minutes q8–12h, depending upon the type and severity of infection.

Drug Preparation/Administration:

- Reconstitute single-dose vial by slowly adding 5 mL of solution or preservative-free sterile water for injection. CAUTION: FURTHER DILUTION IS REQUIRED PRIOR TO ADMINSTRATION.
- According to patient weight, Synercid solution should be added to 250 mL of D5W solution within 30 minutes of initial reconsitution.
- Stability of the prepared infusate is 5 h at room temperature or 54 h under refrigeration at 2–8°C (36–46°F).
- Drug is NOT compatible with 0.9% Sodium Chloride or heparin-containing solutions.
- Desired dose should be administered IV over 60 minutes. If drug is administered through a common IV line, flush with 5% Dextrose prior to and following administration.

Drug Interactions:

- Synercid should not be physically mixed with or added to other drugs since compatibility has not been established.
- Drugs metabolized by CYP450 3A4 isoenzyme system: drug is metabolized by CYP450 3A4 isoenzymes and is an inhibitor of CYP450 3A4, and thus

may increase the serum concentrations of drugs metabolized by this isoenzyme, e.g., nifedipine, cyclosporin. Use together with caution and assess for toxicity.

Lab Effects/Interference:

- Eosinophils, BUN, GGT (gammaglutamyl transferase), LDH, CPK, AST, ALT, blood glucose, alk phos, and creatinine: concentrations may be increased.
- Hemoglobin and hematocrit: may be decreased.
- Serum K+ and platelet count: may be increased or decreased.

Special Considerations:

- Infusion via central line preferred to decrease incidence of local infusion reactions.

Potential Toxicities/Side Effects and the Nursing Process

I. ALTERATION IN NUTRITION related to GI SIDE EFFECTS

Defining Characteristics: Nausea, vomiting, diarrhea, constipation, abdominal pain, dyspepsia, stomatitis, and pseudomembranous enterocolitis may occur.

Nursing Implications: Assess elimination and nutrition pattern, baseline and during therapy. Teach patient to report diarrhea and/or abdominal pain immediately. Discuss drug discontinuance with physician if diarrhea occurs. Guaiac stool for occult blood, and notify physician if positive. If severe diarrhea develops, discuss management plan, including endoscopy, fluid and electrolyte replacement. Assess for nausea/vomiting, and administer prescribed antiemetic medications. Encourage small, frequent feedings as tolerated.

II. ALTERATION IN SKIN INTEGRITY related to HYPERSENSITIVITY

Defining Characteristics: Maculopapular rash and urticaria may occur. Allergic reactions (anaphylacticlike) may rarely occur.

Nursing Implications: Assess baseline allergy history. Assess baseline skin integrity. Teach patient to report rash, pruritus. Teach patient symptomatic management of rash, pruritus. Assess for hypersensitivity reaction: if it occurs, monitor VS, discontinue drug, notify physician, and institute supportive measures.

III. ALTERATION IN COMFORT related to LOCAL ADMINISTRATION EFFECTS

Defining Characteristics: IV administration may cause erythema, pain, swelling, and thrombophlebitis.

Nursing Implications: Assess IV site prior to each dose for phlebitis or swelling, and change site at least q 48 hours. Administer dose slowly over 60 minutes. Apply heat to painful IV sites as ordered. Infuse via central line if possible.

IV. ALTERATION IN COMFORT

Defining Characteristics: Myalgias and arthralgias may occur.

Nursing Implications: Assess baseline T, VS, neurologic status, and comfort level and monitor q4–6 hours if patient in hospital. Teach patient self-care measures, including use of prescribed medications as well as use of heat or cold for myalgias and arthralgias.

V. ALTERATION IN HEPATIC FUNCTION

Defining Characteristics: Transient increases in serum BR, AST (SGOT), alk phos have occurred.

Nursing Implications: Assess baseline LFTs and monitor during therapy.

VI. FUNGAL SUPERINFECTION related to REDISTRIBUTION OF ENDOGENOUS MICROORGANISMS

Defining Characteristics: Vaginal moniliasis, vaginitis, and oral moniliasis may occur as endogenous bacteria are eliminated and normal fungal population expands.

Nursing Implications: Teach female patient to report vaginal itching or discharge. Discuss appropriate antifungal treatment with physician. Teach perineal hygiene and symptomatic management.

Drug: rifaximin (Xifaxan)

Class: anti-infective, antidiarrheals, gastrointestinal, rifamycin.

Mechanism of Action: Acts by binding to the beta-subunit of bacterial DNA-dependent RNA polymerase resulting in inhibition of bacterial RNA synthesis. Structural analog of rifampin. Active against Eschericha coli (enterotoxigenic and enteroaggregative strains).

Metabolism: Well absorbed following PO administration. Poorly absorbed from the gastrointestinal tract. Drug excreted unchanged in the feces.

Dosage/Range:
- Traveler's diarrhea: 200mg orally three times daily for 3 days.

Drug Preparation:
- Oral preparation.

Drug Administration:
- May be taken with or without food.

Drug Interactions:
- Rifaximin has not been shown to significantly affect intestinal or hepatic CYP3A4 activity.
- Rifaximin has not been shown to effect contraceptives containing ethinyl estradiol and norgestimate.

Lab Effects/Interference:
- None reported.

Special Considerations:
- Rifaximin was teratogenic in animal studies. There are no adequate and well-controlled studies in pregnant women.

Potential Toxicities/Side Effects and the Nursing Process

I. ALTERATION IN NUTRITION related to GI SIDE EFFECTS

Defining Characteristics: Gas, abdominal pain, nausea, vomiting, constipation, and pseudomembranous enterocolitis may occur.

Nursing Implications: Assess elimination and nutrition pattern, baseline and during therapy. Teach patient to report changes in diarrhea and/or abdominal pain immediately. Guaiac stool for occult blood, and notify physician if positive. Discuss management plan, including fluid and electrolyte replacement. Assess for nausea/vomiting, and administer prescribed antiemetic medications. Encourage small, frequent feedings as tolerated.

Drug: streptomycin sulfate

Class: Antibacterial; antimyobacterial (systemic).

Mechanism of Action: Synthetic antibiotic derived from *Streptomyces;* bactericidal, most probably by inhibition of protein synthesis; active against *Mycobacterium tuberculosis.* Active as second-line agent against sensitive microorganisms (including *Brucella, Nocardia, M. avium-intracellulare*).

Metabolism: Well absorbed following IM administration. Widely distributed into body fluids; 35% bound to plasma proteins. Readily crosses placenta and into breast milk. Drug excreted unchanged in the urine.

Dosage/Range:
- Antituberculosis regimen: Adults: 15 mg/kg/day or 1 g/day IM × 2–3 months, then 1 g 2–3 × per week. Elderly: dose may be limited to 10 mg/kg (or 750 mg). Desired serum peak is 5–25 μg/mL, and trough < 5 μg/mL.

Drug Preparation:
- Prepare a solution with concentration of ≤ 500 mg/mL, using sterile water for injection or 0.9% Sodium Chloride. Use within 2 days if kept at room temperature, or within 2 weeks if refrigerated at 2–8°C (36–46°F).

Drug Administration:
- Deep IM: into large muscle mass; rotate sites as sterile abscesses may form. DO NOT GIVE IV.

Drug Interactions:
- Increased risk of toxicity with other ototoxic drugs: acyclovir, other aminoglycosides, amphotericin B, bacitracin, cephalosporins, colistin, cisplatin, ethacrynic acid, furosemide, vancomycin.
- Potentiation of neuromuscular blockade when given concurrently with general anesthetics (succinylcholine, tubocurarine)—use cautiously, observe for signs/symptoms of respiratory depression.
- Synergism with extended-spectrum penicillins, but must be administered separately.

Lab Effects/Interference:
- Serum ALT, serum alk phos, serum AST, serum bili, and serum LDH values may be increased.
- BUN and serum creatinine concentrations may be increased.
- Serum Ca++, serum Mg++, serum K+, and serum Na+ concentrations may be decreased.

Special Considerations:
- Used parenterally with at least one other agent in treatment of tuberculosis.
- Use in pregnancy only if infection is life-threatening and no safer drug exists; drug crosses placenta and may cause fetal toxicity.

Potential Toxicities/Side Effects and the Nursing Process

I. ALTERATIONS IN SENSORY/PERCEPTUAL PATTERNS related to OTOTOXICITY

Defining Characteristics: Damage to eighth cranial nerve (auditory) may result in dizziness, nystagmus, vertigo, ataxia (vestibular damage), and more commonly, tinnitus, roaring sound in ears, and impaired hearing (auditory damage). Hearing loss usually begins with high-frequency loss, followed by clinical hearing loss, then permanent hearing loss if damage continues. Increased risk in elderly or renally impaired patients.

Nursing Implications: Assess baseline hearing (ability to hear spoken voice) and continue during therapy. Teach patient potential side effects, and instruct patient to report any hearing/perceptual problems (e.g., tinnitus, vertigo, decreased hearing). Discuss drug discontinuance and audiogram with physician to confirm hearing dysfunction if symptoms arise. Assess for increased risk if given concurrently with other ototoxic medications (e.g., cisplatin, furosemide).

II. ALTERATION IN URINARY ELIMINATION related to NEPHROTOXICITY

Defining Characteristics: Risk of nephrotoxicity is less than with other aminoglycosides. Renal damage characterized by tubular necrosis with increased serum BUN, creatinine; decreased urine creatinine clearance and specific gravity; proteinuria and casts in urine. Azotemia usually not associated with oliguria. Rarely, electrolyte wasting with hypomagnesemia, hypocalcemia, and hypokalemia may occur. Renal dysfunction is usually reversible after drug discontinuance. Increased risk exists in elderly and if there is preexisting renal dysfunction. Risk is low in well-hydrated patients with normal renal function when normal doses are given.

Nursing Implications: Assess baseline renal function and electrolytes, and monitor periodically during therapy. Discuss any abnormalities with physician, as drug should be dose-reduced or discontinued if renal dysfunction develops. Assess baseline total body fluid balance, weight, and monitor periodically during antibiotic therapy. Monitor hydration status to keep patient well hydrated. Assess drug peak and trough levels as ordered so that drug dosage is correctly titrated. Increased risk of toxicity if peak serum concentration >40 μg/mL. Draw blood for peak drug concentration 30 minutes after end of 30-minute infusion or at the end of a 60-minute infusion; draw trough immediately before next dose.

III. ALTERATIONS IN SENSORY/PERCEPTUAL PATTERNS related to CNS EFFECTS, NEUROMUSCULAR BLOCKADE

Defining Characteristics: Headache, tremor, lethargy may occur. Peripheral neuropathy or encephalopathy (numbness, skin tingling, muscle twitching) may occur rarely. Neuromuscular blockade is dose-related, self-limiting, and uncommon. Risk is greater with topical application or when drug is administered to patient with neuromuscular disease (myasthenia gravis) or hypocalcemia.

Nursing Implications: Assess baseline neurologic status. Assess coexisting risk factors, neuromuscular blockade medications. Teach patient about side effects and instruct to report headache, tremor, lethargy. Observe for respiratory depression. If signs/symptoms arise, discuss drug discontinuance with physician.

IV. POTENTIAL FOR INJURY related to HYPERSENSITIVITY

Defining Characteristics: Rash, urticaria, pruritus, fever, eosinophilia have occurred rarely. CROSS-SENSITIVITY between AMINOGLYCOSIDES existsHandling of drug can cause sensitization to the drug.

Nursing Implications: Assess for drug allergies to any aminoglycoside—amikacin, gentamicin, kanamycin, neomycin, netilmicin, streptomycin, tobramycin—prior to drug administration. Instruct patient to report any allergic reactions. Assess for signs/symptoms of allergic reaction after drug dose. Take special care in preparing drug or wear gloves.

V. ALTERATION IN NUTRITION, LESS THAN BODY REQUIREMENTS, related to GI SIDE EFFECTS

Defining Characteristics: Nausea, vomiting, anorexia have occurred rarely. Also, transient hepatomegaly with increased LFTs—AST, ALT, LDH, alk phos—has occurred.

Nursing Implications: Assess baseline nutritional status, preexisting nausea/vomiting, anorexia. Assess baseline LFTs and monitor periodically during treatment. Instruct patient to report side effects. Provide symptomatic interventions if side effects occur; discuss with physician use of alternative drug(s).

VI. POTENTIAL FOR FATIGUE, INFECTION, AND BLEEDING related to BONE MARROW INJURY

Defining Characteristics: Anemia, leukopenia, granulocytopenia, and thrombocytopenia may occur. Also, patients receiving antibiotics are at risk for overgrowth of nonsusceptible microorganisms, such as fungi (superinfection). Rare.

Nursing Implications: Assess baseline CBC, differential, and monitor periodically during treatment. Instruct patient to report signs/symptoms of fatigue, infection, or bleeding immediately. Assess for signs/symptoms of superinfection. Discuss any adverse effects with physician.

VII. ALTERATION IN SKIN INTEGRITY related to IRRITATION AT INJECTION SITE, EXFOLIATIVE DERMATITIS

Defining Characteristics: Exfoliative dermatitis rarely occurs; may develop pain, irritation, and sterile abscesses at injection site.

Nursing Implications: Assess skin integrity and presence of lesions. Monitor for changes during treatment, and instruct patient to report them. Rotate injection sites and give injection deeply into large muscle mass, e.g., upper outer quadrant of buttock. Administer solutions of ≤ 500 mg/mL.

Drug: telithromycin (Ketek)

Class: Antimicrobial agent. This antibiotic is a new structural class called ketolides.

Mechanism of Action: Similar to that of macrolides and is related to the 50S-ribosomal subunit binding with inhibition of bacterial protein synthesis. Telithromycin appears to have greater affinity for the ribosomal binding site than macrolides. Demonstrated efficacy against *Staphylococcus aureus, Streptococcus aureus, Streptococcus pheumoniae, Haemophilus influenzae, Moraxella catarrhalis, Chlamydia pneumoniae*, and *Mycoplasma pneumoniae*.

Metabolism: Absorbed from the GI tract. Eliminated by multiple pathways: 7% of the dose is excreted unchanged by biliary and/or intestinal secretion; 13% of the dose is excreted unchanged in urine; and 37% of the dose is metabolized by the liver. May accumulate in patients with severe hepatic disease.

Dosage/Range:

- Adult: Oral: 800 mg daily for 5–10 days. Duration of therapy depends on indication. Drug dose should be reduced or adjusted in patients with hepatic or renal insufficiency

Drug Preparation/Administration:

- Oral: Administration of telithromycin with food had no significant effect on extent or rate of oral absorption in healthy subjects.

Drug Interactions:

- Class I, IA, & III Anti-arrhythmic Agents: Concomitant use is contraindicated as it may lead to QT prolongation. Serum levels may be increased.
- CYP 3A4 inhibitors: Itraconazole and Ketoconazole: Increases telithromycin levels and AUC by ~54% and 95%, respectively.
- CYP3A4 substrates: Cisapride, Simvastin, and Midazolam: Increases serum concentration of cisapride by 95%; significantly increases serum concentration of simvastin and midazolam. These drugs SHOULD NOT be used when a patient is taking telithromycin.
- CYP 2D6 substrates: Metoprolol: Increases serum concentrations. Administer with caution. Rifampin: Decreases serum concentrations. Digoxin: Increases serum concentration. Theophylline: Increases serum concentrations. Take 1 hour apart to decrease the gastrointestinal side effects. Sotalol: Decreases serum concentrations.

Lab Effects/Interference:

- There are no reported drug-laboratory test interactions. SGPT, alk phos, Amylase, SGOT, and bilirubin: serum concentrations may be increased in patients with pre-existing hepatic disease.

Special Considerations:

- Avoid use in pregnant or lactating women.
- Contraindicated in patients with known hypersensitivity.
- Obtain ordered specimen and send for culture and sensitivity prior to first antibiotic dose.

Potential Toxicities/Side Effects and the Nursing Process

I. ALTERATION IN NUTRITION related to GI SIDE EFFECTS

Defining Characteristics: Anorexia, nausea, vomiting, diarrhea, glossitis, dysphagia, gastroenteritis, gastritis, constipation.

Nursing Implications: Assess baseline nutritional status. Assess for and teach patient to report any symptoms. Administer and teach patient self-administration of prescribed antiemetic or antidiarrheal medication as appropriate.

II. ALTERATION IN PROTECTIVE MECHANISMS

Defining Characteristics: Prolonged PT, prolonged INR, cardiac arrhythmias including atrial arrhythmias, bradycardia, and hypotension.

Nursing Implications: Monitor and teach patient about potential side effects and to report abnormalities such as fainting & dizziness.

III. POTENTIAL FOR INJURY related to VISUAL DISTURBANCES

Defining Characteristics: Blurred vision and difficulty focusing.

Nursing Implications: Assess baseline visual and neurologic status. Teach patient to report any changes in vision. If signs/symptoms arise, discuss discontinuance with physician, and institute supportive measures.

IV. FUNGAL SUPERINFECTION related to REDISTRIBUTION OF ENDOGENOUS MICROORGANISMS

Defining Characteristics: Vaginal moniliasis, vaginitis may occur as endogenous bacteria are eliminated and normal fungal population expands.

Nursing Implications: Teach female patient to report vaginal itching or discharge. Discuss appropriate antifungal treatment with physician. Teach perineal hygiene and symptom management.

Drug: ticarcillin disodium (Ticar); combined with clavulanate potassium (Timentin)

Class: Antibacterial (systemic) (extended spectrum penicillin).

Mechanism of Action: Semisynthetic antibiotic prepared from fungus *Penicillium*. Contains β-lactam ring and is bactericidal by inhibiting cell wall synthesis. Active against most gram-positive (except penicillinase-producing strains) and most gram-negative bacilli. Used in the treatment of serious gram-negative infections, especially *P. aeruginosa*–related infections of lower respiratory tract, urinary tract, and skin. When combined with clavulanate potassium, the drug is protected from breakdown by bacterial β-lactamase enzymes, thus keeping therapeutic antibiotic serum levels.

Metabolism: Poorly absorbed from GI tract, so must be given parenterally. Widely distributed in body tissues and fluids. Crosses placenta and is excreted in breast milk. Excreted via urine and bile.

Dosage/Range:
- IV dosing preferred but drug can be given IM or IV.

Adult:

Ticarcillin disodium:
- 3 g q4–6h (200–300 mg/kg/day in divided doses).
- Dosage modification required if renal insufficiency exists; refer to manufacturer's package insert.

Timentin:
- 3 g ticarcillin plus 0.1 g clavulanic acid (3.1 g) IV q4–6h × 10–14 days if weight < 60 kg: 200–300 mg ticarcillin/kg/d in divided doses q4–6h IV.

Drug Preparation/Administration:
- IV: reconstitute each gram with 4 mL 0.9% Sodium Chloride or 5% Dextrose injection. Further dilute in 50–100 mL IV solution and infuse over 30 minutes to 2 hours.
- IM: reconstitute each gram with 2 mL sterile water for injection or 1% lidocaine HCl (without epinephrine). Ensure patient is NOT ALLERGIC to lidocaine. Inject drug deep IM in large muscle mass (e.g., gluteus maximus). Maximum 2 g at one site.

Drug Interactions:
- Aminoglycosides: synergism.
- Aminoglycosides (e.g., gentamicin): incompatible when mixed together; administer at separate sites at different times. Also, penicillinase-resistant penicillins can inactivate aminoglycoside serum samples from patients receiving both drugs.
- Probenecid: increased serum level of penicillin; may be coadministered to exert this effect.

- Clavulanic acid (β-lactamase inhibitor): Synergistic bactericial effect.

Lab Effects/Interference:

Major clinical significance:

- Urine glucose: high urinary concentrations of a penicillin may produce false-positive or falsely elevated test results with copper sulfate tests (Benedict's, Clinitest, or Fehling's); glucose enzymatic tests (Clinistix or Testape) are not affected.
- PTT and PT: an increase has been associated with ticarcillin.

Clinical significance:

- Coombs' (direct antiglobulin) test: false-positive result may occur during therapy with any penicillin.
- Urine protein: high urinary concentrations of ticarcillin may produce false-positive protein reactions (pseudoproteinuria) with the sulfosalicylic acid and boiling test; bromophenol blue reagent test strips (Multistix) are reportedly unaffected.
- ALT, alk phos, AST, serum LDH values may be increased.
- Serum bili: an increase has been associated with ticarcillin.
- BUN and serum creatinine: increased concentrations have been associated with ticarcillin.
- Serum K+: hypokalemia may occur following administration of parenteral ticarcillin, which may act as a non-reabsorbable anion in the distal tubules; this may cause an increase in pH and result in increased urinary potassium loss. The risk of hypokalemia increases with use of larger doses.
- WBC: leukopenia or neutropenia is associated with the use of all penicillins; the effect is more likely to occur with prolonged therapy and severe hepatic function impairment

Special Considerations:

- Contraindicated in patients with prior hypersensitivity to penicillins. Use with caution in patients sensitive to other β-lactams (e.g., cephalosporins) since partial cross-allergenicity exists.
- Obtain ordered specimen, and send for culture and sensitivity test prior to first antibiotic dose.
- Consider alternative antibiotic therapy if eosinophilia, drug fever or rash, arthralgia, hematuria, or unexplained rise in BUN and serum creatinine occur.
- Monitor electrolytes and renal, hepatic, and hematologic laboratory parameters during extended treatment periods.
- Use with caution in pregnant or nursing women.
- Decreased incidence of hypokalemia, and less salt load, than other extended spectrum penicillins.

Potential Toxicities/Side Effects and the Nursing Process

I. POTENTIAL FOR INJURY related to HYPERSENSITIVITY REACTION

Defining Characteristics: Urticaria, pruritus, rash (maculopapular or erythematous), fever and chills, eosinophilia, myalgia, edema, erythema, angioedema, Stevens-Johnson syndrome, and exfoliative skin reactions occur in 5% of patients. Increased risk in individuals allergic to cephalosporin antibiotics.

Nursing Implications: Assess allergy to cephalosporin antibiotics and penicillin: if patient states "yes," determine actual response, e.g., "swollen lips = angioedema." If angioedema, patient SHOULD NOT receive drug. Discuss other patient responses with physician to determine whether drug should be given. Assess baseline skin condition, including integrity and allergy history to drugs. Instruct patient to report rash, itching, other skin changes. Teach patient skin care and symptomatic measures as appropriate. If skin rash develops, discuss drug discontinuance with physician. If rash progresses, drug should be discontinued, as fatal Stevens-Johnson syndrome may develop. Be prepared to treat severe acute hypersensitivity reactions with airway management, oxygen, epinephrine, corticosteroids, antihistamines as ordered.

II. ALTERATION IN NUTRITION, LESS THAN BODY REQUIREMENTS, related to GI SIDE EFFECTS

Defining Characteristics: Nausea, vomiting, diarrhea may occur; rarely, pseudomembranous colitis caused by *C. difficile* resistant to the antibiotic occurs. Rarely, transient increases in LFTs—AST, ALT, alk phos, bili—may occur.

Nursing Implications: Assess baseline nutritional status. Instruct patient to report GI disturbances. Administer and teach patient to self-administer antiemetics, antidiarrheals as needed and as ordered. Teach patient importance of nutritious diet, and suggest small, frequent, high-calorie, high-protein meals as appropriate. Assess baseline LFTs, and monitor periodically during treatment. Discuss abnormalities and drug interruption with physician.

III. FUNGAL SUPERINFECTION related to REDISTRIBUTION OF ENDOGENOUS MICROORGANISMS

Defining Characteristics: Vaginal candidiasis, vaginitis may occur as endogenous bacteria are eliminated, and normal fungal population expands.

Nursing Implications: Instruct female patient to report vaginal itching or discharge. Discuss appropriate antifungal treatment with physician. Teach perineal hygiene and symptomatic management.

IV. ALTERATIONS IN PROTECTIVE MECHANISMS (RARE) related to TRANSIENT LEUKOPENIA

Defining Characteristics: Rarely, transient leukopenia, lymphocytosis, anemia, eosinophilia may occur. Prolonged PT, prolonged APTT, and hypoprothrombinemia have occurred rarely, especially in elderly or debilitated patients, or in individuals with vitamin K deficiency.

Nursing Implications: Assess baseline laboratory parameters, and monitor periodically during treatment. Assess patient for response to antibiotics. Discuss abnormalities with physician. Assess for signs/symptoms of bleeding.

V. ALTERATIONS IN SENSORY/PERCEPTUAL PATTERNS related to DIZZINESS, SOMNOLENCE

Defining Characteristics: Dizziness, headache, somnolence occur rarely. Neuromuscular irritability and seizures may occur with high drug serum levels.

Nursing Implications: Assess baseline neurologic function and comfort, and monitor during treatment. Instruct patient to report any changes. Discuss any abnormalities with physician. Institute seizure precautions.

VI. ALTERATIONS IN COMFORT related to LOCAL INJECTION IRRITATION

Defining Characteristics: Vein irritation (pain, erythema), phlebitis, and thrombophlebitis may occur at IV administration site.

Nursing Implications: Change IV sites q48h, and assess for signs/symptoms of phlebitis prior to each administration. Administer drug slowly. Apply warm packs to increase comfort. Discuss central line with patient and physician to facilitate administration.

VII. ALTERATION IN FLUID AND ELECTROLYTE BALANCE related to HYPOKALEMIA AND INCREASED SODIUM INTAKE

Defining Characteristics: Prolonged therapy may cause hypokalemia; also, drug is prepared as sodium salt. Frequent IV infusions increase fluid intake.

Nursing Implications: Assess baseline electrolytes, fluid balance, weight, and monitor throughout therapy. Monitor renal function studies, especially if patient has preexisting renal dysfunction.

Drug: tigecycline (Tygacil)

Class: Antimicrobial agent. This antibiotic is the first in a new class called glycylcyclines. This novel IV antibiotic has a broad spectrum of antimicrobial activity, including activity against the drug-resistant bacteria methicillin-resistant Staphylococcus aureus (MRSA).

Mechanism of Action: Inhibits protein transplation in bacteria by binding to the 30Sribosomal subunit and blocking entry of amino-acyl tRNA molecules into the A site of the ribosome. Demonstrated efficacy against methicillin-susceptible and -resistant Staphylococcus aureus (MRSA), Escherichia coli, Enterococcus faecalis (vancomycin-resistant isolates), Streptococcus anginosus, Streptococcus intermedius, and Streptococcus constellatus, Bacteroides fragilis, Bacteroides thetaiotaomicron, Bacteroides uniformis, Bacteroides vulgatus, Clostridium perfringens, and Peptostreptococcus micros.

Metabolism: Is not extensively metabolized. Eliminated by multiple pathways: 7% of the dose is excreted unchanged by biliary and/or intestinal secretion; 59% of the dose is excreted unchanged in bile/feces and 33% of the dose is excreted in the urine. May accumulate in patients with severe hepatic disease.

Dosage/Range:

Adult:

Initial dose 100 mg IV, followed by 50 mg every 12 hours. Duration of therapy depends on indication. Drug dose should be reduced or adjusted in patients with severe hepatic insufficiency.

Drug Preparation/Administration:

- Intravenous injection should be administered over 30–60 minutes every 12 hours.

Drug Interactions:

- Monitor prothrombin time if administered with warfarin.
- Concurrent use of antibacterial drugs with oral contraceptives may render the oral contraceptives less effective.

Lab Effects/Interference:

- There are no reported drug-laboratory test interactions. SGPT, alk phos, Amylase, SGOT, and bilirubin: serum concentrations may be increased in patients with pre-existing hepatic disease.

Special Considerations:

- Avoid use in pregnant or lactating women.
- Contraindicated in patients with known hypersensitivity.
- Obtain ordered specimen and send for culture and sensitivity prior to first antibiotic dose.

Potential Toxicities/Side Effects and the Nursing Process

I. ALTERATION IN NUTRITION related to GI SIDE EFFECTS

Defining Characteristics: Anorexia, nausea, vomiting, diarrhea, glossitis, dysphagia, gastroenteritis, gastritis, constipation.

Nursing Implications: Assess baseline nutritional status. Assess for and teach patient to report any symptoms. Administer and teach patient self-administration of prescribed antiemetic or antidiarrheal medication as appropriate.

II. POTENTIAL FOR INJURY related to HYPERSENSITIVITY REACTION

Defining Characteristics: Urticaria, pruritus, rash (maculopapular or erythematous), fever and chills, eosinophilia, myalgia, edema, erythema, angioedema, Stevens-Johnson syndrome, and exfoliative skin reactions occur.

Nursing Implications: Assess allergy to antibiotics: if patient states "yes," determine actual response, e.g., "swollen lips = angioedema." If angioedema, patient SHOULD NOT receive drug. Discuss other patient responses with physician to determine whether drug should be given. Assess baseline skin condition, including integrity and allergy history to drugs. Instruct patient to report rash, itching, and other skin changes. Teach patient skin care and symptomatic measures as appropriate. If skin rash develops, discuss drug discontinuance with physician. If rash progresses, drug should be discontinued, as fatal Stevens-Johnson syndrome may develop. Be prepared to treat severe acute hypersensitivity reactions with airway management, oxygen, epinephrine, corticosteroids, and antihistamines as ordered.

III. ALTERATIONS IN COMFORT related to LOCAL INJECTION IRRITATION

Defining Characteristics: Vein irritation (pain, erythema), phlebitis, and thrombophlebitis may occur at IV administration site.

Nursing Implications: Change IV sites q48h, and assess for signs/symptoms of phlebitis prior to each administration. Administer drug slowly. Apply warm packs to increase comfort. Discuss central line with patient and physician to facilitate administration.

IV. FUNGAL SUPERINFECTION related to REDISTRIBUTION OF ENDOGENOUS MICROORGANISMS

Defining Characteristics: Vaginal moniliasis, vaginitis may occur as endogenous bacteria are eliminated and normal fungal population expands.

Nursing Implications: Teach female patient to report vaginal itching or discharge. Discuss appropriate antifungal treatment with physician. Teach perineal hygiene and symptom management.

Drug: tobramycin sulfate (Nebcin)

Class: Aminoglycoside antibacterial (systemic).

Mechanism of Action: Synthetic antibiotic derived from *Streptomyces;* bactericidal, most probably by inhibition of protein synthesis. Active against aerobic microorganisms: many sensitive gram-negative (including *Acinetobacter, Citrobacter, Enterobacter, E. coli, Klebsiella, Proteus, Pseudomonas, Salmonella, Serratia,* and *Shigella*) and some sensitive gram-positive organisms (*S. aureus* and *S. epidermidis*). Over time, bacterial resistance may develop, either naturally or acquired.

Metabolism: Well absorbed following parenteral administration, but variability in absorption after IM injection (peak serum level 0.5–2 hours, duration 8–12 hours). Widely distributed into body fluids. Minimally protein-bound. Readily crosses placenta and into breast milk. Drug excreted unchanged in the urine.

Dosage/Range:
- 3 mg/kg/day given in equally divided doses q8h.
- Desired peak serum concentration is 4–10 μg/mL, and trough serum concentration is 1–2 μg/mL.
- May use 5–6 mg/kg/day in three equally divided doses to treat life-threatening infections.
- If loading dose required, 2 mg/kg; usual dosing q8h, but q12 or q24 dosing may also be used.
- DOSE-REDUCE IF RENAL IMPAIRMENT.

Drug Preparation:
- Store unreconstituted vials at 15–30°C (59–86°F).
- Store injections at 25°C (77°F).
- Store reconstituted solution (using sterile water for injection, with final concentration 40 mg/mL) at room temperature (stable 24 hours) or in refrigerator at 2–8°C (36–46°F) (stable 96 hours).

Drug Administration:
- IV: further dilute by adding dose to 50–100 mL in 0.9% Sodium Chloride and administer over 30–60 minutes.

Drug Interactions:

- Increased risk of toxicity with other ototoxic drugs: acyclovir, other aminoglycosides, amphotericin B, bacitracin, cephalosporins, colistin, cisplatin, ethacrynic acid, furosemide, vancomycin.
- Potentiation of neuromuscular blockade when given concurrently with general anesthetics (succinylcholine, tubocurarine); use cautiously; observe for signs/symptoms of respiratory depression.
- Synergism with extended-spectrum penicillins, but must be administered separately.

Lab Effects/Interference:

- Serum ALT, serum alk phos, serum AST, serum bili, and serum LDH values may be increased.
- BUN and serum creatinine concentrations may be increased.
- Serum Ca++, serum Mg++, serum K+, and serum Na+ concentrations may be decreased.

Special Considerations:

- Used as first-line treatment in short-term treatment of serious gram-negative infections (e.g., septicemia, respiratory tract infections).
- Use against gram-positive organisms only as second-line treatment.
- Use in pregnancy only if infection is life-threatening and no safer drug exists; drug crosses placenta and may cause fetal toxicity.

Potential Toxicities/Side Effects and the Nursing Process

I. ALTERATIONS IN SENSORY/PERCEPTUAL PATTERNS related to OTOTOXICITY

Defining Characteristics: Damage to eighth cranial nerve (auditory) may result in dizziness, nystagmus, vertigo, ataxia (vestibular damage), and more commonly, tinnitus, roaring sound in ears, and impaired hearing (auditory damage). Hearing loss usually begins with high-frequency loss, followed by clinical hearing loss, then permanent hearing loss if damage continues. Increased risk in elderly or renally impaired patients.

Nursing Implications: Assess baseline hearing (ability to hear spoken voice) and continue during therapy. Teach patient potential side effects, and instruct patient to report any hearing/perceptual problems (e.g., tinnitus, vertigo, decreased hearing). Discuss drug discontinuance and audiogram with physician to confirm hearing dysfunction if symptoms arise. Assess for increased risk if given concurrently with other ototoxic medications (e.g., cisplatin, furosemide).

II. ALTERATION IN URINARY ELIMINATION related to NEPHROTOXICITY

Defining Characteristics: Risk of nephrotoxicity is less than with other aminoglycosides. Renal damage characterized by tubular necrosis with increased serum BUN, creatinine; decreased urine creatinine clearance and specific gravity; proteinuria and casts in urine. Azotemia usually not associated with oliguria. Rarely, electrolyte wasting with hypomagnesemia, hypocalcemia, and hypokalemia may occur. Renal dysfunction is usually reversible after drug discontinuance. Increased risk exists in elderly and if there is preexisting renal dysfunction. Risk is low in well-hydrated patients with normal renal function when normal doses given.

Nursing Implications: Assess baseline renal function and electrolytes, and monitor periodically during therapy. Discuss any abnormalities with physician, as drug should be dose-reduced or discontinued if renal dysfunction develops. Assess baseline total body fluid balance, weight, and monitor periodically during antibiotic therapy. Monitor hydration status to keep patient well hydrated. Assess drug peak and trough levels as ordered so that drug dosage is correctly titrated. Increased risk of toxicity if peak serum concentration > 10–12 μg/mL. Draw blood for peak drug concentration 30 minutes after end of 30-minute infusion or at the end of a 60-minute infusion; draw trough immediately before next dose.

III. ALTERATIONS IN SENSORY/PERCEPTUAL PATTERNS related to CNS EFFECTS, NEUROMUSCULAR BLOCKADE

Defining Characteristics: Headache, tremor, lethargy may occur. Peripheral neuropathy or encephalopathy (numbness, skin tingling, muscle twitching) may occur rarely. Neuromuscular blockade is dose-related, self-limiting, and uncommon. Risk is greater with topical application or when drug is administered to patient with neuromuscular disease (myasthenia gravis) or hypocalcemia.

Nursing Implications: Assess baseline neurologic status. Assess coexisting risk factors, neuromuscular blockade medications. Teach patient about side effects, and instruct to report headache, tremor, lethargy. Observe for respiratory depression. If signs/symptoms arise, discuss drug discontinuance with physician.

IV. POTENTIAL FOR INJURY related to HYPERSENSITIVITY

Defining Characteristics: Rash, urticaria, pruritus, fever, eosinophilia have occurred rarely. CROSS-SENSITIVITY between AMINOGLYCOSIDES exists!

Nursing Implications: Assess for drug allergies to any aminoglycoside—amikacin, gentamicin, kanamycin, neomycin, netilmicin, streptomycin, tobramycin—prior to drug administration. Instruct patient to report any allergic reactions. Assess for signs/symptoms of allergic reaction after drug dose.

V. ALTERATION IN NUTRITION, LESS THAN BODY REQUIREMENTS, related to GI SIDE EFFECTS

Defining Characteristics: Nausea, vomiting, anorexia have occurred rarely. Also, transient hepatomegaly with increased LFTs—AST, ALT, LDH, alk phos—has occurred.

Nursing Implications: Assess baseline nutritional status, preexisting nausea/vomiting, anorexia. Assess baseline LFTs and monitor periodically during treatment. Instruct patient to report side effects. Provide symptomatic interventions if side effects occur; discuss with physician use of alternative drug(s).

VI. POTENTIAL FOR FATIGUE, INFECTION, AND BLEEDING related to BONE MARROW INJURY

Defining Characteristics: Anemia, leukopenia, granulocytopenia, and thrombocytopenia may occur. Also, patients receiving antibiotics are at risk for overgrowth of nonsusceptible microorganisms, such as fungi (superinfection). Rare.

Nursing Implications: Assess baseline CBC, differential, and monitor periodically during treatment. Instruct patient to report signs/symptoms of fatigue, infection, or bleeding immediately. Assess for signs/symptoms of superinfection. Discuss any adverse effects with physician.

Drug: vancomycin hydrochloride (Vancocin)

Class: Antibacterial (systemic).

Mechanism of Action: Derived from cultures of *Streptomyces orientalis;* drug is bactericidal by binding to bacterial cell wall, thus blocking protein polymerization and cell wall synthesis. Also damages cell membrane and acts at a different site than the penicillins. Bacteriostatic for enterococci. Active against many gram-positive organisms (staphylococci, group A β-hemolytic streptococci, *S. pneumoniae, C. difficile,* enterococci, *Corynebacterium, Clostridium*).

Metabolism: Not well absorbed from the GI tract—except in those patients with colitis—especially if patient has renal compromise. Effective when administered IV and is widely distributed in body tissues and fluid, including bile. Crosses placenta; unknown whether drug is excreted in breast milk;

52–60% bound to plasma proteins. IV dose excreted primarily by kidneys and, to a small degree, in bile; oral dose excreted in feces.

Dosage/Range:

Adult:

- Oral (for use in pseudomembranous colitis): capsules or powder: 0.5–1 g/day in four divided doses × 7–10 days.
- IV: 500 mg or 1 g q12h.
- Desired peak serum concentration is 20 to 40 mg/mL; and trough serum concentration is 5–15 μg/ml.
- Dose reduction necessary if renal dysfunction; see manufacturer's package insert.

Drug Preparation/Administration:

- Oral dose for treatment of *C. difficile* pseudomembranous colitis. Oral dose not recommended for treating systemic infections.
- Reconstituted by adding 10 mL of sterile water to 500-mg vial (20 mL to 1-g vial). Further dilute in at least 100 mL 0.9% Sodium Chloride or 5% Dextrose in water, and infuse over 1 hour (central line).
- For peripheral lines, further dilution in 250 mL is recommended.
- Causes tissue necrosis if given IM; DO NOT ADMINISTER IM.

Drug Interactions:

- Nephrotoxic drugs (aminoglycoside antibiotics, amphotericin B, cisplatin, colistin): increased risk of nephrotoxicity; avoid concurrent use if possible.

Lab Effects/Interference:

- BUN concentrations may be increased.

Special Considerations:

- Use cautiously in patients with renal dysfunction.
- DO NOT USE in patients with hearing loss—or use at reduced doses if necessary in life-threatening infections.
- Contraindicated in patients with known hypersensitivity.
- Obtain ordered specimen for culture and sensitivity prior to first antibiotic dose.
- Use with caution in pregnancy, as fetal effects are unknown, and in lactating mothers, as drug may be excreted in breast milk.

Potential Toxicities/Side Effects and the Nursing Process

I. ALTERATIONS IN SENSORY PERCEPTUAL PATTERNS related to OTOTOXICITY

Defining Characteristics: IV drug appears to damage eighth cranial nerve (auditory). First symptom of ototoxicity is tinnitus and may progress to deafness; may also be associated with vertigo and dizziness (vestibular branch). High risk exists in patients with renal impairment who are receiving concurrent ototoxic drugs (e.g., cisplatin) or prolonged therapy, or those whose age > 60 years old.

Nursing Implications: Assess baseline hearing (ability to hear spoken voice) or audiogram if patient is at high risk—both at baseline and throughout therapy. Monitor serum drug concentrations during therapy if at high risk. Teach patient potential side effects, and instruct patient to report any hearing/perceptual problems (e.g., tinnitus, decreased hearing, vertigo). Discuss drug discontinuance with physician if symptoms arise.

II. ALTERATION IN URINARY ELIMINATION related to NEPHROTOXICITY

Defining Characteristics: Renal damage may occur, characterized by transient increases in serum BUN or creatinine, hyaline casts, and albuminuria. May cause acute interstitial nephritis. High risk in patients with renal impairment who are receiving concurrent nephrotoxic drugs (e.g., cisplatin) or prolonged therapy, or those whose age > 60 years.

Nursing Implications: Assess baseline renal function and electrolytes, and monitor periodically during therapy. Discuss any abnormalities with physician, as drug should be dose-reduced or discontinued if renal dysfunction develops. Assess baseline hydration status, including urinary output, total body balance, daily weights; keep patient well hydrated.

III. ALTERATION IN COMFORT related to LOCAL TISSUE EFFECTS

Defining Characteristics: Vesicant if given IM (causing tissue necrosis). Irritating to veins when given IV, causing pain and thrombophlebitis.

Nursing Implications: Administer drug IV *NOT* IM. Assess IV site prior to each dose and at completion of dose; instruct patient to report pain or burning; change IV site if irritation, phlebitis develop. Change site at least q48h and consider central line for prolonged therapy. AVOID EXTRAVASATION.

IV. ALTERATION IN CARDIAC OUTPUT related to RAPID IV INFUSION

Defining Characteristics: Rapid IV administration may cause histamine release and "red-neck" syndrome, characterized by rapid onset of hypotension, flushing, and erythematous or maculopapular rash of neck, face, chest. May be associated with wheezing, dyspnea, angioedema, urticaria, pruritus. Rarely, seizures and cardiac arrest may occur. Syndrome occurs minutes after beginning infusion, but may occur at end; usually resolves spontaneously over 2+

hours, but may require antihistamines, corticosteroids, or IV fluids. Rare when drug is administered over 1 hour.

Nursing Implications: Monitor temperature, VS at baseline, 5 minutes into IV administration, and at end of infusion, at least with the initial dose; infuse over at least 1 hour, using infusion controller if necessary. Observe patient during first 5 minutes, and instruct patient to report rash, wheezing, itching immediately. If reaction occurs, stop infusion, assess VS, and notify physician. Patient may be treated with antihistamine or IV fluids, or both. Completion of dose and subsequent doses may be ordered at very slow rate. Document episode in medical record and update care plan/medication sheet to reflect change in drug administration.

V. INJURY related to BONE MARROW SUPPRESSION

Defining Characteristics: Rarely, leukopenia, thrombocytopenia, agranulocytosis may occur, especially with cumulative doses > 25 g.

Nursing Implications: Monitor baseline and periodic WBC, differential, platelet count, especially if receiving other bone marrow-suppressive drugs. Discuss abnormalities with physician.

VI. INFECTION related to OVERGROWTH OF NONSUSCEPTIBLE MICROORGANISMS

Defining Characteristics: Normal microflora populations altered by drug, with possible overgrowth by nonsusceptible microorganisms, i.e., fungi, gram-negative bacteria.

Nursing Implications: Assess for signs/symptoms of other infections of skin, mucous membranes. Instruct patient to report signs/symptoms. Discuss further antimicrobial therapy with physician.

ANTIFUNGALS

Drug: amphotericin B (deoxycholate) (Fungizone); amphotericin B lipid complex (Abelcet); amphotericin B cholesteryl sulfate complex (Amphotec); liposomal amphotericin B (AmBisome)

Class: Antifungal (systemic); antiprotozoal.

Mechanism of Action: Produced by *Streptomyces;* binds to sterol molecule in fungal membrane, causing disruption and leakage of intracellular ions. Is fungistatic (prevents replication at normal doses) and fungicidal (kills fungi at high doses). Active against systemic fungal infections (*Aspergillus, Candida,*

Cryptococcus, Histoplasma capsulatum); used to treat fungal meningitis and *Leishmania* (protozoan) infections.

Metabolism: Poorly absorbed from GI tract so must be given IV. Crosses BBB and the placenta; 90–95% bound to serum proteins. Single-dose elimination half-life is 24 hours, while following long-term administration is 15 days.

Dosage/Range:
Adult:
Amphotericin B (deoxycholate):
- Initial: 0.25 mg/kg IV (or first dose of 1 mg IV) over 6-hour period (may use 2–4 hours).
- Gradual increase in daily dosage, (e.g., over 1 week) to dose of 0.5 mg/kg/day to 1 mg/kg/day or 1.5 mg/kg on alternate days (maximum 1.5 mg/kg/day).
- If dose is interrupted for > 1 week, reinstitute at 0.25 mg/kg/day and titrate up.
- Intrathecal: 25 μg (0.1 mL diluted with 10–20 mL CSF) 2–3 × /week.
- Oral: oral candida: amphotericin B oral suspension: 1 mL (100 mg) qid.

Lipid-based amphotericin B (infection refractory or pt has renal impairment):
- Amphotec: test dose 1.6–8.3 mg/10 mL IV over 15–30 min, 3–4 mg/kg/d prepared as a 0.6 mg/mL infusion IV @ 1 mg/kg/hr.
- Abelcet: 5 mg/kg/day (1–2 mg/mL) IV @ 2.5 mg/kg/hr; if infusion time > 2 hr, shake to remix q2h.
- AmBisome: 3–5 mg/kg/day IV (1–2 mg/mL) over 1–2 hrs.
- Bladder irrigation: 50 mcg/mL solution given into bladder intermittently or as a continuous irrigation × 5–20 days.

Drug Preparation: (amphotericin B deoxycholate)
- Use sterile water for injection (NO PRESERVATIVES) to reconstitute drug; for peripheral line only further dilute to a concentration of 0.1 mg/mL using 500 mL of 5% Dextrose injection. Manufacturer recommends protecting from light, but appears to be stable for 24 hours in room light.

Drug Administration:
- Administer slowly over 2–6 hours.
- If an inline filter is used, it must have a mean pore diameter of ≥ 1 μm or drug will be filtered out; no filter for Amphotec, Abelcet.
- Protect from light during infusion.

Drug Interactions:
- Norfloxacin: possible enhanced antifungal action.
- Additive nephrotoxic effects when combined with other nephrotoxic drugs: aminoglycosides, cisplatin, cyclosporine, pentamidine, vancomycin, so concurrent administration should be avoided.

- Enhanced hypokalemic effects when combined with other drugs that lower serum potassium: corticosteroids.
- Enhanced digitoxin: toxicity related to amphotericin-induced hypokalemia.
- Synergism with flucytosine with increased drug effect.
- Antagonism with miconazole: do not use together.
- Nitrogen mustard: increases toxicity (renal, bronchospasm, hypotension)—avoid concurrent administration.
- Granulocyte transfusions: acute pulmonary dysfunction may occur if given concurrently or close together. Time administration far apart and monitor pulmonary function.

Lab Effects/Interference:
- Increased AST, ALT, alk phos, creatinine, BUN.
- Hypomagnesemia, hypokalemia, hypocalcemia.
- Hypoglycemia, hyperglycemia.

Special Considerations:
- Use with caution in patients with renal dysfunction.
- Contraindicated if hypersensitive to amphotericin.
- Safety in pregnancy has not been established—use with caution only if benefits outweigh risks.
- Drug encapsulation in liposome decreases toxicity, including renal toxicity. Amphotericin B lipid complex injection is approved for the treatment of aspergillosis in patients refractory or intolerant to conventional amphotericin B.

Potential Toxicities/Side Effects and the Nursing Process

I. POTENTIAL FOR INJURY related to DRUG ADMINISTRATION

Defining Characteristics: Headache, hypotension, malaise, myalgias, tachypnea, cramping, nausea, and vomiting may occur. Fever and chills usually begin 1–3 hours after infusion is started, and tolerance develops with subsequent doses. Rapid IV administration may cause hypertension and shock, hypokalemia, and arrhythmias.

Nursing Implications: Assess baseline comfort level, temperature, VS. Teach patient potential side effects, and instruct to report any changes. Discuss premedication with physician, such as ibuprofen (inhibits prostaglandin PGE_2) and/or hydrocortisone. Discuss with physician use of IV meperedine HCl (Demerol) for management of rigor if it develops. Administer test dose (e.g., 1 mg/250 mL 5% Dextrose IV over 1–4 hours) and monitor temperature, heart rate, BP, respiratory rate during infusion. Administer drug slowly (over 2–6 hours) and escalate dose slowly. Administer antiemetic agents as needed, then prophylactically.

II. ALTERATION IN URINARY ELIMINATION related to NEPHROTOXICITY

Defining Characteristics: 80% incidence; multiple toxic effects (vasoconstriction, lytic action on renal tubular cell membranes, calcium deposits in distal nephron); hypokalemia may precede azotemia with increased BUN and creatinine, decreased creatinine clearance, and increased excretion of K+, uric acid, and protein. Renal tubular acidosis may occur. Renal impairment usually diminishes after drug discontinuance, but some degree of impairment may be permanent.

Nursing Implications: Assess baseline renal function and electrolytes; monitor every other day during dosage escalation, then at least weekly. Discuss any abnormalities with physician. Drug should be dose-reduced if renal dysfunction develops. Slowly administer initial test dose, then gradually increase doses over first week. Assess fluid status and total body balance closely to keep patient well hydrated. Assess for signs/symptoms of hypokalemia: arthralgia, myalgia, muscle weakness. Administer potassium and magnesium replacements as ordered.

III. FATIGUE related to ANEMIA

Defining Characteristics: High incidence of reversible normocytic, normochromic anemia that rarely requires transfusion.

Nursing Implications: Assess baseline cbc, HCT; monitor Hgb and HCT during treatment. Instruct patient to report fatigue, shortness of breath, headache. Transfuse red blood cells as needed and ordered by physician.

IV. ALTERATION IN COMFORT, PAIN related to PAIN AT INJECTION SITE

Defining Characteristics: Drug may cause pain at injection site, phlebitis, thrombophlebitis; extravasation causes local irritation.

Nursing Implications: Select veins for IV administration distally and then more proximally, avoiding phlebitic veins or small veins. Apply heat to increase comfort. Administer drug slowly.

V. ALTERATION IN CARDIAC OUTPUT related to CARDIOPULMONARY DYSFUNCTION

Defining Characteristics: Rarely, hypertension, ventricular fibrillation, cardiac arrest, failure, pulmonary edema may occur. Pulmonary hypersensitivity may occur with bronchospasm, wheezing, or pulmonary pneumonitis.

Nursing Implications: Monitor VS closely, noting heart rate and rhythm, BP, breath sounds at baseline and during infusion. Instruct patient to report dyspnea, other changes in breathing pattern, or general feeling state ASAP. Discuss any changes, abnormalities with physician. Administer granulocyte transfusions as far apart from amphotericin administration as possible, and monitor pulmonary status closely. Be prepared to provide basic life support/resuscitation if needed.

VI. ALTERATIONS IN SENSORY/PERCEPTUAL PATTERNS related to PERIPHERAL AND CNS DYSFUNCTION

Defining Characteristics: Rarely, hearing loss, tinnitus, transient vertigo, blurred vision or diplopia, peripheral neuropathy, and seizures may occur. Following intrathecal drug administration, headache, lumbar nerves, arachnoiditis, and visual changes may occur.

Nursing Implications: Assess baseline neurologic function and monitor during drug administration and over time, especially when drug is given intrathecally. Notify physician if abnormalities occur. Discuss with physician coadministration of small doses of intrathecal corticosteroids to decrease CNS irritation.

VII. ALTERATION IN NUTRITION, LESS THAN BODY REQUIREMENTS, related to GI TOXICITY

Defining Characteristics: Anorexia, nausea, vomiting, dyspepsia, cramping, epigastric pain, and diarrhea may occur. Rarely, melena and hemorrhagic gastroenteritis may occur. Elevated LFTs may occur.

Nursing Implications: Assess baseline nutritional status, including weight and usual weight. Administer antiemetics as ordered and needed, then prophylactically prior to infusion if nausea and/or vomiting develop. Administer antidiarrheal medicine as ordered and needed. Instruct patient to report any symptoms; teach/reinforce importance of high-calorie, high-protein diet; suggest family/significant other bring in favorite foods from home as appropriate. Assess LFT results at baseline and periodically during treatment as elevated serum aminotransferase, bili, and alk phos may occur. Discuss abnormalities with physician. Encourage patient to eat favorite foods, especially those high in calories, protein, potassium, and magnesium. Monitor daily weight during treatment, and discuss weight loss with dietitian, patient, and physician to revise nutritional plan.

VIII. ALTERATION IN PROTECTIVE MECHANISMS related to BONE MARROW INJURY

Defining Characteristics: Rarely, thrombocytopenia, leukopenia, agranulocytosis, and coagulation defects may occur.

Nursing Implications: Assess baseline CBC, differential. Assess for any signs/symptoms of bleeding or infection, and discuss with physician if they occur. Teach patient general self-assessment guidelines, such as taking temperature and reporting any changes from baseline condition.

Drug: caspofungin (Cancidas)

Class: Echinocandin; glucan synthesis inhibitor.

Mechanism of Action: Caspofungin inhibits the synthesis of β (1, 3)-D-glucan, an integral component of the fungal cell wall of susceptible filamentous fungi. It has demonstrated activity in regions of active cell growth of *Aspergillus fumigatus*.

Metabolism: Caspofungin is slowly metabolized by hydrolysis and N-acetylation. Elimination route is via feces and urine.

Dosage/Range:
- The recommended dose of caspofungin is a 70-mg loading dose on the first day, followed by 50 mg/daily.
- No dosage adjustment is necessary for the elderly.
- No dosage adjustment is necessary for patients with renal insufficiency. Caspofungin is not dialyzable.
- No dosage adjustment is recommended for patients with mild hepatic insufficiency (Child-Pugh score 5 to 6). In those with moderate hepatic insufficiency (Child-Pugh score 7 to 9), a daily dose of 35 mg after the 70-mg loading dose is recommended.

Drug Administration:
- Caspofungin should be given as a slow IV infusion in 250 ml 0.9% Sodium Chloride over 1 hour.
- Caspofungin is not compatible with dextrose-containing solutions.

Drug Interactions:
- Transient increase in AST and ALT have been observed when caspofungin and cyclosporine are coadministered. Therefore, concomitant use of these two agents is not recommended unless the potential benefit outweighs the potential risk.

I. I. ALTERATIONS IN COMFORT related to LOCAL VEIN IRRITATION (IV ADMINISTRATION)

Defining Characteristics: Erythema, irritation, pain, swelling, phlebitis may occur at injection site. Consider use of central line.

Nursing Implications: Assess IV site for patency, irritation prior to each dose. Change IV site at least q 48 hours. Apply warmth/heat to painful area as needed.

II. POTENTIAL FOR INJURY related to HYPERSENSITIVITY REACTION

Defining Characteristics: Fever and erythema. Increased risk in allergic individuals.

Nursing Implications: Assess allergy/allergic potential to drug. Discuss other patient responses with physician to determine whether drug should be given. Assess baseline skin condition, including integrity and allergy history to drugs. Teach patient to report rash, itching, and other skin changes. Teach patient skin care and symptomatic measures as appropriate. If reaction occurs, discuss drug discontinuance with physician.

III. ALTERATION IN NUTRITION, LESS THAN BODY REQUIREMENTS, related to GI SIDE EFFECTS

Defining Characteristics: Nausea and vomiting may occur. Rarely, transient increases in LFTs—AST (SGOT), ALT (SGPT), ALKPHOS, bilirubin (BR)—may occur with coadministration of cyclosporine.

Nursing Implications: Assess baseline nutritional status. Teach patient to report GI disturbances. Administer and teach patient to self-administer antiemetics as needed and as ordered. Teach patient importance of nutritious diet, and suggest small, frequent, high-calorie, high-protein meals as appropriate. Assess baseline LFTs and monitor periodically during treatment. Discuss abnormalities and drug interruption with physician.

IV. SENSORY/PERCEPTUAL ALTERATIONS

Defining Characteristics: Headache.

Nursing Implications: Assess baseline neurological function and comfort, and monitor during treatment. Teach patient to report any changes. Discuss any abnormalities with physician.

Drug: fluconazole (Diflucan)

Class: Azole, antifungal (systemic).

Mechanism of Action: Fungistatic; causes increased permeability of fungal cell membrane, so intracellular nutrients leak out (potassium, amino acids) and cell is unable to take in nutrients to make DNA (precursors for purine, pyrimidines). Active against most fungi, including yeast.

Metabolism: Drug is rapidly and highly absorbed from GI tract, with > 90% of drug bioavailable. GI absorption is unaffected by food or gastric pH. Steady-state plasma levels achieved in 5–10 days, or by second day if loading dose given. Widely distributed in body tissues and fluids, including CSF. There is minimal protein binding. It is unknown whether drug crosses the placenta or is excreted in human milk; 60–80% of drug is excreted unchanged in the urine. Renal dysfunction results in higher circulating serum levels with prolonged drug effect and potential toxicity. Drug elimination in elderly clients may be decreased.

Dosage/Range:

- Oral and parenteral dosages are the same; IV dosage recommended for patients unable to take oral form. Dose is a single daily dose.
- Dosage depends on fungal infection. Candidiasis (oropharyngeal or esophageal): 200 mg day 1, followed by 100 mg/day (may titrate based on patient's response up to 400 mg/day) × 2 weeks (oropharyngeal); × 3 weeks or at least × 2 weeks after symptoms resolve (esophageal). Candidiasis (systemic): 400 mg day 1, followed by 200 mg/day × 4 weeks at least, then × 2 weeks after symptoms resolve (esophageal). Cryptococcal infections: Initial: 400 mg day 1, followed by 200–400 mg/day × 10–12 weeks after CSF cultures for *Cryptococcus* are negative. Maintenance (AIDS patients): 200 mg/day indefinitely.
- DOSE-REDUCE AFTER LOADING DOSE IF RENAL COMPROMISE based on creatinine clearance (e.g., 21–50 mL/min, dose-reduce 50%; if 11–20 mL/min, dose-reduce 75%).

Drug Preparation:

- Oral: store in tight containers at < 30°C (86°F).
- Parenteral: glass vials for injection should be stored at 5–30°C, (41–86°F); protect from freezing. Plastic containers should be stored at 5–25°C (41–77°F). Inspect for any discoloration, particulate matter, or leaks in plastic bags. If found, do not use.

Drug Administration:

- Oral: once daily without regard to food intake.
- IV: once daily at a rate ≤ 200 mg/hour. DO NOT ADD ADDITIVES. DO NOT ADMINISTER IV IN SERIES THAT COULD INTRODUCE AIR EMBOLISM.

Drug Interactions:

- Coumarin anticoagulants: increased PT; monitor PT closely.
- Cyclosporine: increased cyclosporine serum levels; monitor closely and adjust dose.
- Phenytoin: increased phenytoin serum level; monitor closely and reduce phenytoin dose as needed.

- Rifampin: decreased fluconazole serum level; increase fluconazole dose when given concurrently.
- Sulfonylurea antidiabetic agents (tolbutamide, glyburide, glipizide): increased drug serum levels; monitor blood glucose levels closely and decrease dose as needed.
- Thiazide diuretics: increased fluconazole serum level; do not appear to increase fluconazole toxicity so dose adjustment not necessary.
- Rifampin, isoniazid, phenytoin, valproic acid, oral sulfonylurea: increased risk of elevated hepatic transaminases exists.

Lab Effects/Interference:

Major clinical significance:

- ALT, alk phos, AST, and serum bili values may be elevated.

Special Considerations:

- Drug is being studied as a prophylactic antifungal agent in patients at risk for neutropenia and fungal infections (cancer patients receiving myelosuppressive chemotherapy, bone marrow transplant patients).
- Use cautiously in patients with renal dysfunction; dose reduction based on creatinine clearance (see Dosage/Range section).
- Absorption NOT affected by gastric pH or food intake.
- Risk of drug toxicity may be higher in patients with HIV infection.

Potential Toxicities/Side Effects and the Nursing Process

I. ALTERATION IN NUTRITION, LESS THAN BODY REQUIREMENTS, related to GI SIDE EFFECTS

Defining Characteristics: 2–8% incidence of mild-to-moderate nausea, vomiting, abdominal pain, diarrhea is seen; anorexia, dyspepsia, dry mouth, flatus, bloating occur rarely; 5–7% incidence of mild, transient increases in LFTs, which are reversible with drug discontinuance.

Nursing Implications: Assess baseline nutritional and elimination status. Instruct patient to report GI disturbances. Administer and teach patient to selfadminister antiemetics, antidiarrheals as needed and as ordered. Teach patient importance of nutritious diet, and suggest small, frequent, high-calorie, high-protein meals as appropriate. Assess baseline LFTs and monitor periodically during treatment. Discuss abnormalities and drug interruption with physician. Assess whether patient is taking other hepatotoxic drugs (see Special Considerations section).

II. ALTERATION IN SKIN INTEGRITY related to ALLERGY/HYPERSENSITIVITY

Defining Characteristics: 5% incidence is seen of rash, often diffuse, associated with eosinophilia and pruritus; rarely, exfoliative dermatitis and Stevens-Johnson syndrome may occur in patients receiving multiple drugs.

Nursing Implications: Assess baseline skin condition, including integrity and drug allergy history. Instruct patient to report rash, itching, and other skin changes. Teach patient skin care and symptomatic measures as appropriate. If skin rash develops, discuss drug discontinuance with physician. If rash progresses, especially in HIV-infected patients, drug should be discontinued, as fatal Stevens-Johnson syndrome may develop. Be prepared to treat severe acute hypersensitivity reactions with airway management, oxygen, epinephrine, corticosteroids, antihistamines as ordered.

III. ALTERATIONS IN SENSORY/PERCEPTUAL PATTERNS related to CNS EFFECTS

Defining Characteristics: Dizziness and headache occur in 2% of patients. Rarely, somnolence, delirium/coma, dysesthesia, malaise, fatigue, seizure, and psychiatric disturbance may occur.

Nursing Implications: Assess baseline neurologic function and comfort, and monitor during treatment. Instruct patient to report any changes. Discuss any abnormalities with physician.

Drug: flucytosine (Ancobon)

Class: Antifungal (systemic).

Mechanism of Action: Nonantibiotic antifungal; enters fungal cell and undergoes deamination to fluorouracil, which acts as an antimetabolite, preventing RNA and protein synthesis; may also inferfere with DNA synthesis. Active against *Candida* and *Cryptococcus.*

Metabolism: Oral preparation well absorbed from GI tract; decreased rate of absorption when taken with food. Widely distributed into body tissues and fluids, including CSF; 75–90% of dose excreted unchanged by kidneys, with increased serum levels and toxicity in patients with renal dysfunction.

Dosage/Range:
- Oral: 50–150 mg/kg/day in four equally divided doses given q6h × weeks or months until fungal studies are negative. Dose may be 150–250 mg/kg/day in *Cryptococcus* meningitis.
- Dose must be reduced in patients with renal dysfunction:

Dose must be determined by flucytosine levels (therapeutic range is 25–120 μg/mL).

Dose may be determined by creatinine clearance. Individual dose of 12.5–37.5 mg/kg given:

- q12h if creatinine clearance is 20–40 mL/min.
- q24h if creatinine clearance is 10–20 mL/min.
- q24–48h if creatinine clearance is < 10 mL/min.

Drug Preparation/Administration:
- Store in tight, light-resistant container at < 40°C (104°F).
- Oral.

Drug Interactions:
- Amphotericin B: theoretical synergism.
- Norfloxacin: theoretical synergism.

Lab Effects/Interference:
- Rare anemia, leukopenia, agranulocytosis, thrombocytopenia, pancytopenia, eosinophilia.

Special Considerations:
- Use only in severe infections, as drug is toxic.
- Theoretically synergistic with amphotericin, but some studies do not show significant benefit of combination.
- Therapeutic response (negative fungal cultures) may take weeks to months.
- Drug has no antineoplastic activity.
- Drug is teratogenic, capable of causing fetal malformations when given to pregnant women. Risks and benefits should be carefully considered before drug is used in a pregnant patient.

Potential Toxicities/Side Effects and the Nursing Process

I. POTENTIAL FOR INFECTION, BLEEDING, AND FATIGUE related to BONE MARROW DEPRESSION

Defining Characteristics: Anemia, leukopenia, thrombocytopenia may occur; agranulocytosis and aplastic anemia occur rarely. Increased risk exists with increased serum flucytosine levels (100 μg/mL), especially in patients with renal compromise or those receiving concurrent amphotericin B.

Nursing Implications: Assess baseline CBC, differential, BUN, and creatinine, and monitor closely during therapy, especially if receiving concurrent amphotericin B. Assess for signs/symptoms of bleeding, fatigue, infection during therapy. Teach patient to self-assess for signs/symptoms of infection, bleeding, and instruct to report them immediately. Discuss dose with physician; dose modification is needed if renal dysfunction occurs. Monitor flucytosine therapeutic levels (to maintain level of 25–100 μg/mL).

II. ALTERATION IN NUTRITION, LESS THAN BODY REQUIREMENTS, related to MUCOSITIS, NAUSEA, VOMITING

Defining Characteristics: Frequently dividing epithelial cells of GI mucosa are damaged, leading to diarrhea and possible bowel perforation (rare). Nausea, vomiting, anorexia, abdominal bloating may also occur. Elevated LFTs may occur, but are dose-related and reversible; liver enlargement may occur.

Nursing Implications: Assess elimination and nutritional status, baseline and throughout treatment. Assess baseline LFTs. Instruct patient to report diarrhea, nausea, vomiting immediately, and teach self-administration of prescribed antiemetics and antidiarrheal medication. Monitor weight, and teach patient importance of high-protein, high-calorie diet. Instruct patient to administer dose over 15 minutes to decrease nausea and vomiting. If weight loss occurs/persists, refer to dietitian/nutritionist. Monitor LFTs during treatment: AST, ALT, bili, and alk phos.

III. INJURY related to ANAPHYLAXIS

Defining Characteristics: Rare anaphylaxis has occurred in patients with AIDS, characterized by diffuse erythema, pruritus, injection of conjunctiva, fever, tachycardia, hypotension, edema, and abdominal pain.

Nursing Implications: Instruct AIDS patients to report any signs/symptoms of rash, pruritus, conjunctivitis, abdominal pain immediately. Use drug cautiously in AIDS patients. Monitor any adverse sensations over time. Assess for signs/ symptoms.

IV. ALTERATION IN SENSORY/PERCEPTUAL PATTERNS related to CNS CHANGES

Defining Characteristics: Confusion, sedation, hallucinations, and headaches occur infrequently.

Nursing Implications: Assess baseline mental status. Instruct patient to report headaches, abnormal thoughts, mental status changes. Discuss alternative drug if mental status changes occur.

Drug: itraconazole (Sporanox)

Class: Azole; antifungal.

Mechanism of Action: Fungistatic; may be fungicidal, depending on concentration; azole antifungals interfere with cytochrome P-450 activity, which is necessary for the demethylation of 14-α-methylsterols to ergosterol. Ergosterol, the principal sterol in the fungal cell membrance, becomes depleted. This damages the cell membrane, producing alterations in membrane function and permeability. In *Candida albicans,* azole antifungals inhibit transformation of blastospores into invasive mycelial form.

Metabolism: Rapidly absorbed from GI tract in acid environment. Decreased absorption in patients with gastric hypochlorhydria or achlorhydria, or in patients taking medications that raise pH (antacids, H_2 antagonists).

Dosage/Range:
- Oral: 100–200 mg/day × 7–14 days (candidiasis); longer for other infections (400 mg/day in severe infections).
- Although studies did not provide a loading dose, in life-threatening situations a loading dose of 200 mg three times a day (600 mg/day) for the first 3 days is recommended, based on pharmacokinetic data.
- Doses above 200 mg/day should be given in two divided doses.
- IV: 200 mg bid × 4 doses followed by 200 mg qd; gave each dose over 1 hour—do not use for more than 14 days.

Drug Preparation:
- Store in tightly closed container at < 40°C (104°F).
- Itraconazole injection must be diluted prior to IV infusion. The entire 250 mg ampule should be diluted in the 50 mL bag of 0.9% Sodium Chloride provided by the manufacturer. The final concentration of the solution is 3.33 mg/mL (250 mg/75 mL).

Drug Administration:
- Orally in single or split dose, depending on total daily dose.
- Should take with meals to increase absorption of medication.
- Oral solution should be taken on an empty stomach to increase absorption of the medication.
- To administer a 200 mg dose of itraconazole, 60 mL should be given by IV infusion over 60 minutes. The infusion should be given using a controlled-infusion device, the manufacturer-provided infusion set, and a dedicated IV line. When the infusion is complete, the manufacturer recommends that the infusion set be flushed via the 2-way stopcock using 15–20 mL of 0.9% Sodium Chloride over 30 seconds to 15 minutes. The entire IV line should then be discarded.

Drug Interactions:
- Drugs that increase gastric pH: antacids, anticholinergics/antispasmodics, histamine H_2-receptor antagonists, or omeprazole will decrease the absorption of itraconazole.
- Didanosine contains a buffer to increase its absorption; this will decrease the absorption of itraconazole since itraconazole needs an acidic environment.

- Use with oral antidiabetic agents has increased the plasma concentration of these sulfonylurea agents, leading to hypoglycemia.
- Use with carbamazepine may decrease itraconazole plasma concentrations, leading to clinical failure or relapse.
- Itraconazole may increase digoxin concentrations, leading to digoxin toxicity.
- Use with lovastatin or simvastatin may increase the plasma concentrations of these cholesterol-lowering agents and may increase the risk of rhabdomyolysis.
- Use with midazolam or triazolam may potentiate the hyponotic and sedative effects of these benzodiazepines.

Lab Effects/Interference:

Major clinical significance:

- ALT, alk phos, AST, serum bili values may be elevated.
- Serum K+: hypokalemia has occurred in approximately 2–6% of patients treated with itraconazole and has resulted in ventricular fibrillation, especially in higher doses.

Special Considerations:

- High failure rate in HIV-infected patients due to achlorhydria.

Potential Toxicities/Side Effects and the Nursing Process

I. ALTERATION IN NUTRITION, LESS THAN BODY REQUIREMENTS, related to GI SIDE EFFECTS

Defining Characteristics: Increased LFTs may occur: AST, ALT, alk phos. Hepatotoxicity is less common, is usually reversible, and is rarely fatal.

Nursing Implications: Assess baseline nutritional and elimination status. Instruct patient to report GI disturbances. Administer and teach patient to selfadminister antiemetics, antidiarrheals as needed and as ordered. Teach patient importance of nutritious diet, and suggest small, frequent, high-calorie, high-protein meals as appropriate. Assess baseline LFTs and monitor periodically during treatment. Discuss abnormalities and drug interruption with physician. Assess whether taking other hepatotoxic drugs (see Special Considerations section). Assess for increased fatigue, jaundice, dark urine, pale stools (signs of hepatotoxicity), and discuss drug discontinuance immediately with physician.

II. ALTERATION IN SKIN INTEGRITY related to ALLERGIC REACTION

Defining Characteristics: Rash, dermatitis, purpura, urticaria occur; rarely, anaphylaxis may occur.

Nursing Implications: Assess baseline skin condition and integrity. Instruct patient to report itch, rash, other skin changes. Teach patient skin care and symptomatic measures. If rash or dermatitis progresses, discuss drug discontinuance with physician. Assess for signs/symptoms of anaphylaxis.

Drug: ketoconazole (Nizoral)

Class: Azole; antifungal (systemic).

Mechanism of Action: Fungistatic by damaging fungal cell membrane and increasing permeability, altering cell metabolism, and inhibiting cell growth. Fungicidal at high concentrations. Active against mucocutaneous candidiasis, histoplasmosis, coccidioidomycosis, and blastomycosis.

Metabolism: Rapidly absorbed from GI tract in acid environment. Decreased absorption in patients with gastric hypochlorhydria (25% of all AIDS patients) or in patients taking medications that raise pH (antacids, H_2 antagonists). Distributed widely but cerebrospinal penetration is unpredictable. Drug is ~90% protein-bound. Partially metabolized in liver, and mostly excreted in the feces via bile.

Dosage/Range:

- Oral: 200 mg/day × 7–14 days (candidiasis); longer for other infections (400 mg/day in severe infections).

Drug Preparation:

- Store in tightly closed container at < 40°C (104°F).

Drug Administration:

- Orally in single dose.
- May take with meals to decrease GI side effects (unclear if food increases absorption).
- In patients with gastric achlorhydria, patient may be instructed to dissolve ketoconazole in 4 mL aqueous solution of 0.2 N hydrochloric acid and drink through a straw; follow with 4 oz (120 mL) water.

Drug Interactions:

- Drugs that increase gastric pH: antacids, cimetidine, rantidine, famotidine, sucralfate decrease ketoconazole absorption; give these drugs at least 2 hours after ketoconazole.
- Other hepatotoxic drugs: use cautiously, and monitor liver function studies closely.
- Rifampin or rifampin plus isoniazid: decreased ketoconazole levels, especially if isoniazid is taken as well. Increase ketoconazole dose.
- Acyclovir: synergism and increased antiviral action against herpes simplex virus.

- Norfloxacin: theoretically increases antifungal action of ketoconazole, but studies are inconsistent.
- Coumarin anticoagulants: increased PT; monitor patient closely and decrease anticoagulant dose accordingly.
- Cyclosporine: increased cyclosporine serum level; monitor serum level and decrease cyclosporine dose accordingly.
- Phenytoin: may have altered serum levels of phenytoin or ketoconazole; monitor serum levels of each and adjust dosages accordingly.
- Theophylline: may decrease theophylline serum concentrations; monitor serum levels and increase dosage accordingly.
- Corticosteroids: may increase corticosteroid serum level; may need to decrease dosage.

Lab Effects/Interference:

Major clinical significance:

- ALT, alk phos, AST, serum bili values may be elevated.
- ACTH-induced serum corticosteroid concentrations and serum testosterone concentrations may be decreased by doses of 800 mg/day of ketoconazole; serum testosterone concentrations are abolished by values of 1.6 g/day of ketoconazole, but return to baseline values when ketoconazole is discontinued.

Special Considerations:

- Monitor liver function studies.
- High failure rate in HIV-infected patients due to achlorhydria.

Potential Toxicities/Side Effects and the Nursing Process

I. ALTERATION IN NUTRITION, LESS THAN BODY REQUIREMENTS, related to GI SIDE EFFECTS

Defining Characteristics: Nausea, vomiting is seen in 3–10% of patients. Diarrhea, abdominal pain, flatulence, constipation may occur less frequently. Increased LFTs may occur: AST, ALT, alk phos. Hepatotoxicity is less common, is usually reversible, and is rarely fatal.

Nursing Implications: Assess baseline nutritional and elimination status. Instruct patient to report GI disturbances. Administer and teach patient to self-administer antiemetics, antidiarrheals as needed and as ordered. Teach patient importance of nutritious diet, and suggest small, frequent, high-calorie, high-protein meals as appropriate. Assess baseline LFTs and monitor periodically during treatment. Discuss abnormalities and drug interruption with physician. Assess whether taking other hepatotoxic drugs (see Special Considerations section). Assess for increased fatigue, jaundice, dark urine, pale stools (signs of hepatotoxicity), and discuss drug discontinuance immediately with physician.

II. ALTERATION IN COMFORT related to GYNECOMASTIA AND BREAST TENDERNESS

Defining Characteristics: Breast enlargement and tenderness may occur in some men, lasting weeks to duration of therapy.

Nursing Implications: Assess for occurrence in male patients. Assess comfort level, degree of tenderness, and self-care measures used to increase comfort. Assess impact on body image.

III. ALTERATION IN SKIN INTEGRITY related to ALLERGIC REACTION

Defining Characteristics: Rash, dermatitis, purpura, urticaria occur in 1% of patients; rarely, anaphylaxis may occur.

Nursing Implications: Assess baseline skin condition and integrity. Teach patient to report itch, rash, and other skin changes. Teach patient skin care and symptomatic measures. If rash or dermatitis progresses, discuss drug discontinuance with physician. Assess for signs/symptoms of anaphylaxis.

IV. ALTERATIONS IN SENSORY/PERCEPTUAL PATTERNS related to CNS EFFECTS

Defining Characteristics: Dizziness, headache, nervousness, insomnia, lethargy, somnolence, and paresthesia have occurred in ~1% of patients.

Nursing Implications: Assess baseline neurologic function and comfort, and monitor during treatment. Instruct patient to report any changes. Discuss any abnormalities with physician.

Drug: micafungin sodium (Mycamine)

Class: antifungal.

Mechanism of Action: Fungistatic by damaging fungal cell membrane increasing permeability, altering cell metabolism, and inhibiting cell growth. Fungicidal at high concentrations. Inhibits the synthesis of 1,3-β-D-glucan, an integral component of the fungal cell wall.

Metabolism: Metabolized by liver and excreted in urine.

Dosage/Range:
- Esophageal Candidiasis: 150 mg/day × 15 days.
- Prophylaxis of Candida Infections in HSCT recipients 50 mg/day × 19 days.

Drug Preparation/Administration:

- Do not mix or co-infuse with other medications. Mycafungin has been shown to precipitate when mixed directly with a number of other commonly used medications.
- No dose adjustment is required with concomitant use of mycophenolate mofetil, cyclosporine, tacrolimus, prednisolone, Sirolimus, nifedipine, fluconazole, ritonavir, or rifampin.
- A loading dose is not required; typically, 85% of the steady-state is achieved after three daily doses.
- IV: Dilute in 0.9% Sodium Chloride, USP (without a bacteriostatic agent) or 5% Dextrose injection, USP.
- Infuse over 1 hour. Stable × 24 hours at room temperature.

Drug Interactions:

- Coumarin anticoagulants: increased PT. Monitor patient closely and decrease anticoagulant dose accordingly.
- Norfloxacin: may increase antifungal action.
- Cyclosporine: increased cyclosporine serum level. Monitor serum level and decrease cyclosporine dose accordingly.

Lab Effects/Interference: *Major clinical significance:*

- ALT, alk phos, AST, serum bili values may be elevated.

Special Considerations:

- Used in treatment of fungal infections.
- Monitor HCT, Hgb, serum electrolytes, and lipids, as changes may occur during treatment.

Potential Toxicities/Side Effects and the Nursing Process

I. POTENTIAL FOR INJURY related to ANAPHYLAXIS

Defining Characteristics: Anaphylaxis with tachycardia, arrhythmias, and cardiac arrest may occur.

Nursing Implications: Assess baseline VS and monitor throughout infusion. Instruct patient to report signs/symptoms immediately. Assess for signs/symptoms: nausea, generalized itching, crampy abdominal pain, chest tightness, anxiety, agitation, sense of impending doom, wheezing, and dizziness.

II. ALTERATION IN COMFORT related to PRURITUS, PHLEBITIS, SKIN ERUPTIONS, FEVER

Defining Characteristics: Phlebitis, pruritus with or without rash may occur.

Nursing Implications: Assess temperature, skin integrity, and comfort prior to drug administration, and monitor throughout treatment. Discuss with physician use of diphenhydramine to decrease itching. Change IV sites q48h to decrease phlebitis, or discuss with patient and physician use of central line. If rash and pruritus worsen, discuss with physician drug discontinuance.

III. ALTERATION IN NUTRITION, LESS THAN BODY REQUIREMENTS, related to GI SIDE EFFECTS

Defining Characteristics: Nausea, vomiting, diarrhea, and anorexia may occur.

Nursing Implications: Assess baseline nutritional and elimination status. Instruct patient to report GI disturbances. Administer and teach patient to self-administer antiemetics, antidiarrheals as needed and as ordered. Teach patient importance of nutritious diet, and suggest small, frequent, high-calorie, high-protein meals as appropriate.

IV. ALTERATIONS IN SENSORY/PERCEPTUAL PATTERNS related to CNS, ENDOCRINE EFFECTS

Defining Characteristics: Dizziness, headache, and somnolence may occur.

Nursing Implications: Assess baseline neurologic function and comfort, and monitor during treatment. Instruct patient to report any changes. Discuss any abnormalities with physician.

Drug: miconazole nitrate (Monistat)

Class: Azole; antifungal (systemic).

Mechanism of Action: Fungistatic by damaging fungal cell membrane and increasing permeability, altering cell metabolism, and inhibiting cell growth. Fungicidal at high concentrations. Active against most fungi, especially candidiasis, coccidioidomycosis, cryptococcosis.

Metabolism: Limited (50%) oral absorption so usually given parenterally; 91–93% protein-bound to plasma proteins. Unpredictable penetration into CSF, so must be given intrathecally to achieve therapeutic levels. Metabolized by liver and excreted in urine.

Dosage/Range:

IV:

- Coccidioidomycosis: 1.8–3.6 g/day × 3–20+ weeks.
- Cryptococcosis: 1.2–2.4 g/day × 3–12+ weeks.
- Candidiasis: 600 mg–1.8 g/day × 1–20+ weeks.
- Intrathecal: refer to protocol; usually 20 mg q1–2 days, or q3–7 days if given by lumbar puncture.

- Intravesical: 200 mg in dilute solution 2–4 × day or by continuous bladder irrigation.

Drug Preparation/Administration:
- IV: Dilute in 200 mL of 0.9% Sodium Chloride (preferred) or 5% Dextrose injection and infuse over 30–60 min; daily dosage usually given in three divided doses q8h. Stable × 24 hours at room temperature.
- Intrathecal: is administered undiluted.
- Intravesical: as above (dosage) in conjunction with IV drug as well.

Drug Interactions:
- Coumarin anticoagulants: increased PT. Monitor patient closely and decrease anticoagulant dose accordingly.
- Norfloxacin: may increase antifungal action.
- Oral sulfonylureas: increased hypoglycemia effect. Monitor blood glucose and decrease dose of oral sulfonylurea.
- Rifampin or rifampin plus isoniazid: decreased miconazole levels, especially if isoniazid taken as well. Increase miconazole dose.
- Phenytoin: may have altered serum levels of phenytoin or miconazole.
- Monitor serum levels of each and adjust dosages accordingly.
- Cyclosporine: increased cyclosporine serum level. Monitor serum level and decrease cyclosporine dose accordingly.

Lab Effects/Interference:
Major clinical significance:
- ALT, alk phos, AST, serum bili values may be elevated.

Clinical significance:
- Serum lipid profile: hyperlipidemia has occurred in patients receiving intravenous miconazole; this is reportedly due to the vehicle in the miconazole solution, PEG 40 castor oil (Cremophor EL).

Special Considerations:
- Used in treatment of severe fungal infections.
- Initial dose should be in hospital with resuscitation equipment available to determine hypersensitivity (cardiac arrest has occurred with initial dose). Drug is suspended in castor oil base, which stimulates allergic reaction. Subsequent dosing can be safely given to selected patients in ambulatory settings.
- IV push injection of drug may cause arrhythmias, so drug must be diluted (200+ mL) and administered over 30–60 minutes.
- Monitor HCT, Hgb, serum electrolytes, and lipids, as changes may occur during treatment.

Potential Toxicities/Side Effects and the Nursing Process

I. POTENTIAL FOR INJURY related to ANAPHYLAXIS

Defining Characteristics: Anaphylaxis with tachycardia, arrhythmias, and cardiac arrest may occur on first IV dose, probably related to suspension medium of drug (castor oil).

Nursing Implications: Ensure first dose is given in inpatient setting with resuscitation equipment and physician available. Assess baseline VS and monitor throughout infusion. Instruct patient to report signs/symptoms immediately. Assess for signs/symptoms: nausea, generalized itching, crampy abdominal pain, chest tightness, anxiety, agitation, sense of impending doom, wheezing, and dizziness.

II. ALTERATION IN COMFORT related to PRURITUS, PHLEBITIS, SKIN ERUPTIONS, FEVER

Defining Characteristics: Phlebitis, pruritus with or without rash may occur.

Nursing Implications: Assess temperature, skin integrity, and comfort prior to drug administration, and monitor throughout treatment. Discuss with physician use of diphenhydramine to decrease itching. Change IV sites q48h to decrease phlebitis, or discuss with patient and physician use of central line. If rash and pruritus worsen, discuss with physician drug discontinuance.

III. ALTERATION IN NUTRITION, LESS THAN BODY REQUIREMENTS, related to GI SIDE EFFECTS

Defining Characteristics: Nausea, vomiting, diarrhea, anorexia, and bitter taste may occur.

Nursing Implications: Assess baseline nutritional and elimination status. Instruct patient to report GI disturbances. Administer and teach patient to self-administer antiemetics, antidiarrheals as needed and as ordered. Teach patient importance of nutritious diet, and suggest small, frequent, high-calorie, high-protein meals as appropriate.

IV. ALTERATIONS IN SENSORY/PERCEPTUAL PATTERNS related to CNS, ENDOCRINE EFFECTS

Defining Characteristics: Dizziness, flushing, anxiety, increased libido, blurred vision, eye dryness, headache may occur.

Nursing Implications: Assess baseline neurologic function and comfort, and monitor during treatment. Instruct patient to report any changes. Discuss any abnormalities with physician.

Drug: nystatin (Mycostatin, Nilstat)

Class: Antifungal.

Mechanism of Action: Binds to sterol molecule in fungi cell membrane, increasing permeability so that potassium and other intracellular ions are lost. Active against yeast and fungi, especially *Candida.*

Metabolism: Drug is not absorbed from intact skin, mucous membranes, and is poorly absorbed from GI tract. Excreted as unchanged drug in the feces.

Dosage/Range:
- Oral (for treatment of oral or intestinal candidiasis): 500,000–1 million U tid; continue therapy for 48 hours after clinical remission to prevent recurrence.
- Powder: topical for candidal rash infections.
- Vaginal: 100,000 U as vaginal tablet, inserted into vagina qd or bid × 14 days.

Drug Preparation:
- Oral suspension and tablets should be stored in tight, light-resistant containers < 40°C (104°F).

Drug Administration:
- Oral suspension. Instruct patient to:
  - Rinse mouth with oral hygiene solution to clean food debris.
  - Hold suspension in mouth and swish for 1–2 minutes, then swallow or spit solution.
  - Do not rinse mouth or eat for 15–30 minutes.

Drug Interactions:
- None.

Lab Effects/Interference:
- None known.

Special Considerations:
- For patients with oral thrush who have difficulty taking oral suspension:
  - Oral suspension can be frozen in medicine cups so it is easier to administer if the patient has stomatitis.
  - Vaginal suppository may be sucked as this increases mucosal contact with drug.
  - Cannot be used to treat systemic infections.
  - Adverse effects are infrequent.

Potential Toxicities/Side Effects and the Nursing Process

I. ALTERATION IN NUTRITION, LESS THAN BODY REQUIREMENTS, related to GI SIDE EFFECTS

Defining Characteristics: High oral doses may cause nausea, vomiting, diarrhea.

Nursing Implications: Assess baseline nutritional status. Instruct patient to report GI disturbances. Administer and teach patient to self-administer antiemetics, antidiarrheals as needed and as ordered. Teach patient importance of nutritious diet, and suggest small, frequent, high-calorie, high-protein meals as appropriate.

II. KNOWLEDGE DEFICIT related to SELF-ADMINISTRATION OF MEDICATION

Defining Characteristics: Increased compliance when patient is instructed in self-care activities.

Nursing Implications: Assess knowledge about infection and planned treatment. Teach about drug action, potential side effects, and when and how to take drug. Instruct patient to rinse mouth with saline gargle (or other rinse) to remove food debris prior to taking nystatin suspension; solution should be swished in mouth 1–2 minutes, then swallowed or spit out. Patient should not eat or rinse mouth for 15–30 minutes.

Drug: voriconazole (VFEND)

Class: Triazole; antifungal (systemic).

Mechanism of Action: Fungistatic by damaging fungal cell membrane and increasing permeability, altering cell metabolism, and inhibiting cell growth. Fungicidal at high concentrations. Active against invasive aspergillosis fumigatus, Fusarium spp. infection, and Scedosporium apiospermum infection.

Metabolism: Rapidly absorbed from GI tract in acid environment. Partially metabolized in liver, and mostly excreted in the feces via bile.

Dosage/Range:

- Oral: 200 mg q 12 hours for 7–14 days; dose may be increased if there is an inadequate response to infections (300 mg q 12 hours).
- IV preparation is available. The final voriconazole preparation must be infused over 1–2 hours at a maximum rate of 3 mg/kg per hour.

Drug Preparation:
- Once reconstituted, drug should be used immediately, or it can be stored for no longer than 24 hours at 2–8°C (37–46°F).

Drug Administration:
- Orally. May take 1 hour before meals or 1 hour after meals.
- The final voriconazole preparation must be infused over 1–2 hours at a maximum rate of 3 mg/kg per hour.

Drug Interactions:
- Drugs that increase gastric pH: antacids, cimetidine, rantidine have minor or no significant effect on voriconazole.
- Hepatotoxic drugs: use cautiously, and monitor liver function studies closely.
- Rifampin decreases the steady state of voriconazole.
- Coumarin anticoagulants: increases PT; monitor patient closely and decrease anticoagulant dose accordingly.
- Cyclosporine: increases cyclosporine serum level; monitor serum level and decrease cyclosporine dose accordingly.
- Phenytoin: may have altered serum levels of phenytoin or ketoconazole; monitor serum levels of each and adjust dosages accordingly.
- Carbamazepine and long-acting barbiturates and macrolide antibiotics reduce the efficacy of voriconazole.

Lab Effects/Interference:
Major clinical significance:
- ALT, alk phos, AST, serum bili values may be elevated.

Special Considerations:
- Monitor liver function studies.

Potential Toxicities/Side Effects and the Nursing Process

I. ALTERATION IN NUTRITION, LESS THAN BODY REQUIREMENTS, related to GI SIDE EFFECTS

Defining Characteristics: Nausea, vomiting is seen in 3–10% of patients. Diarrhea, abdominal pain, flatulence, constipation may occur less frequently. Increased LFTs may occur: AST, ALT, alk phos. Hepatotoxicity is less common, is usually reversible, and is rarely fatal.

Nursing Implications: Assess baseline nutritional and elimination status. Instruct patient to report GI disturbances. Administer and teach patient to self-administer antiemetics, antidiarrheals as needed and as ordered. Teach patient importance of nutritious diet, and suggest small, frequent, high-calorie, high-protein meals as appropriate. Assess baseline LFTs and monitor periodically during treatment. Discuss abnormalities and drug interruption with physician. Assess whether taking other hepatotoxic drugs (see Special Considerations section). Assess for increased fatigue, jaundice, dark urine, pale stools (signs of hepatotoxicity), and discuss drug discontinuance immediately with physician.

II. ALTERATION IN SENSORY/PERCEPTUAL PATTERNS related to VISUAL DISTURBANCES

Defining Characteristics: Treatment-related visual disturbances are common (30%). Generally mild and rarely result in discontinuing treatment.

Nursing Implications: Assess for occurrence. Assess comfort level. Educate patient about this side effect. Assess impact on body image.

III. ALTERATION IN SKIN INTEGRITY related to ALLERGIC REACTION

Defining Characteristics: Rash, dermatitis, purpura, urticaria occur in 6% of patients.

Nursing Implications: Assess baseline skin condition and integrity. Teach patient to report itch, rash, and other skin changes. Teach patient skin care and symptomatic measures. If rash or dermatitis progresses, discuss drug discontinuance with physician. Assess for signs/symptoms of anaphylaxis.

ANTIVIRALS

Drug: acyclovir (Zovirax)

Class: Antiviral (systemic).

Mechanism of Action: Interferes with DNA synthesis so that viral replication cannot occur. Active against herpes simplex virus (HSV-1, HSV-2), varicella-zoster virus (VZV) (shingles), Epstein-Barr virus (EBV), and cytomegalovirus (CMV).

Metabolism: Variable GI absorption; unaffected by food. Widely distributed in body tissue and fluids, including CSF. Variable protein-binding (9–33%). Crosses placenta and is excreted in breast milk.

Dosage/Range:
Adult:
- Oral: 200 mg PO q4h (genital herpes) to 800 mg PO 5 × /day (acute herpes zoster).
- IV (initial/recurrent infections in immunocompromised patients): 5–10 mg/kg q8h × 7 days; 5 mg/kg q8h × 7–14 days (herpes simplex); 10 mg/kg q8h × 7–14 days (herpes zoster, herpes encephalitis).
- Use ideal body weight for dose calculation.

- Avoid doses greater than 1000 mg/dose.
- Dose modification is required if renal dysfunction is present.

Drug Preparation/Administration:
- Oral: store in tight, light-resistant containers at 15–25°C (59–77°F).
- IV: reconstitute with sterile water for injection per manufacturer's directions and further dilute in 50–100 mL IV fluid; a final concentration of 7 mg/mL or less is recommended to minimize the incidence of phlebitis; infuse over 1 hour.

Drug Interactions:
- Zidovudine: potentiates antiretroviral activity of zidovudine, but may cause increased neurotoxicity (drowsiness, lethargy) in AIDS patients. Monitor for increased neurotoxicity.
- Probenecid: may increase plasma half-life. Monitor for increased acyclovir toxicity.
- Antifungals: potential antiviral synergy.
- Interferon: potential synergistic antiviral effect, potential increased neurotoxicity. Use together with caution.
- Methotrexate (intrathecal): possible increased neurotoxicity. Use together with caution.

Lab Effects/Interference:

Major clinical significance:
- BUN and serum creatinine concentrations required prior to and during therapy, since intravenous acyclovir may be nephrotoxic; if acyclovir is given by rapid intravenous injection or its urine solubility is exceeded, precipitation of acyclovir crystals may occur in renal tubules; renal tubular damage may occur and may progress to acute renal failure.

Clinical significance:
- Pap test: although clear association has not been shown to date, patients with genital herpes may be at increased risk of developing cervical cancer. Pap test should be done at least once a year to detect early cervical changes.

Special Considerations:
- Use cautiously in patients with preexisting renal dysfunction or dehydration; underlying neurologic dysfunction or neurologic reactions to cytotoxic drugs, intrathecal methotrexate, or interferon and in patients with hepatic dysfunction.
- It is imperative that patients be well hydrated, with adequate urine output prior to and for up to 2 hours after IV dosing.
- Administer with caution if patient is receiving other nephrotoxic drugs.
- Contraindicated in patients hypersensitive to drug.
- Minimal injury to normal cells, so few adverse effects exist.

Potential Toxicities/Side Effects and the Nursing Process

I. ALTERATION IN URINARY ELIMINATION related to RENAL TOXICITY

Defining Characteristics: Transient increase is seen in renal function tests (serum BUN, creatinine) and decreased urine creatinine clearance, as drug may precipitate in renal tubules during dehydration or rapid IV drug administration. Increased risk exists if preexisting renal disease or concurrent administration of nephrotoxic drugs.

Nursing Implications: Assess baseline renal function, and monitor periodically during therapy. Notify physician of any abnormalities before administering next dose. Ensure adequate hydration and urine output prior to and for 2 hours after IV drug administration. Administer IV drug slowly over 1 hour.

II. ALTERATIONS IN SENSORY/PERCEPTUAL PATTERNS related to ENCEPHALOPATHY

Defining Characteristics: IV administration: encephalopathy (lethargy, tremors, confusion, agitation, seizures, dizziness) may occur rarely. Oral: headache occurs in 13% of patients receiving chronic suppressive treatment.

Nursing Implications: Assess baseline neurologic function and comfort, and monitor during treatment. Instruct patient to report any changes. Discuss any abnormalities with physician.

III. ALTERATIONS IN COMFORT related to LOCAL VEIN IRRITATION (IV ADMINISTRATION)

Defining Characteristics: Erythema, irritation, pain, swelling, phlebitis may occur at injection site.

Nursing Implications: Assess IV site for patency, irritation prior to each dose. Change IV site at least q48h. Apply warmth/heat to painful area as needed.

IV. ALTERATION IN NUTRITION, LESS THAN BODY REQUIREMENTS, related to GI SIDE EFFECTS (ORAL DOSAGE)

Defining Characteristics: Nausea, vomiting, and diarrhea occur in 2–5% of patients receiving chronic therapy.

Nursing Implications: Assess history of nausea/vomiting, diarrhea, and instruct patient to report any occurrence. Teach patient self-medication of prescribed antinausea or antidiarrheal medicines. Discuss drug discontinuance with physician if symptoms are severe.

V. ALTERATION IN SKIN INTEGRITY related to RASH

Defining Characteristics: Rash, urticaria, pruritus may occur.

Nursing Implications: Assess baseline history of drug allergy and skin integrity. Instruct patient to report any occurrence of rash, pruritus. Teach symptomatic management measures unless severe; if severe, discuss drug discontinuance with physician.

VI. KNOWLEDGE DEFICIT related to (ORAL) DRUG ADMINISTRATION

Defining Characteristics: Patient may not realize drug does not cure viral infection, nor does it prevent spread of virus to others. Prodrome of tingling, itching, or pain can herald mucocutaneous herpes.

Nursing Implications: Teach patient about herpetic infection and goal of therapy to suppress infection. When used to treat recurrent episodes of chronic infection, teach patient to recognize prodromal symptoms and to take prescribed drug then or within two days of onset of lesions. Teach patient about routes of viral spread, and instruct to avoid contacts with others that may lead to viral spread.

Drug: cidofovir (Vistide)

Class: Antiviral (systemic).

Mechanism of Action: Suppresses CMV replication by selective inhibition of viral DNA synthesis.

Metabolism: Less than 6% bound to plasma proteins. Renal clearance is reduced with the concomitant administration of probenecid.

Dosage/Range:
- Weekly induction regimen: 5 mg/kg infused every week × 2 weeks.
- Twice monthly maintenance regimen: 5 mg/kg infused every other week.

Drug Preparation:
- Requires chemotherapy safety handling (drug is mutagenic, tumorogenic, embryotoxic).
- Reconstitute drug (single use, nonpreserved); vial contains 75 mg/mL.
- Further dilute in 100 mL 0.9% Sodium Chloride.

Drug Administration:
- Administer 2 g probenecid (four 500-mg tabs) 3 hours prior to drug infusion.

- Infuse 1 L of 0.9% Sodium Chloride over 1–2 hours immediately prior to drug infusion.
- Infuse IV drug over 1 hour.
- As ordered by physician, may administer second liter of 0.9% Sodium Chloride at the start of the drug infusion, and continue for 1–3 hours.
- 2 hours after end of drug infusion, administer 1 g probenecid (two 500-mg tabs).
- 8 hours after end of the drug infusion, administer 1 g probenecid (two 500-mg tabs).

Drug Interactions:
- Probenecid: interacts with the metabolism or renal tubular excretion of acetaminophen, acyclovir, angiotensin-converting enzyme (ACE) inhibitors, barbiturates, NSAIDS, theophylline, zidovudine.
- Increased nephrotoxicity when combined with other nephrotoxic drugs.

Lab Effects/Interference:
- Serum creatinine levels may be elevated.

Special Considerations:
- Indicated for the treatment of AIDS patients who have newly diagnosed or relapsed CMV retinitis.
- Dose-limiting toxicity is nephrotoxicity evidenced by proteinuria and increased serum creatinine.
- Treatment requires prehydration and posthydration use of concomitant probenecid.
- Drug contraindicated in patients with baseline serum creatinine > 1.5 mg/dL, creatinine clearance ≤ 55 mL/min, proteinuria ≥ 3+, past severe hypersensitivity to probenecid or other sulfa-containing medications, hypersensitivity to cidofovir, and patients who are pregnant or breast-feeding.

DOSE REDUCTIONS:
- (a) Patients with baseline normal renal function:

Renal abnormality	Cidofovir dosage
Serum creatinine 0.3–0.4 mg/dL > baseline	3 mg/kg
Serum creatinine = 0.5 mg/dL above baseline	discontinue cidofovir
Proteinuria ≥ 3+	discontinue cidofovir

- (b) Patients with baseline renal impairment:

Creatinine clearance (mL/min)	Induction (once a week × 2 weeks)	Maintenance (once every 2 weeks)
41–55	2.0 mg/kg	2.0 mg/kg

Creatinine clearance (mL/min)	Induction (once a week × 2 weeks)	Maintenance (once every 2 weeks)
30–40	1.5 mg/kg	1.1 mg/kg
20–29	1.0 mg/kg	1.0 mg/kg
≤ 19	0.5 mg/kg	0.1 mg/kg

- Patient teaching:
  - Encourage increased oral intake of fluids to 1–3 L as tolerated.
  - Return to clinic for appointments (induction: weekly × 2 weeks, maintenance every other week).
  - Report side effects immediately.
  - Ophthalmologic appointments as scheduled for intraocular pressure (IOP), visual acuity monitoring.

Potential Toxicities/Side Effects and the Nursing Process

I. POTENTIAL FOR INJURY related to NEUTROPENIA

Defining Characteristics: Neutropenia (< 750/mm^2) may occur in 28% of patients, and < 500/mm^3 occurred in 20% of patients. Infections occurred in 25% of patients.

Nursing Implications: Monitor WBC and ANC prior to each drug dose, and hold treatment if neutropenic. Discuss with physician use of G-CSF. If the patient is receiving zidovudine, the zidovudine should be temporarily discontinued or dose decreased by 50% on days of probenecid therapy. Instruct patient to monitor temperature and to report fever > 101°F immediately. Discuss use of G-CSF with physician as needed (up to 34% required G-CSF in clinical trials).

II. ALTERATION IN NUTRITION, LESS THAN BODY REQUIREMENTS, related to NAUSEA/VOMITING

Defining Characteristics: Nausea/vomiting occurs in about 65% of patients.

Nursing Implications: Encourage patients to eat food prior to each dose of probenecid. Discuss antiemetic prior to the first dose of probenecid, and then during period of probenecid therapy.

III. ALTERATION IN COMFORT related to FEVER, CHILLS, RASH, HEADACHE FROM PROBENECID

Defining Characteristics: Fever occurs in up to 57% of patients, rash in 30%, headache in 27%, chills in 24%. Asthenia (46% incidence), diarrhea (27%), alopecia (25%), anorexia (22%), dyspnea (22%), abdominal pain (17%), and anemia (20%). In clinical trials, 25% of patients withdrew from treatment due to adverse events.

Nursing Implications: Assess baseline comfort, and instruct patient to report symptoms. Discuss symptom management with physician, such as antihistamine and/or antipyretic (acetaminophen) for fever, and then use prophylactically in subsequent doses.

IV. ALTERATION IN ELIMINATION related to RENAL TOXICITY

Defining Characteristics: Creatinine elevations to > 1.5 mg/dL occur in approximately 17% of patients, proteinuria in 80% of patients, and decreased serum bicarbonate in > 5% of patients.

Nursing Implications: Encourage patients to increase their daily oral fluid intake to 2–3 L. Closely monitor renal function; patients who have received foscarnet are at increased risk for nephrotoxicity. Ensure that patient receives prehydration and posthydration, and is able to take oral fluids. Discuss dose reductions based on alterations in renal function with physician. Check urine for protein. If positive, discuss additional hydration and rechecking of urine for blood with physician.

V. ALTERATIONS IN SENSORY/PERCEPTUAL PATTERNS related to OCULAR HYPOTONY

Defining Characteristics: OCULAR HYPOTONY occurs rarely, may be increased risk for patients with concomitant diabetes mellitus.

Nursing Implications: Patients should see ophthalmologist for IOP assessments and visual acuity periodically.

VI. METABOLIC ACIDOSIS related to DECREASED SERUM BICARBONATE

Defining Characteristics: Occurs rarely (2%).

Nursing Implications: Assess for decreases in serum bicarbonate < 16 mEq/L associated with evidence of renal tubular damage (incidence 9%). Serious metabolic acidosis in association with liver failure, mucormycosis, aspergillus, and disseminated MAC has occurred, with subsequent death in one patient. Monitor baseline chemistries, and review results prior to each treatment.

Drug: famciclovir (Famvir)

Class: Antiviral (systemic).

Mechanism of Action: Rapidly transformed into antiviral penciclovir, which inhibits herpes simplex types HSV-1, HSV-2, or VZV by inhibiting HSV-2 polymerase. Herpes viral DNA synthesis and viral replication are selectively inhibited.

Metabolism: Oral bioavailability is 77%, with peak plasma levels 30–90 minutes after dosing. Plasma half-life is 2.3 hours. In the virus, the active form of the drug has a long intracellular half-life. Low protein binding and rapid and complete elimination in the urine (73%) and feces (27%).

Dosage/Range:
- Herpes zoster: 500 mg q8h × 7 days.
- Genital herpes: 125 mg bid × 5 days.

Drug Preparation:
- Available in 125-, 250-, 500-mg tablets.

Drug Administration:
- Oral, without regard to meals.

Drug Interactions:
- None.

Lab Effects/Interference:
- None known.

Special Considerations:
- Treatment of herpes zoster: viral shedding stopped 50% faster than with placebo, with full crusting in < 1 week, and shorter time to relief from acute pain. In addition, drug significantly reduces the duration of postherpetic neuralgia by two months compared to placebo.
- Dose should be reduced in patients with renal impairment according to schedule below:

Condition	Creatinine clearance cc/min	Dose
Herpes zoster	40–59	500 mg q12h
	20–39	500 mg q24h
	< 20	250 mg q48h
Recurrent genital herpes	20–39	125 mg q24h
	< 20	125 mg q48h

Condition	Creatinine clearance cc/min	Dose

Potential Toxicities/Side Effects and the Nursing Process

I. ALTERATION IN COMFORT related to HEADACHE, NAUSEA

Defining Characteristics: Headache occurred in approximately 22% of patients. Nausea occurred in 12% of patients.

Nursing Implications: Teach patient that side effects may occur and are usually mild. Instruct patient to report headache that does not resolve with acetaminophen, or nausea that does not resolve with diet modification.

Drug: foscarnet sodium (Foscavir)

Class: Antiviral (systemic).

Mechanism of Action: Inhibits binding sites on virus-specific DNA polymerases and reverse transcriptases without affecting cellular DNA polymerases. Thus, prevents viral replication of all known herpes viruses: CMV, HSV-1, HSV-2, EBV, and VZV. Active against resistant herpes simplex viruses that are resistant via thymidine kinase deficiency. Indicated for treatment of CMV retinitis in AIDS patients.

Metabolism: 14–17% bound to plasma proteins, and excreted into urine 80–90% unchanged by kidneys. Variable penetration into CSF.

Dosage/Range:
Adult (normal renal function):
- IV induction: 60 mg/kg IV over 1 hour q8h × 2–3 weeks.
- Maintenance: 90–120 mg/kg/day IV over 2 hours.
- Dose modification is necessary if renal insufficiency. See manufacturer's package insert.

Drug Preparation/Administration:
- Add drug solution (24 mg/mL) to 0.9% Sodium Chloride or 5% Dextrose to achieve a final concentration ≤ 12 mg/mL.
- Administer via rate controller or infusion pump over 1 hour (induction) or 2 hours (maintenance) via peripheral or central vein.
- Do not administer or give concurrently with other drugs or solutions.

Drug Interactions:
- Incompatible with $D_{30}W$, amphotericin B, Ringer's lactate, total parenteral nutrition (TPN), acyclovir, ganciclovir, trimetrexate, pentamidine, vanco-

mycin, trimethoprim/sulfamethoxazole, diazepam, digoxin, phenytoin, leucovorin, prochlorperazine.
- Pentamidine: potentially fatal HYPOCALCEMIA; seizures have occurred; AVOID CONCURRENT USE.
- Nephrotoxic drugs (amphotericin B, aminoglycosides): additive nephrotoxicity; AVOID CONCURRENT USE.
- Hypocalcemic agents: additive hypocalcemia; AVOID CONCURRENT USE.
- Zidovudine: increased anemia; monitor patient closely and transfuse with red blood cells as ordered.

Lab Effects/Interference: Lab Effects/Alterations:
Major clinical significance:
- Serum calcium (ionized), serum calcium (total), and serum phosphate: concentrations of phosphate may be increased or decreased; concentrations of total calcium may be decreased; although the total calcium concentration may also appear normal, the level of ionized calcium may be decreased and result in symptomatic hypocalcemia.
- Serum creatinine concentrations may be increased.
- Serum Mg++ concetrations may be decreased.

Clinical significance:
- ALT, alk phos, AST, and serum bili values may be increased.
- Serum K+ concentrations may be decreased.

Special Considerations:
- Contraindicated in patients hypersensitive to foscarnet.
- DO NOT administer concomitantly with IV pentamidine.
- Avoid use during pregnancy; lactating women should interrupt breast-feeding while receiving the drug.
- Regular monitoring of renal function IMPERATIVE; dose modifications must be made if renal insufficiency exists.
- Use measures for safe handling of cytotoxic drugs (see Appendix 1).

Potential Toxicities/Side Effects and the Nursing Process

I. ALTERATION IN URINARY ELIMINATION related to RENAL TOXICITY

Defining Characteristics: Abnormal renal function occurs commonly; increased serum creatinine, decreased creatinine clearance, acute renal failure may occur.

Nursing Implications: Assess baseline elimination pattern and renal function studies, and monitor closely throughout treatment. Manufacturer suggests creatinine clearance be calculated 2–3 × per week (induction) and q1–2 weeks (maintenance). Creatinine clearance can be calculated from modified Cockcroft and Gault equation:

For males: $$\frac{140 - \text{age}}{\text{serum creatinine} \times 72}$$

For females: $$\frac{140 - \text{age}}{\text{serum creatinine} \times 72} \times 0.085$$

Discuss dose modifications with physician if renal dysfunction occurs. Ensure adequate hydration and urinary output prior to and following dose; administer drug slowly over 1–2 hours, at no more than 1 mg/kg/min. Teach patient to increase oral fluids as tolerated to clear drug from kidneys.

II. ALTERATION IN ELECTROLYTE BALANCE related to METABOLIC ABNORMALITIES

Defining Characteristics: Hypocalcemia, hypophosphatemia, hyperphosphatemia, hypomagnesemia, and hypokalemia occur. Transient decreased ionized calcium may not appear in serum total calcium value. Tetany and seizures may occur, especially in patients receiving foscarnet and IV pentamidine. Increased risk exists if renal impairment or neurologic impairment.

Nursing Implications: Assess baseline calcium, phosphorus, magnesium, potassium, and concurrent drugs that might affect these values. Assess patient for signs/symptoms of hypocalcemia, such as perioral tingling, numbness, or paresthesias during or after infusion. Instruct patient to report these signs/symptoms immediately. If signs/symptoms occur, stop infusion, notify physician, and evaluate serum electrolyte, renal studies. Administer ordered electrolyte repletion.

III. ALTERATIONS IN SENSORY/PERCEPTUAL PATTERNS related to NEUROLOGIC CHANGES

Defining Characteristics: Headache, paresthesia, dizziness, involuntary muscle contractions, hypoesthesia, neuropathy, and seizures (including grand mal) have occurred. Increased risk exists of hypocalcemia (ionized Ca^{++}) and renal insufficiency.

Nursing Implications: Assess baseline risk factors and neurologic status, and monitor during treatment. Assess for and instruct patient to report signs/symptoms. Discuss abnormalities with physician, and possible drug discontinuance.

IV. FATIGUE related to ANEMIA

Defining Characteristics: Anemia occurs in 33% of patients, and in 60% of patients receiving concomitant zidovudine.

Nursing Implications: Assess baseline HCT/Hgb, activity tolerance, cardiopulmonary status, and monitor during therapy. Instruct patient to report increasing fatigue, headache, irritability, shortness of breath, chest pain. Transfuse RBCs as ordered by physician. Discuss with clinic patient self-care ability; refer for home health assistance as needed.

V. ALTERATION IN NUTRITION, LESS THAN BODY REQUIREMENTS, related to GI SIDE EFFECTS

Defining Characteristics: Nausea, vomiting, diarrhea are common; anorexia, abdominal pain may also occur.

Nursing Implications: Assess baseline nutrition, liver function and monitor during therapy. Instruct patient to report GI side effects. Administer or teach patient to self-administer prescribed antiemetic or antidiarrheal medications. Encourage adequate oral or IV hydration. Notify physician of abnormal LFTs. If anorexia occurs, encourage favorite foods and small, frequent meals as tolerated.

VI. INFECTION related to NEUTROPENIA

Defining Characteristics: May occur in 17% of patients; increased risk when receiving concurrent zidovudine.

Nursing Implications: Assess baseline WBC, ANC, and temperature; monitor during therapy. Assess for signs/symptoms of infection and discuss these with physician. Instruct patient to report signs/symptoms of infection.

VII. ALTERATIONS IN COMFORT related to LOCAL VEIN IRRITATION (IV ADMINISTRATION)

Defining Characteristics: Erythema, irritation, pain, swelling, phlebitis may occur at injection site. Consider use of central line.

Nursing Implications: Assess IV site for patency, irritation prior to each dose. Change IV site at least q48h. Apply warmth/heat to painful area as needed.

VIII. ALTERATION IN SKIN INTEGRITY related to RASH

Defining Characteristics: Rash, sweating may occur. Also, rarely, local irritation and ulcerations of penile epithelium in males, and vulvovaginal mucosa in females has occurred—perhaps related to drug in urine.

Nursing Implications: Assess skin integrity baseline and during treatment. Instruct patient to report any irritation or lesions. Teach patient to perform frequent perineal hygiene.

Drug: ganciclovir (Cytovene)

Class: Antiviral (systemic).

Mechanism of Action: Interferes with DNA synthesis so that viral replication cannot occur. Active against HSV-1, HSV-2, VZV (shingles), EBV, and CMV.

Metabolism: Poorly absorbed from GI tract. Appears to be widely distributed, concentrates in kidneys, and is well distributed to the eyes. Crosses BBB. Drug crosses placenta and is excreted in breast milk in animals. Excreted unchanged in urine. Active against CMV infections, especially in the retina.

Dosage/Range:

Adult:

- IV induction: 5 mg/kg IV q12h × 14–21 days.
- Maintenance: 5 mg/kg IV 7 days/week or 6 mg/kg/day × 5 days/week.
- Intravitreous by ophthalmologist (investigational).
- DOSE MUST BE REDUCED IN RENAL IMPAIRMENT.

Drug Preparation/Administration:

- Drug is CARCINOGENIC and TERATOGENIC: use chemotherapy handling precautions (see Appendix 1) when preparing and administering ganciclovir.
- Administer only if ANC is > 500 cells/mm^3 and platelet count > 25,000/mm^3.
- Add 10 mL of sterile water for injection to 500-mg vial. Further dilute dose in 50–250 mL of IV fluid and infuse over at least 1 hour.

Drug Interactions:

- Zidovudine: increased hematologic toxicity (neutropenia, anemia); do not use together if possible. Consider didanosine (ddI) instead of zidovudine (AZT) or concomitant use of neutrophil growth factor (e.g., G-CSF or GM-CSF).
- Foscarnet: additive or synergistic antiviral activity.
- Probenecid: may increase ganciclovir serum levels. Monitor closely and decrease ganciclovir dose as needed.
- Immunosuppressant (corticosteroids, cyclosporine, azathioprine): increased bone marrow suppression; dose reduce or hold immunosuppressants during ganciclovir treatment.
- Interferon: potent synergism against herpes virus, VZV.
- Imipenem/cilastatin: increase neurotoxicity with seizures. AVOID CONCURRENT USE.
- Cytotoxic antineoplastic agents: additive toxicity in bone marrow, gonads, GI epithelium/mucosa.

- Other cytotoxic drugs (dapsone, pentamidine, flucytosine, amphotericin B, trimethoprim-sulfamethoxazole): increase toxicity. Use cautiously if unable to avoid concurrent use.

Lab Effects/Interference:
- Serum ALT, serum alk phos, serum AST, and serum bili values may be increased.
- BUN and serum creatinine values may be increased.

Special Considerations:
- Do not use in pregnancy.
- Patient should be well hydrated; use with caution at reduced doses if renal insufficiency exists.
- Drug is mutagenic; patient should use barrier contraceptive.
- For CMV retinitis patient, should see ophthalmologist at least every 6 weeks during ganciclovir therapy.
- Administer over at least 1 hour.
- Monitor blood counts frequently (3 × per week).

Potential Toxicities/Side Effects and the Nursing Process

I. INFECTION, BLEEDING related to BONE MARROW DEPRESSION

Defining Characteristics: Neutropenia (< 1000/mm^3) occurs in 25–50% of patients, especially in patients with AIDS or those undergoing bone marrow transplant. Thrombocytopenia (< 50,000/mm^3) occurs in 20% of patients. Anemia occurs in 1% of patients.

Nursing Implications: Assess baseline WBC, ANC, and platelet count; monitor throughout therapy (every other day initially, then 3 × per week). Hold ganciclovir if ANC < 500/mm^3, platelet count < 25,000/mm^3. Assess for signs/symptoms of infection or bleeding; instruct patient in signs/symptoms of infection and bleeding, and instruct to report these immediately. Teach patient self-care measures to minimize risk of infection, bleeding, including avoidance of OTC aspirin-containing medicines. Administer or teach patient to self-administer prescribed G-CSF or GM-CSF. Assess Hgb/HCT and signs/symptoms of fatigue. Instruct patient to alternate rest and activity periods.

II. ALTERATIONS IN SENSORY/PERCEPTUAL PATTERNS related to SENSORY CHANGES

Defining Characteristics: Retinal detachment may occur in 30% of patients treated for CMV retinitis. Local reactions (foreign body sensation, conjunctival or vitreal hemorrhage) may occur with intravitreal injection. CNS effects include headache, confusion, altered dreams, ataxia, dizziness, and affect 5–17% of patients.

Nursing Implications: Assess baseline neurologic status, including vision, and monitor during treatment. Patient should see ophthalmologist at least every six weeks. Instruct patient to report any abnormalities and discuss them with physician.

III. ALTERATION IN NUTRITION, LESS THAN BODY REQUIREMENTS, related to GI SIDE EFFECTS

Defining Characteristics: Nausea, vomiting, diarrhea, anorexia may occur in 2% of patients. Elevated LFTs may occur due to drug, but may be difficult to distinguish from CMV infection of liver or biliary tree.

Nursing Implications: Assess baseline nutrition, liver function, and monitor during therapy. Instruct patient to report GI side effects. Administer or teach patient to self-administer prescribed antiemetic or antidiarrheal medications. Encourage adequate oral or IV hydration. Notify physician of abnormal LFTs. If anorexia occurs, encourage favorite foods and small, frequent meals as tolerated.

IV. ALTERATION IN URINARY ELIMINATION related to RENAL TOXICITY

Defining Characteristics: 2% of patients have increased serum BUN, creatinine, hematuria. Increased risk exists in elderly or patients with renal insufficiency.

Nursing Implications: Ensure adequate hydration with urinary output prior to drug administration and infuse drug over at least 1 hour. Dose should be reduced in patients with decreased renal function.

V. ALTERATIONS IN COMFORT related to LOCAL VEIN IRRITATION (IV ADMINISTRATION)

Defining Characteristics: Inflammation, phlebitis, pain occur often at IV infusion site due to high pH of drug.

Nursing Implications: Assess IV site for patency, irritation, prior to each dose. Change IV site at least q48h. Apply warmth/heat to painful area as needed. Assess need for tunneled central line. Avoid drug extravasation.

VI. ALTERATION IN CARDIAC OUTPUT related to CHANGES IN BP

Defining Characteristics: Rarely, hypotension, or hypertension, arrhythmia, myocardial infarction, arrest occur.

Nursing Implications: Assess baseline VS and monitor throughout treatment. Notify physician of any changes from baseline.

VII. ALTERATION IN SEXUALITY/REPRODUCTIVE PATTERNS related to REPRODUCTIVE HAZARD

Defining Characteristics: Drug is carcinogenic, mutagenic, and teratogenic; may produce infertility in males. It is unknown whether drug crosses placenta and is excreted in breast milk.

Nursing Implications: Assess sexuality/reproductive patterns. Teach patient and partner about reproductive hazards; offer contraceptive counseling or refer for counseling, as barrier contraceptive should be used by patient.

Drug: valacyclovir hydrochloride (Valtrex)

Class: Antiviral (systemic).

Mechanism of Action: Drug is well absorbed and rapidly converted to acyclovir. Drug interferes with DNA synthesis so that viral replication cannot occur. Active against HSV-1, HSV-2, VZV (shingles), EBV, and CMV.

Metabolism: Widely distributed in body tissues and fluids including the CNS.

Dosage/Range:
- Herpes zoster: 1 g tid × 7 days.

Drug Preparation/Administration:
- Available in 500-mg caplets.
- Oral, without regard to meals.

Drug Interactions:
- Cimetidine and probenecid decrease renal clearance of valacyclovir.

Lab Effects/Interference:
- None known.

Special Considerations:
- Dose-reduce for renal impairment:

Creatinine Clearance (cc/min)	Dose
≥ 50	1 g q8h
30–49	1 g q12h
10–29	1 g q24h
< 10	500 mg q24h

- Treatment should be started within 48 hours of rash onset.
- AVOID DRUG IN IMMUNOCOMPROMISED PATIENTS, as patients with advanced HIV infection, and those undergoing bone marrow and renal transplants, have developed thrombotic thrombocytopenic purpura/hemolytic uremic syndrome (TTP/HUS).

Potential Toxicities/Side Effects and the Nursing Process

I. ALTERATION IN COMFORT related to HEADACHE, NAUSEA

Defining Characteristics: Headache occurred in approximately 22% of patients. Nausea occurred in 12% of patients.

Nursing Implications: Teach patient that side effects may occur and are usually mild. Patient 1/4 should report headache that does not resolve with acetaminophen or nausea that does not resolve by diet modification.

Chapter 12
Constipation

Constipation is a decreased frequency of defecation that is difficult or uncomfortable (Walsh 1989). Levy (1992) reports five causes of constipation in cancer patients. They include:

1. Disease itself: i.e., primary bowel cancers, paraneoplastic autonomic neuropathy.
2. Disease sequelae: i.e., dehydration, paralysis, immobility, alterations in bowel elimination patterns.
3. Prior history of laxative abuse, hemorrhoids/anal fissures, other diseases.
4. Cancer therapy: chemotherapy (vinca alkaloids, e.g., vincristine, vinblastine); bowel surgery.
5. Medications used to manage symptoms: opioids, antihistamines, tricyclic antidepressants, aluminum antacids.

Complications of constipation can be severe (i.e., bowel perforation), extremely painful, and compromise quality of life. Nurses play an enormous role in preventing morbidity from constipation in patients with cancer. Assessment of the patient's previous and current nutrition and elimination patterns, along with assessment of probable etiology of constipation, are critical, as is patient/ family teaching about constipation management and prevention. Teaching should include dietary modifications to include high-fiber intake (fruits, vegetables, or nutritional supplements high in fiber); fluid intake of 3 L/day; and moderate exercise as tolerated. Patients receiving drugs (i.e., opioids) that are likely to be constipating should also receive a bowel regimen to prevent constipation. Available laxatives include the following types:

- *Bulk-forming* laxatives cause the stool to retain water, and thus increase peristalsis (fiber, bran, psyllium, methylcellulose).
- *Lubricants* coat and soften the stool so it can move more smoothly through the intestines (mineral oil).
- *Saline laxatives* pull water into the gut and into the stool, increasing peristalsis (magnesium citrate, sodium biphosphate, magnesium hydroxide).
- *Osmotic laxatives* work through colonic bacteria that metabolize osmotic laxatives causing increased osmotic pressure gradient, pulling water into the

gut and then into the stool, thus increasing peristalsis (glycerin, lactulose, sorbitol).

- *Detergent laxatives* reduce surface tension of the colonic cells, so water and fats enter the stool; in addition, electrolyte and water absorption is decreased (docusate salts).
- *Stimulant laxatives* irritate the gut, increasing gut motility (senna, bisacodyl).

References

Levy MH. Constipation and Diarrhea in Cancer Patients, Part I. *Prim Care Cancer* 1992;12(4):11–18

Massey RL, Haylock PJ, Curtiss C. *Constipation,* Chapter 27. Yarbro CH, Frogge MH, Goodman M, (eds), *Cancer Symptom Management,* 3rd ed. Sudbury, MA: Jones and Bartlett, 2003

Twycross RG, Harcourt JMV. The Use of Laxatives at a Palliative Care Centre. *Pallia Med* 1991;5:27–33

Walsh TD. Constipation. Walsh TD, (eds), *Symptom Control.* Cambridge: Blackwell Scientific Publications Inc.,1989;331–381

Drug: bisacodyl (Dulcolax)

Class: Stimulant laxative.

Mechanism of Action: Stimulates/irritates smooth muscle of intestines, increasing peristalsis; increases fluid accumulation in colon and small intestines. Indicated for relief of constipation and bowel preparation prior to bowel surgery.

Metabolism: Minimal oral absorption. Evacuation occurs in 6–10 hours when taken orally, or within 15 minutes to 1 hour when administered rectally.

Dosage/Range:

Adult:

- Oral: 5–15 mg at bedtime or early morning. Bowel preparation may use up to 30 mg.
- Suppository: 10 mg PR.

Drug Preparation/Administration:

- Administer oral tablet > 1 hour after antacids or milk.
- Insert suppository as high as possible against wall of rectum.

Drug Interactions:

- None.

Lab Effects/Interference:

- None known.

Special Considerations:

- Contraindicated in patients with signs/symptoms of acute abdomen (nausea, vomiting, abdominal pain), intestinal obstruction, fecal impaction, or ulcerative bowel lesions.

Potential Toxicities/Side Effects and the Nursing Process

I. ALTERATIONS IN BOWEL ELIMINATION related to CHRONIC USE

Defining Characteristics: Removes defecation reflexes when used chronically (laxative dependence). Narcotic analgesics and vinca alkaloid chemotherapy may predispose to constipation.

Nursing Implications: Assess baseline elimination pattern. Teach patient how to self-administer laxative. Encourage patient to normalize bowel habits through adequate fluid intake (2–3 L/day), diet high in fiber and bulk (bran, cereals, fruits, and vegetables), and exercise as tolerated. Teach patient bowel regimen when on narcotics or vinca alkaloids to promote regular evacuation.

II. ALTERATION IN NUTRITION, LESS THAN BODY REQUIREMENTS, related to GI SIDE EFFECTS

Defining Characteristics: Constipation or drug may cause nausea, vomiting, abdominal pain; rectal suppository may cause burning in rectum as it is absorbed.

Nursing Implications: Assess comfort level and GI distress related to constipation. Encourage patient to drink cold fluids or ginger ale as tolerated. Encourage patient to try resting in different positions; warm packs may decrease abdominal pain. Teach patient to expect burning sensation with suppository use; reassure that it will resolve in 5–10 minutes.

III. ALTERATION IN FLUID AND ELECTROLYTE BALANCE related to LAXATIVE ABUSE

Defining Characteristics: Diarrhea resulting from laxative abuse can deplete fluid volume, nutrients, and electrolytes.

Nursing Implications: Teach patient regular bowel regimen when receiving constipating drugs (narcotics, vinca alkaloids). Teach patient to replace lost fluids and electrolytes (encourage chicken soup, sports drink).

Drug: docusate calcium, docusate potassium, docusate sodium (Dioctyl Calcium Sulfosuccinate, Dioctyl Potassium Sulfosuccinate, Dioctyl Sodium Sulfosuccinate, Colace, Diocto-K, Diosuccin, DOK-250, Doxinate, Duosol, Laxinate 100, Regulax SS, Stulex)

Class: Stool softener.

Mechanism of Action: The calcium, sodium, and potassium salts of docusate soften stool by decreasing surface tension, emulsification, and wetting action, thus increasing stool absorption of water in the bowel.

Metabolism: Appears to be absorbed somewhat in the duodenum and jejunum, and excreted in bile. Stool softening occurs in 1–3 days.

Dosage/Range:

Adult:

- Oral: 50–360 mg/day, in single or divided doses, depending on stool-softening response.

Drug Preparation/Administration:

- Oral: store gelatin capsule in tight container; store syrup in light-resistant containers.
- Rectal: according to manufacturer's package insert.

Drug Interactions:

- Mineral oil: increased mineral oil absorption; AVOID CONCURRENT USE.

Lab Effects/Interference:

- None known.

Special Considerations:

- Useful in prevention of straining-at-stool in patients receiving narcotics; when combined with other agents/laxatives, prevents constipation in these patients.
- Does not increase intestinal peristalsis; stop drug if severe abdominal cramping occurs.
- Is effective only in prevention of constipation, not in treating constipation.

Potential Toxicities/Side Effects and the Nursing Process

I. KNOWLEDGE DEFICIT related to BOWEL ELIMINATION

Defining Characteristics: Oncology patients who are receiving narcotic analgesics, vinca alkaloid chemotherapy (vincristine, vinblastine, vindesine), or who are dehydrated or hypercalcemic are at increased risk of constipation.

Nursing Implications: Assess baseline elimination pattern. Teach patient need for bowel movement at least every other day, depending on usual pattern.

Teach patient importance of adequate fluid intake (2–3 L/day), diet high in fiber and bulk (bran, cereals, fruits, vegetables, and supplements with fiber), and exercise as tolerated. Teach self-administration of stool softeners and prescribed laxatives.

Drug: glycerin suppository (Fleet Babylax, Sani-Supp)

Class: Hyperosmotic laxative.

Mechanism of Action: Local irritant, with hyperosmotic action, drawing water from tissues into feces and stimulating fecal evacuation within 15–30 minutes.

Metabolism: Poorly absorbed from rectum.

Dosage/Range:

Adult:

- Rectal suppository: 2–3 g PR.
- Enema: 5–15 mL PR.

Drug Preparation/Administration:

- Rectal administration must be retained for 15 minutes.

Drug Interactions:

- None.

Lab Effects/Interference:

- None known.

Special Considerations:

- Contraindicated in patients with undiagnosed abdominal pain, intestinal obstruction.

Potential Toxicities/Side Effects and the Nursing Process

I. ALTERATIONS IN BOWEL ELIMINATION related to CHRONIC USE

Defining Characteristics: Removes defecation reflexes when used chronically (laxative dependence). Narcotic analgesics and vinca alkaloid chemotherapy may predispose to constipation.

Nursing Implications: Assess baseline elimination pattern. Teach patient how to self-administer laxative. Encourage patient to normalize bowel habits through adequate fluid intake (2–3 L/day), diet high in fiber and bulk (bran, cereals, fruits, and vegetables), and exercise as tolerated. Teach patient bowel regimen when on narcotics or vinca alkaloids to promote regular evacuation.

II. ALTERATION IN FLUID AND ELECTROLYTE BALANCE related to LAXATIVE ABUSE

Defining Characteristics: Diarrhea resulting from laxative abuse can deplete fluid volume, nutrients, and electrolytes.

Nursing Implications: Teach patient regular bowel regimen when receiving constipating drugs (narcotics, vinca alkaloids). Teach patient to replace lost fluids and electrolytes (encourage chicken soup, sports drink).

III. ALTERATION IN COMFORT related to CRAMPING PAIN, RECTAL IRRITATION, OR DISCOMFORT

Defining Characteristics: Cramping pain, rectal irritation, and inflammation or discomfort may occur.

Nursing Implications: Teach patient this may occur. If discomfort is not self-limited, suggest sitz bath, warm or cold packs, and position changes.

Drug: lactulose (Cholac, Constilac, Constulose, Duphalac)

Class: Hyperosmolar sugar.

Mechanism of Action: Delivers osmotically active molecules to intestine, drawing fluid into colon and causing distension; this stimulates peristalsis and evacuation in 24–48 hours. Also used to lower blood ammonia in hepatic encephalopathy.

Metabolism: Less than 3% absorbed; metabolized by bacteria in colon into lactic acid.

Dosage/Range:

Adult:

- Oral: 10–20 g (15–30 mL)/day to 40 g (60 mL)/day.

Drug Preparation/Administration:

- Store solution at 15–30°C (59–86°F).
- Give with juice.

Drug Interactions:

- Antacids: may decrease lactulose effect; avoid administering together.

Special Considerations:

- Diarrhea indicates overdosage; dose should be reduced.

Potential Toxicities/Side Effects and the Nursing Process

I. ALTERATION IN COMFORT related to GI SIDE EFFECTS

Defining Characteristics: Gaseous distension, flatulence, abdominal pain may occur.

Nursing Implications: Encourage patient to find comfortable position; apply warmth to decrease abdominal pain; reassure that symptoms will resolve.

II. ALTERATION IN FLUID AND ELECTROLYTE BALANCE related to DIARRHEA

Defining Characteristics: Diarrhea resulting from laxative abuse can deplete fluid volume, nutrients, and electrolytes.

Nursing Implications: Teach patient regular bowel regimen when receiving constipating drugs (narcotics, vinca alkaloids). Teach patient to replace lost fluids and electrolytes (encourage chicken soup, sports drink).

Drug: magnesium citrate

Class: Saline laxative.

Mechanism of Action: Draws water into small intestinal lumen, stimulating peristalsis and evacuation in 3–6 hours.

Metabolism: 15–30% absorbed, excreted in urine.

Dosage/Range:

Adult:

- Oral: 11–25 g (5–10 oz or 150–300 mL)/day as single or divided dose at bedtime.

Drug Preparation/Administration:

- Refrigerate and serve with ice. Taste can be masked by adding small amount of juice.

Drug Interactions:

- None.

Lab Effects/Interference:

- None known.

Special Considerations:

- Contraindicated in patients with signs/symptoms of acute abdomen (nausea, vomiting, abdominal pain), intestinal obstruction, fecal impaction, or ulcerative bowel lesions.

- Contraindicated in patients with rectal fissures, myocardial infarction, renal disease.

Potential Toxicities/Side Effects and the Nursing Process

I. ALTERATIONS IN BOWEL ELIMINATION related to CHRONIC USE

Defining Characteristics: Removes defecation reflexes when used chronically (laxative dependence). Narcotic analgesics and vinca alkaloid chemotherapy may predispose to constipation.

Nursing Implications: Assess baseline elimination pattern. Teach patient how to self-administer laxative. Encourage patient to normalize bowel habits through adequate fluid intake (2–3 L/day), diet high in fiber and bulk (bran, cereals, fruits, and vegetables), and exercise as tolerated. Teach patient bowel regimen when on narcotics or vinca alkaloids to promote regular evacuation.

II. ALTERATION IN NUTRITION, LESS THAN BODY REQUIREMENTS, related to GI SIDE EFFECTS

Defining Characteristics: Constipation or drug may cause nausea and abdominal pain.

Nursing Implications: Assess comfort level and GI distress related to constipation. Encourage patient to drink cold fluids or ginger ale as tolerated. Encourage patient to try resting in different positions; warm packs may decrease abdominal pain.

III. ALTERATION IN FLUID AND ELECTROLYTE BALANCE related to LAXATIVE ABUSE

Defining Characteristics: Diarrhea resulting from laxative abuse can deplete fluid volume, nutrients, and electrolytes.

Nursing Implications: Teach patient regular bowel regimen when receiving constipating drugs (narcotics, vinca alkaloids). Teach patient to replace lost fluids and electrolytes (encourage chicken soup, sports drink).

Drug: methylcellulose (Citrucel)

Class: Bulk-producing laxative.

Mechanism of Action: Absorbs water; bulk expansion stimulates peristalsis and evacuation in 12–24 hours. May also be used to slow diarrhea.

Metabolism: Not absorbed by GI tract.

Dosage/Range:

Adult:

- Oral: up to 6 g/day PO in 2–3 divided doses.

Drug Preparation/Administration:

- Administer each dose with at least 250 mL of water or juice.

Drug Interactions:

- None.

Lab Effects/Interference:

- None known.

Special Considerations:

- Safest and most physiologically normal laxative.

Potential Toxicities/Side Effects and the Nursing Process

I. ALTERATIONS IN BOWEL ELIMINATION related to CHRONIC USE

Defining Characteristics: Removes defecation reflexes when used chronically (laxative dependence). Narcotic analgesics and vinca alkaloid chemotherapy may predispose to constipation.

Nursing Implications: Assess baseline elimination pattern. Teach patient how to self-administer laxative. Encourage patient to normalize bowel habits through adequate fluid intake (2–3 L/day), diet high in fiber and bulk (bran, cereals, fruits, and vegetables), and exercise as tolerated. Teach patient bowel regimen when on narcotics or vinca alkaloids to promote regular evacuation.

II. ALTERATION IN NUTRITION, LESS THAN BODY REQUIREMENTS, related to GI SIDE EFFECTS

Defining Characteristics: Constipation or drug may cause nausea, vomiting, cramps.

Nursing Implications: Assess comfort level and GI distress related to constipation. Encourage patient to drink cold fluids or ginger ale as tolerated. Encourage patient to try resting in different positions; warm packs may decrease abdominal pain. Teach patient laxative effect may take 12–24 hours, and assess need for other cathartic(s).

Drug: mineral oil (Fleet Mineral Oil)

Class: Lubricant laxative.

Mechanism of Action: Lubricates intestine, preventing fecal fluid from being absorbed in colon; water retention distends colon, stimulating peristalsis and evacuation in 6–8 hours.

Metabolism: Minimal GI absorption occurs following oral or rectal administration.

Dosage/Range:

Adult:

- Oral: 15–45 mL PO in single or divided doses.
- Rectal enemas: 120 mL PR as a single dose.

Drug Preparation/Administration:

- Administer plain mineral oil at bedtime on an empty stomach.
- Administer mineral oil emulsion with food if desired at bedtime.
- May mix with juice to mask taste.

Drug Interactions:

- Docusate salts: increase mineral oil absorption; DO NOT ADMINISTER concurrently.
- Fat-soluble vitamins: decrease absorption with chronic mineral oil administration.

Lab Effects/Interference:

- Decreased fat-soluble vitamins, e.g., vitamins A, D, E, K with chronic drug administration.

Special Considerations:

- Contraindicated in patients with signs/symptoms of acute abdomen (nausea, vomiting, abdominal pain), intestinal obstruction, fecal impaction, or ulcerative bowel lesions.
- Do not use for more than 1 week.

Potential Toxicities/Side Effects and the Nursing Process

I. ALTERATIONS IN BOWEL ELIMINATION related to CHRONIC USE

Defining Characteristics: Removes defecation reflexes when used chronically (laxative dependence). Narcotic analgesics and vinca alkaloid chemotherapy may predispose to constipation.

Nursing Implications: Assess baseline elimination pattern. Teach patient how to self-administer laxative. Encourage patient to normalize bowel habits through adequate fluid intake (2–3 L/day), diet high in fiber and bulk (bran, cereals, fruits, and vegetables), and exercise as tolerated. Teach patient bowel regimen when on narcotics or vinca alkaloids to promote regular evacuation.

II. ALTERATION IN NUTRITION, LESS THAN BODY REQUIREMENTS, related to GI SIDE EFFECTS

Defining Characteristics: Constipation or drug may cause nausea, vomiting, cramps.

Nursing Implications: Assess comfort level and GI distress related to constipation. Encourage patient to drink cold fluids or ginger ale as tolerated. Encourage patient to try resting in different positions; warm packs may decrease abdominal pain. Teach patient to expect burning sensation with suppository use; reassure that it will resolve in 5–10 minutes.

Drug: polyethylene glycol 3350, NF powder (Miralax®)

Class: Osmotic cathartic.

Mechanism of Action: Drug is an osmotic agent that pulls water into the intestines with the stool, softening the stool and causing peristalsis and evacuation in 2–4 days.

Metabolism: Is not fermented by colonic microflora and does not affect intestinal absorption or secretion of glucose or electrolytes.

Dosage/Range:
- 17 g (1 heaping T) (product comes with a measuring cup).

Drug Preparation:
- Mix in 8 oz of water and take orally once a day.

Drug Administration:
- Oral. Available in 14-oz and 26-oz containers.
- Store at room temperature.

Drug Interactions:
- None.

Lab Effects/Interference:
- None.

Special Considerations:
- Contraindicated in patients with bowel obstruction.
- Indicated for the treatment of occasional constipation for up to 2 weeks.
- Use during pregnancy only if clearly needed.
- Excessive or frequent use or use > 2 weeks may result in electrolyte imbalance and dependence on laxatives.

Potential Toxicities/Side Effects and the Nursing Process

I. ALTERATIONS IN BOWEL ELIMINATION related to CHRONIC USE

Defining Characteristics: Removes defecation reflexes when used chronically (laxative dependence). Narcotic analgesics and vinca alkaloid chemotherapy may predispose to constipation.

Nursing Implications: Assess baseline elimination pattern. Teach patient how to self-administer laxative. Encourage patient to normalize bowel habits through adequate fluid intake (2–3 L/day), diet high in fiber and bulk (bran, cereals, fruits, and vegetables), and exercise as tolerated. Teach patient bowel regimen when on narcotics or vinca alkaloids to promote regular evacuation.

II. ALTERATION IN NUTRITION related to GI SIDE EFFECTS

Defining Characteristics: Constipation or drug may cause nausea, cramps, abdominal bloating, flatulence. High doses may cause diarrhea, especially in the elderly. Continued use beyond 2 weeks may cause electrolyte imbalance.

Nursing Implications: Assess comfort level and GI distress related to constipation. Encourage patient to drink cold fluids or ginger ale as tolerated. Encourage patient to try resting in different positions; warm packs may decrease abdominal pain. Teach patient laxative effect may take 2–4 days and assess need for other cathartic(s).

Drug: senna (Senexon, Senokot)

Class: Irritant/stimulant laxative.

Mechanism of Action: Stimulates/irritates smooth muscle of intestines, increasing peristalsis; increases fluid accumulation in colon and small intestines. Indicated for relief of constipation or bowel preparation prior to bowel surgery.

Metabolism: Minimal oral absorption occurs. Evacuation occurs in 6–10 hours when taken orally.

Dosage/Range:
- Senexon: 2 tablets at bedtime (187 mg senna).
- Senokot: 2–4 tablets bid (187 mg senna); 1–2 tsp granules bid (326 mg senna); 1 suppository at bedtime, repeat PRN in 2 hours (652 mg senna).
- Black-Draught: 2 tablets (600 mg senna) or 1/4–1/2 level tsp granules (1.65 gm senna).

Drug Preparation/Administration:
- Store in a tightly closed bottle.

Drug Interactions:

- None.

Lab Effects/Interference:

- None known.

Special Considerations:

- Contraindicated in patients with signs/symptoms of acute abdomen (nausea, vomiting, abdominal pain), intestinal obstruction, fecal impaction, or ulcerative bowel lesions.
- Senna is very effective as part of bowel regimen for patients receiving narcotic analgesic medication.

Potential Toxicities/Side Effects and the Nursing Process

I. ALTERATIONS IN BOWEL ELIMINATION related to CHRONIC USE

Defining Characteristics: Removes defecation reflexes when used chronically (laxative dependence). Narcotic analgesics and vinca alkaloid chemotherapy may predispose to constipation.

Nursing Implications: Assess baseline elimination pattern. Teach patient how to self-administer laxative. Encourage patient to normalize bowel habits through adequate fluid intake (2–3 L/day), diet high in fiber and bulk (bran, cereals, fruits, and vegetables), and exercise as tolerated. Teach patient bowel regimen when on narcotics or vinca alkaloids to promote regular evacuation.

II. ALTERATION IN NUTRITION, LESS THAN BODY REQUIREMENTS, related to GI SIDE EFFECTS

Defining Characteristics: Constipation or drug may cause nausea, vomiting, abdominal pain; rectal suppository may cause burning in rectum as it is absorbed.

Nursing Implications: Assess comfort level and GI distress related to constipation. Encourage patient to drink cold fluids or ginger ale as tolerated. Encourage patient to try resting in different positions; warm packs may decrease abdominal pain. Teach patient to expect burning sensation with suppository use; reassure that it will resolve in 5–10 minutes.

III. ALTERATION IN FLUID AND ELECTROLYTE BALANCE related to LAXATIVE ABUSE

Defining Characteristics: Diarrhea resulting from laxative abuse can deplete fluid volume, nutrients, and electrolytes.

Nursing Implications: Teach patient regular bowel regimen when receiving constipating drugs (narcotics, vinca alkaloids). Teach patient to replace lost fluids and electrolytes (encourage chicken soup, sports drink).

Drug: sorbitol

Class: Hyperosmotic laxative.

Mechanism of Action: Local irritant, with hyperosmotic action, drawing water from tissues into feces and stimulating fecal evacuation within 15–30 minutes.

Metabolism: Poorly absorbed from GI tract.

Dosage/Range:

Adult:

- Oral: 15 mL of 70% solution repeated until diarrhea starts.
- Rectal: 120 mL if a 25–30% solution is used.

Drug Preparation/Administration:

- Keep stored in tightly closed bottle.

Drug Interactions:

- None.

Lab Effects/Interference:

- None known.

Special Considerations:

- Contraindicated in patients with undiagnosed abdominal pain, intestinal obstruction.
- Oral 70% sorbitol may be as effective as lactulose in relieving constipation.

Potential Toxicities/Side Effects and the Nursing Process

I. ALTERATIONS IN BOWEL ELIMINATION related to CHRONIC USE

Defining Characteristics: Removes defecation reflexes when used chronically (laxative dependence). Narcotic analgesics and vinca alkaloid chemotherapy may predispose to constipation.

Nursing Implications: Assess baseline elimination pattern. Teach patient how to self-administer laxative. Encourage patient to normalize bowel habits through adequate fluid intake (2–3 L/day), diet high in fiber and bulk (bran, cereals, fruits, and vegetables), and exercise as tolerated. Teach patient bowel regimen when on narcotics or vinca alkaloids to promote regular evacuation.

II. ALTERATION IN FLUID AND ELECTROLYTE BALANCE related to LAXATIVE ABUSE

Defining Characteristics: Diarrhea resulting from laxative abuse can deplete fluid volume, nutrients, and electrolytes.

Nursing Implications: Teach patient regular bowel regimen when receiving constipating drugs (narcotics, vinca alkaloids). Teach patient to replace lost fluids and electrolytes (encourage chicken soup, sports drink).

III. ALTERATION IN COMFORT related to CRAMPING PAIN, RECTAL IRRITATION OR DISCOMFORT

Defining Characteristics: Cramping pain, rectal irritation, and inflammation or discomfort may occur.

Nursing Implications: Teach patient this may occur. If discomfort is not self-limited, suggest sitz bath, warm or cold packs, and position changes.

Chapter 13
Diarrhea

Rutledge and Engleking (1998) define diarrhea as an abnormal increase in liquidity and frequency, and occurring as acute (within 24–48 hours of a stimulus, resolving in 7–14 days) or chronic (late onset, lasting >2–3 weeks). Diarrhea occurring in patients with cancer is most often related to osmotic, malabsorptive, secretory, exudative, dysmotility-associated, or chemotherapy-induced (Levy, 1992; Engleking, 2003). Engleking (2003) gives examples of each.

- *Osmotic diarrhea* occurs as a result of hyperosmolar or non-absorbable substances, which draw large volumes of fluid into the intestines, producing watery stools that usually resolve with removal of the cause. Causative factors include high osmolality tube feedings, lactulose or sorbital, and gastrointestinal hemorrhage.
- *Malabsorptive diarrhea* results from changes in mucosal integrity causing changes in membrane permeability, or loss of absorptive surfaces, resulting in diarrhea that is large volume, frothy, and foul-smelling (steatorrhea). Causes include deficiency of an enzyme responsible for digestion of fats (lactose intolerance, pancreatic insufficiency) or surgical resection or removal of the intestines.
- *Secretory diarrhea* results from intestinal hypersecretion of large volumes (> 1 L/da) of watery stool with an osmolality equal to that in the plasma. Causes are endocrine tumors (VIPoma and carcinoid), enterotoxin-producing pathogens like c. difficile, acute graft-versus-host disease, and short gut syndrome.
- *Exudative diarrhea* is caused by inflammation or ulceration of the bowel mucosa, resulting in stools containing mucous, blood, and serum protein; the patient experiences frequent stooling, although the total volume is usually < 1 L/da. Unfortunately, this type of diarrhea is associated with hypoalbuminemia and anemia. Causes are radiation to the bowel (radiation enteritis) or opportunistic infection in the denuded bowel, such as with neutropenic typhlitis.
- *Dysmotility-associated diarrhea* is related to factors which increase or decrease normal peristalsis, such as with irritable bowel syndrome, the inges-

tion of food or medication that affects peristalsis, or psychological factors such as anxiety or fear that cause parasympathetic stimulation. Diarrhea of this type is usually semi-solid to liquid, small, and frequent.

- *Chemotherapy-induced diarrhea* occurs as a result of chemotherapy-induced cell death of the intestinal mucosa causing over-stimulation of intestinal water and electrolyte secretion. The patient experiences frequent watery to semi-solid stools within 24–96 hours of chemotherapy administration. With irinotecan chemotherapy, acute diarrhea occurs initially during or soon after administration related to cholinergic stimulation, and then delayed diarrhea occurs about 9–12 days later. In combination with 5-fluorouracil, the delayed diarrhea can lead to dehydration, and together with neutropenia, sepsis. Nurses play a very important role in teaching patients about the potential life-threatening diarrhea that may occur from this chemotherapy, self-adminsitration of anti-diarrheal medicines, increased fluid and diet modifications, and triage if these efforts are not effective.

Nurses are key in the management of diarrhea. Nurses play a significant role in patient assessment and patient/family teaching. Assessment of the patient's previous and current nutrition and elimination patterns, as well as assessment of probable etiology of diarrhea, are critical, as is patient/family teaching about the management and prevention of diarrhea.

Patient teaching includes (Wadler et al, 1998):

1. Diet modification: recommend low-residue foods high in protein and calories; high fluid intake of 3 L/day; avoidance of milk and milk products, foods high in potassium.
2. Care of irritated skin, mucosa in perirectal area; critical in neutropenic or immunocompromised patients.
3. Self-administration of prescribed antidiarrheal medication(s).
4. Need for blood tests to assess electrolyte imbalance and hydration if diarrhea is severe. Diarrhea can lead to severe fluid and electrolyte imbalance, as well as significant patient discomfort. Common electrolyte imbalances related to diarrhea include metabolic acidosis, hypokalemia, hyperchloremia, hypocalcemia, and hypomagnesemia.

Ippoliti (1998) describes antidiarrheal agents as:

- *Intraluminal agents*: decrease water in gut by absorption, increasing bulk of the stool, and protecting intestinal mucosa; includes absorbents such as activated charcoal and mucilloid preparations, and adsorbents such as psyllium, kaolin and pectate; less commonly used as more effective agents available without possible drug interactions or difficulty ingesting them.
- *Intestinal transit inhibitors*: Primarily anti-cholinergic (atropine sulfate and scopolamine) and opiate agonists (DTO and the synthetic opioids diphenox-

ylate and loperamide) which slow intestinal peristalsis and increasing fluid absorption.
- *Proabsorptive agents*: Intraluminal absorbent agents as above.
- *Antisecretory agents*: Octreotide (Sandostatin) is a synthetic somatostatin analogue that inhibits the secretion of gut hormones like serotonin and motilin, and thus slows transit time and improves regulation of water and electolyte movement in the gut. Bismuth subsalicylate (Pepto-Bismol) also works to decrease gut mucosal inflammation and hypermotility by binding to toxins and inhibition of prostaglandin synthesis.

References

Engleking C. Diarrhea, Chapter 28. Yarbro CH, Frogge MH, Goodman M, (eds), *Cancer Symptom Management,* 3rd ed. Sudbury, MA: Jones and Bartlett Publishers, 2003

Harris AG. Consensus Statement Recommendations: Octreotide Dose Titration in Secretory Diarrhea. *Dig Dis Sci* 1995;40(7):1464–1473

Ippoliti C. Antidiarrheal Agents for the Management of Treatment-related Diarrhea in Cancer Patients. *Am J Health Syst Pharm* 1998;55(15):1573–80

Levy MH. Constipation and Diarrhea, Part II. *Prim Care Cancer* 1992;12(5):53–58

Rutledge D, Engleking C. Cancer-related Diarrhea: Selected Findings of a National Survey of Oncology nurse experiences. *Oncol Nurs Forum* 1998;25:861–878

Wadler S, Benson AB, Engelking C, et al. Recommended Guidelines for the Treatment of Chemotherapy-Induced Diarrhea. *J Clin Oncol* 1998;16(9):3169–3178

Drug: deodorized tincture of opium (DTO, Laudanum)

Class: Opium antidiarrheal agent.

Mechanism of Action: Increases GI smooth muscle tone and inhibits GI motility, delaying movement of intestinal contents; water is absorbed from fecal contents, decreasing diarrhea.

Metabolism: Variable absorption from GI tract; metabolized by liver and excreted in urine.

Dosage/Range:

Adult:
- Oral: 0.3–1 mL qid (maximum 6 mL/day).

Drug Preparation/Administration:
- Store in tight, light-resistant bottle. Administer with water or juice.

Drug Interactions:
- None.

Lab Effects/Interference:
- None known.

Special Considerations:
- DTO contains 25 times more morphine than paregoric.
- Physical dependence may develop if drug is used chronically (e.g., colitis).
- Controlled substance.
- May be used in combination with kaolin and pectin mixtures.
- Do not use in diarrhea that results from poisoning until poison is removed (e.g., by lavage or cathartics).

Potential Toxicities/Side Effects and the Nursing Process

I. ALTERATION IN NUTRITION, LESS THAN BODY REQUIREMENTS, related to GI SIDE EFFECTS

Defining Characteristics: Nausea, vomiting may occur.

Nursing Implications: Assess baseline nutrition, GI status. If nausea/vomiting appears to follow dose administration, administer DTO with juice to disguise taste.

Drug: diphenoxylate hydrochloride and atropine (Lomotil)

Class: Antidiarrheal agent.

Mechanism of Action: Diphenoxylate is a synthetic opiate agonist that inhibits intestinal smooth muscle activity, thereby slowing peristalsis so that excess water is absorbed from feces. Atropine discourages deliberate overdosage.

Metabolism: Well absorbed from GI tract. Metabolized in liver. Excreted principally via feces in bile. Onset of action 45 minutes to 1 hour; duration 3–4 hours.

Dosage/Range:
Adult:
- Oral: 5 mg PO qid then titrate to response × 2 days (if no response in 48 hours, drug ineffective).

Drug Preparation/Administration:
- Oral: one tablet contains 2.5 mg diphenoxylate HCl and 0.025 mg atropine sulfate.

Drug Interactions:
- CNS depressants (alcohol, barbiturates): potentiate CNS depressant action; use together cautiously.

- MAOIs: may cause hypertensive crisis (similar structure to meperidine); use together cautiously.

Lab Effects/Interference:
- None known.

Special Considerations:
- May be habit-forming when used in high doses (40–60 mg); physical dependence.
- Use with extreme caution in patients with hepatic cirrhosis, as drug may precipitate hepatic coma, and in patients with acute ulcerative colitis.
- Contraindicated in patients with jaundice, diarrhea resulting from poisoning or pseudomembranous colitis caused by antibiotics.

Potential Toxicities/Side Effects and the Nursing Process

I. ALTERATION IN NUTRITION, LESS THAN BODY REQUIREMENTS, related to GI SIDE EFFECTS

Defining Characteristics: Nausea, vomiting, abdominal distension or discomfort, anorexia, mouth dryness, and (rarely) paralytic ileus may occur.

Nursing Implications: Assess baseline nutrition and elimination status. Instruct patient to report signs and symptoms. Discuss drug discontinuance with physician. Instruct patient that drug should be used for two days and physician notified if diarrhea persists.

II. ALTERATIONS IN SENSORY/PERCEPTUAL PATTERNS related to SEDATION

Defining Characteristics: Sedation, dizziness, lethargy, restlessness or insomnia, headache, paresthesia occur rarely with higher doses and prolonged therapy. Blurred vision may occur due to mydriasis.

Nursing Implications: Teach patient that drug is for short-term relief of diarrhea. Assess for and instruct patient to report signs/symptoms. Discuss drug discontinuance with physician if symptoms are severe.

III. ALTERATION IN SKIN INTEGRITY related to RASH, SENSITIVITY

Defining Characteristics: Pruritus, angioedema (swelling of lips, face, gums), giant urticaria may occur.

Nursing Implications: Assess for and instruct patient to report signs/symptoms immediately. Drug should be discontinued if angioedema or giant urticaria occur.

Drug: kaolin/pectin (Kaodene, K-P, Kaopectate, K-Pek)

Class: Antidiarrheal agent.

Mechanism of Action: Drug acts as absorbent and protectant; decreases stool fluidity but not total amount of fluid excreted.

Metabolism: Not absorbed from GI tract and excreted in stool.

Dosage/Range:

Adult:

- Oral: 60–120 mL regular or 45–90 mL concentrated suspension after each loose bowel movement < 48 hours.

Drug Preparation/Administration:

- Shake well prior to administration.

Drug Interactions:

- Oral lincomycin: decreases lincomycin absorption; administer kaolin/pectin at least 2 hours before or 3–4 hours after lincomycin dose.
- Oral digoxin: decreases digoxin absorption; administer kaolin/pectin 2 hours after digoxin dose.

Lab Effects/Interference:

- None known.

Special Considerations:

- Few adverse effects.
- Used for temporary relief of diarrhea.

Potential Toxicities/Side Effects and the Nursing Process

I. KNOWLEDGE DEFICIT related to SELF-ADMINISTRATION

Defining Characteristics: Transient constipation may occur.

Nursing Implications: Assess understanding of medication and self-administration schedule. Instruct patient in self-administration and to notify nurse/physician if diarrhea persists beyond 48 hours or fever develops. Reinforce need to drink fluids, especially in elderly or debilitated patients, to prevent constipation.

Drug: loperamide hydrochloride (Imodium)

Class: Antidiarrheal agent.

Mechanism of Action: Slows intestinal motility by inhibiting peristalsis (direct effect on circular and longitudinal intestinal muscles); increases stool bulk and viscosity.

Metabolism: Well absorbed from GI tract. Metabolized and small amounts are excreted in urine and feces as intact drug.

Dosage/Range:

Adult:

- Oral: 4 mg followed by 2 mg after each unformed stool (maximum 16 mg or higher if under direction of a physician; 8 mg per 24-hour period if self-medicating).

Drug Preparation/Administration:

- Oral.

Drug Interactions:

- None.

Lab Effects/Interference:

- None known.

Special Considerations:

- Reduces electrolyte and fluid loss from intestines; may be used to reduce volume of ileostomy drainage. 2–3 times more potent than diphenoxylate.
- Use cautiously in patients with acute ulcerative colitis; drug should be discontinued if abdominal distension occurs (risk of megacolon).
- Intended for self-medication × 48 hours; patients should be taught to notify nurse/physician if symptoms persist or fever occurs.
- Contraindicated in diarrhea due to pseudomembranous colitis (antibioticrelated), in acute diarrhea caused by mucosal-penetrating organisms (*Shigella, E. coli, Salmonella*), or if hypersensitivity to drug exists.
- Use cautiously in pregnant or nursing women.

Potential Toxicities/Side Effects and the Nursing Process

I. ALTERATION IN NUTRITION, LESS THAN BODY REQUIREMENTS, related to GI SIDE EFFECTS

Defining Characteristics: Less frequent adverse reactions occur than with diphenoxylate/atropine. Nausea, vomiting, abdominal pain, and distension may occur.

Nursing Implications: Assess baseline nutrition and elimination status. Instruct patient to report signs and symptoms. Discuss drug discontinuance with physician. Instruct patient that drug should be used for two days and physician notified if diarrhea persists.

II. ALTERATIONS IN SENSORY/PERCEPTUAL PATTERNS related to DROWSINESS

Defining Characteristics: Drowsiness, dizziness, fatigue may occur.

Nursing Implications: Teach patient that drug is for short-term relief of diarrhea. Assess for and instruct patient to report signs/symptoms. Discuss drug discontinuance with physician if symptoms are severe.

III. ALTERATION IN SKIN INTEGRITY related to RASH, SENSITIVITY

Defining Characteristics: Rarely, rash may develop.

Nursing Implications: Assess baseline skin integrity. Instruct patient to report rash. Discuss drug discontinuance with physician.

Drug: octreotide acetate (Sandostatin)

Class: Cyclic cotapeptide that mimics the pharmacologic actions of the natural hormone somatostatin and is long-acting.

Mechanism of Action: Drug is a more potent inhibitor than somatostatin of growth hormone, glucagon, insulin; also suppresses LH (luteinizine hormone) response to GnRH (gonadotropin-releasing hormone); decreases splanchnic blood flow; and inhibits release of serotonin, gastrin, vasoactive intestinal peptide (VIP), secretin, motilin, and pancreatic polypeptide like somatostatin. Stimulates fluid and electrolyte absorption from GI tract, and lengthens transit time of intestinal contents. Controls symptoms associated with carcinoid syndrome (e.g., flushing, levels of serotonin metabolite 5-HIAA), and VIP-secreting adenomas (e.g., watery diarrhea).

Metabolism: Absorbed rapidly and completely after injection, with peak concentrations after 24 minutes. Protein binding 65%, and eliminated from plasma with a half-life of 1.7 hours (natural hormone is 1–3 minutes). Duration of action approximately 12 hours depending upon tumor type. Excreted in urine, with decreased clearance by 26% in the elderly. LAR Depot consists of biodegradable microspheres that slowly release octreotide from the injection site over 4 weeks. After IM injection, serum octreotide concentration reaches a transient initial peak within 1 hour, then declines over the next 3–5 days, then slowly increases to plateau 2–3 weeks post-injection. Steady state is reached by the 3rd monthly injection.

Dosage/Range:

Adult (immediate release injection):

- Carcinoid: Starting dose of 100–600 mcg/day (median 450 mcg/day) in 2–4 divided doses SQ.
- VIPoma: 200–300 mcg/day SQ in 2–4 divided doses during initial 2 weeks, then titrated to response with range of 150–750 mcg/day to control symptoms.
- Acromegaly: 50 mcg SQ tid, titrated to need every 2 weeks based on IGF (somatomedin C) levels.
- AIDS-related diarrhea: 500 mcg SQ q8h.
- Chemotherapy-induced diarrhea (high dose): 300 mcg/day continuous infusion.
- Radiation-induced diarrhea: 50 mcg SQ q8h.
- Graft-versus-host disease (GVHD): 100 mcg IV q8h.
- Short bowel syndrome: 50 mcg SQ q8h.
- Chronic idiopathic secretory diarrhea: 100 mcg SQ q8h.

Sandostatin LAR Depot:

- Renal failure: drug half-life may be increased requiring dosage adjustment.

Carcinoid Tumors and VIPomas

- If patient is not currently on octreotide acetate, begin therapy with immediate release dosing for 2 weeks: Carcinoid: 100–600 mcg/da SQ in 2–4 divided doses (mean daily dose 300 mcg) although some patients may require up to 1500 mcg/da; VIPoma: 200–300 mcg/da SQ in 2–4 divided doses (range 150–750 mcg) and dosage may be individualized to control symptoms, but usually does not exceed 450 mcg/da.
- For patients who respond to the initial 2 week therapy, switch to Sandostatin LAR Depot 20 mg IM q4 weeks × 2 months. In addition, since it will take at least 2 weeks to achieve steady state, the patient should ALSO continue to receive Sandostatin immediate release dosing SQ for atleast 2 weeks at the same dose as in the first 2 weeks. After 2 months of Sandostatin LAR Depot 20 mg, the dose may be increased to 30 mg q4 weeks if symptoms are not controlled. Some patients who have their symptoms controlled on 20 mg q4 weeks, may be decreased to 10 mg q4 weeks.
- Some patients may have exacerbation of symptoms and require temporary additional immediate release in addition to the LAR Depot to control the increase in symptoms.

Acromegaly

- If patient is not currently on octreotide acetate, begin therapy with immediate release dosing q8h at an initial dose of 50 mcg tid, and gradually increase as needed (based on growth hormone (GH) levels) as the goal is to normalize GH and IGF-1 (somatomedin C) levels. After 2 weeks, tolerance and response should be evident, so that patient can be changed to LAR Depot at a dose of 20 mg q4 weeks if tolerance and effectiveness positive.

- For patients currently on octreotide, they can be changed directly to LAR Depot q4 weeks, and at the end of 3 months, the LAR Depot dose should be titrated based on growth hormone level:
  - —GH ≤ 2.5 ng/mL, IGF-1 (somatomedin C) normal and controlled symptoms, 20 mg IM (intragluteally) q4 weeks.
  - —GH > 2.5 ng/mL, IGF-1 elevated and/or uncontrolled symptoms, increase dose to 30 mg IM q4 weeks.
  - —GH ≤ 1 ng/mL, IGF-1 normal and controlled symptoms, reduce dose to 10 mg IM q4 weeks.

Drug Preparation/Administration:

- Available in 1-mL ampules and 5-mL (5 mg) multidose vials. Immediate release injection: administer SQ, IV over 15–30 minutes, or IVP over 3 minutes.
- Stable in solution in 0.9% sodium chloride or 5% dextrose in water for 24 hours; dilute drug in 50–200 mL of 0.9% sodium chloride or 5% dextrose for IV infusions over 15–30 minutes.
- Patient may develop pain, stinging, tingling, or burning sensation at injection site, with redness and swelling.

LAR Depot:

- Available in (5-mL) vials containing 10, 20, or 30 mg octreotide free peptide; injection kit includes a syringe containing 2.5 mL of diluent, 2 sterile 1.5 inch 19 gauge needles, and 2 alcohol wipes as well as instruction booklet.
- Allow drug vial and diluent-filled syringe to reach room temperature (30–60 minutes) prior to preparation of drug suspension.
- Drug must be administered immediately after mixing.
- Tap vial to ensure drug has settled to bottom of vial; asceptically inject diluent slowly down the inside wall of the vial while rotating the vial to evenly distribute the diluent using one of the needles. Allow to sit for 5 minutes or longer to assure full saturation of the drug powder; once saturated, swirl the vial gently for 30–60 seconds until a milky uniform suspension appears (DO NOT shake vigorously or invert the vial). Asceptically withdraw the ordered dose, holding the vial at 45 degrees. There will be some remaining suspension as the vial has over-fill. Add a small amount of air into the syringe, and gently rock back and forth until the patient is given the injection (DO NOT invert syringe). Eliminate air from the syringe.
- Replace needle with second needle, and asceptically administer drug immediately.
- Administer IM in gluteal muscle as other sites too painful (never give IV or SC) q28 days.

- Record injection site and rotate sites.

Drug Interactions:
- May affect absorption of orally administered drugs.
- Cyclosporine: decreased serum levels of cyclosporine, resulting in transplant rejection.
- Insulin, oral hypoglycemic agents, beta-blockers, calcium channel blockers: assess patient response and need for dosage adjustment of these drugs.

Lab Effects/Interference:
- Hypoglycemia or hyperglycemia: suppression of TSH may result in hypothyroidism and decreased total/free T_4 (generally patients with acromegaly receiving long-term therapy).
- Decreased vitamin B_{12} levels (Shilling's test).

Special Considerations:
- Sandostatin LAR Depot is indicated for patients in whom initial treatment with Sandostatin Injection has been shown to be effective and tolerated, 1) carcinoid tumors: the long-term treatment of severe diarrhea and flushing episodes, 2) VIPomas: long-term treatment of profuse watery diarrhea, 3) acromegaly: long-term maintenance therapy who require medical treatment.
- Octreotide acetate is appropriate when other conventional antidiarrheal medications have failed, and other treatable causes of diarrhea have been excluded (e.g., obstruction, infection).
- Patient should be taught sterile SQ injection technique for immediate release preparations.
- Laboratory test monitoring (efficacy) based on treatment intent:
  - Carcinoid: 5-HIAA (urinary 5-hydroxyindoleacetic acid), plasma substance P and serotonin.
  - VIPoma: VIP (plasma vasoactive intestinal peptide).
  - Acromegaly: growth hormone, IGF-1 (somatomedin C).
- Adverse reactions of diabetes mellitus, hypothyroidism, and cardiovascular disease occur in patients treated for acromegaly.
- May change to long-acting depot if already controlled on immediate-release preparation, or in a new patient, after response is assessed after 2 weeks of immediate-release dosing.
- Drug inhibits gallbladder contraction and decreases bile secretion in 63% of patients with acromegaly or psoriasis when treated for long periods of time.

Potential Toxicities/Side Effects and the Nursing Process

I. ALTERATION IN NUTRITION, LESS THAN BODY REQUIREMENTS, related to CARBOHYDRATE METABOLISM

Defining Characteristics: Rarely, transient hypoglycemia or hyperglycemia due to altered balance between hormones regulating serum glucose (insulin, glucagon, growth hormone). Rarely, diarrhea, nausea and vomiting, abdominal pain or discomfort. Incidence 3–10%.

Nursing Implications: Assess baseline nutritional balance. Instruct patient to report any changes, and assess for hyperglycemia (drowsiness, dry mouth, flushing, dry skin, fruity breath, polyuria, polydipsia, polyphagia, weight loss, stomach ache, nausea/vomiting, fatigue), hypoglycemia (anxiety, chills, cool/pale skin, difficulty concentrating, headache, hunger, shakiness, diaphoresis, fatigue, weakness, nausea). If patient is hypoglycemic, teach patient to carry candy. Monitor serum glucose, and discuss alterations with physician. Treat nausea and vomiting symptomatically, and discuss need for antiemetic if significant.

II. ALTERATION IN COMFORT related to HEADACHE, FLUSHING

Defining Characteristics: Rarely (1–3%) patient may experience lightheadedness, dizziness, fatigue, pedal edema, headache, flushing of the face, weakness.

Nursing Implications: Assess baseline comfort, and instruct patient to report any changes. Assess safety, and manage symptoms symptomatically. If unrelieved or significant, discuss with physician.

Appendix 1

Controlling Occupational Exposure to Hazardous Drugs

A. Introduction

In response to numerous inquiries,[1] OSHA published guidelines for the management of cytotoxic (antineoplastic) drugs in the workplace in 1986.[106] At that time, surveys indicated little standardization in the use of engineering controls and personal protective equipment (PPE).[56,73] Although practices have improved in subsequent years, problems still exist.[111] In addition, the occupational management of these chemicals has been further clarified. These trends, in conjunction with many information requests, have prompted OSHA to revise its recommendations for hazardous drug handling. In addition, some of these agents are covered under the Hazard Communication Standard (HCS) [29 CFR 1910.1200].[107] In order to provide recommendations consistent with current scientific knowledge, this informational guidance document has been expanded to cover hazardous drugs (HD), in addition to the cytotoxic drugs (CD) that were covered in the 1986 guidelines. The recommendations apply to all settings where employees are occupationally exposed to HDs, such as hospitals, physicians' offices, and home health care agencies. This review will:

- provide criteria for classifying drugs as hazardous,
- summarize the evidence supporting the management of HDs as an occupational hazard,
- discuss the equipment and worker education recommended as well as the legal requirements of standards for the protection of workers exposed and potentially exposed to HDs,
- update the important aspects of medical surveillance and,
- list some common HDs currently in use.

Anesthetic agents have not been considered in this review. However, exposure to some of these agents is a recognized health hazard,[104] and they have been considered in a separate Technical Manual Chapter.

B. Categorization of Drugs as Hazardous

The purpose of this section is to describe the biological effects of those pharmaceuticals that are considered hazardous. A number of pharmaceuticals in the health care setting may pose occupational risk to employees through acute and chronic workplace exposure. Past attention focused on drugs used to treat cancer. However, it is clear that many other agents also have toxicity profiles of concern. This recognition prompted the American Society of Hospital Pharmacists (ASHP) to define a class of agents as "hazardous drugs."[3] That report specified concerns about antineoplastic and nonantineoplastic hazardous drugs in use in most institutions throughout the country. OSHA shares this concern. The ASHP Technical Assistance

Bulletin (TAB) described four drug characteristics, each of which could be considered hazardous:

- genotoxicity,
- carcinogenicity,
- teratogenicity or fertility impairment, and
- serious organ or other toxic manifestation at low doses in experimental animals or treated patients.

Table A.1 of this review lists some common drugs that are considered hazardous by the above criteria. There is no standardized reference for this information nor is there complete consensus on all agents listed. Professional judgment by personnel trained in pharmacology/toxicology is essential in designating drugs as hazardous, and reference 65 provides information regarding the development of such a list at one institution. Some drugs, which have a long history of safe use in humans despite *in vitro* or animal evidence to toxicity, may be excluded by the institution's experts by considerations such as those used to formulate GRAS *(Generally Regarded as Safe)* lists by the FDA under the Food, Drug, and Cosmetics Act.

Table A.1 is not all inclusive, should not be construed as complete, and represents an assessment of some, but not all, marketed drugs at a fixed point in time. Table A.1 was developed through consultation with institutions that have assembled teams of pharmacists and other health care personnel to determine which drugs should be used with caution. These teams reviewed product literature and drug information when considering each product.

Sources for this appendix are the *Physicians' Desk Reference,* Section 10:00 in the American Hospital Formulary Service Drug Information,[68] IARC publications (particularly volume 50),[43] the Johns Hopkins Hospital, and the National Institutes of Health, Clinical Center Nursing Department. No attempt to include investigational drugs was made, but they should be prudently handled as hazardous drugs until adequate information becomes available to exclude them. Any determination of the hazard status of drug should be periodically reviewed and updated as new information becomes available. Importantly, new drugs should routinely undergo a hazard assessment.

Table A.1 Some Common Drugs Considered Hazardous

Chemical/Generic Name	Source*
ALTRETAMINE	C
AMINOGLUTETHIMIDE	A
AZATHIOPRINE	ACE
L-ASPARAGINASE	ABC
BLEOMYCIN	ABC
BUSULFAN	ABC
CARBOPLATIN	ABC
CARMUSTINE	ABC
CHLORAMBUCIL	ABCE
CHLORAMPHENICOL	E
CHLOROTRIANISENE	B
CHLOROZOTOCIN	E
CYCLOSPORIN	E
CISPLATIN	ABCE

Table A.1 *(continued)*

Chemical/Generic Name	Source*
CYCLOPHOSPHAMIDE	ABCE
CYTARABINE	ABC
DACARBAZINE	ABC
DACTINOMYCIN	ABC
DAUNORUBICIN	ABC
DIETHYLSTILBESTROL	BE
DOXORUBICIN	ABCE
ESTRADIOL	B
ESTRAMUSTINE	AB
ETHINYL ESTRADIOL	B
ETOPOSIDE	ABC
FLOXURIDINE	AC
FLUOROURACIL	ABC
FLUTAMIDE	BC
GANCICLOVIR	AD
HYDROXYUREA	ABC
IDARUBICIN	AC
IFOSFAMIDE	ABC
INTERFERON-α	BC
ISOTRETINOIN	D
LEUPROLIDE	BC
LEVAMISOLE	C
LOMUSTINE	ABCE
MECHLORETHAMINE	BC
MEDROXYPROGESTERONE	B
MEGESTROL	BC
MELPHALAN	ABCE
MERCAPTOPURINE	ABC
METHOTREXATE	ABC
MITOMYCIN	ABC
MITOTANE	ABC
MITOXANTRONE	ABC
NAFARELIN	C
PIPOBROMAN	C
PLICAMYCIN	BC
PROCARBAZINE	ABCE
RIBAVIRIN	D
STREPTOZOCIN	AC
TAMOXIFEN	BC
TESTOLACTONE	BC
THIOGUANINE	ABC
THIOTEPA	ABC
URACIL MUSTARD	ACE

Table A.1 *(continued)*

Chemical/Generic Name	Source*
VIDARABINE	D
VINBLASTINE	ABC
VINCRISTINE	ABC
ZIDOVUDINE	D

*Sources:
A The National Institutes of Health, Clinical Center Nursing Department
B Antineoplastic drugs in the *Physicians' Desk Reference*
C American Hospital Formulary, Antineoplastics
D Johns Hopkins Hospital E International Agency for Research on Cancer

List of Abbreviations

ANSI	American National Standards Institute
ASHP	American Society of Hospital Pharmacists
BSC	Biological Safety Cabinet
CD	Cytotoxic Drug
EPA	Environmental Protection Agency
HD	Hazardous Drug
HCS	Hazard Communication Standard
HEPA	High Efficiency Particulate Air
IARC	International Agency for Research on Cancer
MSDS	Material Safety Data Sheet
NIOSH	National Institute for Occupational Safety and Health
NTP	National Toxicology Program
OSHA	Occupational Safety and Health Administration
PPE	Personal Protective Equipment

In contrast, investigational drugs are new chemicals for which there is often little information on potential toxicity. Structure or activity relationships with similar chemicals and in vitro data can be considered in determining potential toxic effects. Investigational drugs should be prudently handled as HDs unless adequate information becomes available to exclude them.

Some major considerations by professionals trained in pharmacology/toxicology[65] in designating a drug as hazardous are:

- Is the drug designated as Therapeutic Category 10:00 (Antineoplastic Agent) in the American Hospital Formulary Service Drug Information?[68]
- Does the manufacturer suggest the use of special isolation techniques in its handing, administration, or disposal?
- Is the drug known to be a human mutagen, carcinogen, teratogen, or reproductive toxicant?
- Is the drug known to be carcinogenic or teratogenic in animals (drugs known to be mutagenic in multiple bacterial systems or animals should also be considered hazardous)?
- And, is the drug known to be acutely toxic to an organ system?

C. Background: Hazardous Drugs as Occupational Risk

Preparation, administration, and disposal of HDs may expose pharmacists, nurses, physicians, and other health care workers to potentially significant workplace levels of these chemicals. The literature establishing these agents as occupational hazards deals primarily with CDs; however, documentation of adverse exposure effects from other HDs is rapidly accumulating.[15,40,41,42,43,59] The degree of absorption that takes place during work and the significance of secondary early biological effects on each individual encounter are difficult to assess and may vary depending on the HD. As a result, it is difficult to set safe levels of exposure on the basis of current scientific information.

However, there are several lines of evidence supporting the toxic potential of these drugs if handled improperly. Therefore, it is essential to minimize exposure to all HDs. Summary tables of much of the data presented below can be found in Sorsa[95] and Rogers.[84]

1. Mechanism of Action

Most HDs either bind directly to genetic material in the cell nucleus or affect cellular protein synthesis. Cytotoxic drugs may not distinguish between normal and cancerous cells. The growth and reproduction of the normal cells are often affected during treatment of cancerous cells.

2. Animal Data

Numerous studies document the carcinogenic, mutagenic, and teratogenic effects of HD exposure in animals. They are well summarized in the pertinent IARC publications.[37–43] Alkylating agents present the strongest evidence of carcinogenicity (e.g., *cyclophosphamide, mechlorethamine hydrochloride [nitrogen mustard]*). However, other classes, such as some antibiotics, have been implicated as well. Extensive evidence for mutagenic and reproductive effects can be found in all antineoplastic classes. The antiviral agent *ribavirin* has additionally been shown to be teratogenic in all rodent species tested.[31,49] The ASHP recommends that all pharmaceutical agents that are animal carcinogens be handled as if human carcinogens.

3. Human Data at Therapeutic Levels

Many HDs are known human carcinogens, for which there is no safe level of exposure. The development of secondary malignancies is a well-documented side effect of chemotherapy treatment.[52,86,90,115] Leukemia has been most frequently observed. However, other secondary malignancies, such as bladder cancer and lymphoma, have been documented in patients treated for other, usually solid, primary malignancies.[52,114] Chromosomal aberrations can result from chemotherapy treatment as well. One study, on *chlorambucil,* reveals chromosomal damage in recipients to be cumulative and related to both dose and duration of therapy.[77]

Numerous case reports have linked chemotherapeutic treatment to adverse reproductive outcomes.[7,88,91,98] Testicular and ovarian dysfunction, including permanent sterility, have occurred in male and female patients who have received CDs either singly or in combination.[14] In addition, some antineoplastic agents are known or suspected to be transmitted to infants through breast milk.[79]

The literature also documents the effects of these drugs on other organ systems. Extravasation of some agents can cause severe soft-tissue injury, consisting of necrosis and sloughing of exposed areas.[23,78,87] Other HDs, such as *pentamidine* and *zidovudine* (formerly AZT), are known to have significant side effects (i.e., hematologic abnormalities), in treated patients.[4,33] Serum transaminase elevation has also been reported in treated patients.[4,33]

4. Occupational Exposure—Airborne Levels

Monitoring efforts for cytotoxic drugs have detected measurable air levels when exhaust biological safety cabinets (BSC) were not used for preparation or when monitoring was performed inside the BSC.[50,73]

Concentrations of *fluorouracil* ranging from 0.12 to 82.26 ng/m^3 have been found during monitoring of drug preparation without a BSC implying an opportunity for respiratory exposure.[73] Elevated concentrations of *cyclophosphamide* were found by these authors as well. *Cyclophosphamide* has also been detected on the HEPAfilters of flow hoods used in HDpreparation, demonstrating aerosolization of the drug and an exposure opportunity mitigated by effective engineering controls.[81]

A recent study has reported wipe samples of *cyclophosphamide,* one of the Class I IARC carcinogens, on surfaces of work stations in an oncology pharmacy and outpatient treatment areas (sinks and countertops). Concentrations ranged from 0.005 to 0.03 μg/cm^2, documenting opportunity for dermal exposure.[60]

Administration of drugs via aerosolization can lead to measurable air concentrations in the breathing zone of workers providing treatment. Concentrations up to 18 μg/m^3 have been found by personal air sampling of workers administering *pentamidine.*[67] Similar monitoring for *ribavirin* has found concentrations as high as 316 μg/m[331]

5. Occupational Exposure—Biological Evidence of Absorption

Urinary Mutagenicity

Falk et al. were the first to note evidence of mutagenicity in the urine of nurses who handled cytotoxic drugs.[26] The extent of this effect increased over the course of the work week. With improved handling practices, a decrease in mutagenic activity was seen.[27] Researchers have also studied pharmacy personnel who reconstitute antineoplastic drugs. These employees showed increasingly mutagenic urine over the period of exposure; when they stopped handling the drugs, activity fell within 2 days to the level of unexposed controls.[5,76] They also found mutagenicity in workers using horizontal laminar flow BSCs that decreased to control levels with the use of vertical flow containment BSCs.[76] Other studies have failed to find a relationship between exposure and urine mutagenicity.[25] Sorsa[95] summarizes this information and discusses the factors, such as differences in urine collection timing and variations in the use of PPE, which could lead to disparate results. Differences may also be related to smoking status; smokers exposed to CDs exhibit greater urine mutagenicity than exposed non-smokers or control smokers, suggesting contamination of the work area by CDs and some contribution of smoking to their mutagenic profile.[9]

Urinary Thioethers

Urinary thioethers are glutathione conjugated metabolites of alkylating agents that have been evaluated as an indirect means of measuring exposure. Workers who handle cytotoxic drugs have been reported to have increased levels compared to controls and also have increasing thioether levels over a five-day work week.[44,48] Other studies of nurses who handle CDs and of treated patients have yielded variable results that could be due to confounding by smoking, PPE, and glutathione-S-transferase activity.[11]

Urinary Metabolites

Venitt[112] assayed the urine of pharmacy and nursing personnel handling cisplatin and found platinum concentrations at or below the limit of detection for both workers and controls.

Hirst[35] found *cyclophosphamide* in the urine of two nurses who handled the drug, documenting worker absorption. (Hirst also documented skin absorption in human volunteers by using gas chromatography after topical application of the drug.) Urinary *pentamidine* recovery has also been reported in exposed health care workers.[94]

6. Occupational Exposure—Human Effects

Cytogenetic Effects

A number of studies have examined the relationship of exposure to CDs in the workplace to chromosomal aberrations. These studies have looked at a variety of markers for damage, including sister chromatid exchanges (SCE), structural aberrations (e.g., gaps, breaks, translocations), and micronuclei in peripheral blood lymphocytes. The results have been somewhat conflicting. Several authors found increases in one or more markers.[74,75,88,113] Increased mutilation frequency has been reported as well.[17] Other studies have failed to find a significant difference between workers and controls.[99,101] Some researchers have found higher individual elevations[28] or a relationship between number of drugs handled and SCEs.[8] These disparate results are not unexpected. The difficulties in quantitating exposure have resulted in different exposure magnitudes between studies; workers in several negative studies appear to have a lower overall exposure.[10] In addition, differences in the use of PPE and work technique will alter absorption of CDs and resultant biologic effects.

Finally, techniques for SCE measurement may not be optimal. A recent study that looked at correlation of phosphoramide-induced SCE levels with duration of anticancer drug handling found a statistically significant correlation coefficient of 0.[63,66]

Taken together, the evidence indicates an excess of markers of mutagenic exposure in unprotected workers.

Reproductive Effects

Reproductive effects associated with occupational exposure to CDs have been well documented. Hemminki et al.[32] found no difference in exposure between nurses who had spontaneous abortions and those who had normal pregnancies. However, the study group consisted of nurses who were employed in surgical or medical floors of a general hospital. When the relationship between CD exposure and congenital malformations was explored, the study group was expanded to include oncology nurses, among others, and an odds ratio of 4:7 was found for exposures of more than once per week. This observed odds ratio is statistically significant. Selevan et al.[39] found a relationship between CD exposure and spontaneous abortion in a case-control study of Finnish nurses. This well-designed study reviewed the reproductive histories of 568 women (167 cases) and found a statistically significant odds ratio of 2:3. Similar results were obtained in another large casecontrol study of French nurses,[102] and a study of Baltimore area nurses found a significantly higher proportion of adverse pregnancy outcomes when exposure to antineoplastic agents occurred during the pregnancy.[85] The nurses involved in these studies usually prepared and administered the drugs. Therefore, workplace exposure of these groups of professionals to such products has been associated with adverse reproductive outcomes in several investigations.

Other Effects

Hepatocellular damage has been reported in nurses working in an oncology ward; the injury appeared to be related to intensity and duration of work exposure to CDs.[96] Symptoms such as light-headedness, dizziness, nausea, headache, and allergic reactions have also been described in employees after the preparation and administration of antineoplastic drugs in unventilated areas.[22,96] In occupational settings, these agents are known to be toxic to the skin and mucous membranes, including the cornea.[69,82]

Pentamidine has been associated with respiratory damage in one worker who administered the aerosol. The injury consisted of a decrease in diffusing capacity that improved after exposure ceased.[29] The onset of bronchospasm in a pentamidine-exposed worker has also been reported.[22] Employees involved in the aerosol administration of *ribavirin* have noted symptoms of respiratory tract irritation.[55] A number of medications including *psyllium* and various antibiotics are known respiratory and dermal sensitizers. Exposure in susceptible individuals can lead to asthma or allergic contact dermatitis.

D. Work Areas

Risks to personnel working with HDs are a function of the drugs' inherent toxicity and the extent of exposure. The main routes of exposure are: inhalation of dusts or aerosols, dermal absorption, and ingestion. Contact with contaminated food or cigarettes represents the primary means of ingestion. Opportunity for exposure to HDs may occur at many points in the handling of these drugs.

1. Pharmacy or Other Preparation Areas

In large oncology centers, HDs are usually prepared in the pharmacy. However, in small hospitals, outpatient treatments areas, and physicians' offices they have been prepared by physicians or nurses without appropriate engineering controls and protective apparel.[16,20] Many HDs must be reconstituted, transferred from one container to another, or manipulated before administration to patients. Even if care is taken, opportunity for absorption through inhalation or direct skin contact can occur.[35,36,73,116] Examples of manipulations that can cause splattering, spraying, and aerosolization include:

- withdrawal of needles from drug vials,
- drug transfer using syringes and needles or filter straws,
- breaking open of ampules, and
- expulsion of air from a drug-filled syringe.

Evaluation of these preparation techniques, using fluorescent dye solutions, has shown contamination of gloves and the sleeves and chest of gowns.[97]

Horizontal airflow work benches provide an aseptic environment for the preparation of injectable drugs. However, these units provide a flow of filtered air originating at the back of the workspace and exiting toward the employee using the unit. Thus, they increase the likelihood of drug exposure for both the preparer and other personnel in the room. As a result, the use of horizontal BSCs is contraindicated in the preparation of HDs. Smoking, drinking, applying cosmetics, and eating where these drugs are prepared, stored, or used also increase the chance of exposure.

2. Administration of Drugs to Patients

Administration of drugs to patients is generally performed by nurses or physicians. Drug injection into the IV line, clearing of air from the syringe or infusion line, and leakage at the tubing, syringe, or stopcock connection present opportunities for skin contact and aerosol generation. Clipping used needles and crushing used syringes can produce considerable aerosolization as well.

Such techniques where needles and syringes are contaminated with blood or other potentially infectious material are prohibited by the Bloodborne Pathogens Standard.[109] Prohibition of clipping or crushing of any needle or syringe is sound practice.

Excreta from patients who have received certain antineoplastic drugs may contain high concentrations of the drug or its hazardous metabolites. For example, patients receiving *cyclophosphamide* excrete large amounts of the drug and its mutagenic metabolites.[46,92] Patients treated with *cisplatin* have been shown to excrete potentially hazardous amounts of the drug.[112] Unprotected handling of urine or urine-soaked sheets by nursing or housekeeping personnel poses a source of exposure.

3. Disposal of Drugs and Contaminated Materials

Contaminated materials used in the preparation and administration of HDs, such as gloves, gowns, syringes, and vials, present a hazard to support and housekeeping staff. The use of properly labeled, sealed, and covered disposal containers, handled by trained and protected personnel, should be routine, and is required under the Bloodborne Pathogens Standard[109] if such items are contaminated with blood or other potentially infectious materials. HDs and contaminated materials should be disposed of in accordance with federal, state, and local laws. Disposal of some of these drugs is regulated by the EPA. Those drugs that are unused commercial chemical products and are considered by the EPA to be toxic wastes must be disposed of in accordance with 40 CFR part 261.33.[24] Spills can also represent a hazard; the employer should ensure that all employees are familiar with appropriate spill procedures.

4. Survey of Current Work Practices

Surveys of U.S. cancer centers and oncology clinics reveal wide variation in work practices, equipment, or training for personnel preparing CDs.[56,73] This lack of standardization results in a high prevalence of potential occupational exposure to CDs. One survey found that 40% of hospital pharmacists reported a skin exposure to CDs at least once a month, and only 28% had medical surveillance programs in their workplace.[16] Nurses, particularly those in outpatient settings, were found to be even less well protected than pharmacists.[111] Such findings emphasize current lack of protection for all personnel who risk potential exposure to HDs.

E. Prevention of Employee Exposure

1. Hazardous Drug Safety and Health Plan

Where hazardous drugs, as defined in this review, are used in the workplace, sound practice would dictate that a written *Hazardous Drug Safety and Health Plan* be developed. Such a plan assists in:

- protecting employees from health hazards associated with HDs, and
- keeping exposures as low as reasonably achievable.

When a *Hazardous Drug Safety and Health Plan* is developed, it should be readily available and accessible to all employees, including temporary employees, contractors, and trainees.

The ASHP recommends that the Plan include each of the following elements and indicate specific measures that the employer is taking to ensure employee protection:[3]

- standard operating procedures relevant to safety and health considerations to be followed when health care workers are exposed to hazardous drugs,

- criteria that the employer uses to determine and implement control measures to reduce employee exposure to hazardous drugs including engineering controls, the use of personal protective, equipment, and hygiene practices,
- a requirement that ventilation systems and other protective equipment function properly, and specific measures to ensure proper and adequate performance of such equipment,
- provision for information and training,
- the circumstances under which the use of specific HDs (that is, FDA investigational drugs) require prior approval from the employer before implementation,
- provision for medical examinations of potentially exposed personnel, and
- designation of personnel responsible for implementation of the *Hazardous Drug Safety and Health Plan,* including the assignment of Hazardous Drug Officer (who is an industrial hygienist, nurse, or pharmacist health and safety representative); and, if appropriate, establishment of a Hazardous Drug Committee or a joint Hazardous Drug Committee/Chemical Committee.

The ASHP further recommends that specific consideration of the following provisions be included where appropriate:

- establishment of a designated HD handling area,
- use of containment devices such as biological safety cabinets,
- procedures for safe removal of contaminated waste, and
- decontamination procedures.

The ASHP recommends that the *Hazardous Drug Safety and Health Plan* be reviewed and its effectiveness reevaluated at least annually and updated as necessary.

A comparison of OSHA 200 log entries to employee medical clinic appointment or visit rosters can be made[3] to establish if there is evidence of disorders that could be hazardous drug-related.

Previous health and safety inspections by local health departments, fire departments, regulatory or accrediting agencies may be helpful for the facility's planning purposes as well as any OSHA review of hazards and programs in the facility. Joint Commission on Accreditation of Healthcare Organizations (JCAHO), or College of American Pathologists (CAP) review of facilities may contain information on hazardous drugs used in the facility.

2. Drug Preparation Precautions

Work Area

The ASHP recommends that HD preparation be performed in a restricted, preferably centralized, area. Signs restricting the access of unauthorized personnel are to be prominently displayed. Eating, drinking, smoking, chewing gum, applying cosmetics, and storing food in the preparation area should be prohibited.[71] The ASHP recommends that procedures for spills and emergencies, such as skin or eye contact, be available to workers, preferably posted in the area.[3]

Biological Safety Cabinets

Class II or III Biological Safety Cabinets (BSC) that meet the current National Sanitation Foundation Standard[49,70,72] should minimize exposure to HDs during preparation. Although these cabinets are designed for biohazards, several studies have documented reduced urine mutagenicity in CDexposed workers or reduce environmental levels after the institution of BSCs.[5,51,61] If a BSC is unavailable, for example in private practice office, accepted medical practice is the sharing of a cabinet (e.g., several medical offices share a cabinet) or sending the patient to a center where HDs can be prepared in a BSC. Alternatively, preparation can be performed in a facility with a BSC and the drugs transported to the area of administration. Use of a dedicated BSC, where only HDs are prepared, is prudent medical practice.

Types of BSCs

Four main types of Class II BSCs are available. They all have downward airflow and HEPA filters. They are differentiated by the amount of air recirculated within the cabinet, whether this air is vented to the room or the outside, and whether contaminated ducts are under positive or negative pressure. These four types are:

- Type A cabinets recirculate approximately 70% of cabinet air through HEPA filters back into the cabinet; the rest is discharged through a HEPA filter into the preparation room. Contaminated ducts are under positive pressure.
- Type B1 cabinets have higher velocity air inflow, recirculate 30% of the cabinet air, and exhaust the rest to the outside through HEPA filters. They have negative pressure contaminated ducts and plenums.
- Type B2 systems are similar to Type B1 except that no air is recirculated.
- Type B3 cabinets are similar to Type A in that they recirculate approximately 70% of cabinet air. However, the other 30% is vented to the outside and the ducts are under negative pressure.

Class III cabinets are totally enclosed with gas-tight construction. The entire cabinet is under negative pressure, and operations are performed through attached gloves. All air is HEPA filtered.

Class II, type B, or Class III BSCs are recommended since they vent to the outside.[3] Those without air recirculation are the most protective. If the BSC has an outside exhaust, it should be vented away from air intake units.

The blower on the vertical airflow hood should be on at all times. If the BSC is turned off, it should be decontaminated and covered in plastic until airflow is resumed.[3,72] Each BSC should be equipped with a continuous monitoring device to allow confirmation of adequate air flow and cabinet performance. The cabinet should be in an area with minimal air turbulence; this will reduce leakage to the environment.[6,70] Additional information on design and performance testing of BSCs can be found in papers by Avis and Levchuck,[6] Bryan and Marback,[10] and the National Sanitation Foundation.[70] Practical information regarding space needs and conversion possibilities is contained in the ASHP's 1990 technical assistance bulletins.[3]

Ventilation and biosafety cabinets installed should be maintained and evaluated for proper performance in accordance with the manufacturer's instructions.

Decontamination

The cabinet should be cleaned according to the manufacturer's instructions. Some manufacturers have recommended weekly decontamination as well as whenever spills occur or when the cabinet requires moving, service, or certification.

Decontamination should consist of surface cleaning with water and detergent, followed by thorough rinsing. The use of detergent is recommended because there is no single accepted method of chemical deactivation for all agents involved.[13,45] Quaternary ammonium cleaners should be avoided due to the possibility of vapor build-up in recirculated air.[3] Ethyl alcohol or 70% isopropyl alcohol may be used with the cleaner if the contamination is soluble only in alcohol.[3] Alcohol vapor build-up has also been a concern, so the use of alcohol should be avoided in BSCs where air is recirculated.[3] Spray cleaners should also be avoided due to the risk of spraying the HEPA filter. Ordinary decontamination procedures, which include fumigation with a germicidal agent, are inappropriate in a BSC used for HDs because such procedures do not remove or deactivate the drugs.

Removable work trays, if present, should be lifted in the BSC, so the back and the sump below can be cleaned. During cleaning, the worker should wear PPE similar to that used for spills. *Ideally, the sash should remain down during cleaning; however, a NIOSH-approved respirator appropriate for the hazard must be worn by the worker if the sash will be lifted during the process.* The exhaust fan/blower should be left on. Cleaning should proceed from least to most contaminated areas. The drain spillage trough area should be cleaned twice since it can be heavily contaminated. All materials from the decontamination process should be handled as HDs and disposed of in accordance with federal, state, and local laws.

Service and Certification

The ASHP recommends that BSCs be serviced and certified by a qualified technician every 6 months or any time the cabinet is moved or repaired.[3,71] Technicians servicing these cabinets or changing the HEPA filters should be aware of HD risk through hazard communication training from their employers and should use the same personal protective equipment as recommended for large spills. Certification of the BSC includes performance testing as outlined in the procedures of the National Sanitation Foundation's Standard Number 49.[70] Helpful information on such testing can be found in the ASHP 1990 technical assistance bulletins,[3] the BSC manufacturer's equipment manuals, and Bryan and Marback's paper.[10] HEPA filters should be changed when they restrict air flow or if they are contaminated by an accidental spill. They should be bagged in plastic and disposed of as HDs. Any time the cabinet is turned off or transported, it should be sealed with plastic.

Personal Protective Equipment

1. Gloves

Research indicates that the thickness of gloves used in handling HDs is more important than the type of material, since all materials tested have been found to be permeable to some HDs.[3,19,53] The best results are seen with latex gloves. Therefore, latex gloves should be used for the preparation of HDs unless the drug-product manufacturer specifically stipulates that some other glove provides better protection.[19,53,72,93,100] Thicker, longer latex gloves that cover the gown cuff are recommended for the use with HDs. *Individuals with latex allergy should consider the use of vinyl or nitrile gloves or glove liners.* Gloves with minimal or no powder are preferred since the powder may absorb contamination.[3,104]

The above referenced sources have noted great variability in permeability within and between glove lots. Therefore, double gloving is recommended if it does not interfere with an individual's technique.[3] Because all gloves are permeable to some extent and their permeability increases with time, they should be changed regularly (hourly) or immediately if they are torn, punctured, or contaminated with a spill. Hands should always be washed before gloves are put on and after they are removed. Employees need thorough training in proper methods for contaminated glove removal.

2. Gowns

A protective disposable gown made of lint-free, low-permeability fabric with a closed front, long sleeves, and elastic or knit closed cuff should be worn. The cuffs should be tucked under the gloves. If double gloves are worn, the outer glove should be over the gown cuff and the inner glove should be under the gown cuff. When the gown is removed, the inner glove should be removed last. Gowns and gloves in use in the HD preparation area should not be used outside the HD preparation area.[3]

As with gloves, there is no ideal material. Research has found non-porous Tyvek and Kaycel to be more permeable than Saranex-laminated Tyvek and polyethylene-coated Tyvek after 4 hours of exposure to the CDs tested.[54] However, little airflow is allowed with the latter materials. As a result, manufacturers have produced gowns with Saranex or polyethylene reinforced sleeves and front in an effort to decrease permeability in the most exposure-prone areas, but little data exists on decreasing exposure.

3. Respiratory Protection

A BSC is essential for the preparation of HDs. Where a BSC is not currently available, a *NIOSH-approved respirator* appropriate for the hazard must be worn to afford protection until the BSC is installed.* The use of respirators must comply with OSHA's Respiratory Protection Standard,[105] which outlines the aspects of a respirator program, including selection, fit testing, and worker training. Surgical masks are *not appropriate* since they *do not prevent* aerosol inhalation. Permanent respirator use, in lieu of BSCs, is imprudent practice and should not be a substitute for engineering controls.

4. Eye and Face Protection

Whenever splashes, sprays, or aerosols of HDs may be generated, which can result in eye, nose, or mouth contamination, chemical barrier face and eye protection must be provided and used in accordance with 29 CFR 1910.133. Eye glasses with temporary side shields are inadequate protection.

When a respirator is used to provide temporary protection as described above, and splashes, sprays, or aerosols are possible, employee protection should be:

- a respirator with a full face piece, or
- a plastic face shield or splash goggles complying with ANSI standards[2] when using a respirator of less than full face piece design.

Eyewash facilities should also be made available.

5. PPE Disposal and Decontamination

All gowns, gloves, and disposable materials used in preparation should be disposed of according to the hospital's hazardous drug waste procedures and as described under this review's section on Waste Disposal. Goggles, face shields, and respirators may be cleaned with mild detergent and water for reuse.

Work Equipment

NIH has recommended the work with HDs be carried out in a BSC on a disposable, plastic-backed paper liner. The liner should be changed after preparation is completed for the day, or after a shift. whichever comes first. Liners should also be changed after a spill.[103]

*NIOSH recommendation at the time of this publication is for a respirator with a high-efficiency filter, preferably a powered air-purifying respirator.

Syringes and IV sets with Luer-Lok fittings should be used for HDs. Syringe size should be large enough so that they are not full when the entire drug dose is present.

A covered disposable container should be used to contain excess solution. A covered sharps container should be in the BSC.

The ASHP recommends that HD-labeled plastic bags be available for all contaminated materials (including gloves, gowns, and paper liners), so that contaminated material can be immediately placed in them and disposed of in accordance with ASHP recommendations.[3]

Work Practices

Correct work practices are essential to worker protection. *Aseptic technique* is assumed as a standard practice in drug preparation. The general principles of aseptic technique, therefore, will not be detailed here. It should be noted, however, that BSC benches differ from horizontal flow units in several ways that require special precautions. Manipulations should not be performed close to the work surface of a BSC. Unsterilized items, including liners and hands, should be kept downstream from the working area. Entry and exit of the cabinet should be perpendicular to the front. Rapid lateral hand movements should be avoided. Additional information can be found in the National Sanitation Foundation Standard 49 for Class II (Laminar Flow) Biohazard Cabinetry[70] and Avis and Levchuck's paper.[6] All operators should be trained in these containment-area protocols.

All PPE should be donned before work is started in the BSC. All items necessary for drug preparation should be placed within the BSC before work is begun. Extraneous items should be kept out of the work area.

1. Labeling

In addition to standard pharmacy labeling practices, all syringes and IV bags containing HDs should be labeled with a distinctive warning label such as

SPECIAL HANDLING/Disposal Precautions

In addition, those HDs covered under HCS must have labels in accordance with section (f) of the standard to warn employees handling the drug(s) of the hazards.

2. Needles

The ASHP recommends that all syringes and needles used in the course of preparation be placed in *"sharps"* containers for disposal without being crushed, clipped, or capped.[3,103]

3. Priming

Prudent practice dictates that drug administration sets be attached and primed within the BSC, prior to addition of the drug. This eliminates the need to prime the set in a less well-controlled environment and ensures that any fluid that escapes during priming contains no drug. If priming must occur at the site of administration, the intravenous line should be primed with non-drug containing fluid, or backflow closed system should be used.[3]

4. Handling Vials

Extremes of positive and negative pressure in medication vials should be avoided, e.g., attempting to withdraw 10 mL of fluid from a 10-mL vial or placing 10 mL of a fluid into an air filled 10-mL vial. The use of large-bore needles, #18 or #20, avoids *high-pressure syring-*

ing of solutions. However, some experienced personnel believe that large-bore needles are more likely to drip. Multi-use dispensing pins are recommended to avoid these problems.

Venting devices such as filter needles or dispensing pins permit outside air to replace the withdrawn liquid. Proper worker education is essential before using these devices.[3] Although venting devices are recommended, another technique is to add diluent slowly to the vial by alternately injecting small amounts and allowing displaced air to escape into the syringe. When all diluent has been added, a small amount of additional air may be withdrawn to create a slight negative pressure in the vial. This should not be expelled into room air because it may contain drug residue. It should either be injected into a vacuum vial or remain in the syringe to be discarded.

If any negative pressure must be applied to withdraw a dosage from a stoppered vial and handling safety is compromised, an air-filled syringe should be used to equalize pressure in the stoppered vial. The volume of drug to be withdrawn can be replaced by injecting small amounts of air into the vial and withdrawing equal amounts of liquid until the required volume is withdrawn. The drug should be cleared from the needle and hub (neck) of the syringe before separating to reduce spraying on separation.

5. Handling Ampules

Prudent practice requires that ampules with dry material should be "*gently tapped down*" before opening to move any material in the top of the ampule to the bottom quantity. A sterile gauze pad should be wrapped around the ampule neck before breaking the top.[3] This can protect against cuts and catch airborne powder or aerosol. If diluent is to be added, it should be injected slowly down the inside wall of the ampule. The ampule should be tilted gently to ensure that all the powder is wet before agitating it to dissolve the contents.

After the solution is withdrawn from the ampule with a syringe, the needle should be cleared of solution by holding it vertically with the point upwards; the syringe should be tapped to remove air bubbles. Any bubbles should be expelled into a closed container.

6. Packaging HDs for Transport

The outside of bags or bottles containing the prepared drug should be wiped with moist gauze.

Entry ports should be wiped with moist alcohol pads and capped. Transport should occur in sealed plastic bags and in containers designed to avoid breakage.

HDs that are shipped and which are subject to EPA regulation as hazardous waste are also subject to Department of Transportation (DOT) regulations as specified in 49 CFR part 172.101.

7. Non-liquid HDs

The handling of non-liquid forms of HDs requires special precautions as well. Tablets that may produce dust or potential exposure to the handler should be counted in a BSC. Capsules, i.e., gel caps or coated tablets, are unlikely to produce dust unless broken in handling.

These are counted in a BSC on equipment designated for HDs only, because even manual counting devices may be covered with dust from the drugs handled. Automated counting machines should not be used unless an enclosed process isolates the hazard from the employee(s).

Compounding should also occur in a BSC. A gown and gloves should be worn. *(If a BSC is unavailable, an appropriate NIOSH-approved respirator must be worn.)*

Drug Administration

1. Personal Protective Equipment

The National Study Commission on Cytotoxic Exposure has recommended that personnel administering HDs wear gowns, latex gloves, and chemical splash goggles or equivalent safety glasses as described under the PPE section, preparation.[71] *NIOSH-approved respirators should be worn when administering aerosolized drugs.*

2. Administration Kit

Protective and administration equipment may be packaged together and labeled as an HD administration kit. Such a kit should include:

- personal protective equipment,
- gauze (4 × 4) for cleanup,
- alcohol wipes,
- disposable plastic-backed absorbent liner,
- puncture-resistant container for needles and syringes,
- a thick sealable plastic bag (with warning label), and
- accessory warning labels.

3. Work Practices

Safe work practices when handling HDs should include:

- Hands should be washed before donning and after removing gloves. Gowns or gloves that become contaminated should be changed immediately. Employees should be trained in proper methods to remove contaminated gloves and gowns. After use, gloves and gowns should be disposed of in accordance with ASHP recommendations.
- Infusion sets and pumps, which should have Luer-Lok fittings, should be observed for leakage during use. A plastic-backed absorbent pad should be placed under the tubing during administration to catch any leakage. Sterile gauze should be placed around any push sites; IV tubing connection sites should be taped.
- Priming IV sets or expelling air from syringes should be carried out in a BSC. If done at the administration site, ASHP recommends that the line be primed with non-drug-containing solution or that a backflow closed system be used. IV containers with venting tubes should not be used.[3]
- Syringes, IV bottles and bags, and pumps should be wiped clean of any drug contamination with sterile gauze. Needles and syringes should not be crushed or clipped. They should be placed in a puncture-resistant container then into the HD disposal bag with all other HD contaminated materials. Administration sets should be disposed of intact. Disposal of the waste bag should follow HD disposal requirements. Unused drugs should be returned to the pharmacy.
- Protective goggles should be cleaned with detergent and properly rinsed. All protective equipment should be disposed of upon leaving the patient care area.
- Nursing stations where these drugs will be administered should have spill and emergency skin and eye decontamination kits available and relevant MSDSs for guidance. The HCS requires MSDSs to be readily available in the workplace to all employees working with hazardous chemicals.
- PPE should be used during the administration of oral HDs if splashing is possible.

A large number of investigational HDs are under clinical study in health care facilities. Personnel not directly involved in the investigation should not administer these drugs unless they have received adequate instructions regarding safe handling procedures. Literature regarding potential toxic effects of investigational drugs should be evaluated prior to the drug's introduction into the workplace.[65]

The increased use of HDs in the home environment necessitates special precautions. Employees involved in home care delivery should follow the above work practices, and employers should make administration and spill kits available. Home health care workers should have emergency protocols with them as well as phone numbers and addresses in the event emergency care becomes necessary.[3] Waste disposal for drugs delivered for home use and other home-contaminated material should also be considered by the employer and should follow applicable regulations.

4. Aerosolized Drugs

The administration of aerosolized HDs requires special engineering controls to prevent exposure to health care workers and others in the vicinity. In the case of *pentamidine,* these controls include treatment booths with local exhaust ventilation designed specifically for its administration. A variety of ventilation methods have also been used for the administration of *ribavirin.* These include isolation rooms with separate HEPA-filtered ventilation systems and administration via endotracheal tube.[30,47] Engineering controls used to manage employee exposure to anesthetic gases is a traditional example of occupational chemical management. Both isolation and ventilation are used for these volatile HDs.

Caring for Patients Receiving HDs

In accordance with the Bloodborne Pathogens Standard, universal precautions must be observed to prevent contact with blood or other potentially infectious materials. Under circumstances in which differentiation between body fluid types is difficult or impossible, all body fluids should be considered potentially infectious materials and must be managed as dictated in the Bloodborne Pathogens Standard.[109]

1. Personal Protective Equipment

Personnel dealing with excreta, primarily urine, from patients who have received HDs in the last 48 hours should be provided with and wear latex or other appropriate gloves and disposable gowns, to be discarded after each use or whenever contaminated, as detailed under Waste Disposal. Eye protection should be worn if splashing is possible. Such excreta contaminated with blood, or other potentially infectious materials as well, should be managed according to the Bloodborne Pathogen Standard. Hands should be washed after removal of gloves or after contact with the above substances.

2. Linen

Linen contaminated with HDs or excreta from patients who have received HDs in the past 48 hours is a potential source of exposure to employees. Linen soiled with blood or other potentially infectious materials as well as contaminated with excreta must also be managed according to the Bloodborne Pathogens Standard.[109] Linen contaminated with HDs should be placed in specially marked laundry bags and then placed in a labeled, impervious bag. The laundry bag and its contents should be prewashed, and then the linens added to other laundry for a second wash. Laundry personnel should wear latex gloves and gowns while handling prewashed material.

3. Reusable Items

Glassware or other contaminated reusable items should be washed twice with detergent by a trained employee wearing double latex gloves and a gown.

Waste Disposal

1. Equipment

Thick, leakproof plastic bags, colored differently from other hospital trash bags, should be used for routine accumulation and collection of used containers, discarded gloves, gowns, and any other disposable material. Bags containing hazardous chemicals (as defined by Section C of HCS), shall be labeled in accordance with Section F of the Hazard Communication Standard where appropriate. Where the Hazard Communication Standard does not apply, labels should indicate that bags contain HD-related wastes.

Needles, syringes, and breakable items not contaminated with blood or other potentially infectious materials should be placed in a *"sharps"* container before they are stored in the waste bag. Such items that are contaminated with blood or other potentially infectious material *must* be placed in a *"sharps"* container. Similarly, needles should not be clipped or capped nor syringes crushed. If contaminated by blood or other potentially infectious material, such needles/syringes *must not* be clipped, capped, or crushed (except as on a rare instance where a *medical* procedure requires recapping). The waste bag should be kept inside a covered waste container clearly labeled "HD Waste Only." At least one such receptacle should be located in every area where the drugs are prepared or administered. Waste should not be moved from one area to another. The bag should be sealed when filled and the covered waste container taped.

2. Handling

Prudent practice dictates that every precaution be taken to prevent contamination of the exterior of the container. Personnel disposing of HD waste should wear gowns and protective gloves when handling waste containers with contaminated exteriors. Prudent practice further dictates that such a container with a contaminated exterior be placed in a second container in a manner that eliminates contamination of the second container. HD waste handlers should also receive hazard communication training as discussed below in Section H.

3. Disposal

Hazardous drug-related wastes should be handled separately from other hospital trash and disposed of in accordance with applicable EPA, state, and local regulations for hazardous waste.[24,110] This disposal can occur at either an incinerator or a licensed sanitary landfill for toxic wastes, as appropriate. Commercial waste disposal is performed by a licensed company. While awaiting removal, the waste should be held in a secure area in covered, labeled drums with plastic liners.

Chemical inactivation traditionally has been a complicated process that requires specialized knowledge and training. The MSDS should be consulted regarding specific advice on cleanup. IARC13 and Lunn et al.[56] have validated inactivation procedures for specific agents that are effective. However, these procedures vary from drug to drug and may be impractical for small amounts. Care must be taken because of unique problems presented by the cleanup of some agents, such as byproduct formation.[57] Serious consideration should be given to alternative disposal methods.

Spills

Emergency procedures to cover spills or inadvertent release of hazardous drugs should be included in the facility's overall health and safety program.

Incidental spills and breakages should be cleaned up immediately by a properly protected person trained in the appropriate procedures. The area should be identified with a warning sign to limit access to the area. Incident Reports should be filed to document the spill and those exposed.

1. Personnel Contamination

Contamination of protective equipment or clothing, or direct skin or eye contact should be treated by:

- Immediately removing the gloves or gown,
- Immediate cleansing of the affected skin with soap and water,
- Flooding an affected eye at an eyewash fountain or with water or isotonic eyewash designated for that purpose for at least 15 minutes, for eye exposure,
- Obtaining medical attention [Protocols for emergency procedures should be maintained at the designated sites for such medical care. Medical attention should also be sought for inhalation of HDs in powder form.],
- Documenting the exposure in the employee's medical record.

2. Cleanup of Small Spills

The ASHP considers small spills to be those less than 5 mL. The 5 mL volume of material should be used to categorize spills as large or small. Spills of less than 5 mL or 5 gm outside a BSC should be cleaned up immediately by personnel wearing gowns, double latex gloves, and splash goggles. *An appropriate NIOSH-approved respirator should be used for either powder or liquid spills where airborne powder or aerosol is or has been generated.*

- Liquids should be wiped with absorbent gauze pads; solids should be wiped with wet absorbent gauze. The spill areas should then be cleaned three times using a detergent solution followed by clean water.
- Any broken glass fragments should be picked up using a small scoop (never the hands) and placed in a "sharps" container. The container should then go into a HD disposal bag, along with used absorbent pads and any other contaminated waste.
- Contaminated reusable items, for example glassware and scoops, should be treated as outlined above under Reusable Items.

3. Cleanup of Large Spills

When a large spill occurs, the area should be isolated and aerosol generation avoided. For spills larger than 5 mL, liquid spread is limited by gently covering with absorbent sheets or spill-control pads or pillows. If a powder is involved, damp cloths or towels should be used. Specific individuals should be trained to clean up large spills.

- Protective apparel, including respirators, should be used as with small spills when there is any suspicion of airborne powder or that an aerosol has been or will be generated. Most

CDs are not volatile; however, this may not be true for all HDs. The volatility of the drug should be assessed in selecting the type of respiratory protection.

- As discussed under Waste Disposal, chemical inactivation should be avoided in this setting.
- All contaminated surfaces should be thoroughly cleaned three times with detergent and water.
- All contaminated absorbent sheets and other materials should be placed in the HD disposal bag.

4. Spills in BSCs

Extensive spills within a BSC necessitate decontamination of all interior BSC surfaces after completion of the spill cleanup. The ASHP3 recommends this action for spills larger than 150 mL or the contents of one vial. If the HEPA filter of a BSC is contaminated, the unit should be labeled and sealed in plastic until the filter can be changed and disposed of properly by trained personnel wearing appropriate protective equipment.

5. Spill Kits

Spill kits, clearly labeled, should be kept in or near preparation and administrative areas. The MSDSs include sections on emergency procedures, including appropriate personal protective equipment. The ASHP recommends that kits include: chemical splash goggles, two pairs of gloves, utility gloves, a low-permeability gown, two sheets (12″ × 12″) of absorbent material, 250-mL and liter spill control pillows, a *"sharps"* container, a small scoop to collect glass fragments, and two large HD waste-disposal bags.[3]

Prior to cleanup, appropriate protective equipment should be donned. Absorbent sheets should be incinerable. Protective goggles and respirators should be cleaned with mild detergent and water after use.

Storage and Transport

1. Storage Areas

Access to areas where HDs are stored should be limited to authorized personnel with signs restricting entry.[72] A list of drugs covered by HD policies and information on spill and emergency contact procedures should be posted or easily available to employees. Facilities used for storing HDs should not be used for other drugs, and should be designed to prevent containers from falling to the floor, e.g., bins with barrier fronts. Warning labels should be applied to all HD containers, as well as the shelves and bins where these containers are permanently stored.

2. Receiving Damaged HD Packages

Damaged shipping cartons should be opened in an isolated area or a BSC by a designated employee wearing double gloves, a gown, goggles, and appropriate respiratory protection. Individuals must be trained to process damaged packages as well.

The ASHP recommends that broken containers and contaminated packaging mats be placed in a *"sharps"* container and then into HD disposal bags.[3] The bags should then be closed and placed in receptacles as described under Waste Disposal.

The appropriate protective equipment and waste disposal materials should be kept in the area where shipments are received, and employees should be trained in their use and the risks of exposure to HDs.

3. Transport

HDs should be securely capped or sealed, placed in sealed clear plastic bags, and transported in containers designed to avoid breakage.

Personnel involved in transporting HDs should be trained in spill procedures, including sealing off the contaminated area and calling for appropriate assistance.

All HD containers should be labeled as noted in Drug Preparation Work Practices. If transport methods that produce stress on contents, such as pneumatic tubes are used, guidance from the OSHA clarification of 1910.1030 with respect to transport (M.4.b.(8)(c)) should be followed. This clarification provides for use of packaging material inside the tube to prevent breakage. These recommendations that pertain to the Bloodborne Pathogens Standard are prudent practice for HDs, e.g., padded inserts for carriers.

F. Medical Surveillance

Workers who are potentially exposed to chemical hazards should be monitored in a systematic program or medical surveillance intended to prevent occupational injury and disease.[3,7] The purpose of surveillance is to identify the earliest reversible biologic effects so that exposure can be reduced or eliminated before the employee sustains irreversible damage. The occurrence of exposure-related disease or other adverse health effects should prompt immediate re-evaluation of primary preventive measures (e.g., engineering controls, personal protective equipment). In this manner, medical surveillance acts as a check on the appropriateness of controls already in use.[62]

For detection and control of work-related health effects, *job-specific* medical evaluations should be performed:

- before job placement,
- periodically during employment,
- following acute exposures, and
- at the time of job termination or transfer (exit examination).

This information should be collected and analyzed in a systematic fashion to allow early detection of disease patterns in individual workers and groups of workers.

1. Pre-placement Medical Examinations

Sound medical practice dictates that employees who will be working with HDs in the workplace have an initial evaluation consisting of a history, physical exam, and laboratory studies.

Information made available, by the employer, to the examining physician should be:

- a description of the employee's duties as they relate to the employee's exposure,
- the employee's exposure levels or anticipated exposure levels,
- a description of any personal protective equipment used or to be used, and
- information from previous medical examinations of the employee, which is not readily available to the examining physician.

The history details the individual's medical and reproductive experience with emphasis on potential risk factors, such as past hematopoietic, malignant, or hepatic disorders. It also includes a complete occupational history with information on extent of past exposures (including environmental sampling data, if possible) and use of protective equipment. Surrogates for worker exposure, in the absence of environmental sampling data, include:

- records of drugs and quantities handled,

- hours spent handling these drugs per week,
- number of preparations/administrations per week.

The physical examination should be complete, but the skin, mucous membranes, cardiopulmonary, lymphatic system, and liver should be emphasized. An evaluation for respirator use must be performed in accordance with 29 CFR 1910.134, if the employee will wear a respirator. The laboratory assessment may include a complete blood count with differential, liver function tests, blood urea nitrogen, creatinine, and a urine dipstick. Other aspects of the physical and laboratory evaluation should be guided by known toxicities of the HD of exposure. Due to poor reproducibility, interindividual variability, and lack of prognostic value regarding disease development, no biological monitoring tests (e.g., genotoxic markers) are currently recommended for routine use in employee surveillance. Biological marker testing should be performed only within the context of a research protocol.

2. Periodic Medical Examinations

Recognized occupational medicine experts in the HD area recommend these exams to update the employee's medical, reproductive, and exposure histories. They are recommended on a yearly basis or every 2–3 years. The interval between exams is a function of the opportunity for exposure, duration of exposure, and possibly the age of the worker at the discretion of the occupational medicine physician, guided by the worker's history. Careful documentation of an individual's routine exposure and any acute accidental exposures are made. The physical examination and laboratory studies follow the format outlined in the pre-placement examination.[54]

3. Post-exposure Examinations

Post-exposure evaluation is tailored to the type of exposure (e.g., spills or needle sticks from syringes containing HDs). An assessment of the extent of exposure is made and included in the confidential database (discussed below) and in an incident report. The physical examination focuses on the involved area as well as other organ systems commonly affected (i.e., for CDs the skin and mucous membranes; for aerosolized HDs the pulmonary system). Treatment and laboratory studies follow as indicated and should be guided by emergency protocols.

4. Exit Examinations

The exit examination completes the information on the employee's medical, reproductive and exposure histories. Examination and laboratory evaluation should be guided by the individual's history of exposures and follow the outline of the periodic evaluation.

5. Exposure/Health Outcome Linkage

Exposure assessment of all employees who have worked with HDs is important, and the maintenance of records is required by 29 CFR 1910.20. The use of previously outlined exposure surrogates is acceptable, although actual environmental or employee monitoring data is preferable. An MSDS can serve as an exposure record. Details of the use of personal protective equipment and engineering controls present should be included. A confidential database should be maintained with information regarding the individual's medical and reproductive history, with linkage to exposure information to facilitate epidemiologic review.

6. Reproductive Issues

The examining physician should consider the reproductive status of employees and inform them regarding relevant reproductive issues. The reproductive toxicity of hazardous drugs should be carefully explained to all workers who will be exposed to these chemicals, and is required for those chemicals covered by the HCS. Unfortunately, no information is available regarding the reproductive risks of HD handling with the current use of BSCs and PPE. However, as discussed earlier, both spontaneous abortion and congenital malformation excesses have been documented among workers handling some of these drugs without currently recommended engineering controls and precautions. The facility should have a policy regarding reproductive toxicity of HDs and worker exposure in male and female employees and should follow that policy.

G. Hazard Communication

> *This section is for informational purposes only and is not a substitute for the requirements of the Hazard Communication Standard.*

The Hazard Communication Standard (HCS),107 is applicable to some drugs. It defines a hazardous chemical as *any chemical that is a physical hazard or a health hazard.*

Physical hazard refers to characteristics such as combustibility or reactivity. A health hazard is defined as *a chemical for which there is statistically significant evidence based on at least one study conducted in accordance with established scientific principles that acute or chronic health effects may occur in exposed employees.* Appendixes A and B of the HCS outline the criteria used to determine whether an agent is hazardous.

According to HCS Appendix A, agents with any of the following characteristics would be considered hazardous:

- carcinogens,
- corrosives,
- toxic or highly toxic (defined on the basis of median lethal doses),
- irritants,
- sensitizers, or
- target organ effectors, including reproductive toxins, hepatotoxins, nephrotoxins, neurotoxins, agents that act on the hematopoietic system, and agents that damage the lungs, skin, eyes, or mucous membranes.

Both human and animal data are to be used in this determination. HCS Appendix C lists sources of toxicity information.

As a result of the February 21, 1990 Supreme Court decision,21 all provisions of the Hazard Communication Standard [29 CFR 1910.1200]107 are now in effect for all industrial segments. This includes the coverage of drugs and pharmaceuticals in the non-manufacturing sector. On February 9, 1994, OSHA issued a revised Hazard Communication Final Rule with technical clarification regarding drugs and pharmaceutical agents.

The Hazard Communication Standard (HCS) requires that drugs posing a health hazard (with the exception of those in solid, final form for direct administration to the patient, i.e., tablets or pills) be included on lists of hazardous chemicals to which employees are exposed.[107] Their storage and use locations can be confirmed by reviewing purchasing office records of currently used and past used agents such as those in Table I.1. Employee exposure records, including workplace monitoring, biological monitoring, and MSDSs, as well as employee medical records related to drugs posing a health hazard must be maintained and access to them provided to employees in accordance with 29 CFR 1910.20. Training required under the HCS should include all employees potentially exposed to these agents, not only health care professional staff, but also physical plant, maintenance, or support staff.

MSDSs are required to be prepared and transmitted with the initial shipment of all hazardous chemicals including covered drugs and pharmaceutical products. This excludes drugs defined by the Federal Food, Drug and Cosmetic Act, which are in solid, final form for direct administration to the patient (e.g., tablets, pills, or capsules) or which are packaged for sale to consumers in a retail establishment. Package inserts and the *Physicians' Desk Reference* are not acceptable in lieu of requirements of MSDSs under the Standard. Items mandated by the Standard will use the term *shall* instead of *should.*

1. Written Hazard Communication Program

Employers shall develop, implement, and maintain at the workplace, a written hazard communication program for employees handling or otherwise exposed to chemicals, including drugs that represent a health hazard to employees. The written program will describe how the criteria specified in the Standard concerning labels and other forms of warning, MSDSs, and employee information and training will be met. This also includes the following:

- a list of the covered hazardous drugs known to be present using an identity that is referenced on the appropriate MSDS,
- the methods the employer will use to inform employees of the hazards of non-routine tasks in their work areas, and
- the methods the employer will use to inform employees of other employers of hazards at the worksite.

The employer shall make the written hazard communication program available, upon request, to employees, their designated representatives, and the Assistant Secretary of OSHA in accordance with requirements of the HCS.

2. MSDSs

In accordance with requirements in the Hazard Communication Standard, the employer must maintain MSDSs accessible to employees for all covered HDs used in the hospital. Specifics regarding MSDS content are contained in the Standard. Essential information includes: health hazards, primary exposure routes, carcinogenic evaluations, acute exposure treatment, chemical inactivators, solubility, stability, volatility, PPE-required and spill procedures for each covered HD. MSDSs shall also be made readily available upon request to employees, their designated representatives, or the Assistant Secretary of OSHA.

H. Training and Information Dissemination

In compliance with the Hazard Communication Standard, all personnel involved in any aspect of the handling of covered HDs (physicians, nurses, pharmacists, housekeepers, employees involved in receiving, transport, or storage) must receive information and training to appraise them of the hazards of HDs present in the work area.[71] Such information should be provided at the time of an employee's initial assignment to a work area where HDs are present and prior to assignments involving new hazards. The employer should provide annual refresher information and training.

The National Study Commission on Cytotoxic Exposure has recommended that knowledge and competence of personnel be evaluated after the first orientation or training session, and then yearly, or more often if a need is perceived.[71] Evaluation may involve direct observation of an individual's performance on the job. In addition, non-HD solutions should be used for evaluation of preparation technique; quinine, which will fluoresce under ultraviolet light, provides an easy mechanism for evaluation of technique.

1. Employee Information

Employees must be informed of the requirements of the Hazard Communication Standard, 29 CFR 1910.1200

- any operation/procedure in their work area where drugs that present a hazard are present, and
- the location and availability of the written hazard communication program.

In addition, they should be informed regarding:

- any operations or procedure in their work area where other HDs are present, and
- the location and availability of any other plan regarding HDs.

2. Employee Training

Employee training must include at least:

- methods of observations that may be used to detect the presence or release of a HCS-covered hazardous drug in the work area (such as monitoring conducted by the employer, continuous monitoring devices, visual appearance, or odor of covered HDs being released, etc.),
- the physical and health hazards of the covered HDs in the area,
- the measures employees can take to protect themselves from these hazards. This includes specific procedures that the employer has implemented to protect the employees from exposure to such drugs, such as identification of covered drugs and those to be handled as hazardous, appropriate work practices, emergency procedures (for spills or employee exposure), and personal protective equipment, and
- the details of the hazard communication program developed by the employer, including an explanation of the labeling system and the MSDS, and how employees can obtain and use the appropriate hazard information.

It is essential that workers understand the carcinogenic potential and reproductive hazards of these drugs. Both females and males should understand the importance of avoiding exposure, especially early in pregnancy, so they can make informed decisions about the hazards involved. In addition, the facility's policy regarding reproductive toxicity of HDs should be explained to workers. Updated information should be provided to employees on a regular basis and whenever their jobs involve new hazards. Medical staff and other personnel who are not hospital employees should be informed of hospital policies and of the expectation that they will comply with these policies.

I. Record Keeping

Any workplace-exposure record created in connection with HD handling shall be kept, transferred, and made available for at least thirty years and medical records shall be kept for the duration of employment plus thirty years in accordance with the Access to Employee Exposure and Medical Records Standard (29 CFR 1910.20).[108] In addition, sound practice dictates that training records should include the following information:

- the dates of the training sessions,
- the contents or a summary of the training sessions,
- the names and qualifications of the persons conducting the training, and
- the names and job titles of all persons attending the training sessions.

Training records should be maintained for three years from the date on which the training occurred.

Position Statement

For the handling of cytotoxic agents by women who are pregnant, attempting to conceive, or breastfeeding. There are substantial data regarding the mutagenic, teratogenic, and abortifacient properties of certain cytotoxic agents both in animals and humans who have received therapeutic doses of these agents. Additionally, the scientific literature suggests a possible association of occupational exposure to certain cytotoxic agents during the first trimester of pregnancy with fetal loss or malformation. These data suggest the need for caution when women who are pregnant, or attempting to conceive, handle cytotoxic agents. Incidentally, there is no evidence relating male exposure to cytotoxic agents with adverse fetal outcome. There are no studies that address the possible risk associated with the occupational exposure to cytotoxic agents and the passage of these agents into breast milk. Nevertheless, it is prudent that women who are breast-feeding should exercise caution in handling cytotoxic agents.

If all procedures for safe handling, such as those recommended by the Commission, are complied with, the potential for exposure will be minimized. Personnel should be provided with information to make an individual decision. This information should be provided in written form, and it is advisable that a statement of understanding be signed. It is essential to refer to individual state right-to-know laws to ensure compliance.

Approved by the National Study Commission on Cytotoxic Exposure, September 1987.

References

1. American Medical Association Council on Scientific Affairs. Guidelines for handling parenteral antineoplastics. *JAMA* 1985;253:1590–2
2. American National Standards Institute. Occupational and Educational Eye and Face Protection. *ANSI* 1968;Z87:1
3. American Society of Hospital Pharmacists. ASHP Technical Assistance Bulletin on Handling Cytotoxic and Hazardous Drugs. *Am. J. Hosp. Pharm.* 1990;47:1033–49
4. Andersen R, Boedicker M, Ma M, Goldstein EJC. Adverse Reactions Associated with Pentamidine Isethionate in AIDS Patients: Recommendations for Monitoring Therapy. *Drug Intell. Clin. Pharm.* 1986;20:862–8
5. Anderson RW, Puckett WH, Dana WJ, et al. Risk of handling injectable antineoplastic agents. *Am. J. Hosp. Pharm.* 1982;39:1881–87
6. Avis KE, Levchuck JW. Special considerations in the use of vertical laminar flow workbenches. *Am. J. Hosp. Pharm.* 1984;41:81–7
7. Barber RK. Fetal and neonatal effects of cytotoxic agents. *Obstet. Gynecol.* 1981;51: 41S–47S

8. Benhamou S, Pot-Deprun J, Sancho-Garnier H, Chouroulinkov I. Sister chromatid exchanges and chromosomal aberrations in lymphocytes of nurses handling cytostatic drugs. *Int. J. Cancer* 1988;41:350–3
9. Bos RP, Leenars AO, Theuws JL, Henderson PT. Mutagenicity of urine from nurses handling cytostatic drugs, influence of smoking. *Int. Arch. Occ. Envir. Health* 1982; 50:359–69
10. Bryan D, Marback RC. Laminar-airflow equipment certification: What the pharmacist needs to know. *Am. J. Hosp. Pharm.* 1984;41:1343–9
11. Burgaz S, Ozdamar YN, Karakaya AE. A signal assay for the detection of toxic compounds: Application on the urines of cancer patients on chemotherapy and of nurses handling cytotoxic drugs. *Human Toxicol.* 1988;7:557–60
12. California Department of Health Services Occupational Health Surveillance and Evaluation Program. *Health care worker exposure to ribavirin aerosol: field investigation FI-86-009.* Berkeley: California Department of Health Services. 1986
13. Castegnaro M, Adams J, Armour MA, eds, et al. *Laboratory decontamination and destruction of carcinogens in laboratory wastes: Some antineoplastic agents.* International Agency for Research on Cancer. Scientific Publications No. 73. Lyons, France: IARC 1985
14. Chapman RM. Effect of cytotoxic therapy on sexuality and gonadal function. Perry MC, Yarbro JW, (eds), *Toxicity of Chemotherapy* Orlando: Grune & Stratton.1984; 343–363
15. Chen CH, Vazquez-Padua M, Cheng YC. Effect of antihuman immunodeficiency virus nucleoside analogs on mDNA and its implications for delayed toxicity. *Mol. Pharm.* 1990;39:625–628
16. Christensen CJ, Lemasters GK, Wakeman MA. Work practices and policies of hospital pharmacists preparing antineoplastic agents. *J. Occup. Med.* 1990;32:508–12
17. Chrysostomou A, Morley AA, Seshadri R. Mutation frequency in nurses and pharmacists working with cytotoxic drugs. *Aust. N. Z. J. Med.* 1984;14:831–4
18. Connor JD, Hintz M, Van Dyke R. Ribavirin pharmacokinetics in children and adults during therapeutic trials. Smith RA, Knight V, Smith JAD, (eds), *In Clinical Applications of Ribavirin* Orlando: Academic Press, 1984
19. Connor TH, Laidlaw JL, Theiss JC, et al. Permeability of latex and polyvinyl chloride gloves to carmustine. *Am. J. Hosp. Pharm.* 1984;41:676–9
20. Crudi CB. A compounding dilemma: I've kept the drug sterile but have I contaminated myself? *Nat. Intra. Therapy J.* 1980;3:77–80
21. Dole *v.* United Steelworkers. 1990;494 U.S.26.
22. Doll C. Aerosolised pentamidine. *Lancet* 1989;ii:1284–5
23. Duvall E, Baumann B. An unusual accident during the administration of chemotherapy. *Cancer Nurs.* 1980;3:305–6
24. Environmental Protection Agency. *Discarded commercial chemical products, off specification species, container residues, and spill residues thereof.* 40 CFR:1991; 261.33(f)
25. Everson RB, Ratcliffe JM, Flack PM, et al. Detection of low levels of urinary mutagen excretion by chemotherapy workers which was not related to occupational drug exposures. *Cancer Research* 1985;45:6487–97
26. Falck K, Grohn P, Sorsa M, et al. Mutagenicity in urine of nurses handling cytostatic drugs. *Lancet* 1979;i:1250–1
27. Falck K, Sorsa M, Vainio H. Use of the bacterial fluctuation test to detect mutagenicity in urine of nurses handling cytostatic drugs (abstract). *Mutation Res.* 1981;85: 236–7

28. Ferguson LR, Everts R, Robbie MA, et al. The use within New Zealand of cytogenetic approaches to monitoring of hospital pharmacists for exposure to cytotoxic drugs: Report of a pilot study in Auckland. *Aust J Hosp Pharm.* 1988;18:228–33
29. Gude JK. Selective delivery of pentamidine to the lung by aerosol. *Am. Rev. Resp. Dis.* 1989;139:1060
30. Guglielmo BJ, Jacobs RA, Locksley RM. The exposure of health care workers to ribavirin aerosol. *JAMA* 1989;261:1880–1
31. Harrison R, Bellows J, Rempel D, et al. Assessing exposures of health-care personnel to aerosols of ribavirin—California. *Morbidity and Mortality Weekly Report* 1988;37:560–3
32. Hemminki K, Kyyronen P, Lindbohm ML. Spontaneous abortions and malformations in the offspring of nurses exposed to anaesthetic gases, cytostatic drugs, and other potential hazards in hospitals, based on registered information of outcome. *J. Epidem. Comm. Health* 1985;39:141–7
33. Henderson DK, Gerberding JL. Prophylactic zidovudine after occupational exposure to the human immunodeficiency virus: An interim analysis. *J. Infectious Diseases* 1989;160:321–7
34. Hillyard IW. The preclinical toxicology and safety of ribavirin. Smith RA, Kirkpatrick W, (eds), *In Ribavirin: a broad spectrum antiviral agent.* New York: Academic Press 1980
35. Hirst M, Tse S, Mills DG, et al. Occupational exposure to cyclophosphamide. *Lancet* 1984;i:186–8
36. Hoy RH, Stump LM. Effect of an air-venting filter device on aerosol production from vials. *Am. J. Hosp. Pharm.* 1984;41:324–6
37. International Agency for Research on Cancer. *IARC Monographs on the Evaluation of the Carcinogenic Risk of Chemicals to Man: Some Aziridines, N-, S-, and O-mustards and selenium. Lyons, France.* 1975;Vol. 9
38. International Agency for Research on Cancer. *IARC Monographs on the Evaluation of the Carcinogenic Risk of Chemicals to Man: Some naturally occurring substances.* Lyons, France: IARC. 1976;Vol. 10
39. International Agency for Research on Cancer. *IARC Monographs on the Evaluation of the Carcinogenic Risk of Chemicals to Humans: Some Antineoplastic and Immunosuppressive Agents.* Lyons, France: IARC. 1981;Vol. 26
40. International Agency for Research on Cancer. *IARC Monographs on the Evaluation of the Carcinogenic Risk of Chemicals to Humans: Chemicals, Industrial Processes and Industries Associated with Cancer in Humans.* Lyons, France: IARC. 1982;Vol. 1–29 (Suppl. 4)
41. International Agency for Research on Cancer. *IARC Monographs on the Evaluation of the Carcinogenic Risk of Chemicals to Humans: Genetic and related effects: An updating of selected IARC Monographs from Volumes 1–42.* Lyons, France: IARC. 1987;Vol. 1–42 (Suppl. 6)
42. International Agency for Research on Cancer. *IARC Monographs on the Evaluation of the Carcinogenic Risk of Chemicals to Humans; Overall evaluations of carcinogenicity: An updating of IARC Monographs Volumes 1 to 42.* Lyons, France: IARC. 1987;Vol. 1–42 (Suppl. 7)
43. International Agency for Research on Cancer. *IARC Monographs on the Evaluation of the Carcinogenic Risk of Chemicals to Humans: Pharmaceutical Drugs.* Lyons, France: IARC.
44. Jagun O, Ryan M, Waldron HA. Urinary thioether excretion in nurses handling cytotoxic drugs. *Lancet* 1982;i:443–4

45. Johnson EG, Janosik JE. Manufacturer's recommendations for handling spilled antineoplastic agents. *Am. J. Hosp. Pharm.* 1989;46:318–9
46. Juma FD, Rogers HJ, Trounce JR, Bradbrook ID. Pharmacokinetics of intravenous cyclophosphamide in man, estimated by gas-liquid chromatography. *Cancer Chemother. Pharmacol.* 1978;1:229–31
47. Kacmarek RM. Ribavirin and pentamidine aerosols: Caregiver beware! *Respiratory Care* 1990;35:1034–6
48. Karakaya AE, Burgaz S, Bayhan A. The significance of urinary thioethers as indicators of exposure to alkylating agents. *Arch. Toxicol.* 1989;13(suppl):117–9
49. Kilham L, Ferm VH. Congenital anomalies induced in hamster embryos with ribavirin. *Science* 1977;195:413–4
50. Kleinberg ML, Quinn MJ. Airborne drug levels in a laminar-flow hood. *Am. J. Hosp. Pharm.* 1981;38:1301–3
51. Kolmodin-Hedman B, Hartvig P, Sorsa M, Falck K. Occupational handling of cytostatic drugs. *Arch. Toxicol.* 1983;54:25–33
52. Kyle RA. Second malignancies associated with chemotherapy. Perry MC, Yarbro JW, (eds), *Toxicity of Chemotherapy.* Orlando: Grune & Stratton.1984;479–506
53. Laidlaw JL, Connor TH, Theiss JC, et al. Permeability of latex and polyvinyl chloride gloves to 20 antineoplastic drugs. *Am. J. Hosp. Pharm.* 1984;41:2618–23
54. Laidlaw JL, Connor TH, Theiss JC, et al. Permeability of four disposable protective clothing materials to seven antineoplastic drugs. *Am. J. Hosp. Pharm.* 1985;42: 2449–54
55. Lee SB. Ribavirin—Exposure to health care workers. *Am. Ind. Hyg. Assoc.* 1988;49: A13–A14
56. LeRoy ML, Roberts MJ, Theisen JA. Procedures for handling antineoplastic injections in comprehensive cancer centers. *Am. J. Hosp. Pharm.* 1983;40:601–3
57. Lunn G, Sansone EB. Validated methods for handling spilled antineoplastic agents. *Am. J. Hosp. Pharm.* 1989;46:1131
58. Lunn G, Sansone EB, Andrews AW, Hellwig LC. Degradation and disposal of some antineoplastic drugs. *J. Pharm. Sciences.* 1989;78:652–9
59. Matthews T, Boehme R. Antiviral activity and mechanism of action of ganciclovir. *Rev. Infect. Diseases* 1988;10 (suppl 3):S490–94
60. McDevitt JJ, Lees PSJ, McDiarmid MA. Exposure of hospital pharmacists and nurses to antineoplastic agents. *J. Occup. Med.* 1993;35:57–60
61. McDiarmid MA, Egan T, Furio M, et al. Sampling for airborne fluorouracil in a hospital drug preparation area. *Am. J. Hosp. Pharm.* 1988;43:1942–5
62. McDiarmid MA, Emmett EA. Biological monitoring and medical surveillance of workers exposed to antineoplastic agents. *Seminars in Occup. Med.* 1987;2:109–17
63. McDiarmid MA, Jacobson-Kram D. Aerosolized pentamidine and public health. *Lancet* 1989;ii:863
64. McDiarmid MA. Medical surveillance for antineoplastic-drug handlers. *Am. J. Hosp. Pharm.* 1990;47:1061–6
65. McDiarmid MA, Gurley HT, Arrington D. Pharmaceuticals as hospital hazards: Managing the risks. *J. Occup. Med.* 1991;33:155–8
66. McDiarmid MA, Kolodner K, Humphrey F, et al. Baseline and phosphoramide mustard-induced sister chromatid exchanges in pharmacists handling anti-cancer drugs. *Mutation Research* 1992;279:199–204
67. McDiarmid MA, Schaefer J, Richard CL, Chaisson RE, Tepper BS. Efficacy of engineering controls in reducing occupational exposure to aerosolized pentamidine. *Chest* 1992;102:1764–6

68. McEvoy GK, ed. *American Hospital Formulary Service Drug Information.* Bethesda: American Society of Hospital Pharmacists, 1993
69. McLendon BF, Bron AF. Corneal toxicity from vinblastine solution. *Br. J. Ophthalmol.* 1978;62:97–9
70. National Sanitation Foundation. *Standard No. 49 for Class II (Laminar Flow) Biohazard Cabinetry.* Ann Arbor: National Sanitation Foundation, 1990
71. National Study Commission on Cytotoxic Exposure. Louis P Jeffrey Sc.D Chairman, (eds), *Recommendations for Handling Cytotoxic Agents.* Providence, Rhode Island: Rhode Island Hospital, 1983
72. National Study Commission on Cytotoxic Exposure. Consensus Responses to Unresolved Questions Concerning Cytotoxic Agents. Louis P Jeffrey Sc. D, (eds), Providence, Rhode Island. Chairman, Rhode Island Hospital, 1984
73. Neal AD, Wadden RA, Chiou WL. Exposure of hospital workers to airborne antineoplastic agents. *Am. J. Hosp. Pharm.* 1983;40:597–601
74. Nikula E, Kiviniitty K, Leisti J, Taskinen P. Chromosome aberrations in lymphocytes of nurses handling cytostatic agents. *Scand. J. Work Environ. Health.* 1984;10:71–4
75. Norppa H, Sorsa M, Vainio H, et al. Increased sister chromatid exchange frequencies in lymphocytes of nurses handling cytostatic drugs. *Scand. J. Work Environ. Health* 1980;6:299–301
76. Nguyen TV, Theiss JC, Matney TS. Exposure of pharmacy personnel to mutagenic antineoplastic drugs. *Cancer Research* 42:4792–6
77. Palmer RG, Dore CJ, Denman AM. Chlorambucil-induced chromosome damage to human lymphocytes is dose-dependent and cumulative. *Lancet* 1984;i:246–9
78. Perry MC, Yarbro JW, eds. *Toxicity of Chemotherapy.* Orlando: Grune & Stratton. 1984
79. Physician's Desk Reference. Barnhart ER, (eds), *Physician's Desk Reference,* 45th ed. Oradell, New Jersey: Medical Economics Data.1991;730
80. Pohlova H, Cerna M, Rossner P. Chromosomal aberrations, SCE and urine mutagenicity in workers occupationally exposed to cytostatic drugs. *Mutation Res.* 1986;174: 213–7
81. Pyy L, Sorsa M, Hakala E. Ambient monitoring of cyclophosphamide in manufacture and hospitals. *Am. Ind. Hyg. Assoc. J.* 1988;49:314–7
82. Reich SD, Bachur NR. Contact dermatitis associated with adriamycin (NSC-123127) and daunorubicin (NSC-82151). *Cancer Chemotherap. Reports* 1975;59:677–8
83. Reynolds RD, Ignoffo R, Lawrence J, et al. Adverse reactions to AMSA in medical personnel. *Cancer Treat. Rep.* 1982;66:1885
84. Rogers B. Health hazards to personnel handling antineoplastic agents. *Occupational Medicine: State of the Art Reviews* 1987;2:513–24
85. Rogers B, Emmett EA. Handling antineoplastic agents: Urine mutagenicity in nurses. *IMAGE Journal of Nursing Scholarship.* 1987;19:108–113
86. Rosner F. Acute leukemia as a delayed consequence of cancer chemotherapy. *Cancer* 1976;37:1033–6
87. Rudolph R, Suzuki M, Luce JK. Experimental skin necrosis produced by adriamycin. *Cancer Treat. Reports* 1979;63:529–37
88. Schafer AI. Teratogenic effects of antileukemic therapy. *Arch. Int. Med.* 1981;141: 514–5
89. Selevan SG, Lindbolm ML, Homung RW, Hemminki K. A study of occupational exposure to antineoplastic drugs and fetal loss in nurses. *New Engl. J. Med.* 1985;313: 1173–8
90. Sieber SM. Cancer chemotherapeutic agents and carcinogenesis. *Cancer Chemotherap. Reports* 1975;59:915–8

91. Sieber SM, Adamson RH. Toxicity of antineoplastic agents in man: Chromosomal aberrations, antifertility effects, congenital malformations, and carcinogenic potential. *Adv. Cancer Res.* 1975;22:57–155
92. Siebert D, Simon U. Cyclophosphamide: Pilot study of genetically active metabolites in the urine of a treated human patient. *Mutat. Res.* 1973;19:65–72
93. Slevin ML, Ang LM, Johnston A, Turner P. The efficiency of protective gloves used in the handling of cytotoxic drugs. *Cancer Chemo. Pharmacol.* 1984;12:151–3
94. Smaldone GC, Vincicuerra C, Marchese J. Detection of inhaled pentamidine in health care workers. *New Engl. J. Med.* 1991;325:891–2
95. Sorsa M, Hemminki K, Vanio H. Occupational exposure to anticancer drugs—Potential and real hazards. *Mut. Res.* 1985;154:135–49
96. Sotaniemi EA, Sutinen S, Arranto AJ, et al. Liver damage in nurses handling cytostatic agents. *Acta Med. Scand.* 1983;214:181–9
97. Stellman JM. The spread of chemotherapeutic agents at work: Assessment through stimulation. *Cancer Investigation* 1987;5:75–81
98. Stephens JD, Golbus MS, Miller TR, et al. Multiple congenital abnormalities in a fetus exposed to 5-fluorouracil during the first trimester. *Am. J. Obstet. Gynecol.* 1980;137:747–9
99. Stiller A, Obe G, Bool I, Pribilla W. No elevation of the frequencies of chromosomal aberrations as a consequence of handling cytostatic drugs. *Mut. Res.* 1983;121:253–9
100. Stoikes ME, Carlson JD, Farris FF, Walker PR. Permeability of latex and polyvinyl chloride gloves to fluorouracil and methotrexate. *Am. J. Hosp. Pharm.* 1987;44: 1341–6
101. Stucker I, Hirsch A, Doloy T, et al. Urine mutagenicity, chromosomal abnormalities and sister chromatid exchanges in lymphocytes of nurses handling cytostatic drugs. *Int. Arch. Occup. Environ. Health* 1986;57:195–205
102. Stucker I, Caillard JF, Collin R, et al. Risk of spontaneous abortion among nurses handling antineoplastic drugs. *Scand. J. Work Environ. Health* 1990;16:102–7
103. U.S. Department of Health and Human Services. Public Health Service. National Institutes of Health. *Recommendations for the Safe Handling of Cytotoxic Drugs.* NIH Publication No. 92-2621. 1992
104. U.S. Department of Health and Human Services. Public Health Service. Centers for Disease Control. National Institute for Occupational Safety and Health. *Guidelines for Protecting the Safety and Health of Health Care Workers.* DHHS (NIOSH) Publication No. 88-119. 1988
105. U.S. Department of Labor, Occupational Safety and Health Administration. *Respiratory Protection Standard.* 1984;29 CFR 1910.134
106. U.S. Department of Labor, Occupational Safety and Health Administration. *Work practice guidelines for personnel dealing with cytotoxic (antineoplastic) drugs.* OSHA Publication #8-1.1. 1986
107. U.S. Department of Labor, Occupational Safety and Health Administration. *Hazard Communication Standard.* 1989;29 CFR 1910.1200, as amended February 9, 1994.
108. U.S. Department of Labor, Occupational Safety and Health Administration. *Access to Employee and Medical Records Standard.* 1990;29 CFR 1910.20
109. U.S. Department of Labor, Occupational Safety and Health Administration. *Occupational Exposure to Bloodborne Pathogens Standard.* 1991;29 CFR 1910.1030
110. Vaccari FL, Tonat K, DeChristoforo R, et al. Disposal of antineoplastic waste at the NIH. *Am. J. Hosp. Pharm.* 1984;41:87–92
111. Valanis B, Vollmer WM, Labuhn K, Glass A, Corelle C. Antineoplastic drug handling protection after OSHA guidelines: Comparison by profession, handling activity, and work site. *J. Occup. Med.* 1992;34:149–55

112. Venitt S, Crofton-Sleigh C, Hunt J, et al. Monitoring exposure of nursing and pharmacy personnel to cytotoxic drugs. Urinary mutation assays and urinary platinum as markers of absorption. *Lancet* 1984;i:74:6
113. Waksvik H, Klepp O, Brogger A. Chromosome analyses of nurses handling cytostatic agents. *Cancer Treat. Reports* 1981;65:607–10
114. Wall RL, Clausen KP. Carcinoma of the urinary bladder in patients receiving cyclophosphamide. *New Engl. J. Med.* 1975;293:271–3
115. Weisburger JH, Griswold DP, Prejean JD, et al. Tumor induction by cytostatics. The carcinogenic properties of some of the principal drugs used in clinical cancer chemotherapy. *Recent Results Cancer Res.* 1975;52:1–17
116. Zimmerman PF, Larsen RK, Barkley EW, Gallelli JF. Recommendations for the safe handling of injectable antineoplastic drug products. *Am. J. Hosp. Pharm.* 1981; 38:1693–5

Appendix 2

Common Toxicity Criteria for Adverse Events v. 3.0 (CTCAE)

Source: From *National Cancer Institute Common Toxicity Criteria, Version 2.0* [Online], revised March 23, 1998. Available: http:/ ctep.info.nih.gov/CTC3/ctc.htm

Appendix 2

ALLERGY/IMMUNOLOGY						
		Grade				
Adverse Event	**Short Name**	**1**	**2**	**3**	**4**	**5**
Allergic reaction/hypersensitivity (including drug fever)	Allergic reaction	Transient flushing or rash; drug fever <38°C (<100.4°F)	Rash; flushing; urticaria; dyspnea; drug fever ≥38°C (≥100.4°F)	Symptomatic bronchospasm, with or without urticaria; parenteral medication(s) indicated; allergy-related edema/ angioedema; hypotension	Anaphylaxis	Death
REMARK: Urticaria with manifestations of allergic or hypersensitivity reaction is graded as Allergic reaction/hypersensitivity (including drug fever). ALSO CONSIDER: Cytokine release syndrome/acute infusion reaction.						
Allergic rhinitis (including sneezing, nasal stuffiness, postnasal drip)	Rhinitis	Mild, intervention not indicated	Moderate, intervention indicated	—	—	—
REMARK: Rhinitis associated with obstruction or stenosis is graded as Obstruction/stenosis of airway – *Select* in the PULMONARY/UPPER RESPIRATORY CATEGORY.						
Autoimmune reaction	Autoimmune reaction	Asymptomatic and serologic or other evidence of autoimmune reaction, with normal organ function and intervention not indicated	Evidence of autoimmune reaction involving a nonessential organ or function (e.g., hypothyroidism)	Reversible autoimmune reaction involving function of a major organ or other adverse event (e.g., transient colitis or anemia)	Autoimmune reaction with life-threatening consequences	Death
ALSO CONSIDER: Colitis; Hemoglobin; Hemolysis (e.g., immune hemolytic anemia, drug-related hemolysis); Thyroid function, low (hypothyroidism).						

(continued)

Appendix 2 *(continued)*

			Grade			
Adverse Event	**Short Name**	**1**	**2**	**3**	**4**	**5**
Serum sickness	Serum sickness	—	—	Present	—	Death
NAVIGATION NOTE: Splenic function is graded in the BLOOD/BONE MARROW CATEGORY.						
NAVIGATION NOTE: Urticaria as an isolated symptom is graded as Urticaria (hives, welts, wheals) in the DERMATOLOGY/SKIN CATEGORY.						
Vasculitis	Vasculitis	Mild, intervention not indicated	Symptomatic, nonsteroidal medical intervention indicated	Steroids indicated	Ischemic changes; amputation indicated	Death
Allergy/Immunology – Other (Specify, ______)	Allergy – Other (Specify)	Mild	Moderate	Severe	Life-threatening; disabling	Death

AUDITORY/EAR

			Grade			
Adverse Event	**Short Name**	**1**	**2**	**3**	**4**	**5**
NAVIGATION NOTE: Earache (otalgia) is graded as Pain – *Select* in the PAIN CATEGORY.						

(continued)

Appendix 2 *(continued)*

		Grade				
Adverse Event	**Short Name**	**1**	**2**	**3**	**4**	**5**
Hearing: patients with/without baseline audiogram and enrolled in a monitoring program [1]	Hearing (monitoring program)	Threshold shift or loss of 15 – 25 dB relative to baseline, averaged at 2 or more contiguous test frequencies in at least one ear; or subjective change in the absence of a Grade 1 threshold shift	Threshold shift or loss of >25 – 90 dB, averaged at 2 contiguous test frequencies in at least one ear	Adult only: Threshold shift of >25 – 90 dB, averaged at 3 contiguous test frequencies in at least one ear Pediatric: Hearing loss sufficient to indicate therapeutic intervention, including hearing aids (e.g., ≥20 dB bilateral HL in the speech frequencies; ≥30 dB unilateral HL; and requiring additional speech-language related services)	Adult only: Profound bilateral hearing loss (>90 dB) Pediatric: Audiologic indication for cochlear implant and requiring additional speech-language related services	—
REMARK: Pediatric recommendations are identical to those for adults, unless specified. For children and adolescents (≤18 years of age) without a baseline test, pre-exposure/pretreatment hearing should be considered to be <5 dB loss.						
Hearing: patients without baseline audiogram and not enrolled in a monitoring program[1]	Hearing (without monitoring program)	—	Hearing loss not requiring hearing aid or intervention (i.e., not interfering with ADL)	Hearing loss requiring hearing aid or intervention (i.e., interfering with ADL)	Profound bilateral hearing loss (>90 dB)	—

(continued)

Appendix 2 *(continued)*

		Grade				
Adverse Event	**Short Name**	**1**	**2**	**3**	**4**	**5**
REMARK: Pediatric recommendations are identical to those for adults, unless specified. For children and adolescents (≤18 years of age) without a baseline test, pre-exposure/pretreatment hearing should be considered to be <5 dB loss.						
Otitis, external ear (non-infectious)	Otitis, external	External otitis with erythema or dry desquamation	External otitis with moist desquamation, edema, enhanced cerumen or discharge; tympanic membrane perforation; tympanostomy	External otitis with mastoiditis; stenosis or osteomyelitis	Necrosis of soft tissue or bone	Death
ALSO CONSIDER: Hearing: patients with/without baseline audiogram and enrolled in a monitoring program[1]; Hearing: patients without baseline audiogram and not enrolled in a monitoring program[1].						
Otitis, middle ear (non-infectious)	Otitis, middle	Serous otitis	Serous otitis, medical intervention indicated	Otitis with discharge; mastoiditis	Necrosis of the canal soft tissue or bone	Death
Tinnitus	Tinnitus	—	Tinnitus not interfering with ADL	Tinnitus interfering with ADL	Disabling	—
ALSO CONSIDER: Hearing: patients with/without baseline audiogram and enrolled in a monitoring program[1]; Hearing: patients without baseline audiogram and not enrolled in a monitoring program[1].						
Auditory/Ear – Other (Specify, ______)	Auditory/Ear – Other (Specify)	Mild	Moderate	Severe	Life-threatening; disabling	Death

[1] Drug-induced ototoxicity should be distinguished from age-related threshold decrements or unrelated cochlear insult. When considering whether an adverse event has occurred, it is first necessary to classify the patient into one of two groups. (1) The patient is under standard treatment/enrolled in a clinical trial <2.5 years, and has a 15 dB or greater threshold shift averaged across two contiguous frequencies; or (2) The patient is under standard treatment/enrolled in a clinical trial >2.5 years, and the difference between the expected agerelated and the observed threshold shifts is 15 dB or greater averaged across two contiguous frequencies. Consult standard references for appropriate age- and gender-specific

(continued)

Appendix 2 *(continued)*

hearing norms, e.g., Morrell, et al. Age- and gender-specific reference ranges for hearing level and longitudinal changes in hearing level. Journal of the Acoustical Society of America 100:1949-1967, 1996; or Shotland, et al. Recommendations for cancer prevention trials using potentially ototoxic test agents. Journal of Clinical Oncology 19:1658-1663, 2001.

In the absence of a baseline prior to initial treatment, subsequent audiograms should be referenced to an appropriate database of normals. ANSI. (1996)

American National Standard: Determination of occupational noise exposure and estimation of noise-induced hearing impairment, ANSI S 3.44-1996. (Standard S 3.44). New York: American National Standards Institute. The recommended ANSI S3.44 database is Annex B.

BLOOD/BONE MARROW

		Grade				
Adverse Event	**Short Name**	**1**	**2**	**3**	**4**	**5**
Bone marrow cellularity	Bone marrow cellularity	Mildly hypocellular or ≤25% reduction from normal cellularity for age	Moderately hypocellular or >25 – ≤50% reduction from normal cellularity for age	Severely hypocellular or >50 – ≤75% reduction cellularity from normal for age	—	Death
CD4 count	CD4 count	<LLN – 500/mm³ <LLN – 0.5 × 10^9/L	<500 – 200/mm³ <0.5 – 0.2 × 10^9/L	<200 – 50/mm³ <0.2 × 0.05 – 10^9/L	<50/mm³ <0.05 × 10^9/L	Death
Haptoglobin	Haptoglobin	<LLN	—	Absent	—	Death
Hemoglobin	Hemoglobin	<LLN – 10.0 g/dL <LLN – 6.2 mmol/L <LLN – 100 g/L	<10.0 – 8.0 g/dL <6.2 – 4.9 mmol/L <100 – 80g/L	<8.0 – 6.5 g/dL <4.9 – 4.0 mmol/L <80 – 65 g/L	<6.5 g/dL <4.0 mmol/L <65 g/L	Death
Hemolysis (e.g., immune hemolytic anemia, drugrelated hemolysis)	Hemolysis	Laboratory evidence of hemolysis only (e.g., direct antiglobulin test [DAT, Coombs'] schistocytes)	Evidence of red cell destruction and ≥2 gm decrease in hemoglobin, no transfusion	Transfusion or medical intervention (e.g., steroids) indicated	Catastrophic consequences of hemolysis (e.g., renalfailure, hypotension, bronchospasm, emergency splenectomy)	Death
ALSO CONSIDER: Haptoglobin; Hemoglobin.						

(continued)

Appendix 2 *(continued)*

Adverse Event	Short Name	Grade 1	Grade 2	Grade 3	Grade 4	Grade 5
Iron overload	Iron overload	—	Asymptomatic iron overload, intervention not indicated	Iron overload, intervention indicated	Organ impairment (e.g., endocrinopathy, cardiopathy)	Death
Leukocytes (total WBC)	Leukocytes	<LLN – 3000/mm^3 <LLN – 3.0 × 10^9/L	<3000 – 2000/mm^3 <3.0 – 2.0 × 10^9/L	<2000 – 1000/mm^3 <2.0 – 1.0 × 10^9/L	<1000/mm^3 <1.0 × 10^9/L	Death
Lymphopenia	Lymphopenia	<LLN – 800/mm^3 <LLN × 0.8 – 10^9/L	<800 – 500/mm^3 <0.8 – 0.5 × 10^9/L	<500 – 200 mm^3 <0.5 – 0.2 × 10^9/L	<200/mm^3 <0.2 × 10^9/L	Death
Myelodysplasia	Myelodysplasia	—	—	Abnormal marrow cytogenetics (marrow blasts ≤5%)	RAEB or RAEB-T (marrow blasts >5%)	Death
Neutrophils/granulocytes (ANC/AGC)	Neutrophils	<LLN – 1500/mm^3 <LLN – 1.5 × 10^9/L	<1500 – 1000/mm^3 <1.5 – 1.0 × 10^9/L	<1000 – 500/mm^3 <1.0 – 0.5 × 10^9/L	<500/mm^3 <0.5 × 10^9/L	Death
Platelets	Platelets	<LLN – 75,000/mm^3 <LLN – 75.0 × 10^9/L	<75,000 – 50,000/mm^3 <75.0 – 50.0 × 10^9/L	<50,000 – 25,000/mm^3 <50.0 – 25.0 × 10^9/L	<25,000/mm^3 <25.0 × 10^9/L	Death
Splenic function	Splenic function	Incidental findings (e.g., Howell-Jolly bodies)	Prophylactic antibiotics indicated	—	Life-threatening consequences	Death
Blood/Bone Marrow–Other (Specify, ______)	Blood – Other (Specify)	Mild	Moderate	Severe	Life-threatening; disabling	Death

(continued)

Appendix 2 *(continued)*

CARDIAC ARRHYTHMIA

		Grade				
Adverse Event	**Short Name**	**1**	**2**	**3**	**4**	**5**
Conduction abnormality/atrioventricular heart block – *Select*: – Asystole – AV Block-First degree – AV Block-Second degree Mobitz Type I (Wenckebach) – AV Block-Second degree Mobitz Type II – AV Block-Third degree (Complete AV block) – Conduction abnormality NOS – Sick Sinus Syndrome – Stokes-Adams Syndrome – Wolff-Parkinson-White Syndrome	Conduction abnormalit – *Select*	Asymptomatic, intervention not indicated	Non-urgent medical intervention indicated	Incompletely controlled medically or controlled with device (e.g., pacemaker)	Life-threatening (e.g., arrhythmia associated with CHF, hypotension, syncope, shock)	Death
Palpitations	Palpitations	Present	Present with associated symptoms (e.g., lightheadedness, shortness of breath)	—	—	—

REMARK: Grade palpitations only in the absence of a documented arrhythmia.

(continued)

Appendix 2 *(continued)*

		Grade				
Adverse Event	**Short Name**	**1**	**2**	**3**	**4**	**5**
Prolonged QTc interval	Prolonged QTc	QTc >0.45 – 0.47 second	QTc >0.47 – 0.50 second; ≥0.06 second above baseline	QTc >0.50 second	QTc >0.50 second; lifethreatening signs or symptoms (e.g., arrhythmia, CHF, hypotension, shock syncope); Torsade de pointes	Death
Supraventricular and nodal arrhythmia – *Select*:	Supraventricular arrhythmia – *Select*	Asymptomatic, intervention not indicated	Non-urgent medical intervention indicated	Symptomatic and incompletely controlled medically, or controlled with device (e.g., pacemaker)	Life-threatening (e.g., arrhythmia associated with CHF, hypotension, syncope, shock)	Death
–Atrial fibrillation –Atrial flutter –Atrial tachycardia/Paroxysmal Atrial Tachycardia –Nodal/Junctional –Sinus arrhythmia –Sinus bradycardia –Sinus tachycardia –Supraventricular arrhythmia NOS –Supraventricular extrasystoles (Premature Atrial Contractions; Premature Nodal/Junctional Contractions) –Supraventricular tachycardia						
NAVIGATION NOTE: Syncope is graded as Syncope (fainting) in the NEUROLOGY CATEGORY.						
Vasovagal episode	Vasovagal episode	—	Present without loss of consciousness	Present with loss of consciousness	Life-threatening consequences	Death

(continued)

Appendix 2 *(continued)*

		Grade				
Adverse Event	**Short Name**	**1**	**2**	**3**	**4**	**5**
Ventricular arrhythmia – *Select:* – Bigeminy – Idioventricular rhythm – PVCs – Torsade de pointes – Trigeminy – Ventricular arrhythmia NOS – Ventricular fibrillation – Ventricular flutter – Ventricular tachycardia	Ventricular arrhythmia– Select	Asymptomatic, no intervention indicated	Non-urgent medical intervention indicated	Symptomatic and incompletely controlled medically or controlled with device (e.g., defibrillator)	Life-threatening (e.g., arrhythmia associated with CHF, hypotension, syncope, shock)	Death
Cardiac Arrhythmia – Other (Specify, ______)	Cardiac Arrhythmia – Other (Specify)	Mild	Moderate	Severe	Life-threatening; disabling	Death

CARDIAC GENERAL

		Grade				
Adverse Event	**Short Name**	**1**	**2**	**3**	**4**	**5**
NAVIGATION NOTE: Angina is graded as Cardiac ischemia/infarction in the CARDIAC GENERAL CATEGORY.						
Cardiac ischemia/ infarction	Cardiac ischemia/ infarction	Asymptomatic arterial narrowing without ischemia	Asymptomatic and testing suggesting ischemia; stable angina	Symptomatic and testing consistent with ischemia; unstable angina; intervention indicated	Acute myocardial infarction	Death

(continued)

Appendix 2 *(continued)*

		Grade				
Adverse Event	**Short Name**	**1**	**2**	**3**	**4**	**5**
Cardiac troponin I (cTnI)	cTnI	—	—	Levels consistent with unstable angina as defined by the manufacturer	Levels consistent with myocardial infarction as defined by the manufacturer	Death
Cardiac troponin T (cTnT)	cTnT	0.03 – <0.05 ng/mL	0.05 – <0.1 ng/mL	0.1 – <0.2 ng/mL	0.2 ng/mL	Death
Cardiopulmonary arrest, cause unknown (non-fatal)	Cardiopulmonary arrest	—	—	—	Life-threatening	—

REMARK: Grade 4 (non-fatal) is the only appropriate grade. CTCAE provides three alternatives for reporting Death:

1. A CTCAE term associated with Grade 5.
2. A CTCAE 'Other (Specify, ______)' within any CATEGORY.
3. Death not associated with CTCAE term – *Select* in the DEATH CATEGORY.

NAVIGATION NOTE: Chest pain (non-cardiac and non-pleuritic) is graded as Pain – *Select* in the PAIN CATEGORY.

NAVIGATION NOTE: CNS ischemia is graded as CNS cerebrovascular ischemia in the NEUROLOGY CATEGORY.

(continued)

Appendix 2 *(continued)*

		Grade				
Adverse Event	**Short Name**	**1**	**2**	**3**	**4**	**5**
Hypertension	Hypertension	Asymptomatic, transient (<24 hrs) increase by >20 mmHg (diastolic) or to >150/100 if previously WNL; intervention not indicated Pediatric: Asymptomatic, transient (<24 hrs) BP increase >ULN; intervention not indicated	Recurrent or persistent (≥24 hrs) or symptomatic increase by >20 mmHg (diastolic) or to >150/100 if previously WNL; monotherapy may be indicated Pediatric: Recurrent or persistent (≥24 hrs) BP >ULN; monotherapy may be indicated	Requiring more than one drug or more intensive therapy than previously Pediatric: Same as adult	Life-threatening consequences (e.g., hypertensive crisis) Pediatric: Same as adult	Death
REMARK: Use age and gender-appropriate normal values >95th percentile ULN for pediatric patients.						
Hypotension	Hypotension	Changes, intervention not indicated	Brief (<24 hrs) fluid replacement or other therapy; no physiologic consequences	Sustained (≥24 hrs) therapy, resolves without persisting physiologic consequences	Shock (e.g., acidemia; impairment of vital organ function)	Death
ALSO CONSIDER: Syncope (fainting).						

(continued)

Appendix 2 *(continued)*

		Grade				
Adverse Event	**Short Name**	**1**	**2**	**3**	**4**	**5**
Left ventricular diastolic dysfunction	Left ventricular diastolic dysfunction	Asymptomatic diagnostic finding; intervention not indicated	Asymptomatic, intervention indicated	Symptomatic CHF responsive to intervention	Refractory CHF, poorly controlled; intervention such as ventricular assist device or heart transplant indicated	Death
Left ventricular systolic dysfunction	Left ventricular systolic dysfunction	Asymptomatic, resting ejection fraction (EF) <60 – 50%; shortening fraction (SF) <30 – 24%	Asymptomatic, resting EF <50 – 40%; SF <24 – 15%	Symptomatic CHF responsive to intervention; EF <40 – 20% SF <15%	Refractory CHF or poorly controlled; EF <20%; intervention such as ventricular assist device, ventricular reduction surgery, or heart transplant indicated	Death
NAVIGATION NOTE: Myocardial infarction is graded as Cardiac ischemia/infarction in the CARDIAC GENERAL CATEGORY.						
Myocarditis	Myocarditis	—	—	CHF responsive to intervention	Severe or refractory CHF	Death
Pericardial effusion (non-malignant)	Pericardial effusion	Asymptomatic effusion	—	Effusion with physiologic consequences	Life-threatening consequences (e.g., tamponade); emergency intervention indicated	Death

(continued)

Appendix 2 *(continued)*

		Grade				
Adverse Event	**Short Name**	**1**	**2**	**3**	**4**	**5**
Pericarditis	Pericarditis	Asymptomatic, ECG or physical exam (rub) changes consistent with pericarditis	Symptomatic pericarditis (e.g., chest pain)	Pericarditis with physiologic consequences (e.g., pericardial constriction)	Life-threatening consequences; emergency intervention indicated	Death
NAVIGATION NOTE: Pleuritic pain is graded as Pain – *Select* in the PAIN CATEGORY.						
Pulmonary hypertension	Pulmonary hypertension	Asymptomatic without therapy	Asymptomatic, therapy indicated	Symptomatic hypertension, responsive to therapy	Symptomatic hypertension, poorly controlled	Death
Restrictive cardiomyopathy	Restrictive cardiomyopathy	Asymptomatic, therapy not indicated	Asymptomatic, therapy indicated	Symptomatic CHF responsive to intervention	Refractory CHF, poorly controlled; intervention such as ventricular assist device, or heart transplant indicated	Death
Right ventricular dysfunction (cor pulmonale)	Right ventricular dysfunction	Asymptomatic without therapy	Asymptomatic, therapy indicated	Symptomatic cor pulmonale, responsive to intervention	Symptomatic cor pulmonale poorly controlled; intervention such as ventricular assist device, or heart transplant indicated	Death

(continued)

Appendix 2 *(continued)*

		Grade				
Adverse Event	**Short Name**	**1**	**2**	**3**	**4**	**5**
Valvular heart disease	Valvular heart disease	Asymptomatic valvular thickening with or without mild valvular regurgitation or stenosis; treatment other than endocarditis prophylaxis not indicated	Asymptomatic; moderate regurgitation or stenosis by imaging	Symptomatic; severe regurgitation or stenosis; symptoms controlled with medical therapy	Life-threatening; disabling; intervention (e.g., valve replacement, valvuloplasty) indicated	Death
Cardiac General – Other (Specify, ______)	Cardiac General – Other (Specify)	Mild	Moderate	Severe	Life-threatening; disabling	Death

COAGULATION

		Grade				
Adverse Event	**Short Name**	**1**	**2**	**3**	**4**	**5**
DIC (disseminated intravascular coagulation)	DIC	—	Laboratory findings with no bleeding	Laboratory findings and bleeding	Laboratory findings, lifethreatening or disabling consequences (e.g., CNS hemorrhage, organ damage, or hemodynamically significant blood loss)	Death

REMARK: DIC (disseminated intravascular coagulation) must have increased fibrin split products or D-dimer.
ALSO CONSIDER: Platelets.

(continued)

Appendix 2 *(continued)*

		Grade				
Adverse Event	**Short Name**	**1**	**2**	**3**	**4**	**5**
Fibrinogen	Fibrinogen	<1.0 – 0.75 × LLN or <25% decrease from baseline	<0.75 – 0.5 × LLN or 25 – <50% decrease from baseline	<0.5 – 0.25 × LLN or 50 – <75% decrease from baseline	<0.25 × LLN or 75% decrease from baseline or absolute value <50 mg/dL	Death
REMARK: Use % decrease only when baseline is <LLN (local laboratory value).						
INR (International Normalized Ratio of prothrombin time)	INR	>1 – 1.5 × ULN	>1.5 – 2 × ULN	>2 × ULN	—	—
ALSO CONSIDER: Hemorrhage, CNS; Hemorrhage, GI – *Select*; Hemorrhage, GU – *Select*; Hemorrhage, pulmonary/upper respiratory – *Select*.						
PTT (Partial Thromboplastin Time)	PTT	>1 – 1.5 × ULN	>1.5 – 2 × ULN	>2 × ULN	—	—
ALSO CONSIDER: Hemorrhage, CNS; Hemorrhage, GI – *Select*; Hemorrhage, GU – *Select*; Hemorrhage, pulmonary/upper respiratory – Select.						
Thrombotic microangiopathy (e.g., thrombotic thrombocytopenic purpura [TTP] or hemolytic uremic syndrome [HUS])	Thrombotic microangiopathy	Evidence of RBC destruction (schistocytosis) without clinical consequences	—	Laboratory findings present with clinical consequences (e.g., renal insufficiency, petechiae)	Laboratory findings and life-threatening or disabling consequences, (e.g., CNS hemorrhage/ bleeding or thrombosis/ embolism or renal failure)	Death
REMARK: Must have microangiopathic changes on blood smear (e.g., schistocytes, helmet cells, red cell fragments). ALSO CONSIDER: Creatinine; Hemoglobin; Platelets.						
Coagulation – Other (Specify, ______)	Coagulation – Other (Specify)	Mild	Moderate	Severe	Life-threatening; disabling	Death

(continued)

Appendix 2 *(continued)*

CONSTITUTIONAL SYMPTOMS

		Grade				
Adverse Event	**Short Name**	**1**	**2**	**3**	**4**	**5**
Fatigue (asthenia, lethargy, malaise)	Fatigue	Mild fatigue over baseline	Moderate or causing difficulty performing some ADL	Severe fatigue interfering with ADL	Disabling	—
Fever (in the absence of neutropenia, where neutropenia is defined as ANC $<1.0 \times 10^9/L$)	Fever	38.0 – 39.0°C (100.4 – 102.2°F)	>39.0 – 40.0°C (102.3 – 104.0°F)	>40.0°C (>104.0°F) for ≤24 hrs	>40.0°C (>104.0°F) for >24 hrs	Death
REMARK: The temperature measurements listed are oral or tympanic.						
ALSO CONSIDER: Allergic reaction/hypersensitivity (including drug fever).						
NAVIGATION NOTE: Hot flashes are graded as Hot flashes/flushes in the ENDOCRINE CATEGORY.						
Hypothermia	Hypothermia	—	35 – >32°C 95 – >89.6°F	32 – >28°C 89.6 – >82.4° F	≤28 °C 82.4°F or life-threatening consequences (e.g., coma, hypotension, pulmonary edema, acidemia, ventricular fibrillation)	Death
Insomnia	Insomnia	Occasional difficulty sleeping, not interfering with function	Difficulty sleeping, interfering with function but not interfering with ADL	Frequent difficulty sleeping, interfering with ADL	Disabling	—
REMARK: If pain or other symptoms interfere with sleep, do NOT grade as insomnia. Grade primary event(s) causing insomnia.						

(continued)

Appendix 2 *(continued)*

		Grade				
Adverse Event	**Short Name**	**1**	**2**	**3**	**4**	**5**
Obesity[2]	Obesity	—	BMI 25 – 29.9 kg/m^2	BMI 30 – 39.99 kg/m^2	BMI ≥40 kg/m^2	—
REMARK: BMI = (weight [kg])/ (height [m])^2						
Odor (patient odor)	Patient odor	Mild odor	Pronounced odor	—	—	—
Rigors/chills	Rigors/chills	Mild	Moderate, narcotics indicated	Severe or prolonged, not responsive to narcotics	—	—
Sweating (diaphoresis)	Sweating	Mild and occasional	Frequent or drenching	—	—	—
ALSO CONSIDER: Hot flashes/flushes.						
Weight gain	Weightgain	5 – <10% of baseline	10 – <20% of baseline	≥20% of baseline	—	—
REMARK: Edema, depending on etiology, is graded in the CARDIAC GENERAL or LYMPHATICS CATEGORIES.						
ALSO CONSIDER: Ascites (non-malignant); Pleural effusion (non-malignant).						
Weight loss	Weight loss	5 to <10% from baseline; intervention not indicated	10 – <20% from baseline; nutritional support indicated	≥20% from baseline; tube feeding or TPN indicated	—	—
Constitutional Symptoms – Other (Specify, ______)	Constitutional Symptoms – Other (Specify)	Mild	Moderate	Severe	Life-threatening; disabling	Death

[2] NHLBI Obesity Task Force. Clinical Guidelines on the Identification, Evaluation, and Treatment of Overweight and Obesity in Adults, *The Evidence Report,* Obes Res 6:51S-209S, 1998.

(continued)

Appendix 2 *(continued)*

DEATH

		Grade				
Adverse Event	**Short Name**	**1**	**2**	**3**	**4**	**5**
Death not associated with CTCAE term – *Select*: – Death NOS – Disease progression NOS – Multi-organ failure – Sudden death	Death not associated with CTCAE term – Select	—	—	—	—	Death

REMARK: Grade 5 is the only appropriate grade. 'Death not associated with CTCAE term – *Select'* is to be used where a death:

1. Cannot be attributed to a CTCAE term associated with Grade 5.
2. Cannot be reported within any CATEGORY using a CTCAE 'Other (Specify, ______)'.

DERMATOLOGY/SKIN

		Grade				
Adverse Event	**Short Name**	**1**	**2**	**3**	**4**	**5**
Atrophy, skin	Atrophy, skin	Detectable	Marked	—	—	—
Atrophy, subcutaneous fat	Atrophy, subcutaneous fat	Detectable	Marked	—	—	—
ALSO CONSIDER: Induration/fibrosis (skin and subcutaneous tissue).						
Bruising (in absence of Grade 3 or 4 thrombocytopenia)	Bruising	Localized or in a dependent area	Generalized	—	—	—

(continued)

Appendix 2 *(continued)*

		Grade				
Adverse Event	**Short Name**	**1**	**2**	**3**	**4**	**5**
Burn	Burn	Minimal symptoms; intervention not indicated	Medical intervention; minimal debridement indicated	Moderate to major debridement or reconstruction indicated	Life-threatening consequences	Death
REMARK: Burn refers to all burns including radiation, chemical, etc.						
Cheilitis	Cheilitis	Asymptomatic	Symptomatic, not interfering with ADL	Symptomatic, interfering with ADL	—	—
Dry skin	Dry skin	Asymptomatic	Symptomatic, not interfering with ADL	Interfering with ADL	—	—
Flushing	Flushing	Asymptomatic	Symptomatic	—	—	—
Hair loss/alopecia (scalp or body)	Alopecia	Thinning or patchy	Complete	—	—	—
Hyperpigmentation	Hyperpigmentation	Slight or localized	Marked or generalized	—	—	—
Hypopigmentation	Hypopigmentation	Slight or localized	Marked or generalized	—	—	—

(continued)

Appendix 2 *(continued)*

		Grade				
Adverse Event	**Short Name**	**1**	**2**	**3**	**4**	**5**
Induration/fibrosis (skin and subcutaneous tissue)	Induration	Increased density on palpation	Moderate impairment of function not interfering with ADL; marked increase in density and firmness on palpation with or without minimal retraction	Dysfunction interfering with ADL; very marked density, retraction or fixation	—	—
ALSO CONSIDER: Fibrosis-cosmesis; Fibrosis-deep connective tissue.						
Injection site reaction/extravasation changes	Injection site reaction	Pain; itching; erythema	Pain or swelling, with inflammation or phlebitis	Ulceration or necrosis that is severe; operative intervention indicated	—	—
ALSO CONSIDER: Allergic reaction/hypersensitivity (including drug fever); Ulceration.						
Nail changes	Nail changes	Discoloration; ridging (koilonychias); pitting	Partial or complete loss of nail(s); pain in nailbed(s)	Interfering with ADL	—	—
NAVIGATION NOTE: Petechiae is graded as Petechiae/purpura (hemorrhage/bleeding into skin or mucosa) in the HEMORRHAGE/BLEEDING CATEGORY.						
Photosensitivity	Photosensitivity	Painless erythema	Painful erythema	Erythema with desquamation	Life-threatening; disabling	Death
Pruritus/itching	Pruritus	Mild or localized	Intense or widespread	Intense or widespread and interfering with ADL	—	—

(continued)

Appendix 2 *(continued)*

		Grade				
Adverse Event	**Short Name**	**1**	**2**	**3**	**4**	**5**
ALSO CONSIDER: Rash/desquamation.						
Rash/desquamation	Rash	Macular or papular eruption or erythema without associated symptoms	Macular or papular eruption or erythema with pruritus or other associated symptoms; localized desquamation or other lesions covering <50% of body surface area (BSA)	Severe, generalized erythroderma or macular, papular or vesicular eruption; desquamation covering ≥50% BSA	Generalized exfoliative, ulcerative, or bullous dermatitis	Death
REMARK: Rash/desquamation may be used for GVHD.						
Rash: acne/ acneiform	Acne	Intervention not indicated	Intervention indicated	Associated with pain, disfigurement, ulceration, or desquamation	—	Death
Rash: dermatitis associated with radiatio – *Select*: – Chemoradiation – Radiation	Dermatitis – *Select*	Faint erythema or dry desquamation	Moderate to brisk erythema; patchy moist desquamation, mostly confined to skin folds and creases; moderate edema	Moist desquamation other than skin folds and creases; bleeding induced by minor trauma or abrasion	Skin necrosis or ulceration of full thickness dermis; spontaneous bleeding from involved site	Death

(continued)

Appendix 2 *(continued)*

		Grade				
Adverse Event	**Short Name**	**1**	**2**	**3**	**4**	**5**
Rash: erythema multiforme (e.g., Stevens-Johnson syndrome, toxic epidermal necrolysis)	Erythema multiforme	—	Scattered, but not generalized eruption	Severe (e.g., generalized rash or painful stomatitis); IV fluids, tube feedings, or TPN indicated	Life-threatening; disabling	Death
Rash: hand-foot skin reaction	Hand-foot	Minimal skin changes or dermatitis (e.g., erythema) without pain	Skin changes (e.g., peeling, blisters, bleeding, edema) or pain, not interfering with function	Ulcerative dermatitis or skin changes with pain interfering with function	—	—
Skin breakdown/ decubitus ulcer	Decubitus	—	Local wound care; medical intervention indicated	Operative debridement or other invasive intervention indicated (e.g., hyperbaric oxygen)	Life-threatening consequences; major invasive intervention indicated (e.g., tissue reconstruction, flap, or grafting)	Death
REMARK: Skin breakdown/decubitus ulcer is to be used for loss of skin integrity or decubitus ulcer from pressure or as the result of operative or medical intervention.						
Striae	Striae	Mild	Cosmetically significant	—	—	—
Telangiectasia	Telangiectasia	Few	Moderate number	Many and confluent	—	—

(continued)

Appendix 2 *(continued)*

		Grade				
Adverse Event	**Short Name**	**1**	**2**	**3**	**4**	**5**
Ulceration	Ulceration	—	Superficial ulceration <2 cm size; local wound care; medical intervention indicated	Ulceration ≥2 cm size; operative debridement, primary closure or other invasive intervention indicated (e.g., hyperbaric oxygen)	Life-threatening consequences; major invasive intervention indicated (e.g., complete resection, tissue reconstruction, flap, or grafting)	Death
Urticaria (hives, welts, wheals)	Urticaria	Intervention not indicated	Intervention indicated for <24 hrs	Intervention indicated for ≥24 hrs	—	—
ALSO CONSIDER: Allergic reaction/hypersensitivity (including drug fever).						
Wound complication, non-infectious	Wound complication, non-infectious	Incisional separation of ≤25% of wound, no deeper than superficial fascia	Incisional separation >25% of wound with local care; asymptomatic hernia	Symptomatic hernia without evidence of strangulation; fascial disruption/dehiscence without evisceration; primary wound closure or revision by operative intervention indicated; hospitalization or hyperbaric oxygen indicated	Symptomatic hernia with evidence of strangulation; fascial disruption with evisceration; major reconstruction flap, grafting, resection, or amputation indicated	Death
REMARK: Wound complication, non-infectious is to be used for separation of incision, hernia, dehiscence, evisceration, or second surgery for wound revision.						

(continued)

Appendix 2 *(continued)*

		Grade				
Adverse Event	**Short Name**	**1**	**2**	**3**	**4**	**5**
Dermatology/Skin – Other (Specify, ______)	Dermatology – Other (Specify)	Mild	Moderate	Severe	Life-threatening; disabling	Death

ENDOCRINE

		Grade				
Adverse Event	**Short Name**	**1**	**2**	**3**	**4**	**5**
Adrenal insufficiency	Adrenal insufficiency	Asymptomatic, intervention not indicated	Symptomatic, intervention indicated	Hospitalization	Life-threatening; disabling	Death
REMARK: Adrenal insufficiency includes any of the following signs and symptoms: abdominal pain, anorexia, constipation, diarrhea, hypotension, pigmentation of mucous membranes, pigmentation of skin, salt craving, syncope (fainting), vitiligo, vomiting, weakness, weight loss. Adrenal insufficiency must be confirmed by laboratory studies (low cortisol frequently accompanied by low aldosterone). ALSO CONSIDER: Potassium, serum-high (hyperkalemia); Thyroid function, low (hypothyroidism).						
Cushingoid appearance (e.g., moon face, buffalo hump, centripetal obesity, cutaneous striae)	Cushingoid	—	Present	—	—	—
ALSO CONSIDER: Glucose, serum-high (hyperglycemia); Potassium, serum-low (hypokalemia).						
Feminization of male	Feminization of male	—	—	Present	—	—
NAVIGATION NOTE: Gynecomastia is graded in the SEXUAL/REPRODUCTIVE FUNCTION CATEGORY.						
Hot flashes/flushes[3]	Hot flashes	Mild	Moderate	Interfering with ADL	—	—

(continued)

Appendix 2 *(continued)*

		Grade				
Adverse Event	**Short Name**	**1**	**2**	**3**	**4**	**5**
Masculinization of female	Masculinization of female	—	—	Present	—	—
Neuroendocrine: ACTH deficiency	ACTH	Asymptomatic	Symptomatic, not interfering with ADL; intervention indicated	Symptoms interfering with ADL; hospitalization indicated	Life-threatening consequences (e.g., severe hypotension)	Death
Neuroendocrine: ADH secretion abnormality (e.g., SIADH or low ADH)	ADH	Asymptomatic	Symptomatic, not interfering with ADL; intervention indicated	Symptoms interfering with ADL	Life-threatening consequences	Death
Neuroendocrine: gonadotropin secretion abnormality	Gonadotropin	Asymptomatic	Symptomatic, not interfering with ADL; intervention indicated	Symptoms interfering with ADL; osteopenia; fracture; infertility	—	—
Neuroendocrine: growth hormone secretion abnormality	Growth hormone	Asymptomatic	Symptomatic, not interfering with ADL; intervention indicated	—	—	—
Neuroendocrine: prolactin hormone secretion abnormality	Prolactin	Asymptomatic	Symptomatic, not interfering with ADL; intervention indicated	Symptoms interfering with ADL; amenorrhea; galactorrhea	—	Death

(continued)

Appendix 2 *(continued)*

		Grade				
Adverse Event	**Short Name**	**1**	**2**	**3**	**4**	**5**
Pancreatic endocrine: glucose intolerance	Diabetes	Asymptomatic, intervention not indicated	Symptomatic; dietary modification or oral agent indicated	Symptoms interfering with ADL; insulin indicated	Life-threatening consequences (e.g., ketoacidosis, hyperosmolar nonketotic coma)	Death
Parathyroid function, low (hypoparathyroidism)	Hypoparathyroidism	Asymptomatic, intervention not indicated	Symptomatic; intervention indicated	—	—	—
Thyroid function, high (hyperthyroidism, thyrotoxicosis)	Hyperthyroidism	Asymptomatic, intervention not indicated	Symptomatic, not interfering with ADL; thyroid suppression therapy indicated	Symptoms interfering with ADL; hospitalization indicated	Life-threatening consequences (e.g., thyroid storm)	Death
Thyroid function, low (hypothyroidism)	Hypothyroidism	Asymptomatic, intervention not indicated	Symptomatic, not interfering with ADL; thyroid replacement indicated	Symptoms interfering with ADL; hospitalization indicated	Life-threatening myxedema coma	Death
Endocrine – Other (Specify, ______)	Endocrine – Other (Specify)	Mild	Moderate	Severe	Life-threatening; disabling	Death

[3] Sloan JA, Loprinzi CL, Novotny PJ, Barton DL, Lavasseur BI, Windschitl HJ. Methodologic Lessons Learned from Hot Flash Studies, *J Clin Oncol* 2001;19(23):4280-90

(continued)

Appendix 2 *(continued)*

GASTROINTESTINAL

		Grade				
Adverse Event	**Short Name**	**1**	**2**	**3**	**4**	**5**
NAVIGATION NOTE: Abdominal pain or cramping is graded as Pain – *Select* in the PAIN CATEGORY.						
Anorexia	Anorexia	Loss of appetite without alteration in eating habits	Oral intake altered without significant weight loss or malnutrition; oral nutritional supplements indicated	Associated with significant weight loss or malnutrition (e.g., inadequate oral caloric and/or fluid intake); IV fluids, tube feedings or TPN indicated	Life-threatening consequences	Death
ALSO CONSIDER: Weight loss.						
Ascites (non-malignant)	Ascites	Asymptomatic	Symptomatic, medical intervention indicated	Symptomatic, invasive procedure indicated	Life-threatening consequences	Death
REMARK: Ascites (non-malignant) refers to documented non-malignant ascites or unknown etiology, but unlikely malignant, and includes chylous ascites.						
Colitis	Colitis	Asymptomatic, pathologic or radiographic findings only	Abdominal pain; mucus or blood in stool	Abdominal pain, fever, change in bowel habits with ileus; peritoneal signs	Life-threatening consequences (e.g., perforation, bleeding, ischemia, necrosis, toxic megacolon)	Death
ALSO CONSIDER: Hemorrhage, GI – *Select*.						

(continued)

Appendix 2 *(continued)*

		Grade				
Adverse Event	**Short Name**	**1**	**2**	**3**	**4**	**5**
Constipation	Constipation	Occasional or intermittent symptoms; occasional use of stool softeners, laxatives, dietary modification, or enema	Persistent symptoms with regular use of laxatives or enemas indicated	Symptoms interfering with ADL; obstipation with manual evacuation indicated	Life-threatening consequences (e.g., obstruction, toxic megacolon)	Death
ALSO CONSIDER: Ileus, GI (functional obstruction of bowel, i.e., neuroconstipation); Obstruction, GI – *Select*.						
Dehydration	Dehydration	Increased oral fluids indicated; dry mucous membranes; diminished skin turgor	IV fluids indicated $<$24 hrs	IV fluids indicated $\geq$24 hrs	Life-threatening consequences (e.g., hemodynamic collapse)	Death
ALSO CONSIDER: Diarrhea; Hypotension; Vomiting.						
Dental: dentures or prosthesis	Dentures	Minimal discomfort, no restriction in activities	Discomfort preventing use in some activities (e.g., eating), but not others (e.g., speaking)	Unable to use dentures or prosthesis at any time	—	—
Dental: periodontal disease	Periodontal	Gingival recession or gingivitis; limited bleeding on probing; mild local bone loss	Moderate gingival recession or gingivitis; multiple sites of bleeding on probing; moderate bone loss	Spontaneous bleeding; severe bone loss with or without tooth loss; osteonecrosis of maxilla or mandible	—	—
REMARK: Severe periodontal disease leading to osteonecrosis is graded as Osteonecrosis (avascular necrosis) in the MUSCULOSKELETAL CATEGORY.						

(continued)

Appendix 2 *(continued)*

		Grade				
Adverse Event	**Short Name**	**1**	**2**	**3**	**4**	**5**
Dental: teeth	Teeth	Surface stains; dental caries; restorable, without extractions	Less than full mouth extractions; tooth fracture or crown amputation or repair indicated	Full mouth extractions indicated	—	—
Dental: teeth development	Teeth development	Hypoplasia of tooth or enamel not interfering with function	Functional impairment correctable with oral surgery	Maldevelopment with functional impairment not surgically correctable	—	—
Diarrhea	Diarrhea	Increase of <4 stools per day over baseline; mild increase in ostomy output compared to baseline	Increase of 4 – 6 stools per day over baseline; IV fluids indicated <24hrs; moderate increase in ostomy output compared to baseline; not interfering with ADL	Increase of ≥ 7 stools per day over baseline; incontinence; IV fluids ≥ 24 hrs; hospitalization; severe increase in ostomy output compared to baseline; interfering with ADL	Life-threatening consequences (e.g., hemodynamic collapse)	Death
REMARK: Diarrhea includes diarrhea of small bowel or colonic origin, and/or ostomy diarrhea. ALSO CONSIDER: Dehydration; Hypotension.						
Distension/bloating, abdominal	Distension	Asymptomatic	Symptomatic, but not interfering with GI function	Symptomatic, interfering with GI function	—	—
ALSO CONSIDER: Ascites (non-malignant); Ileus, GI (functional obstruction of bowel, i.e., neuroconstipation); Obstruction, GI – *Select*.						

(continued)

Appendix 2 *(continued)*

		Grade				
Adverse Event	**Short Name**	**1**	**2**	**3**	**4**	**5**
Dry mouth/salivary gland (xerostomia)	Dry mouth	Symptomatic (dry or thick saliva) without significant dietary alteration; unstimulated saliva flow >0.2 ml/min	Symptomatic and significant oral intake alteration (e.g., copious water, other lubricants, diet limited to purees and/or soft, moist foods); unstimulated saliva 0.1 to 0.2 ml/min	Symptoms leading to inability to adequately aliment orally; IV fluids, tube feedings, or TPN indicated; unstimulated saliva <0.1 ml/min	—	—
REMARK: Dry mouth/salivary gland (xerostomia) includes descriptions of grade using both subjective and objective assessment parameters. Record this event consistently throughout a patient's participation on study. If salivary flow measurements are used for initial assessment, subsequent assessments must use salivary flow. ALSO CONSIDER: Salivary gland changes/saliva.						
Dysphagia (difficulty swallowing)	Dysphagia	Symptomatic, able to eat regular diet	Symptomatic and altered eating/swallowing (e.g., altered dietary habits, oral supplements); IV fluids indicated <24 hrs	Symptomatic and severely altered eating/swallowing (e.g., inadequate oral caloric or fluid intake); IV fluids, tube feedings, or TPN indicated ≥24 hrs	Life-threatening consequences (e.g., obstruction, perforation)	Death
REMARK: Dysphagia (difficulty swallowing) is to be used for swallowing difficulty from oral, pharyngeal, esophageal, or neurologic origin. Dysphagia requiring dilation is graded as Stricture/stenosis (including anastomotic), GI – *Select*. ALSO CONSIDER: Dehydration; Esophagitis.						

(continued)

Appendix 2 *(continued)*

		Grade				
Adverse Event	**Short Name**	**1**	**2**	**3**	**4**	**5**
Enteritis (inflammation of the small bowel)	Enteritis	Asymptomatic, pathologic or radiographic findings only	Abdominal pain; mucus or blood in stool	Abdominal pain, fever, change in bowel habits with ileus; peritoneal signs	Life-threatening consequences (e.g., perforation, bleeding, ischemia, necrosis)	Death
ALSO CONSIDER: Hemorrhage, GI – *Select*; Typhlitis (cecal inflammation).						
Esophagitis	Esophagitis	Asymptomatic pathologic, radiographic, or endoscopic findings only	Symptomatic; altered eating/swallowing (e.g., altered dietary habits, oral supplements); IV fluids indicated <24 hrs	Symptomatic and severely altered eating/swallowing (e.g., inadequate oral caloric or fluid intake); IV fluids, tube feedings, or TPN indicated ≥24 hrs	Life-threatening consequences	Death
REMARK: Esophagitis includes reflux esophagitis. ALSO CONSIDER: Dysphagia (difficulty swallowing).						

(continued)

Appendix 2 *(continued)*

		Grade				
Adverse Event	**Short Name**	**1**	**2**	**3**	**4**	**5**
Fistula, GI – *Select*: – Abdomen NOS – Anus – Biliary tree – Colon/cecum/appendix – Duodenum – Esophagus – Gallbladder – Ileum – Jejunum – Oral cavity – Pancreas – Pharynx – Rectum – Salivary gland – Small bowel NOS – Stomach	Fistula, GI – *Select*	Asymptomatic, radiographic findings only	Symptomatic; altered GI function (e.g., altered dietary habits, diarrhea, or GI fluid loss); IV fluids indicated <24 hrs	Symptomatic and severely altered GI function (e.g., altered dietary habits, diarrhea, or GI fluid loss); IV fluids, tube feedings, or TPN indicated ≥24 hrs	Life-threatening consequences	Death
REMARK: A fistula is defined as an abnormal communication between two body cavities, potential spaces, and/or the skin. The site indicated for a fistula should be the site from which the abnormal process is believed to have originated. For example, a tracheo-esophageal fistula arising in the context of a resected or irradiated esophageal cancer is graded as Fistula, GI – esophagus.						
Flatulence	Flatulence	Mild	Moderate	—	—	—

(continued)

Appendix 2 *(continued)*

		Grade				
Adverse Event	**Short Name**	**1**	**2**	**3**	**4**	**5**
Gastritis (including bile reflux gastritis)	Gastritis	Asymptomatic radiographic or endoscopic findings only	Symptomatic; altered gastric function (e.g., inadequate oral caloric or fluid intake); IV fluids indicated <24 hrs	Symptomatic and severely altered gastric function (e.g., inadequate oral caloric or fluid intake); IV fluids, tube feedings, or TPN indicated ≥24 hrs	Life-threatening consequences; operative intervention requiring complete organ resection (e.g., gastrectomy)	Death
ALSO CONSIDER: Hemorrhage, GI – *Select*; Ulcer, GI – *Select*.						
NAVIGATION NOTE: Head and neck soft tissue necrosis is graded as Soft tissue necrosis – *Select* in the MUSCULOSKELETAL/SOFT TISSUE CATEGORY.						
Heartburn/dyspepsia	Heartburn	Mild	Moderate	Severe	—	—
Hemorrhoids	Hemorrhoids	Asymptomatic	Symptomatic; banding or medical intervention indicated	Interfering with ADL; interventional radiology, endoscopic, or operative intervention indicated	Life-threatening consequences	Death
Ileus, GI (functional obstruction of bowel, i.e., neuroconstipation)	Ileus	Asymptomatic, radiographic findings only	Symptomatic; altered GI function (e.g., altered dietary habits); IV fluids indicated <24 hrs	Symptomatic and severely altered GI function; IV fluids, tube feeding, or TPN indicated ≥24 hrs	Life-threatening consequences	Death
REMARK: Ileus, GI is to be used for altered upper or lower GI function (e.g., delayed gastric or colonic emptying). ALSO CONSIDER: Constipation; Nausea; Obstruction, GI – *Select*; Vomiting.						

(continued)

Appendix 2 *(continued)*

		Grade				
Adverse Event	**Short Name**	**1**	**2**	**3**	**4**	**5**
Incontinence, anal	Incontinence, anal	Occasional use of pads required	Daily use of pads required	Interfering with ADL; operative intervention indicated	Permanent bowel diversion indicated	Death
REMARK: Incontinence, anal is to be used for loss of sphincter control as sequelae of operative or therapeutic intervention.						
Leak (including anastomotic), GI – *Select*: – Biliary tree – Esophagus – Large bowel – Leak NOS – Pancreas – Pharynx – Rectum – Small bowel – Stoma – Stomach	Leak, GI – *Select*	Asymptomatic radiographic findings only	Symptomatic; medical intervention indicated	Symptomatic and interfering with GI function; invasive or endoscopic intervention indicated	Life-threatening consequences	Death
REMARK: Leak (including anasomotic), GI – *Select* is to be used for clinical signs/symptoms or radiographic confirmation of anastomotic or conduit leak (e.g., biliary, esophageal, intestinal, pancreatic, pharyngeal, rectal), but without development of fistula.						
Malabsorption	Malabsorption	—	Altered diet; oral therapies indicated (e.g., enzymes, medications, dietary supplements)	Inability to aliment adequately via GI tract (i.e., TPN indicated)	Life-threatening consequences	Death

(continued)

Appendix 2 *(continued)*

		Grade				
Adverse Event	**Short Name**	**1**	**2**	**3**	**4**	**5**
Mucositis/stomatitis (clinical exam) – *Select*: – Anus – Esophagus – Large bowel – Larynx – Oral cavity – Pharynx – Rectum – Small bowel – Stomach – Trachea	Mucositis (clinical exam) – *Select*	Erythema of the mucosa	Patchy ulcerations or pseudomembranes	Confluent ulcerations or pseudomembranes; bleeding with minor trauma	Tissue necrosis; significant spontaneous bleeding; life-threatening consequences	Death
REMARK: Mucositis/stomatitis (functional/symptomatic) may be used for mucositis of the upper aero-digestive tract caused by radiation, agents, or GVHD.						

(continued)

Appendix 2 *(continued)*

		Grade				
Adverse Event	**Short Name**	**1**	**2**	**3**	**4**	**5**
Mucositis/stomatitis (functional/symptomatic) – *Select*: – Anus – Esophagus – Large bowel – Larynx – Oral cavity – Pharynx – Rectum – Small bowel – Stomach – Trachea	Mucositis (functional/symptomatic) – *Select*	*Upper aerodigestive tract sites:* Minimal symptoms, normal diet; minimal respiratory symptoms but not interfering with function *Lower GI sites:* Minimal discomfort, intervention not indicated	*Upper aerodigestive tract sites:* Symptomatic but can eat and swallow modified diet; respiratory symptoms interfering with function but not interfering with ADL *Lower GI sites:* Symptomatic, medical intervention indicated but not interfering with ADL	*Upper aerodigestive tract sites:* Symptomatic and unable to adequately aliment or hydrate orally; respiratory symptoms interfering with ADL *Lower GI sites:* Stool incontinence or other symptoms interfering with ADL	Symptoms associated with life-threatening consequences	Death
Nausea	Nausea	Loss of appetite without alteration in eating habits	Oral intake decreased without significant weight loss, dehydration or malnutrition; IV fluids indicated <24 hrs	Inadequate oral caloric or fluid intake; IV fluids, tube feedings, or TPN indicated ≥24 hrs	Life-threatening consequences	Death
ALSO CONSIDER: Anorexia; Vomiting.						

(continued)

Appendix 2 *(continued)*

		Grade				
Adverse Event	**Short Name**	**1**	**2**	**3**	**4**	**5**
Necrosis, GI – *Select*: – Anus – Colon/cecum/appendix – Duodenum – Esophagus – Gallbladder – Hepatic – Ileum – Jejunum – Oral – Pancreas – Peritoneal cavity – Pharynx – Rectum – Small bowel NOS – Stoma – Stomach	Necrosis, GI – *Select*	—	—	Inability to aliment adequately by GI tract (e.g., requiring enteral or parenteral nutrition); interventional radiology, endoscopic, or operative intervention indicated	Life-threatening consequences; operative intervention requiring complete organ resection (e.g., total colectomy)	Death
ALSO CONSIDER: Visceral arterial ischemia (non-myocardial).						

(continued)

Appendix 2 *(continued)*

		Grade				
Adverse Event	**Short Name**	**1**	**2**	**3**	**4**	**5**
Obstruction, GI – *Select*: – Cecum – Colon – Duodenum – Esophagus – Gallbladder – Ileum – Jejunum – Rectum – Small bowel NOS – Stoma – Stomach	Obstruction, GI – *Select*	Asymptomatic radiographic findings only	Symptomatic; altered GI function (e.g., altered dietary habits, vomiting, diarrhea, or GI fluid loss); IV fluids indicated <24 hrs	Symptomatic and severely altered GI function (e.g., altered dietary habits, vomiting, diarrhea, or GI fluid loss); IV fluids, tube feedings, or TPN indicated ≥24 hrs; operative intervention indicated	Life-threatening consequences; operative intervention requiring complete organ resection (e.g., total colectomy)	Death

NAVIGATION NOTE: Operative injury is graded as Intra-operative injury – *Select Organ or Structure* in the SURGERY/INTRA-OPERATIVE INJURY CATEGORY.

NAVIGATION NOTE: Pelvic pain is graded as Pain – *Select* in the PAIN CATEGORY.

(continued)

Appendix 2 *(continued)*

		Grade				
Adverse Event	**Short Name**	**1**	**2**	**3**	**4**	**5**
Perforation, GI – *Select*: – Appendix – Biliary tree – Cecum – Colon – Duodenum – Esophagus – Gallbladder – Ileum – Jejunum – Rectum – Small bowel NOS – Stomach	Perforation, GI – *Select*	Asymptomatic radiographic findings only	Medical intervention indicated; IV fluids indicated <24 hrs	IV fluids, tube feedings, or TPN indicated ≥24 hrs; operative intervention indicated	Life-threatening consequences	Death
Proctitis	Proctitis	Rectal discomfort, intervention not indicated	Symptoms not interfering with ADL; medical intervention indicated	Stool incontinence or other symptoms interfering with ADL; operative intervention indicated	Life-threatening consequences (e.g., perforation)	Death
Prolapse of stoma, GI	Prolapse of stoma, GI	Asymptomatic	Extraordinary local care or maintenance; minor revision indicated	Dysfunctional stoma; major revision indicated	Life-threatening consequences	Death

REMARK: Other stoma complications may be graded as Fistula, GI – *Select*; Leak (including anastomotic), GI – *Select*; Obstruction, GI – *Select;* Perforation, GI – *Select*; Stricture/stenosis (including anastomotic), GI – *Select*.

(continued)

Appendix 2 *(continued)*

		Grade				
Adverse Event	**Short Name**	**1**	**2**	**3**	**4**	**5**
NAVIGATION NOTE: Rectal or perirectal pain (proctalgia) is graded as Pain – *Select* in the PAIN CATEGORY.						
Salivary gland changes/saliva	Salivary gland changes	Slightly thickened saliva; slightly altered taste (e.g., metallic)	Thick, ropy, sticky saliva; markedly altered taste; alteration in diet indicated; secretioninduced symptoms not interfering with ADL	Acute salivary gland necrosis; severe secretion-induced symptoms interfering with ADL	Disabling	—
ALSO CONSIDER: Dry mouth/salivary gland (xerostomia); Mucositis/stomatitis (clinical exam) – *Select*; Mucositis/stomatitis (functional/symptomatic) – *Select*; Taste alteration (dysgeusia).						
NAVIGATION NOTE: Splenic function is graded in the BLOOD/BONE MARROW CATEGORY.						

(continued)

Appendix 2 *(continued)*

		Grade				
Adverse Event	**Short Name**	**1**	**2**	**3**	**4**	**5**
Stricture/stenosis (including anastomotic), GI – *Select*: – Anus – Biliary tree – Cecum – Colon – Duodenum – Esophagus – Ileum – Jejunum – Pancreas/pancreatic duct – Pharynx – Rectum – Small bowel NOS – Stoma – Stomach	Stricture, GI – *Select*	Asymptomatic radiographic findings only	Symptomatic; altered GI function (e.g., altered dietary habits, vomiting, bleeding, diarrhea); IV fluids indicated <24 hrs	Symptomatic and severely altered GI function (e.g., altered dietary habits, diarrhea, or GI fluid loss); IV fluids, tube feedings, or TPN indicated ≥24 hrs; operative intervention indicated	Life-threatening consequences; operative intervention requiring complete organ resection (e.g., total colectomy)	Death
Taste alteration (dysgeusia)	Taste alteration	Altered taste but no change in diet	Altered taste with change in diet (e.g., oral supplements); noxious or unpleasant taste; loss of taste	—	—	—

(continued)

Appendix 2 *(continued)*

		Grade				
Adverse Event	**Short Name**	**1**	**2**	**3**	**4**	**5**
Typhlitis (cecal inflammation)	Typhlitis	Asymptomatic, pathologic or radiographic findings only	Abdominal pain; mucus or blood in stool	Abdominal pain, fever, change in bowel habits with ileus; peritoneal signs	Life-threatening consequences (e.g., perforation, bleeding, ischemia, necrosis); operative intervention indicated	Death
ALSO CONSIDER: Colitis; Hemorrhage, GI – *Select* ; Ileus, GI (functional obstruction of bowel, i.e., neuroconstipation).						
Ulcer, GI – *Select*: – Anus – Cecum – Colon – Duodenum – Esophagus – Ileum – Jejunum – Rectum – Small bowel NOS – Stoma – Stomach	Ulcer, GI – *Select*	Asymptomatic, radiographic or endoscopic findings only	Symptomatic; altered GI function (e.g., altered dietary habits, oral supplements); IV fluids indicated <24 hrs	Symptomatic and severely altered GI function (e.g., inadequate oral caloric or fluid intake); IV fluids, tube feedings, or TPN indicated ≥24 hrs	Life-threatening consequences	Death
ALSO CONSIDER: Hemorrhage, GI – *Select*.						
Vomiting	Vomiting	1 episode in 24 hrs	2 – 5 episodes in 24 hrs; IV fluids indicated <24 hrs	≥6 episodes in 24 hrs; IV fluids, or TPN indicated ≥24 hrs	Life-threatening consequences	Death

(continued)

Appendix 2 *(continued)*

		Grade				
Adverse Event	**Short Name**	**1**	**2**	**3**	**4**	**5**
ALSO CONSIDER: Dehydration.						
Gastrointestinal – Other (Specify, ______)	GI – Other (Specify)	Mild	Moderate	Severe	Life-threatening; disabling	Death
GROWTH AND DEVELOPMENT						
		Grade				
Adverse Event	**Short Name**	**1**	**2**	**3**	**4**	**5**
Bone age (alteration in bone age)	Bone age	—	±2 SD (standard deviation) from normal	—	—	—
Bone growth: femoral head; slipped capital femoral epiphysis	Femoral head growth	Mild valgus/varus deformity	Moderate valgus/varus deformity, symptomatic, interfering with function but not interfering with ADL	Mild slipped capital femoral epiphysis; operative intervention (e.g., fixation) indicated; interfering with ADL	Disabling; severe slipped capital femoral epiphysis >60%; avascular necrosis	—
Bone growth: limb length discrepancy	Limb length	Mild length discrepancy <2 cm	Moderate length discrepancy 2 – 5 cm; shoe lift indicated	Severe length discrepancy >5 cm; operative intervention indicated; interfering with ADL	Disabling; epiphysiodesis	—

(continued)

Appendix 2 *(continued)*

		Grade				
Adverse Event	**Short Name**	**1**	**2**	**3**	**4**	**5**
Bone growth: spine kyphosis/lordosis	Kyphosis/lordosis	Mild radiographic changes	Moderate accentuation; interfering with function but not interfering with ADL	Severe accentuation; operative intervention indicated; interfering with ADL	Disabling (e.g., cannot lift head)	—
Growth velocity (reduction in growth velocity)	Reduction in growth velocity	10 – 29% reduction in growth from the baseline growth curve	30 – 49% reduction in growth from the baseline growth curve	≥50% reduction in growth from the baseline growth curve	—	—
Puberty (delayed)	Delayed puberty	—	No breast development by age 13 yrs for females; no Tanner Stage 2 development by age 14.5 yrs for males	No sexual development by age 14 yrs for girls, age 16 yrs for boys; hormone replacement indicated	—	—
REMARK: Do not use testicular size for Tanner Stage in male cancer survivors.						
Puberty (precocious)	Precocious puberty	—	Physical signs of puberty <7 years for females, <9 years for males	—	—	—
Short stature	Short stature	Beyond two standard deviations of age and gender mean height	Altered ADL	—	—	—
REMARK: Short stature is secondary to growth hormone deficiency.						

(continued)

Appendix 2 *(continued)*

		Grade				
Adverse Event	**Short Name**	**1**	**2**	**3**	**4**	**5**
ALSO CONSIDER: Neuroendocrine: growth hormone secretion abnormality.						
Growth and Development – Other (Specify, ______)	Growth and Development – Other (Specify)	Mild	Moderate	Severe	Life-threatening; disabling	Death

HEMORRHAGE/BLEEDING

		Grade				
Adverse Event	**Short Name**	**1**	**2**	**3**	**4**	**5**
Hematoma	Hematoma	Minimal symptoms, invasive intervention not indicated	Minimally invasive evacuation or aspiration indicated	Transfusion, interventional radiology, or operative intervention indicated	Life-threatening consequences; major urgent intervention indicated	Death
REMARK: Hematoma refers to extravasation at wound or operative site or secondary to other intervention. Transfusion implies pRBC.						
ALSO CONSIDER: Fibrinogen; INR (International Normalized Ratio of prothrombin time); Platelets; PTT (Partial Thromboplastin Time).						
Hemorrhage/bleeding associated with surgery, intra-operative or postoperative	Hemorrhage with surgery	—	—	Requiring transfusion of 2 units non-autologous (10 cc/kg for pediatrics) pRBCs beyond protocol specification; postoperative interventional radiology, endoscopic, or operative intervention indicated	Life-threatening consequences	Death

(continued)

Appendix 2 *(continued)*

		Grade				
Adverse Event	**Short Name**	**1**	**2**	**3**	**4**	**5**
REMARK: Postoperative period is defined as ≤72 hours after surgery. Verify protocol-specific acceptable guidelines regarding pRBC transfusion.						
ALSO CONSIDER: Fibrinogen; INR (International Normalized Ratio of prothrombin time); Platelets; PTT (Partial Thromboplastin Time).						
Hemorrhage, CNS	CNS hemorrhage	Asymptomatic, radiographic findings only	Medical intervention indicated	Ventriculostomy, ICP monitoring, intraventricular thrombolysis, or operative intervention indicated	Life-threatening consequences; neurologic deficit or disability	Death
ALSO CONSIDER: Fibrinogen; INR (International Normalized Ratio of prothrombin time); Platelets; PTT (Partial Thromboplastin Time).						

(continued)

Appendix 2 *(continued)*

		Grade				
Adverse Event	**Short Name**	**1**	**2**	**3**	**4**	**5**
Hemorrhage, GI – *Select*: – Abdomen NOS – Anus – Biliary tree – Cecum/appendix – Colon – Duodenum – Esophagus – Ileum – Jejunum – Liver – Lower GI NOS – Oral cavity – Pancreas – Peritoneal cavity – Rectum – Stoma – Stomach – Upper GI NOS – Varices (esophageal) – Varices (rectal)	Hemorrhage, GI – *Select*	Mild, intervention (other than iron supplements) not indicated	Symptomatic and medical intervention or minor cauterization indicated	Transfusion, interventional radiology, endoscopic, or operative intervention indicated; radiation therapy (i.e., hemostasis of bleeding site)	Life-threatening consequences; major urgent intervention indicated	Death
REMARK: Transfusion implies pRBC.						
ALSO CONSIDER: Fibrinogen; INR (International Normalized Ratio of prothrombin time); Platelets; PTT (Partial Thromboplastin Time).						

(continued)

Appendix 2 *(continued)*

		Grade				
Adverse Event	**Short Name**	**1**	**2**	**3**	**4**	**5**
Hemorrhage, GU – *Select*: – Bladder – Fallopian tube – Kidney – Ovary – Prostate – Retroperitoneum – Spermatic cord – Stoma – Testes – Ureter – Urethra – Urinary NOS – Uterus – Vagina – Vas deferens	Hemorrhage, GU – *Select*	Minimal or microscopic bleeding; intervention not indicated	Gross bleeding, medical intervention, or urinary tract irrigation indicated	Transfusion, interventional radiology, endoscopic, or operative intervention indicated; radiation therapy (i.e., hemostasis of bleeding site)	Life-threatening consequences; major urgent intervention indicated	Death
REMARK: Transfusion implies pRBC.						
ALSO CONSIDER: Fibrinogen; INR (International Normalized Ratio of prothrombin time); Platelets; PTT (Partial Thromboplastin Time).						

(continued)

Appendix 2 *(continued)*

		Grade				
Adverse Event	**Short Name**	**1**	**2**	**3**	**4**	**5**
Hemorrhage, pulmonary/upper respiratory – *Select*: – Bronchopulmonary NOS – Bronchus – Larynx – Lung – Mediastinum – Nose – Pharynx – Pleura – Respiratory tract NOS – Stoma – Trachea	Hemorrhage pulmonary – *Select*	Mild, intervention not indicated	Symptomatic and medical intervention indicated	Transfusion, interventional radiology, endoscopic, or operative intervention indicated; radiation therapy (i.e., hemostasis of bleeding site)	Life-threatening consequences; major urgent intervention indicated	Death
REMARK: Transfusion implies pRBC.						
ALSO CONSIDER: Fibrinogen; INR (International Normalized Ratio of prothrombin time); Platelets; PTT (Partial Thromboplastin Time).						
Petechiae/purpura (hemorrhage/bleeding into skin or mucosa)	Petechiae	Few petechiae	Moderate petechiae; purpura	Generalized petechiae or purpura	—	—
ALSO CONSIDER: Fibrinogen; INR (International Normalized Ratio of prothrombin time); Platelets; PTT (Partial Thromboplastin Time).						
NAVIGATION NOTE: Vitreous hemorrhage is graded in the OCULAR/VISUAL CATEGORY.						

(continued)

Appendix 2 *(continued)*

		Grade				
Adverse Event	**Short Name**	**1**	**2**	**3**	**4**	**5**
Hemorrhage/Bleeding – Other (Specify, ______)	Hemorrhage – Other (Specify)	Mild without transfusion	—	Transfusion indicated	Catastrophic bleeding, requiring major nonelective intervention	Death

HEPATOBILIARY/PANCREAS

		Grade				
Adverse Event	**Short Name**	**1**	**2**	**3**	**4**	**5**
NAVIGATION NOTE: Biliary tree damage is graded as Fistula, GI – *Select*; Leak (including anastomotic), GI – *Select*; Necrosis, GI – *Select*; Obstruction, GI – *Select*; Perforation, GI – *Select*; Stricture/stenosis (including anastomotic), GI – *Select* in the GASTROINTESTINAL CATEGORY.						
Cholecystitis	Cholecystitis	Asymptomatic, radiographic findings only	Symptomatic, medical intervention indicated	Interventional radiology, endoscopic, or operative intervention indicated	Life-threatening consequences (e.g., sepsis or perforation)	Death
ALSO CONSIDER: Infection (documented clinically or microbiologically) with Grade 3 or 4 neutrophils – *Select*; Infection with normal ANC or Grade 1 or 2 neutrophils – *Select*; Infection with unknown ANC – *Select*.						
Liver dysfunction/failure (clinical)	Liver dysfunction	—	Jaundice	Asterixis	Encephalopathy or coma	Death
REMARK: Jaundice is not an AE, but occurs when the liver is not working properly or when a bile duct is blocked. It is graded as a result of liver dysfunction/failure or elevated bilirubin. ALSO CONSIDER: Bilirubin (hyperbilirubinemia).						
Pancreas, exocrine enzyme deficiency	Pancreas, exocrine enzyme deficiency	—	Increase in stool frequency, bulk, or odor; steatorrhea	Sequelae of absorption deficiency (e.g., weight loss)	Life-threatening consequences	Death

(continued)

Appendix 2 *(continued)*

		Grade				
Adverse Event	**Short Name**	**1**	**2**	**3**	**4**	**5**
ALSO CONSIDER: Diarrhea.						
Pancreatitis	Pancreatitis	Asymptomatic, enzyme elevation and/or radiographic findings	Symptomatic, medical intervention indicated	Interventional radiology or operative intervention indicated	Life-threatening consequences (e.g., circulatory failure, hemorrhage, sepsis)	Death
ALSO CONSIDER: Amylase.						
NAVIGATION NOTE: Stricture (biliary tree, hepatic or pancreatic) is graded as Stricture/stenosis (including anastomotic), GI – *Select* in the GASTROINTESTINAL CATEGORY.						
Hepatobiliary/Pancreas – Other (Specify, ______)	Hepatobiliary – Other (Specify)	Mild	Moderate	Severe	Life-threatening; disabling	Death

INFECTION

		Grade				
Adverse Event	**Short Name**	**1**	**2**	**3**	**4**	**5**
Colitis, infectious (e.g., Clostridium difficile)	Colitis, infectious	Asymptomatic, pathologic or radiographic findings only	Abdominal pain with mucus and/or blood in stool	IV antibiotics or TPN indicated	Life-threatening consequences (e.g., perforation, bleeding, ischemia, necrosis or toxic megacolon); operative resection or diversion indicated	Death
ALSO CONSIDER: Hemorrhage, GI – *Select*; Typhlitis (cecal inflammation).						

(continued)

Appendix 2 *(continued)*

		Grade				
Adverse Event	**Short Name**	**1**	**2**	**3**	**4**	**5**
Febrile neutropenia (fever of unknown origin without clinically or microbiologically documented infection) (ANC $<1.0 \times 10^9$/L, fever $\geq$38.5°C)	Febrile neutropenia	—	—	Present	Life-threatening consequences (e.g., septic shock, hypotension, acidosis, necrosis)	Death
ALSO CONSIDER: Neutrophils/granulocytes (ANC/AGC).						
Infection (documented clinically or microbiologically) with Grade 3 or 4 neutrophils (ANC $<1.0 \times 10^9$/L) – *Select* *'Select'* AEs appear at the end of the CATEGORY.	Infection (documented clinically) – *Select*	—	Localized, local intervention indicated	IV antibiotic, antifungal, or antiviral intervention indicated; interventional radiology or operative intervention indicated	Life-threatening consequences (e.g., septic shock, hypotension, acidosis, necrosis)	Death
REMARK: Fever with Grade 3 or 4 neutrophils in the absence of documented infection is graded as Febrile neutropenia (fever of unknown origin without clinically or microbiologically documented infection).						
ALSO CONSIDER: Neutrophils/granulocytes (ANC/AGC).						

(continued)

Appendix 2 *(continued)*

		Grade				
Adverse Event	**Short Name**	**1**	**2**	**3**	**4**	**5**
Infection with normal ANC or Grade 1 or 2 neutrophils – *Select* '*Select*' AEs appear at the end of the CATEGORY.	Infection with normal ANC – *Select*	—	Localized, local intervention indicated	IV antibiotic, antifungal, or antiviral intervention indicated; interventional radiology or operative intervention indicated	Life-threatening consequences (e.g., septic shock, hypotension, acidosis, necrosis)	Death
Infection with unknown ANC – *Select* '*Select*' AEs appear at the end of the CATEGORY.	Infection with unknown ANC – *Select*	—	Localized, local intervention indicated	IV antibiotic, antifungal, or antiviral intervention indicated; interventional radiology or operative intervention indicated	Life-threatening consequences (e.g., septic shock, hypotension, acidosis, necrosis)	Death
REMARK: Infection with unknown ANC – *Select* is to be used in the rare case when ANC is unknown.						
Opportunistic infection associated with ≥Grade 2 Lymphopenia	Opportunistic infection	—	Localized, local intervention indicated	IV antibiotic, antifungal, or antiviral intervention indicated; interventional radiology or operative intervention indicated	Life-threatening consequences (e.g., septic shock, hypotension, acidosis, necrosis)	Death
ALSO CONSIDER: Lymphopenia.						

(continued)

Appendix 2 *(continued)*

		Grade				
Adverse Event	**Short Name**	**1**	**2**	**3**	**4**	**5**
Viral hepatitis	Viral hepatitis	Present; transaminases and liver function normal	Transaminases abnormal, liver function normal	Symptomatic liver dysfunction; fibrosis by biopsy; compensated cirrhosis	Decompensated liver function (e.g., ascites, coagulopathy, encephalopathy, coma)	Death
REMARK: Non-viral hepatitis is graded as Infection – *Select.*						
ALSO CONSIDER: Albumin, serum-low (hypoalbuminemia); ALT, SGPT (serum glutamic pyruvic transaminase); AST, SGOT (serum glutamic oxaloacetic transaminase); Bilirubin (hyperbilirubinemia); Encephalopathy.						
Infection – Other (Specify, ______)	Infection – Other (Specify)	Mild	Moderate	Severe	Life-threatening; disabling	Death

INFECTION – *SELECT*

AUDITORY/EAR
- External ear (otitis externa)
- Middle ear (otitis media)

CARDIOVASCULAR
- Artery
- Heart (endocarditis)
- Spleen
- Vein

DERMATOLOGY/SKIN
- Lip/perioral
- Peristomal
- Skin (cellulitis)
- Ungual (nails)

GENERAL
- Blood
- Catheter-related
- Foreign body (e.g., graft, implant, prosthesis, stent)
- Wound

HEPATOBILIARY/PANCREAS
- Biliary tree
- Gallbladder (cholecystitis)
- Liver
- Pancreas

LYMPHATIC
- Lymphatic

PULMONARY/UPPER RESPIRATORY
- Bronchus
- Larynx
- Lung (pneumonia)
- Mediastinum NOS
- Mucosa
- Neck NOS
- Nose
- Paranasal
- Pharynx
- Pleura (empyema)
- Sinus
- Trachea

(continued)

Appendix 2 *(continued)*

GASTROINTESTINAL
- Abdomen NOS
- Anal/perianal
- Appendix
- Cecum
- Colon
- Dental-tooth
- Duodenum
- Esophagus
- Ileum
- Jejunum
- Oral cavity-gums (gingivitis)
- Peritoneal cavity
- Rectum
- Salivary gland
- Small bowel NOS
- Stomach

MUSCULOSKELETAL
- Bone (osteomyelitis)
- Joint
- Muscle (infection myositis)
- Soft tissue NOS

NEUROLOGY
- Brain (encephalitis, infectious)
- Brain + Spinal cord (encephalomyelitis)
- Meninges (meningitis)
- Nerve-cranial
- Nerve-peripheral
- Spinal cord (myelitis)

OCULAR
- Conjunctiva
- Cornea
- Eye NOS
- Lens
- Upper aerodigestive NOS
- Upper airway NOS

RENAL/GENITOURINARY
- Bladder (urinary)
- Kidney
- Prostate
- Ureter
- Urethra
- Urinary tract NOS

SEXUAL/REPRODUCTIVE FUNCTION
- Cervix
- Fallopian tube
- Pelvis NOS
- Penis
- Scrotum
- Uterus
- Vagina
- Vulva

LYMPHATICS

		Grade				
Adverse Event	**Short Name**	**1**	**2**	**3**	**4**	**5**
Chyle or lymph leakage	Chyle or lymph leakage	Asymptomatic, clinical or radiographic findings	Symptomatic, medical intervention indicated	Interventional radiology or operative intervention indicated	Life-threatening complications	Death

ALSO CONSIDER: Chylothorax.

(Continued)

Appendix 2 *(continued)*

		Grade				
Adverse Event	**Short Name**	**1**	**2**	**3**	**4**	**5**
Dermal change lymphedema, phlebolymphedema	Dermal change	Trace thickening or faint discoloration	Marked discoloration; leathery skin texture; papillary formation	—	—	—
REMARK: Dermal change lymphedema, phlebolymphedema refers to changes due to venous stasis. ALSO CONSIDER: Ulceration.						
Edema: head and neck	Edema: head and neck	Localized to dependent areas, no disability or functional impairment	Localized facial or neck edema with functional impairment	Generalized facial or neck edema with functional impairment (e.g., difficulty in turning neck or opening mouth compared to baseline)	Severe with ulceration or cerebral edema; tracheotomy or feeding tube indicated	Death

(Continued)

Appendix 2 *(continued)*

		Grade				
Adverse Event	**Short Name**	**1**	**2**	**3**	**4**	**5**
Edema: limb	Edema: limb	5 – 10% inter-limb discrepancy in volume or circumference at point of greatest visible difference; swelling or obscuration of anatomic architecture on close inspection; pitting edema	>10 – 30% inter-limb discrepancy in volume or circumference at point of greatest visible difference; readily apparent obscuration of anatomic architecture; obliteration of skin folds; readily apparent deviation from normal anatomic contour	>30% inter-limb discrepancy in volume; lymphorrhea; gross deviation from normal anatomic contour; interfering with ADL	Progression to malignancy (i.e., lymphangiosarcoma); amputation indicated; disabling	Death
Edema: trunk/genital	Edema: trunk/genital	Swelling or obscuration of anatomic architecture on close inspection; pitting edema	Readily apparent obscuration of anatomic architecture; obliteration of skin folds; readily apparent deviation from normal anatomic contour	Lymphorrhea; interfering with ADL; gross deviation from normal anatomic contour	Progression to malignancy (i.e., lymphangiosarcoma); disabling	Death

(Continued)

Appendix 2 *(continued)*

		Grade				
Adverse Event	**Short Name**	**1**	**2**	**3**	**4**	**5**
Edema:viscera	Edema: viscera	Asymptomatic; clinical or radiographic findings only	Symptomatic; medical intervention indicated	Symptomatic and unable to aliment adequately orally; interventional radiology or operative intervention indicated	Life-threatening consequences	Death
Lymphedema-related fibrosis	Lymphedema-related fibrosis	Minimal to moderate redundant soft tissue, unresponsive to elevation or compression, with moderately firm texture or spongy feel	Marked increase in density and firmness, with or without tethering	Very marked density and firmness with tethering affecting ≥40% of the edematous area	—	—
Lymphocele	Lymphocele	Asymptomatic, clinical or radiographic findings only	Symptomatic; medical intervention indicated	Symptomatic and interventional radiology or operative intervention indicated	—	—
Phlebolymphatic cording	Phlebolymphatic cording	Asymptomatic, clinical findings only	Symptomatic; medical intervention indicated	Symptomatic and leading to contracture or reduced range of motion	—	—
Lymphatics – Other (Specify, ______)	Lymphatics – Other (Specify)	Mild	Moderate	Severe	Life-threatening; disabling	Death

(Continued)

Appendix 2 *(continued)*

METABOLIC/LABORATORY

		Grade				
Adverse Event	**Short Name**	**1**	**2**	**3**	**4**	**5**
Acidosis (metabolic or respiratory)	Acidosis	pH <normal, but ≥7.3	—	pH <7.3	pH <7.3 with lifeth-reatening consequences	Death
Albumin, serum-low (hypoalbuminemia)	Hypoalbuminemia	<LLN – 3 g/dL <LLN – 30 g/L	<3 – 2 g/dL <30 – 20 g/L	<2 g/dL <20 g/L	—	Death
Alkaline phosphatase	Alkaline phosphatase	>ULN – 2.5 × ULN	>2.5 – 5.0 × ULN	>5.0 – 20.0 × ULN	>20.0 × ULN	—
Alkalosis (metabolic or respiratory)	Alkalosis	pH >normal, but ≥7.5	—	pH >7.5	pH >7.5 with lifeth-reatening consequences	Death
ALT, SGPT (serum glutamic pyruvic transaminase)	ALT	>ULN – 2.5 × ULN	>2.5 – 5.0 × ULN	>5.0 – 20.0 × ULN	>20.0 × ULN	—
Amylase	Amylase	>ULN – 1.5 × ULN	>1.5 – 2.0 × ULN	>2.0 – 5.0 × ULN	>5.0 × ULN	—
AST, SGOT (serum glutamic oxaloacetic transaminase)	AST	>ULN – 2.5 × ULN	>2.5 – 5.0 × ULN	>5.0 – 20.0 × ULN	>20.0 × ULN	—
Bicarbonate, serum-low	Bicarbonate, serum-low	<LLN – 16 mmol/L	<16 – 11 mmol/L	<11 – 8 mmol/L	<8 mmol/L	Death
Bilirubin (hyperbilirubinemia)	Bilirubin	>ULN – 1.5 × ULN	>1.5 – 3.0 × ULN	>3.0 – 10.0 × ULN	>10.0 × ULN	—

(Continued)

Appendix 2 *(continued)*

		Grade				
Adverse Event	**Short Name**	**1**	**2**	**3**	**4**	**5**
REMARK: Jaundice is not an AE, but may be a manifestation of liver dysfunction/failure or elevated bilirubin. If jaundice is associated with elevated bilirubin, grade bilirubin.						
Calcium, serum-low (hypocalcemia)	Hypocalcemia	<LLN – 8.0 mg/dL <LLN – 2.0 mmol/L Ionized calcium: <LLN – 1.0 mmol/L	<8.0 – 7.0 mg/dL <2.0 – 1.75 mmol/L Ionized calcium: <1.0 – 0.9 mmol/L	<7.0 – 6.0 mg/dL <1.75 – 1.5 mmol/L Ionized calcium: <0.9 – 0.8 mmol/L	<6.0 mg/dL <1.5 mmol/L Ionized calcium: <0.8 mmol/L	Death
REMARK: Calcium can be falsely low if hypoalbuminemia is present. Serum albumin is <4.0 g/dL, hypocalcemia is reported after the following corrective calculation has been performed: Corrected Calcium (mg/dL) = Total Calcium (mg/dL) – 0.8 [Albumin (g/dL) – 4][4]. Alternatively, direct measurement of ionized calcium is the definitive method to diagnose metabolically relevant alterations in serum calcium.						
Calcium, serum-high (hypercalcemia)	Hypercalcemia	>ULN – 11.5 mg/dL >ULN – 2.9 mmol/L Ionized calcium: >ULN – 1.5 mmol/L	>11.5 – 12.5 mg/dL >2.9 – 3.1 mmol/L Ionized calcium: >1.5 – 1.6 mmol/L	>12.5 – 13.5 mg/dL >3.1 – 3.4 mmol/L Ionized calcium: >1.6 – 1.8 mmol/L	>13.5 mg/dL >3.4 mmol/L Ionized calcium: >1.8 mmol/L	Death
Cholesterol, serum-high (hypercholesteremia)	Cholesterol	>ULN – 300 mg/dL >ULN – 7.75 mmol/L	>300 – 400 mg/dL >7.75 – 10.34 mmol/L	>400 – 500 mg/dL >10.34 – 12.92 mmol/L	>500 mg/dL >12.92 mmol/L	Death
CPK (creatine phosphokinase)	CPK	>ULN – 2.5 × ULN	>2.5 × ULN – 5 × ULN	>5 × ULN – 10 × ULN	>10 × ULN	Death
Creatinine	Creatinine	>ULN – 1.5 × ULN	>1.5 – 3.0 × ULN	>3.0 – 6.0 × ULN	>6.0 × ULN	Death
REMARK: Adjust to age-appropriate levels for pediatric patients. ALSO CONSIDER: Glomerular filtration rate.						
GGT (γ-Glutamyltranspeptidase)	GGT	>ULN – 2.5 × ULN	>2.5 – 5.0 × ULN	>5.0 – 20.0 × ULN	>20.0 × ULN	—

(Continued)

Appendix 2 *(continued)*

		Grade				
Adverse Event	**Short Name**	**1**	**2**	**3**	**4**	**5**
Glomerular filtration rate	GFR	<75 – 50% LLN	<50 – 25% LLN	<25% LLN, chronic dialysis not indicated	Chronic dialysis or renal transplant indicated	Death
ALSO CONSIDER: Creatinine.						
Glucose, serum-high (hyperglycemia)	Hyperglycemia	>ULN – 160 mg/dL >ULN – 8.9 mmol/L	>160 – 250 mg/dL >8.9 – 13.9 mmol/L	>250 – 500 mg/dL >13.9 – 27.8 mmol/L	>500 mg/dL >27.8 mmol/L or acidosis	Death
REMARK: Hyperglycemia, in general, is defined as fasting unless otherwise specified in protocol.						
Glucose, serum-low (hypoglycemia)	Hypoglycemia	<LLN – 55 mg/dL <LLN – 3.0 mmol/L	<55 – 40 mg/dL <3.0 – 2.2 mmol/L	<40 – 30 mg/dL <2.2 – 1.7 mmol/L	<30 mg/dL <1.7 mmol/L	Death
Hemoglobinuria	Hemoglobinuria	Present	—	—	—	Death
Lipase	Lipase	>ULN – 1.5 × ULN	>1.5 – 2.0 × ULN	>2.0 – 5.0 × ULN	>5.0 × ULN	—
Magnesium, serum-high (hypermagnesemia)	Hypermagnesemia	>ULN – 3.0 mg/dL >ULN – 1.23 mmol/L	—	>3.0 – 8.0 mg/dL >1.23 – 3.30 mmol/L	>8.0 mg/dL >3.30 mmol/L	Death
Magnesium, serum-low (hypomagnesemia)	Hypomagnesemia	<LLN – 1.2 mg/dL <LLN – 0.5 mmol/L	<1.2 – 0.9 mg/dL <0.5 – 0.4 mmol/L	<0.9 – 0.7 mg/dL <0.4 – 0.3 mmol/L	<0.7 mg/dL <0.3 mmol/L	Death
Phosphate, serum-low (hypophosphatemia)	Hypophosphatemia	<LLN – 2.5 mg/dL <LLN – 0.8 mmol/L	<2.5 – 2.0 mg/dL <0.8 – 0.6 mmol/L	<2.0 – 1.0 mg/dL <0.6 – 0.3 mmol/L	<1.0 mg/dL <0.3 mmol/L	Death
Potassium, serum-high (hyperkalemia)	Hyperkalemia	>ULN – 5.5 mmol/L	>5.5 – 6.0 mmol/L	>6.0 – 7.0 mmol/L	>7.0 mmol/L	Death

(Continued)

Appendix 2 *(continued)*

		Grade				
Adverse Event	**Short Name**	**1**	**2**	**3**	**4**	**5**
Potassium, serum-low (hypokalemia)	Hypokalemia	<LLN – 3.0 mmol/L	—	<3.0 – 2.5 mmol/L	<2.5 mmol/L	Death
Proteinuria	Proteinuria	1+ or 0.15 – 1.0 g/24 hrs	2+ to 3+ or >1.0 – 3.5 g/24 hrs	4+ or >3.5 g/24 hrs	Nephrotic syndrome	Death
Sodium, serum-high (hypernatremia)	Hypernatremia	>ULN – 150 mmol/L	>150 – 155 mmol/L	>155 – 160 mmol/L	>160 mmol/L	Death
Sodium, serum-low (hyponatremia)	Hyponatremia	<LLN – 130 mmol/L	—	<130 – 120 mmol/L	<120 mmol/L	Death
Triglyceride, serum-high (hypertriglyceridemia)	Hypertriglyceridemia	>ULN – 2.5 × ULN	>2.5 – 5.0 × ULN	>5.0 – 10 × ULN	>10 × ULN	Death
Uric acid, serum-high (hyperuricemia)	Hyperuricemia	>ULN – 10 mg/dL ≤0.59 mmol/L without physiologic consequences	—	>ULN – 10 mg/dL ≤0.59 mmol/L with physiologic consequences	>10 mg/dL >0.59 mmol/L	Death
ALSO CONSIDER: Creatinine; Potassium, serum-high (hyperkalemia); Renal failure; Tumor lysis syndrome.						
Metabolic/Laboratory – Other (Specify, ______)	Metabolic/Lab – Other (Specify)	Mild	Moderate	Severe	Life-threatening; disabling	Death

[4]Crit Rev Clin Lab Sci 1984;21(1):51-97

(Continued)

Appendix 2 *(continued)*

MUSCULOSKELETAL/SOFT TISSUE

		Grade				
Adverse Event	**Short Name**	**1**	**2**	**3**	**4**	**5**
Arthritis (non-septic)	Arthritis	Mild pain with inflammation, erythema, or joint swelling, but not interfering with function	Moderate pain with inflammation, erythema, or joint swelling interfering with function, but not interfering with ADL	Severe pain with inflammation, erythema, or joint swelling and interfering with ADL	Disabling	Death
REMARK: Report only when the diagnosis of arthritis (e.g., inflammation of a joint or a state characterized by inflammation of joints) is made. Arthralgia (sign or symptom of pain in a joint, especially non-inflammatory in character) is graded as Pain – *Select* in the PAIN CATEGORY.						
Bone: spine-scoliosis	Scoliosis	≤20 degrees; clinically undetectable	>20 – 45 degrees; visible by forward flexion; interfering with function but not interfering with ADL	>45 degrees; scapular prominence in forward flexion; operative intervention indicated; interfering with ADL	Disabling (e.g., interfering with cardiopulmonary function)	Death
Cervical spine-range of motion	Cervical spine ROM	Mild restriction of rotation or flexion between 60 – 70 degrees	Rotation <60 degrees to right or left; <60 degrees of flexion	Ankylosed/fused over multiple segments with no C-spine rotation	—	—
REMARK: 60 – 65 degrees of rotation is required for reversing a car; 60 – 65 degrees of flexion is required to tie shoes.						
Exostosis	Exostosis	Asymptomatic	Involving multiple sites; pain or interfering with function	Excision indicated	Progression to malignancy (i.e., chondrosarcoma)	Death

(Continued)

Appendix 2 *(continued)*

		Grade				
Adverse Event	**Short Name**	**1**	**2**	**3**	**4**	**5**
Extremity-lower (gait/walking)	Gait/walking	Limp evident only to trained observer and able to walk ≥1 kilometer; cane indicated for walking	Noticeable limp, or limitation of limb function, but able to walk ≥0.1 kilometer (1 city block); quad cane indicated for walking	Severe limp with stride modified to maintain balance (widened base of support, marked reduction in step length); ambulation limited to walker; crutches indicated	Unable to walk	—
ALSO CONSIDER: Ataxia (incoordination); Muscle weakness, generalized or specific area (not due to neuropathy) – *Select*.						
Extremity-upper (function)	Extremity-upper (function)	Able to perform most household or work activities with affected limb	Able to perform most household or work activities with compensation from unaffected limb	Interfering with ADL	Disabling; no function of affected limb	—
Fibrosis-cosmesis	Fibrosis-cosmesis	Visible only on close examination	Readily apparent but not disfiguring	Significant disfigurement; operative intervention indicated if patient chooses	—	—
Fibrosis-deep connective tissue	Fibrosis-deep connective tissue	Increased density, "spongy" feel	Increased density with firmness or tethering	Increased density with fixation of tissue; operative intervention indicated; interfering with ADL	Life-threatening; disabling; loss of limb; interfering with vital organ function	Death

(Continued)

Appendix 2 *(continued)*

		Grade				
Adverse Event	**Short Name**	**1**	**2**	**3**	**4**	**5**
ALSO CONSIDER: Induration/fibrosis (skin and subcutaneous tissue); Muscle weakness, generalized or specific area (not due to neuropathy) – *Select*; Neuropathy: motor; Neuropathy: sensory.						
Fracture	Fracture	Asymptomatic, radiographic findings only (e.g., asymptomatic rib fracture on plain x-ray, pelvic insufficiency fracture on MRI, etc.)	Symptomatic but nondisplaced; immobilization indicated	Symptomatic and displaced or open wound with bone exposure; operative intervention indicated	Disabling; amputation indicated	Death
Joint-effusion	Joint-effusion	Asymptomatic, clinical or radiographic findings only	Symptomatic; interfering with function but not interfering with ADL	Symptomatic and interfering with ADL	Disabling	Death
ALSO CONSIDER: Arthritis (non-septic).						
Joint-function[5]	Joint-function	Stiffness interfering with athletic activity; ≤25% loss of range of motion (ROM)	Stiffness interfering with function but not interfering with ADL; >25 – 50% decrease in ROM	Stiffness interfering with ADL; >50 – 75% decrease in ROM	Fixed or non-functional joint (arthrodesis); >75% decrease in ROM	—
ALSO CONSIDER: Arthritis (non-septic).						

(Continued)

Appendix 2 *(continued)*

		Grade				
Adverse Event	**Short Name**	**1**	**2**	**3**	**4**	**5**
Local complication – device/prosthesis-related	Device/prosthesis	Asymptomatic	Symptomatic, but not interfering with ADL; local wound care; medical intervention indicated	Symptomatic, interfering with ADL; operative intervention indicated (e.g., hardware/device replacement or removal, reconstruction)	Life-threatening; disabling; loss of limb or organ	Death
Lumbar spine-range of motion	Lumbar spine ROM	Stiffness and difficulty bending to the floor to pick up a very light object but able to do activity	Some lumbar spine flexion but requires a reaching aid to pick up a very light object from the floor	Ankylosed/fused over multiple segments with no L-spine flexion (i.e., unable to reach to floor to pick up a very light	—	—

(Continued)

Appendix 2 *(continued)*

		Grade				
Adverse Event	**Short Name**	**1**	**2**	**3**	**4**	**5**
Muscle weakness, generalized or specific area (not due to neuropathy) – *Select*: – Extraocular – Extremity-lower – Extremity-upper – Facial – Left-sided – Ocular – Pelvic – Right-sided – Trunk – Whole body/generalized	Muscle weakness – *Select*	Asymptomatic, weakness on physical exam	Symptomatic and interfering with function, but not interfering with ADL	Symptomatic and interfering with ADL	Life-threatening; disabling	Death
ALSO CONSIDER: Fatigue (asthenia, lethargy, malaise).						
Muscular/skeletal hypoplasia	Muscular/skeletal hypoplasia	Cosmetically and functionally insignificant hypoplasia	Deformity, hypoplasia, or asymmetry able to be remediated by prosthesis (e.g., shoe insert) or covered by clothing	Functionally significant deformity, hypoplasia, or asymmetry, unable to be remediated by prosthesis or covered by clothing	Disabling	—

(Continued)

Appendix 2 *(continued)*

		Grade				
Adverse Event	**Short Name**	**1**	**2**	**3**	**4**	**5**
Myositis (inflammation/damage of muscle)	Myositis	Mild pain, not interfering with function	Pain interfering with function, but not interfering with ADL	Pain interfering with ADL	Disabling	Death
REMARK: Myositis implies muscle damage (i.e., elevated CPK). ALSO CONSIDER: CPK (creatine phosphokinase); Pain – *Select*.						
Osteonecrosis (avascular necrosis)	Osteonecrosis	Asymptomatic, radiographic findings only	Symptomatic and interfering with function, but not interfering with ADL; minimal bone removal indicated (i.e., minor sequestrectomy)	Symptomatic and interfering with ADL; operative intervention or hyperbaric oxygen indicated	Disabling	Death
Osteoporosis[6]	Osteoporosis	Radiographic evidence of osteoporosis or Bone Mineral Density (BMD) t-score –1 to –2.5 (osteopenia) and no loss of height or therapy indicated	BMD t-score < -2.5; loss of height <2 cm; antiosteoporotic therapy indicated	Fractures; loss of height ≥ 2 cm	Disabling	Death
Seroma	Seroma	Asymptomatic	Symptomatic; medical intervention or simple aspiration indicated	Symptomatic, interventional radiology or operative intervention indicated	—	—

(Continued)

Appendix 2 *(continued)*

		Grade				
Adverse Event	**Short Name**	**1**	**2**	**3**	**4**	**5**
Soft tissue necrosis – *Select*: – Abdomen – Extremity-lower – Extremity-upper – Head – Neck – Pelvic – Thorax	Soft tissue necrosis – *Select*	—	Local wound care; medical intervention indicated	Operative debridement or other invasive intervention indicated (e.g., hyperbaric oxygen)	Life-threatening consequences; major invasive intervention indicated (e.g., tissue reconstruction, flap, or grafting)	Death
Trismus (difficulty, restriction or pain when opening mouth)	Trismus	Decreased range of motion without impaired eating	Decreased range of motion requiring small bites, soft foods or purees	Decreased range of motion with inability to adequately aliment or hydrate orally	—	—
NAVIGATION NOTE: Wound-infectious is graded as Infection – *Select* in the INFECTION CATEGORY.						
NAVIGATION NOTE: Wound non-infectious is graded as Wound complication, non-infectious in the DERMATOLOGY/SKIN CATEGORY.						
Musculoskeletal/Soft Tissue – Other (Specify, ______)	Musculoskeletal – Other (Specify)	Mild	Moderate	Severe	Life-threatening; disabling	Death

[5] Adapted from the *International SFTR Method of Measuring and Recording Joint Motion, International Standard Orthopedic Measurements (ISOM),* Jon J. Gerhardt and Otto A.
[6] Assessment of Fracture Risk and its Application to Screening for Postmenopausal Osteoporosis, Report of a *WHO Study Group Technical Report Series*, No. 843, 1994, v + 129

(Continued)

Appendix 2 *(continued)*

NEUROLOGY

Adverse Event	**Short Name**	**Grade 1**	**Grade 2**	**Grade 3**	**Grade 4**	**Grade 5**
NAVIGATION NOTE: ADD (Attention Deficit Disorder) is graded as Cognitive disturbance.						
NAVIGATION NOTE: Aphasia, receptive and/or expressive, is graded as Speech impairment (e.g., dysphasia or aphasia).						
Apnea	Apnea	—	—	Present	Intubation indicated	Death
Arachnoiditis/meningismus/radiculitis	Arachnoiditis	Symptomatic, not interfering with function; medical intervention indicated	Symptomatic (e.g., photophobia, nausea) interfering with function but not interfering with ADL	Symptomatic, interfering with ADL	Life-threatening; disabling (e.g., paraplegia)	Death
ALSO CONSIDER: Fever (in the absence of neutropenia, where neutropenia is defined as ANC $<1.0 \times 10^9/L$); Infection (documented clinically or microbiologically) with Grade 3 or 4 neutrophils (ANC $<1.0 \times 10^9/L$) – *Select*; Infection with normal ANC or Grade 1 or 2 neutrophils – *Select*; Infection with unknown ANC – *Select*; Pain – *Select*; Vomiting.						
Ataxia (incoordination)	Ataxia	Asymptomatic	Symptomatic, not interfering with ADL	Symptomatic, interfering with ADL; mechanical assistance indicated	Disabling	Death
REMARK: Ataxia (incoordination) refers to the consequence of medical or operative intervention.						
Brachial plexopathy	Brachial plexopathy	Asymptomatic	Symptomatic, not interfering with ADL	Symptomatic, interfering with ADL	Disabling	Death
CNS cerebrovascular ischemia	CNS ischemia	—	Asymptomatic, radiographic findings only	Transient ischemic event or attack (TIA) ≤24 hrs duration	Cerebral vascular accident (CVA, stroke), neurologic deficit >24 hrs	Death

(Continued)

Appendix 2 *(continued)*

		Grade				
Adverse Event	**Short Name**	**1**	**2**	**3**	**4**	**5**
NAVIGATION NOTE: CNS hemorrhage/bleeding is graded as Hemorrhage, CNS in the HEMORRHAGE/BLEEDING CATEGORY.						
CNS necrosis/cystic progression	CNS necrosis	Asymptomatic, radiographic findings only	Symptomatic, not interfering with ADL; medical intervention indicated	Symptomatic and interfering with ADL; hyperbaric oxygen indicated	Life-threatening; disabling; operative intervention indicated to prevent or treat CNS necrosis/cystic progression	Death
Cognitive disturbance	Cognitive disturbance	Mild cognitive disability; not interfering with work/school/life performance; specialized educational services/devices not indicated	Moderate cognitive disability; interfering with work/school/life performance but capable of independent living; specialized resources on part-time basis indicated	Severe cognitive disability; significant impairment of work/school/life performance	Unable to perform ADL; full-time specialized resources or institutionalization indicated	Death
REMARK: Cognitive disturbance may be used for Attention Deficit Disorder (ADD).						
Confusion	Confusion	Transient confusion, disorientation, or attention deficit	Confusion, disorientation, or attention deficit interfering with function, but not interfering withC ADL	Confusion or delirium interfering with ADL	Harmful to others or self; hospitalization indicated	Death
REMARK: Attention Deficit Disorder (ADD) is graded as Cognitive disturbance.						
NAVIGATION NOTE: Cranial neuropathy is graded as Neuropathy-cranial – *Select*.						

(Continued)

Appendix 2 *(continued)*

		Grade				
Adverse Event	**Short Name**	**1**	**2**	**3**	**4**	**5**
Dizziness	Dizziness	With head movements or nystagmus only; not interfering with function	Interfering with function, but not interfering with ADL	Interfering with ADL	Disabling	—
REMARK: Dizziness includes disequilibrium, lightheadedness, and vertigo.						
ALSO CONSIDER: Neuropathy: cranial – *Select*; Syncope (fainting).						
NAVIGATION NOTE: Dysphasia, receptive and/or expressive, is graded as Speech impairment (e.g., dysphasia or aphasia).						
Encephalopathy	Encephalopathy	—	Mild signs or symptoms; not interfering with ADL	Signs or symptoms interfering with ADL; hospitalization indicated	Life-threatening;disabling	Death
ALSO CONSIDER: Cognitive disturbance; Confusion; Dizziness; Memory impairment; Mental status; Mood alteration – *Select*; Psychosis (hallucinations/delusions); Somnolence/depressed level of consciousness.						
Extrapyramidal/involuntary movement/ restlessness	Involuntary movement	Mild involuntary movements not interfering with function	Moderate involuntary movements interfering with function, but not interfering with ADL	Severe involuntary movements or torticollis interfering with ADL	Disabling	Death
NAVIGATION NOTE: Headache/neuropathic pain (e.g., jaw pain, neurologic pain, phantom limb pain, post-infectious neuralgia, or painful neuropathies) is graded as Pain – *Select* in the PAIN CATEGORY.						
Hydrocephalus	Hydrocephalus	Asymptomatic, radiographic findings only	Mild to moderate symptoms not interfering with ADL	Severe symptoms or neurological deficit interfering with ADL	Disabling	Death

(Continued)

Appendix 2 *(continued)*

		Grade				
Adverse Event	**Short Name**	**1**	**2**	**3**	**4**	**5**
Irritability (children <3 years of age)	Irritability	Mild; easily consolable	Moderate; requiring increased attention	Severe; inconsolable	—	—
Laryngeal nerve dysfunction	Laryngeal nerve	Asymptomatic, weakness on clinical examination/testing only	Symptomatic, but not interfering with ADL; intervention not indicated	Symptomatic, interfering with ADL; intervention indicated (e.g., thyroplasty, vocal cord injection)	Life-threatening; tracheostomy indicated	Death
Leak, cerebrospinal fluid (CSF)	CSF leak	Transient headache; postural care indicated	Symptomatic, not interfering with ADL; blood patch indicated	Symptomatic, interfering with ADL; operative intervention indicated	Life-threatening; disabling	Death
REMARK: Leak, cerebrospinal fluid (CSF) may be used for CSF leak associated with operation and persisting >72 hours.						
Leukoencephalopathy (radiographic findings)	Leukoencephalopathy	Mild increase in subarachnoid space (SAS); mild ventriculomegaly; small (+/− multiple) focal T2 hyperintensities, involving periventricular white matter or <1/3 of susceptible areas of cerebrum	Moderate increase in SAS; moderate ventriculomegaly; focal T2 hyperintensities extending into centrum ovale or involving 1/3 to 2/3 of susceptible areas of cerebrum	Severe increase in SAS; severe ventriculomegaly; near total white matter T2 hyperintensities or diffuse low attenuation (CT)	—	—
REMARK: Leukoencephalopathy is a diffuse white matter process, specifically NOT associated with necrosis. Leukoencephalopathy (radiographic findings) does not include lacunas, which are areas that become void of neural tissue.						

(Continued)

Appendix 2 *(continued)*

		Grade				
Adverse Event	**Short Name**	**1**	**2**	**3**	**4**	**5**
Memory impairment	Memory impairment	Memory impairment not interfering with function	Memory impairment interfering with function, but not interfering with ADL	Memory impairment interfering with ADL	Amnesia	—
Mental status[7]	Mental status	—	1 – 3 point below age and educational norm in Folstein Mini-Mental Status Exam (MMSE)	>3 point below age and educational norm in Folstein MMSE	—	—
Mood alteration – *Select*: – Agitation – Anxiety – Depression – Euphoria	Mood alteration – *Select*	Mild mood alteration not interfering with function	Moderate mood alteration interfering with function, but not interfering with ADL; medication indicated	Severe mood alteration interfering with ADL	Suicidal ideation; danger to self or others	Death
Myelitis	Myelitis	Asymptomatic, mild signs (e.g., Babinski's or Lhermitte's sign)	Weakness or sensory loss not interfering with ADL	Weakness or sensory loss interfering with ADL	Disabling	Death

NAVIGATION NOTE: Neuropathic pain is graded as Pain – *Select* in the PAIN CATEGORY.

(Continued)

Appendix 2 *(continued)*

		Grade				
Adverse Event	**Short Name**	**1**	**2**	**3**	**4**	**5**
Neuropathy: cranial – *Select*: – CN I Smell – CN II Vision – CN III Pupil, upper eyelid, extra ocular movements – CN IV Downward, inward movement of eye – CN V Motor-jaw muscles; Sensory-facial – CN VI Lateral deviation of eye – CN VII Motor-face; Sensory-taste – CN VIII Hearing and balance – CN IX Motor-pharynx; Sensory-ear, pharynx, tongue – CN X Motor-palate; pharynx, larynx – CN XI Motor-sternomastoid and trapezius – CN XII Motor-tongue	Neuropathy: cranial – *Select*	Asymptomatic, detected on exam/testing only	Symptomatic, not interfering with ADL	Symptomatic, interfering with ADL	Life-threatening; disabling	Death
Neuropathy: motor	Neuropathy-motor	Asymptomatic, weakness on exam/testing only	Symptomatic weakness interfering with function, but not interfering with ADL	Weakness interfering with ADL; bracing or assistance to walk (e.g., cane or walker) indicated	Life-threatening; disabling (e.g., paralysis)	Death

REMARK: Cranial nerve *motor* neuropathy is graded as Neuropathy: cranial – *Select*.
ALSO CONSIDER: Laryngeal nerve dysfunction; Phrenic nerve dysfunction.

(Continued)

Appendix 2 *(continued)*

		Grade				
Adverse Event	**Short Name**	**1**	**2**	**3**	**4**	**5**
Neuropathy: sensory	Neuropathy-sensory	Asymptomatic; loss of deep tendon reflexes or paresthesia (including tingling) but not interfering with function	Sensory alteration or paresthesia (including tingling), interfering with function, but not interfering with ADL	Sensory alteration or paresthesia interfering with ADL	Disabling	Death
REMARK: Cranial nerve *sensory* neuropathy is graded as Neuropathy: cranial – *Select*.						
Personality/ behavioral	Personality	Change, but not adversely affecting patient or family	Change, adversely affecting patient or family	Mental health intervention indicated	Change harmful to others or self; hospitalization indicated	Death
Phrenic nerve dysfunction	Phrenic nerve	Asymptomatic weakness on exam/ testing only	Symptomatic but not interfering with ADL; intervention not indicated	Significant dysfunction; intervention indicated (e.g., diaphragmatic plication)	Life-threatening respiratory compromise; mechanical ventilation indicated	Death
Psychosis (hallucinations/delusions)	Psychosis	—	Transient episode	Interfering with ADL; medication, supervision or restraints indicated	Harmful to others or self; life-threatening consequences	Death
Pyramidal tract dysfunction (e.g., ↑ tone, hyperreflexia, positive Babinski, ↓ fine motor coordination)	Pyramidal tract dysfunction	Asymptomatic, abnormality on exam or testing only	Symptomatic; interfering with function but not interfering with ADL	Interfering with ADL	Disabling; paralysis	Death

(Continued)

Appendix 2 *(continued)*

		Grade				
Adverse Event	**Short Name**	**1**	**2**	**3**	**4**	**5**
Seizure	Seizure	—	One brief generalized seizure; seizure(s) well controlled by anticonvulsants or infrequent focal motor seizures not interfering with ADL	Seizures in which consciousness is altered; poorly controlled seizure disorder, with breakthrough generalized seizures despite medical intervention	Seizures of any kind which are prolonged, repetitive, or difficult to control (e.g., status epilepticus, intractable epilepsy)	Death
Somnolence/depressed level of consciousness	Somnolence	—	Somnolence or sedation interfering with function, but not interfering with ADL	Obtundation or stupor; difficult to arouse; interfering with ADL	Coma	Death
Speech impairment (e.g., dysphasia or aphasia)	Speech impairment	—	Awareness of receptive or expressive dysphasia, not impairing ability to communicate	Receptive or expressive dysphasia, impairing ability to communicate	Inability to communicate	—
REMARK: Speech impairment refers to a primary CNS process, not neuropathy or end organ dysfunction. ALSO CONSIDER: Laryngeal nerve dysfunction; Voice changes/dysarthria (e.g., hoarseness, loss, or alteration in voice, laryngitis).						
Syncope (fainting)	Syncope (fainting)	—	—	Present	Life-threatening consequences	Death
ALSO CONSIDER: CNS cerebrovascular ischemia; Conduction abnormality/atrioventricular heart block – *Select*; Dizziness; Supraventricular and nodal arrhythmia – *Select*; Vasovagal episode; Ventricular arrhythmia – *Select*.						
NAVIGATION NOTE: Taste alteration (CN VII, IX) is graded as Taste alteration (dysgeusia) in the GASTROINTESTINAL CATEGORY.						

(Continued)

Appendix 2 *(continued)*

		Grade				
Adverse Event	**Short Name**	**1**	**2**	**3**	**4**	**5**
Tremor	Tremor	Mild and brief or intermittent but not interfering with function	Moderate tremor interfering with function, but not interfering with ADL	Severe tremor interfering with ADL	Disabling	—
Neurology – Other (Specify, ______)	Neurology – Other (Specify)	Mild	Moderate	Severe	Life-threatening; disabling	Death

[7] Folstein MF, Folstein SE, and McHugh PR 1975; Mini-Mental State: A Practical Method for Grading the State of Patients for the Clinician, *Journal of Psychiatric Research*, 12:189-198.

OCULAR/VISUAL

		Grade				
Adverse Event	**Short Name**	**1**	**2**	**3**	**4**	**5**
Cataract	Cataract	Asymptomatic, detected on exam only	Symptomatic, with moderate decrease in visual acuity (20/40 or better); decreased visual function correctable with glasses	Symptomatic with marked decrease in visual acuity (worse than 20/40); operative intervention indicated (e.g., cataract surgery)	—	—

(Continued)

Appendix 2 *(continued)*

		Grade				
Adverse Event	**Short Name**	**1**	**2**	**3**	**4**	**5**
Dry eye syndrome	Dry eye	Mild, intervention not indicated	Symptomatic, interfering with function but not interfering with ADL; medical intervention indicated	Symptomatic or decrease in visual acuity interfering with ADL; operative intervention indicated	—	—
Eyelid dysfunction	Eyelid dysfunction	Asymptomatic	Symptomatic, interfering with function but not ADL; requiring topical agents or epilation	Symptomatic; interfering with ADL; surgical intervention indicated	—	—
REMARK: Eyelid dysfunction includes canalicular stenosis, ectropion, entropion, erythema, madarosis, symblepharon, telangiectasis, thickening, and trichiasis.						
ALSO CONSIDER: Neuropathy: cranial – *Select*.						
Glaucoma	Glaucoma	Elevated intraocular pressure (EIOP) with single topical agent for intervention; no visual field deficit	EIOP causing early visual field deficit (i.e., nasal step or arcuate deficit); multiple topical or oral agents indicated	EIOP causing marked visual field deficits (i.e., involving both superior and inferior visual fields); operative intervention indicated	EIOP resulting in blindness (20/200 or worse); enucleation indicated	—

(Continued)

Appendix 2 *(continued)*

		Grade				
Adverse Event	**Short Name**	**1**	**2**	**3**	**4**	**5**
Keratitis (corneal inflammation/corneal ulceration)	Keratitis	Abnormal ophthalmologic changes only; intervention not indicated	Symptomatic and interfering with function, but not interfering with ADL	Symptomatic and interfering with ADL; operative intervention indicated	Perforation or blindness (20/200 or worse)	—
NAVIGATION NOTE: Ocular muscle weakness is graded as Muscle weakness, generalized or specific area (not due to neuropathy) – *Select* in the MUSCULOSKELETAL/SOFT TISSUE CATEGORY.						
Night blindness (nyctalopia)	Nyctalopia	Symptomatic, not interfering with function	Symptomatic and interfering with function but not interfering with ADL	Symptomatic and interfering with ADL	Disabling	—
Nystagmus	Nystagmus	Asymptomatic	Symptomatic and interfering with function but not interfering with ADL	Symptomatic and interfering with ADL	Disabling	—
ALSO CONSIDER: Neuropathy: cranial – *Select*; Ophthalmoplegia/diplopia (double vision).						
Ocular surface disease	Ocular surface disease	Asymptomatic or minimally symptomatic but not interfering with function	Symptomatic, interfering with function but not interfering with ADL; topical antibiotics or other topical intervention indicated	Symptomatic, interfering with ADL; operative intervention indicated	—	—

(Continued)

Appendix 2 *(continued)*

		Grade				
Adverse Event	**Short Name**	**1**	**2**	**3**	**4**	**5**
REMARK: Ocular surface disease includes conjunctivitis, keratoconjunctivitis sicca, chemosis, keratinization, and palpebral conjunctival epithelial metaplasia.						
Ophthalmoplegia/ diplopia (double vision)	Diplopia	Intermittently symptomatic, intervention not indicated	Symptomatic and interfering with function but not interfering with ADL	Symptomatic and interfering with ADL; surgical intervention indicated	Disabling	—
ALSO CONSIDER: Neuropathy: cranial – *Select*.						
Optic disc edema	Optic disc edema	Asymptomatic	Decreased visual acuity (20/40 or better); visual field defect present	Decreased visual acuity (worse than 20/40); marked visual field defect but sparing the central 20 degrees	Blindness (20/200 or worse)	—
ALSO CONSIDER: Neuropathy: cranial – *Select*.						
Proptosis/ enophthalmos	Proptosis/ enophthalmos	Asymptomatic, intervention not indicated	Symptomatic and interfering with function, but not interfering with ADL	Symptomatic and interfering with ADL	—	—
Retinal detachment	Retinal detachment	Exudative; no central vision loss; intervention not indicated	Exudative and visual acuity 20/40 or better but intervention not indicated	Rhegmatogenous or exudative detachment; operative intervention indicated	Blindness (20/200 or worse)	—

(Continued)

Appendix 2 *(continued)*

		Grade				
Adverse Event	**Short Name**	**1**	**2**	**3**	**4**	**5**
Retinopathy	Retinopathy	Asymptomatic	Symptomatic with moderate decrease in visual acuity (20/40 or better)	Symptomatic with marked decrease in visual acuity (worse than 20/40)	Blindness (20/200 or worse)	—
Scleral necrosis/melt	Scleral necrosis	Asymptomatic or symptomatic but not interfering with function	Symptomatic, interfering with function but not interfering with ADL; moderate decrease in visual acuity (20/40 or better); medical intervention indicated	Symptomatic, interfering with ADL; marked decrease in visual acuity (worse than 20/40); operative intervention indicated	Blindness (20/200 or worse); painful eye with enucleation indicated	—
Uveitis	Uveitis	Asymptomatic	Anterior uveitis; medical intervention indicated	Posterior or pan-uveitis; operative intervention indicated	Blindness (20/200 or worse)	—
Vision-blurred vision	Blurred vision	Symptomatic not interfering with function	Symptomatic and interfering with function, but not interfering with ADL	Symptomatic and interfering with ADL	Disabling	—
Vision-flashing lights/floaters	Flashing lights	Symptomatic not interfering with function	Symptomatic and interfering with function, but not interfering with ADL	Symptomatic and interfering with ADL	Disabling	—

(Continued)

Appendix 2 *(continued)*

		Grade				
Adverse Event	**Short Name**	**1**	**2**	**3**	**4**	**5**
Vision-photophobia	Photophobia	Symptomatic not interfering with function	Symptomatic and interfering with function, but not interfering with ADL	Symptomatic and interfering with ADL	Disabling	—
Vitreous hemorrhage	Vitreous hemorrhage	Asymptomatic, clinical findings only	Symptomatic, interfering with function, but not interfering with ADL; intervention not indicated	Symptomatic, interfering with ADL; vitrectomy indicated	—	—
Watery eye (epiphora, tearing)	Watery eye	Symptomatic, intervention not indicated	Symptomatic, interfering with function but not interfering with ADL	Symptomatic, interfering with ADL	—	—
Ocular/Visual – Other (Specify, ______)	Ocular – Other (Specify)	Symptomatic not interfering with function	Symptomatic and interfering with function, but not interfering with ADL	Symptomatic and interfering with ADL	Blindness (20/200 or worse)	Death

(Continued)

Appendix 2 *(continued)*

PAIN

		Grade				
Adverse Event	**Short Name**	**1**	**2**	**3**	**4**	**5**
Pain – *Select*: '*Select*' AEs appear at the end of the CATEGORY.	Pain – *Select*	Mild pain not interfering with function	Moderate pain; pain or analgesics interfering with function, but not interfering with ADL	Severe pain; pain or analgesics severely interfering with ADL	Disabling	—
Pain – Other (Specify, ______)	Pain – Other (Specify)	Mild pain not interfering with function	Moderate pain; pain or analgesics interfering with function, but not interfering with ADL	Severe pain; pain or analgesics severely interfering with ADL	Disabling	—

PAIN – *SELECT*

AUDITORY/EAR	HEPATOBILIARY/PANCREAS	PULMONARY/UPPER RESPIRATORY
– External ear	– Gallbladder	– Chest wall
– Middle ear	– Liver	– Chest/thorax NOS
CARDIOVASCULAR	LYMPHATIC	– Larynx
– Cardiac/heart	– Lymph node	– Pleura
– Pericardium	MUSCULOSKELETAL	– Sinus
DERMATOLOGY/SKIN	– Back	– Throat/pharynx/larynx
– Face	– Bone	RENAL/GENITOURINARY
– Lip	– Buttock	– Bladder
– Oral-gums	– Extremity-limb	– Kidney
– Scalp	– Intestine	SEXUAL/REPRODUCTIVE FUNCTION
– Skin	– Joint	– Breast

(Continued)

Appendix 2 *(continued)*

GASTROINTESTINAL
- Abdomen NOS
- Anus
- Dental/teeth/peridontal
- Esophagus
- Oral cavity
- Peritoneum
- Rectum
- Stomach

GENERAL
- Pain NOS
- Tumor pain

- Muscle
- Neck
- Phantom (pain associated with missing limb)

NEUROLOGY
- Head/headache
- Neuralgia/peripheral nerve

OCULAR
- Eye

- Ovulatory
- Pelvis
- Penis
- Perineum
- Prostate
- Scrotum
- Testicle
- Urethra
- Uterus
- Vagina

PULMONARY/UPPER RESPIRATORY

		Grade				
Adverse Event	**Short Name**	**1**	**2**	**3**	**4**	**5**
Adult Respiratory Distress Syndrome (ARDS)	ARDS	—	—	Present, intubation not indicated	Present, intubation indicated	Death
ALSO CONSIDER: Dyspnea (shortness of breath); Hypoxia; Pneumonitis/pulmonary infiltrates.						

(Continued)

Appendix 2 *(continued)*

		Grade				
Adverse Event	**Short Name**	**1**	**2**	**3**	**4**	**5**
Aspiration	Aspiration	Asymptomatic (''silent aspiration''); endoscopy or radiographic (e.g., barium swallow) findings	Symptomatic (e.g., altered eating habits, coughing or choking episodes consistent with aspiration); medical intervention indicated (e.g., antibiotics, suction or oxygen)	Clinical or radiographic signs of pneumonia or pneumonitis; unable to aliment orally	Life-threatening (e.g., aspiration pneumonia or pneumonitis)	Death
ALSO CONSIDER: Infection (documented clinically or microbiologically) with Grade 3 or 4 neutrophils (ANC <1.0 × 10^9/L) – *Select;* Infection with normal ANC or Grade 1 or 2 neutrophils – *Select;* Infection with unknown ANC – *Select;* Laryngeal nerve dysfunction; Neuropathy: cranial – *Select*; Pneumonitis/pulmonary infiltrates.						
Atelectasis	Atelectasis	Asymptomatic	Symptomatic (e.g., dyspnea, cough), medical intervention indicated (e.g., bronchoscopic suctioning, chest physiotherapy, suctioning)	Operative (e.g., stent, laser) intervention indicated	Life-threatening respiratory compromise	Death
ALSO CONSIDER: Adult Respiratory Distress Syndrome (ARDS); Cough; Dyspnea (shortness of breath); Hypoxia; Infection (documented clinically or microbiologically) with Grade 3 or 4 neutrophils (ANC <1.0 × 10^9/L) – *Select*; Infection with normal ANC or Grade 1 or 2 neutrophils – *Select*; Infection with unknown ANC – *Select*; Obstruction/stenosis of airway – *Select*; Pneumonitis/pulmonary infiltrates; Pulmonary fibrosis (radiographic changes).						

(Continued)

Appendix 2 *(continued)*

		Grade				
Adverse Event	**Short Name**	**1**	**2**	**3**	**4**	**5**
Bronchospasm, wheezing	Bronchospasm	Asymptomatic	Symptomatic not interfering with function	Symptomatic interfering with function	Life-threatening	Death
ALSO CONSIDER: Allergic reaction/hypersensitivity (including drug fever); Dyspnea (shortness of breath).						
Carbon monoxide diffusion capacity (DL_{CO})	DL_{CO}	90 – 75% of predicted value	<75 – 50% of predicted value	<50 – 25% of predicted value	<25% of predicted value	Death
ALSO CONSIDER: Hypoxia; Pneumonitis/pulmonary infiltrates; Pulmonary fibrosis (radiographic changes).						
Chylothorax	Chylothorax	Asymptomatic	Symptomatic; thoracentesis or tube drainage indicated	Operative intervention indicated	Life-threatening (e.g., hemodynamic instability or ventilatory support indicated)	Death
Cough	Cough	Symptomatic, non-narcotic medication only indicated	Symptomatic and narcotic medication indicated	Symptomatic and significantly interfering with sleep or ADL	—	—
Dyspnea (shortness of breath)	Dyspnea	Dyspnea on exertion, but can walk 1 flight of stairs without stopping	Dyspnea on exertion but unable to walk 1 flight of stairs or 1 city block (0.1km) without stopping	Dyspnea with ADL	Dyspnea at rest; intubation/ventilator indicated	Death
ALSO CONSIDER: Hypoxia; Neuropathy: motor; Pneumonitis/pulmonary infiltrates; Pulmonary fibrosis (radiographic changes).						

(Continued)

Appendix 2 *(continued)*

		Grade				
Adverse Event	**Short Name**	**1**	**2**	**3**	**4**	**5**
Edema, larynx	Edema, larynx	Asymptomatic edema by exam only	Symptomatic edema, no respiratory distress	Stridor; respiratory distress; interfering with ADL	Life-threatening airway compromise; tracheotomy, intubation, or laryngectomy indicated	Death
ALSO CONSIDER: Allergic reaction/hypersensitivity (including drug fever).						
FEV_1	FEV_1	90 – 75% of predicted value	<75 – 50% of predicted value	<50 – 25% of predicted value	<25% of predicted	Death
Fistula, pulmonary/upper respiratory – *Select*: – Bronchus – Larynx – Lung – Oral cavity – Pharynx – Pleura – Trachea	Fistula, pulmonary – *Select*	Asymptomatic, radiographic findings only	Symptomatic, tube thoracostomy or medical management indicated; associated with altered respiratory function but not interfering with ADL	Symptomatic and associated with altered respiratory function interfering with ADL; or endoscopic (e.g., stent) or primary closure by operative intervention indicated	Life-threatening consequences; operative intervention with thoracoplasty, chronic open drainage or multiple thoracotomies indicated	Death
REMARK: A fistula is defined as an abnormal communication between two body cavities, potential spaces, and/or the skin. The site indicated for a fistula should be the site from which the abnormal process is believed to have arisen. For example, a tracheo-esophageal fistula arising in the context of a resected or irradiated esophageal cancer should be graded as Fistula, GI – esophagus in the GASTROINTESTINAL CATEGORY.						
NAVIGATION NOTE: Hemoptysis is graded as Hemorrhage, pulmonary/upper respiratory – *Select* in the HEMORRHAGE/BLEEDING CATEGORY.						
Hiccoughs (hiccups, singultus)	Hiccoughs	Symptomatic, intervention not indicated	Symptomatic, intervention indicated	Symptomatic, significantly interfering with sleep or ADL	—	—

(Continued)

Appendix 2 *(continued)*

		Grade				
Adverse Event	**Short Name**	**1**	**2**	**3**	**4**	**5**
Hypoxia	Hypoxia	—	Decreased O_2 saturation with exercise (e.g., pulse oximeter <88%); intermittent supplemental oxygen	Decreased O_2 saturation at rest; continuous oxygen indicated	Life-threatening; intubation or ventilation indicated	Death
Nasal cavity/paranasal sinus reactions	Nasal/paranasal reactions	Asymptomatic mucosal crusting, blood-tinged secretions	Symptomatic stenosis or edema/narrowing interfering with airflow	Stenosis with significant nasal obstruction; interfering with ADL	Necrosis of soft tissue or bone	Death
ALSO CONSIDER: Infection (documented clinically or microbiologically) with Grade 3 or 4 neutrophils (ANC <1.0 × 10^9/L) – *Select;* Infection with normal ANC or Grade 1 or 2 neutrophils – *Select;* Infection with unknown ANC – *Select.*						
Obstruction/stenosis of airway – *Select*: – Bronchus – Larynx – Pharynx – Trachea	Airway obstruction – *Select*	Asymptomatic obstruction or stenosis on exam, endoscopy, or radiograph	Symptomatic (e.g., noisy airway breathing), but causing no respiratory distress; medical management indicated (e.g., steroids)	Interfering with ADL; stridor or endoscopic intervention indicated (e.g., stent, laser)	Life-threatening airway compromise; tracheotomy or intubation indicated	Death
Pleural effusion (non-malignant)	Pleural effusion	Asymptomatic	Symptomatic, intervention such as diuretics or up to 2 therapeutic thoracenteses indicated	Symptomatic and supplemental oxygen, >2 therapeutic thoracenteses, tube drainage, or pleurodesis indicated	Life-threatening (e.g., causing hemodynamic instability or ventilatory support indicated)	Death

(Continued)

Appendix 2 *(continued)*

		Grade				
Adverse Event	**Short Name**	**1**	**2**	**3**	**4**	**5**
ALSO CONSIDER: Atelectasis; Cough; Dyspnea (shortness of breath); Hypoxia; Pneumonitis/pulmonary infiltrates; Pulmonary fibrosis (radiographic changes).						
NAVIGATION NOTE: Pleuritic pain is graded as Pain – *Select* in the PAIN CATEGORY.						
Pneumonitis/pulmonary infiltrates	Pneumonitis	Asymptomatic, radiographic findings only	Symptomatic, not interfering with ADL	Symptomatic, interfering with ADL; O_2 indicated	Life-threatening; ventilatory support indicated	Death
ALSO CONSIDER: Adult Respiratory Distress Syndrome (ARDS); Cough; Dyspnea (shortness of breath); Hypoxia; Infection (documented clinically or microbiologically) with Grade 3 or 4 neutrophils (ANC <1.0 × 10^9/L) – *Select;* Infection with normal ANC or Grade 1 or 2 neutrophils – *Select;* Infection with unknown ANC – *Select*; Pneumonitis/pulmonary infiltrates; Pulmonary fibrosis (radiographic changes).						
Pneumothorax	Pneumothorax	Asymptomatic, radiographic findings only	Symptomatic; intervention indicated (e.g., hospitalization for observation, tube placement without sclerosis)	Sclerosis and/or operative intervention indicated	Life-threatening, causing hemodynamic instability (e.g., tension pneumothorax); ventilatory support indicated	Death
Prolonged chest tube drainage or air leak after pulmonary resection	Chest tube drainage or leak	—	Sclerosis or additional tube thoracostomy indicated	Operative intervention indicated (e.g., thoracotomy with stapling or sealant application)	Life-threatening; debilitating; organ resection indicated	Death
Prolonged intubation after pulmonary resection (>24 hrs after surgery)	Prolonged intubation	—	Extubated within 24 – 72 hrs postoperatively	Extubated >72 hrs postoperatively, but before tracheostomy indicated	Tracheostomy indicated	Death

(Continued)

Appendix 2 *(continued)*

		Grade				
Adverse Event	**Short Name**	**1**	**2**	**3**	**4**	**5**
NAVIGATION NOTE: Pulmonary embolism is graded as Grade 4 either as Thrombosis/embolism (vascular access-related) or Thrombosis/thrombus/embolism in the VASCULAR CATEGORY.						
Pulmonary fibrosis (radiographic changes)	Pulmonary fibrosis	Minimal radiographic findings (or patchy or bibasilar changes) with estimated radiographic proportion of total lung volume that is fibrotic of <25%	Patchy or bi-basilar changes with estimated radiographic proportion of total lung volume that is fibrotic of 25 – <50%	Dense or widespread infiltrates/consolidation with estimated radiographic proportion of total lung volume that is fibrotic of 50 – <75%	Estimated radiographic proportion of total lung volume that is fibrotic is ≥75%; honeycombing	Death
REMARK: Fibrosis is usually a ''late effect'' seen >3 months after radiation or combined modality therapy (including surgery). It is thought to represent scar/fibrotic lung tissue. It may be difficult to distinguish from pneumonitis that is generally seen within 3 months of radiation or combined modality therapy. ALSO CONSIDER: Adult Respiratory Distress Syndrome (ARDS); Cough; Dyspnea (shortness of breath); Hypoxia; Infection (documented clinically or microbiologically) with Grade 3 or 4 neutrophils (ANC <1.0 × 10^9/L) – *Select;* Infection with normal ANC or Grade 1 or 2 neutrophils – *Select;* Infection with unknown ANC – *Select.*						
NAVIGATION NOTE: Recurrent laryngeal nerve dysfunction is graded as Laryngeal nerve dysfunction in the NEUROLOGY CATEGORY.						
Vital capacity	Vital capacity	90 – 75% of predicted value	<75 – 50% of predicted value	<50 – 25% of predicted value	<25% of predicted value	Death

(Continued)

Appendix 2 *(continued)*

		Grade				
Adverse Event	**Short Name**	**1**	**2**	**3**	**4**	**5**
Voice changes/dysarthria (e.g., hoarseness, loss or alteration in voice, laryngitis)	Voice changes	Mild or intermittent hoarseness or voice change, but fully understandable	Moderate or persistent voice changes, may require occasional repetition but understandable on telephone	Severe voice changes including predominantly whispered speech; may require frequent repetition or face-to-face contact for understandability; requires voice aid (e.g., electrolarynx) for ≤50% of communication	Disabling; nonunderstandable voice or aphonic; requires voice aid (e.g., electrolarynx) for >50% of communication or requires >50% written communication	Death
ALSO CONSIDER: Laryngeal nerve dysfunction; Speech impairment (e.g., dysphasia or aphasia).						
Pulmonary/Upper Respiratory – Other (Specify, ________)	Pulmonary – Other (Specify)	Mild	Moderate	Severe	Life-threatening; disabling	Death

RENAL/GENITOURINARY

		Grade				
Adverse Event	**Short Name**	**1**	**2**	**3**	**4**	**5**
Bladder spasms	Bladder spasms	Symptomatic, intervention not indicated	Symptomatic, antispasmodics indicated	Narcotics indicated	Major surgical intervention indicated (e.g., cystectomy)	—

(Continued)

Appendix 2 *(continued)*

		Grade				
Adverse Event	**Short Name**	**1**	**2**	**3**	**4**	**5**
Cystitis	Cystitis	Asymptomatic	Frequency with dysuria; macroscopic hematuria	Transfusion; IV pain medications; bladder irrigation indicated	Catastrophic bleeding; major non-elective intervention indicated	Death
ALSO CONSIDER: Infection (documented clinically or microbiologically) with Grade 3 or 4 neutrophils (ANC <1.0 × 10^9/L) – *Select*; Infection with normal ANC or Grade 1 or 2 neutrophils – *Select*; Infection with unknown ANC – *Select*; Pain – *Select*.						
Fistula, GU – *Select*: – Bladder – Genital tract-female – Kidney – Ureter – Urethra – Uterus – Vagina	Fistula, GU – *Select*	Asymptomatic, radiographic findings only	Symptomatic; noninvasive intervention indicated	Symptomatic interfering with ADL; invasive intervention indicated	Life-threatening consequences; operative intervention requiring partial or full organ resection; permanent urinary diversion	Death
REMARK: A fistula is defined as an abnormal communication between two body cavities, potential spaces, and/or the skin. The site indicated for a fistula should be the site from which the abnormal process is believed to have originated.						
Incontinence, urinary	Incontinence, urinary	Occasional (e.g., with coughing, sneezing, etc.), pads not indicated	Spontaneous, pads indicated	Interfering with ADL; intervention indicated (e.g., clamp, collagen injections)	Operative intervention indicated (e.g., cystectomy or permanent urinary diversion)	—

(Continued)

Appendix 2 *(continued)*

		Grade				
Adverse Event	**Short Name**	**1**	**2**	**3**	**4**	**5**
Leak (including anastomotic), GU – *Select*: – Bladder – Fallopian tube – Kidney – Spermatic cord – Stoma – Ureter – Urethra – Uterus – Vagina – Vas deferens	Leak, GU – *Select*	Asymptomatic, radiographic findings only	Symptomatic; medical intervention indicated	Symptomatic, interfering with GU function; invasive or endoscopic intervention indicated	Life-threatening	Death
REMARK: Leak (including anastomotic), GU – *Select* refers to clinical signs and symptoms or radiographic confirmation of anastomotic leak but without development of fistula.						

(Continued)

Appendix 2 *(continued)*

		Grade				
Adverse Event	**Short Name**	**1**	**2**	**3**	**4**	**5**
Obstruction, GU – *Select*: – Bladder – Fallopian tube – Prostate – Spermatic cord – Stoma – Testes – Ureter – Urethra – Uterus – Vagina – Vas deferens	Obstruction, GU – *Select*	Asymptomatic, radiographic or endoscopic findings only	Symptomatic but no hydronephrosis, sepsis or renal dysfunction; dilation or endoscopic repair or stent placement indicated	Symptomatic and altered organ function (e.g., sepsis or hydronephrosis, or renal dysfunction); operative intervention indicated	Life-threatening consequences; organ failure or operative intervention requiring complete organ resection indicated	Death

NAVIGATION NOTE: Operative injury is graded as Intra-operative injury – *Select Organ or Structure* in the SURGERY/INTRA-OPERATIVE INJURY CATEGORY.

(Continued)

Appendix 2 *(continued)*

		Grade				
Adverse Event	**Short Name**	**1**	**2**	**3**	**4**	**5**
Perforation, GU – *Select*: – Bladder – Fallopian tube – Kidney – Ovary – Prostate – Spermatic cord – Stoma – Testes – Ureter – Urethra – Uterus – Vagina – Vas deferens	Perforation, GU – *Select*	Asymptomatic radiographic findings only	Symptomatic, associated with altered renal/GU function	Symptomatic, operative intervention indicated	Life-threatening consequences or organ failure; operative intervention requiring organ resection indicated	Death
Prolapse of stoma, GU	Prolapse stoma, GU	Asymptomatic; special intervention, extraordinary care not indicated	Extraordinary local care or maintenance; minor revision under local anesthesia indicated	Dysfunctional stoma; operative intervention or major stomal revision indicated	Life-threatening consequences	Death
REMARK: Other stoma complications may be graded as Fistula, GU – *Select*; Leak (including anastomotic), GU – *Select*; Obstruction, GU – *Select;* Perforation, GU – *Select*; Stricture/stenosis (including anastomotic), GU – *Select*.						
Renal failure	Renal failure	—	—	Chronic dialysis not indicated	Chronic dialysis or renal transplant indicated	Death

(Continued)

Appendix 2 *(continued)*

		Grade				
Adverse Event	**Short Name**	**1**	**2**	**3**	**4**	**5**
ALSO CONSIDER: Glomerular filtration rate.						
Stricture/stenosis (including anastomotic), GU – *Select*: – Bladder – Fallopian tube – Prostate – Spermatic cord – Stoma – Testes – Ureter – Urethra – Uterus – Vagina – Vas deferens	Stricture, anastomotic, GU – *Select*	Asymptomatic, radiographic or endoscopic findings only	Symptomatic but no hydronephrosis, sepsis or renal dysfunction; dilation or endoscopic repair or stent placement indicated	Symptomatic and altered organ function (e.g., sepsis or hydronephrosis, or renal dysfunction); operative intervention indicated	Life-threatening consequences; organ failure or operative intervention requiring organ resection indicated	Death
ALSO CONSIDER: Obstruction, GU – *Select*.						
Urinary electrolyte wasting (e.g., Fanconi's syndrome, renal tubular acidosis)	Urinary electrolyte wasting	Asymptomatic, intervention not indicated	Mild, reversible and manageable with replacement	Irreversible, requiring continued replacement	—	—
ALSO CONSIDER: Acidosis (metabolic or respiratory); Bicarbonate, serum-low; Calcium, serum-low (hypocalcemia); Phosphate, serum-low (hypophosphatemia).						

(Continued)

Appendix 2 *(continued)*

		Grade				
Adverse Event	**Short Name**	**1**	**2**	**3**	**4**	**5**
Urinary frequency/ urgency	Urinary frequency	Increase in frequency or nocturia up to 2 × normal; enuresis	Increase $>2 \times$ normal but $<$hourly	≥ 1 x/hr; urgency; catheter indicated	—	—
Urinary retention (including neurogenic bladder)	Urinary retention	Hesitancy or dribbling, no significant residual urine; retention occurring during the immediate postoperative period	Hesitancy requiring medication; or operative bladder atony requiring indwelling catheter beyond immediate postoperative period but for <6 weeks	More than daily catheterization indicated; urological intervention indicated (e.g., TURP, suprapubic tube, urethrotomy)	Life-threatening consequences; organ failure (e.g., bladder rupture); operative intervention requiring organ resection indicated	Death
REMARK: The etiology of retention (if known) is graded as Obstruction, GU – *Select*; Stricture/stenosis (including anastomotic), GU – *Select*.						
ALSO CONSIDER: Obstruction, GU – *Select*; Stricture/stenosis (including anastomotic), GU – *Select*.						
Urine color change	Urine color change	Present	—	—	—	—
REMARK: Urine color refers to change that is not related to other dietary or physiologic cause (e.g., bilirubin, concentrated urine, and hematuria).						
Renal/Genitourinary – Other (Specify, ________)	Renal – Other (Specify)	Mild	Moderate	Severe	Life-threatening; disabling	Death

(Continued)

Appendix 2 *(continued)*

SECONDARY MALIGNANCY

		Grade				
Adverse Event	**Short Name**	**1**	**2**	**3**	**4**	**5**
Secondary Malignancy – possibly related to cancer treatment (Specify, ________)	Secondary Malignancy (possibly related to cancer treatment)	—	—	Non-life-threatening basal or squamous cell carcinoma of the skin	Solid tumor, leukemia or lymphoma	Death

REMARK: Secondary malignancy excludes metastasis from initial primary. Any malignancy possibly related to cancer treatment (including AML/MDS) should be reported via the routine reporting mechanisms outlined in each protocol. Important: Secondary Malignancy is an exception to NCI Expedited Adverse Event Reporting Guidelines. Secondary Malignancy is ''Grade 4, present'' but NCI does not require AdEERS Expedited Reporting for any (related or unrelated to treatment) Secondary Malignancy. A diagnosis of AML/MDS following treatment with an NCI-sponsored investigational agent is to be reported using the form available from the CTEP Web site at http://ctep.cancer.gov. Cancers not suspected of being treatment-related are not to be reported here.

SEXUAL/REPRODUCTIVE FUNCTION

		Grade				
Adverse Event	**Short Name**	**1**	**2**	**3**	**4**	**5**
Breast function/lactation	Breast function	Mammary abnormality, not functionally significant	Mammary abnormality, functionally significant	—	—	—
Breast nipple/areolar deformity	Nipple/areolar	Limited areolar asymmetry with no change in nipple/areolar projection	Asymmetry of nipple areolar complex with slight deviation in nipple projection	Marked deviation of nipple projection	—	—

(Continued)

Appendix 2 *(continued)*

		Grade				
Adverse Event	**Short Name**	**1**	**2**	**3**	**4**	**5**
Breast volume/ hypoplasia	Breast	Minimal asymmetry; minimal hypoplasia	Asymmetry exists, ≤1/3 of the breast volume; moderate hypoplasia	Asymmetry exists, >1/3 of the breast volume; severe hypoplasia	—	—
REMARK: Breast volume is referenced with both arms straight overhead.						
NAVIGATION NOTE: Dysmenorrhea is graded as Pain – *Select* in the PAIN CATEGORY.						
NAVIGATION NOTE: Dyspareunia is graded as Pain – *Select* in the PAIN CATEGORY.						
NAVIGATION NOTE: Dysuria (painful urination) is graded as Pain – *Select* in the PAIN CATEGORY.						
Erectile dysfunction	Erectile dysfunction	Decrease in erectile function (frequency/ rigidity of erections) but erectile aids not indicated	Decrease in erectile function (frequency/ rigidity of erections), erectile aids indicated	Decrease in erectile function (frequency/ rigidity of erections) but erectile aids not helpful; penile prosthesis indicated	—	—
Ejaculatory dysfunction	Ejaculatory dysfunction	Diminished ejaculation	Anejaculation or retrograde ejaculation	—	—	—
NAVIGATION NOTE: Feminization of male is graded in the ENDOCRINE CATEGORY.						
Gynecomastia	Gynecomastia	—	Asymptomatic breast enlargement	Symptomatic breast enlargement; intervention indicated	—	—
ALSO CONSIDER: Pain – *Select*.						

(Continued)

Appendix 2 *(continued)*

		Grade				
Adverse Event	**Short Name**	**1**	**2**	**3**	**4**	**5**
Infertility/sterility	Infertility/sterility	—	Male: oligospermia/ low sperm count Female: diminished fertility/ovulation	Male: sterile/azoospermia Female: infertile/ anovulatory	—	—
Irregular menses (change from baseline)	Irregular menses	1 – 3 months without menses	>3 – 6 months without menses but continuing menstrual cycles	Persistent amenorrhea for >6 months	—	—
Libido	Libido	Decrease in interest but not affecting relationship; intervention not indicated	Decrease in interest and adversely affecting relationship; intervention indicated	—	—	—
NAVIGATION NOTE: Masculinization of female is graded in the ENDOCRINE CATEGORY.						
Orgasmic dysfunction	Orgasmic function	Transient decrease	Decrease in orgasmic response requiring intervention	Complete inability of orgasmic response; not responding to intervention	—	—
NAVIGATION NOTE: Pelvic pain is graded as Pain – *Select* in the PAIN CATEGORY.						
NAVIGATION NOTE: Ulcers of the labia or perineum are graded as Ulceration in DERMATOLOGY/SKIN CATEGORY.						
Vaginal discharge (non-infectious)	Vaginal discharge	Mild	Moderate to heavy; pad use indicated	—	—	—

(Continued)

Appendix 2 *(continued)*

		Grade				
Adverse Event	**Short Name**	**1**	**2**	**3**	**4**	**5**
Vaginal dryness	Vaginal dryness	Mild	Interfering with sexual function; dyspareunia; intervention indicated	—	—	—
ALSO CONSIDER: Pain – *Select.*						
Vaginal mucositis	Vaginal mucositis	Erythema of the mucosa; minimal symptoms	Patchy ulcerations; moderate symptoms or dyspareunia	Confluent ulcerations; bleeding with trauma; unable to tolerate vaginal exam, sexual intercourse or tampon placement	Tissue necrosis; significant spontaneous bleeding; life-threatening consequences	—
Vaginal stenosis/length	Vaginal stenosis	Vaginal narrowing and/or shortening not interfering with function	Vaginal narrowing and/or shortening interfering with function	Complete obliteration; not surgically correctable	—	—
Vaginitis (not due to infection)	Vaginitis	Mild, intervention not indicated	Moderate, intervention indicated	Severe, not relieved with treatment; ulceration, but operative intervention not indicated	Ulceration and operative intervention indicated	—
Sexual/Reproductive Function – Other (Specify, ________)	Sexual – Other (Specify)	Mild	Moderate	Severe	Disabling	Death

(Continued)

Appendix 2 *(continued)*

SURGERY/INTRA-OPERATIVE INJURY

		Grade				
Adverse Event	**Short Name**	**1**	**2**	**3**	**4**	**5**
NAVIGATION NOTE: Intra-operative hemorrhage is graded as Hemorrhage/bleeding associated with surgery, intra-operative or postoperative in the HEMORRHAGE/BLEEDING CATEGORY.						
Intra-operative injury – *Select Organ or Structure* *'Select'* AEs appear at the end of the CATEGORY.	Intraop injury – *Select*	Primary repair of injured organ/structure indicated	Partial resection of injured organ/structure indicated	Complete resection or reconstruction of injured organ/structure indicated	Life threatening consequences; disabling	—
REMARK: The *'Select'* AEs are defined as significant, unanticipated injuries that are recognized at the time of surgery. These AEs do not refer to additional surgical procedures that must be performed because of a change in the operative plan based on intra-operative findings. Any sequelae resulting from the intra-operative injury that result in an adverse outcome for the patient must also be recorded and graded under the relevant CTCAE Term.						
Intra-operative Injury – Other (Specify, ________)	Intraop Injury – Other (Specify)	Primary repair of injured organ/structure indicated	Partial resection of injured organ/structure indicated	Complete resection or reconstruction of injured organ/structure indicated	Life threatening consequences; disabling	—
REMARK: Intra-operative Injury – Other (Specify, ______)is to be used only to report an organ/structure not included in the *'Select'* AEs found at the end of the CATEGORY. Any sequelae resulting from the intra-operative injury that result in an adverse outcome for the patient must also be recorded and graded under the relevant CTCAE Term.						

(Continued)

Appendix 2 *(continued)*

SURGERY/INTRA-OPERATIVE INJURY – *SELECT*

AUDITORY/EAR
- Inner ear
- Middle ear
- Outer ear NOS
- Outer ear-Pinna

CARDIOVASCULAR
- Artery-aorta
- Artery-carotid
- Artery-cerebral
- Artery-extremity (lower)
- Artery-extremity (upper)
- Artery-hepatic
- Artery-major visceral artery
- Artery-pulmonary
- Artery NOS
- Heart
- Spleen
- Vein-extremity (lower)
- Vein-extremity (upper)
- Vein-hepatic
- Vein-inferior vena cava
- Vein-jugular
- Vein-major visceral vein
- Vein-portal vein
- Vein-pulmonary
- Vein-superior vena cava
- Vein NOS

GASTROINTESTINAL
- Abdomen NOS
- Anal sphincter
- Anus
- Appendix
- Cecum
- Colon
- Duodenum
- Esophagus
- Ileum
- Jejunum
- Oral
- Peritoneal cavity
- Rectum
- Small bowel NOS
- Stoma (GI)
- Stomach

HEPATOBILIARY/ PANCREAS
- Biliary tree-common bile duct
- Biliary tree-common hepatic duct
- Biliary tree-left hepatic duct
- Biliary tree-right hepatic duct
- Biliary tree NOS
- Gallbladder
- Liver
- Pancreas
- Pancreatic duct

NEUROLOGY *(Continued)*

NERVES:
- CN IX (glossopharyngeal) sensory ear-pharynx-tongue
- CN X (vagus)
- CN XI (spinal accessory)
- CN XII (hypoglossal)
- Cranial nerve or branch NOS
- Lingual
- Lung thoracic
- Peripheral motor NOS
- Peripheral sensory NOS
- Recurrent laryngeal
- Sacral plexus
- Sciatic
- Thoracodorsal

OCULAR
- Conjunctiva
- Cornea
- Eye NOS
- Lens
- Retina

PULMONARY/UPPER RESPIRATORY
- Bronchus
- Lung

(Continued)

Appendix 2 *(continued)*

DERMATOLOGY/SKIN
- Breast
- Nails
- Skin

ENDOCRINE
- Adrenal gland
- Parathyroid
- Pituitary
- Thyroid

HEAD AND NECK
- Gingiva
- Larynx
- Lip/perioral area
- Face NOS
- Nasal cavity
- Nasopharynx
- Neck NOS
- Nose
- Oral cavity NOS
- Parotid gland
- Pharynx
- Salivary duct
- Salivary gland
- Sinus
- Teeth
- Tongue
- Upper aerodigestive NOS

MUSCULOSKELETAL
- Bone
- Cartilage
- Extremity-lower
- Extremity-upper
- Joint
- Ligament
- Muscle
- Soft tissue NOS
- Tendon

NEUROLOGY
- Brain
- Meninges
- Spinal cord

NERVES:
- Brachial plexus
- CN I (olfactory)
- CN II (optic)
- CN III (oculomotor)
- CN IV (trochlear)
- CN V (trigeminal) motor
- CN V (trigeminal) sensory
- CN VI (abducens)
- CN VII (facial) motor-face
- CN VII (facial) sensorytaste
- CN VIII (vestibulocochlear)
- CN IX (glossopharyngeal) motor pharynx
- Mediastinum
- Pleura – Thoracic duct
- Trachea
- Upper airway NOS

RENAL/GENITOURINARY
- Bladder
- Cervix
- Fallopian tube
- Kidney
- Ovary
- Pelvis NOS
- Penis
- Prostate
- Scrotum
- Testis
- Ureter
- Urethra
- Urinary conduit
- Urinary tract NOS
- Uterus
- Vagina
- Vulva

Appendix 2 *(continued)*

SYNDROMES

		Grade				
Adverse Event	**Short Name**	**1**	**2**	**3**	**4**	**5**
NAVIGATION NOTE: Acute vascular leak syndrome is graded in the VASCULAR CATEGORY.						
NAVIGATION NOTE: Adrenal insufficiency is graded in the ENDOCRINE CATEGORY.						
NAVIGATION NOTE: Adult Respiratory Distress Syndrome (ARDS) is graded in the PULMONARY/UPPER RESPIRATORY CATEGORY.						
Alcohol intolerance syndrome (antabuse-like syndrome)	Alcohol intolerance syndrome	—	—	Present	—	Death
REMARK: An antabuse-like syndrome occurs with some new anti-androgens (e.g., nilutamide) when patient also consumes alcohol.						
NAVIGATION NOTE: Autoimmune reaction is graded as Autoimmune reaction/hypersensitivity (including drug fever) in the ALLERGY/IMMUNOLOGY CATEGORY.						
Cytokine release syndrome/acute infusion reaction	Cytokine release syndrome	Mild reaction; infusion interruption not indicated; intervention not indicated	Requires therapy or infusion interruption but responds promptly to symptomatic treatment (e.g., antihistamines, NSAIDS, narcotics, IV fluids); prophylactic medications indicated for ≤24 hrs	Prolonged (i.e., not rapidly responsive to symptomatic medication and/or brief interruption of infusion); recurrence of symptoms following initial improvement; hospitalization indicated for other clinical sequelae (e.g., renal impairment, pulmonary infiltrates)	Life-threatening; pressor or ventilatory support indicated	Death

(Continued)

Appendix 2 *(continued)*

		Grade				
Adverse Event	**Short Name**	**1**	**2**	**3**	**4**	**5**
REMARK: Cytokine release syndromes/acute infusion reactions are different from Allergic/hypersensitive reactions, although some of the manifestations are common to both AEs. An acute infusion reaction may occur with an agent that causes cytokine release (e.g., monoclonal antibodies or other biological agents). Signs and symptoms usually develop during or shortly after drug infusion and generally resolve completely within 24 hrs of completion of infusion. Signs/symptoms may include: Allergic reaction/hypersensitivity (including drug fever); Arthralgia (joint pain); Bronchospasm; Cough; Dizziness; Dyspnea (shortness of breath); Fatigue (asthenia, lethargy, malaise); Headache; Hypertension; Hypotension; Myalgia (muscle pain); Nausea; Pruritis/itching; Rash/desquamation; Rigors/chills; Sweating (diaphoresis); Tachycardia; Tumor pain (onset or exacerbation of tumor pain due to treatment); Urticaria (hives, welts, wheals); Vomiting. ALSO CONSIDER: Allergic reaction/hypersensitivity (including drug fever); Bronchospasm, wheezing; Dyspnea (shortness of breath); Hypertension; Hypotension; Hypoxia; Prolonged QTc interval; Supraventricular and nodal arrhythmia – *Select*; Ventricular arrhythmia – *Select*.						
NAVIGATION NOTE: Disseminated intravascular coagulation (DIC) is graded in the COAGULATION CATEGORY.						
NAVIGATION NOTE: Fanconi's syndrome is graded as Urinary electrolyte wasting (e.g., Fanconi's syndrome, renal tubular acidosis) in the RENAL/ GENITOURINARY CATEGORY.						
Flu-like syndrome	Flu-like syndrome	Symptoms present but not interfering with function	Moderate or causing difficulty performing some ADL	Severe symptoms interfering with ADL	Disabling	Death
REMARK: Flu-like syndrome represents a constellation of symptoms which may include cough with catarrhal symptoms, fever, headache, malaise, myalgia, prostration, and is to be used when the symptoms occur in a cluster consistent with one single pathophysiological process.						
NAVIGATION NOTE: Renal tubular acidosis is graded as Urinary electrolyte wasting (e.g., Fanconi's syndrome, renal tubular acidosis) in the RENAL/ GENITOURINARY CATEGORY.						

(Continued)

Appendix 2 *(continued)*

		Grade				
Adverse Event	**Short Name**	**1**	**2**	**3**	**4**	**5**
Retinoic acid syndrome	Retinoic acid syndrome	Fluid retention; less than 3 kg of weight gain; intervention with fluid restriction and/or diuretics indicated	Mild to moderate signs/symptoms; steroids indicated	Severe signs/symptoms; hospitalization indicated	Life-threatening; ventilatory support indicated	Death
REMARK: Patients with acute promyelocytic leukemia may experience a syndrome similar to ''retinoic acid syndrome'' in association with other agents such as arsenic trioxide. The syndrome is usually manifested by otherwise unexplained fever, weight gain, respiratory distress, pulmonary infiltrates and/or pleural effusion, with or without leukocytosis. ALSO CONSIDER: Acute vascular leak syndrome; Pleural effusion (nonmalignant); Pneumonitis/pulmonary infiltrates.						
NAVIGATION NOTE: SIADH is graded as Neuroendocrine: ADH secretion abnormality (e.g., SIADH or low ADH) in the ENDOCRINE CATEGORY.						
NAVIGATION NOTE: Stevens-Johnson syndrome is graded as Rash: erythema multiforme (e.g., Stevens-Johnson syndrome, toxic epidermal necrolysis) in the DERMATOLOGY/SKIN CATEGORY.						
NAVIGATION NOTE: Thrombotic microangiopathy is graded as Thrombotic microangiopathy (e.g., thrombotic thrombocytopenic purpura [TTP] or hemolytic uremic syndrome [HUS]) in the COAGULATION CATEGORY.						
Tumor flare	Tumor flare	Mild pain not interfering with function	Moderate pain; pain or analgesics interfering with function, but not interfering with ADL	Severe pain; pain or analgesics interfering with function and interfering with ADL	Disabling	Death
REMARK: Tumor flare is characterized by a constellation of signs and symptoms in direct relation to initiation of therapy (e.g., anti-estrogens/androgens or additional hormones). The symptoms/signs include tumor pain, inflammation of visible tumor, hypercalcemia, diffuse bone pain, and other electrolyte disturbances. ALSO CONSIDER: Calcium, serum-high (hypercalcemia).						

(Continued)

Appendix 2 *(continued)*

		Grade				
Adverse Event	**Short Name**	**1**	**2**	**3**	**4**	**5**
Tumor lysis syndrome	Tumor lysis syndrome	—	—	Present	—	Death
ALSO CONSIDER: Creatinine; Potassium, serum-high (hyperkalemia).						
Syndromes – Other (Specify, ________)	Syndromes – Other (Specify)	Mild	Moderate	Severe	Life-threatening; disabling	Death

VASCULAR

		Grade				
Adverse Event	**Short Name**	**1**	**2**	**3**	**4**	**5**
Acute vascular leak syndrome	Acute vascular leak syndrome	—	Symptomatic, fluid support not indicated	Respiratory compromise or fluids indicated	Life-threatening; pressor support or ventilatory support indicated	Death
Peripheral arterial ischemia	Peripheral arterial ischemia	—	Brief (<24 hrs) episode of ischemia managed nonsurgically and without permanent deficit	Recurring or prolonged (≥24 hrs) and/or invasive intervention indicated	Life-threatening, disabling and/or associated with end organ damage (e.g., limb loss)	Death
Phlebitis (including superficial thrombosis)	Phlebitis	—	Present	—	—	—
ALSO CONSIDER: Injection site reaction/extravasation changes.						

(Continued)

Appendix 2 *(continued)*

		Grade				
Adverse Event	**Short Name**	**1**	**2**	**3**	**4**	**5**
Portal vein flow	Portal flow	—	Decreased portal vein flow	Reversal/retrograde portal vein flow	—	—
Thrombosis/embolism (vascular access-related)	Thrombosis/embolism (vascular access)	—	Deep vein thrombosis or cardiac thrombosis; intervention (e.g., anticoagulation, lysis, filter, invasive procedure) not indicated	Deep vein thrombosis or cardiac thrombosis; intervention (e.g., anticoagulation, lysis, filter, invasive procedure) indicated	Embolic event including pulmonary embolism or life-threatening thrombus	Death
Thrombosis/thrombus/embolism	Thrombosis/thrombus/embolism	—	Deep vein thrombosis or cardiac thrombosis; intervention (e.g., anticoagulation, lysis, filter, invasive procedure) not indicated	Deep vein thrombosis or cardiac thrombosis; intervention (e.g., anticoagulation, lysis, filter, invasive procedure) indicated	Embolic event including pulmonary embolism or life-threatening thrombus	Death
Vessel injury-artery – *Select*: – Aorta – Carotid – Extremity-lower – Extremity-upper – Other NOS – Visceral	Artery injury – *Select*	Asymptomatic diagnostic finding; intervention not indicated	Symptomatic (e.g., claudication); not interfering with ADL; repair or revision not indicated	Symptomatic interfering with ADL; repair or revision indicated	Life-threatening; disabling; evidence of end organ damage (e.g., stroke, MI, organ or limb loss)	Death

(Continued)

Appendix 2 *(continued)*

		Grade				
Adverse Event	**Short Name**	**1**	**2**	**3**	**4**	**5**
NAVIGATION NOTE: Vessel injury to an artery intra-operatively is graded as Intra-operative injury – *Select Organ or Structure* in the SURGERY/INTRA-OPERATIVE INJURY CATEGORY.						
Vessel injury-vein – *Select*: – Extremity-lower – Extremity-upper – IVC – Jugular – Other NOS – SVC – Viscera	Vein injury — *Select*	Asymptomatic diagnostic finding; intervention not indicated	Symptomatic (e.g., claudication); not interfering with ADL; repair or revision not indicated	Symptomatic interfering with ADL; repair or revision indicated	Life-threatening; disabling; evidence of end organ damage	Death
NAVIGATION NOTE: Vessel injury to a vein intra-operatively is graded as Intra-operative injury – *Select Organ or Structure* in the SURGERY/INTRA-OPERATIVE INJURY CATEGORY.						
Visceral arterial ischemia (non-myocardial)	Visceral arterial ischemia	—	Brief (<24 hrs) episode of ischemia managed medically and without permanent deficit	Prolonged (≥24 hrs) or recurring symptoms and/or invasive intervention indicated	Life-threatening; disabling; evidence of end organ damage	Death
ALSO CONSIDER: CNS cerebrovascular ischemia.						
Vascular – Other (Specify, ________)	Vascular – Other (Specify)	Mild	Moderate	Severe	Life-threatening; disabling	Death

Appendix 3

Cancer Chemotherapeutic Regimens (Adult)

The use of cancer chemotherapeutic agents in combination is well established. The knowledge of cell kinetics and the pharmacology of antitumor agents have allowed the clinician to use combination therapy to maximize tumor cell kill with minimal or acceptable toxicity to the patient. The basic principles of combination therapy are to use agents that are individually active against a given tumor, in a dosage as close as possible to that used in single-agent therapy; agents with different mechanisms of action; and agents with different or minimally overlapping toxicities.

This review lists some of the common combination regimens and doses used in the cancers noted. It also lists selected single-agent regimens. The included regimens and doses were selected based on the following criteria: regimens published in 2 tertiary references; regimens positively evaluated in Phase II or III trials published in major English language journals; or regimens/agents that have received approval by the Food and Drug Administration with or without published literature. The accuracy of all regimens in this review has been checked against and matched with findings in the scientific literature. Therefore, in each case, references are provided.

This review should serve as a general reference only, as variations of many of the combinations exist, and the dose and frequency of administration may be altered because of tumor response or patient toxicity. These regimens may vary from institution to institution and from physician to physician. *Source:* Modified from Adams VR, DeRemer D, Holdsworth MT. Guide to Cancer Chemotherapy Regimens 2005. *Oncology Special Edition,* volume 7. NY: McMahon Publishing 2005

Adenocarcinoma—Unknown Primary

Carbo-Tax	**Carboplatin** dose targeted by Calvert equation to AUC 6 mg/mL/min I.V. **FOLLOWED BY** **Paclitaxel*** 200 mg/m² I.V. over 3 hours, day 1 **G-CSF** 300 mcg/d SQ, days 5–12 *Repeat cycle every 21 days*
EP	**Cisplatin** 60–100 mg/m² I.V., day 1

	Etoposide 80–120 mg/m²/d I.V., days 4, 6, 8, or 3, 5, 7 *Repeat cycle every 21–28 days*
Paclitaxel/Carboplatin/ Etoposide	**Paclitaxel*** 200 mg/m² I.V. over 1 hour, day 1 **FOLLOWED BY** **Carboplatin** dose targeted by Calvert equation to AUC 6 mg/mL/min I.V. **Etoposide** 50 mg/d PO alternated with 100 mg/d PO, days 1–10 *Repeat cycle every 21 days*

References

Carbo-Tax

Briasoulis E, Kalofonos H, Bafaloukos D, et al. Carboplatin plus paclitaxel in unknown primary carcinoma: a phase II Hellenic Cooperative Oncology Group Study. *J Clin Oncol.* 2000;18:3101–3107.

EP

Longeval E, Klastersky J. Combination chemotherapy with cisplatin and etoposide in bronchogenic squamous cell carcinoma and adenocarcinoma. *Cancer.* 1982;50: 2751–2756.

Shepherd FA Treatment of advanced non-small cell lung cancer. *Semin Oncol.* 1994; 21(Suppl 7):7–18.

Paclitaxel, Carboplatin, Etoposide

Hainsworth JD, Erland JB, Kalman LA, et al. Carcinoma of unknown primary site: treatment with 1-hour paclitaxel, carboplatin, and extended-schedule etoposide. *J Clin Oncol.* 1997;15:2385–2393.

AIDS-Related Kaposi's Sarcoma

Single-Agent Regimens

Alitretinoin	Apply generous coat to cutaneous Kaposi's sarcoma lesions bid initially, then gradually increase to tid or qid according to individual lesion tolerance.
Liposomal daunorubicin	**Liposomal daunorubicin** 40 mg/m² I.V. over 60 minutes *Repeat cycle every 14 days*
Pegylated liposomal doxorubicin	**Pegylated liposomal doxorubicin** 20 mg/m² I.V. over 30 minutes *Repeat cycle every 21 days*

Single-Agent Regimen (2nd Line)

Paclitaxel	**Paclitaxel*** 135 mg/m² I.V. over 3 hours *Repeat cycle every 21 days*

OR
Paclitaxel* 100 mg/m^2 I.V. over 3 hours
Repeat cycle every 14 days

References

Alitretinoin

Panretin Gel 0.1% (alitretinoin) (package insert). San Diego, CA: Ligand Pharmaceuticals Inc., 2001.

Liposomal daunorubicin

DaunoXome (package insert). San Dimas, CA: Gilead Sciences; 2002.

Pegylated liposomal doxorubicin

Doxil (package insert). Raritan, NJ: Ortho Biotech Products, LP; 2003.

Paclitaxel

Taxol (package insert). Princeton, NJ: Bristol-Myers Squibb Oncology; 2003.

AIDS-Related Lymphoma

CDE	**Cyclophosphamide** 200 mg/m^2/d I.V. Cl for 96 hours **Doxorubicin** 12.5 mg/m^2/d I.V. CI for 96 hours **Etoposide** 60 mg/m^2/d I.V. CI for 96 hours *Repeat cycle every 28 days*
CHOP	**Cyclophosphamide** 750 mg/m^2 I.V., day 1 **Doxorubicin** 50 mg/m^2 I.V., day 1 **Vincristine#** 1.4 mg/m^2 I.V., day 1 **Prednisone** 100 mg/d PO, days 1–5 Doses of doxorubicin/cyclophosphamide may be reduced by up to 50% in high-risk patients *Repeat cycle every 21 days*
m-BACOD	**Methotrexate** 200 mg/m^2 I.V., day 15 **Bleomycin** 4 units/m^2 I.V., day 1 **Doxorubicin** 25 mg/m^2 I.V., day 1 **Cyclophosphamide** 300 mg/m^2 I.V., day 1 **Vincristine#** 1.4 mg/m^2 I.V., day 1 **Dexamethasone** 3 mg/m^2/d PO, days 1–5 **GM-CSF** 5 mcg/kg/d SQ, days 4–13 *Repeat cycle when ANC ≥1,000/mm^3 but not earlier than day 22*

References

CDE

Sparano JA, Wiernik PH, Hu X, et al. Pilot trial of infusional cyclophosphamide, doxorubicin, and etoposide plus didanosine and filgrastim in patients with human immunodeficiency virus-associated non-Hodgkin's lymphoma. *J Clin Oncol.* 1996;14: 3026–3035.

CHOP

Ratner L, Lee J, Tang S, et al. Chemotherapy for human immunodeficiency virus-associated non-Hodgkin's lymphoma in combination with highly active antiretroviral therapy. *J Clin Oncol.* 2001;19:2171–2178.

Levine AM Acquired immunodeficiency syndrome–related lymphoma: clinical aspects. *Semin Oncol.* 2000;27:442–453.

m-BACOD

Kaplan LD, Straus DJ, Testa MA, et al. Low-dose compared with standard-dose m-BACOD chemotherapy for non-Hodgkin's lymphoma associated with human immunodeficiency virus infection. *N Engl J Med.* 1997;336:1641–1648.

Breast Cancer

Combination Regimens

AC	**Doxorubicin** 60 mg/m^2 I.V., day 1 **Cyclophosphamide** 600 mg/m^2 I.V., day 1 *Repeat cycle every 21 days*
AT	**Doxorubicin** 50 mg/m^2 I.V., day 1 **FOLLOWED 24 HOURS LATER BY** **Paclitaxel*** 220 mg/m^2 I.V. over 3 hours, day 2 *Repeat cycle every 21 days for up to 8 cycles*
A→T→C→ (dose dense)	**Doxorubicin** 60 mg/m^2 I.V. q 2 wk × 4 cycles (dose dense) **FOLLOWED BY** **Paclitaxel** 175 mg/m^2 I.V. q 2 wk × 4 cycles **FOLLOWED BY** **Cyclophosphamide** 600 mg/m^2 I.V. q 2 wk × 4 cycles *Administer filgrastim 5 mcg/kg SQ on days 3-10 of each 2 week cycle*
CAF	**Cyclophosphamide** 500 mg/m^2 I.V., day 1 **Doxorubicin** 50 mg/m^2 I.V., day 1 **Fluorouracil** 500 mg/m^2 I.V., day 1 *Repeat cycle every 21 days*
CEF (FEC)	**Cyclophosphamide** 75 mg/m^2/d PO, days 1–14 **Epirubicin** 60 mg/m^2/d I.V., days 1, 8 **Fluorouracil** 500 mg/m^2/d I.V., days 1, 8

	Repeat cycle every 28 days for 6 cycles
	OR
	Cyclophosphamide 500 mg/m² I.V., day 1
	Epirubicin 100 mg/m² I.V., day 1
	Fluorouracil 500 mg/m² I.V., day 1
	Repeat cycle every 21 days for 4 cycles
CFM (CNF, FNC)	**Cyclophosphamide** 600 mg/m² I.V., day 1
	Fluorouracil 600 mg/m² I.V., day 1
	Mitoxantrone 12 mg/m² I.V., day 1
	Repeat cycle every 21 days
CMF	**Cyclophosphamide** 100 mg/m²/d PO, days 1–14 or 600 mg/m²/d I.V., days 1, 8
	Methotrexate 40 mg/m²/d I.V., days 1, 8 (for patients >60 years, 30 mg/m²)
	Fluorouracil 600 mg/m²/d I.V., days 1, 8 (for patients >60 years, 400 mg/m²)
	Repeat cycle every 28 days
	OR
	Cyclophosphamide 600 mg/m² I.V., day 1
	Methotrexate 40 mg/m² I.V., day 1
	Fluorouracil 600 mg/m² I.V., day 1
	Repeat cycle every 21 days
Gem/Tax	**Gemcitabine** 1,250 mg/m² I.V. over 30 min. days 1,8
	Paclitaxel 175 mg/m² I.V. over 3 hr. before gemcitabine day 1
	Repeat cycle every 21 days
HEC	**Epirubicin** 100 mg/m² I.V., day 1
	Cyclophosphamide 830 mg/m² I.V., day 1
	Repeat cycle every 21 days for up to 8 cycles
NA	**Vinorelbine** 25 mg/m²/d I.V., days 1, 8
	Doxorubicin 50 mg/m² I.V., day 1
	Repeat cycle every 21 days
NFL	**Mitoxantrone** 10 mg/m² I.V., day 1
	Fluorouracil 1,000 mg/m²/d I.V. CI, days 1–3
	Leucovorin 100 mg/m²/d I.V. over 15 minutes, days 1–3
	Repeat cycle every 21 days
	OR
	Mitoxantrone 12 mg/m² I.V., day 1
	Fluorouracil 350 mg/m²/d I.V. bolus, days 1–3 after leucovorin
	Leucovorin 300 mg/d I.V. over 30–60 minutes, days 1–3
	Repeat cycle every 21 days

Paclitaxel/Virorelbine

Paclitaxel* 135 mg/m^2 I.V. CI over 3 hours, starting 1 hour after vinorelbine, day 1
Vinorelbine 30 $mg/m^2/d$ I.V. over 20 minutes, days 1, 8
Repeat cycle every 28 days

Sequential AC/ Paclitaxel

Doxorubicin 60–90 mg/m^2 I.V., day 1
Cyclophosphamide 600 mg/m^2 I.V., day 1
Repeat cycle every 21 days for 4 cycles,
FOLLOWED BY
Paclitaxel* 175 mg/m^2 I.V.
Repeat cycle every 21 days for 4 cycles

Sequential Dox-CMF

Doxorubicin 75 mg/m^2 I.V. every 21 days for 4 cycles,
FOLLOWED BY
21- or 28-day CMF *(see previous page)* for 8 cycles

TAC

Doxorubicin 50 mg/m^2 as a 15-minute I.V. bolus,
FOLLOWED IMMEDIATELY BY
Cyclosphosphamide 500 mg/m^2 as 15-minute I.V. bolus,
FOLLOWED 1 HOUR AFTER COMPLETION OF THE DOXORUBICIN INFUSION BY
Docetaxel 75 mg/m^2 I.V. over 1 hour

Tamoxifen/Epirubicin Epirubicin

Tamoxifen 20 mg/d PO for 4 years
Epirubicin 50 $mg/m^2/d$ I.V., days 1, 8
Repeat epirubicin cycle every 28 days for 6 cycles

Trastuzumab/Paclitaxel

Trastuzumab 4 mg/kg I.V. loading dose over 90 minutes,
FOLLOWED BY
Trastuzumab 2 mg/kg I.V. over 30 minutes, weekly
Paclitaxel* 175 mg/m^2 over 3 hours, every 21 days for at least 6 cycles

X + T

Capecitabine 1,250 mg/m^2 PO bid, days 1–14
Docetaxel 75 mg/m^2 as a 1-hour I.V. infusion, day 1
Repeat cycle every 21 days

Monoclonal Antibody Regimen

Trastuzumab

Trastuzumab 4 mg/kg I.V. loading dose over 90 minutes,
FOLLOWED BY
2 mg/kg I.V. over 30 minutes, weekly

Single-Agent Regimens

Abraxane

Paclitaxel protein-bound particles for injectable suspension 260 mg/m^2 I.V. every 3 weeks

Anastrozole	**Anastrozole** 1 mg/d PO
Capecitabine	**Capecitabine** 1,250–1,255 mg/m² PO bid, days 1–14, followed by 7 days rest *Repeat cycle every 21 days*
Docetaxel	**Docetaxel** 60–100 mg/m² I.V., over 1 hour, every 21 days All patients should be premedicated with oral corticosteroids such as dexamethasone 16 mg/d (e.g., 8 mg bid) for 3 days starting 1 day prior to docetaxel administration. **Docetaxel** 40 mg/m² q wk × 6, repeated q 8 weeks
Exemestane	**Exemestane** 25 mg/d PO
Fulvestrant	**Fulvestrant** 250 mg IM into the buttock every month
Gemcitabine	**Gemcitabine** 725 mg/m²/d I.V. over 30 minutes, days 1, 8, 15 *Repeat cycle every 28 days*
Letrozole	**Letrozole** 2.5 mg/d PO
Megestrol	**Megestrol** 40 mg PO qid
Paclitaxel	**Paclitaxel*** 250 mg/m² I.V. over 3 or 24 hours, every 21 days **OR** **Paclitaxel*** 175 mg/m² I.V. over 3 hours, every 21 days
Tamoxifen	**Tamoxifen** 20–40 mg/d, dosages >20 mg/d should be given in divided doses (morning and evening)
Toremifene	**Toremifene** 60 mg/d PO
Vinorelbine	**Vinorelbine** 30 mg/m² I.V. every 7 days

References

AC

Fisher B, Brown AM, Dimitrov NV, et al. Two months of doxorubicin–cyclophosphamide with and without interval reinduction therapy compared with 6 months of cyclophosphamide, methotrexate, and fluorouracil in positive-node breast cancer patients with tamoxifen-nonresponsive tumors: results from the National Surgical Adjuvant Breast and Bowel Project B-15. *J Clin Oncol.* 1990;8:1483–1496.

ATC

Citron ML, Berry DA, Cirrincione C, et al. Randomized trial of dose-dense versus conventionally scheduled and sequential versus concurrent combination chemotherapy as postoperative adjuvant treatment of node-positive primary breast cancer: First report of intergroup trial C9741/Cancer and Leukemia Group B Trial 9741 *Clin J Oncol* 2003;21:1431–1439.

AT

Jassem J, Pienkowski T, Pluzanska A, et al. Doxorubicin and paclitaxel versus fluorouracil, doxorubicin, and cyclophosphamide as first-line therapy for women with metastatic breast cancer: final results of a randomized phase III multicenter trial. *J Clin Oncol.* 2001;19:1707–1715.

CAF

Smalley RV, Lefante J, Bartolucci A, et al. A comparison of cyclophosphamide, adriamycin, and 5-fluorouracil (CAF) and cyclophosphamide, methotrexate, 5-fluorouracil, vincristine, and prednisone (CMFVP) in patients with advanced breast cancer. *Breast Cancer Res Treat.* 1983;3:209–220.

CEF (FEC)

Levine MN, Bramwell VH, Pritchard KI, et al. Randomized trial of intensive cyclophosphamide, epirubicin, and fluorouracil chemotherapy compared with cyclophosphamide, methotrexate, and fluorouracil in premenopausal women with node-positive breast cancer. *J Clin Oncol.* 1998;16:2651–2658.

French Epirubicin Study Group. Epirubicin-based chemotherapy in metastatic breast cancer patients: role of dose intensity and duration of treatment. *J Clin Oncol.* 2000;18:3115–3124.

CFM (CNF, FNC)

Alonso MC, Tabernero JM, Ojeda B, et al. A phase III randomized trial of cyclophosphamide, mitoxantrone and 5-fluorouracil (CNF) versus cyclophosphamide, adriamycin, and 5-fluorouracil (CAF) in patients with metastatic breast cancer. *Breast Cancer Res Treat.* 1995;34:15–24.

CMF

Bonadonna G, Valagussa P, Moliterni A, Zambetti M, Brambilla C. Adjuvant cyclophosphamide, methotrexate, and fluorouracil in node-positive breast cancer: the results of 20 years of follow-up. *N Engl J Med.* 1995;332:901–906.

Bonadonna G, Zambetti M, Valagussa P. Sequential or alternating doxorubicin and CMF regimens in breast cancer with more than three positive nodes: ten year results. *JAMA.* 1995;273:542–547.

Gemcitabine/Paclitaxel

Gemzar [package insert]. Indianapolis, IN: Eli Lilly and Company; 2004

HEC

Piccart MJ, Di Leo A, et al. Phase III trial comparing two dose levels of epirubicin combined with cyclophosphamide with cyclophosphamide, methotrexate, and fluorouracil in node-positive breast cancer. *J Clin Oncol.* 2001;19:3103–3110.

NA

Blajman C, Balbiani L, Block J, et al. A prospective, randomized Phase III trial comparing combination chemotherapy with cyclophosphamide, doxorubicin, and 5-fluorouracil with vinorelbine plus doxorubicin in the treatment of advanced breast carcinoma. *Cancer.* 1999;85:1091–1097.

NFL

Jones SE, Mennel RG, Brooks B, et al. Phase II study of mitoxantrone, leucovorin, and infusional fluorouracil for treatment of metastatic breast cancer. *J Clin Oncol.* 1991;9:1736–1739.

Hainsworth JD, Jolivet J, Birch R, et al. Mitoxantrone, 5-fluorouracil, and high-dose leucovorin (NFL) versus intravenous cyclophosphamide, methotrexate, and 5-fluorouracil (CMF) in first-line chemotherapy for patients with metastatic breast carcinoma: a randomized phase II trial. *Cancer.* 1997;79:740–748.

Paclitaxel/Vinorelbine

Acuña LR, Langhi M, Pérez J, et al. Vinorelbine and paclitaxel as first-line chemotherapy in metastatic breast cancer. *J Clin Oncol.* 1999;17:74–81.

Sequential AC/Paclitaxel

Henderson IC, Berry DA, Demetri GD, et al. Improved outcomes from adding sequential paclitaxel but not from escalating doxorubicin dose in an adjuvant chemotherapy regimen for patients with node-positive primary breast cancer. *J Clin Oncol.* 2003;21:976–983.

Taxol (package insert). Princeton, NJ: Bristol-Myers Squibb Oncology; 2003.

Sequential Dox-CMF

Bonadonna G, Zambetti M, Valagussa P. Sequential or alternating doxorubicin and CMF regimens in breast cancer with more than three positive nodes: ten year results. *JAMA.* 1995;273:542–547.

TAC

Nabholtz JM, Pienkowski T, Mackey J, et al. Phase III trial comparing TAC (docetaxel, doxorubicin, cyclophosphamide) with FAC (5-fluorouracil, doxorubicin, cyclophosphamide) in the adjuvant treatment of node-positive breast cancer (BC) patients: interim analysis of the BCIRG 001 study (abstract). *Proc Am Soc Clin Oncol.* 2002;21:36a. Abstract 141.

Tamoxifen/Epirubicin

Wils JA, Bliss JM, Marty M, et al. Epirubicin plus tamoxifen versus tamoxifen alone in node-positive postmenopausal patients with breast cancer: a randomized trial of the International Collaborative Cancer Group. *J Clin Oncol.* 1999;17:1988–1998.

Trastuzumab/Paclitaxel

Slamon D, Leyland-Jones B, Shak S, et al. Use of chemotherapy plus a monoclonal antibody against HER2 for metastatic breast cancer that overexpresses HER2. *N Engl J Med.* 2001;344:783–792.

Herceptin (package insert). South San Francisco, CA: Genentech, Inc; 2003.

X + T

Xeloda (package insert). Nutley, NJ: Roche Pharmaceuticals; 2003.

Trastuzumab

Herceptin (package insert). South San Francisco, CA: Genentech, Inc; 2003.

Abraxane

(package insert). South San Francisco, CA: Genentech, Inc; 2004.

Anastrozole

Arimidex (package insert). Wilmington, DE: AstraZeneca Pharmaceuticals; 2003.

Capecitabine

Blum JL, Jones SE, Buzdar AU, et al. Multicenter phase II study of capecitabine in paclitaxel-refractory metastatic breast cancer. *J Clin Oncol.* 1999;17:485–493.

Xeloda (package insert). Nutley, NJ: Roche Pharmaceuticals; 2003.

Docetaxel

Burstein HJ, Manol J, Younger J, et al. Docetaxel administered on a weekly basis for metastatic breast cancer. *J Clin Oncol.* 2001;18(6):1212–1219.

Chan S, Friedrichs K, Noel D, et al. Prospective randomized trial of docetaxel versus doxorubicin in patients with metastatic breast cancer. *J Clin Oncol.* 1999;17: 2341–2354.

Nabholtz JM, Senn HJ, Bezwoda WR, et al. Prospective randomized trial of docetaxel versus mitomycin plus vinblastine in patients with metastatic breast cancer progressing despite previous anthracycline-containing chemotherapy. *J Clin Oncol.* 1999;17: 1413–1424.

Taxotere (package insert). Bridgewater, NJ: Aventis Pharmaceuticals; 2003.

Exemestane

Lønning PE, Bajetta E, Murray R, et al. Activity of exemestane in metastatic breast cancer after failure of nonsteroidal aromatase inhibitors: a phase II trial. *J Clin Oncol.* 2000;18:2234–2244.

Kaufmann M, Bajetta E, Dirix LY, et al. Exemestane is superior to megestrol acetate after tamoxifen failure in postmenopausal women with advanced breast cancer: results of a phase III randomized double-blind trial. The Exemestane Study Group. *J Clin Oncol.* 2000;18:1399–1411.

Coombes RC, Hall E, Gibson LJ, et al. A randomized trial of exemestane after two to three years of tamoxifen therapy in postmenopausal women with primary breast cancer. *N Engl J Med.* 2004;350:1081–1092.

Aromasin (package insert). New York, NY: Pfizer; 2003.

Fulvestrant

Faslodex (package insert). Wilmington, DE: AstraZeneca Pharmaceuticals LP; 2003.

Gemcitabine

Carmichael J, Possinger K, Phillip P, et al. Advanced breast cancer: a phase II trial with gemcitabine. *J Clin Oncol.* 1995;13:2731–2736.

Letrozole

Dombernowsky P, Smith I, Falkson G, et al. Letrozole, a new oral aromatase inhibitor for advanced breast cancer: double-blind randomized trial showing a dose effect and improved efficacy and tolerability compared with megestrol acetate. *J Clin Oncol.* 1998; 16:453–461.

Ingle JN, et al. A randomized phase II trial of two dosage levels of letrozole as third-line hormonal therapy for women with metastatic breast cancer. *Cancer.* 1997;80: 218–224.

Goss PE, Ingle JN, Martino S, et al. A randomized trial of letrozole in postmenopausal women after five years of tamoxifen therapy for early-stage breast cancer. *N Engl J Med.* 2003;349:1793–1802.

Megestrol

Megace (package insert). Princeton, NJ: Bristol-Myers Squibb Oncology; 2002.

Paclitaxel

Seidman AD, Tiersten A, Hudis C, et al. Phase II trial of paclitaxel by 3-hour infusion as initial and salvage chemotherapy for metastatic breast cancer. *J Clin Oncol.* 1995;13:2575–2581.

Smith RE, et al. Randomized trial of 3-hour versus 24-hour infusion of high-dose paclitaxel in patients with metastatic or locally advanced breast cancer: National Surgical Adjuvant Breast and Bowel Project Protocol B-26. *J Clin Oncol.* 1999;17:3403–3411.

Tamoxifen

Nolvadex (package insert). Wilmington, DE: AstraZeneca; 2003.

Toremifene

Hayes DF, Van Zyl JA, Hacking A, et al. Randomized comparison of tamoxifen and two separate doses of toremifene in postmenopausal patients with metastatic breast cancer. *J Clin Oncol.* 1995;13:2556–2566.

Fareston (package insert). Newport, KY: Shire Pharmaceuticals; 1999.

Vinorelbine

Weber BL, Vogel C, Jones S, et al. Intravenous vinorelbine as first-line and second-line therapy in advanced breast cancer. *J Clin Oncol.* 1995;13:2722–2730.

Colorectal Cancer

Combination Regimens

Cetuximab/Irinotecan	**Cetuximab** 400 mg/m^2 I.V. initial dose, then 250 mg/m^2 I.V. every 7 days **Irinotecan** 350 mg/m^2 I.V. every 21 days **OR** 180 mg/m^2 I.V. every 14 days **OR** 125 mg/m^2 I.V. every 7 days × 4 doses every 6 weeks
Fluorouracil/Leucovorin (Mayo regimen)	**Fluorouracil** 370 mg/m^2/d I.V. bolus 1 hour after start of leucovorin, days 1–5 **Leucovorin** 200 mg/m^2/d I.V. bolus, days 1–5 *Repeat cycle at 4 and 8 weeks, and every 5 weeks thereafter*
Fluorouracil/Leucovorin (Roswell Park regimen)	**Fluorouracil** 600 mg/m^2/d I.V. bolus 1 hour after start of leucovorin, days 1, 8, 15, 22, 29, 35 **Leucovorin** 500 mg/m^2/d I.V. over 2 hours, days 1, 8, 15, 22, 29, 35 *Repeat cycle every 8 weeks*
IFL (Saltz regimen)	**Irinotecan** 125 mg/m^2/d I.V. over 90 minutes, days 1, 8, 15, 22 **Leucovorin** 20 mg/m^2/d I.V. bolus, days 1, 8, 15, 22 **Fluorouracil** 500 mg/m^2/d I.V. bolus, days 1, 8, 15, 22 *Repeat cycle every 6 weeks*

IFL/BV	**IFL** (see above) **Bevacizumab** 5 mg/kg I.V. every 14 days
Douillard regimen	**Irinotecan** 180 mg/m² I.V., day 1 **Leucovorin** 200 mg/m²/d I.V., days 1, 2 **Fluorouracil** 400 mg/m² I.V. bolus and **Fluorouracil** 600 mg/m² I.V. over 22 hours, day 1 *Repeat cycle every 14 days*
Oxaliplatin/ Fluorouracil/ Leucovorin (FOLFOX4)	**Oxaliplatin** 85 mg/m² I.V. and Leucovorin 200 mg/m² I.V. over 120 minutes at same time (separate bags, Y-line), day 1, **FOLLOWED BY** **Fluorouracil** 400 mg/m² I.V. bolus over 2–4 minutes, day 1, **FOLLOWED BY** **Fluorouracil** 600 mg/m² I.V. CI over 22 hours, day 1 **Leucovorin** 200 mg/m² I.V. over 120 minutes, day 2, **FOLLOWED BY** **Fluorouracil** 400 mg/m² I.V. bolus over 2–4 minutes, day 2, **FOLLOWED BY** **Fluorouracil** 600 mg/m² I.V. CI over 22 hours, day 2 *Repeat cycle every 14 days*
(FOLFOX6)	**Oxaliplatin** 85-100 mg/m² I.V. and Leucovorin 200 mg/m² I.V. over 120 minutes at same time (separate bags, Y-line), day 1, **FOLLOWED BY** **Fluorouracil** 400 mg/m² I.V. bolus day 1 **FOLLOWED BY** **Fluorouracil** 2,400-3,000 mg/m² I.V. CI over 46 hours *Repeat cycle every 14 days*
FOLFOX+BV	**FOLFOX regimen as above** **Bevacizumab** 5 mg/kg I.V. over 90 min then repeated q 2 wk; if well tolerated, next infusion is over 60 min; if this goes well; subsequent infusions are over 30 min
XELIRI	**Irinotecan** 250 mg/m² I.V. day 1 **Capecitabine** 1,000 mg/m² PO bid from the evening of day 1 to morning of day 15. *Repeat cycle every 21 days*
XELOX	**Oxaliplatin** 130 mg/m² I.V. day 1 **Capecitabine** 1,000 mg/m² PO bid from the evening of day 1 to morning of day 15. *Repeat cycle every 21 days*

Single-Agent Regimens

Capecitabine	**Capecitabine** 2,500 mg/m^2/d PO in 2 divided doses, days 1–14, followed by 7 days rest *Repeat cycle every 21 days*
Cetuximab	**Cetuximab** 400 mg/m^2 I.V. initial dose, then 250 mg/m^2 I.V. every 7 days *For irinotecan-intolerant patients*
5-Fluorouracil	**5-Fluorouracil** 1,000 mg/m^2/d I.V. CI, days 1–5 *Repeat cycle every 28 days*
Irinotecan	**Irinotecan** 125 mg/m^2/d I.V. over 90 minutes, days 1, 8, 15, 22 *Repeat cycle every 6 weeks* **OR** **Irinotecan** 350 mg/m^2 I.V. over 90 minutes, day 1 *Repeat cycle every 21 days*

References

Cetuximab/Irinotecan

Erbitux (package insert). Branchburg, NJ and Princeton, NJ: ImClone Systems/Bristol-Myers Squibb; 2004.

Fluorouracil/Leucovorin (Mayo regimen)

Poon MA, O'Connell MJ, Moertel CG. Biochemical modulation of fluorouracil: evidence of significant improvement of survival and quality of life in patients with advanced colorectal carcinoma. *J Clin Oncol.* 1989;7:1407–1418.

Fluorouracil/Leucovorin (Roswell Park regimen)

Petrelli N, et al. The modulation of fluorouracil with leucovorin in metastatic colorectal carcinoma: a prospective randomized phase III trial. *J Clin Oncol.* 1989;7:1419–1426.

Petrelli N, Herrera L, Rustum Y, et al. A prospective randomized trial of 5-fluorouracil versus 5-fluorouracil and high-dose leucovorin versus 5-fluorouracil and methotrexate in previously untreated patients with advanced colorectal carcinoma. *J Clin Oncol.* 1987;5:1559–1565.

IFL (Saltz regimen)

Saltz LB, Cox JV, Blanke C, et al. Irinotecan plus fluorouracil and leucovorin for metastatic colorectal cancer. *N Engl J Med.* 2000;343:905–914.

IFL/BV and FOLFOX/BV

Avastin (package insert). South San Francisco, CA: Genentech, Inc; 2004.

Hurwitz H, Fehrenbacher L, Cartwright T, et al. Bevacizumab prolongs survival in first-line colorectal cancer: results of a phase III trial of bevacizumab in combination with bolus IFL as first-line therapy in subjects with metastatic CRC. Abstract presented at: The 39th Annual Meeting of the American Society of Clinical Oncology. May 31, June 3, 2003; Chicago, Ill. Abstract 3646.

Douillard

Douillard JY, Cunningham D, Roth AD, et al. Irinotecan combined with fluorouracil compared with fluorouracil alone as first-line treatment for metastatic colorectal cancer: a multicentre randomised trial. *Lancet.* 2000;355:1041–1047.

Oxaliplatin/Fluorouracil/Leucovorin (FOLFOX4)

Eloxatin (package insert). New York, NY: Sanofi Aventis; 2004.

FOLFOX6

Tournigand C, Andre T, Achille E, et al. FOLFIRI followed by FOLFOX6 on the reverse sequence in advanced colorectal cancer: a randomized GERCOR study. *J Clin Oncol.* 2004;22:229–237.

XELOX

Cassidy J, Tabernero J, Twelves C, et al. XELOX (capecitabine plus oxaliplatin): active first-line therapy for patients with metastatic colorectal cancer. *J Clin Oncol.* 2004;22: 2084–2091.

Capecitabine

Cox JV, Pazdur R, Thibault A, et al. A phase III trial of Xeloda (capecitabine) in previously untreated advanced/metastatic colorectal cancer (abstract). *Proc Am Soc Clin Oncol.* 1999;18:265a. Abstract 1016.

Patt YZ, Liebmann J, Diamandidis D, et al. Capecitabine (X) plus irinotecan (XELIRI) as first-line treatment for metastatic colorectal cancer (MCRC): Final safety findings from a phase II trial [Abstract 3602]. *Proc Am Soc Clin Oncol.* 23:271.

Van Cutsem E, Findlay M, Osterwalder B, et al. Capecitabine, an oral fluoropyrimidine carbamate with substantial activity in advanced colorectal cancer: results of a randomized phase II study. *J Clin Oncol.* 2000;18:1337–1345.

Cetuximab

Erbitux (package insert). Branchburg, NJ and Princeton NJ: ImClone Systems; Bristol-Myers Squibb; 2004.

5-Fluorouracil

Kemeny N, Israel K, Neidzweiki D, et al. Randomized study of continuous-infusion fluorouracil versus fluorouracil plus cisplatin in patients with metastatic colorectal cancer. *J Clin Oncol.* 1990;8:313–318.

Schmoll HJ. Development of treatment for advanced colorectal cancer: infusional 5-FU and the role of new agents. *Eur J Cancer.* 1996;32A(suppl 5):S18–S22.

Irinotecan

Rougier P, Bugat R, Douillard JY, et al. Phase II study of irinotecan in the treatment of advanced colorectal cancer in chemotherapy-naïve patients and patients pretreated with fluorouracil-based chemotherapy. *J Clin Oncol.* 1997;15:251–260.

Camptosar (package insert). New York, NY: Pfizer; 2002.

Conti JA, Kemeny NE, Saltz LB, et al. Irinotecan is an active agent in untreated patients with metastatic colorectal cancer. *J Clin Oncol.* 1996;14:709–715.

Cunningham D, Pyrhönen S, James RD, et al. Randomised trial of irinotecan plus supportive care versus supportive care alone after fluorouracil failure for patients with metastatic colorectal cancer. *Lancet.* 1998;352:1413–1418.

Gastric Cancer

Docetaxel/Cisplatin	**Docetaxel** 85 mg/m² I.V. over 1 hour, day 1, **FOLLOWED BY** **Cisplatin** 75 mg/m² I.V. over 1 hour, day 1 *Repeat cycle every 21 days for a maximum of 8 cycles*
ECF	**Epirubicin** 50 mg/m² I.V., day 1 **Cisplatin** 60 mg/m² I.V., day 1 *Repeat cycle every 21 days for a maximum of 8 cycles* **WITH** **Fluorouracil** 200 mg/m²/d I.V. CI, for up to 6 months
ELF	**Leucovorin** 150 mg/m²/d I.V. over 10 minutes, **FOLLOWED BY** **Etoposide** 120 mg/m²/d I.V. over 30 minutes, **FOLLOWED BY** **Fluorouracil** 500 mg/m²/d I.V. over 10 minutes *Give all agents on days 1–3; repeat cycle every 3 weeks* **OR** **Leucovorin** 300 mg/m²/d I.V. over 10 minutes, **FOLLOWED BY** **Etoposide** 120 mg/m²/d I.V. over 50 minutes, **FOLLOWED BY** **Fluorouracil** 500 mg/m²/d I.V. bolus *Give all agents on days 1–3; repeat cycle every 3 weeks*
FAMTX	**Methotrexate** 1,500 mg/m² I.V., day 1, **FOLLOWED 1 HOUR LATER BY** **Fluorouracil** 1,500 mg/m² I.V., day 1, FOLLOWED 24 HOURS AFTER METHOTREXATE DOSE BY **Leucovorin** 15 mg/m² PO every 6 hours for 48 hours **Doxorubicin** 30 mg/m² I.V., day 15 *Repeat cycle every 28 days*
5-FU/LV	**Fluorouracil** 425 mg/m²/d for 5 days **Leucovorin** 20 mg/m²/d for 5 days **FOLLOWED BY** **Radiation** 4,500 cGy (180 cGy/d), 5 days a week for 5 weeks **Fluorouracil** 400 mg/m²/d I.V., on the first 4 and last 3 days of radiation **Leucovorin** 20 mg/m²/d, on the first 4 and last 3 days of radiation **FOLLOWED 1 AND 2 MONTHS LATER BY** **Fluorouracil** 425 mg/m²/d for 5 days

	Leucovorin 20 mg/m²/d for 5 days
FUP	**Fluorouracil** 1,000 mg/m²/d I.V. CI, days 1–5
	Cisplatin 100 mg/m² I.V. over 1 hour, day 2
	Repeat cycle every 4 weeks

References

Docetaxel/Cisplatin

Roth AD, Maibach R, Martinelli G, et al. Docetaxel (Taxotere)-cisplatin (TC): an effective drug combination in gastric carcinoma. *Ann Oncol.* 2000;11:301–306.

ECF

Waters JS, Norman A, Cunningham D, et al. Long-term survival after epirubicin, cisplatin and fluorouracil for gastric cancer: results of a randomized trial. *Br J Cancer.* 1999;80:269–272.

ELF

di Bartolomeo M, Bajetta E, de Braud F, et al. Phase II study of the etoposide, leucovorin and fluorouracil combination for patients with advanced gastric cancer unsuitable for aggressive chemotherapy. *Oncology.* 1995;52:41–44.

Vanhoefer U, Rougier P, Wilke H, et al. Final results of a randomized phase III trial of sequential high-dose methotrexate, fluorouracil, and doxorubicin versus etoposide, leucovorin, and fluorouracil versus infusional fluorouracil and cisplatin in advanced gastric cancer: a trial of the European Organization for Research and Treatment of Cancer Gastrointestinal Tract Cancer Cooperative Group. *J Clin Oncol.* 2000;18: 2648–2657.

FAMTX

Wils J, Bleiberg H, Dalesio O, et al. An EORTC Gastrointestinal Group evaluation of the combination of sequential methotrexate and 5-fluorouracil, combined with adriamycin in advanced measurable gastric cancer. *J Clin Oncol.* 1986;4:1799–1803.

5-FU/LV

Macdonald JS, Smalley SR, Benedetti J, et al. Chemoradiotherapy after surgery compared with surgery alone for adenocarcinoma of the stomach or gastroesophageal junction. *N Engl J Med.* 2001;345:725–730.

FUP

Vanhoefer U, Rougier P, Wilke H, et al. Final results of a randomized phase III trial of sequential high-dose methotrexate, fluorouracil, and doxorubicin versus etoposide, leucovorin, and fluorouracil versus infusional fluorouracil and cisplatin in advanced gastric cancer: a trial of the European Organization for Research and Treatment of Cancer Gastrointestinal Tract Cancer Cooperative Group. *J Clin Oncol.* 2000;18: 2648–2657.

Genitourinary Malignancy—Bladder

Combination Regimens

CISCA	**Cyclophosphamide** 650 mg/m^2 I.V. over 15 minutes, day 1 **Doxorubicin** 50 mg/m^2 I.V. over 15 minutes, day 1 **Cisplatin** 100 mg/m^2 I.V. over 2 hours, day 2 *Repeat cycle every 21 days*
Cisplatin/Docetaxel	**Cisplatin** 30 mg/m^2/d I.V. over 30 minutes, days 1, 8, 15, 22, 29, 36, 43, 50 **Docetaxel** 40 mg/m^2/d I.V. over 1 hour, days 4, 11, 18, 25, 32, 39, 46, 53 with radiation **OR** **Cisplatin** 75 mg/m^2 I.V., day 1 **Docetaxel** 75 mg/m^2 I.V. over 1 hour, day 1 *Repeat cycle every 21 days*
CMV	**Cisplatin** 100 mg/m^2 I.V. over 4 hours, day 2 (12 hours after methotrexate and vinblastine) **Methotrexate** 30 mg/m^2/d I.V., days 1, 8 **Vinblastine** 4 mg/m^2/d I.V., days 1, 8 *Repeat cycle every 21 days*
Gemcitabine/Cisplatin	**Gemcitabine** 1,000 mg/m^2/d I.V. over 30–60 minutes, days 1, 8, 15
Cisplatin	**Cisplatin** 70 mg/m^2 I.V., day 2 *Repeat cycle every 28 days*
MVAC	**Methotrexate** 30 mg/m^2/d I.V., days 1, 15, 22 **Vinblastine** 3 mg/m^2/d I.V., days 2, 15, 22 **Doxorubicin** 30 mg/m^2 I.V., day 2 **Cisplatin** 70 mg/m^2 I.V., day 2 *Repeat cycle every 28 days*
PC	**Paclitaxel*** 200 mg/m^2 or 150–225 mg/m^2 over 3 hours, day 1 **Carboplatin** targeted by Calvert equation to AUC 5 or 6 mg/mL/min I.V., after paclitaxel, day 1 *Repeat cycle every 21 days*

Single-Agent Regimens

Gemcitabine	**Gemcitabine** 1,200 mg/m^2/d I.V. over 30 minutes, days 1, 8, 15 *Repeat cycle every 28 days*
Paclitaxel	**Paclitaxel*** 250 mg/m^2 I.V. over 24 hours, day 1 *Repeat cycle every 21 days*

References

CISCA

Sternberg JJ, Bracken RB, Handel PB, Johnson DE. Combination chemotherapy (CISCA) for advanced urinary tract carcinoma: a preliminary report. *JAMA.* 1977;238: 2282–2287.

Cisplatin/Docetaxel

Varveris H, Delakas D, Anezinis P, et al. Concurrent platinum and docetaxel chemotherapy and external radical radiotherapy in patients with invasive transitional cell bladder carcinoma: a preliminary report of tolerance and local control. *Anticancer Res.* 1997; 17:4771–4780.

Sengelov L, Kamby C, Lund B, Engelholm SA. Docetaxel and cisplatin in metastatic urothelial cancer: a phase II study. *J Clin Oncol.* 1998;16:3392–3397.

CMV

Harker WG, Meyers FJ, Freiha FS, et al. Cisplatin, methotrexate, and vinblastine (CMV): an effective chemotherapy regimen for metastatic transitional cell carcinoma of the urinary tract: a Northern California Oncology Group study. *J Clin Oncol.* 1985;3: 1463–1470.

Gemcitabine/Cisplatin

von der Maase H, Hansen SW, Roberts JT, et al. Gemcitabine and cisplatin versus methotrexate, vinblastine, doxorubicin, and cisplatin in advanced or metastatic bladder cancer: results of a large, randomized, multinational, multicenter, phase III study. *J Clin Oncol.* 2000;17:3068–3077.

MVAC

von der Maase H, Hansen SW, Roberts JT, et al. Gemcitabine and cisplatin versus methotrexate, vinblastine, doxorubicin, and cisplatin in advanced or metastatic bladder cancer: results of a large, randomized, multinational, multicenter, phase III study. *J Clin Oncol.* 2000;17:3068–3077.

PC

Redman BG, Smith DC, Flaherty L, Du W, Hussain M. Phase II trial of paclitaxel and carboplatin in the treatment of advanced urothelial carcinoma. *J Clin Oncol.* 1998;16: 1844–1848.

Vaughn DJ, Malkowicz SB, Zoltick B, et al. Paclitaxel plus carboplatin in advanced carcinoma of the urothelium: an active and tolerable outpatient regimen. *J Clin Oncol.* 1998;16:255–260.

Gemcitabine

Moore MJ, Tannock IF, Ernst DS, Huan S, Murray N. Gemcitabine: a promising new agent in the treatment of advanced urothelial cancer. *J Clin Oncol.* 1997;15: 3441–3445.

Stadler WM, Kuzel T, Roth B, Roghavan D, Dorr FA. Phase II study of single-agent gemcitabine in previously untreated patients with metastatic urothelial cancer. *J Clin Oncol.* 1997;15:3394–3398.

Paclitaxel

Roth BJ, Dreicer R, Einhorn LH, et al. Significant activity of paclitaxel in advanced transitional cell carcinoma of the urothelium: a phase II trial of the Eastern Cooperative Oncology Group. *J Clin Oncol.* 1994;12:2264–2270.

Genitourinary Malignancy—Prostate

Combination Regimens

Docetaxel/Estramustine	**Docetaxel** 70 mg/m² I.V. over 1 hour, 12 hours after first dose of estramustine **Estramustine** 280 mg PO every 6 hours for 5 doses *Repeat cycle every 21 days for maximum of 6 cycles*
Docetaxel/prednisone	**Docetaxel** 75 mg/m² I.V. over 1 hr, day 1 **Prednisone** 5 mg PO bid, days 1–21 *Repeat cycle every 21 days*
Estramustine/ Vinblastine	**Estramustine** 600 mg/m²/d PO bid or tid, days 1–42 **Vinblastine** 4 mg/m² I.V. weekly for 6 weeks, begin day 1 *Repeat cycle every 8 weeks*
FL	**Flutamide** 250 mg PO tid **WITH** **Leuprolide** 1 mg/d SQ **OR** **Leuprolide depot** 7.5 mg IM every 28 days
FZ	**Flutamide** 250 mg PO tid **WITH** **Goserelin implant** 3.6 mg SQ every 28 days, beginning 8 weeks prior to radiotherapy for 4 cycles **OR** **Goserelin implant** 3.6 mg SQ 8 weeks prior to radiotherapy **Goserelin implant** 10.8 mg SQ 4 weeks prior to radiotherapy
Mitoxantrone/ Prednisone	**Mitoxantrone** 12 mg/m² I.V., day 1 **Prednisone** 5 mg PO bid *Repeat cycle every 21 days*
No Known Acronym	**Bicalutamide** 50 mg/d PO **WITH** **Leuprolide depot** 7.5 mg IM every 28 days **OR** **Goserelin implant** 3.6 mg SQ every 28 days
PE	**Paclitaxel*** 120 mg/m² by 96-hour I.V. infusion, days 1–4 **Estramustine** 600 mg/m²/d PO in 2 or 3 divided doses, starting 24 hours before paclitaxel *Repeat cycle every 21 days*

Single-Agent Regimens

Estramustine	**Estramustine** 14 mg/kg/d PO in 3 or 4 divided doses
Goserelin	**Goserelin implant** 3.6 mg SQ every 28 days or 10.8 mg SQ every 12 weeks
Leuprolide	**Leuprolide depot** 7.5 mg IM every 28 days, 22.5 mg IM every 3 months, or 30 mg IM every 4 months
Nilutamide	**Nilutamide** 300 mg/d PO, days 1–30, then 150 mg/d PO, in combination with surgical castration; begin on same day or day after castration
Prednisone	**Prednisone** 5 mg PO bid
Triptorelin	**Triptorelin** 3.75 mg IM every 28 days

References

Docetaxel/Estramustine

Sinibaldi VJ, Carducci MA, Moore-Cooper S, Laufer M, Zahurak M, Eisenberger MA. Phase II evaluation of docetaxel plus one-day oral estramustine phosphate in the treatment of patients with androgen independent prostate carcinoma. *Cancer.* 2002;94: 1457–1465.

Docetaxel/Predinisone

Tannock IF, de Wit R, Berry WR, et al. Docetaxel plus prednisone or mitoxantrone plus prednisone for advanced prostate cancer. *New Engl J Med.* 2004;351:1502–1512.

Estramustine/Vinblastine

Hudes G, Einhorn L, Ross E, et al. Vinblastine versus vinblastine plus oral estramustine phosphate for patients with hormone-refractory prostate cancer: a Hoosier Oncology Group and Fox Chase Network phase III trial. *J Clin Oncol.* 1999;17:3160–3166.

FL

Fischer DS, Knobf MT, Durivage HJ, eds. *The Cancer Chemotherapy Handbook*, 5th ed. St. Louis, MO: CV Mosby1997;369.

Sarosdy MF, Schellhammer PF, Johnson R, Carroll K, Kolvenbag GJCM. Does prolonged combined androgen blockade have survival benefits over short-term combined androgen blockade therapy? *Urology.* 2000;15:391–396.

FZ

Zoladex 3.6 mg, Zoladex 10.8 mg (package inserts). Wilmington, DE: AstraZeneca; 2003.

Jurincic CD, Horlbeck R, Klippel KF. Combined treatment (goserelin plus flutamide) versus monotherapy (goserelin alone) in advanced prostate cancer: a randomized study. *Semin Oncol.* 1991;18(suppl 6):21–25.

Mitoxantrone/Prednisone

Tannock IF, Osoba D, Stockler MR, et al. Chemotherapy with mitoxantrone plus prednisone or prednisone alone for symptomatic hormone-resistant prostate cancer: a Canadian randomized trial with palliative endpoints. *J Clin Oncol.* 1996;14:1756–1764.

No Known Acronym

Schellhammer P, Sharifi R, Block N, et al. A controlled trial of bicalutamide versus flutamide, each in combination with luteinizing hormone-releasing hormone analogue therapy, in patients with advanced prostate cancer. *Urology.* 1995;45:745–752.

PE

Hudes GR, Nathan F, Khater C, et al. Phase II trial of 96-hour paclitaxel plus oral estramustine phosphate in metastatic hormone-refractory prostate cancer. *J Clin Oncol.* 1997;15:3156–3163.

Estramustine

Emcyt (package insert). New York, NY: Pfizer; 2003.

Goserelin

Zoladex 3.6 mg, Zoladex 10.8 mg (package inserts). Wilmington, DE: AstraZeneca; 2003.

Leuprolide

Lupron Depot 7.5 mg, Lupron Depot 22.5 mg, Lupron Depot 30 mg (package inserts.) Lake Forest, IL: TAP Pharmaceuticals; 2003.

Nilutamide

Nilandron (package insert). New York, NY: Pfizer; 2004.

Prednisone

Tannock IF, Osoba D, Stockler MR, et al. Chemotherapy with mitoxantrone plus prednisone or prednisone alone for symptomatic hormone-resistant prostate cancer: a Canadian randomized trial with palliative endpoints. *J Clin Oncol.* 1996;14:1756–1764.

Triptorelin

Kuhn JM, Abourachid H, Brucher P, et al. A randomized comparison of the clinical and hormonal effects of two GnRH agonists in patients with prostate cancer. *Eur Urol.* 1997;32:397–403.

Genitourinary Malignancy—Renal

Combination Regimens

Interleukin-2/ Interferon alfa	**Interleukin-2** 18 million units/m²/d I.V. CI, days 1–5, × 2, separated by 6 days rest (induction) **THEN, AFTER 3 WEEKS** 18 million units/m²/d I.V. CI, days 1–5 (maintenance) *Repeat maintenance cycle for 4 cycles, with 3 weeks rest after each cycle* **WITH**

	Interferon alfa-2a 6 million units SQ, 3 times per week during each interleukin-2 cycle (induction and maintenance)
Vinblastine/ Interferon alfa	**Vinblastine** 0.1 mg/kg I.V. every 3 weeks **Interferonalfa-2a** 3 million units SQ, 3 times per week for the first week, then 18 million units 3 times per week for subsequent weeks (9 million units for those unable to tolerate higher dose)

Single-Agent Regimens

Interferon alfa	**Interferon alfa-2b** 10 million units SQ, 3 times per week for 12 weeks (first week: 5, 5, and 10 million units)
Interleukin-2	**Interleukin-2** **High Dose:** 600,000–720,000 units/kg I.V. over 15 minutes, every 8 hours until toxicity or 14 doses; administer 2 courses separated by 5–9 days *Repeat 2-course cycle every 6–12 weeks* **Low Dose:** 18 million units/d SQ, days 1–5, week 1 **THEN,** 9 million units/d SQ, days 1, 2 and 18 million units/d, days 3–5, weeks 2–6 *Cycle may be repeated after 3 weeks rest* **OR** 3 million units/m^2/d I.V. CI, days 1–5 and 12–17; *repeat cycle on day 35* **THEN,** 3 million units/m^2/d I.V. CI, days 1–5 *Repeat second cycle every 28 days for 4 cycles*

References

Interleukin-2/Interferon alfa

Negrier S, Escudier B, Lasset C, et al. Recombinant human interleukin-2, recombinant human interferon alfa-2a, or both in a metastatic renal-cell carcinoma. *N Engl J Med.* 1998;338:1272–1278.

Vinblastine/Interferon alfa

Pyrhönen S, Salminen E, Ruutu M, et al. Prospective randomized trial of interferon alfa-2a plus vinblastine versus vinblastine alone in patients with advanced renal cell cancer. *J Clin Oncol.* 1999;17:2859–2867.

Interferon alfa

Medical Research Council Renal Cancer Collaborators.. Interferon-α and survival in metastatic renal carcinoma: early results of a randomised controlled trial. *Lancet.* 1999; 353:14–17.

Interleukin-2

Fyfe G, Fisher RI, Rosenberg SA, Sznol M, Parkinson DR, Louie AC. Results of treatment of 255 patients with metastatic renal cell carcinoma who received high-dose recombinant interleukin-2 therapy. *J Clin Oncol.* 1995;13:688–696.

Sleijfer DT, Janssen RAJ, Buter J, et al. Phase II study of subcutaneous interleukin-2 in unselected patients with advanced renal cell cancer on an outpatient basis. *J Clin Oncol.* 1992;10:1119–1123.

Stoter G, Fossa SD, Rugarli C, et al. Metastatic renal cell cancer treated with low-dose interleukin-2: a phase II multicentre study. *Cancer Treat Rev.* 1989;16(suppl A): 111–113.

Genitourinary Malignancy—Testicular

BEP	**Bleomycin** 30 units I.V. bolus, weekly for 12 weeks **Etoposide** 100 mg/m²/d I.V. over 30–60 minutes, days 1–5 **Cisplatin** 20 mg/m²/d I.V. over 30–60 minutes, days 1–5 *Repeat cycle every 21 days*
EP	**Etoposide** 100 mg/m²/d I.V., days 1–5 **Cisplatin** 20 mg/m²/d I.V., days 1–5 *Repeat cycle once after 21 days*
PVB	**Cisplatin** 20 mg/m²/d I.V. over 15–30 minutes, days 1–5 **Vinblastine** 0.15 mg/kg/d I.V. bolus, days 1, 2 **Bleomycin** 30 units/d I.V. bolus, days 2, 9, 16 *Repeat cycle every 21 days*
VIP	**Vinblastine** 0.11 mg/kg/d I.V., days 1, 2 **OR** **Etoposide** 75 mg/m²/d I.V., days 1–5 AND **Ifosfamide** 1,200 mg/m²/d I.V., days 1–5 **Cisplatin** 20 mg/m²/d I.V., days 1–5 **Mesna** 400 mg I.V. 15 minutes prior to ifosfamide, then 1,200 mg/d I.V. CI, days 1–5 *Repeat cycle every 21 days for 4 cycles*

References

BEP

Nichols CR, Catalano PJ, Crawford ED, et al. Randomized comparison of cisplatin and etoposide and either bleomycin or ifosfamide in treatment of advanced disseminated germ cell tumors: an Eastern Cooperative Oncology Group, Southwest Oncology Group, and Cancer and Leukemia Group B Study. *J Clin Oncol.* 1998;16:1287–1293.

EP

Motzer RJ, Sheinfeld J, Mazumdar M, et al. Etoposide and cisplatin adjuvant therapy for patients with pathologic stage II germ cell tumors. *J Clin Oncol.* 1995;13:2700–2704.

PVB

Williams SD, Birch R, Einhorn LH, et al. Treatment of disseminated germ cell tumors with cisplatin, bleomycin, and either vinblastine or etoposide. *N Engl J Med.* 1987;316:1435–1440.

VIP

Loehrer PJ, Lauer R, Roth BJ, et al. Salvage therapy in recurrent germ cell cancer: ifosfamide and cisplatin plus either vinblastine or etoposide. *Ann Intern Med.* 1988;109:540–546.

Gynecologic Malignancy—Cervical

Combination Regimens

Cisplatin/Fluorouracil	**Cisplatin** 75 mg/m² I.V. over 4 hours, day 1, given within 16 hours of the first dose of radiotherapy
	Fluorouracil 4,000 mg/m² I.V. CI over 96 hours, days 2–5
	Repeat cycle every 21 days for 3 cycles
	OR
	Cisplatin 50 mg/m²/d I.V., days 1, 29, given 4 hours before the first dose of radiotherapy
	Fluorouracil 1,000 mg/m²/d I.V., days 2–5, 30–33
C-P	**Cisplatin** 50 mg/m² I.V. day 1, IMMEDIATELY AFTER
	Paclitaxel 135 mg/m² I.V. over 24 hours, day 1
	Repeat cycle every 21 days for 6 cycles
Cisplatin/Vinorelbine	**Cisplatin** 80 mg/m² I.V., day 1
	Vinorelbine 25 mg/m²/d, days 1, 8
	Repeat cycle every 21 days for 3 to 6 cycles

Single-Agent Regimen

Cisplatin	**Cisplatin** 40 mg/m² I.V. once per week during radiation therapy for up to 6 doses, followed by hysterectomy 3–6 weeks later; do not exceed 70 mg per dose

References

Cisplatin/Fluorouracil

Morris M, Eifel PJ, Lu J, et al. Pelvic radiation with concurrent chemotherapy compared with pelvic and para-aortic radiation for high-risk cervical cancer. *N Engl J Med.* 1999;340:1137–1143.

Whitney CW, Sause W, Bundy BN, et al. Randomized comparison of fluorouracil plus cisplatin versus hydroxyurea as an adjunct to radiation therapy in stage IIB-IVA carcinoma of the cervix with negative para-aortic lymph nodes: a Gynecologic Oncology Group and Southwest Oncology Group study. *J Clin Oncol.* 1999;17:1339–1348.

Cisplatin/Paclitaxel

Moore DH, Blessing JA, McQuellon RP, et al. Phase III study of cisplatin with or without paclitaxel in stage IV, recurrent or persistent squamous cell carcinoma of the cervix: A Gynecologic Oncology Study Group study. *J Clin Oncol.* 2004;22:3113–3119.

Cisplatin/Vinorelbine

Pignata S, Silvestro G, Ferrari E, et al. Phase II study of cisplatin and vinorelbine as first-line chemotherapy in patients with carcinoma of the uterine cervix. *J Clin Oncol.* 1999;17:756–760.

Cisplatin

Keys HM, Bundy BN, Stehman FB, et al. Cisplatin, radiation, and adjuvant hysterectomy compared with radiation and adjuvant hysterectomy for bulky stage IB cervical carcinoma. *N Engl J Med.* 1999;340:1154–1161.

Gynecologic Malignancy—Endometrial

Combination Regimen

TAP	**Doxorubicin** 45 mg/m² I.V. day 1 **Cisplatin** 50 mg/m² I.V. day 1 **Paclitaxel*** 160 mg/m² I.V. over 3 hours, day 2 **Filgrastim** 5 mcg/kg SQ, days 3–21 *Repeat cycle every 21 days for a maximum of 7 cycles*

Single-Agent Regimens

Doxorubicin	**Doxorubicin** 60 mg/m² I.V. every 21 days (maximum cumulative dose, 500 mg/m²)
Medroxyprogesterone	**Medroxyprogesterone acetate** 200 mg/d PO

References

TAP

Fleming GF, Brunetto VL, Cella D, et al. Phase III trial of doxorubicin plus cisplatin with or without paclitaxel plus filgrastim in advanced endometrial carcinoma: a Gynecologic Oncology Study Group. *J Clin Oncol.* 2004;22:2159–2166.

Doxorubicin

Morrow CP, Bundy BN, Homesley HD, et al. Doxorubicin as an adjuvant following surgery and radiation therapy in patients with high-risk endometrial carcinoma, stage I and occult stage II: a Gynecologic Oncology Group study. *Gynecol Oncol.* 1990;36:166–171.

Medroxyprogesterone

Thigpen JT, Brady MF, Alvarez RD, et al. Oral medroxyprogesterone acetate in the treatment of advanced or recurrent endometrial carcinoma: a dose-response study by the Gynecological Oncology Group. *J Clin Oncol.* 1999;17:1736–1744.

Gynecologic Malignancy—Ovarian/Epithelial

Combination Regimens

Carbo-Docetaxel	**Docetaxel** 75 mg/m^2 I.V. over 1 hour, day 1 **FOLLOWED BY** **Carboplatin** AUC 5 I.V. over 1 hour, day 1 *Repeat cycle every 21 days*
Carbo-Tax	**Paclitaxel*** 175 mg/m^2 I.V. over 3 hours, day 1 **Carboplatin** dose targeted by Calvert equation to AUC 5 units, I.V., day 1 *Repeat cycle every 21 days*
CT**	**Paclitaxel*** 135 mg/m^2 I.V. over 24 hours, day 1 **Cisplatin** 75 mg/m^2 I.V., day 1 *Repeat cycle every 21 days* **OR** **Paclitaxel*** 175 mg/m^2 I.V. over 3 hours, day 1 **Cisplatin** 75 mg/m^2 I.V., day 1 *Repeat cycle every 21 days*

Single-Agent Regimens

Altretamine	**Altretamine** 260 mg/m^2/d PO in 4 divided doses after meals and at bedtime for 14 days *Repeat cycle every 28 days*
Gemcitabine	**Gemcitabine** 800 mg/m^2/d I.V., days 1, 8, 15 *Repeat cycle every 28 days*
Paclitaxel	**Paclitaxel*** 175 mg/m^2 I.V. over 3 hours, every 21 days
Pegylated liposomal doxorubicin	**Pegylated liposomal doxorubicin** 50 mg/m^2 I.V. every 28 days at an initial rate of 1 mg/min; if no infusion-related adverse events are observed, the infusion rate can be increased to complete administration over 1 hour
Topotecan	**Topotecan** 1.5 mg/m^2/d I.V. over 30 minutes, days 1–5 *Repeat cycle every 21 days*

References

Carbo-Docetaxel

Vasey PA, Jayson GC, Gordon A, et al. Phase III randomized trial of docetaxel-carboplatin versus paclitaxel-carboplatin as first-line chemotherapy for ovarian carcinoma. *J Natl Cancer Instit.* 2004;96:1682–1691.

Carbo-Tax

Neijt JP, Engelholm SA, Tuxen MK, et al. Exploratory phase III study of paclitaxel and cisplatin versus paclitaxel and carboplatin in advanced ovarian cancer. *J Clin Oncol.* 2000;18:3084–3092.

CT

McGuire WP, Hoskins WJ, Brady MF, et al. Cyclophosphamide and cisplatin compared with paclitaxel and cisplatin in patients with stage III and stage IV ovarian ancer. *N Engl J Med.* 1996;334:1–6.

Neijt JP, Engelholm SA, Tuxen MK, et al. Exploratory phase III study of paclitaxel and cisplatin versus paclitaxel and carboplatin in advanced ovarian cancer. *J Clin Oncol.* 2000;18:3084–3092.

Altretamine

Markman M, Blessing JA, Moore D, Ball H, Lentz SS. Altretamine (hexamethylmelamine) in platinum-resistant and platinum-refractory ovarian cancer: a Gynecologic Oncology Group phase II trial. *Gynecol Oncol.* 1998;69:226–229.

Gemcitabine

Lund B, Hansen OP, Theilade K, et al. Phase II study of gemcitabine (2',2' difluorodeoxycitidine) in previously treated ovarian cancer patients. *J Natl Cancer Instit.* 1994;86: 1530–1533.

Paclitaxel

ten Bokkel Huinink W, Gore M, Carmichael J, et al. Topotecan versus paclitaxel for the treatment of recurrent epithelial ovarian cancer. *J Clin Oncol.* 1997;15:2183–2193.

Pegylated liposomal doxorubicin

Gordon AN, Granal CO, Rose PG, et al. Phase II study of liposomal doxorubicin in platinum- and paclitaxel-refractory epithelial ovarian cancer. *J Clin Oncol.* 2000;18: 3093–3100.

Doxil (package insert). Bridgewater, NJ: Tibotec Therapeutics, Division of Ortho Biotech Products, LP; 2005.

Topotecan

ten Bokkel Huinink W, Gore M, Carmichael J, et al. Topotecan versus paclitaxel for the treatment of recurrent epithelial ovarian cancer. *J Clin Oncol.* 1997;15:2183–2193.

Head and Neck/Esophageal Malignancies

Carboplatin/ Fluorouracil	**Carboplatin** 400 mg/m² I.V. CI over 24 hours, day 1 **Fluorouracil** 5,000 mg/m² I.V. CI over 120 hours *Repeat cycle every 21 days*

Cisplatin/Fluorouracil	**Cisplatin** 100 mg/m^2 I.V., day 1 **Fluorouracil** 5,000 mg/m^2 I.V. CI over 120 hours *Repeat cycle every 21 days*

References

Carboplatin/Fluorouracil

De Andrés L, Brunt J, López-Pousa A, et al. Randomized trial of neoadjuvant cisplatin and fluorouracil versus carboplatin and fluorouracil in patients with stage IV-M0 head and neck cancer. *J Clin Oncol.* 1995;13:1493–1500.

Cisplatin/Fluorouracil

De Andrés L, Brunt J, López-Pousa A, et al. Randomized trial of neoadjuvant cisplatin and fluorouracil versus carboplatin and fluorouracil in patients with stage IV-M0 head and neck cancer. *J Clin Oncol.* 1995;13:1493–1500.

Leukemia—AML

Combination Regimens (Induction)

Idarubicin/Cytarabine/ Etoposide	**Idarubicin** 5 mg/m^2/d slow I.V. push, days 1–5 **Cytarabine** 2 g/m^2 every 12 hours as 3-hour infusion, days 1–5 **Etoposide** 100 mg/m^2/d as 1-hour infusion, days 1–5 **OR** **Idarubicin** 6 mg/m^2/d I.V. bolus, days 1–5 **Cytarabine** 600 mg/m^2/d I.V. over 2 hours, days 1–5 **Etoposide** 150 mg/m^2/d over 2 hours, days 1–3
5 + 2	**Cytarabine** 100 mg/m^2/d I.V. CI, days 1–5 **WITH** **Daunorubicin** 45 mg/m^2/d I.V., days 1–2 **OR** **Mitoxantrone** 12 mg/m^2/d I.V., days 1–2 For reinduction or consolidation
7 + 3	**Cytarabine** 100 mg/m^2/d I.V. CI, days 1–7 **WITH** **Daunorubicin** 45 mg/m^2/d I.V., days 1–3 **OR** **Idarubicin** 12 mg/m^2/d I.V., days 1–3 **OR** **Mitoxantrone** 12 mg/m^2/d I.V., days 1–3
7 + 3 + 7	**Cytarabine** 100 mg/m^2/d I.V. CI, days 1–7 **Daunorubicin** 50 mg/m^2/d I.V., days 1–3 **Etoposide** 75 mg/m^2/d I.V. over 1 hour, days 1–7

Monoclonal Antibody Regimen

Gemtuzumab	**Gemtuzumab** 2 doses of 9 mg/m^2 I.V., each as a 2-hour infusion, separated by 14 days

Single-Agent Regimens (Induction)

Arsenic	**Arsenic trioxide** 0.15 mg/kg I.V. daily until remission, not to exceed 50 doses
ATRA	**All-*trans*-retinoic acid (ATRA)** 45 mg/m^2/d PO

Single-Agent Regimens (Post-Remission)

Arsenic	**Arsenic trioxide** 0.15 mg/kg/d I.V., days 1–5 *Repeat cycle every week for 5 weeks (25 doses)*
Cytarabine	**Cytarabine** 100 mg/m^2/d I.V. CI, days 1–5 For patients ≥ 60 years of age *Repeat cycle every 28 days*
HiDAC	**Cytarabine** 3,000 mg/m^2 I.V. over 3 hours, every 12 hours, days 1, 3, 5 For patients <60 years of age *Repeat cycle every 28 days*

References

Idarubicin/Cytarabine/Etoposide

Mehta J, Powles R, Singhai S, et al. Idarubicin, high-dose cytarabine, and etoposide for induction of remission in acute leukemia. *Semin Hematol.* 1996;33(suppl 3):18–23.

Carella AM, Carlier P, Pungolino E, et al. Idarubicin in combination with intermediate-dose cytarabine and VP-16 in the treatment of refractory or rapidly relapsed patients with acute myeloid leukemia. *Leukemia.* 1993;7:196–199.

5 + 2

Skeel RT, Lachant NA, eds. *Handbook of Cancer Chemotherapy*, 4th ed. Boston, MA: Little, Brown and Co;1995:400.

7 + 3

Preisler H, Davis RB, Kirshner J, et al. Comparison of three remission induction regimens and two post-induction strategies for the treatment of acute nonlymphocytic leukemia: a cancer and leukemia group B study. *Blood.* 1987;69:1441–1449.

Skeel RT, Lachant NA, eds. *Handbook of Cancer Chemotherapy*, 4th ed. Boston, MA: Little, Brown and Co; 1995:400.

7 + 3 + 7

Bishop JF, Lowenthal RM, Joshua D, et al. Etoposide in acute nonlymphocytic leukemia. *Blood.* 1990;75:27–32.

Gemtuzumab

Mylotarg (package insert). Philadelphia, PA: Wyeth-Ayerst Pharmaceuticals; 2004.

Arsenic

Trisenox (package insert). Seattle, WA: Cell Therapeutics, Inc; 2003.

ATRA

Degos L, Dombret H, Chomienne C, et al. All-*trans*-retinoic acid as a differentiating agent in the treatment of acute promyelocytic leukemia. *Blood.* 1995;85:2643–2653.

Single-Agent Regimens (Post-Remission)

Arsenic

Trisenox (package insert). Seattle, WA: Cell Therapeutics, Inc; 2003.

Cytarabine

Stone RM. Leukemia in the elderly. LAR Depot consists of biodegradable microspheres which slowly release octreotide from the injection site over 4 weeks. After IM injection, serum octreotide concentration reaches a transient initial peak within 1 hour, then declines over the next 3–5 days, then slowly increases to plateau 2–3 weeks post-injection. Steady state is reached by the 3rd monthly injection. *Hematology.* Washington, DC: American Society of Hematology. 1999;510–516. Available at www.hematology.org/education/hema99/stone.pdf

HiDAC

Mayer RJ, Davis RB, Schiffer CA, et al. Intensive postremission chemotherapy in adults with acute myeloid leukemia. *N Engl J Med.* 1994;331:896–903.

Leukemia—Chronic Lymphocytic

Alemtuzumab	**Alemtuzumab** 3 mg/d I.V. over 2 hours initial dose, increasing to maintenance dose of 30 mg/d I.V. over 2 hours, 3 times per week on alternating days for up to 12 weeks. Do not exceed 30 mg per single dose or 90 mg per week.
Chlorambucil	**Chlorambucil** 0.1–0.2 mg/kg/d PO for 3–6 weeks as required **THEN** (as intermittent therapy) **Chlorambucil** 0.4 mg/kg PO *Repeat intermittent therapy every 14–28 days, increasing dose by 0.1 mg/kg until control of lymphocytosis or toxicity is observed*
Cyclophosphamide	**Cyclophosphamide** 2–3 mg/kg/d PO **OR** **Cyclophosphamide** 20 mg/kg I.V. every 2–3 weeks
Fludarabine	**Fludarabine** 25 mg/m^2/d I.V. over 30 minutes, days 1–5 *Repeat cycle every 28 days*
Prednisone	**Prednisone** 60–100 mg/m^2/d PO for 3–6 weeks

Use if patient symptomatic with autoimmune hemolytic anemia or immune thrombocytopenia

References

Alemtuzumab

Campath (package insert). Richmond, CA: Berlex Laboratories; 2004.

Chlorambucil

Leukeran (package insert). Research Triangle Park, NC: GlaxoSmithKline; 2004.

Cyclophosphamide

Han T, Rai KR. Management of chronic lymphocytic leukemia. *Hematol Oncol Clin North Am.* 1990;4:431–445.

Fludarabine

The French Cooperative Group on CLL., Johnson S, Smith AG, Löffler H, et al. Multicentre prospective randomised trial of fludarabine versus cyclophosphamide, doxorubicin, and prednisone (CAP) for treatment of advanced-stage chronic lymphocytic leukemia. *Lancet.* 1996;347:1432–1438.

Prednisone

Skeel RT, Lachant NA, eds. *Handbook of Cancer Chemotherapy,* 4th ed. Boston, MA: Little, Brown and Co;1995;430–431.

Leukemia—Chronic Myelogenous

Combination Regimen (Induction)

Interferon alfa-2b/ Hydroxyurea/ Cytarabine	**Interferon alfa-2b** 5 million units/m²/d SQ qd (dose dependent on granulocyte and platelet count) **Hydroxyurea** 50 mg/kg/d (dose dependent on WBC count) **Cytarabine** 20 mg/m²/d SQ for 10 days starting 2 weeks after initiation of induction (interferon alfa-2b + hydroxyurea) therapy, repeating every month (dose dependent on WBC, granulocyte, and platelet count)

Single-Agent Regimens (Post-Remission)

Hydroxyurea	**Hydroxyurea** 20–30 mg/kg/d PO
Imatinib mesylate	**Imatinib mesylate** 400–800 mg/d PO
Interferon alfa-2a	**Interferon alfa-2a** 9 million units/d SQ or IM 120 Tolerance dose: 3 million units/d for 3 days, then 6 million units/d to a target dose of 9 million units/d for the duration of the treatment period

References

Interferon alfa-2b/Hydroxyurea/Cytarabine

Guilhot F, Chastang C, Michallet M, et al. Interferon alfa-2b combined with cytarabine versus interferon alone in chronic myelogenous leukemia. *N Engl J Med.* 1997;337: 223–229.

Hydroxyurea

Hydrea (package insert). Princeton, NJ: Bristol-Myers Squibb; 2001.

Imatinib mesylate

Gleevec (package insert). East Hanover, NJ: Novartis; 2004.

Interferon alfa-2a

Roferon-A (package insert). Nutley, NJ: Roche Pharmaceuticals; 2004.

Leukemia—Hairy Cell

Cladribine	**Cladribine** 0.09 mg/kg/d I.V. CI, days 1–7 *Administer 1 cycle only*
Interferon alfa-2a	**Interferon alfa-2a** 3 million units SQ 3 times per week for 6 months
Pentostatin	**Pentostatin** 4 mg/m^2 I.V. every 14 days

References

Cladribine

Leustatin (package insert). Raritan, NJ; Ortho Biotech Products, LP; 1996.

Interferon alfa-2a

Grever M, Kopecky K, Foucar MK, et al. Randomized comparison of pentostatin versus interferon alfa-2a in previously untreated patients with hairy cell leukemia: an intergroup study. *J Clin Oncol.* 1995;13:974–982.

Pentostatin

Grever M, Kopecky K, Foucar MK, et al. Randomized comparison of pentostatin versus interferon alfa-2a in previously untreated patients with hairy cell leukemia: an intergroup study. *J Clin Oncol.* 1995;13:974–982.

Lung Cancer-Small Cell

Combination Regimens

CAE	**Cyclophosphamide** 1,000 mg/m^2 I.V., day 1 **Doxorubicin** 45 mg/m^2 I.V., day 1 **Etoposide** 50 mg/m^2/d I.V., days 1–5 *Repeat cycle every 21 days*

Carboplatin/Paclitaxel/ Etoposide	**Carboplatin** dose targeted by Calvert equation to AUC 6 units I.V., day 1 **Paclitaxel*** 200 mg/m² I.V. over 1 hour, day 1 **Etoposide** 50 mg alternating with 100 mg PO, days 1–10 *Repeat cycle every 21 days for 4 cycles*
CAV	**Cyclophosphamide** 800–1,000 mg/m² I.V., day 1 **Doxorubicin** 45–50 mg/m² I.V., day 1 **Vincristine#** 1.4–2.0 mg/m² I.V., day 1 *Repeat cycle every 21–28 days*
CAV/EP	**CAV:** **Cyclophosphamide** 1,000 mg/m² I.V., day 1 **Doxorubicin** 50 mg/m² I.V., day 1 **Vincristine#** 1.2 mg/m² I.V., day 1 **EP:** **Etoposide** 100 mg/m²/d I.V., days 1–3 **Cisplatin** 25 mg/m²/d I.V., days 1–3 *Alternate regimens every 21 days*
CDDP + CPT-11	**Cisplatin** 60 mg/m², day 1 **Irinotecan** 60 mg/m²/d, days 1, 8, 15 *Repeat cycle every 28 days*
EC	**Etoposide** 100 mg/m²/d I.V., days 1–3 **Carboplatin** 450 mg/m² I.V., day 1 *Repeat cycle every 28 days*
EP (PE)	**Etoposide** 80 mg/m²/d I.V., days 1–3 **Cisplatin** 80 mg/m² I.V., day 1 (standard dose) *Repeat cycle every 21 days* **OR** **Etoposide** 80 mg/m²/d I.V., days 1–5 **Cisplatin** 27 mg/m²/d I.V., days 1–5 (high dose) *Repeat cycle every 21 days*
VIP	**Etoposide** 75 mg/m²/d I.V., days 1–4 **Ifosfamide** 1,200 mg/m²/d I.V., days 1–4 **Cisplatin** 20 mg/m²/d I.V., days 1–4 **Mesna** 300 mg/m² I.V. bolus before the first dose of ifosfamide, then 1,200 mg/m²/d I.V. CI, days 1–4 *Repeat cycle every 21 days for 4 cycles*

Single-Agent Regimens

Etoposide	**Etoposide** 160 mg/m²/d PO, days 1–5 *Repeat cycle every 28 days* **OR** **Etoposide** 50 mg PO, bid for 14 days

	Repeat cycle every 21 days
Paclitaxel	**Paclitaxel*** 250 mg/m^2 I.V. over 24 hours, every 21 days
Topotecan	**Topotecan** 1.5 mg/m^2/d I.V. over 30 minutes, days 1–5
	Repeat cycle every 21 days

References

CAE

Bunn PA Jr, Greco FA, Einhorn L. *Cyclophosphamide, doxorubicin, and etoposide as first-line therapy in the treatment of small-cell lung cancer. Semin Oncol.* 1986;13(3 suppl 3):45–53.

Fischer DS, Knobf MT, Durivage HJ, eds. *The Cancer Chemotherapy Handbook,* 5th ed. St. Louis, MO: CV Mosby;1997;370–371.

Carboplatin/Paclitaxel/Etoposide

Hainsworth JD, Gray JR, Stroup SL, et al. Paclitaxel, carboplatin, and extended-schedule etoposide in the treatment of small cell lung cancer: comparison of sequential Phase II trials using different dose intensities. *J Clin Oncol.* 1997;15:3464–3470.

CAV

Fukuoka M, Furuse K, Saijo N, et al. Randomized trial of cyclophosphamide, doxorubicin, and vincristine versus cisplatin and etoposide versus alternation of these regimens in small cell lung cancer. *J Natl Cancer Inst.* 1991;83:855–861.

DeVita VT, Hellman S, Rosenberg SA, eds. *Cancer: Principles and Practice of Oncology,* 5th ed. Philadelphia, PA: JB Lippincott Co; 1997;911–949.

CAV/EP

Murray N, Livingston RB, Shepherd FA, et al. Randomized study of CODE versus alternating CAV/EP for extensive-stage small cell lung cancer: an intergroup study of the National Cancer Institute of Canada Clinical Trials Group and the Southwest Oncology Group. *J Clin Oncol.* 1999;17:2300–2308.

CDDP + CPT-11

Noda K, Nishiwaki Y, Kawahara M, et al. Irinotecan plus cisplatin compared with etoposide plus cisplatin for extensive small-cell lung cancer. *N Engl J Med.* 2002;346: 85–91.

EC

Viren M, Liippo K, Ojala A, et al. Carboplatin and etoposide in extensive small-cell-lung cancer. *Acta Oncol.* 1994;33:921–924.

EP (PE)

Ihde DC, Mulshine JL, Kramer BS, et al. Prospective randomized comparison of high-dose and standard-dose etoposide and cisplatin chemotherapy in patients with extensive-stage small-cell lung cancer. *J Clin Oncol.* 1994;12:2022–2034.

VIP

Loehrer PJ Sr, Rynard S, Ansari R, et al. Etoposide, ifosfamide, and cisplatin in extensive small-cell lung cancer. *Cancer.* 1992;69:669–673.

Etoposide

Johnson DH. Recent developments in chemotherapy treatment of small-cell lung cancer. *Semin Oncol.* 1993;20:315–325.

Paclitaxel

Ettinger DS, Finkelstein DM, Sarma RP, Johnson DH. Phase II study of paclitaxel in patients with extensive-disease small-cell lung cancer: an Eastern Cooperative Oncology Group study. *J Clin Oncol.* 1995;13:1430–1435.

Kirschling RJ, Grill JP, Marks RS, et al. Paclitaxel and G-CSF in previously untreated patients with extensive-stage small-cell lung cancer: a phase II study of the North Central Cancer Treatment Group. *Am J Clin Oncol.* 1999;22:517–522.

Topotecan

Adrizzoni A, Hansen H, Dombernowsky P, et al. Topotecan, a new active drug in the second-line treatment of small-cell lung cancer: a phase II study in patients with refractory and sensitive disease. *J Clin Oncol.* 1997;15:2090–2096.

von Pawel J, Schiller JH, Shepherd FA, et al. Topotecan versus cyclophosphamide, doxorubicin, and vincristine for the treatment of recurrent small-cell lung cancer. *J Clin Oncol.* 1999;17:658–667.

Lung Cancer—Non-Small Cell

Combination Regimens

Carbo-Tax	**Paclitaxel*** 225 mg/m² I.V. over 3 hours, day1
	Carboplatin dose targeted by Calvert equation to AUC 6 mg/mL/min, day 1
	Repeat cycle every 21 days
Docetaxel/Cisplatin**	**Docetaxel** 75 mg/m² I.V., day 1
	Cisplatin 75 mg/m² I.V., day 1
	Repeat cycle every 21 days
Gemcitabine/Cisplatin**	**Gemcitabine** 1,000 mg/m²/d I.V., days 1, 8, 15
	Cisplatin 100 mg/m² I.V., day 1
	Repeat cycle every 28 days
	OR
	Gemcitabine 1,250 mg/m²/d I.V., days 1, 8
	Cisplatin 100 mg/m² I.V., day 1
	Repeat cycle every 21 days
Gemcitabine/Docetaxel	**Gemcitabine** 1,100 mg/m²/d I.V., days 1, 8
	Docetaxel 100 mg/m² I.V., day 8
	Filgrastim 150 mcg/m²/d SQ, days 9-15
	Repeat cycle every 21 days
Gemcitabine/Paclitaxel	**Paclitaxel*** 200 mg/m² I.V. over 3 hours, day 1
	Repeat cycle every 21 days

Gemcitabine/ Vinorelbine	**Gemcitabine** 1,200 mg/m²/d I.V., days 1, 8 **Vinorelbine** 30 mg/m²/d I.V., days 1, 8 *Repeat cycle every 21 days* **OR** **Gemcitabine** 800–1,000 mg/m²/d I.V., days 1, 8, 15 **Vinorelbine** 20 mg/m²/d I.V., days 1, 8, 15 *Repeat cycle every 28 days*
PC**	**Paclitaxel*** 135 mg/m² over 24 hours, day 1 **Cisplatin** 75 mg/m² I.V., day 1 *Repeat cycle every 21 days* **OR** **Paclitaxel*** 175 mg/m² over 3 hours, day 1 **Cisplatin** 80 mg/m² I.V., day 1 *Repeat cycle every 21 days*
Vinorelbine/ Cisplatin**	**Vinorelbine** 30 mg/m² I.V. over 20 minutes, every 7 days **Cisplatin** 120 mg/m² I.V. over 1 hour, days 1, 29, then every 6 weeks

Single-Agent Regimens

Docetaxel	**Docetaxel** 75 mg/m² I.V. over 1 hour, every 21 days
Erlotinib	**Erlotinib** 150 mg PO qd at least 1 hour before or 2 hours after eating
Gefitinib	**Gefitinib** 250 mg PO daily
Gemcitabine	**Gemcitabine** 1,000 mg/m²/d I.V. over 30 minutes, days 1, 8, 15 *Repeat cycle every 28 days*
Vinorelbine	**Vinorelbine** 30 mg/m² I.V. over 20 minutes, every 7 days

References

Carbo-Tax

Schiller JH, Harrington D, Belani CP, et al. Comparision of four chemotherapy regimens for advanced non-small-cell lung cancer. *N Engl J Med.* 2002;346:92–98.

Docetaxel/Cisplatin**

Schiller JH, Harrington D, Belani CP, et al. Comparision of four chemotherapy regimens for advanced non-small-cell lung cancer. *N Engl J Med.* 2002;346:92–98.

Gemcitabine/Cisplatin**

Schiller JH, Harrington D, Belani CP, et al. Comparision of four chemotherapy regimens for advanced non-small-cell lung cancer. *N Engl J Med.* 2002;346:92–98.

Cardenal F, López-Cabrerizo MP, Anton A, et al. Randomized phase III study of gemcitabinecisplatin versus etoposide-cisplatin in the treatment of locally advanced or metastatic non-small cell lung cancer. *J Clin Oncol.* 1999;17:12–18.

Gemcitabine/Docetaxel

Georgoulias V, Papadakis E, Alexopoulos A, et al. Platinum-based and non-platinum based chemotherapy in advanced non-small-cell-lung-cancer: A randomized multicentre trial. *Lancet.* 2001;357:1478–1484.

Gemcitabine/Paclitaxel

Kosmidis P, Mylonakis N, Nicolaides C, et al. Paclitaxel plus carboplatin versus gemcitabine plus paclitaxel in advanced non-small-cell-lung-cancer: A phase III randomized trial. *J Clin Oncol.* 2002;20:3578–3585.

Gemcitabine/Vinorelbine

Frasci G, Lorusso V, Panza N, et al. Gemcitabine plus vinorelbine versus vinorelbine alone in elderly patients with advanced non-small cell lung cancer. *J Clin Oncol.* 2000;18:2529–2536.

Chen YM, Perng RP, Young KY, et al. A multicenter phase II trial of vinorelbine plus gemcitabine in previously untreated inoperable (stage IIIB/IV) non-small-cell lung cancer. *Chest.* 2000;117:1583–1589.

Hainsworth JD, Burris HA 3rd, Litchy S, et al. Gemcitabine and vinorelbine in the secondline treatment of non-small cell lung carcinoma patients: a Minnie Pearl Cancer Research Network phase II trial. *Cancer.* 2000;88:1353–1358.

PC**

Schiller JH, Harrington D, Belani CP, et al. Comparision of four chemotherapy regimens for advanced non-small-cell lung cancer. *N Engl J Med.* 2002;346:92–98.

Smit EF, van Meerbeeck JP, Lianes P, et al. Three-arm randomized study of two cisplatin-based regimens and paclitaxel plus gemcitabine in advanced non-small-cell lung cancer: a phase III trial of the European Organization for Research and Treatment of Cancer Lung Cancer Group—EORTC 08975. *J Clin Oncol.* 2003;21:3909–3917.

Vinorelbine/Cisplatin**

Le Chevalier T, Brisgand D, Douillard JY, et al. Randomized study of vinorelbine and cisplatin versus vindesine and cisplatin versus vinorelbine alone in advanced non-small-cell lung cancer: results of a European multicenter trial including 612 patients. *J Clin Oncol.* 1994;12:360–367.

Docetaxel

Shepherd FA, Dancey J, Ramlau R, et al. Prospective randomized trial of docetaxel versus best supportive care in patients with non-small-cell lung cancer previously treated with platinum-based chemotherapy. *J Clin Oncol.* 2000;18:2095–2103.

Fossella FV, DeVore R, Kerr RN, et al. Randomized phase III trial of docetaxel versus vinorelbine or ifosfamide in patients with advanced non-small cell lung cancer previously treated with platinum-containing chemotherapy regimens. *J Clin Oncol.* 2000; 18:2354–2362.

Erlotinib

Tarceva (package insert). Melville NY and South San Francisco, CA: OSI Pharmaceuticals Inc and Genentech Inc; 2004

Gefitinib

Iressa (package insert). Wilmington, DE: AstraZeneca Pharmaceuticals LP; 2004.

Gemcitabine

Crinò L, Mosconi AM, Scagliotti G, et al. Gemcitabine as second-line treatment for advanced non-small-cell lung cancer: a phase II trial. *J Clin Oncol.* 1999;17:2081–2085.

Ricci S, Antonuzzo A, Galli L, et al. Gemcitabine monotherapy in elderly patients with advanced non-small-cell lung cancer: a multicenter phase II study. *Lung Cancer.* 2000;27:75–80.

Vinorelbine

Le Chevalier T, Brisgand D, Douillard JY, et al. Randomized study of vinorelbine and cisplatin versus vindesine and cisplatin versus vinorelbine alone in advanced non-small-cell lung cancer: results of a European multicenter trial including 612 patients. *J Clin Oncol.* 1994;12:360–367.

Lymphoma—Hodgkin's

ABVD	**Doxorubicin** 25 mg/m^2 I.V., days 1, 15 **Bleomycin** 10 mg/m^2 I.V., days 1, 15 **Vinblastine** 6 mg/m^2 I.V., days 1, 15 **Dacarbazine** 375 mg/m^2 I.V., days 1, 15 *Repeat cycle every 28 days*
ChlVPP	**Chlorambucil** 6 mg/m^2/d PO (maximum, 10 mg/d), days 1–14 **Vinblastine** mg/m^2/d I.V. (maximum, 10 mg/single dose), days 1, 8 **Procarbazine** mg/m^2/d PO (maximum, 150 mg/d), days 1–14 **Prednisolone** 40 mg/d PO, days 1–14 *Repeat cycle every 28 days*
MOPP	**Mechlorethamine** 6 mg/m^2/d I.V., days 1, 8 **Vincristine**[#] 1.4 mg/m^2/d I.V., days 1, 8 **Procarbazine** 100 mg/m^2/d PO, days 1–14 **Prednisone** 40 mg/m^2/d PO, days 1–14, cycles 1 and 4 *Repeat cycle every 28 days*
MOPP/ABVD	Refer to MOPP and ABVD regimens *Alternating months of MOPP and ABVD*
Stanford V	**Doxorubicin** 25 mg/m^2/d I.V., days 1 and 15 **Vinblastine**[a] 6 mg/m^2/d I.V., days 1 and 15 **Mechlorethamine** 6 mg/m^2 I.V., day **Vincristine**[#] 1.4 mg/m^2/d I.V., days 8 and 22 **Bleomycin** 5 units/m^2/d I.V., days 8 and 22 **Etoposide** 60 mg/m^2/d I.V., days 15 and 16 **Prednisone**[b] 40 mg/m^2 PO qod; *repeat regimen every 28 days for 3 cycles*

[a]For patients &gte;50 years old, decrease dose to 4 mg/m^2 and 1mg/m^2 for vinblastine and vincristine, respectively, during cycle 3

[b] Tapered by 10 mg qod starting at week 10

References

ABVD

Harker WG, Kushlan P, Rosenberg SA. Combination chemotherapy for advanced Hodgkin's disease after failure of MOPP: ABVD and B-CAVe. *Ann Intern Med.* 1984;101: 440–446.

Longo DL. The use of chemotherapy in the treatment of Hodgkin's disease. *Semin Oncol.* 1990;17:716–735.

ChlVPP

Selby P, Patel P, Milan S, et al. ChlVPP combination chemotherapy for Hodgkin's disease: long-term results. *Br J Cancer.* 1990;62:279–285.

MOPP

DeVita VT Jr, Serpick AA, Carbone PP. Combination chemotherapy in the treatment of advanced Hodgkin's disease. *Ann Intern Med.* 1970;73:881–895.

Longo D. The use of chemotherapy in the treatment of Hodgkin's disease. *Semin Oncol.* 1990;17:716–735.

MOPP/ABVD

DeVita VT Jr, Hellman S, Rosenberg SA, eds. *Cancer: Principles & Practices of Oncology,* 5th ed. Philadelphia, PA: JB Lippincott Co;1997:1839.

Longo DL. The use of chemotherapy in the treatment of Hodgkin's disease. *Semin Oncol.* 1990;17:716–735.

Stanford V

Bartlett NL, Rosenberg SA, Hoppe RT, Hancock SL, Hornig SJ. Brief chemotherapy, Stanford V, and adjuvant radiotherapy for bulky or advanced-stage Hodgkin's disease: a preliminary report. *J Clin Oncol.* 1995;13:1080–1088.

Lymphoma—Non-Hodgkin's

Combination Regimens

CHOP	**Cyclophosphamide** 750 mg/m^2 I.V., day 1
	Doxorubicin 50 mg/m^2 I.V., day 1
	Vincristine[#] 1.4 mg/m^2 I.V., day 1
	Prednisolone 50 mg/m^2/d PO, days 1–5
	Repeat cycle every 21 days
CHOP + Rituximab	**Cyclophosphamide** 750 mg/m^2 I.V., day 1
	Doxorubicin 50 mg/m^2 I.V., day 1
	Vincristine[#] 1.4 mg/m^2 I.V., day 1
	Prednisone 40 mg/m^2/d PO, days 1–5

Rituximab 375 mg/m^2 I.V., day 1
Repeat cycle every 21 days for 8 cycles (diffuse large B-cell lymphoma)

OR

Cyclophosphamide 750 mg/m^2 I.V., day 1
Doxorubicin 50 mg/m^2 I.V., day 1
Vincristine[#] 1.4 mg/m^2 I.V., day 1
Prednisone 100 mg/m^2/d PO, days 1–5
Rituximab 375 mg/m^2 I.V., given 7 and 2 days before 1st CHOP cycle; then 2 days before 3rd and 5th CHOP cycles; then 134 and 141 days after 6th CHOP cycle
Repeat CHOP cycle every 21 days for 6 cycles (follicular or low-grade lymphoma)

CNOP

Cyclophosphamide 750 mg/m^2 I.V., day 1
Mitoxantrone 10 mg/m^2 I.V., day 1
Vincristine[#] 1.4 mg/m^2 I.V., day 1
Prednisolone 50 mg/m^2/d PO, days 1–5
Repeat cycle every 21 days

COP

Cyclophosphamide 800 mg/m^2 I.V., day 1
Vincristine[#] 2 mg (total dose) I.V., day 1
Prednisone 60 mg/m^2/d PO, days 1–5, then taper over 3 days
Repeat cycle every 14 days

CVP

Cyclophosphamide 300 mg/m^2/d PO, days 1–5
Vincristine[#] 1.2 mg/m^2 (maximum, 2 mg) I.V., day 1
Prednisone 40 mg/m^2/d PO, days 1–5
Repeat cycle every 21 days for 8 cycles

DHAP

Dexamethasone 40 mg/d PO or I.V. over 24 hours, days 1–4
Cisplatin 100 mg/m^2 I.V. CI, day 1
Cytarabine 2,000 mg/m^2 I.V. over 3 hours every 12 hours for 2 doses, day 2
Repeat cycle every 21–28 days for 6–10 cycles

ESHAP

Etoposide 40 mg/m^2/d I.V., days 1–4
Methylprednisolone 500 mg/d I.V., days 1–5
Cytarabine 2,000 mg/m^2 I.V. over 2–3 hours, day 5
Cisplatin 25 mg/m^2/d I.V. CI, days 1–4

OR

Etoposide 60 mg/m^2/d I.V., days 1–4
Methylprednisolone 500 mg/d I.V., days 1–4
Cisplatin 25 mg/m^2/d I.V. CI, days 1–4

Cytarabine 2,000 mg/m^2 I.V. over 2 hours, day 5, immediately following completion of cisplatin
Repeat cycle every 21–28 days

Hyper-CVAD/ MTX-Ara-C

Course 1: Cyclophosphamide 300 mg/m^2 over 3 hours every 12 hours × 6 doses, days 1–3
Doxorubicin 50 mg/m^2 over 48 hours after cyclophosphamide, days 4–5
Vincristine# 2 mg administered 12 hours after last cyclophosphamide dose, repeated on day 11
Dexamethasone 40 mg/d I.V. or PO, days 1–4 and days 11–14
Filgrastim 5 mcg/kg I.V. or SQ beginning 24 hours after doxorubicin is complete
Course 2 (begin after clinical and hermatologic recovery from Course 1):
Methotrexate 200 mg/m^2 I.V. bolus, day 1,
FOLLOWED BY
Methotrexate 800 mg/m^2 over 24 hours, day 1,
FOLLOWED BY
Cytarabine 3,000 mg/m^2 I.V. every 12 hours × 4 doses, days 2–3 (dose reduced to 1,000 mg/m2 in patients older than 60 years or with serum creatinine > 1.5 mg/dL)
Leucovorin 50 mg PO 24 hours after end of MTX infusion, FOLLOWED 6 HOURS LATER BY
Leucovorin 15 mg PO every 6 hours × 8 doses (dose adjusted for MTX concentration at 24 and 48 hours after completion of MTX infusion)
Filgrastim 5 mcg/kg I.V. or SQ beginning 24 hours after cytarabine
Repeat courses every 21 days

MINE-ESHAP

Mesna 1,330 mg/m^2/d I.V. over 1 hour, administered at same time as ifosfamide, then 500 mg/d PO 4 hours after ifosfamide, days 1–3
Ifosfamide 1,330 mg/m^2/d I.V. over 1 hour, days 1–3
Mitoxantrone 8 mg/m^2 I.V., day 1
Etoposide 65 mg/m^2/d I.V., days 1–3
Repeat cycle every 21 days for 6 cycles, followed by 3–6 cycles of ESHAP

ProMACE/cytaBOM

Prednisone 60 mg/m^2/d PO, days 1–14
Doxorubicin 25 mg/m^2 I.V., day 1
Cyclophosphamide 650 mg/m^2 I.V., day 1

	Etoposide 120 mg/m^2 I.V., day 1
	Cytarabine 300 mg/m^2 I.V., day 8
	Bleomycin 5 units/m^2 I.V., day 8
	Vincristine# 1.4 mg/m^2 I.V. (no cap at 2 mg total dose), day 8
	Methotrexate 120 mg/m^2 I.V., day 8
	Leucovorin 25 mg/m^2 PO every 6 hours for 4 doses, beginning 24 hours after methotrexate
	Repeat cycle every 21 days

Monoclonal Antibody Regimens

Ibritumomab tiuxetan	**Ibritumomab tiuxetan** is administered in 2 steps: **Step 1: Rituximab** 250 mg/m2 infusion followed within 4 hours by a fixed 5.0 mCi (1.6 mg total antibody dose) of **In-111 Ibritumomab tiuxetan** administered as a 10-minute I.V. push **Step 2 (7–9 days after step 1): Rituximab** 250 mg/m^2 infusion followed within 4 hours by **Y-90 Ibritumomab tiuxetan** 0.4 mCi/kg (maximum 32 mCi) administered as a 10-minute I.V. push
Rituximab	**Rituximab** 375 mg/m^2/d I.V., days 1, 8, 15, 22 Infuse at 50 mg/h initially; increase rate if tolerated
Tositumomab	**Dosimetric step: Tositumomab** 450 mg infused over 60 minutes **Iodine I^{131} tositumomab** (35 mg tositumomab containing 5.0 mCi I^{131}) infused over 20 minutes **Therapeutic step: Tositumomab** 450 mg infused over 60 minutes **Iodine I^{131} tositumomab** (dose individualized for each patient based on results of dosimetric step)

Single-Agent Regimens

Bexarotene	**Bexarotene** 300 mg/m^2/d PO with a meal until benefit is no longer derived
Denileukin diftitox	**Denileukin diftitox** 9 or 18 mcg/kg/d I.V. over 15–60 minutes, days 1–5 *Repeat cycle every 21 days*
Fludarabine	**Fludarabine** 25 mg/m^2/d I.V. over 10 minutes, days 1–5 *Repeat cycle every 21–28 days*

Lymphoma–Primary CNS

MTX

Methotrexate 2.5 g/m^2 I.V. over 2–3 hours every other wk × 5 doses (weeks 1, 3, 5, 7, 9)

Leucovorin 20 mg PO q 6 hours × 12 doses (weeks 1, 3, 5, 7, 9)

Methotrexate 12 mg IT via Ommaya reservoir (weeks 2, 4, 6, 8, 10)

FOLLOWED BY

Leucovorin 10 mg PO bid × 8 doses beginning the evening after Methotrexate administration

Vincristine 1.4 mg/m^2 I.V. (max 2.8 mg) every other wk × 5 doses (week 1, 3, 5, 7, 9)

Procarbazine 100 mg/m^2 PO × 7 days (weeks 1, 5, 9)

Dexamethasone 16 mg/d PO week 1, 12 mg/d week 2, 8 mg/d week 3, 6 mg/d week 4, 4 mg/d week 5, and 2 mg/d week 6.

Whole-brain RT 1.20 Gy fractions, bid × 15 days (if CR after week 10)

Cytarabine 3 mg/m ^{2}/d I.V. over 3 hr × 2 days × 2 cycles (begin after RT on weeks 16, 19)

References

CHOP

Bezwoda W, Ristogi RB, Erazo Valla A, et al. Long-term results of a multicentre randomised, comparative phase III trial of CHOP versus CNOP regimens in patients with intermediate and high-grade non-Hodgkin's lymphomas. *Eur J Cancer.* 1995;31A: 903–911.

CHOP+ Rituximab

Coiffier B, Lepage E, Brière J, et al. CHOP chemotherapy plus rituximab compared with CHOP alone in elderly patients with diffuse large B-cell lymphoma. *N Engl J Med.* 2002;346:235–242.

Czuczman MS, Grillo-López AJ, White CA, et al. Treatment of patients with low-grade B-cell lymphoma with the combination of chimeric anti-CD20 monoclonal antibody and CHOP chemotherapy. *J Clin Oncol.* 1999;17:268–276.

CNOP

Bezwoda W, Ristogi RB, Erazo Valla A, et al. Long-term results of a multicentre randomised, comparative phase III trial of CHOP versus CNOP regimens in patients with intermediate and high-grade non-Hodgkin's lymphomas. *Eur J Cancer.* 1995;31A: 903–911.

COP

Luce JK, Gamble JF, Wilson HE, et al. Combined cyclophosphamide, vincristine, and prednisone therapy of malignant lymphoma. *Cancer.* 1971;28:306–317.

CVP

Hagenbeek A, Carde P, Meerwaldt JH, et al. Maintenance of remission with human recombinant interferon alfa-2a in patients with stages III and IV low-grade malignant non-Hodgkin's lymphoma. *J Clin Oncol.* 1998;16:41–47.

DHAP

Velasquez WS, Cabanillas F, Salvador P, et al. Effective salvage therapy for lymphoma with cisplatin in combination with high-dose Ara-C and dexamethasone (DHAP). *Blood.* 1988;71:117–122.

ESHAP

Velasquez WS, McLaughlin P, Tucker S, et al. ESHAP—an effective chemotherapy regimen in refractory and relapsing lymphoma: a 4-year follow-up study. *J Clin Oncol.* 1994;12:1169–1176.

Rodriguez MA, Cabanillas FC, Velasquez W, et al. Results of a salvage treatment program for relapsing lymphoma: MINE consolidated with ESHAP. *J Clin Oncol.* 1995; 13:1734–1741.

Fischer DS, Knobf MT, Durivage HJ, eds. *The Cancer Chemotherapy Handbook,* 5th ed. St. Louis, MO: CV Mosby;1997;397.

Casciato CA, Lowitz BB, eds. *Manual of Clinical Oncology*, 4th ed. Boston, MA: Little, Brown and Co; 2000;379.

Hyper-CVAD/MTX-Ara-C

Khouri IF, Romaguera J, Kantarjian H, et al. Hyper-CVAD and high-dose methotrexate/cytarabine followed by stem-cell transplantation: an active regimen for aggressive mantle-cell lymphoma. *J Clin Oncol.* 1998;16:3803–3809.

MINE-ESHAP

Velasquez WS, McLaughlin P, Tucker S, et al. ESHAP—an effective chemotherapy regimen in refractory and relapsing lymphoma: a 4-year follow-up study. *J Clin Oncol.* 1994;12:1169–1176.

Rodriguez MA, Cabanillas FC, Velasquez W, et al. Results of a salvage treatment program for relapsing lymphoma: MINE consolidated with ESHAP. *J Clin Oncol.* 1995; 13:1734–1741.

Fischer DS, Knobf MT, Durivage HJ, eds. *The Cancer Chemotherapy Handbook,* 5th ed. St. Louis, MO: CV Mosby;1997;397.

Casciato CA, Lowitz BB, eds. *Manual of Clinical Oncology*, 4th ed. Boston, MA: Little, Brown and Co;2000;379.

ProMACE/cytaBOM

Longo DL, DeVita VT Jr, Duffey PL, et al. Superiority of ProMACE-CytaBOM over ProMACE-MOPP in the treatment of advanced diffuse aggressive lymphoma: results of a prospective randomized trial. *J Clin Oncol.* 1991;9:25–38.

Ibritumomab tiuxetan

Zevalin (package insert). San Diego, CA: IDEC Pharmaceutical Corporation; 2003.

Wiseman GA, White CA, Sparks RB, et al. Biodistribution and dosimetry results from a phase III prospectively randomized controlled trial of Zevalin radioimmunotherapy for low-grade, follicular, or transformed B-cell non-Hodgkin's lymphoma. *Crit Rev Oncol Hematol.* 2001;39:181–194.

Rituximab

McLaughlin P, Grillo-López AJ, Link BK, et al. Rituximab chimeric anti-CD20 monoclonal antibody therapy for relapsed indolent lymphoma: half of patients respond to a four-dose treatment program. *J Clin Oncol.* 1998;16:2825–2833.

Maloney DG, Grillo-López AJ, White CA, et al. IDEC-C2B8 (rituximab) anti-CD20 monoclonal antibody therapy in patients with relapsed low-grade non-Hodgkin's lymphoma. *Blood.* 1997;90:2188–2195.

Tositumomab

Bexxar (package insert). Seattle, WA, and Philadelphia, PA: Corixa Corp and GlaxoSmithKline; 2003.

Bexarotene

Targretin (package insert). San Diego, CA: Ligand Pharmaceuticals, Inc; 2001.

Denileukin diftitox

Olsen E, Duvic M, Frankel A, et al. Pivotal phase III trial of two dose levels of denileukin diftitox for the treatment of cutaneous T-cell lymphoma. *J Clin Oncol.* 2001;19: 376–388.

Fludarabine

Pigaditou A, Rohantiner AZS, Whelan JS, et al. Fludarabine in low-grade lymphoma. *Semin Oncol.* 1993;20(suppl 7):24–27.

MTX

DeAngelis LM, Seiferheld W, Schold SC, et al. Combination chemotherapy and radiotherapy for primary central nervous system lymphoma: Radiation Oncology Group Study 93-10. *J Clin Oncol.* 2002;20(suppl 7):2643–4648.

Melanoma

Combination Regimens

Cisplatin/Dacarbazine/ Carmustine/Tamoxifen	**Cisplatin** 25 mg/m²/d I.V., days 1–3
	Dacarbazine 220 mg/m²/d I.V., days 1–3
	Carmustine 150 mg/m² I.V., day 1 of every odd 21-day cycle
	Tamoxifen 10 mg PO bid
	Repeat cycle every 21 days
CVD	**Cisplatin** 20 mg/m²/d I.V., days 2–5
	Vinblastine 1.6 mg/m²/d I.V., days 1–5
	Dacarbazine 800 mg/m² I.V., day 1
	Repeat cycle every 21 days
CVD + IL-2	**Cisplatin** 20 mg/m²/d I.V., days 1–4
	Vinblastine 1.6 mg/m²/d I.V., days 1–4
	Dacarbazine 800 mg/m² I.V., day 1

	Interleukin-2 9 million units/m²/d I.V. CI, days 1–4
	Interferon alfa 5 million units/m²/d SQ, days 1–5, 7, 9, 11, 13
	Repeat cycle every 21 days

Single-Agent Regimens

Aldesleukin	**Aldesleukin** 0.037 mg/kg I.V. over 15 minutes, every 8 hours (maximum, 14 doses)
	Repeat cycle after 9 days; treatment course (28 doses) may be repeated following rest period of at least 7 weeks
Dacarbazine	**Dacarbazine** 2.0–4.5 mg/kg/d I.V., days 1–10
	Repeat cycle every 28 days
	OR
	Dacarbazine 250 mg/m²/d I.V., days 1–5
	Repeat cycle every 21 days
Interferon alfa-2a	**Interferon alfa-2a** 20 million units/m² IM 3 times a week for 12 weeks
Interferon alfa-2b	**Interferon alfa-2b** 20 million units/m²/d I.V., days 1–5 for 4 weeks, then 10 million units/m² SQ 3 times a week for 48 weeks
Temozolomide	**Temozolomide** 200 mg/m²/d PO under fasting conditions, days 1–5
	Repeat cycle every 28 days

References

Cisplatin/Dacarbazine/Carmustine/Tamoxifen

Chapman PB, Einhorn LH, Meyers ML, et al. Phase III multicenter randomized trial of the Dartmouth regimen versus dacarbazine in patients with metastatic melanoma. *J Clin Oncol.* 1999;17:2745–2751.

CVD

Legha SS, Ring S, Papadopoulos N, et al. A prospective evaluation of a triple drug regimen containing cisplatin, vinblastine, and dacarbazine (CVD) for metastatic melanoma. *Cancer.* 1989;64:2024–2029.

CVD + IL-2

Legha SS, Ring S, Eton O, et al. Development of a biochemotherapy regimen with concurrent administration of cisplatin, vinblastine, dacarbazine, interferon alfa, and interleukin-2 for patients with metastatic melanoma. *J Clin Oncol.* 1998;16:1752–1759.

Aldesleukin

Proleukin (package insert). Emeryville, CA: Chiron Corporation; 2000.

Dacarbazine

Middleton MR, Grob JJ, Aaronson N, et al. Randomized phase III study of temozolomide versus dacarbazine in the treatment of patients with advanced metastatic malignant melanoma. *J Clin Oncol.* 2000;18:158–166.

DTIC-Dome (package insert). West Haven, CT: Bayer Corporation; 1998.

Interferon alfa-2a

Creagan ET, Dalton RJ, Ahmann DL, et al. Randomized, surgical adjuvant clinical trial of recombinant interferon alfa-2a in selected patients with malignant melanoma. *J Clin Oncol.* 1995;13:2776–2783.

Interferon alfa-2b

Kirkwood JM, Strawderman MH, Ernstoff MS, et al. Interferon alfa-2b adjuvant therapy of high-risk resected cutaneous melanoma: the Eastern Cooperative Oncology Trial EST 1684. *J Clin Oncol.* 1996;14:7–17.

Intron A (package insert). Kenilworth, NJ: Schering Corporation; 2002.

Temozolomide

Middleton MR, Grob JJ, Aaronson N, et al. Randomized phase III trial study of temozolomide versus dacarbazine in the treatment of patients with advanced metastatic malignant melanoma. *J Clin Oncol.* 2000;18:158–166.

Multiple Myeloma

Combination Regimens

M2	**Vincristine**# 0.03 mg/kg I.V., day 1
	Carmustine 0.5 mg/kg I.V., day 1
	Cyclophosphamide 10 mg/kg I.V., day 1
	Melphalan 0.25 mg/kg/d PO, days 1–4 OR 0.1 mg/kg/d PO, days 1–7 or 1–10
	Prednisone 1 mg/kg/d PO, days 1–7, then taper and discontinue on day 21, unless continued therapy is warranted
	Repeat cycle every 35 days
MP	**Melphalan** 10 mg/m²/d PO, days 1–4
	Prednisone 60 mg/m²/d PO, days 1–4
	Repeat cycle every 42 days
Thalidomide/ Dexamethasone	**Thalidomide** 200 mg/d PO
	Dexamethasone 40 mg/d PO d 1–4, 9–12, 17–20 during odd cycles, and 40 mg PO d 1–4 during even cycles
VAD	**Vincristine**# 0.4 mg/d I.V. CI, days 1–4
	Doxorubicin 9 mg/m²/d I.V. CI, days 1–4
	Dexamethasone 40 mg PO, days 1–4, 9–12, 17–20
	Repeat cycle every 25 days
VBMCP	**Vincristine**# 1.2 mg/m² I.V., day 1

Carmustine 20 mg/m² I.V., day 1
Melphalan 8 mg/m²/d PO, days 1–4
Cyclophosphamide 400 mg/m² I.V., day 1
Prednisone 40 mg/m²/d PO, days 1–7 (all cycles), and 20 mg/m²/d PO, days 8–14 (first 3 cycles only)
Repeat cycle every 35 days for 10 cycles (induction), then every 42 days for 3 cycles, then every 56 days until relapse

Single-Agent Regimens

Bortezomib	**Bortezomib** 1.3 mg/m²/d I.V. bolus, days 1, 4, 8, 11 *Repeat cycle every 21 days*
Dexamethasone	**Dexamethasone** 20 mg/m²/d PO, days 1–4, 9–12, and 17–20 *Repeat cycle after 14–day rest period*
Interferon alfa-2b	**Interferon alfa-2b** 2 million units/m² SQ 3 times per week for maintenance therapy in selected patients with significant response to initial melphalan treatment. Continue until evidence of relapse.
Melphalan	**Melphalan** 90–200 mg/m² I.V. *Administer 1 cycle*
Thalidomide	**Thalidomide** 200 mg/d PO at hs with dose escalation q 2 weeks over 6 weeks to target dose of 800 mg/d

References

M2

Case DC Jr, Lee DJ 3rd, Clarkson BD. Improved survival times in multiple myeloma treated with melphalan, prednisone, cyclophosphamide, vincristine and BCNU: M-2 protocol. *Am J Med.* 1977;63:897–903.

MP

Southwest Oncology Group Study.. Remission maintenance therapy for multiple myeloma. *Arch Intern Med.* 1975;135:147–152.

Fischer DS, Knobf MT, Durivage HJ, eds. *The Cancer Chemotherapy Handbook,* 5th ed. St. Louis, MO: CV Mosby; 1997;408.

Thalidomide/Dexamethasone

Rajkumar SV, Hayman S, Gertz MA, et al. Combination therapy with thalidomide plus dexamethasone for newly diagnosed myeloma. *J Clin Oncol* 2002;20:4319–4323

VAD

Barlogie B, Smith L, Alexanian R. Effective treatment of advanced multiple myeloma refractory to alkylating agents. *N Engl J Med.* 1984;310:1353–1356.

VBMCP

Oken MM, Harrington DP, Abramson N, et al. Comparison of melphalan and prednisone with vincristine, carmustine, melphalan, cyclophosphamide, and prednisone in the treatment of multiple myeloma: results of Eastern Cooperative Oncology Group study E2479. *Cancer.* 1997;79:1561–1567.

Bortezomib

Richardson PG, Barlogie B, Berenson J, et al. A phase 2 study of bortezomib in relapsed, refractory myeloma. *N Engl J Med.* 2003;348:2609–2617.

Dexamethasone

Alexanian R, Dimopoulos MA, Delasalle K, Barlogie B. Primary dexamethasone treatment of multiple myeloma. *Blood.* 1992;80:887–890.

Interferon alfa-2b

Browman GP, Bergsagel D, Sicheri D, et al. Randomized trial of interferon maintenance in multiple myeloma: a study of the National Cancer Institute of Canada Clinical Trials Group. *J Clin Oncol.* 1995;13:2354–2360.

Melphalan

Cunningham D, Paz-Ares L, Gore ME, et al. High-dose melphalan for multiple myeloma: long-term follow-up data. *J Clin Oncol.* 1994;12:764–768.

Vesole DH, Barlogie B, Jagannath S, et al. High-dose therapy for refractory multiple myeloma: improved prognosis with better supportive care and double transplants. *Blood.* 1994;84:950–956. Thalidomide

Singhal S, Mehta J, Desikan R, et al. Antitumor activity of thalidomide in refractory multiple myeloma. *N Engl J Med.* 1999;341:1565–1571.

Pancreatic Cancer

Combination Regimens

GEMOX	**Gemcitabine** 1 g/m^2, day 1 as 100-minute infusion **Oxaliplatin** 100 mg/m^2, day 2 as 2-hour infusion
SMF	**Streptozocin** 1,000 mg/m^2/d I.V. over 10–20 minutes, days 1, 8, 29, 36 **Mitomycin-C** 10 mg/m^2 I.V., day 1 **Fluorouracil** 600 mg/m^2/d I.V., days 1, 8, 29, 36 *Repeat cycle every 56 days*

Single-Agent Regimen

Gemcitabine	**Gemcitabine** 1,000 mg/m^2 I.V. over 30 minutes once weekly for 7 weeks, followed by a 1-week rest period *Subsequent cycles once weekly for 3 consecutive weeks out of every 4 weeks*

References

GEMOX

Louvet C, Labianca R, Hammel P. Gemcitabine versus GEMOX (gemcitabine + oxaloplatin) in nonresectable pancreatic adenocarcinoma: interim results of GERCOR/GISCAD Intergroup Phase III. Abstract presented at: American Society for Clinical Oncology 39th Annual Meeting;. May 31–June 1, 2003; Chicago, Ill. Abstract 1004.

SMF

The Gastrointestinal Tumor Study Group,. Phase II studies of drug combinations in advanced pancreatic carcinoma: fluorouracil plus doxorubicin plus mitomycin C and two regimens of streptozotocin plus mitomycin C plus fluorouracil. *J Clin Oncol.* 1986;4:1794–1798.

Gemcitabine

Burris HA, Moore MJ, Andersen J, et al. Improvements in survival and clinical benefit with gemcitabine as first-line therapy for patients with advanced pancreas cancer: a randomized trial. *J Clin Oncol.* 1997;15:2403–2413.

Pleural Mesothelioma

Pemetrexed/Cisplatin	**Pemetrexed** 500 mg/m^2 I.V. over 10 minutes, day 1
Cisplatin	**Cisplatin** 75 mg/m^2 I.V. over 2 hours, 30 minutes after pemetrexed dose Premedications: **Dexamethasone** 4 mg PO day 0, day 1, day 2 **Folic acid** 400 &microg; PO qd starting 7 days prior to pemetrexed dose (Cycle 1), continuing qd during treatment, then for 21 days following last cycle of pemetrexed **Vit B12** 1000 &microg; IM/SQ beginning week prior to cycle 1, and continuing q 3 cycles during pemetrexed therapy *Repeat cycle every 21 days*

References

Pemetrexed/Cisplatin

Alimta (package insert). Indianapolis, IN: Eli Lilly and Company; 2004.

Sarcoma

Combination Regimens

AD	**Doxorubicin** 15 mg/m^2/d I.V. CI, days 1–4

	Dacarbazine 250 mg/m²/d I.V. CI, days 1–4 *Repeat cycle every 21 days*
DI	**Doxorubicin** 50 mg/m² I.V. bolus, day 1 **Ifosfamide** 5,000 mg/m² I.V. CI following doxorubicin, day 1 **Mesna** 600 mg/m² I.V. bolus before ifosfamide, followed by 2,500 mg/m² I.V. CI with ifosfamide, and 1,250 mg/m² I.V. over 12 hours following ifosfamide *Repeat cycle every 21 days*
MAID	**Mesna** 2,500 mg/m²/d I.V. CI, days 1–4 **Doxorubicin** 15 mg/m²/d I.V. CI, days 1–4 **Ifosfamide** 2,500 mg/m²/d I.V. CI, days 1–3 **Dacarbazine** 250 mg/m²/d I.V. CI, days 1–4 *Repeat cycle every 21 days*

Single-Agent Regimen

Doxorubicin	**Doxorubicin** 75 mg/m² I.V. every 21 days

References

AD

Antman K, Crowley J, Balcerzak SP, et al. An intergroup phase III randomized study of doxorubicin and dacarbazine with or without ifosfamide and mesna in advanced soft tissue and bone sarcomas. *J Clin Oncol.* 1993;11:1276–1285.

DI

Santoro A, Tursz T, Mouridsen H, et al. Doxorubicin versus CYVADIC versus doxorubicin plus ifosfamide in first-line treatment of advanced soft tissue sarcomas: a randomized study of the European Organization for Research and Treatment of Cancer Soft Tissue and Bone Sarcoma Group. *J Clin Oncol.* 1995;13:1537–1545.

MAID

Antman K, Crowley J, Balcerzak SP, et al. An intergroup phase III randomized study of doxorubicin and dacarbazine with or without ifosfamide and mesna in advanced soft tissue and bone sarcomas. *J Clin Oncol.* 1993;11:1276–1285.

Doxorubicin

Nielsen OS, Dombernowsky P, Mouridsen H, et al. High-dose epirubicin is not an alternative to standard-dose doxorubicin in the treatment of advanced soft tissue sarcomas: a study of the EORTC soft tissue and bone sarcoma group. *Br J Cancer.* 1998;78: 1634–1639.

---

*All patients should be premedicated with dexmethasone, diphenhydramine, and either ranitidine or cimetidine prior to paclitaxel administration. See paclitaxel package insert for dosages.

#Maximum vincristine dose should never exceed 2 mg.

**Amifostine 910 mg/m²/d I.V. over 15 min can be administered 30 min prior to chemotherapy with cisplatin to reduce cumulative renal toxicity in patients with ovarian cancer or non-small-cell lung cancer.

Index

Note: Page numbers followed by f indicate figures; those followed by t indicate tables. Generic drug names are in boldface type.